CURRENT ISSUES IN NURSING

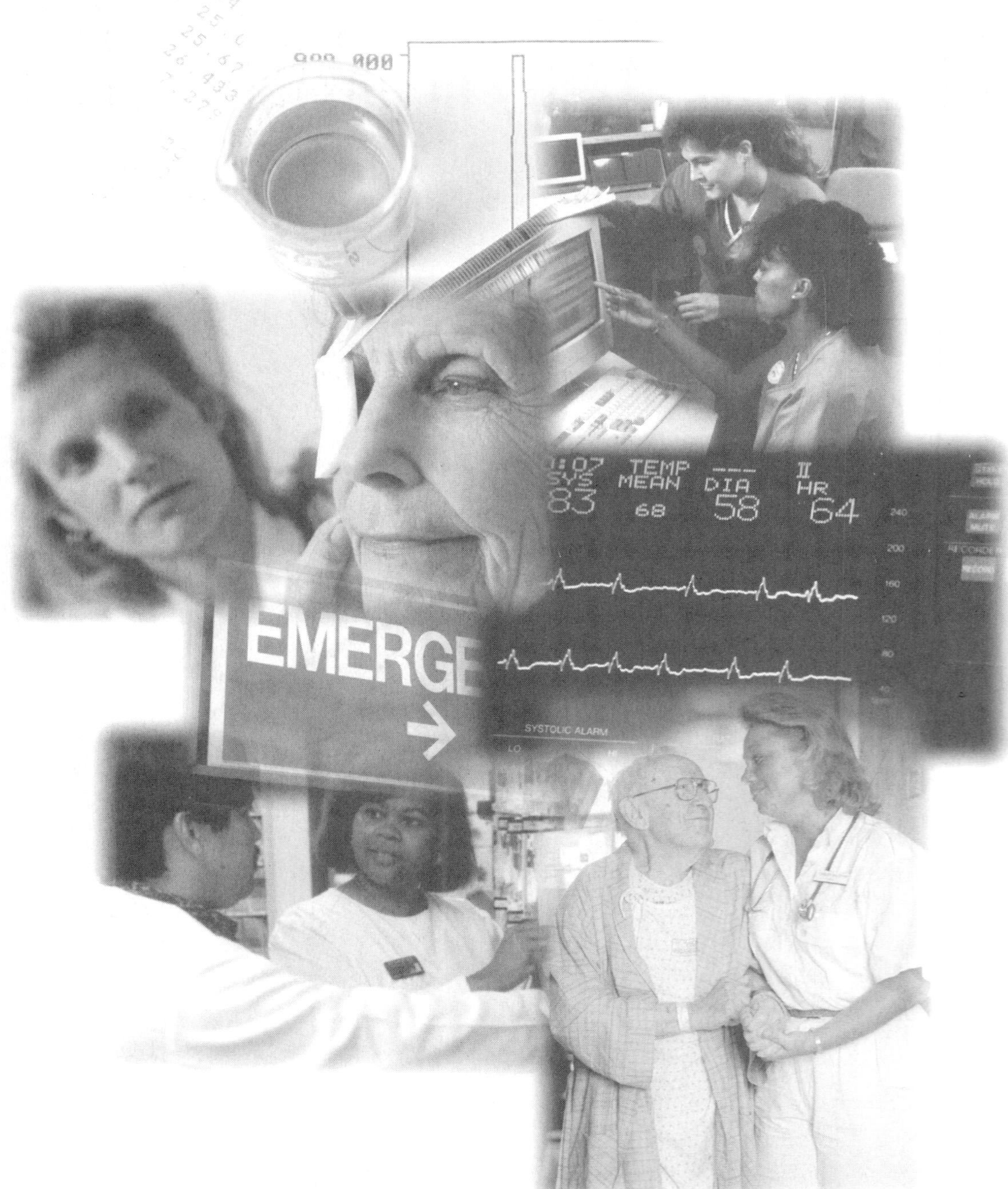
TEMP
SYS MEAN DIA HR
83 68 58 64
EMERGE
SYSTOLIC ALARM

CURRENT ISSUES IN NURSING

Fifth Edition

EDITED BY

Joanne Comi McCloskey, PhD, RN, FAAN

Distinguished Professor, College of Nursing
The University of Iowa
Adjunct Associate Director of Nursing
The University of Iowa Hospitals and Clinics
Iowa City, Iowa

Helen Kennedy Grace, PhD, RN, FAAN

Special Assistant to the President
W.K. Kellogg Foundation
Battle Creek, Michigan

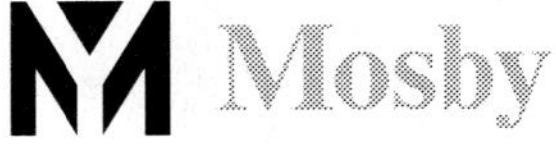

St. Louis Baltimore Boston Carlsbad Chicago Naples New York Philadelphia Portland
London Madrid Mexico City Singapore Sydney Tokyo Toronto Wiesbaden

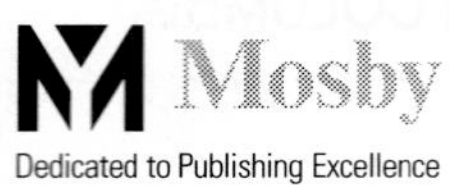

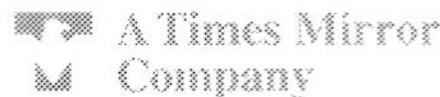

Publisher: Nancy L. Coon
Executive Editor: N. Darlene Como
Senior Developmental Editor: Laurie Sparks
Associate Developmental Editor: Lisa P. Newton
Project Manager: Chris Baumle
Production Editor: Stacy M. Loonstyn
Design Manager: Nancy McDonald
Cover: Sheriff Design
Manufacturing Manager: William A. Winneberger, Jr.

FIFTH EDITION

Printed in the United States of America
Composition by Graphic Composition, Inc.
Printing/binding by Maple-Vail–Binghamton

Mosby–Year Book, Inc.
11830 Westline Industrial Drive
St. Louis, Missouri 63146

Library of Congress Cataloging-in-Publication Data

Current issues in nursing / edited by Joanne Comi McCloskey, Helen Kennedy Grace. — 5th ed.
p. cm.
Includes bibliographical references and index.
ISBN 0-8151-8594-4
1. Nursing. 2. Nursing—United States. 3. Nursing—Social aspects. 4. Nursing—Social aspects—United States. 5. Nursing—Practice. 6. Nursing—Practice—United States.
I. McCloskey, Joanne Comi. II. Grace, Helen K.
[DNLM: 1. Nursing. 2. Nursing Theory. 3. Education, Nursing. 4. Ethics, Nursing. WY 16 C976 1997]
RT63.C87 1997
610.73—dc20
DNLM/DLC
for Library of Congress 96-35126
CIP

97 98 99 00 / 9 8 7 6 5 4 3 2 1

Contributors

Tonia D. Aiken, BSN, RN, JD
President, The American Association of Nurse Attorneys Foundation
President, RN Development, Inc., Metairie, Louisiana

Cathy A. Alessi, MD
Geriatric Research, Education, & Clinical Center (GRECC)
Sepulveda VA Medical Center, Sepulveda, California

Ferial A.M. Aly, PhD, RN
Dean and Professor
Faculty of Nursing
University of Alexandria, Alexandria, Egypt

Carole A. Anderson, PhD, RN, FAAN
Dean and Professor
College of Nursing
The Ohio State University, Columbus, Ohio

Ida M. Androwich, PhD, RN, FAAN
Professor
Community, Mental Health, and Administrative Nursing
Niehoff School of Nursing
Loyola University, Chicago, Illinois

JoAnn Appleyard, PhD, RN
Director of Ambulatory Nursing
FHP, Inc., Cerritos, California

Harriet Udin Aronow, PhD
Multicampus Program in Geriatric Medicine and Gerontology
UCLA School of Medicine
University of California, Los Angeles, California
and Senior Health & Peer Counseling
Santa Monica, California
and Nursing Research & Development
Cedars-Sinai Medical Center, Los Angeles, California

Susan M. Awbrey, PhD
Department Chair and Associate Professor
School of Education and Human Services
Oakland University, Rochester, Michigan

Judith Gedney Baggs, PhD, RN
Clinical Nurse Researcher, Strong Memorial Hospital
Assistant Professor of Clinical Nursing
School of Nursing
University of Rochester, Rochester, New York

John C. Beck, MD
Multicampus Program in Geriatric Medicine and Gerontology
UCLA School of Medicine
University of California, Los Angeles, California

Geraldine Polly Bednash, PhD, RN, FAAN
Executive Director
American Association of Colleges of Nursing
Washington, DC

Jennifer Maria Ann Bichel, MPH, RN
Lecturer
School of Nursing
Queensland University of Technology
Brisbane, Queensland
Australia

Leah F. Binder, MGA, MA
Senior Project Advisor
Health & Hospitals Corporation of New York City
New York, New York

Mary A. Blegen, PhD, RN
Associate Professor
and Area Chair for Theory and Health Promotion
College of Nursing
The University of Iowa, Iowa City, Iowa

Carol J. Boyd, PhD, RN
Associate Professor
School of Nursing/Women's Studies
University of Michigan, Ann Arbor, Michigan

Dorothy Brooten, PhD, RN, FAAN
Associate Dean for Research and Graduate Studies
Case Western Reserve University
Francis Payne Bolton School of Nursing
Cleveland, Ohio

Ginette Budreau, MA, MBA, RN
Clinical Nurse Specialist
Pediatric/Ob-Gyn Nursing Division
The University of Iowa Hospitals and Clinics
Iowa City, Iowa

Peter I. Buerhaus, PhD, RN, FAAN
Director, Harvard Nursing Research Institute
and Assistant Professor
Harvard School of Public Health
Department of Health Policy and Management
Boston, Massachusetts

Vern L. Bullough, PhD, RN, FAAN
Visiting Professor, Nursing
University of Southern California
Los Angeles, California

Paulette Burns, PhD, RN
Associate Professor
and Coordinator, Tulsa Campus
University of Oklahoma
College of Nursing, Tulsa, Oklahoma

Dorothy D. Camilleri, PhD, RN
Assistant Professor
and Executive Associate Dean, Emerita
College of Nursing
University of Illinois at Chicago, Chicago, Illinois

Cecelia Capuzzi, PhD, RN
Associate Professor
Oregon Health Sciences University
Community Health Care Systems, Portland, Oregon

Lynda Juall Carpenito, MSN, RN
President
LJC Consultants, Inc., Mickleton, New Jersey

Patricia T. Castiglia, PhD, RN-C, PNP
Dean
College of Nursing and Health Sciences
University of Texas at El Paso, El Paso, Texas

Helen Castillo, PhD, RN, FAAN
Associate Professor
and Chair, Nursing Department
College of Nursing and Health Sciences
University of Texas at El Paso, El Paso, Texas

Peggy L. Chinn, PhD, RN, FAAN
Professor of Nursing
University of Colorado Health Sciences Center
Denver, Colorado

Roseni Rosangela Chompré, MS, RN
Assistant Professor
School of Nursing
University Federal of Minas Gerais
Minas Gerais, Brasil

Maria Auxiliadora Cardova Christofaro, RN
Assistant Professor
School of Nursing
University Federal of Minas Gerais
Minas Gerais, Brasil

Charlene E. Clark, MEd, RN, FAAN
Professor of Nursing
and Assistant Dean, Instructional Resources
Intercollegiate Center for Nursing Education
Learning Resources Unit, Spokane, Washington

June Clark, DBE, PhD, RN, RHV, FRCN
Professor of Nursing
Middlesex University, Queensway
London, England

Laurel Archer Copp, PhD, RN, FAAN
Honorary Doctor of Letters
Editor *Journal of Professional Nursing*
and Professor, Dean Emeritus
University of North Carolina
Chapel Hill, North Carolina

Mori Costantino, MS, RN
Doctoral Student
University of California, San Francisco
School of Nursing, San Francisco, California

Perle Slavik Cowen, PhD, RN
Assistant Professor
The University of Iowa
College of Nursing, Iowa City, Iowa

Shelly Crow, MS, RN
Second Chief
Muscogee (Creek) National, Okmulgee, Oklahoma

Connie Curran, EdD, RN, FAAN
President
CurranCare, North Riverside, Illinois

Susan L. Dean-Baar, PhD, RN, CRRN, FAAN
Assistant Professor
University of Wisconsin–Milwaukee
School of Nursing
Department of Health Restoration
Milwaukee, Wisconsin

Betty Pierce Dennis, DrPH, RN
Associate Professor
Department of Nursing
North Carolina Central University
Durham, North Carolina

Donna Diers, MSN, RN, FAAN
The Annie W. Goodrich Professor
Yale University School of Nursing
and Lecturer
Department of Epidemiology and Public Health
Yale University School of Medicine
New Haven, Connecticut

Laura Duckett, PhD, RN
Associate Professor
School of Nursing
University of Minnesota, Minneapolis, Minnesota

Dawn A. Duncan, MSN, RN
Patient Care Manager
University of Nebraska Medical Center
Omaha, Nebraska

Joellen B. Edwards, PhD, RN, CS
Dean and Professor
College of Nursing
East Tennessee State University, Johnson City, Tennessee

Claire M. Fagin, PhD, RN, FAAN
Leadership Professor, Dean Emeritus
University of Pennsylvania School of Nursing
Philadelphia, Pennsylvania

Sharon Farley, PhD, RN
Interim Dean
and Director, Kellogg Project
School of Nursing
Auburn University at Montgomery
Montgomery, Alabama

Mary V. Fenton, DrPH, RN
Dean and Professor
University of Texas Medical Branch
School of Nursing, Galveston, Texas

Marilyn S. Fetter, PhD, RN, CS
Assistant Professor
Villanova University, Villanova, Pennsylvania

Lyndia Flanagan, MA
Workplace Consultant, Kansas City, Missouri

Patricia R. Forni, PhD, RN, FAAN
Dean and Professor
University of Oklahoma
College of Nursing, Oklahoma City, Oklahoma

Virginia Kliner Fowkes, FNP, MHS
Director, Primary Care Associate Program
and Stanford Area Health Education Center
Division of Family and Community Medicine
Palo Alto, California

Latrell P. Fowler, PhD, RN
Assistant Professor
College of Nursing
Medical University of South Carolina
Charleston, South Carolina

Sara T. Fry, PhD, RN, FAAN
Henry R. Luce Professor of Nursing Ethics
Boston College School of Nursing
Chestnut Hill, Massachusetts

Mohan L. Garg, ScD
Professor
Department of Medical Education
University of Illinois at Chicago
College of Medicine, Chicago, Illinois

Marcia N. Gold, MSN, RN-C
Multicampus Program in Geriatric Medicine
and Gerontology
UCLA School of Medicine
University of California, Los Angeles, California
and Eichenbaum Health Center
Jewish Family Service, Los Angeles, California

Helen Kennedy Grace, PhD, RN, FAAN
Special Assistant to the President
W.K. Kellogg Foundation, Battle Creek, Michigan

Cecelia Gatson Grindel, PhD, RN
Assistant Professor
Northeastern University, Boston, Massachusetts

Carole A. Gutt, EdD, RN, CCM
Director, Graduate Nursing
Assistant Chairperson, Nursing Division
D'Youville College, Buffalo, New York

Sheila A. Haas, PhD, RN
Professor and Chair
Community, Mental Health, and Administrative Nursing
Niehoff School of Nursing, Loyola University
Chicago, Illinois

Donna Sullivan Havens, PhD, RN
Program Director and Assistant Professor
Nursing Systems Administration Graduate Program
Duke University School of Nursing
Durham, North Carolina

Susan O. Hendricks, MA, MS
Quality Officer
University of Nebraska Medical Center
Omaha, Nebraska

Ann Henrick, PhD, RN, FAAN
Clinical Nurse Specialist
Edward Hines Junior Hospital, Hines, Illinois
and Clinical Associate Professor
Neihoff School of Nursing
Loyola University, Chicago, Illinois

Suzanne Bakken Henry, DNSc, RN, FAAN
Assistant Professor
University of California, San Francisco
School of Nursing, San Francisco, California

JoAnne Herman, PhD, RN
Associate Professor
College of Nursing
University of South Carolina, Columbia, South Carolina

Tonda L. Hughes, PhD, RN
Assistant Professor
Department of Public Health, Mental Health, and Administrative Nursing
University of Illinois at Chicago, Chicago, Illinois

Marguerite McMillian Jackson, PhD, RN, CIC, FAAN
Administrative Director
Medical Center Epidemiology Unit
University of California, San Diego
San Diego, California

Sonia Jaimovich, MPH, RN
Associate Professor
School of Nursing
Pontifical Catholic University of Chile
Santiago, Chile

Lucille A. Joel, EdD, RN, FAAN
Professor
Rutgers-The State University of New Jersey
College of Nursing, Newark, New Jersey

Karlene Kerfoot, PhD, RN, CNAA, FAAN
Executive Vice President, Patient Care
Chief Nursing Officer
Chief Quality Officer
St. Luke's Episcopal Hospital
Texas Medical Center, Houston, Texas

Janet C. Ross Kerr, PhD, RN
Professor, Faculty of Nursing and Division of Bioethics
Faculty of Medicine
University of Alberta, Edmonton, Canada

Shaké Ketefian, EdD, RN, FAAN
Professor, and Director of the Doctoral Program
University of Michigan
School of Nursing, Ann Arbor, Michigan

Diane K. Kjervik, JD, RN, FAAN
Professor and
Associate Dean for Community Outreach and Practice
The University of North Carolina at Chapel Hill
School of Nursing, Chapel Hill, North Carolina

Kathleen Krichbaum, PhD, RN
Assistant Professor
School of Nursing
University of Minnesota, Minneapolis, Minnesota

Phyllis Beck Kritek, PhD, RN, FAAN
Chair and Professor
University of Texas Medical Branch
School of Nursing, Galveston, Texas

Jody L. Kurtt, MA, RN, CPNP, CNAA
Clinical Director
Pediatric/Ob-Gyn Nursing Division
The University of Iowa Hospitals and Clinics
Iowa City, Iowa

Susan Park Kyzer, MS, RN
Senior Consultant
The Center for Case Management
South Natick, Massachusetts

Bernadine M. Lacey, EdD, RN, FAAN
Associate Professor and Director
School of Nursing
Western Michigan University, Kalamazoo, Michigan

Ilta Lange, MS, RN
Associate Professor and Director
School of Nursing
Pontifical Catholic University of Chile, Santiago, Chile

Marlene Lawrence, BSN, RN
Program Manager
Calhoun County Health Improvement Program
Battle Creek Community Foundation
Battle Creek, Michigan

Scott Leighty
Associate
APM, Inc., Chicago, Illinois

Marsha Lewis, PhD, RN
Assistant Professor
School of Nursing
University of Minnesota, Minneapolis, Minnesota

Sally Peck Lundeen, PhD, RN, FAAN
Associate Professor
University of Wisconsin–Milwaukee
School of Nursing, Milwaukee, Wisconsin

Meridean L. Maas, PhD, RN, FAAN
Professor
The University of Iowa
College of Nursing, Iowa City, Iowa

Cynthia MacLeod, BSN, RN
Master's Student
School of Public Health
University of Illinois at Chicago, Chicago, Illinois

Beverly L. Malone, PhD, RN, FAAN
Professor
North Carolina A&T State University
Greensboro, North Carolina
and President
American Nurses Association
Washington, DC

Diann L. Martin, DNSc, RN
Vice President and Chief Operating Officer
Visiting Nurse Association of Chicago, Chicago, Illinois

Karen S. Martin, MSN, RN, FAAN
Health Care Consultant, Omaha, Nebraska

Mary N. McAlindon, EdD, RN, CNAA
Clinical Informatics Manager
McLaren Health Care Corporation, Flint, Michigan

Joanne Comi McCloskey, PhD, RN, FAAN
Distinguished Professor of Nursing
College of Nursing
The University of Iowa, Iowa City, Iowa
and Adjunct Associate Director of Nursing
The University of Iowa Hospitals and Clinics
Iowa City, Iowa

Diana C. McPherson, RN, BSN, CIC
Senior Nurse Epidemiologist
Medical Center Epidemiology Unit
University of California, San Diego
San Diego, California

Anamaria Vaz de Assis Medina, MS
Consultant
Minas Gerais, Brasil

Afaf I. Meleis, PhD, RN, DrPS (hon), FAAN
Professor
Department of Mental Health, Community, and Administrative Nursing
School of Nursing
University of California, San Francisco
San Francisco, California

Andrea Mengel, PhD, RN
Professor, Department of Nursing
Community College of Philadelphia
Philadelphia, Pennsylvania

Janet Mentink, PhD, FNP, MHS
Director, Family Nurse Practitioner and Physician Assistant Program
Department of Family Medicine
School of Medicine
University of California at Davis, Davis, California

Patricia Maguire Meservey, PhD, RN
Executive Director
Center for Community Health Education, Research, and Service
and Associate Professor
Northeastern University
College of Nursing, Boston, Massachusetts

Mary Etta Mills, ScD, RN, CNAA
Department Chair and Associate Professor
Department of Education, Administration, Health Policy, and Informatics
University of Maryland School of Nursing
Baltimore, Maryland

Maria Mitchell, MS, RN, PNP
Mayor's Special Advisor on Health Policy
New York, New York

Margo C. Neal, MN, RN
Vice President and Publisher
Nursecom, Inc., Malibu, California

Virginia M. Ohlson, PhD, RN, FAAN
Professor Emeritus
University of Illinois at Chicago
College of Nursing, Chicago, Illinois

Daniel J. Pesut, PhD, RN, FAAN
Associate Professor
College of Nursing
University of South Carolina, Columbia, South Carolina

Adele W. Pike, MSN, RN
Clinical Nurse
Visiting Nurse Association of Boston
Boston, Massachusetts

Eve Pinsker, PhD
Research Associate
Department of Medical Education
University of Illinois at Chicago
College of Medicine, Chicago, Illinois

Cheryl L. Ramler, PhD, RN
Nurse Anesthesia Student
The University of Iowa
College of Nursing, Iowa City, Iowa

Marilyn J. Rantz, PhD, RN, FAAN
Assistant Professor and
University Hospital and Clinics Professor of Nursing
University of Missouri-Columbia
Sinclair School of Nursing, Columbia, Missouri

Richard W. Redman, PhD, RN
Associate Professor and
Director, Division of Nursing and Health Systems Administration
The University of Michigan
School of Nursing, Ann Arbor, Michigan

Marilyn Rice, MPA, RN, CEN, CNAA
New Business Development Representative
Sterling Healthcare Group, Toledo, Ohio
and Past President
Emergency Nurses Association

Barbara Robertson, D.Litt et Phil RNRM
Professor and Head
Department of Nursing Education
University of the Witwatersrand
Johannesburg, South Africa

Marilyn L. Rothert, PhD, RN, FAAN
Dean and Professor
Michigan State University
College of Nursing, East Lansing, Michigan

Marla E. Salmon, ScD, RN, FAAN
Director
Division of Nursing
U.S. Department of Health & Human Services
Public Health Service, Rockville, Maryland

Susan Sherman, MA, RN
Professor and Head
Department of Nursing
Community College of Philadelphia
Philadelphia, Pennsylvania

Carolyn Hope Smeltzer, EdD, RN, FAAN, FACHE
Principal, Coopers & Lybrand
Integrated Health Care Consulting Services
Chicago, Illinois
and Professor
Niehoff School of Nursing
Loyola University, Chicago, Illinois

Deborah S. Smith, MS, MBA, RN
Assistant Administrator Nursing Services
St. Joseph Medical Center, Bloomington, Illinois

Linda S. Smith, MSN, RN
Assistant Professor of Nursing
State University of West Georgia, Carrollton, Georgia
and Founder of the US-Russian Nurse Exchange Consortium, Racine, Wisconsin
and Special Government Employee
Department of Health and Human Services
Food and Drug Administration, Rockville, Maryland

Susan M. Sparks, PhD, RN, FAAN
Senior Education Specialist
Extramural Programs
National Library of Medicine, Bethesda, Maryland

Janet P. Specht, PhD, RN
Program Assistant, Family Involvement in Care
The University of Iowa
College of Nursing, Iowa City, Iowa

Richard Splane, CM, PhD, LLD
Professor Emeritus
University of British Columbia
and Consultant, Social Policy
Vancouver, British Columbia, Canada

Verna Huffman Splane, OC, RN, MPH, LLD
Consultant, Health Policy
Vancouver, British Columbia, Canada

Dulcelina Albano Stahl, PhD, RN, CNAA
President
D. A. Stahl & Associates, Northbrook, Illinois

Victoria M. Steelman, MA, RN, CNOR
Advanced Practice Nurse
Intensive and Surgical Services
The University of Iowa Hospitals and Clinics
Iowa City, Iowa
and Doctoral Candidate, Nursing, The University of Iowa

Nancy A. Stotts, EdD, RN
Associate Professor
Department of Physiological Nursing
School of Nursing
University of California, San Francisco
San Francisco, California

Gail W. Stuart, PhD, RN, CS, FAAN
Administrator, Institute of Psychiatry
Professor, College of Nursing
Associate Professor, College of Medicine
Medical University of South Carolina
Charleston, South Carolina

Margretta Madden Styles, EdD, RN, FAAN
President, International Council of Nurses
Geneva, Switzerland

Elaine Tagliareni, MSN
Independence Chair in Community Based Nursing Education
Community College of Philadelphia
Philadelphia, Pennsylvania

Geraldine J. Talarczyk, EdD, RN
Associate Professor and Associate Dean for Academic Affairs
Michigan State University
College of Nursing, East Lansing, Michigan

Barbara Volk Tebbitt, MS, RN
Consultant in Organizational Service Integration
Shoreview, Minnesota

Marita G. Titler, PhD, RN, FAAN
Director, Nursing Research and Quality Management
The University of Iowa Hospitals and Clinics
Iowa City, Iowa

Linda Titus, MSN, RN, CNA
Associate Chief, Nursing Service
VA Connecticut, West Haven Campus
West Haven, Connecticut

Sara Torres, PhD, RN, CS, FAAN
Associate Professor and Department Chair
Department of Community Nursing
College of Nursing
University of North Carolina at Charlotte
Charlotte, North Carolina

Pamela Klauer Triolo, PhD, RN
Chief Nursing Officer and Associate Dean
University of Nebraska Medical Center
Omaha, Nebraska

Toni Tripp-Reimer, PhD, RN, FAAN
Professor and
Director, Office for Nursing Research, Development, and Utilization
College of Nursing
The University of Iowa, Iowa City, Iowa

Michelle Vruwink, MPA
Assistant Director
Mayor's Office of Health Services
Medical Managed Care, New York, New York

Patricia Hinton Walker, PhD, RN, FAAN
Kate Hanna Harvey Visiting Professor
Frances Payne Bolton School of Nursing
Case Western Reserve University
Cleveland, Ohio
and Associate Professor of Clinical Nursing
University of Rochester
School of Nursing, Rochester, New York

Verle Waters, MA, RN
Dean Emeritus
Ohlone College, Fremont, California

Kay Weiler, MA, RN, JD
Associate Professor
The University of Iowa
College of Nursing, Iowa City, Iowa

Ruth Williams-Brinkley, MSN, RN
Wharton Fellow
Senior Associate
APM, Inc., Atlanta, Georgia

Karen S. Wulff, EdD, MN, RN
Assistant Administrator, Patient Care Services
Fred Hutchinson Cancer Research Center
and Clinical Assistant Professor
School of Nursing
University of Washington, Seattle, Washington

Carolyn J. Yocom, PhD, RN, FAAN
Director of Research Services
National Council of State Boards of Nursing
Chicago, Illinois

Karen E. Yuhas, MPH, RN-C
Adventist Home Health Services
Silver Spring, Maryland

Polly Gerber Zimmermann, MS, MBA, RN, CEN
Staff Nurse III (Emergency Room)
Swedish Covenant Hospital, Chicago, Illinois
and Consulting Editor, *Journal of Emergency Nursing*
and Consultant, International Healthcare
Consulting Group

Margo R. Zink, EdD, RN, CNAA
Healthcare Consultant
Baltimore, Maryland

Laurie Zoloth-Dorfman, PhD
Ethicist and Associate Professor
Children's Hospital, Oakland, California
and San Francisco State University
San Francisco, California

Mary Zwygart-Stauffacher, PhD, RN
Associate Professor and Coordinator
Gerontological Nurse Practitioner Program
College of St. Catherine, St. Paul, Minnesota
and Gerontological Nurse Practitioner
Red Cedar Clinic/Mayo Health System
Menomonie, Wisconsin

Preface

Previous editions of this book were published in 1981, 1985, 1990, and 1994—every 4 or 5 years. This edition published in 1997, comes only 3 years after the previous edition. We were asked to increase the frequency of the editions by users of the book and by our publisher due to the many changes in health care and the need to keep current with the changes. Initially we were reluctant to do this given our busy work schedules and the fact that each edition takes approximately two years to produce, but we agree with the need and have tried to produce this volume in a timely manner.

Given the rapidity of changes in the health care environment, we believe that a book such as ours that attempts to describe and discuss all the current issues in nursing is important. In periods of rapid change, decisions must often be made quickly. With many issues confronting such a large and diverse profession, there is danger that decisions will be made without full knowledge or without sufficient opportunity to discuss and debate. Or worse yet, issues may be ignored and decisions not made. **The purpose of this book is to provide a forum for knowledgeable debate on the important issues that concern all of today's nurses so that intelligent decision making can occur.**

As in the previous editions, the issues are identified and addressed in sections. Previous editions had 12 sections but this edition has 11: definitions of nursing, changing information, changing education, changing practice, quality improvement, governance, health care systems, health care costs, role transitions, cultural diversity, and ethics and legal issues. The previous sections on personal and professional assertiveness and role conflict were combined to form our current section called role transitions. The last section on ethics has been expanded to include legal issues. One of the other major changes in format compared with previous editions is the nature of the chapters in section four on changing practice. Each of the viewpoints in this section relates to changes and issues in specific areas of specialty practice. We expanded the usual number of chapters in this section to include ten viewpoints, nine about areas of specialty practice plus an international chapter.

As in previous editions, each section includes an **overview** of the section, a **debate** chapter, and several **viewpoint** chapters. In the first edition, we had 75 chapters, in the second 84, and in the third 89, in the fourth 103, and in this edition 92. We made a conscious attempt in this edition to reduce the number of chapters as the size of the book was becoming unmanageable. Of the 92 chapters in this edition, only 1 is a reprint from the fourth edition, 39 are updates from the fourth edition, and 52 are totally new. Most of the updated chapters are so much revised that they are not comparable to the previous versions. All of the chapters are original pieces written for this book and none, to our knowledge, are published elsewhere. We have continued a feature that was introduced in the third edition, the conclusion of each section with a chapter written from an international perspective.

Among the new content topics for this edition are: benchmarking, the internet, critical thinking, distance learning, community-based nursing education, clinical pathways, coalition building, academic health centers, home care costs, legal implications for professional practice, sexual and verbal harassment, and nursing ethics committees. We have kept the fourth edition format of section one, Definitions of Nursing, where the section overviews the facts and issues about specific groups of nurses and serves as an introduction to the rest of the book. A new chapter in this section discusses the role of the nurse informaticist as this is a new, rapidly growing, and important role in nursing. As mentioned previously, section four on Changing Practice has totally new content. Changes and issues are addressed related to various specialties: ambulatory nursing, community nursing, emergency nursing, gerontological nursing, medical-surgical nursing, pediatric nursing, perinatal nursing, perioperative nursing, and psychiatric nursing. These chapters are among the most exciting in the book and demonstrate the impact of health care changes on nursing. Section ten, Cultural Diversity, also looks at changes and issues related to three specific cultures: Native Americans, African Americans, and Hispanics/Latinos.

Each section begins with an **overview** where we briefly introduce the section and "overview" each of the chapters in it. The sections' overviews, which highlight some of the important points in each chapter and raise some related issues, assist readers to select chapters for in-depth reading.

Following the overview, each section has a **debate** chapter, featuring the differing perspectives on one of the problematic issues in nursing. A listing of the titles of debate chapters in the edition gives some idea of the scope of the issues:

- What is nursing?
- Nursing theory, nursing research, and nursing practice: Connected or separate?
- Nursing education for the 21st century: Old traditions and new challenges
- Moving the care site from hospital to home: Whose turf?
- Improving quality of care: Can managed care make a difference?
- The increasing use of unlicensed assistive personnel: The erosion or elevation of nursing?
- From a medical care system for a few to a comprehensive health care system for all
- Controlling health care costs: Regulation versus competition
- Collaboration between nurses and physicians: What is it? Does it exist? Why does it matter?
- Why isn't nursing more diversified?
- The ethics of health care reform: Should rationing strategies target the elderly?

In the first edition, the debate chapters were a result of master's students participation in an issues course at the University of Illinois College of Nursing. The chapters were based on actual oral debates that took place in class. For each debate a small group of students (anywhere from two to five) were asked to choose a topic, make up a reading list for advance distribution, and present all sides of the issue in the debate format to the rest of the class. Each group was instructed to stress the facts and research findings and to be as creative in presentation as they could. The approach was intellectual but the mood was fun. Several groups conducted their own surveys of class knowledge and options prior to class. Others dressed for and acted out parts. For example, in one class there was a physician's assistant and a nurse practitioner who dressed exactly alike in their lab coats and stethoscopes. In another, the students played the parts of nursing deans to argue out the merits of a PhD or a DN program.

Each group was required to state its debate topic in a debate form; the same topic could lead to several debates. For example, the topic, expanded role, resulted in one group in a debate entitled, "Should Nurses Practice Dependently, Independently, or Interdependently?" and in another group resulted in a debate entitled "Nurse Practitioners or Physician Assistants?" In a two-hour class, one hour was allocated for the debate presentation and one hour for questions and debate with the rest of the class.

Some of the class debates were written up and published in the first edition. In ensuing editions we have kept the same format as we think debates are an excellent teaching mode for this content. Students who debate the material as well as their audience are involved in sorting out the complicated issues surrounding the debate. Many times just knowing all the facts leads to effective decision making; other times, it leads to the knowledge of what further research is needed before effective decision making can occur.

The bulk of the book is composed of **viewpoint** chapters. In these chapters, each author gives her or his own view and critical analysis of one particular aspect of the section's general topic. Viewpoints are those of the individual authors and may involve their taking a controversial stand, presenting a case study or results of some research, reviewing the past and current status of a topic, or outlining problems and future decisions. The viewpoint chapters differ from the debate chapters in offering only one side or a piece of an issue. It is hoped that the viewpoint chapters provide material and ideas for other debates, that readers will agree or take issue, that after reading a viewpoint they will be stimulated to think and seek out more information. It is impossible to list all the many viewpoints here but a sample list of titles will, we hope, make you eager to read these and more.

- Clinical nurse specialists and nurse practitioners: Who are they, what do they do, and what challenges do they face?
- Toward a revolution in thinking: The OPT model of clinical reasoning
- Decreasing nursing education costs: Where is the bottom line?
- Recent changes and current issues in community nursing
- Ensuring quality in a managed care system
- Shared governance models in nursing: What is shared, who governs, and who benefits?
- Nursing practice in a political era
- How changes in payment systems are affecting nurses
- Collaboration between medical and nursing education in community-based settings
- Minority representation in nursing educational programs: Increasing cultural awareness
- Working with drug users: Is abstinence the best policy?

Each of the sections ends with an **international** chapter. Reading these chapters will expand the horizons of all nurses. Their titles are:

- International nursing leaders past and present
- The international classification for nursing practice
- Development of models of international exchange to upgrade nursing education
- Reflections on primary health care in developing countries
- Self-care nursing as a contribution to quality improvement in health: A Latin American experience
- International nursing: The role of the International Council of Nurses and the World Health Organization
- The Canadian health care system: Overview and issues
- Financing health care costs in Australia
- Traditional roles for women and the impact on nursing services in Brazil
- Women's health: A global perspective
- Nursing in Russia: Impact of recent political changes

This edition of Current Issues in Nursing, as others in the past, offer a fairly complete analysis of all of today's important nursing issues. Careful reading, thought, and debate today can result in good decisions, actions, and achievements tomorrow.

Who is this book for?

This book is appropriate for several audiences. First, it is an ideal book to use in a senior level undergraduate or graduate level issues course. Faculty who are teaching courses designed to help associate degree and diploma RNs make the transition to the university will also find this book particularly useful. A teacher using this book could easily have her or his class orally present the debates written here or could structure a whole new set of debates using the readings as source material.

Second, it is a good book to use as a core book for a graduate curriculum. There is something here that will fit with most graduate nursing courses. For example, the section on changing information is useful in theory and informatics courses, the section on education for education courses, the sections on practice, quality improvement, and health care systems for advanced practice and nursing administration courses, the section on governance and role transitions for leadership classes, and so on. By picking and choosing from the numerous viewpoints, every class in the graduate curriculum can benefit from the use of this book. By using one text throughout the curriculum, there is financial savings for the individual student and consistency in expectations from the faculty.

Third, the book is of interest to all nurses or nonnurses interested about the profession of nursing. The book is an excellent source of information about nursing and about the issues confronting the profession. The chapters are written by experts in the area and include many well known nursing leaders. The book is stimulating and invigorating and the challenges within will revitalize and energize the reader. It would make a good gift for a new RN or for a nurse going back to graduate school.

Acknowledgments

For help with the fifth edition, we wish to thank the following people:

- Darlene Como, Executive Editor, Mosby–Year Book, who urged us to begin this edition earlier and who has been supportive of the process throughout.
- Jeff Burnham, Editor, Mosby–Year Book, who took over the book from Darlene in the summer of 1996.
- Stacy Loonstyn, Production Editor, Mosby–Year Book, who helped transform the manuscript into this final product.
- Maureen McNally, who did a great job copyediting this textbook.
- Jennifer Clougherty, Program Associate at the University of Iowa, who did most of the administrative detail work related to the book.
- Janet Anderson, Secretary at the University of Iowa, who substituted for Jennifer in the spring of 1995 while she was on maternity leave.
- Sherri Douglas, Executive Secretary at W. K. Kellogg Foundation who worked with Jennifer to coordinate the review of chapters by the editors.

We also want to thank all of our authors for taking the time from busy schedules to think and write about their topics in an interesting and helpful manner. This book is only as good as their contributions.

We are grateful for the continued support and enthusiasm for this book from the nursing community, both in the United States and other countries. We hope that this edition continues to meet your needs.

Finally, we both want to acknowledge the support of our immediate families as well as close friends. Both of us lost our husbands during the production of this edition but with the support of others we were able to finish the preparation of this book.

Joanne Comi McCloskey
and Helen Kennedy Grace

Contents

Section Four
CHANGING PRACTICE

Section Five
QUALITY IMPROVEMENT

Section One

DEFINITIONS OF NURSING

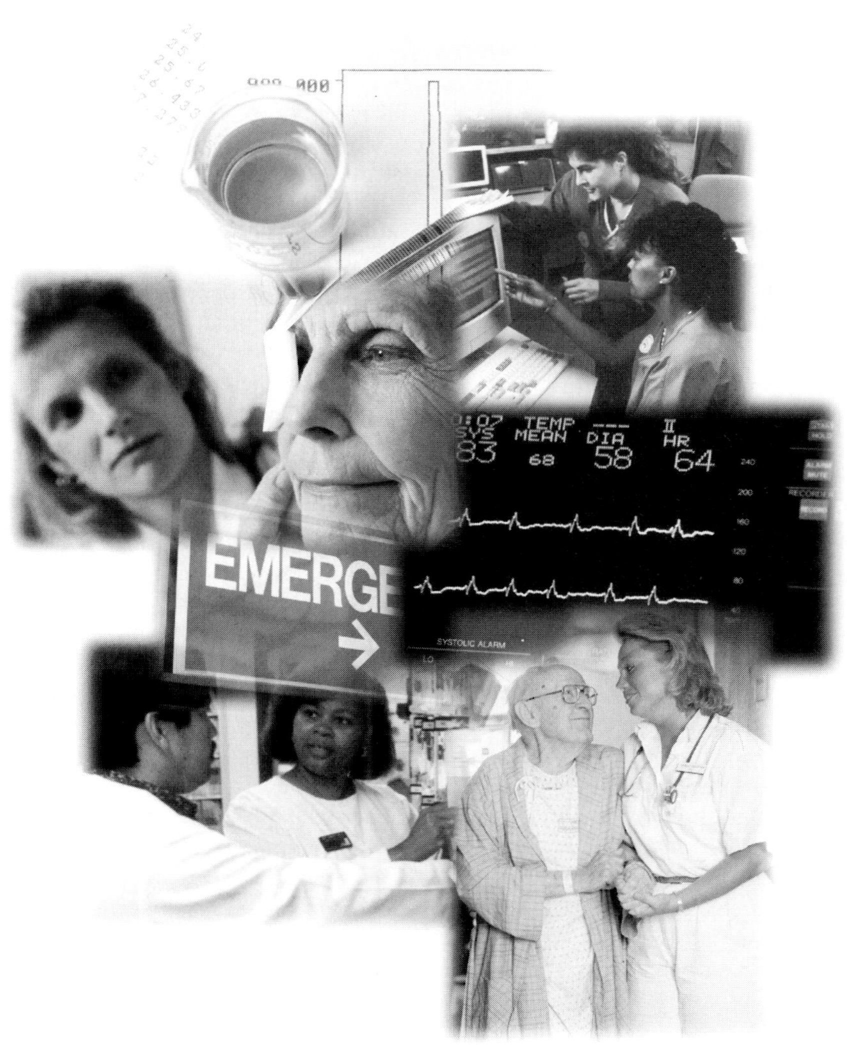

OVERVIEW

The richness of nursing

JOANNE COMI McCLOSKEY, HELEN KENNEDY GRACE

Nursing is a career rich in opportunity and variety. Entering the profession provides an enormous choice of work and setting. Nurses work in hospitals, homes, hospices, nursing homes, industries, doctors' offices, neighborhood health centers, private practices, schools, universities, government agencies, professional associations, and insurance companies. Education levels among nurses are as varied as the work settings, ranging from a 2-year associate degree and a 3-year diploma to master's and doctoral degrees. Most nurses remain in the profession and change jobs several times over the course of their professional careers. The incredible variety among work and workers is the source of many of the important issues that confront the profession. This section serves as an introduction to the issues discussed in the rest of the book. Many of the key positions in nursing are discussed in separate chapters in this section.

What is nursing? In the opening chapter, Diers examines nursing's long-time search for a definition of nursing. She begins by examining dictionary definitions then definitions in law, illustrating the need to evaluate definitions according to the purpose and times for which they are written. Diers then examines the nursing definitions of Nightingale and Henderson because these are important background works. Nursing theories are then reviewed as another source of nursing definitions. Later theorists do not attempt to define nursing; rather they try to understand what works in practice. Diers concludes that the definitional question is a political and legal one, and, increasingly, an economic one—not a conceptual one. She addresses advanced practice as a definitional problem as well as the current challenge that comes from the managed care environment and consulting firms that are downsizing hospitals. Diers says that a description of our ever-changing and complex role goes further to answer the question of what is nursing than any of the definitions put forth over the years. Her chapter is a rich and thoughtful description of the history of various approaches in nursing to capture the nature of our discipline.

In the first viewpoint chapter, Flanagan overviews the roles and challenges of the staff nurse. Approximately two thirds of the 2 million nurses in the United States work in hospitals, mostly as staff nurses. Today's typical staff nurse is older, however, and has more education than in the past. This more stable and mature workforce is more vocal in expressing the frustrations of the job. Flanagan indicates that numerous studies have confirmed that staff nurses want to provide the best nursing care possible but circumstances make it difficult. Nurses today function in a more stressful environment than earlier generations of nurses did. Flanagan overviews the recent changes in the health care marketplace. Patients now have more power and are more knowledgeable, less trusting, and more demanding of higher-quality care. Hospitals are retooling in response to managed care, and nurses, the largest employee group, have become a primary target for redesign measures. Flanagan lists 11 consequences of redesign for the hospital-employed nurse, each of which increases concerns for job security and flexibility. Job security concerns for job are particularly stressful for many nurses who are typically security-oriented and entered nursing for a secure wage. Flanagan ends her chapter with future challenges, including a better understanding of the managed care environment, a need to define services and use information systems, development of stronger leadership skills, strengthening of the professional self-concept, and more attention to career development.

Challenged by their jobs, many staff nurses return to school to get advanced degrees and more knowledge that will help them make needed reforms in their work settings. Many nurses who go on to receive advanced degrees become specialized in a clinical area of practice. Two types of advance practice nurses are the clinical nurse specialist and the nurse practitioner. Henrick and

Appleyard review the origins and outline the functions and roles of each of these advance practitioners. Profiles of six clinical specialists who function in different specialties demonstrate their wide variety of depth and expertise. Henrick and Appleyard then discuss recent trends that may lead to the merger of the two roles with the single title of "advanced practitioner." Clinical nurse specialists and nurse practitioners face many challenges, but their potential impact as a united group should be strong enough to both meet the challenges and make a valuable contribution to health care.

Next, Tebbitt discusses the challenging job of the nurse administrator, which has been made more complex by recent changes and cutbacks in hospitals and other health care organizations. A brief look at the past begins with Nightingale, who defined the major role of the nurse administrator as that of an educator and caretaker for the acutely ill. As time went on, the roles of education and administration were separated. Today's nurse executive has 10 major roles: figurehead, leader, liaison, monitor, disseminator, spokesperson, entrepreneur, disturbance handler, resource allocator, and negotiator. Tebbitt also discusses six functions of the nurse executive: planner, implementer, coordinator, arbitrator, guide, and image setter. She provides an overview of the nurse executive's opportunities, salary ranges, turnover data, academic preparation, and experience. She concludes with four challenges that face tomorrow's nurse executives. The job dimensions of tomorrow's nurse executive will include business acumen, program planning, change management, rapid problem solving, team building, communication skills, conflict management, negotiation skills, and community relationships. This role is not for the faint of heart or the poorly prepared; more than ever it is filled with difficult challenges and responsibilities.

Nursing faculty and the challenges they face are addressed next. Anderson profiles the estimated 19,000 nursing faculty members working in more than 1,400 programs across the country. Nursing, she says, has two types of faculty members, those who are master's prepared teaching mostly clinical instruction in a diploma or associate degree program, and those who are more likely to possess a doctorate degree employed by a college or university and expected to integrate teaching, research, and service. While progress has been made in doctoral preparation of nursing faculty, still only half of those teaching in baccalaureate- and higher-degree programs have doctorates. Anderson says that this noncomparability of credentials, coupled with the lower status of a female occupation, marginalizes academic nurses. Without power and influence women academic nurses become angry and distrustful, which in turn causes academic men in other disciplines to isolate them further. Anderson overviews the various faculty roles and identifies the challenges facing nursing faculty. One challenge is the need for new models for undergraduate clinical teaching. Another is to ensure that our programs meet the needs of students but are rigorous and of high quality. She challenges faculty to work to eliminate practices that do not enhance the goal of becoming full participants in the academy. Among the poor practices she lists are team teaching and harsh treatment of students. This chapter raises many issues that need to be discussed and debated widely. It is an excellent introduction to issues in changing education.

In the next chapter, Stotts overviews the role of the nurse researcher. This is an excellent overview of the various research positions held by nurses and the issues related to the conduction of nursing research. Stotts reviews the roles of research assistant, research nurse, project director, coinvestigator, and principal investigator. The wide variety of methods in nursing research include surveys, interviews, clinical trials, evaluation research, and laboratory research. Time and funding for research are essential. Myriad challenges face nurse researchers including defining why nursing research is important, supporting other nurse researchers whose focus and methods are different from their own, conducting health systems research, getting access to subjects, and obtaining funding. Stotts does a good job of describing this diverse group of nurses who conduct research, and her chapter reflects the diversity of the profession of nursing.

Perhaps the most nontraditional role in nursing is that of the entrepreneur. Carpenito and Neal say that nurse entrepreneurs include a variety of people who are self-employed or pursuing careers that include consulting, writing, editing, owning staffing agencies, giving workshops, or providing patient care. Entrepreneurs seek to "make a difference for a profit." They say that the growth of entrepreneurship in nursing parallels the women's movement. Using their own experience as successful entrepreneurs and those of 19 colleagues whom they queried, Carpenito and Neal discuss a number of issues, including the pros and cons of being self-employed. The pros include the freedom to "do one's own thing" and the flexible work hours. The cons include financial worries and isolation from colleagues. Excellent tips are provided for starting your own business. The chapter provides a very helpful orientation to the work and concerns of nurse entrepreneurs.

Another new role in nursing is the emerging group of nurse specialists who are informaticists. McAlindon begins her chapter with an overview of the history of nursing informatics and goes on to review the titles, roles, and characteristics of this person. The role responsibilities are varied and challenging and require computer skills as well as people skills. Nursing is more in need of data than ever before and more well-trained nurses with computer skills are needed to help us build knowledge from data. The challenges for the nurse informaticist outlined by McAlindon include keeping abreast of the numerous hardware and software changes, determining the appropriate level and type of education and other credentials, and deciding on reporting arrangements that facilitate both the individual, the nursing department, and the organization. In addition, there are other issues related to privacy and confidentiality of data. This is a good introductory chapter to an important role that is growing rapidly in nursing.

The last chapter in the section focuses on nurses in leadership positions at the international level. In 1985 Splane and Splane set out to study chief nursing officers (CNOs) in national health ministries. They traveled to more than 50 countries and interviewed over 90 CNOs. Building on this study of current nurse leaders they then delved into an analysis of past international nursing leaders. In this chapter they discuss past and present international nursing leaders and their leadership within three organizations: the International Council of Nurses, the Red Cross, and the World Health Organization. All nurses in all countries should know about these organizations and the nurses who work in them. Splane and Splane do an excellent job of identifying past and present international nursing leaders. Collaboration among these leaders has been common and, despite obstacles, Splane and Splane show that nursing has provided a good deal of leadership in health care at the international level.

Around the world, it is the nursing leaders who are shaping the future of nursing and health care. Nurse leaders can be found working in a variety of positions and places. Nurse practitioners, administrators, faculty members, researchers, entrepreneurs, informaticists, and other nurses are joining hands to better define nursing's impact on health care. They continually face new challenges, which are discussed in the rest of this book, but their united efforts will keep nursing strong.

What is nursing?

DONNA DIERS

Nursing does not suffer from lack of attempted definition.

In this chapter, the search for a proper definition is examined. The intent is neither to resolve the question by providing a new definition nor to debate old ones. Rather, the purposes, parameters, and consequences of this search are examined with a beady eye. Why define nursing? To what end?

If we do not know what nursing is, how can we justify teaching or studying it or making decisions about it in a policy framework?

DICTIONARY DEFINITIONS

Dictionaries are nothing more than published reports of common usage. In the first edition of the *Random House Dictionary* (1966), the verb "to nurse" means to foster or cherish ("to nurse one's meager talents"); to treat or handle with adroit care ("to nurse one's nest egg"); to bring up, train, or nurture; to clasp or handle carefully or fondly ("to nurse a memento"); to preserve ("to nurse a drink") (p. 990). "Nurse" suggests attendance and service; its antonym is neglect.

Note that these definitions are of the transitive verb form. Because the word *nursing* derives from it, there is no definition of "nursing." In the noun form in this dictionary, a nurse is "a person, especially a woman [sic] who takes care of the sick or infirm; a woman who has the general care of a child or children; a woman employed to suckle an infant; or any fostering agency or influence" (p. 990). A delightfully obscure meaning in billiards says a "nurse" is the act of maintaining the position of billiard balls in preparation for a carom.

Since dictionaries record common meaning, that meaning can and does change. It is encouraging to note that in the 1995 *Random House Collegiate Dictionary,* the first meaning of "nurse" is now "a person formally educated in the care of the sick or infirm, especially a registered nurse" (p. 1061)—surely progress even if they have not learned to capitalize the title.

Congress weighed in when the staff to the Subcommittee on Health and the Environment of the House Committee on Interstate and Foreign Commerce produced *A Discursive Dictionary of Health Care* (1976; never updated) to help members of Congress find their way through the minefield of healthspeak. Here, a nurse is "an individual whose primary responsibility is the provision of nursing care;" and nursing care is

> care intended to assist an individual, sick or well, in the performance of those activities contributing to health or its recovery (or to peaceful death) that he would perform unaided if he had the necessary strength, will or knowledge. (p. 111)

This definition borrows from Virginia Henderson, to whom we will return shortly.

The purpose of dictionary definitions is simply to record common usage, not to distinguish nursing from anything else or to isolate core concepts. There is no political agenda for dictionary definitions, except to the extent common meaning reflects the perspective of those who write the definitions.

DEFINITION IN THE LAW

Legal definitions in Nurse Practice Acts exist to protect the public and to protect the *title*. These laws define (more or less vaguely) authorized practice and qualifications for using the legal title Registered Nurse (RN; or licensed practical [vocational] nurse (LP[V]N), Advanced Practice RN (APRN or ARNP), or nurse-midwife, depending on state law). Licensing laws and their definitions are regula-

Acknowledgement: Sharon Eck, RN, MS, doctoral student, Yale School of Nursing gave valuable assistance in the revision of this chapter.

tory. They do not protect the nurse's practice from the challenge of practicing medicine without a license nor malpractice, although with clever legal assistance the language of practice acts may be used to *win* a court case.

Practice acts are interpreted by state agencies and boards of nursing by interpretive statements, in regulations or declaratory rulings, and by *ad hoc* interpretations by the board or staff in court or less formally. For example, performing a genital examination in a case of suspected child abuse or first-assisting at surgery may be within the authorized practice of nursing in one state but not in another, depending on how expert and liberal the interpreter and the law are. Further refinement of definitions of nursing come from Attorneys General rulings when requested by the board of nursing or another state agency. The extent to which Attorneys General understand modern nursing practice or consult with practicing nurses will determine how conservative or liberal an interpretation of the nurse practice act will emerge.

North Carolina was the first state to pass a licensing law, in 1903, and like many subsequent acts in other states, it was intended to protect the title, not to define the practice. The early statutes were certification laws, permissive rather than mandatory, and in general permitted anyone to perform legally the functions of a nurse, even for compensation, but only those who were licensed could use the RN title (Hadley, 1989).

The early acts were criticized by organized medicine and hospital associations for creating a nursing shortage by requiring registration and restricting the use of the title. Connecticut's legislature dealt with this problem interestingly. An amendment to the Nurse Practice Act in 1907 created a board of appeals to which nurses denied certification by the nursing board could turn. The appeals board consisted entirely of physicians and their decisions were binding on the nursing board. As Hadley (1989) notes, ". . . the appeal board allowed the medical establishment to ensure that there would be an ample supply of nurses able to work at lower wages . . ." (p. 255).

New York state was the first to incorporate a definition of nursing, in 1938. The New York State Nurses Association (NYSNA) argued that "No practice can be controlled unless it is defined" (Driscoll, 1976, p. 46). The control that was sought was over unlicensed or otherwise unqualified individuals who were trading on the title "nurse" and, it could be assumed, taking work away from those who could demand higher wages because of the license.

In this regard, nursing is not different from other licensed professions including medicine. Licensure is usually sought by the profession to protect its own interests, as a study by Andrews (1983) of medical licensure laws often amusingly points out. By defining medicine very broadly, practically anyone's work including a mother's may be captured within it. See, for example, the Michigan definition of medical practice:

> "Practice of medicine" means the diagnosis, treatment, prevention, cure or relieving of a human disease, ailment, defect, complaint or other physical or mental condition, by attendance, advice, device, diagnostic test, or other means, or offering, undertaking, attempting to do, or holding oneself out as able to do, any of those acts. (Andrews, 1983, p. 21, citing Michigan Comp. Laws, 1980)

Medical licensing laws were written long before those of any other profession. This "first mover" advantage has meant that all other personal health care professions have had to contend with the fact that medicine defined the territory first (Safreit, 1993).

The act of defining the work of a profession within the law, then, is a political act, and the resulting definitions must be read in that context. A compelling instance is the way in which the notion of diagnosis has been inserted into nurse practice acts. Idaho slipped the diagnosing function into its practice act first by legislating an exception to the part of the statute that prohibited unauthorized diagnosis and treatment (Bullough, 1980). It was New York, however, that redefined nursing:

> The practice of the profession of nursing . . . is defined as diagnosing and treating human responses to actual or potential health problems through such services as casefinding, health teaching, health counseling and provision of care supportive to and restorative of life and well-being. (Driscoll, 1976, p. 59)

The New York State Nurses Association was advised by its counsel that the diagnostic privilege was the *sine qua non* of independent practice (Driscoll, 1976, p. 59). The "human responses" phrase slips around "disease," which is central to medical practice acts. As a legislative memorandum (drafted by NYSNA) that accompanied the original bill notes,

> Inclusion . . . of the diagnostic function would authorize the nursing practitioner to make *nursing diagnoses, not* medical diagnoses. Whereas the diagnostic function as an intellectual process is central to the practice of any number of professions, including medicine and nursing, the *focus* of this function varies among these professions. For example, the focus in medicine is the nature and degree of pathology or deviation from normalcy; within nursing the focus is the *individual's response* to an actual or potential health problem and the nursing needs arising from such responses. (Driscoll, 1976, p. 61; emphasis in original)

Thus, the attempt to broaden the definition of nursing to include diagnosis had, on the advice of one person, to consider the reality of physician opposition to *independent* practice, and what emerged was a semantic slight of hand. The political reality was the need to build a fence between medicine and nursing; the problem is that this very real concern translates to defining the core of nursing in a way ("human responses") that limits expansion and economic progress. Once "diagnosis" was defined as a nursing function, then obviously there had to be a taxonomy of things nurses could name or diagnose that were not the same as "medical" diagnoses. Without reviewing the entire nursing diagnosis movement, a topic for another whole book, suffice it to say that the attempt to create new language for old things ("pain" as "alteration in comfort") follows from the political agenda to separate nursing from medicine.

The publication and wide distribution of the American Nurses Association (ANA) monograph, *Nursing—A Social Policy Statement* (1980) has had the effect of codifying a definition of nursing based on New York's: "Nursing is the diagnosis and treatment of human responses to actual or potential health problems" (ANA, 1980, p. 9), as if there was some national consensus. The slippage from one political agenda in one state to ANA's own agenda underscores the need to examine definitions according to their purpose. The purpose of the ANA document was to define the nature and scope of nursing practice to serve as a basis for ANA policy regarding credentialing and establishment of qualifications for entry into nursing practice (ANA, 1980, p. v). ANA has another agenda, however, which is to position the Association to speak to and for all kinds of registered nurses, resisting the notion of a second license for specialized practice. Despite the publication of the *Social Policy Statement* and its new language in 1980, in 1981, the ANA's suggested language for nurse practice acts did not mention "human responses" or "actual or potential health problems." But the purpose of these statements is different. The *Social Policy Statement* was exactly that, a statement of organizational policy cast as more general policy. The suggested language for state law is much more operational, because law always is. Thus, in keeping with the above agenda, the suggested language reads:

> The practice of nursing means the performance for compensation of professional services requiring substantial specialized knowledge of the biological, physical, behavioral, psychological and sociological sciences and of nursing theory as the basis for assessment, diagnosis, planning, intervention and evaluation in the promotion and maintenance of health; the casefinding and management of illness, injury or infirmity; the restoration of optimum function; or the achievement of a dignified death. Nursing practice includes but is not limited to administration, teaching, counseling, supervision, delegation, and evaluation of practice and execution of the medical regimen including the administration of medications and treatments prescribed by any person authorized by state law to prescribe. Each registered nurse is directly accountable and responsible to the consumer for quality of nursing care rendered. (ANA, 1981, p. 6)

The landmark case *Sermchief v. Gonzales* (1983) turned on the language of the Missouri Nurse Practice Act, which is very close to the ANA suggested language. In *Sermchief*, the Supreme Court of Missouri determined that the acts of two nurse practitioners did indeed constitute the practice of nursing under Missouri law, including prescribing under standing orders and protocols, not the practice of medicine, overturning a ruling by the Circuit Court. In arriving at this decision, the Court did its own research and noted that many states had by then revised their nurse practice acts to broaden nursing's function. The Court explicitly refused to "draw the elusive line between medicine and nursing," saying that the "hallmark of the professional" is knowing the limits of one's knowledge (Wolff, 1984, p. 26).

By 1990, ANA's suggested language had changed in an interestingly subtle way. Now, "the practice of nursing means the performance of services for compensation in the provision of diagnosis and treatment of human responses to health or illness" (ANA, 1990, p. 8). This change from "health problems" in the *Social Policy Statement* to "health and illness" broadens the target of nursing practice and still slithers away from boldly stating that nurses diagnose and treat disease (a "human response" to health could . . . er . . . be disease). The 1990 version also widens nursing's scope to include case management, establishing standards of practice, directing practice, and collaboration, again following from ANA's wish to be representative of all nurses.

As advanced or specialized practice has grown in nursing with the roles of nurse practitioner,[1] nurse-midwife, and nurse anesthetist increasingly codified in law, the question of the extent to which such advanced practice is really nursing, and thus encompassed in a Nurse Practice Act, or requires some other legal authorization or license has heated up. While the ANA holds firmly to the posi-

[1]The 1995 *Random House Collegiate Dictionary* (p. 1061) defines nurse practitioner as a registered nurse with additional training that prepares the nurse to *diagnose and treat* minor or common diseases. The lay definition is ahead of the legal and professional definitions, recognizing what is now common practice.

tion that if the nurse practice act is worded correctly, a second license (and by implication another organization for practitioners) is not necessary, several states have passed laws or regulations to define various kinds of advanced practice. Florida wins the prize for the most complex and intricate law with some 27 different categories of advanced practice nurses.

The legal challenges to the definition of nursing may also bring into question a particular act or task. One interesting case in Texas that went all the way to the Supreme Court cracked open a door that swings both ways for nursing. In *Irving Independent School District v. Tatro* (1984), the Supreme Court ruled that performing clean intermittent catheterization did not require a medical license and could be performed by a school nurse or "other qualified person." The background of this case illuminates why the context of definition is important. The Tatros are parents of a child with spina bifida. They wished their child, who is fine aside from having this neurological problem, to go to public grade school, but the child required catheterization every 4 hours. Under federal law—the Education for all Handicapped Children Act of 1975 (PL 94-142)—with provisions that bind the states, public education systems must provide free, accessible education for handicapped children, but are not obliged to provide health services (diagnosis, evaluation) by a licensed physician, which was thought to be expensively beyond the intent of the law. The Court explicitly interpreted clean intermittent catheterization as "a simple procedure that can be performed in a few minutes by a layperson with less than an hour's training" (p. 883). Thus the Irving School District was obligated to arrange for the provision of this service so that Amelia Tatro could benefit from free public education. Advocates for disabled persons hailed the decision as broadening the provisions of the law and making education available even when a special service was required. Some in the nursing community cheered that catheterization was interpreted not to need physician supervision. Others were concerned that if this one task could be performed by a layperson, the school nurse's definition of practice was compromised (Vitello, 1987). This piecemeal task-oriented interpretation of what is or isn't nursing has contemporary consequences as we shall see later.

NIGHTINGALE AND HENDERSON

A careful examination of Florence Nightingale's and Virginia Henderson's "definitions" of nursing is in order because they are so often consulted when the nature of nursing is in question.

In *Notes on Nursing—What it is and What it is Not* (1859/1946), Florence Nightingale wrote, "I use the word nursing for want of a better" (p. 6) and "a nurse means any person in charge of the personal health of another" (p. 79).

Miss Nightingale wrote *Notes on Nursing* as a kind of Red Cross handbook for home nursing, to explain the laws of the human body as she understood them and thus how nursing functions could affect health and comfort. She wrote to make conscious the implicit knowledge that women in particular had, especially of diet and cleanliness, so that all women who "nursed" could be better prepared. But she was also writing a political treatise to enlist others in her ideas.

The often-quoted "definition" of nursing comes late in the book in a discussion of what medicine or surgery can do and what nature can do (better) if just left alone:

> It is often thought that medicine is the curative process. It is no such thing; medicine is the surgery of functions, as surgery proper is that of limbs and organs. Neither can do anything but remove obstructions; neither can cure; nature alone cures. (p. 74)

And then, "what nursing has to do . . . is put the patient in the best condition for nature to act upon him" (p. 75). But this is not a definition of nursing. Read in context, it is a somewhat off-handed statement of nursing's function or goal in the context of Miss Nightingale's notions about the causes of illness and her reservations about medicine with its suspicious germ theory.

Virginia Henderson's definition is of the unique *function* of the nurse, which she deliberately calls not a definition, but a "personal concept":

> The unique function of the nurse is to assist the individual sick or well, in the performance of those activities contributing to health or its recovery (or to peaceful death) that he would perform unaided if he had the necessary strength, will or knowledge. And to do this in such a way as to help him gain independence as rapidly as possible. (Henderson, 1961, p. 2)

Miss Henderson is careful to say in the immediately following sentences that this is not all there is to nursing, and thus this definition was never intended to define either the entire discipline or the entire field of practice. The statement is about the *unique* function of the nurse, "this aspect of her work . . . she initiates and controls; of this she is master" (Henderson, 1991, p. 21). For Miss Henderson, this unique function is the core of nursing which must be protected. "No one . . . should make such heavy demands on another member [of the medical team] that any one of them is unable to perform his or her unique function" (p. 42).

In these activities, the nurse is, and, as Miss Henderson argues, should be, an independent practitioner, "able to make independent judgments as long as he, or she, is not diagnosing, prescribing treatment for disease, or making a prognosis, for these are the physician's functions" (p. 22). Reflecting on these statements 30 years later, Miss Henderson revised her emphasis:

> Today I see the role of nurses as givers of "primary health care," as those who diagnose and treat when a doctor is unavailable, even as the midwife functions in the absence of an obstetrician. Nurses may be the general (medical) practitioners of tomorrow. (Henderson, 1991, p. 33)

> The modification in my concept of nursing since I wrote in 1966 suggests a different emphasis. . . . I recognize now, as I think the majority of health care providors recognize, that registered nurses . . . are the major providers of primary care. Obstetrical nurses, or midwives, have been universally recognized worldwide as the providers of primary care for mothers and newborns. They diagnose and treat as well as "care." (p. 98)

Both Nightingale's and Henderson's "definitions" go not to what nursing "is" but rather what nurses *do*. That is a distinction to keep in mind as we dig deeper into the definitional trench.

THEORIES AND DEFINITIONS

This is neither the time nor the place to analyze fully the various theoretical perspectives on nursing that might constitute another source of definition. That work has been done (and done and done again) and is usefully summarized by Afaf Meleis (1991).

Most of the work on the nature of nursing in theory was done by the first wave of nurses either seeking or profiting from doctoral degrees in education or in other disciplines, since there were few doctoral programs in nursing. Most of the theorists came of nursing age before there was the degree of specialist immersion that is now common in practice. Further, the nursing theories emerged at a time when nursing was moving rapidly into the universities. It was important for nursing faculties to justify what was particularly and peculiarly nursing. Thus the search for ways of conceiving of nursing and its knowledge that would mark it as intellectual and as different from simply "applied" anything else (Wald & Leonard, 1964). What resulted was what Virginia Henderson actually advocated—personal conceptions—but those conceptions were not about the work or the practice of nursing, they were about the *discipline*.

These were the content theories: Martha Rogers' "science of unitary man;" Sr. Callista Roy's adaptation theory; Dorothea Orem's theory of self-care deficits, and so on. These theories were really conceptual models, as Fawcett (1980) points out, and they all had the same domains: person, environment, health, and nursing. "Nursing" was more or less the glue that held the whole thing together, often without much specificity as the theories dealt more with the nature of human beings in sickness and health than about what we are supposed to do about sickness and health. Thus, for Martha Rogers, the goal of nursing is to "strengthen the coherence and integrity of the human field and to direct and redirect patterning of the human and environmental fields" (Rogers, 1970, p. 122). And nursing is simply the "learned profession" that does that, whatever that is. For Imogene King, nursing is called for when individuals cannot function in their roles and is "a process of human interaction between nurse and client whereby each perceives the other in the situation and, through communication, they set goals, explore means and agree on means to achieve goals" (King, 1981, p. 144).

The purpose of these grand theories or conceptual models was to develop the discipline (particularly the academic part of the discipline), to provide some structure to the research, and perhaps to stake out turf that would be uniquely nursing, not in opposition to medicine, but as different from applied social science. There was, however, a less-than-explicit agenda that if we would all just do the research guided by whatever conceptual model under whatever theoretical emphasis, when it was all added up we would know what nursing *is*.

The grand theories can be contrasted to another set of "practice theories" that evolved about the same time. The ones most often cited are Ida Orlando's (1961, 1972), Ernestine Weidenbach's (1964), and Joyce Travelbee's (1966). There are two important differences between the grand theories and these: these are about *practice*, not about the nature of the discipline, and their authors were all nurses prepared in specialist or advanced practice (Orlando and Travelbee in psychiatric nursing, Weidenbach in nurse-midwifery).

With the possible exception of Travelbee, these latter theorists did not even attempt to define nursing. For them there is an assumption that we know what nursing *is*, we just need to understand what within it works (i.e., produces desired changes in patient state). The purpose of the theories here was to guide practice and practice-based research, not to fight the definitional battles. For these theorists, nursing was already an independently practicing profession, as their experience in specialized practice roles had taught them. The present effort to create categories of nursing intervention (Iowa Intervention Project, 1995; McCloskey & Bulechek, 1996) follow from the ideas of practice theory, if not explicitly from the theorists. The developing taxonomy of nursing interventions is about practice and the relationship of nursing work to patient outcomes, not about definitions of nursing or nursing diagnoses.

ADVANCED PRACTICE AS A DEFINITIONAL PROBLEM

When nursing roles began to expand beginning in the 1960s with critical care, nursing's outer boundaries, which no one had worried much about before, both loosened and sharpened, again depending on the purpose of definition.

Expanding the nursing role was made legitimate by the *Report of the Secretary's Commission to Study the Extended Role of Nurses* (1971), chaired by Rozella Schlotfeldt. This report defined "primary care" as first contact, continuing, and coordinated care that nurses surely could provide. The expansion of nursing's boundaries was twofold: into independent functioning without physician direction, and into providing services, especially physical examination, diagnosis, and treatment that had been "formerly medicine" (Diers & Molde, 1983).

By this time, nurse-midwives and nurse anesthetists were already firmly established in primary practice roles (Diers, 1992), but with much the same internal and external controversy about whether what they did was "really" nursing. Martha Rogers was moved to write that nurse practitioners ought to just admit that they were filling in for doctors (Rogers, 1975); her argument was not that nurses should not do this work, but that it should be acknowledged as nursing. Loretta Ford (1982) has written poignantly of the discrimination from both nursing and medicine against her pediatric nurse practitioner program.

Ford was clear from the beginning that the nurse practitioner role grew from a base in community health nursing in which nurses had long functioned independently and managed illness alone. Very soon, research showed that nurses could do the work and, over time, enough evidence accumulated to conclude that the performance of nurse practitioners, in productivity and quality, was at least equal to if not better than that of physicians (Brown & Grimes, 1993; Office of Technology Assessment, 1986; Safreit, 1993).

Yet questions remain about whether the work of advanced practice, as it has come to be called (Cronenwett, 1995), is delegated medical functions or within nursing's boundaries. The definitional question, however, is a political and legal one, not a conceptual one, and it is increasingly becoming an economic question as well.

Nurse practitioners grew up in an era of physician shortage, so it was alright for nurses to substitute. When there is a need, it is okay for nurses to do almost anything, as even Virginia Henderson wrote. Where there is competition, challenges to the definition of nursing surface and are very difficult to defend against because the problem is not whether or not this is nursing, but whether we ought to get paid for it.

Advanced practice nursing grew up outside of the professional organization (ANA) for the most part because ANA's priorities have been occupied by economic and general welfare and entry into practice. Without the strong leadership of a national organization representing the breadth of nurse practice roles, both the roles and their definitions have had to turn to the legal system or to specialized nursing associations. In the United States, the regulation of practice is done state by state and there are now over 40 specialized nursing associations, many of which are quite professional with journals, newsletters, annual conventions, lawyers, and lobbyists. There is such a patchwork of nursing specialties that it has become a political problem for nursing at the federal level. It is not the lack of definition that has led to this confusion, however; it is the absence of leadership from a professional association consumed with other issues.

OTHER DEFINITIONAL CHALLENGES

The contemporary challenge to the definition of nursing practice comes from the managed care environment and the consulting firms, which advise hospitals that the fragmentation of patient care in more than 600 categories of hospital workers, as well as the downtime for professional nurses, can be fixed if only hospitals would realize that a good deal of what nurses do (and have to do) is not "really" nursing. Of course it isn't. It does not require a license to call a physician to question a medication order (but it requires knowledge of clinical care), nor is a license required to get the housekeeping department to mop a

EXAMPLES OF NURSING TASKS

Transport patients
Check patient restraints
Keep interior windows clean
Handle red bag waste
Inspect and clean equipment
Assist patients with bathing
Change bed linen
Lift patients
Perform Basic Cardiac Life Support (BCLS)
Collect urine specimens
Feed patients
Handle patient valuables and clothing
Ambulate patients
Request assistance from other team members
Sit with patients in need of comforting
Provide information to visitors
Ensure discharge orders are entered
Complete patient assessment on admission
Develop a realistic written plan of care
Document response to interventions
Integrate research findings into practice
Perform venipuncture
Order office supplies and forms
Process patient charge cards
Facilitate self-care as possible
Replace light bulbs
Perform EKG
Accompany patients to other areas of the hospital

floor (but that requires knowledge of the system of care). Hospital reengineering is pernicious because it leaps to a definition of clinical work, which is not the problem. The problem is the unappreciated role of nursing in tending the environment within which care happens; this does not require a license but does require credit.

The argument goes that there are any number of tasks that nurses do (did) that could be done by others because the tasks do not, of themselves, require a nursing license. The box shows excerpts from a typical list of tasks. The list of tasks did not include those things that are, by state definition, done only by licensed nurses, such as administering medications by any route. Those that did not require a license were determined delegable to unlicensed assistive personnel.

Here, the purpose of the definition of nursing gets very complicated. On the one hand, adding up tasks is neither the way to define the work that RNs do nor the way to define the discipline. Turning tasks over to unlicensed personnel smacks of eroding nursing. Tasks themselves are just that, but this isn't about tasks or nursing work; it is about trying to decrease hospital expenses by substituting lesser prepared and lower paid personnel for professional nurses, while substituting nurses for more expensive people such as physicians or administrators on the off shifts and at unpopular times.

If professional nursing seizes the opportunity to define and supervise the work for these new others (the ANA definition in practice act language might help), then "nursing," as the field expands, and nurses actually might get some help.

USES OF DEFINITION

It should be clear that there is no one agreed upon definition of nursing as the work, the discipline, the profession, or the public image. There isn't one of any other discipline either, if one probes deeply enough. Why, then, do we worry so much about definition in nursing?

It should also be clear that different purposes require different approaches to definition.

If the purpose is to define nursing in order to guide research, then an operational definition—an outline of the work—is in order.

If the purpose is to change the law, then a politically feasible definition that will fit existing law is required.

If the purpose is to convince Congress or a state or federal agency of the value of nursing, then definition is irrelevant; data on increasing access to care, decreasing cost, and improving outcomes will make the case, and those who do it—nurses—win.

If the purpose is to explain what nursing is to a lay audience, then no definition will work, because what the audience will relate to is a *description* of the work, not a definition.

> . . . when a person says, "I am going to *nurse* my cold," he hastens to arrange the environment so that he can be as free as possible from stress and takes all means at his disposal to increase his comfort. On the other hand, when he says, "I am *doctoring* my cold," we know that he is not only relying on his own inner natural resources, but also on the products of medical science—pills, inhalers and the like. (Orlando, 1961, p. 5)

That description works better than definition because everyone has had a cold. People who have never nursed have no way to understand what the work is like and what it takes to do it, it is so personal and intimate a service and so fiendishly difficult to describe.

Finally, if the purpose is to explain to one's extended family what one does for a living as a nurse, one might start with Virginia Henderson's translation of her own "personal concept":

[The nurse] is temporarily the consciousness of the unconscious, the love of life for the suicidal, the leg of the amputee, the eyes of the newly blind, a means of locomotion for the infant, knowledge and confidence for the young mother, the [voice] for those too weak or withdrawn to speak. (Henderson, 1964, pp. 63-64)

REFERENCES

American Nurses Association. (1980). *Nursing—A social policy statement.* Kansas City: Author.

American Nurses Association. (1981). *Suggested state legislation.* Kansas City: Author.

American Nurses Association. (1990). *Suggested state legislation.* Washington, DC: Author.

Andrews, L.B. (1983). *Deregulating doctoring.* Emmaus, PA: People's Medical Society.

Brown, S.A., & Grimes, D.E. (1993). *Nurse practitioners and certified nurse-midwives: A meta-analysis of studies on nurses in primary care roles.* Washington, DC: American Nurses Publishing.

Bullough, B. (Ed.). (1980). *The law and the expanding nursing role* (1st ed.). Philadelphia: FA Davis.

Cronenwett, L.R. (1995). Molding the future of advanced practice nursing. *Nursing Outlook, 43,* 112-118.

Diers, D., & Molde, S. (1983). Nurses in primary care: The new gatekeepers. *American Journal of Nursing, 83,* 742-745.

Diers, D. (1992). Nurse-midwives and nurse anesthetists: The cutting edge in specialist practice. In L.H. Aiken (Ed.), *Charting nursing's future: Nursing in the '90's* (pp. 159-180). Philadelphia: Lippincott.

Driscoll, V.M. (1976). *Legitimizing the profession of nursing: The distinct mission of the New York State Nurses Association.* Albany, NY: Foundation of NYSNA.

Fawcett, J. (1980). A framework for analysis and evaluation of conceptual models of nursing. *Nurse Educator, 5,* 10-14.

Ford, L.C. (1982). Nurse practitioners: History of a new idea and predictions for the future. In L.H. Aiken (Ed.), *Nursing in the 1980's: Crises, challenges, opportunities* (pp. 231-248). Philadelphia: Lippincott.

Hadley, E.H. (1989). Nurses and prescriptive authority: A legal and economic analysis. *American Journal of Law and Medicine, 15,* 245-300.

Henderson, V.A. (1964). The nature of nursing. *American Journal of Nursing, 64,* 62-68.

Henderson, V.A. (1961). *Basic principles of nursing care.* Geneva: International Council of Nurses.

Henderson, V.A. (1991). *The nature of nursing: Reflections after 25 years.* New York: National League for Nursing.

Iowa Intervention Project. (1995). Validation and coding of the NIC taxonomy structure. *Image, 27,* 43-49.

Irving Independent School District v. Tatro, No. SC 3371. S. Ct. (1984).

King, I.M. (1981) *A theory for nursing: Systems, concepts, process.* New York: Wiley.

McCloskey, J.C., & Bulechek, G. (Eds.). (1996). *Nursing Interventions Classification* (2nd ed.). St Louis: Mosby.

Meleis, A.I. (1991). *Theoretical nursing: Development and progress* (2nd ed.). Philadelphia: Lippincott.

Nightingale, F. (1859/1946). *Notes on nursing—What it is and what it is not.* Philadelphia: Lippincott.

Office of Technology Assessment, US Congress. (1986). *Nurse practitioners, physician assistants and Certified Nurse-Midwives: A policy analysis.* (OTA-HCS-37) Washington, DC: U.S. Government Printing Office.

Orlando, I.J. (1961). *The dynamic nurse-patient relationship.* New York: G.P. Putnam's Sons.

Orlando, I.J. (1972). *The discipline and teaching of nursing process.* New York: G.P. Putnam's Sons.

Random House dictionary. (1966). New York: Random House.

Random House collegiate dictionary. (1995). New York: Random House.

Secretary's Commission to Study the Extended Role of Nurses. (1971). *Extending the scope of nursing practice* (DHEW Pub. HSM 73-2037). Washington, DC: U.S. Government Printing Office.

Rogers, M. (1970). *An introduction to the theoretical basis of nursing.* Philadelphia: Lippincott.

Rogers, M. (1975). Euphemisms in nursing's future. *Image, 7,* 3-9.

Safreit, B.J. (1993). Health care dollars and regulatory sense: The role of advanced practice nursing. *Yale Journal on Regulation, 9*(2), 417-488.

Sermchief v. Gonzales, 660 S.W.2d 683 (1983).

Subcommittee on Health and the Environment, US House of Representatives. (1976). *A discursive dictionary of health care.* (59-892O) Washington, DC: U.S. Government Printing Office.

Travelbee, J. (1966). *Interpersonal aspects of nursing.* Philadelphia: Lippincott.

Vitello, S.J. (1987). School health services after *Tatro. Journal of School Health, 57,* 77-80.

Wald, F.S., & Leonard, R.C. (1964). Towards development of nursing practice theory. *Nursing Research, 23,* 309-313.

Weidenbach, E. (1964). *Clinical nursing: A helping art.* New York: Springer.

Wolff, M.A. (1984, February). Court upholds expanded practice roles for nurses. *Law, Medicine & Health Care,* 26-29.

Staff nurses

Who are they, what do they do, and what challenges do they face?

LYNDIA FLANAGAN

Over the past 25 years, there have been profound changes in both the demands for health care services and the ways in which these services are financed and delivered. Most notably, hospitalization has come to be viewed as part of a continuum of care rather than as the primary site of treatment. While the emergence of alternative delivery systems has created new and different career and employment opportunities for nurses, hospitals have remained the primary worksite for registered nurses (RNs). Approximately two thirds of RNs are employed in hospitals. Moreover, about two thirds of all employed RNs hold staff nurse positions or "general duty" nursing jobs.

WORK FORCE PROFILE

Many observers contend that today's staff nurse population represents a workforce with greater experience, expertise, and efficiency than in earlier generations. A number of factors influence this assessment, including the average age and education level of nurses.

The RN population is growing older. Like the general population, the RN workforce seems to mirror the pattern of the baby boom generation (McKibbin, 1990). It is worth noting that the first of the baby boomers will reach age 50 in 1996.

Thirty years ago, the largest portion of staff nurses (RNs performing direct patient care) was under 30 years of age. By 1977, the median age of employed RNs had climbed to 38 years of age. The average age of RNs had reached 42 by 1988 (U.S. Department of Health and Human Services, 1990). A variety of more recent surveys place the median age of today's staff nurses between 38 and 45. It has been suggested that the older-age profile of RNs allows for nursing services to build a more highly expert and stable work force (Young, 1989).

While the staff nurse population has been aging, the level of education has also changed. In 1977, for example, the nursing diploma was the highest nursing-related educational credential achieved by the majority of nurses (67%). Only 18% held baccalaureates in nursing and 11% held associate degrees. By 1988, however, fewer than 40% of nurses reported a nursing diploma as the highest level of their educational preparation (McKibbin, 1990). Today, the majority of RNs hold either an associate degree or a baccalaureate in nursing.

While demographics such as age and educational preparation are fundamental to any workforce profile, such data reflect only one dimension of a population's characteristics. To understand today's staff nurses fully, it is equally important to take a closer look at what motivates these individuals to enter nursing and what is most important to them in their work.

In 1991, the American Nurses Association (ANA) enlisted the assistance of the Opinion Research Division of Fleishman-Hillard, Inc. to conduct a survey of RNs. The survey targeted hospital nurses located in all 50 states and the District of Columbia. Staff nurses and special assignment nurses (emergency room, intensive care unit, operating room) comprised 91% of the sample. This nationwide mail survey resulted in the first major examination of staff nurse attitudes about nursing and workplace issues in the 1990s (ANA, 1991). Among the insight gleaned from this survey is basic information about why staff nurses enter the profession and what is most and least important to them in their work as nurses.

The motivation for choosing a career in nursing has

not changed dramatically over the years. A desire to help people (71%) and an interest in health care (63%) were the leading reasons that survey respondents became nurses. The prospect of job opportunities was reported almost twice as often as income as a primary reason (44% vs. 23%). The desire to be a professional was selected by 43% of the respondents as their primary reason for becoming an RN (Yeast, 1991).

Given this perspective, it is not surprising that the survey also revealed that patient care and professional issues dominate the list of workplace concerns. From a list of 19 work-related factors, respondents assigned the greatest importance to the following: providing quality patient care (89%); caring about patients' best interests (77%); being treated as a professional (65%); adequate staffing (60%); safe working environment (57%); and letting RNs do what they are taught to do (56%). Far less importance was assigned to such considerations as working with new technology, health care benefits, time off on holidays, child care and elder care assistance, and opportunities for overtime (Fleishman-Hillard, Inc., 1991).

Numerous studies have confirmed that the highest priority of staff nurses is quality patient care. Most of these studies also document the growing challenges and frustrations staff nurses are experiencing in an industry that is undergoing dramatic changes (Kramer, 1974; Kramer & Schmalenberg, 1991a; Kramer & Schmalenberg, 1991b; McClure et al., 1983; Schmalenberg & Kramer, 1979; Wandelt, Pierce, & Widdowson, 1981). This type of information provides insight into yet another dimension of the profile of today's staff nurses—the roles they perform and the level of professional security and job satisfaction they experience.

A DIFFERENT WORK ENVIRONMENT

When asked about how they feel about the work they are doing, staff nurses respond with one common theme: Although they want to provide the best nursing care possible, circumstances make it extremely difficult. Within the span of a very few years, the health care industry (and the hospital setting, in particular) has changed dramatically—creating a work environment for nurses that is far more complex and challenging.

The availability of new technologies in nonhospital settings enables more patients to receive their care outside of the hospital in a way that was not possible before. Patients who are hospitalized are admitted at a later point in their illness and discharged earlier (the "sicker and quicker" reality of the prospective payment system). Patients are generally no longer admitted a day early for preoperative diagnostic procedures, nor do they remain nearly as long following surgery. Patients who would have been cared for in intensive care units only a few years ago are now assigned to regular medical-surgical units. Older patients, who are more critically ill than ever before, are requiring increased nursing skill and nursing time, and patients with medical illnesses are discharged earlier to nursing homes, subacute care facilities, home health agencies, or to follow-up through clinics or the private offices of health care practitioners.

Further compounding the demands placed on staff nurses today is the shift in focus from caring for a patient to providing a service to a customer. There is general consensus within the industry that patients are acting more like customers and that this change represents a significant shift in the patient's power. Nurses describe patients as more questioning, less trusting, more knowledgeable, more demanding of high-quality service and care, more cost-conscious, more willing to shop around, and quicker to sue.

While demands for a new and different type of health care were emerging, hospital executives were focusing more attention on ways to cut costs while expanding services and increasing staff productivity. The need to strengthen market forces in the late 1980s led many health care institutions to restructure (horizontally and vertically) or diversify. As a result, nurses once employed by small, private hospitals now find themselves working for national chains or regional integrated systems. In many instances, this is only one of many changes in the employer-employee relationship. Many hospitals have contracted with outside services to provide entire management teams or to oversee certain clinical services. Some hospitals have devised arrangements whereby two or more organizations share certain staff, services, and facilities (Flanagan, 1995).

According to some experts, hospitals have now entered into a second phase of "retooling." In the first phase, the focus was on developing an outpatient infrastructure. In this second, more complex phase of retooling, hospital executives are said to be addressing critical structure issues, such as the organization of the physical plant, the roles and responsibilities of caregivers, and the process of decision making. While many employers claim to be instituting quality management measures, it is apparent that their efforts at workplace redesign are really directed at cutting costs, not improving care (Solovy, 1993).

THE TARGET OF WORK REDESIGN

Because nurses are the largest employee group in hospitals, they have become a primary target for redesign measures. Many hospitals have increased the work responsibilities of RNs while simultaneously increasing their substitution with less-skilled workers. Based on information gathered by the ANA, work redesign is likely to include some combination of the following (Ketter, 1994):

- Consolidation of management services and reduction in management layers through management layoffs, reducing labor costs, and streamlining the organization
- Early retirement programs and buyout for staff with seniority
- Implementation of nursing care models that change the nursing skill mix, lowering labor costs by replacing more costly RNs with less-skilled and lower paid ancillary staff
- Reassignment of RNs or a reduction in the workforce
- Substitution of RNs by paramedical staff, and replacing RN full-time equivalents with lesser-paid employees
- Increased use of licensed practical nurses, further decreasing the number of RN full-time equivalents and increasing the RN's role of responsibility
- Cross-training of RNs to other nursing specialities and to nonnursing clinical tasks
- Cross-training of ancillary staff
- An increase in part-time positions with a corresponding decrease in full-time positions
- Elimination of preferential staffing and scheduling systems
- Reduced hours of operation for ancillary departments with a corresponding shift to the nursing units

Significant issues have been raised regarding such measures. These issues focus on potentially unsafe staffing levels, inappropriate use of assistive personnel and aides, and potential or actual layoffs.

In an effort to collect more concrete data on workplace conditions, the ANA distributed a survey questionnaire to its members in *The American Nurse* in September 1994. This self-administered survey dealt with a number of issues concerning staffing and service cutbacks that had been implemented or were planned by facilities that employ RNs and the impact of those actions on RNs and the patients they serve.

A total of 1,835 responses were received, reflecting input from all 50 states and the District of Columbia in rough proportion to the population distribution in the United States. Nearly three fourths of the survey respondents were employed in hospitals, two thirds of whom indicated that they were staff nurses. In analyzing survey responses, Decision Data Collection, Inc. (1994) reported the following findings:

- More than two thirds (68.4%) of respondents said that the number of RNs employed in their facilities had been reduced in the past 12 months. The most frequently reported explanations for nurse cutbacks were economic reasons (60%) and a decrease in patient census (58.2%).
- More than three fourths of respondents who reported a reduction in RN staff indicated that the quality of patient care had, in their estimation, been degraded as a result of those cutbacks. Nearly two thirds of this group (64.0%) said they felt that patient safety had been affected adversely as well. Two factors were identified as contributing to the deterioration of safety and quality of care: Nurses are "taking care of more patients than before" (53.9%) and "there is less time to provide patient care" (53.7%) (p. 13).
- Increased use of unlicensed assistive personnel to provide direct patient care was reported by 44.7% of all respondents.

While it would not be appropriate to suggest that these survey findings are representative of the entire nurse population, there is a growing body of data substantiating changes in nursing roles, nurse:patient ratios, and the use of assistive personnel. As Curtain noted in a July 1995 editorial in *Nursing Management,* "Hospitals are undergoing traumatic downsizing and wrenching reorganization, and nurses—always at the heart of health care—are finding out just exactly what it means to be downsized, rightsized, restructured, reengineered and redesigned" (Curtain, 1995, p. 7).

HIGH LEVEL OF STRESS

So what does all of this mean with regard to a profile of the staff nurse population? No explanation would be complete without the acknowledgment that today's staff nurses function in a *much more* stressful environment than did nurses in earlier generations.

According to Jaffe and Scott (1984), the majority of life stresses fall into four categories, which are best described by the words *loss, threat, frustration,* and *uncertainty.* Unfortunately, these are the very words many nurses use to describe their reactions to the massive changes occurring in the health care industry (Decision Data Collections, Inc., 1994).

"This situation with no jobs is appalling and frustrating. I have been a nurse for 19 years and *never* has it been this bad."

"I started in nursing in 1954. This is the first time I've seen nursing as I know it being phased out."

"With all the changes in my hospital, floating to areas where I don't have experience (or any interest), I am considering changing careers."

"Bottom line for hospital employed nurses is: Lower patient census, less need for nurses. What I want to know . . . is where do we go from here for employment?"

For many staff nurses, job security is a growing concern. In *Job Satisfaction Strategies for Health Care Professionals,* Leebov (1991) notes that many people over the years chose health care careers because they traditionally offered job security. Given the "turbulent" state of health care, Leebov points out that "life has become very uncomfortable for such security-oriented people" (p. 20).

Studies have also shown that individuals entering the nursing field tend to have similar personality traits. According to Gallagher (1989), they are action-oriented, attentive to detail, set high standards for themselves, have difficulty accepting work that is less than perfect, and "are giving to the point that their own health and relationships tend to rank second to patient care" (p. 59). She concludes, "The qualities that provide an unusually high level of dedication and good quality patient care are also the source of potential burnout" (p. 59).

There is no question that today's staff nurses are concerned about quality of care and patient safety as well as their own job security. It is not surprising then that they frequently report feelings of being "used up" at the end of the day, emotionally drained from work, frustrated by work, fatigued when having to get up and go to work, and burned out (ANA, 1991). How staff nurses cope with these feelings and other symptoms of job stress will greatly affect how this segment of the workforce is perceived in the future.

FUTURE CHALLENGES

Clearly, staff nurses must become more sophisticated about survival and growth in an industry playing under different rules. Foremost, they must understand what it means to operate in an environment of managed care and capitation. More attention is being focused on providing health care services within a defined network of health care providers who are given the responsibility to manage and provide quality, cost-effective care. These providers accept a fixed amount of payment per subscriber, per period of time, in return for providing specified services over a specified time period (capitation).

Nurses must learn to define their roles within a continuum of care in relation to other providers in a variety of settings. They will need to be able to talk about their services in terms of process and outcomes as well as cost and benefits. In addition, they will be expected to use centralized information systems that integrate financial information with clinical and statistical data.

Staff nurses must also develop stronger leadership skills. More and more frequently, staff nurses are delivering patient care in models that use multi-skilled teams of workers. In the past, leadership and management education were reserved for nurses assuming administrative roles. As a result, most staff nurses are facing work redesign without the tools they need to function effectively as team leaders. Attention needs to focus on the cultivation of skills in delegation, critical thinking, problem solving, prioritization, and conflict resolution. Staff nurses must also possess a clear understanding of the legal implications of delegation.

Moreover, staff nurses must identify a range of creative and unique resources to cultivate and strengthen a positive professional self-concept. Today, a positive professional self-concept is as important as clinical competency. The degree of attention paid to *professional self-enhancement* is becoming much more of a key factor in achieving job satisfaction and long-term career success. Unfortunately, while nurses have been oriented to seek out educational opportunities to update and fine tune clinical expertise, much less attention has been focused on such topics as values clarification, career planning, change management, stress management, and assertive communication. Staff nurses should be encouraged to use a broad range of resources, including self-help books, training videos, audiotapes, seminars and workshops, organizational affiliation, mentors, discussion groups, inservice education, and so on.

Finally, staff nurses must be open to new and innovative approaches to more traditional roles. They must also look beyond their current employment situation and past experiences to potential opportunities in a range of areas. Job advertisements provide a starting point for identifying potential employers, the types of nursing openings available, and job requirements. However, a more effective way to find out about employment opportunities is through personal contacts, i.e., by cultivating a network. An effective network draws from a variety of sources, including employers and supervisors; coworkers; instructors and fellow students; fellow members of civic, religious, and social groups; and family, friends, and neighbors (Flanagan, 1995).

In a time when the environment seems so chaotic and ever-changing, it is crucial for all nurses to seek out stimuli that help to put things into perspective, are energizing and thought-provoking, and lend a sense of support and understanding.

REFERENCES

American Nurses Association. (1991, July 1). Inadequate staffing threatens patient care, nurses say. *American Nurses Association News,* 1-3.

Curtain, L.L. (1995). Job security: Is nothing sacred anymore? *Nursing Management, 26*(7), 7-9.

Decision Data Collections, Inc. (1994, November). *Report of survey results: The 1994 ANA layoffs survey, a report submitted to the American Nurses Association.*

Flanagan, L. (1995). *What you need to know about today's workpace: A survival guide for nurses.* Washington, DC: American Nurses Publishing.

Fleishman-Hillard, Inc. (1991, May). *Opportunities for growth: A report to the American Nurses Association.*

Gallagher, D. (1989). Is stress ripping nurses apart? *Imprint, 36*(2), 59-63.

Jaffe, D.T., & Scott, C.D. (1984). *From burnout to balance: A workbook for peak performance and self renewal.* New York: McGraw-Hill.

Ketter, J. (1994). What restructuring may mean to nurses. *The American Nurse, 26*(5), 1, 14.

Kramer, M. (1974). *Reality shock: Why nurses leave nursing.* St. Louis: Mosby.

Kramer, M., & Schmalenberg, C. (1991a). Job satisfaction and retention, insights for the 90s: Part 1. *Nursing 91, 21*(3), 50-55.

Kramer, M., & Schmalenberg, C. (1991b). Job satisfaction and retention, insights for the 90s: Part 2. *Nursing 91, 21*(4), 51-55.

Leebov, W. (1991). *Job satisfaction strategies for health care professionals.* Chicago: American Hospital Publishing, Inc.

McClure, M.L., Poulin, M.A., Sovie, M.D., & Wandelt, M.A. (1983). *Magnet hospitals: Attraction and retention of professional nurses.* Kansas City, MO: American Nurses Association.

McKibbin, R.C. (1990). *The nursing shortage and the 1990s.* Kansas City, MO: American Nurses Association.

Schmalenberg, C., & Kramer, M. (1979). *Coping with reality shock: The voices of experience.* Rockville, MD: Aspen Systems Corporation.

Solovy, A.T. (1993). Retooling the hospital: Moving into the second phase. *Hospitals, 67*(5), 18-19.

U.S. Department of Health and Human Services. (1990). *The registered nurse population—1988.* Washington, DC: Author.

Wandelt, M.A., Pierce, P.M., & Widdowson, R.R. (1981). Why nurses leave nursing and what can be done about it. *American Journal of Nursing, 81*(1), 72-77.

Yeast, C. (1991). Nurses—who are we and what motivates us. *The American Nurse, 23*(9), 10.

Clinical nurse specialists and nurse practitioners

Who are they, what do they do, and what challenges do they face?

ANN HENRICK, JOANN APPLEYARD

Specialization has been articulated as "a mark of the advancement of the nursing profession" (American Nurses Association [ANA], 1992b, p. 21). The clinical nurse specialist (CNS) and nurse practitioner (NP) roles were developed in response to this advancement; the profession needed clinical practitioners who could focus on a specific segment of the whole of nursing, seeking in-depth knowledge and advanced skills in a defined area of practice (ANA, 1992b, p. 21).

Historically, there are two significant differences between the prototype CNS and NP: the primary reasons for their becoming and the educational requirements for their respective roles (Elder & Bullough, 1990; Hockenberry & Hodgson, 1991). On the other hand, they share a common element: a continuing commitment to clinical practice—a practice that demands expert knowledge and skill and includes the direct and continuous care of sick patients, as well as health promotion for clients who are well.

Major related issues that currently affect the CNS and NP are being debated, such as (a) their merger (of sorts) into one entity; (b) the regulatory process that legitimizes their advanced practice; (c) prescriptive authority; and (d) compensation for their services. This chapter profiles the CNS and NP,[1] identifying their impact on the health care system and discussing related concepts and issues.

This chapter is an update of a previous chapter in the 4th edition of *Current Issues in Nursing* authored by Margaret Stafford and JoAnn Appleyard and entitled "Clinical Nurse Specialists and Nurse Practitioners."

[1]The ANA lists 25,000 to 30,000 NPs and "about" 40,000 CNSs with advanced degrees.

HISTORICAL ORIGIN OF THE CLINICAL NURSE SPECIALIST

There have always been "specialists" in nursing who acquired specialized knowledge and skill through practice and on-the-job instruction. During the 1930s and 1940s, many nurses also attended short-term postgraduate educational programs sponsored by hospitals and became the specialists in their particular fields (Donahue, 1985; Hamrick, 1989). The modern CNS emerged, however, in response to the recognized need to improve the quality of patient care and the clinical *practice* of professional nursing, primarily in the acute care setting (Berlinger, 1973; Georgopulous & Christman, 1970; Koetters, 1989; Padilla, 1973; Reiter, 1961; Vaughan, 1968).

Nursing care had deteriorated seriously during and immediately after World War II, due in large part to the dramatic decrease in the number of registered nurses (RNs) practicing in hospitals (Sample, 1987). Many nurses returning from the war used the GI bill to go back to school and become teachers or administrators, and a number of nurses were no longer content to work in the paternalistic environment of the hospital, where low salaries and substandard working conditions were the norm (Donahue, 1985).

The "quick fix" (replacing RNs with less-qualified health care providers) to the acute nursing shortage and substandard patient care failed to address the nurses' concerns. Despite emerging technology and increased complexity of care, hospitals continued to use wartime measures to fill the gap: volunteers became paid nurses' aides and vocational (practical) nurses were introduced to provide the major portion of the direct care for patients (Berlinger, 1973; Donahue, 1985; McClure, 1990; Reiter, 1966; Stafford, 1988). Team nursing was introduced, but it further fragmented patient care and frustrated the RNs, who continued to leave the hospital (Donahue, 1985). The RN felt devalued because others with less education and professionalism took over the nursing care of patients, while the professional nurse "nursed" the desk. In addition, the development of shortened programs in hospital diploma schools as well as associate degree programs in community colleges contributed little to the recognized need for *increased* knowledge and skill at the bedside.

In 1947, a National Nursing Council (representing the ANA and other health care organizations) obtained a grant from the Carnegie Foundation and commissioned Esther Lucille Brown to study and determine how professional nursing schools could meet the demand for nursing services. One result of the study was Brown's (1948) publication on *Nursing for the Future,* in which she strongly proposed that basic schools of nursing be a part of universities and colleges but that:

> . . . provisions for the development of some specialists within clinical nursing has been viewed in this report as necessary, if the base on which nursing service rests is to be strengthened, and if the profession is to look forward to a sound healthy development. (Brown, 1948)

The now famous Williamsburg Conference of nurse educators, which put into motion the first master's-prepared psychiatric CNS (National League for Nursing, 1958), followed this report. In 1961, Frances Reiter presented a paper enunciating her concept of the nurse clinician, which is virtually synonymous with the CNS of today: "one . . . who consistently demonstrates a high degree of clinical judgement and an advanced level of competence in the performance of nursing care in a clinical area of specialization" (Reiter, 1961).

During the 1960s, publications expressing the need for clinical nursing to keep abreast of the knowledge explosion in both technological and behavioral sciences (Berlinger, 1973) flourished. Federal funding was obtained to support this "need," and by the early 1960s programs to prepare CNSs were in place in many areas of clinical practice (Hoeffer & Murphy, 1984). In 1966, a change in the structure of the ANA to include divisions of clinical practice gave further impetus to the development of master's-prepared clinicians (Donahue, 1985; Hoeffer & Murphy, 1984).

PROFILES OF THE CLINICAL NURSE SPECIALIST

The criteria for specialists in nursing practice were identified in the ANA's *Social Policy Statement* as "a nurse who, through study and supervised practice at the graduate level (master's or doctorate), has become expert in a defined area of knowledge and practice in a selected clinical area of nursing" (ANA, 1980). Hamrick and Taylor (1989) suggest that the development of this "expert" results from a "complex and emotional process." Their study describes seven identifiable phases of development but indicates that movement from phase to phase occurs in a highly fluid, individual fashion (Hamrick & Taylor, 1989). For purposes of this discussion, the focus is on the experienced CNS who has reached an advanced phase of practice and has successfully integrated the various components of the role.

Organizational placement of the clinical nurse specialist

Although CNSs work primarily in institutional settings, typically in staff positions, many and varied organizational arrangements have been described in the literature (Sample, 1987). The advantages and disadvantages of "line" versus staff accountability have been discussed elsewhere (Baird & Prouty, 1989; Hamrick, 1989), and are not dealt with here other than to present a bias predicated on years of successful experience as a CNS in a staff position and dialogue with CNSs in line positions. The success of this staff role, however, is contingent on reciprocal trust and respect and, as identified by Brown (1989), a sharing of responsibility and authority between the CNS and the person to whom he or she is accountable administratively.

Regardless of organizational placement and reporting mechanisms, the CNS usually works from a "home base" and is available for consultation from other units (Koetters, 1989). Many CNSs have clinical faculty appointments and some full-time faculty members carry part-time CNS appointments. The common element, however, is the direct and continuous involvement with patients and families with emphasis on a nursing versus a medical care model.

Functions of the clinical nurse specialist

Expert clinical practice is the *sine qua non* of the CNS. Practice (i.e., actual ongoing experience with patients and families) provides the content and directs participation in various subroles such as clinical research, consultation, teaching, and leadership and administration (Hamrick,

1989). This concept is exemplified by the following CNS leaders with excerpts from their activities. These examples, gleaned for the most part from personal contact and interaction, are not intended to be all-inclusive but rather to provide the reader with some insight into what Fralic (1988) refers to as "nursing's precious resource."

• Nancy Burke is a CNS in psychiatric mental health nursing. She maintains a private practice, is a consultant to the department of psychiatry in a university hospital, has an adjunct appointment in the college of nursing, and maintains a collaborative practice with her psychiatrist husband. Her activities include liaison work with family members of hospitalized patients, seeing them in the hospital and office, and calling them at least weekly to keep them apprised of the patient's progress and involving them as indicated in the plans for therapy. As a certified psychodramatist, Nancy conducts four psychodrama groups per week. In her group at the university, she has medical residents, nursing students, and myriad others as participant observers, ". . . who never fail to get involved."

• Sandra Cunningham, a CNS in cardiovascular surgery, is a case manager for patients in a large teaching hospital. She coordinates and integrates the delivery of patient care with a dominant focus on nursing care given to the surgical patient (Gibbs, Lonowski, Meyer, & Newlin, 1995). Inherent in the CNS role from its inception, case management, as practiced by Sandy, is initiated when the patient is admitted to the hospital, throughout the surgical experience, the postoperative period, discharge planning, and finally to outpatient clinic visits. Sandy is a constant presence in the process, caring for patients as needed and guiding and coaching others who give care or provide related services. She is instrumental in developing critical pathways for patients, by constantly updating and evaluating them and by using the critical pathways as guides rather than rules.

• Kristin Kleinschmidt was, until recently, the CNS for the cardiac care unit and cardiac arrhythmia and pacemaker clinic of a large Veterans Administration hospital. She has moved from that role to that of an arrhythmia CNS in a large cardiology practice that encompasses three private hospitals. Her well-honed skills as teacher, provider of high-level comprehensive follow-up care for persons with complex arrhythmias, cardiac pacemakers, and automatic internal cardiac defibrillators, as well as consultant to nurses, physicians, and others who care for these patients, serve her well in her new role. Kris works in collaboration with two electrophysiology cardiologists to give complete care to these patients. In her practice, which is outpatient focused, Kris assesses patients independently and in collaboration with the physicians to provide patients with the best possible outcomes and an enhanced quality of life.

• Donna Murphy is a diabetes CNS whose practice has a dual focus in both the outpatient and inpatient arenas within the hospital. Donna acts as a mentor to staff nurses caring for persons with diabetes, helping these nurses to feel more confident in their roles as caregivers, teachers, and coaches of new as well as seasoned diabetics. Occasionally she will act as consultant in the care of a hospitalized diabetic patient with complex human responses to this illness. Donna works with nurses throughout the hospital to upgrade standards of care and gives regular group inservices to update nurses on the latest research in diabetic care. Donna has a diabetic self-management education clinic within the outpatient setting. She works outside the speciality endocrine clinic focusing on those patients cared for by the generalist physician. Her practice centers on coaching, teaching, and performing high-level assessments of these patients, helping them to monitor their own progress and effecting positive patient outcomes.

• Kathleen Perry functions in a hospital-based home care program, giving nursing care to four or five elderly patients and their families on an ongoing basis. She has explored and studied the diagnostic statement, Knowledge Deficit, a recurring problem for this patient population. She likewise has identified the potential for serious negative patient outcomes in the presence of caregiver stress, a phenomenon she currently is addressing as a PhD candidate in nursing. She believes her involvement as a clinical preceptor offers students a "knowledge embedded in practice" that enhances their ability to function in the CNS role. Kathy advises staff nurses in her agency on ethical and professional issues as they move forward in their state nurses' association's professional bargaining unit activities.

• Joyce Waterman Taylor is a CNS emerita in neuroscience. Joyce has not only implemented all of the subroles in a highly qualitative fashion, but she has also expanded and incorporated additional competencies. She believes strongly that primary nursing ("my patient, my nurse") is the way to improve care for all patients and to provide job satisfaction for nurses. In all of her work settings, she has introduced and taught the concepts of primary nursing within a holistic framework. For Joyce, collaborative practice also is an article of faith; she consistently develops and nurtures collaborative relationships with physicians and other disciplines. Her widely published work on the outcomes of care and outcome standards led to her appointment to several national and local committees and task forces. Joyce has been singled out by her peers and colleagues as the quintessential CNS.

ORIGINS OF THE NURSE PRACTITIONER ROLE

The 1960s were characterized by social change, including a political emphasis on health care as a right for all citizens. Access to all levels of health care services was seen as a particular problem, and the NP role was developed to help meet the demand for primary care services. The first formal education program for NPs was established in 1965 at the University of Colorado School of Nursing to prepare RNs to deliver primary care to children in underserved communities (Ford & Silver, 1967; "Interview with Co-founder of Nurse Practitioner Movement," 1995). By 1975, practitioner programs had proliferated, and NPs were being trained in a variety of medical fields, including obstetrics and gynecology, internal medicine, pediatrics, geriatrics, and family practice. During that first decade, educational programs tended to be nondegree certificate programs that were 1 year or less in length. Many of these programs were funded by the federal government in an effort to prepare more primary care providers for underserved populations. Since 1975, the number of nondegree programs has decreased substantially, and most NPs are now educated in graduate programs leading to a master's degree in nursing (Office of Technology Assessment [OTA], 1986).

National certification for NPs was first established in the mid-1970s by the National Certification Board of Pediatric Nurse Practitioners and Nurses. The ANA (American Nurses Credentialing Center) soon followed suit, establishing national certification for NPs in gerontology, pediatrics, adult health, family health, and school health. NPs in neonatology, obstetrics, and gynecology are certified by the National Certification Corporation for Obstetric, Gynecologic, and Neonatal Nursing Specialties. Most NPs today are certified by one of these national organizations. Increasingly, certification is a requirement for employment, and in some states, it is a requirement by the state licensing board.

Who are nurse practitioners and what do they do?

Nurse practitioners are educated to perform a broad spectrum of primary care interventions, including health assessment, risk appraisal, health education and counseling, diagnosis and management of acute minor illnesses and injuries, and management of chronic conditions. Although most NPs work in primary care settings such as physicians' offices, health maintenance organizations, and community or public health clinics, increasing numbers are employed in hospitals, nursing homes, schools, colleges, industrial settings, and home health agencies (OTA, 1986). In all of these settings, NPs provide the essential health care services described above with emphasis on health promotion and disease prevention activities (Lewis & Resnik, 1985).

Taking into account the basic primary care practice divisions of internal medicine, pediatrics, family practice, obstetrics and gynecology, and geriatrics, NPs tend to perform as generalists rather than as specialists in terms of clinical practice. This means that they focus on broad health concerns within a given division of practice rather than concentrating on a particular body system or a set of related diseases. Exceptions to this are NPs who work as employees or as partners to physicians in specialty practice. In these specialty settings, the roles of NPs and CNSs are quite similar and may be considered interchangeable.

Specific role issues for nurse practitioners

The literature on NPs is voluminous, and a review by Koch, Pazaki, and Campbell (1992) categorizes five major topics: NP roles, educational issues, evaluation, legal issues, and the evolving health care crisis. One major concern that has been debated repeatedly over the past 20 years is whether NPs function as physician substitutes or as nurses in advanced practice roles (Bates, 1974a; Bates, 1974b; Edmunds, 1979; Edmunds and Ruth, 1991; "Interview with Co-Founder of Nurse Practitioner Movement," 1995; Mauksch & Rogers, 1975; Weston, 1975). The differences between physician and nursing roles involve issues of nursing autonomy as well as paradigm disparities about the nature of health care (Allen, 1977; "Interview with Co-founder of Nurse Practitioner Movement," 1995).

Historically, nurses have tended to view their focus as "caring," while physicians have directed their efforts toward "curing" (Linn, 1974). Traditionally, nurses have assisted physicians in the cure of patients by following orders and using their nursing skills and knowledge to care for patients and their families. Caring involved activities such as bathing, feeding, and providing skin care and passive exercise for a bedridden patient. It also involved listening, counseling, teaching, and coordinating interventions from multiple health care providers. Curing involved specific activities directed toward the diagnosis and treatment of disease. When nurses followed physician orders in carrying out diagnostic tests or in administering treatments to patients, they were participating in the curative aspect of health care. When they assessed and provided for patient and family needs for emotional support and health teaching or guidance, they were participating in the caring component.

The historical view was that nursing practice was both dependent on medical practice and independent from it, and the independent functions tended to be those on the caring end of the continuum. Thus nursing autonomy was more related to caring interventions than to curative ones. The development of advanced nursing practice roles has changed this circumstance. NPs perform interventions aimed at curing acute minor illnesses and injuries daily. While carrying out these interventions, they assess their patients' responses to their health problems and initiate appropriate teaching and counseling to help them manage treatment plans and prevent recurrences or secondary problems.

As indicated earlier, caring and curing are not mutually exclusive concepts. Rather, they are part of a continuum, and both physicians and nurses carry out activities in these arenas. Both caring and curative interventions are necessary in primary care, and there is convincing evidence that NPs effectively combine these practice components in their roles (Leininger, Little, & Carnevali, 1972; Simborg, Starfield, & Horn, 1978; Yedida, 1981). Although NPs carry out health care activities that used to be primarily in the physician's domain, they are performing these activities as nurses with significant emphasis on the responses and needs of the whole patient and his or her family.

THE CLINICAL NURSE SPECIALIST AND NURSE PRACTITIONER IN TRANSITION

Merging the two councils

Several studies, papers, and intense dialogue with members of the ANA's CNS and NP councils have elucidated more similarities than differences between the CNS and NP (Forbes, 1990; Forbes, Rafson, Spross, & Kozlowski, 1990; Hockenberry & Hodgson, 1991; Kitzman, 1989; Sparacino & Denand, 1986). Thus, the two councils merged into a single Council of Nurses in Advanced Practice (Pokorny & Barnard, 1992). The educational requirements (master's or doctorate) and role development now are well established (ANA, 1980), and although the issue of a singular title at this time is still being debated (Kitzman, 1989), the concept of both groups being identified as advanced practitioners is widely accepted (Forbes et al., 1990).

Regulation and reimbursement issues

The inconsistencies of the regulation and professional certification of nurses in advanced practice prompted the National Council of State Boards of Nursing (NCSBN) in March 1992 to propose a second license for nurses seeking reimbursement and prescriptive authority (NCSBN, 1992). The profession's historical view (which is still valid) is that the responsibility and accountability for defining specialty nursing practice and its qualifications rest with the profession (ANA, 1980; "Interview with Cofounder of Nurse Practitioner Movement," 1995). Formal meetings between the NCSBN and the ANA continue to take place to examine alternative mechanisms (other than licensure) to regulate *advanced* practice.

In addition, the ANA is completing a deliberate process with organized nursing through the Nursing Organization Liaison Forum and other specialty organizations to revisit *Nursing: A Social Policy Statement* as it pertains specifically to specialization (ANA, 1992a; Cronenwett, 1992; Pokorny & Bernard, 1992). It is incumbent on all advanced practitioners to be involved actively and cohesively in the ANA's and the state nurses' associations' collaborative efforts to:

- Protect the public's and nursing's autonomous control of advanced nursing practice
- Increase the adherence of nurses in advanced practice to national standards of certification and peer review
- Introduce requirements for uniform mandatory reimbursement to reflect adequately advanced practitioners' worth
- Eliminate barriers that restrict consumer access to services of qualified advanced practitioners
- Build a national and state database on advanced practitioners including their scope of practice, location, cost, and the outcome of this care (ANA, 1992a).

CURRENT MANDATES AND CHALLENGES

There are substantial barriers to the practice of NP and some CNS roles because of the overlap between traditional medical and nursing functions. This is especially true in settings in which nurses attempt to provide comprehensive primary care services. Although most state nursing practice acts enacted during the past 20 years have been updated to include some kind of legal authority for advanced nursing practice, the statutory language varies widely, from very broad mention of specialty practice to specific definitions of scope of practice (Pearson, 1995). By 1995, NPs in 47 states had some legal authority to prescribe medications, but again the language varies widely (Pearson, 1995). In many states NPs may prescribe independently all kinds of drugs, including controlled substances. The only states in which NPs have no statutory prescribing authority are Alabama, Illinois, and Oklahoma (Pearson, 1995).

The issue of independence is a major problem for both NPs and physicians. From the inception of the NP role, it was intended that some of the interventions involving diagnosis and treatment of disease be carried out in collaboration with physicians or, as organized medicine asserts, *under physician supervision*.

The independent practice of nurses is a politically charged arena, with organized medicine firmly against all efforts of nurses to be recognized as independent health care providers who receive direct reimbursement for their services. When regulatory agencies and state and federal legislative bodies use the term *supervision* rather than *collaboration* to describe the interdependent relationship between physicians and nurses, organized medicine can claim that nursing practice is completely dependent on medical practice and that physicians should receive all direct reimbursement for health care services delivered by nurses outside of institutional settings. Nurses must continue to work diligently to educate legislators, regulators, and the public about the independent aspects of nursing practice that are defined broadly in all nursing practice acts. It is also necessary to remind these groups that nurses do practice under their own licenses and that nurses' licenses are not contingent on physicians' licenses.

An operational definition of the concept of collaboration was adopted in 1992 by the ANA Congress on Nursing Practice:

> Collaboration means a collegial working relationship with another health care provider in the provision of (to supply) patient care. Collaborative practice requires (may include) the discussion of patient diagnosis and cooperation in the management and delivery of care. Each collaborator is available to the other for consultation either in person or by communication device, but need not be physically present on the premises at the time the actions are performed. The patient-designated health care provider is responsible for the overall direction and management of patient care. (ANA, 1992b, p. 104)

This definition should be used as a basis in all discussions or negotiations in which the issue is "physician supervision" of nursing practice.

The individual accomplishments of CNSs and NPs are a prelude to their potential collective positive impact on the health care of individuals and families and on health care policy in general. To this end, they must sustain and enhance their significant roles in the following initiatives:

- State and local health care reform efforts
- Federal government's agenda to improve the effectiveness and appropriateness of health care services through their Agency for Health Care Policy and Research
- Nursing's taxonomy development and related scientific studies

It is likewise crucial that nurses in advanced practice: (a) continue to demonstrate their cost-effectiveness in cost-driven hospital and clinic environments; (b) increase their presence in extended care or nursing home facilities; (c) advance theory- and research-based clinical practice models that demonstrate a high quality of patient care and reflect measurable, nurse-sensitive patient outcomes; and (d) help other health professionals, health care consumers, and public servants recognize the contribution being made by nurses in advanced practices (Donovan, 1985; Wright, 1990).

REFERENCES

Allen, M. (1977). Comparative theories of the expanded role in nursing and implications for nursing practice: A working paper. *Nursing Papers, 9*(2), 38-45.

American Nurses Association. (1980). *Nursing: A social policy statement.* Kansas City, MO: Author.

American Nurses Association. (1992a). *House of Delegates report: 1992 Convention, Las Vegas, Nevada* (pp. 235-240). Kansas City, MO: Author.

American Nurses Association. (1992b). *House of Delegates report: 1992 Convention, Las Vegas, Nevada* (pp. 104-120). Kansas City, MO: Author.

Baird, S.B., & Prouty, M.P. (1989). Administratively enhancing CNS contribution. In A.B. Hamrick & J.A. Spross (Eds.), *The clinical nurse specialist in theory and practice* (2nd ed., pp. 262-264). Philadelphia: W.B. Saunders.

Bates, B. (1974). Doctor and nurse: changing roles and relations. *New England Journal of Medicine, 283*(3), 129-134.

Bates, B. (1974). Twelve paradoxes: A message for nurse practitioners, *Nursing Outlook, 22*(11), 686-688.

Berlinger, M.R. (1973). The preparation and roles of the clinical nurse specialist. In J.P. Riehl & J.W. McVay (Eds.), *The clinical nurse specialist: Interpretations* (pp. 100-107). New York: Appleton Century Croft.

Brown, E.L. (1948). *Nursing for the future.* New York: Russel Sage Foundation.

Brown, S.J. (1989). Supportive supervision of the CNS. In A.B. Hamrick & J.A. Spross (Eds.), *The clinical nurse specialist in theory and practice* (2nd ed., pp. 285–298). Philadelphia: Saunders.

Cronenwett, L.R. (1992, July 14). *A report to CNAP members from the chairperson, Congress of Nursing Practice.* Kansas City, MO: American Nurses Association.

Donahue, M.P. (1985). *Nursing: The finest art.* St. Louis: Mosby.

Donovan, C.T. (1985). Clinical nurse specialist practice in an acute care setting. In K.E. Barnard & G.R. Smith, (Eds.), *Faculty practice in action.* Kansas City, MO: American Academy of Nursing.

Elder, R.G., & Bullough, B. (1990). Nurse practitioners and clinical nurse specialists: Are the roles merging? *Clinical Nurse Specialist,* 4(2), 78-84.

Edmunds, M. (1979, September/October). Junior doctoring. *Nurse Practitioner,* 8-46.

Edmunds, M.W., & Ruth, M.V. (1991). NP's who replace physicians: Role expansion or exploitation? *Nurse Practitioner, 16*(9), 46, 49.

Forbes, K.E. (1990). Merge!!! *Momentum, 8*(31).

Forbes, K.E., Rafson, J., Spross, J.A., & Kozlowski, I. (1990). The clinical nurse specialist and nurse practitioner: Core curriculum survey results. *Clinical Nurse Specialist* 4(2), 63-66.

Ford, L.C., & Silver, H.K. (1967). The expanded role of the nurse in child care. *Nursing Outlook, 15*(8), 43–45.

Fralic, M.F. (1988). Executive development, nursing's precious resource: The clinical nurse specialist. *Journal of Nursing Administration, 18*(2), 5-6.

Georgopulous, B., & Christman, L. (1970). The clinical nurse specialist: A role model, *American Journal of Nursing, 70*(5), 1030-1039.

Gibbs, B., Lonowski, L., Meyer, P.J., & Newlin, P.J. (1995). The role of the clinical nurse specialist and the nurse manager in case management. *Journal of Nursing Administration, 25*(5), 28-34.

Hamrick, A.B. (1989). History and overview of the CNS role. In A.M. Hamrick & J.A. Spross (Eds.), *The clinical nurse specialist in theory and practice* (2nd ed., pp. 3-18). Philadelphia: Saunders.

Hamrick, A.B., & Taylor, J.W. (1989). Role development of the CNS. In A.B. Hamrich & J.A. Spross (Eds.), *The clinical nurse specialist in theory and practice,* (2nd ed., pp. 6-39). Philadelphia: Saunders.

Hockenberry, E.M., & Hodgson, W. (1991). Merging advanced practice roles: The NP and CNS. *Journal of Pediatric Health, 5*(3), 158-159.

Hoeffer, B., & Murphy, S. (1984). Specialization in nursing practice. In *Issues in professional nursing practice, part 2* (pp. 1-5). Kansas City, MO: American Nurses Association.

Interview with Co-founder of Nurse Practitioner Movement. (1995). *Nurse Practitioner News, 3*(4), 8-12.

Kitzman, H.J. (1989). The CNS and NP. In A.B. Hamrick & J.A. Spross (Eds.), *The clinical nurse specialist in theory and practice* (2nd ed., pp. 379–394). Philadelphia: Saunders.

Koch, L.W., Pazaki, S.H., & Campbell, J.D. (1992). The first 20 years of nurse practitioner literature: An evolution of joint practice issues. *Nurse Practitioner, 17*(2), 62-71.

Koetters, L. (1989). Clinical practice and direct patient care. In A.B. Hamrick & J.A. Spross (Eds.), *The clinical nurse specialist in theory and practice* (2nd ed., pp. 107–123). Philadelphia: Saunders.

Leininger, M.M., Little, D.E., & Carnevali, D. (1972). Primex the professional nurse, responsible, accountable, reaching out and taking an active, frontline position in primary health care. *American Journal of Nursing, 72*(7), 1274-1277.

Lewis, C.E., & Resnik, B.A. (1985). Nurse clinics and progressive ambulatory patient care. *New England Journal of Medicine, 277*(23), 1236-1241.

Linn, L.S. (1974). Care vs cure: How the nurse practitioner views the patient. *Nursing Outlook, 22*(10), 641-644.

Mauksch, I.G., & Rogers, M.E. (1975). Nursing is coming of age . . . through the practitioner movement. *American Journal of Nursing, 75*(10), 1834-1943.

McClure, M.L. (1990, October 14-15). Introduction. In I.E. Goertzen (Ed.), *Differentiating nursing practice into the twenty-first century.* Selected papers from the 18th annual meeting and 1990 conference of the American Academy of Nursing, Charleston, SC. Kansas City, MO., American Academy of Nursing.

National Council of State Boards of Nursing, Inc. (1992). Position paper on the licensure of Advanced Nursing Practice, May 18, 1992, Chicago, IL.

National League for Nursing. (1958). *The education of the clinical specialist in psychiatric nursing.* New York: Author.

Office of Technology Assessment. (1986). Nurse practitioners, physician assistants, and certified nurse-midwives: A policy analysis. *Health Technology Case Study 37,* Washington, DC: U.S. Congress.

Padilla, G. (1973). Clinical specialist research: Evaluation and recommendations, conclusions and implications. In J.P. Riehl & J.W. McVay (Eds.), *The clinical nurse specialist: Interpretations* (pp. 283-334). New York: Appleton Century Croft.

Pearson, L.J. (1995). Annual update of how each state stands on legislative issues affecting advanced nursing practice. *Nurse Practitioner, 20*(1), 13-18.

Pokorny, B.E., & Barnard, K.E. (1992). ANA to revise nursing statement. *The American Nurse, 24*(5), 6.

Reiter, F. (1961). Improvement of nursing practice. In J.P. Riehl & J.W. McVay (Eds.), *The clinical nurse specialist: interpretation.* New York: Appleton Century Croft.

Reiter, F. (1966). The clinical nursing approach. *Nursing Forum, 5*(1), 39–44.

Sample, S.A. (1987). Justifying and structuring the CNS role within a nursing organization. In A.B. Hamrick & J.A. Spross (Eds.), *The clinical nurse specialist in theory and practice* (2nd ed., pp. 251-260). Philadelphia: Saunders.

Simborg, D.W., Starfield, B.H., & Horn, S.D. (1978). Physicians and non-physician health practitioners: The characteristics of their practices and their relationships, *American Journal of Public Health, 68*(1), 44-48.

Sparacino, P., & Denand, A. (1986). Specialization in advanced nursing practice [editorial]. *Council of Primary Health Care Nurse Practitioners/Council of Clinical Nurse Specialists Newsletter,* 4(2).

Stafford, M.J. (1988). Margaret Stafford. In T.M. Schorr & A. Zimmerman, (Eds.), *Making choices, taking chances: Nurse leaders tell their stories* (p. 330). St. Louis: Mosby.

Vaughan, M. (1968). Difficult task: Defining role of the clinical specialist. *Hospital Topics, 5*(18), 93-94.

Weston, J. (1975). Whither the "nurse" in nurse practitioner? *Nursing Outlook, 23*(3), 148-152.

Wright, J.E. (1990). Joining forces for the good of our clients. *Clinical Nurse Specialist,* 4(2), 76-77.

Yedida, M.J. (1981). *Delivering primary health care nurse practitioners at work.* Boston: Auburn House.

Nurse executives

Who are they, what do they do, and what challenges do they face?

BARBARA VOLK TEBBITT

Nurse executives come in assortments ranging from rare Stradivarius to country fiddles; from vintage wines to home-brew; and from vibrating VWs to reticent Rolls Royces. Top level nurse executives demonstrate behavioral patterns ranging from the classical X pattern of being business-like, efficient, and responsible to the Y pattern of being understanding, warm, and friendly and on down the alphabet to the Z pattern of being imaginative, responsible, stimulating, enthusiastic, and resurgent. (Anonymous, 1990)

Major economic, political, social, technoscientific, human resource, and market-driven forces have changed health care services dramatically throughout the United States in the last decade. An increasing number of hospitals are facing declining revenues, the prospect of delaying or sacrificing building replacement or renovation, technology enhancement, and wage and benefit competitiveness. Inflationary price increases higher than the national average have added pressure from consumers, third-party payers, and regulators to reduce expenses and system inefficiencies, to increase productivity through work redesign, to manage materials and inventory control, and to reduce personnel and capital expenditures. As a result of these forces, health care organizations are taking on new cost-conscious forms (Allred et al., 1994; Mills, 1990).

This uncertain, pressure-filled environment is negatively affecting health care access, cost, and quality, creating an urgent need for rethinking values, causing increased complexity in relationships, requiring rapid change in the restructuring of service delivery, and necessitating a redefinition of roles. The ever-evolving and dynamic role of executive nursing leadership is essential to this change process and cannot be over-emphasized in the survival and prospering of health care organizations (Mills, 1990).

To better understand both the role and functions of the nurse executive today as well as the future challenges individuals in these positions will face, it is helpful to take a brief look at our past.

HOW THE ROLE OF NURSE EXECUTIVE CAME TO BE

"Nightingale's Perspective of Nursing Administration" reflects the applicability of Nightingale's mid-1880s concepts and theories to nurse executives today (Henry, Woods, & Nagelkerk, 1990). In her time, Nightingale defined the major role of a nurse executive (then called superintendent) to be the education of others in the care of the acutely ill. She espoused the individual characteristics of conciseness and decisiveness along with imagination and wit. Nightingale was committed to intelligent discipline and strength of character for superintendents, also acknowledging a need for collaboration, tact, and sensibility. Her emphasis was on the need for personal lifelong learning.

In her writing Nightingale spoke to the need for the superintendent to have authority for all clinical or nursing practice, administration, and education. She understood effective administration to begin with knowledge of disease, health, and the nursing needs of those requiring care. She used data and statistics to monitor and improve patient outcomes continuously with the understanding and belief that such diligence would eventually ensure health and wellness in society. She introduced the first principles of personnel administration and had an acute awareness of the economics of health care prevalent in her time. Nightingale's prolific writings synchronize the practical and theoretical, qualitative and quantitative data, and clinical practice and administration (Henry, Woods, & Nagelkerk, 1990). This sense of harmonizing and balancing care delivery, program development, and resource management was Nightingale's philosophy on administration and continues to be true today.

Perhaps the major change in nursing administration between the mid-1800s and the early to mid-1900s was differentiating the roles of administration and education, which resulted in separate individuals to direct schools of nursing, their educational standards, and accrediting practices (Erickson, 1980).

Since the mid-1950s numerous national projects and studies have addressed the changing societal, economic, and environmental demands on the roles and functions of the nurse executive. These changes stimulated the evolution of numerous profiles of nurse executive roles and administrative titles and refocused required and desirable nursing leadership knowledge, skills, and behaviors (Erickson, 1980). As responsibilities and priorities for the role and position of the nurse executive have evolved, the criteria for preparation have been addressed and revised by multiple accrediting agencies and professional organizations, most notably the Joint Commission on Accreditation of Healthcare Organizations (JCAHO) and the American Organization of Nurse Executives (AONE).

THE NURSE EXECUTIVE TODAY

The JCAHO and AONE agree that the nurse executive for the 1990s will:

- Be a currently licensed registered nurse qualified by advanced education and management practice
- Be responsible for the administration and management of the nursing organization, whether that be a department or division that is centralized or decentralized in structure
- Have the authority, responsibility, and accountability for defining the discipline of nursing and for establishing and approving written nursing practice standards, policies, and procedures, to be developed consistent with current research findings and nationally recognized professional standards, and adhered to wherever nursing is practiced throughout the organization
- Be an active member of the organization's leadership team and as such be responsible for participating in setting the strategic direction for the organization as well as collaborating with other organizational leaders in designing and providing patient care and services
- Participate with leaders from the governing board, management, medical staff, and clinical areas in planning, promoting, and conducting organization-wide performance-improvement activities (American Hospital Association, 1990; Joint Commission on Accreditation of Health Care Organizations, 1994).

ROLES OF THE NURSE EXECUTIVE

The 10 major roles nurse executives assume in health care today remain as initially identified for those of any executive by Mintzberg (1975) and specifically applied to nurse executive by Stevens (1995). Those roles are:

1. *Figurehead,* serving as both the symbolic and formal head of nursing and patient care in the organization
2. *Leader,* by directing associates to goal achievement through provision of a self-motivating environment
3. *Liaison,* through building communications networks both within and outside of the organization
4. *Monitor,* by continually scanning the external and internal environments to keep abreast of changes in health care that may require redirection of planning or work efforts
5. *Disseminator,* in sharing and distributing information relating to nursing and patient care throughout the organization or community
6. *Spokesperson,* by addressing the key publics in speaking for nursing and patients
7. *Entrepreneur,* in looking for improvement opportunities in the workplace and taking initiative in new projects, programs, and services
8. *Disturbance handler,* by mediating and resolving disagreements among health care teams or work groups
9. *Resource allocator,* by determining how nursing and patient care resources will be distributed
10. *Negotiator,* by managing formal and informal work-related issues with both internal and external groups

FUNCTIONS OF THE NURSE EXECUTIVE

These 10 major role components for the nurse executive hold true regardless of the job or title held or the size or location of the health care institution. These role components may and do differ in specific activities and time requirements from large to small institutions; however, there is great similarity in the overall role functions of nurse executives (Pilette & Kirby, 1991; Sorrentino, 1992; Ulrich, 1985). This similarity minimally includes specific functions as *planner, implementer, coordinator, arbitrator, guide* and *image setter* (Tebbitt, 1990). Activities and expectations within these individual functions are delineated under each area; however, they are not meant to be all-inclusive.

As *planner,* the nurse executive

- Participates in developing, implementing, and evaluating the organization's vision, values, strategic initiatives, goals, and objectives and interprets the role of nursing and patient care in the organization's strategic plan. In so doing, the nurse executive speaks the language of multiple disciplines such as medicine, administration, and nursing and is aware of public policy's influence on the organization's financial well-being
- Participates in the organization's financial forecasting and planning and articulates nursing's contributions to the organization's financial viability as well as the resources necessary for effective patient care delivery
- Formulates nursing's mission, vision, values, goals, and objectives, integrates them with those of the organization, and establishes and executes a financial plan for the same
- Defines nursing standards of care and practice wherever nursing is provided within the organization; and develops, implements, and evaluates nursing's policies and programs to determine and allocate the financial, human, material, and informational resources required
- Is knowledgeable about information technology and its potential; participates in the organization-wide assessment of information and database needs to select and maintain an information system for clinical, management, and administrative decision making; and ensures the most beneficial and affordable integration of nursing's information system into the organization's
- Provides mechanisms for staff to participate in planning, finances, quality improvement, and education activities and processes within both the organization and nursing
- Participates in fundamentally rethinking and redesigning processes and systems to achieve improvements in organizational performance including cost, quality, service, and time by eliminating duplication, nonvalued activities, inefficient methods, and unnecessary tasks (Strasen, 1994)

As *implementer,* the nurse executive

- Works with nursing, medical, and administrative staff by providing the context, structure, systems, and resources to preserve and enhance the integrity of high-quality patient care systems (Fralic, 1993)
- Interprets the standards of care into the nursing process both by establishing and maintaining a suitable, caring environment and by designing, evaluating, and supporting an effective nursing practice model and care delivery system
- Maintains policies, procedures, standards, and programs based on regular evaluation for relevance, practicality, and success by incorporating criteria for quality, productivity, and customer and staff satisfaction

As *coordinator* the nurse executive

- Assumes responsibility for universal quality of nursing care and practice rendered within the organization
- Links nursing and patient care services vertically and horizontally by seeking opportunities for cooperative efforts with other programs, disciplines, and agencies
- Ensures prudent utilization of all resources while ensuring patient safety and that adequate resources are available for providing patient care
- Provides direction in analyzing and maintaining nursing's compliance with regulations and legislation

As *arbitrator* the nurse executive

- Relates to groups and significant individuals such as nurses, medical staff, managers, and administrators to reach mutually beneficial outcomes
- Contributes directly to administrative problem solving and decision making
- Defines and negotiates dependent, interdependent, and independent roles and functions for nursing practice within the organization
- Identifies and negotiates staffing requirements in type and amount
- Responds to nursing staff concerns regarding biomedical, ethical, and legal issues
- Works interdependently with payers, consumers, government officials, and others to meet common goals
- Translates health care delivery programs and services for a variety of constituencies

As *guide* the nurse executive

- Adapts leadership style to changing situations and competencies of staff
- Solves problems with staff, makes decisions, and delegates authority

- Sets expectations for, coaches, counsels, develops, disciplines, or terminates staff (may do so for select positions only, depending on the size and complexity of the organization)
- Encourages and rewards staff for participation in development, implementation, and evaluation of nursing services, programs, and policies
- Develops effective evaluation mechanisms and systems
- Demonstrates commitment to lifelong and accelerated learning for staff to remain flexible, responsive, cost-effective, and outcome-oriented in times of change (Fralic, 1993)

As *image setter* the nurse executive

- Creates and acts as a role model for the values and culture of the nursing organization (Miller, 1987; Brown & Schultz, 1991)
- Defines the characteristics or qualifications for desired applicants
- Develops policies and programs consistent with the recruitment and retention of qualified nursing staff, considering factors both internal and external to the organization
- Employs and deploys staff (may do so for select positions only)
- Earns support, respect, and recognition of the chief executive officer (CEO), colleagues, and the community (Henderson, 1995)

ROLE BEHAVIORS OF THE NURSE EXECUTIVE

Role behaviors of the nurse executive, which are distinct from functions, are unique to the individual nurse executive and are frequently contingent on the following:

- The health care organization's environment (i.e., economic base [profit or nonprofit]; capital and operating funds; life stage of the facility [new or old]; available technology and staff; bed size and percent occupancy; types of patients [acuity and mix]; organizational structure and relationships; and medical staff, governing body, and community involvement) (Fralix, 1989)
- The clinical practice setting (i.e., existing nursing standards, roles, responsibilities, and functions)
- The personal constitution of the nurse executive (i.e., aptitude, attitude, maturation, values, motivation, needs, personality, and past experiences) (Adams, 1990)

Most nurse executives today would agree that the more positive and supportive the organizational environment and practice setting, the greater the opportunity for the nurse executive to achieve personal effectiveness in the most conscientious, efficient, responsible, and responsive manner possible.

JOB OPPORTUNITIES, SALARY RANGES, AND TURNOVER DATA FOR NURSE EXECUTIVES

There are approximately 6,500 hospitals in the United States today, about half of which have under 100 beds and are located in more rural areas. In addition, there are over 30,000 nursing homes and almost 10,000 skilled nursing facilities (Statistical Abstract of the United States, 1994). Well over 500 acute care hospitals have closed since the mid-1980s due to the shrinking health care dollar, constrained human resources, and consumer demands for more effective systems (Mills, 1990). In addition, each year approximately 10% of hospitals are actively engaged in or finalizing mergers or acquisitions (Burda, 1995). This trend is not only projected to continue but also to increase into the year 2000. The rate of change is rapid and uneven with different results in various parts of the country. Great emphasis is being placed on incremental and state-specific approaches to changes in the health care environment (Beyers, 1995).

By their very nature, restructuring, corporate reorganizations, or closures diminish the number of senior nurse executive, middle, and first-line manager positions that will exist into the next decade. However, the opportunities available will be very challenging—requiring considerable management expertise, significant flexibility, and independent, results-oriented personal qualities (Minnick, 1993).

Salary ranges for senior nurse executives vary widely throughout the United States and are usually based on hospital size (number of beds), number of care delivery sites, program or service responsibilities within and outside of nursing, educational preparation, amount of previous managerial experience, and the region of the country (Burda, 1992). In a 1994 survey the average base salary nationwide for participating senior nurse executives was $91,800, with a range from $46,000 to $200,000 (Witt/Kieffer, 1994).

In a study of hospitals over a 10-year period, hospitals averaged 2.5 senior nurse executives, with almost 20% having four or more during that 10-year period. Fewer than 20% of the senior nurse executives remained in the same position for the entire 10 years of the study. Senior nurse executive turnover usually resulted from the following: termination/requested resignation (40%), retirement/personal/family (27%), promotion or better job (17%), and low job satisfaction (12%). Approximately 12% of the newly appointed CEOs terminated their senior nurse executives within 1 year of their arrival, usually because of complex organizational factors or contingencies and environmental uncertainties. In a significant number of cases (40%) disagreement with the CEO was cited, as were "power struggles," lack of support from the CEO, conflict with physicians, and/or CEOs who did not support innovative nursing administration strategies. Senior nurse executive turnover rates were higher in rural hospitals, smaller hospitals, hospitals that were investor-owned, those that belonged to a system of hospitals, and those located in the West. These hospitals usually had lower operating margins with higher costs, had fewer admissions with lower occupancy rates, and derived a higher proportion of their revenue from Medicaid and Medicare. Annual turnover rates ranged from about 14% to 27%, with the average turnover rate at approximately 20% (Kippenbrock & May, 1994).

Retirement, advancement, and career shifts are expected and acceptable reasons for attrition and resignation for the senior nurse executive. Resignation or termination resulting from job dissatisfaction, power struggles, or conflict with the CEO or physicians reflects serious problems within an organization. Factors such as personal values and aspiration, competence, and the intricacies of organizational culture undoubtedly also influence the tenure of senior nurse executives (Kippenbrock & May, 1994).

ACADEMIC PREPARATION AND MANAGERIAL EXPERIENCE FOR THE NURSE EXECUTIVE

There is considerable debate today about what type of advanced educational preparation individuals interested in nursing administration as a career should pursue. Should they seek specialized administrative education in a school of nursing, a generalist management degree such as a master's in business or hospital administration, or a "hybrid" or "dual" graduate degree (i.e., MSN/MBA or MHA) (Sanford, 1994)? There are more than 200 master's degree programs in nursing in the United States today, an increase of over 50% since the 1980s (The nursing profession, 1993). Of these 200 programs, slightly more than 100 offer a degree concentration in nursing administration ("The guide to graduate programs," 1992). In addition, over 30 graduate schools are offering alternative options that enable students to earn a degree in nursing and business or hospital administration simultaneously (Minnick, 1993).

This debate of nursing administration versus a multidisciplinary master's program stems from the fact that nurse executives are reporting a greater span of control and related responsibilities, are administering for care in multiple sites, and are assuming responsibility for other areas in addition to acute care nursing such as home health, ambulatory care, health information, quality improvement, social services, and support services, including admissions, environmental services, and so on (Anderson, 1993). In addition, mergers, affiliations, consolidations, purchases, and other innovative ways to capture market share have necessitated a need to eliminate most, if not all, duplication of services and roles. Indications are that this trend will continue. Some futurists predict that departments of nursing per se will cease to exist and will be replaced by patient care divisions employing a variety of health care professionals and technicians (Sanford, 1994).

This expansion of role responsibilities has resulted in further developmental needs for the nurse executive to balance administrative, clinical, and financial goals in new ways, to allocate resources, to build staff members' self-esteem, to prioritize, and to demonstrate an appreciation for diversity (Beyers, 1995). Consolidation activities, by whatever name or type, are placing on many nurse executives throughout the nation greater accountability, more emphasis on teamwork, more intense involvement with people, greater ambiguity of authority, greater emphasis on one's individuality, more stress, and a new mix of an intellectual and action orientation (Vaill, 1989).

It is important to note that as many nurse executives have assumed expanded roles they have also been given concomitant title changes to vice president of patient care services or chief operating officer to more appropriately reflect these added responsibilities (Anderson, 1993).

Regardless of the program or degree, the job dimensions for the nurse executive over the next 10 years will require knowledge, skill, and experience in the following areas: business acumen, particularly in strategic and financial review and planning, developing, and implementing programs and services; improved work processes and practices; change in times of chaos; rapid problem-solving and decision-making abilities; teamwork and teambuilding; interpersonal and intergroup communication; personnel practices and resource allocation; conflict management and resolution; negotiation and consensus building; and developing employee potential and community-organization relations. Individuals interested in pursuing nursing administration as a career would benefit from checking these job dimensions with the curriculum content in the academic program they are pursing (Sanford, 1994).

Regarding the amount and type of managerial experience necessary before assuming the role of nurse executive, the recommended criteria identified by focus groups of current nurse executives suggest at least 4 to 5 years of experience in first or middle management positions, or both, before assuming the role of nurse executive (Smith et al., 1994).

THE PROFESSIONAL ORGANIZATION FOR NURSE EXECUTIVES

The approximately 6,000-member AONE is the national organization of nurse executives and managers. AONE serves its members by:

- Providing vision and actions for nursing leadership to meet the health care needs of society
- Influencing legislation and public policy related to nursing and patient care issues
- Facilitating and supporting research and development efforts that advance nursing administration practice and quality patient care
- Offering member services that support and enhance the management, leadership, education, and professional development of nursing leaders.

Full membership in AONE is open to any RN who holds an organizational role in administration or management and is accountable for strategic, operational, or management outcomes in a health care delivery setting; serves as dean, director, or faculty in a graduate nursing administration program; serves as a consultant in a nursing administration or management practice; is employed by the JCAHO; serves as an editor of a professional nursing journal; is an executive director of an AONE chapter; or is a retired AONE member. Associate membership in AONE is open to RNs who are students in a relevant degree program with a career path in nursing administration ("AONE: Shaping the future through nursing leadership," 1995).

CHALLENGES FOR NURSE EXECUTIVES INTO THE NEXT MILLENIUM

Never before in the history of health care or nursing has there been such an emphasis on quality, performance, productivity, results, and consumer and employee satisfaction. Competence and commitment, a sense of collegiality, social presence, personal integrity, confidence, composure, courage in risk-taking, a keen sense of humor, well-being, and self-actualization will be keys to success for future nurse executives.

Tomorrow's nurse executives will be more entrepreneurial, catalytic, proactive, and innovative as they search for potential and opportunities for new products, programs, and services that support excellence in patient care in the face of constant environmental uncertainty and ambiguity (Bolster & Petit, 1990; Fralic, 1992; Johnson, 1989; Johnson & Bergmann, 1988).

Daily functions of the nurse executive will include interacting with the health care marketplace; expanding the political influence of nursing; refining, stabilizing, and harmonizing the interests and demands of nursing's constituencies; brokering, bridging, and linking organizational and patient care gaps by anticipating both short- and long-term actions and decisions; and continually assessing the internal and external environments for factors that will potentially affect the organization's policies, programs, and services. Nurse executives will need to formulate their message carefully not only to gain attention but also to result in outcomes. In addition, nurse executives will need to find the best possible means of persuasion, to learn about specific motives behind issues and actions, and to seek insight from a variety of sources (Beyers, 1995). Being appropriately credentialed will be essential for legitimacy and access to arenas of power and influence[1] (Fralic, 1993).

The personal characteristics, roles, and functions identified here will be essential to meet the following environmental and organizational challenges facing nurse executives into the next millenium.

Challenge 1: *Setting the organization's agenda for the future*

Complex social and health-related issues will demand greater social accountability in providing seamless care along a lifelong continuum and across care settings. This will include areas of wellness and prevention; primary, subacute, long-term, ambulatory, home and hospice care; as well as occupational and school health services. Every health care organization and nurse executive within it will need to generate a process to integrate information and

[1]In a December, 1994 survey of nurse executives the following percentages were cited as the highest academic degree earned: 83% had a master's degree; 9% had a bachelor's degree; 5% had a PhD; 2% had an associate degree or nursing school diploma, and fewer than 1% had a law degree. Fourteen percent of respondents were pursuing an additional degree (Witt/Kieffer et al., 1994).

translate its applicability to the organization's internal and external environments quickly and reliably to add cohesion, validity, and viability to management and administrative functions.

Nurse executives will serve a key role in collecting and assessing data to determine the health status of community members, the epidemiology of populations to be served, what individuals and groups in the community need from health services, and the resources currently available. Units of analysis will need to be defined for population types, indicators of quality will need to be agreed upon, parameters of utilization will need to be set, and a database will need to be established to determine (a) the frequency with which patients access care, (b) how quality, cost, and clinical outcomes interrelate, and (c) how services can best be designed and delivered. Nurse executives will make their presence known by designing and directing holistic patient-driven systems that make a significant contribution to the organization and the community (Beyers, 1995).

For the nurse executive this will mean developing a macro- or systems perspective resulting in a "unified, total organizational approach" that is leaner in human and fiscal resource utilization. It also means searching to find the most appropriate and best fit for nursing and patient care within the organization and the community. This will require the ability to move organizations of individuals rapidly by changing perspectives rather than purpose and by optimizing opportunities (Johnson, 1990; Murphy, 1988).

Challenge 2: *Understanding the interrelationships and patterns in solving complex problems*

As primary care, specialization, and diversification continue to be integrated in health care, little will remain straightforward and simple.

Nurse executives will need to apply defined and clear methods, models, plans, and strategies carefully to implement and accomplish goals. Greater consideration will need to be given to interrelationships among programs, products, and services and organizational structure, culture, administrative style, work climate, management practices, and community needs. The effectiveness of forecasting and planning will depend heavily on what kind of fiscal and human resources are available; how clearly roles of individuals and teams are defined; how standards for responsibility, accountability, and authority are set; and the degree to which systems are supportive of work methods necessary for goal achievement.

Information alone will no longer be sufficient to generate alternatives in problem solving as it was in the past. The nurse executive's personal capabilities and claimant groups' expectations, experience, and interest in, knowledge of, and skill in problem solving as well as organizational constraints, needs, resources, and priorities will be critical factors for understanding interrelationships and patterns in solving complex problems.

Challenge 3: *Facilitating and supporting research to maximize human potential and fiscal resources*

Health care delivery will become even more complex, challenging, and difficult in the next decade and century. Confronted with this rapidly changing economic environment and practice setting, the nurse executive will have a newly found responsibility to improve the quality, cost-effectiveness, and efficiency of patient care through research of systems, services, programs, and policies (Rosswurm, 1992).

Critical dimensions of care provided by nurses, and those influenced by and related to nursing, will surface. Opportunities will exist for introducing interactive models of research investigating technological innovations in patient care delivery, health promotion, health maintenance, illness prevention, and holistic care. Continuous quality improvement efforts, policy issues, and ethics will reveal additional opportunities for collaboration and cooperative research efforts with other services or agencies. Discussion, study, analysis, and controlled comparisons of nursing care and management as well as their importance in health care delivery will necessitate the introduction of multisite studies to a much greater degree than has been true in the past (McDaniel, 1990).

Research in nursing and nursing administration will need to set a futuristic course of action to maximize the creative potential of scarce human and fiscal resources. In setting such a course, researchers in nursing will need to move away from the past emphasis on identifying traits and studying the interrelationships of those traits for personal effectiveness, and move toward participation of nursing staff in cooperative inquiry and action research for the purpose of bringing about improvements and change not only in care delivery, but also in the workplace and the organization as a whole (Parker, Gordon, & Brannon, 1992).

Challenge 4: *Creating an empowered work environment—making and implementing decisions through others*

Although decisions are no longer made arbitrarily or autonomously by effective nurse executives today, the need for collaboration through staff involvement in the planning and problem-solving processes will be even more imperative in the future. Leadership will not be measured in terms of the leadership exercised, but rather in the leadership evoked, because it is through a philosophy of caring, a sense of fairness and openness, and valuing others that many of the nurse executive's responsibilities will be met. Leadership will not be measured in the power exercised over others, but rather in terms of the power released in others through the nurse executive's ability to influence the structure in which staff work and thereby facilitate change in their attitudes and behaviors, gain their commitment, and set examples for personal and professional excellence. Leadership will not be measured in goals defined and direction given by the nurse executive, but rather in terms of the plan of action and goals staff members work out for themselves with the nurse executive's help. Lastly, leadership will not be measured by service and projects completed by the nurse executive, but in terms of growth in competence and a sense of autonomy, responsibility, and personal satisfaction felt among the staff. The end result will be a staff who cares and shares a common purpose led by a nurse executive who creates a climate of creativity that translates theoretical verbiage into "how to's" and bridges the gap between what the staff knows and does. Through this process the nurse executive will become a role model and mentor not only of nursing, but also of the organization at large.

In conclusion, the success of the nurse executive in the future will depend on the following:

- Thinking and linking micro (individual), macro (organizational), and mega (societal) needs and results, moving beyond what is known, found acceptable or comfortable, and conventional (Kaufman, 1992)
- Defining and sharing a vision and values that stretch the thoughts, actions, and capacities of the staff beyond today's realities
- Discerning and articulating opportunities and threats facing the organization; concentrating on strengths rather than limitations; and focusing efforts on performance that will yield the greatest competitive advantages, role clarity, and staff satisfaction
- Focusing on results that are essential, strategic, and advantageous both personally and organizationally by identifying outcomes to be accomplished, defining specifically what is needed to achieve the desired outcomes, and demonstrating what accomplishment will mean and the conditions under which accomplishment will be observed by others
- Forsaking the idea of stability and remaining fluid enough to shift structures and systems constantly in response to the changing environment
- Most importantly (Borman, 1993), presenting oneself as authentic, confidence-inspiring, approachable, predictable, accountable, and professional

REFERENCES

Adams, C. (1990). Leadership behavior of chief nurse executives. *Nursing Management, 21*(8), 36-39.

Allred, C.A., Michel, Y., Arford, P.H., Carter, V., Veitch, J.S., Dring, R., Beason, S., Hiott, B.J., & Finch, N.J. (1994). Environmental uncertainty: Implications for practice model redesign. *Nursing Economic$, 12*(6), 318-326.

American Hospital Association. (1990). Role and function of the hospital nurse executive. In *Management Advisory* (pp. 1-3). Chicago, IL: American Organization of Nurse Executives.

Anderson, R. (1993). Nursing leadership and healthcare reform. Part III: Nurse executive role in a reformed healthcare system. *The Journal of Nursing Administration, 23*(12), 8-9.

AONE. (1995). *Shaping the future of health care through innovative nursing leadership.* [Brochure]. Chicago, IL: Author.

Beyers, M. (1995). Health care networks, public policy and the nurse administrator. *Nursing Policy Forum, 1*(1), 28-33.

Bolster, C.J., & Petit, B. (1990). Quest for health care value will drive nontraditional opportunities for patient care executives. *Aspen's Advisor For Nurse Executives, 5*(7), 4-7.

Borman, J.S. (1993). Women and nurse executives finally, some advantages. *The Journal of Nursing Administration, 23*(10), 34-40.

Brown, C.L., & Schultz, P.R. (1991). Outcomes of power development in work relationships. *The Journal of Nursing Administration, 21*(2), 35-39.

Burda, D. (1995, April 24). 14.3% of CEO posts turned over in 1994. *Modern Healthcare,* 8.

Burda, D. (1992, July 6). Top nurse execs net top pay hikes. *Modern Healthcare,* 26-30.

Erickson, E. (1980). The nursing service director 1880-1980. *The Journal of Nursing Administration, 10*(4), 6-12.

Fralic, M.F. (1992). Nurse executive practice—into the next millennium: From limbo dancer to pole vaulter. *The Journal of Nursing Administration, 22(2),* 15-16.

Fralic, M.F. (1993). The new era nurse executive: Centerpiece characteristics. *The Journal of Nursing Administration, 23*(1), 7-8.

Fralix, P. (1989). Administrative positioning of the nurse executive. *Aspen's Advisor For Nurse Executives, 4*(11), 5-6.

Henderson, M.C. (1995). Nurse executives leadership motivation and leadership effectiveness. *The Journal of Nursing Administration, 25*(4), 45-51.

Henry, B., Woods, S., & Nagelkerk, J. (1990). Nightingale's perspective of nursing administration. *Nursing & Health Care, 11*(4), 201-205.

Joint Commission on Accreditation of Health Care Organizations. (1994). *A comprehensive accreditation manual for hospitals* (pp. 521-528). Chicago, IL: Author.

Johnson, J., & Bergmann, C.L. (1988). Nursing managers at the broker's table: The nurse executive's role. *The Journal of Nursing Administration, 18*(6), 18-21.

Johnson, L. (1990). Strategic management: A new dimension of the nurse executive's role. *The Journal of Nursing Administration, 20*(9), 7-10.

Johnson, P.T. (1989). Normative power of chief executive nurses. *IMAGE: Journal of Nursing Scholarship, 21*(3), 162-167.

Kaufman, R. (1992). 6 steps to strategic success. *Training & Development Journal, 46*(5), 107-112.

Kippenbrock, T.A., & May, F.E. (1994). Turnover at the top: CNO's and hospital characteristics. *Nursing Management, 25*(9), 54-57.

McDaniel, C. (1990). Nursing administration research as a paradigm reflection. *Nursing & Health Care, 11*(4), 191-193.

Miller, K.L. (1987). The human care perspective in nursing administration. *The Journal of Nursing Administration, 17*(2), 10-12.

Mills, M.E. (1990). Operations improvement. *The Journal of Nursing Administration, 22*(6), 40-44.

Minnick, A. (1993). MSN in nursing administration & the dual degree. *Nursing and Health Care, 14*(1), 22-26.

Mintzberg, H. (1975). The manager's job: Folklore and fact. *Harvard Business Review, 53*(4), 49-61.

Murphy, M. (1988). Nurse executives: Becoming first-string players. *Aspen's Advisor For Nurse Executives, 3*(9), 7-8.

Nyberg, J. Teaching caring to the nurse administrator. *The Journal of Nursing Administration, 23*(1), 11-17.

Parker, M.E., Gordon, S.C., & Brannon, P.T. (1992). Involving nursing staff in research a non-traditional approach. *The Journal of Nursing Administration, 22*(4), 58-63.

Pilette, P.C., & Kirby, K.K. (1991). Expectations and responsibilities of the nursing director role. *Nursing Management, 22*(3), 77-80.

Rosswurm, M.A. (1992). A research-based practice model in a hospital setting. *The Journal of Nursing Administration, 22*(3), 57-60.

Sanford, K. (1994). Future education: what do nurse executives need? *Nursing Economic$, 12*(3), 126-130.

Smith, P.M., Parsons, R.J., Murray, B.P., Dwore, R.B., Vorderer, L.H., & Okerlund, V.W. (1994). The New Nurse Executive An Emerging Role. *The Journal of Nursing Administration, 24*(11), 56-62.

Sorrentino, E.A. (1992). Profiling a chief nursing officer. *Nursing Management, 23*(3), 32-34.

Statistical abstract of the United States (114th ed., pp. 125, 132). (1994). Washington, DC: U.S. Government Printing Office.

Stevens, B.J. (1995). The role of the nurse executive. In *The nurse as executive* (4th ed., pp. 235-242). Gaithersburg, MD: Aspen Publications.

Strasen, L. (1994). Reengineering hospitals using the "function follows form" model. *The Journal of Nursing Administration, 24*(12), 59-63.

Tebbitt, B.V. (1990). *Nursing services: Internal functions and responsibilities* (pp. 56-62). Course I, Unit 8 Hospital Administration. Minneapolis, MN: University of Minnesota.

The guide to graduate programs in nursing administration (pp. 1-49). (1992). Council on Graduate Education for Administration in Nursing.

The nursing profession. (1993). In *Pew Health Professions Commission: Schools in service to the nation* (pp. 83-90). Durham, North Carolina.

Ulrich, B. (1985). Time management for the nurse executive. *Nursing Economics$, 3*(4), 318-323.

Vaill, P.B. (1989). *Managing as a performing art: New ideas for a world of chaotic change.* San Francisco: Jossey-Bass Publishers.

Witt/Kieffer, Ford, Hadelman, Lloyd. (1994). *Senior nurse executives in transition: New roles and new challenges.* [Co-sponsored by AONE]. Oak Brook, IL.

Nursing faculty

Who are they, what do they do, and what challenges do they face?

CAROLE A. ANDERSON

WHO ARE THE FACULTY?

In 1993 there were 1,493 nursing programs (507 baccalaureate, 857 associate degree, and 129 diploma) in this country (National League for Nursing [NLN], 1995). In 1990 (the latest year for which data are available) they employed an estimated 22,000 full-time (N = 18,853) and part-time (N = 3488) faculty members (National League for Nursing [NLN], 1992). In 1990, 9.8% worked in diploma programs, 50.5% in associate degree programs, 39.7% in baccalaureate and higher degree programs (NLN, 1992). Most faculty work full time, but there is an increasing trend toward the use of part-time faculty.

The doctoral degree is the commonly expected and accepted entry-level credential for teaching in colleges and universities, but in nursing, faculty still fall far short of all being doctorally prepared. Nevertheless, there is a growing trend toward a more educated faculty. In 1995, 49% of nursing faculty in colleges and universities were doctorally prepared, a favorable improvement compared with only 15% in 1978 and 28% in 1984 (American Association of Colleges of Nursing [AACN], 1996). Yet these numbers are still far lower than the percentage of doctorally prepared faculty in other academic disciplines. Not surprisingly, there are significant differences in education levels among types of nursing programs, with the largest percentage of doctorally prepared faculty (49% in 1995-96) being found in baccalaureate and higher-degree programs (AACN, 1996); this is twice the percentage from 1983-84.

The majority of nursing faculty are women and only 8.5% are members of a minority group (AACN, 1996). Interestingly, in colleges and universities, only 37% of the faculty are tenured; this is a low tenure density when compared with other departments and colleges (AACN, 1996).

The reasons for a less-educated nursing faculty can be found in our heritage and history. Nursing education's heritage began in hospitals, not in colleges and universities. Hospital-based (diploma) educational programs were the norm for the first half of the century, and although the first baccalaureate program was started in the early 1900s, for the first half of this century the vast majority of nurses continued to be prepared in diploma schools. Vocational education (diploma) was perhaps appropriate for those earlier times when society deemed the education of women unnecessary and even undesirable.

However, times and women have changed. Women now constitute well over half of the college students in the United States, and in 1993 were awarded 54% of the bachelor's degrees, 54% of the master's degrees, and 38% of the PhD degrees (Chronicle of Higher Education, 1995). Nursing education, however, developed relatively slowly in colleges and universities and even today continues to lag far behind other major professions. It was not until the time of World War II that the number of baccalaureate programs began to increase significantly.

A new type of nursing education program was developed in junior and community colleges during the 1950s: the associate degree. This program was designed to prepare a technical nurse to complement the professional nurse who was prepared in a college or university. In 1993, associate degree programs represented a majority (60%) of all nursing programs. In 1992-93, 70% of graduates were from associate degree programs.

For the past 30 years, considerable discussion has centered on what "entry" credential is needed for beginning nursing practice. The debate persists today despite official resolutions from all of the major nursing organizations declaring that the baccalaureate *should* be the entry-level preparation for professional practice. Nurses continue to have the lowest level of required educational preparation of *all* health professionals. As illustrations, medicine, optometry, dentistry, and veterinary medicine all require a minimum of 4 years of post-baccalaureate education plus additional years in specialty training. Pharmacy is quickly moving from the baccalaureate to the doctoral degree (PharmD) as the entry-level preparation. Occupational and physical therapy, dietetics, and medical technology all require the baccalaureate degree.

Given our history and the present-day reality that only 35% of nursing's educational programs are located in colleges and universities, it is easy to understand why nursing's faculty profile, even today, would most likely parallel that found in vocational and technical institutions, rather than that found in colleges and universities. This may be appropriate for diploma and associate degree programs, given the goals of the parent institution, but the situation in colleges and universities is quite different. In these institutions, nursing programs are seriously compromised because their faculties are so dissimilar from other faculties on their campuses. Furthermore, within the nursing unit itself, the faculty is split into two factions: those with and those without doctorates—a divisive and provocative arrangement. There is currently increased emphasis on nurse practitioner education, hence the need for nurse practitioner faculty. Yet a small percentage of nurse practitioner faculty are doctorally prepared, creating the potential for reducing the percentage of doctorally prepared faculty on any campus.

In colleges and universities, faculty who are not doctorally prepared typically teach at the undergraduate level and are especially involved in undergraduate clinical teaching. Historically, the relatively small number of faculty with doctorates were assigned to the graduate program because most universities require the doctorate for the granting of graduate-level faculty status. A growing exception has been and will be nurse practitioner faculty.

Doctoral education for nurse faculty has an interesting history. Until very recently, most nurses obtained their doctoral work in nonnursing fields (primarily education). But the numbers are changing, and in 1995 almost 3,000 students were enrolled in doctoral programs in nursing. This fact is most likely a function of the increase in the number of doctoral programs in nursing from 14 in 1973 to 62 in 1995 (AACN, 1996).

How do all of these facts and figures combine to make a profile of nursing faculty that answers the question: Who are the faculty in nursing education? Perhaps there is also a more important question: What are the implications of that profile for the future of nursing education?

To begin, nursing doesn't have a single "typical" faculty member because of the diversity of parent institutions in which nursing programs reside. Rather, two faculty profiles emerge. The typical nurse faculty member teaching in a diploma or associate degree program is a nonminority woman prepared at the master's level who devotes the majority of her time to teaching undergraduates in both the classroom and clinical settings. The faculty role in these institutions is confined to only one dimension of the academic role: teaching (Aisenberg & Harrington, 1988).

Conversely, a "typical" faculty member teaching in a college or university is also a nonminority woman but is much more likely to possess the doctorate degree (49%). If the faculty member is doctorally prepared, teaching is most likely concentrated in the graduate program, and the expectation is to fulfill all three requirements of the academic role: teaching, research/scholarship, and service. As the number of doctorally prepared faculty has increased, teaching responsibilities are in both the undergraduate and graduate programs. (In 1994-95, 46% taught at both levels [AACN, 1990].)

Unlike other disciplines, then, nursing as an academic discipline is characterized by wide variation in the types of faculty teaching in our various programs. Today, it is likely that only in the research and comprehensive universities that offer the full range of academic programs including the doctorate ($N = 62$) is there greater uniformity of academic preparation found among the nursing faculty; and these faculty also enjoy greater comparability to their faculty colleagues in other academic disciplines. However, far too many nursing faculty *do not* possess the terminal degree, i.e., the minimal requirement for faculty status. Several implications emerge from the current faculty profile in nursing and are centered around two major factors: noncomparability of credentials and female dominance.

Noncomparability of credentials

Because nursing faculty on the whole are not as fully and comparably prepared as faculty in other academic disciplines they, *de facto,* occupy a marginal social status within the college or university. Faculty with marginal status are not full participants in the life of the academeme and are denied a reference group that represents the diversity of the institution. Furthermore, knowing that they are less qualified than their colleagues, nursing faculty tend to isolate themselves in their own department or college and become further removed from valuable sources of information and opportunities to influence campus decisions.

Higher education is uniquely characterized by its system of faculty governance. Colleges and universities are, in their essence, a collection of people: the faculty and students. The lifeblood of the institution is the faculty. It is the faculty who generates the reputation, attracts the best students, and whose opinions guide the course of action within the institution. Faculty who do not fully participate in this governance are, by definition, set apart from institutional life. To the extent that this is true for nursing faculty, the nursing program is rendered vulnerable because it lacks a strong, fully empowered faculty.

Female dominance

Nursing has always been and continues to be a female-dominated profession. In a very real sense, nursing as a profession can be viewed as a microcosm of women's issues in this country. Women's history is nursing's history! Nursing's development both as a profession and as an academic discipline has been shaped by this powerful fact. Yet, ironically, we in the profession do not directly address this issue and how it influences our professional development and behaviors. Furthermore, nurses do not consistently identify with the goals, objectives, and strategies of the women's rights movement. Additionally, rarely do nurses utilize a feminist paradigm to analyze issues and circumstance. Rather, the tendency is to think more parochially, viewing situations in a particular or local context rather than to analyze events or situations in light of women's deemed social status. The most recent data on women in higher education (Chronicle of Higher Education, 1995) indicate that although the number of women faculty is growing, women represent only about one third of the total college and university faculty, with 42% of them at the entry, assistant professor level. Compared with their male colleagues, women are clustered in the lower academic ranks, a smaller percentage achieve tenure, and they earn lower average salaries at every rank. The most disheartening fact is that precious little has changed in this profile over the last 20 years. The overall conclusion is that it is still difficult for women to succeed in the academe. Why? Based on a review of relevant research, Tierney and Rhoads (1994) describe women faculty as being caught in a "revolving door" phenomenon as a result of such things as inadequate anticipatory socialization, weak mentoring, fewer networking opportunities, divergent priorities, and additional demands, especially families.

Aisenberg and Harrington (1988) studied two groups of academic women: those who were off the academic track and tenured women. They found similar themes in both groups:

> Essentially, they are themes that depict an experience of professional marginality and of exclusion from the centers of professional authority. Taken together, the stories reveal a continuum of outsideness—literal in the case of the deflected women but nonetheless real for the tenured women as well. (Aisenberg and Harrington, 1988, p. xii)

Central to Aisenberg and Harrington's (1988) explanation of what happens to academic women is what they call the "marriage plot," which defines marriage as being the goal for all women and, in turn, the ways in which a woman should behave in order to meet her goal. Because this has been the paradigm for women for so long, it has been argued that women cannot ignore it or rid themselves of it as a guide for their behavior and as a measure of their success (Aisenberg & Harrington, 1988). As a result, women, like men, face the same overall task of becoming expert professionals, but, women must also deal with a whole set of other demands and expectations that relegate the pursuit of a woman's career secondary to her other roles of wife/mother as well as to her male partner's career.

This conflict is carried into the daily lives of many female faculty, and they find themselves faced with a continuous struggle rooted in the desire to be "womanly" as society defines "woman" and "successful" as her profession defines "success." Couple this personal conflict with the reality that the typical academic institution's policies and practices, the very fabric of the culture of higher education, have been crafted by and for men. The result is a climate in which women find it difficult to thrive and achieve. Recent studies on various campuses across this country attest to a climate that makes it difficult for women to advance within professorial ranks and to high-level administrative posts that offer the opportunity to influence policy and improve the climate.

In a profound way then, this marginal status for academic women is compounded for nursing faculty who do not possess the same credentials as other women faculty. Quite realistically, their disenfranchisement and marginality are made even greater.

Interesting behavior patterns emerge when individuals who are dominated by groups that deny them membership and are placed in positions without power and influence. Anger, resentment, and distrust are common as is a sense of futility and frustration and diminished pleasure derived from one's work. At times, these sentiments generate negative behaviors, such as a sense of entitlement, the so-called "queen-bee syndrome," and generalized anger and hostility to compensate for the oppression. Men react to these discomforting behaviors in negative ways that cause them to isolate women further.

Because nursing faculty are predominately women, slightly different patterns of behavior emerge internal to the academic unit. In many ways these patterns parallel those described above: doctorally prepared faculty are the "privileged class," and nondoctorally prepared faculty are marginalized and made ineligible for membership in the elite group. To the extent that this situation exists then, negative behaviors are directed toward one's female colleagues and students. Master's-prepared faculty are often motivated to pursue doctoral education in order to gain membership in the more prestigious group, which, more often than not, also means that they would not have to teach undergraduate, especially clinical, courses. Ironically, undergraduate students constitute the largest percentage of the student body. If teaching them is viewed as undesirable by the most qualified faculty, it not only sends a peculiar message to them, the future of the profession, but it also places the nursing unit at odds with a renewed interest in undergraduate instruction on many university campuses today.

WHAT DO FACULTY DO?

In differing proportions faculty teach, research, publish, and provide service to the institution and the profession. To accomplish these varied tasks, faculty need to acquire the very best graduate education. Ideally they should also possess the desire to develop and strengthen further a set of personal characteristics that Schoenfeld and Magnon (1992; in a delightful and enormously useful book called *Mentor in a Manual*) identify as being necessary to succeed in academe. These characteristics include knowledge (information, data, theories, concepts, facts); skills (technical, scientific, communication, information retrieval, analysis and synthesis); insight (wisdom, vision); and values (Schoenfeld & Magnon, 1992).

Teaching

A successful teacher possesses a thorough command of the subject matter being taught, which requires that faculty must strive continuously to expand their knowledge base in a world of rapidly changing information. This requires a commitment to continuous learning that goes beyond rhetoric to the investment of substantial time, energy, and money in one's own development as a teacher. For nursing faculty that includes staying abreast of contemporary clinical practice.

Successful teachers are those who convey a liking and deep respect for students that in turn creates an environment that is conducive to learning. Good teachers are able to present material in an objective and well-organized manner, convey a sense of excitement for the material, and stimulate students to want to learn more. Successful teachers vary their teaching methodologies according to the characteristics of the class (e.g., large lecture, seminar), understand and use state-of-the-art teaching methods, and evaluate student learning in an objective manner. The very best teachers truly enjoy teaching and their students and have learned to balance their teaching duties with their other responsibilities. Teachers also help students through the advising process to identify their interests and make decisions about their futures.

Research and scholarship

Some institutions claim teaching to be their primary and almost exclusive mission, which means that very little research or scholarship is required of faculty. However, even these institutions are increasingly requiring at least a modest level of research and scholarship. Junior faculty are wise to devote considerable effort in determining the precise expectations for teaching, research, and scholarship to be used as a guide for setting priorities.

Research training is the primary objective of doctoral education. Although nursing typically has required knowledge of the research process as part of the required courses in the master's program, the depth of knowledge and skills necessary to actually conduct research are acquired in a doctoral program. Research in nursing is focused on the development of knowledge that provides the foundation for clinical practice. Consequently, research should focus on clinical phenomena. In 1988, the National Center for Nursing Research (NCNR) was established within the National Institutes for Health (NIH) to provide nursing with increased access to federal support for research. In 1993, NCNR's status was upgraded to an institute (National Institute of Nursing Research [NINR]) within the NIH.

In 1991, the U.S. Surgeon General published *Health Care 2000,* the objectives for the nation's health for the year 2000. These objectives serve as guiding principles for the delineation of research priorities within the NIH (including the NINR) for the rest of the decade. Essentially, this document outlines the nation's most pressing health care problems and sets out objectives to improve the nation's health. Nursing research has the potential to make significant contributions to this agenda, and nursing faculty need to focus their research programs in these areas as a way of establishing nursing as a research discipline capable of making a difference in the lives of those for whom we care: our patients. Between 1989 and 1992, the research agenda set for the NINR by expert panels determined the following areas as priorities for study: low-birth-weight infants, information systems, symptom management, nursing care delivery systems, long-term care, health promotion, and AIDS. Phase II of this process designated the following study priorities for 1995 through 1999: community-based nursing models, health-promoting behaviors and HIV/AIDS, remediation of cognitive impairment, living with chronic illness, and biobehavioral factors related to immunocompetence (NINR, 1994).

Service

Faculty provide service to the nursing department or college, the parent institution, and the profession itself. This service takes many forms but a major mechanism for the provision of service is through a system of faculty governance that is operationalized through a committee structure.

In its simplest form, faculty governance is the authority and control possessed by the faculty to make decisions about curriculum, degree requirements, subject matter and methods of instruction, student policies as they relate to the educational process, and faculty status including appointments, promotion, and tenure. Faculty governance is a critical part of the faculty role and one that should not be taken lightly because it is, in its truest sense, the heart of the university.

Faculty contribute to the profession in a variety of ways. Faculty are members of professional organizations and provide service to them in the form of membership on committees and boards. Faculty also provide continuing education through different organizations that serve the profession.

Nursing faculty may also provide service to the institution through clinical practice. Such service may be part of the faculty role, but it may also be undertaken on a volunteer basis. The extent to which faculty do or do not practice affects their credibility as teachers. Unfortunately, many nursing faculty have become far removed from the realities of contemporary practice, which diminishes not only their teaching ability but also their research because they are not well positioned to identify relevant and significant clinical problems to investigate. This reality is one of the most important challenges facing nursing faculty today.

Although service is an expected part of the faculty role, faculty must guard against spending too much time doing it. Committee work can be very seductive and can also consume inordinate amounts of time. Faculty must remember that their *primary* mission is teaching and research and strive to limit their service activities not only to that which is expected but also to that which informs their teaching and scholarship.

CHALLENGES FACING NURSING FACULTY

The greatest challenge facing nursing faculty in colleges and universities is to become full participants in the academy by contributing fully to the goals of the institution through teaching, research, and service. Nursing faculty need to design and teach in excellent academic programs that are based on a knowledge of higher education and its standards, the discipline of nursing, and the needs of a health care system of both today *and* tomorrow.

Nursing, as a relative newcomer to higher education, can ill afford the risk of mediocre- or poor-quality educational programs. The decade of the 1990s is a time in which higher education faces particularly difficult fiscal challenges. In this type of environment, only the *very best* will survive. Decisions will be made to preserve quality programs that will in the long run preserve and enhance the institution. Nursing programs in major research universities may be particularly vulnerable; on the whole, their research profile does not parallel that of their colleagues, and, in looking at the data, it is apparent that the associate degree is *really* the entry level for nursing.

In the mid-1980s nursing programs were faced with dramatic declines in enrollment. In response to these declines many nursing programs very quickly designed a variety of program offerings as a means of attracting students, thereby preserving themselves. Many of these programs are quite innovative and long overdue, but many also challenge commonly accepted educational standards. As much as these can, in the short run, preserve nursing programs, they will contribute to their demise in the long run if they lack quality that is comparable to the parent institution. As an example, Leininger (1985) writes of her concern that doctoral programs in nursing may reflect a culture of mediocrity. Her concern derives from the fact that there has been a rapid proliferation in the number of doctoral programs but that many of them lack sufficient numbers of qualified faculty, are without a foundation of faculty research, and suffer from unstable leadership. Leininger's concerns, to the extent that they are true, should raise considerable alarm because the products of these programs are our future faculty. A culture of mediocrity will handicap them enormously in their ability to fulfill a faculty role.

Nursing faculty need to learn the norms that guide faculty work, particularly those related to self-governance. Faculty must become knowledgeable by reading widely and regularly about higher education (e.g., *Chronicle of Higher Education*), fully understanding the goals of their own institution, and knowing its system for advancement (knowing what is expected). Faculty especially must understand that colleges and universities are a meritocracy and that the *products* of their research and scholarship are what are valued and rewarded. Nursing faculty must make substantial efforts to bridge the historical schism between nursing service and nursing education. Collaborative efforts contribute to the enhancement of quality in both sectors. Nursing faculty must also increase and keep their knowledge of current clinical practice in order to design and implement high-quality programs, especially at the baccalaureate and master's levels.

Finding ways to stay abreast of current clinical care without having to spend 14 to 16 hours per week teaching undergraduate clinical practice is especially challenging for faculty who teach in major research universities. Because these universities define themselves by their heavy involvement in research, their standards for promotion expect faculty to be active scholars and researchers. For many years, nursing faculty were treated as an exception to this requirement, but this is no longer true. Doctorally prepared faculty must develop and maintain programs of research and scholarship. However, this becomes very difficult to do if a faculty member is assigned to undergraduate clinical teaching on a regular basis. The time commitment is just too great. New models must be developed that utilize other types of instructional personnel. Such models include teaching assistants, clinical faculty, clinical specialists, and staff nurse preceptors. The challenge is to find a way to utilize doctoral faculty effectively in the teaching of undergraduates without burdening them with the direct clinical supervision aspect of that teaching. Nursing's success as a research discipline is unequivocally linked to meeting this challenge.

Nursing faculty are challenged to develop insight into their own history as nurses, faculty, and women and to confront the conflicts derived from each in order to be successful in their careers and personal lives. As identified by Schoenfeld and Magnan (1994), traits related to achievement in a faculty role include integrity, maturity, will, self-discipline, flexibility, confidence, endurance, decisiveness, coolness under stress, initiative, justice, compassion, sense of humor, creativity, humility, and tact. Developing these characteristics and traits may present substantial challenges for nursing faculty because some are counter to traits that are considered desirable for women and because models are lacking for others that have not been part of nursing's culture.

Finally, nursing faculty must actively pursue the elimination of those policies, practices, values, and norms that interfere with their personal goals as well as goals for excellence. Examples of practices that need elimination include large, cumbersome committee structures; commitment to the *process* of education at the expense of the *product;* teaching facts rather than principles and concepts; harsh and punitive treatment of students contributing to a reputation for "eating our young," the absence of a norm for postdoctoral training; devaluing undergraduate instruction; and, finally, team teaching that makes it difficult for individuals to develop strong pedagogical skills and a sense of accountability and responsibility.

Being a faculty member is not an easy job. It requires the very best that one has to offer. It also affords a wealth of opportunity especially to shape the future of the profession and to contribute in meaningful ways to the solution of major health care problems. Becoming a faculty member is not for everyone. It should be reserved for the very best, brightest, and most promising. Our students, our future, deserve no less.

REFERENCES

Aisenberg, N., & Harrington, M. (1988). *Women of academe: Outsiders in the sacred grove.* Amherst, MA: University of Massachusetts Press.

American Association of Colleges of Nursing. (1990). *A data base for graduate education in nursing.* Washington, DC: Author.

American Association of Colleges of Nursing. (1996). *1995-1996 Faculty salaries.* Washington, DC: Author.

American Association of Colleges of Nursing. (1996). *1995-1996 enrollment and graduations.* Washington, DC: Author.

Chronicle of higher education: Almanac issue. (1995, September). Washington, DC: The Chronicle of Higher Education.

Leininger, M. (1985). Current doctoral nursing education: A culture of mediocrity or excellence? In J.C. McCloskey & H.K. Grace (Eds.), *Current issues in nursing education* (2nd ed., pp. 219-235). St. Louis: Mosby.

National League for Nursing. (1992). *Nursing data review: 1992.* New York: Author.

National League for Nursing. (1995). *Nursing data review.* New York: Author.

National Institute for Nursing Research. (1994). *Nursing research at the National Institute of Health: Fiscal years 1989-1992.* Bethesda, MD: Author.

Schoenfeld, A.C., & Magnon, R. (1994). *Mentor in a manual* (2nd ed.). Madison, WI: Magna.

Tierney, W.G., & Rhoads, R.A. (1994). *Faculty socialization as cultural process: A mirror of institutional commitment.* (ASHE-ERIC Higher Education Rep. No. 93-6). Washington, DC: The George Washington University, School of Education and Human Development.

Nurse researchers

Who are they, what do they do, and what challenges do they face?

NANCY A. STOTTS

Nurse researchers are scientists who seek to find answers to questions through methodical observation and experimentation. They design studies, conduct research, and disseminate findings at professional meetings and in peer-reviewed journals.

Nurse researchers seek to understand the science of care through systematic investigation, and the work they do is quite diverse. The design of the studies ranges from qualitative to quantitative research, encompassing interviews, epidemiological surveys, controlled clinical trials, and laboratory experiments. The topics addressed by their research are broad and divergent, reflecting the vast scope of the practice of nursing as well as the rich heritage of nursing in both the biological and the social sciences. Nurse researchers study individuals, families, and communities as well as the health care delivery system. They also are basic scientists who work in the laboratory. There is a great deal of variety in the cluster of persons who call themselves nurse researchers and in the nature of their work (Stotts, 1994).

This chapter is designed to introduce you to the world of nurse researchers. It will answer the following questions: Who are nurse researchers? What do they do? What challenges do they face?

WHO ARE NURSE RESEARCHERS?

In the most encompassing definition, *nurse researchers* are nurses who participate in the systematic study of topics related to nursing. They seek to develop the science behind evidence-based practice and understand the fundamental cellular and humanistic laws that have implications for health and illness.

Most nurse researchers begin their careers as staff nurses and progress up the clinical ladder. Several pathways can lead to the role of the nurse researcher. Some have always dreamed of being a faculty member in a school of nursing, and research is an integral part of that role in major institutions. Others realize they cannot progress in the clinical nursing arena because they do not want to take on administrative responsibilities and so turn to research as another way to progress in nursing. Another group is overcome with a desire to understand "why" and "what is the mechanism," and they use research to find the answers. A fourth group just happens into a job and falls in love with the work of research.

Doctoral preparation is required to be a scientist in nursing as well as most other disciplines. The degree usually obtained is a PhD with a major in nursing, or a doctorate of nursing science (DNS or DNSc). Some nurses earn a PhD in another discipline (e.g., statistics) or in an allied field such as education. In the purest sense, the PhD is designed to prepare a researcher and the DNS is conceptualized as an advanced practice degree, parallel to the MD but with the substantive focus being nursing. In practice, however, there is often little difference between the curriculum in the PhD program and that in the DNS program. Thus, doctorally prepared nurses are able to carry out all aspects of the research process. They have been taught and have actually carried out the process of conceptualizing a problem, formulating a question or hypothesis, designing the study, collecting the data, analyzing the data, and reporting the findings. This process is encompassed in their dissertation research.

Usually as nurses progress through the academic system, they begin to learn the research process by working initially as a research assistant. Classically, the research assistant is an undergraduate or graduate student who is working for a faculty member, doing a library search as the basis for the literature review, collecting data, or putting data into the computer for later analysis. In the most ideal world, the research assistant is an integral member of the research team, learning both process and content through this paid position.

The next level of researcher is a research nurse. This nurse is usually master's-prepared and is hired to collect data, direct and coordinate data collection, or carry out all aspects of the research that have been planned by the researcher who wrote the grant. The project director is the research nurse who assumes responsibility for carrying out the research study.

Coinvestigators are researchers who have expertise in a specific area and share in the responsibilities of conceptualizing and conducting the study. They are asked to participate because they have substantive expertise (e.g., social support), exceptional knowledge in a particular research method (e.g., phenomenological research), or are recognized for understanding analysis technique (e.g., survival analysis). There may be one or more coinvestigators on a grant, depending on the nature of the project and the expertise of the various team members. Consultants also have expertise in a specific area, but their contribution is more circumscribed than that of a coinvestigator.

The leader of the research team is the principal investigator, the person who is responsible for seeing that the grant is written and ultimately for its scientific conduct. This researcher needs to bring the team together, help members define their roles, see that the conceptual work is completed, and later see that the study is conducted and the data analyzed. The tone for how the team works together is set by the principal investigator. The research team may be run with either a democratic or autocratic style. One approach is not better than the other; they just produce different dynamics and each style has its own strengths and limitations. The principal investigator also initiates discussions about authorship of articles and plans with team members the nature of publications and order of authorship. This proactive negotiation sets a tone for fairness and parity in the team. When students are part of the research team, their contributions and roles need to be addressed in the negotiations.

It is important to recognize that many research teams are interdisciplinary. The nurse may be the principal investigator, a coinvestigator, or have any of the other roles described here. It is a rich experience to work on an interdisciplinary team, especially when all members of the team leave their titles behind and bring the full measure of their expertise to the research.

In summary, nurse researchers are nurses who do research. They usually are doctorally prepared. They may design and conduct the entire project or be responsible for only a portion of the research. They perform surveys, interviews, clinical trials, evaluation research, and laboratory research. They function with a variety of titles and roles and the work they accomplish is diverse and reflects the heterogeneity of nursing. The role a specific researcher occupies depends on the nature of the study, the various personalities of the team members, the expertise of the researcher, and timing or serendipity.

WHAT DO NURSE RESEARCHERS DO?

The research process outlines the type of thinking and activities in which nurse researchers engage. For a study to take place, a problem needs to be identified and the researcher must have sufficient interest and expertise in the problem to address it. Seasoned researchers have an identified area of research and know the literature in that substantive area. They often have a long list of questions that they would like to answer. They need only time and funding to address them.

Knowledge of funding sources is an integral part of the role of the researcher because research cannot be conducted without funding. One important source is the National Institute of Nursing Research, which is part of the National Institutes of Health. There also are grants from foundations and professional organizations. Each has its own priorities, funding limits, and application process. In the library there are books that specifically address funding sources and those data are available increasingly by computer on the World Wide Web. The contracts and grants department in some universities also provides assistance in understanding the multiple sources for financial support for research. A specific funding source is usually targeted early in the proposal development process so that the specific criteria for a given funding source can be incorporated into the proposal.

Writing the grant involves analyzing the literature to understand what has been done in the field. Normally, the researcher critically analyzes the literature and puts the proposed study in the context of work that has already been reported. Reviewing the literature also helps in the development of the study procedures because using established approaches and instruments increases the accuracy of the data obtained in the study. When a new area of study is embarked on, pilot work often needs to be undertaken. The process for grant application for pilot work is the same as applying for a major grant; however, because pilot work can often be done more inexpensively, the sources of funding are often different than those used for a larger grant.

A crucial aspect of grant writing is the development of a budget, which involves determining the costs for conducting the research. The researcher must "step through" the entire research process and estimate costs for personnel, equipment, data collection tools, data analysis, and reporting. While this sounds relatively easy to do, it is a sophisticated skill that requires knowledge of the population. For example, in calculating staff costs, one item to consider is recruitment of subjects. The researcher must know the number of subjects who meet the study criteria and have some estimate of how many will consent and in what time period. The researcher also must include in the calculation the number of subjects who will consent and later drop out or die. Part of the consideration is also how sick the potential subjects are, the amount of burden that the study imposes, and what the subject will gain by participating. All of these factors must be considered when calculating the amount of time it will take to recruit subjects and the level of personnel required to do the job.

Thus far, the general activities of the nurse researcher have been discussed. It is important to recognize that what the nurse researcher does is determined in part by the researcher's employer. Researchers are employed by colleges and universities, by industry, or they may be self-employed and work by contract or do consultation.

In the college or university community, researchers serve in an academic position or in a research position. The person in the academic position classically is in a tenure-track position where research or creative work is one criterion for progression in rank. Research needs to be completed but time also needs to be devoted to teaching, professional competence, and university and public service. Thus, most nurse researchers in the academic position are not solely researchers. The nurse researcher who is in the academic position is usually on "hard money" (i.e. university or college funds), and part of his or her salary is offset when he or she receives a research grant that is large enough to include a salary. It also is important to realize that some colleges and universities allow their faculty little time to devote to research, but this depends on the school's philosophy and how it is implemented.

In a peer research position, the researcher is hired specifically to conduct his or her own studies or to be employed on someone else's research. Persons in the research position are funded entirely on grant money or "soft money." Successful nurses in this position are flexible and creative because their position lasts as long as their research is funded.

Nurse researchers employed by industry are often hired because they bridge the gap between clinical practice and the basic sciences. They are often responsible for the clinical research testing of the company's products, locating places to conduct the studies, identifying a principal investigator, setting up multisite studies, and ensuring that the protocol is conducted consistently and that findings are recorded in a manner that allows for analysis by site as well as across settings. Often the nurse researcher employed by industry must understand the requirements of the Federal Drug Administration for testing new products, so that the protocol developed and data gathered will meet the scrutiny required for ultimate approval of the product.

Nurse researchers who are self-employed contract with other people who need their specific services. The type of services offered and the cost vary widely. Some do primarily data analysis, others assist with study design, and others combine their substantive nursing expertise (e.g., cardiovascular nursing of adults) with research skills. Their income depends on developing a set of clients with ongoing needs or being so well known that new clients are consistently referred to them; without clients, the income of the self-employed nurse researcher does not exist.

In summary, nurse researchers are prepared to actualize all aspects of the research process. They may be responsible for the entire study or a portion of it. They may work in academia, industry, or be self-employed. There is much heterogeneity in what nurse researchers do.

WHAT CHALLENGES DO NURSE RESEARCHERS FACE?

Nurse researchers face a myriad of challenges, including defining why nursing research is important to nursing practice; developing intradiscipline respect for nurse researchers whose substantive focus or research methods differ from their own; continuing to define the discipline of nursing through nursing research in a changing health care arena; gaining access to subjects because most nurse researchers do not have their own caseload; and obtaining funding in a world of shrinking fiscal resources.

Both within and outside of nursing there is limited appreciation of the need for nursing research. Research in nursing has been viewed as an activity of nursing students—as one of the hoops to jump through to graduate rather than being important to the development of the practice of nursing. This conclusion does not seem overwhelmingly surprising because in the past, few nurses have conducted research. Only recently have researchers in nursing been recognized for their program of research. Dodd and Dibble's work in self-care (1993) and Braden and Bergstrom's work in pressure ulcer risk assessment (1994) are examples of the substantive content produced by nurse researchers that have important consequences in clinical care. One of the challenges nurse researchers face is to show their worth to nursing practice.

Within the nurse researcher community, there seems to be a lack of support for nurse researchers whose substantive content or research methods differ from one's own (Drew, 1988; Strickland, 1993). There are battles between quantitative versus qualitative methods and bench research versus clinical studies. While some of it is honest discussion in an effort to understand by comparing and contrasting, it often is divisive and detracts from nursing research. A kindlier and more broad-minded approach that encourages understanding of differences and an appreciation of the types of knowledge that can be produced with different approaches would allow nurse researchers to focus their energies on generating knowledge rather than defending their substantive content or research method.

Another challenge for nurse researchers is to continue to define the discipline of nursing through research in a changing health care arena. The nature of nursing is changing due to economic forces and quality is often being exchanged for more inexpensive care. Nursing has not defined well its unique contribution to health care and the discipline is in jeopardy of being destroyed in this period when interventions are linked tightly to outcomes. It would behoove nurse researchers to attend to this serious issue so nursing as a discipline and practice can continue to exist.

Nurse researchers seldom have their own caseload of patients and access to patients of other providers may be a challenge when recruiting subjects for studies. In this instance, access to patients is dependent on the openness of the patient's primary physician to having the patient studied and the collaborative relationship that the nurse researcher has established with the physician. Other considerations that affect access to patients are the numbers of studies being conducted at a particular site, the direct potential financial benefit of the study to the health care team, and whether the researcher is seen as someone who might "steal" patients from the primary care physician's practice to the researcher's.

Another challenge is limited funding. With the current federal fiscal crisis, money from the National Institutes of Health for nursing studies is increasingly limited. When funds are limited, nurse researchers compete directly with each other and with scientists in other institutes. The benefit for research to the consumer needs more emphasis to help leverage funding from both the public and private sectors. One approach to this challenge is to focus for a period on translational research, in which the emphasis is on research utilization and the effects research findings have on outcomes. However, there must be a fine balance between creating knowledge and finding ways to use it, and funding for the pipeline of knowledge must not be sacrificed to the god of immediate utilization.

Thus nurse researchers face many challenges in their work. Knowing what the challenges are assists the researcher in consciously devising approaches to mitigate them in order to focus their energies on the generation of knowledge.

SUMMARY

Nurse researchers are a hearty group who seek to develop an understanding of the basis for clinical care. For the most part they are doctorally prepared persons who initiate or participate in all phases of the research process. They are engaged in diverse methods of research whose substantive content addresses the full life span and the health and illness spectrum as well as the health care system. Nurse researchers face numerous challenges in their daily work. It is critical, however, to recognize that their work is pivotal to the profession and discipline because it lays the foundation of the future of nursing.

REFERENCES

Braden, B.J., & Bergstrom, N. (1994). Predictive validity of the Braden Scale for pressure sore risk in a nursing home population. *Research in Nursing and Health, 17*(6), 459-470.

Dodd, M.J., & Dibble, S.L. (1993). Predictors of self-care: A test of Orem's model. *Oncology Nursing Forum, 20*(6), 895-901.

Drew, B.J. (1988). Devaluation of biological knowledge. *Image—the Journal of Nursing Scholarship, 20*(1), 25-27.

Stotts, N.A. (1994). Nurse researchers: Who are they, what do they do, and what challenges do they face? In J.C. McCloskey & H.K. Grace (Eds.), *Current issues in nursing* (4th ed., pp. 38-42). St. Louis, MO: Mosby.

Strickland, O.L. (1993). Qualitative or quantitative: so what's your religion [editorial; comment]? *Journal of Nursing Measurement, 1*(2), 103-105.

Nurse entrepreneurs

Who are they, what do they do, and what challenges do they face?

LYNDA JUALL CARPENITO, MARGO C. NEAL

What is an entrepreneur? *Webster's New Collegiate Dictionary* (1993) defines an entrepreneur as "one who organizes, manages, and assumes the risks of a business or enterprise" (p. 477). Herron and Herron (1994) see the essence of entrepreneurship as "innovation through reallocation or reconfiguration of resources . . . [and] an awareness of or alertness to the opportunity to do so for the purpose of creating benefit" (p. 310).

A "common sense" of nurse entrepreneurs has not included the traditional role of "private duty nurse" or even nurse therapists. Certainly, nurses in these roles were and are entrepreneurial. Today, the commonly accepted definition of nurse entrepreneur refers to someone who is self-employed in either a nonclinical mode—e.g., consultant, educator, editor, writer—or in a clinical role—e.g., nurse practitioner or nurse therapist.

Nurse entrepreneurs have grown and developed over the past decade, although there were a few nurses who pursued nontraditional careers in the 1970s. For example, Steele set up a joint practice in Boston, and Neal was one of the first nurses to provide continuing education workshops nationally. In the late 1970s and early 1980s, nurse entrepreneurs were a relatively new phenomenon; in the 1990s, they have become a permanent part of the nursing landscape. This nontraditional role for nurses is supported by many graduate schools that invite nurse entrepreneurs to speak to their students. Another indication of the permanence of this role is its listing as a role option in nursing in a survey conducted by Aydelotte, Hardy, and Hope (1988), which was published by the American Nurses Association. The growth of nurse entrepreneurs appears to parallel the women's movement toward greater equality of the genders. It also parallels the increasing number of men and nurses with advanced degrees in the profession.

Where are the outlets for nurses who are highly educated to do specialized assessments, identify and evaluate patient outcomes, and make treatment decisions? Universities take the majority; hospitals and other health agencies take fewer; and managed care agencies are hiring an increasing number. The emphasis on cost containment is providing opportunities in health maintenance organizations for nurse practitioners.

Shoultz, Hatcher, and Hurrell (1992) state that the growing edges of a new paradigm in nursing "are to be found not within the well-developed or established boundaries of the profession, the old paradigm, but on the edges, at the point of interprofessional and community contact" (p. 57). Chaos and needed change still predominate in the health care system. This is a time to focus on preventive care, and nurses, with emphasis on the wellness model, can find opportunities in the present and evolving health care system.

WHO ARE THEY, WHAT DO THEY DO?

In a guest editorial in the *Journal of Continuing Education*, Keough (1977) wrote, "In a field as diversified as nursing, each of us should be able to find career satisfaction" (p. 4). A career is an occupation that one follows as one's life's work. It represents a progressive course of action a person takes to achieve one's professional goals. Entrepreneurs organize, manage, and assume the risk to achieve their goals. They seek to make a difference for a profit.

The exact number of entrepreneurs in nursing is unknown. What is known is that the group is very diverse

EXAMPLES OF SERVICES PROVIDED BY CONSULTANTS

Accreditation and regulatory compliance

Organizational development
Case management
Communications
Computer information management
Cost containment
Evaluation
Quality management
Planning & forecasting
Home health services
Discharge planning
Resource management
Educational programs

Employee relations

Classification systems
Risk management
Recruitment & retention
Staff development
Delivery systems
Documentation systems
Research program development
Staffing & scheduling
Standards
Management development
Fiscal management

From "Directory of Consultants," 1995, *Journal of Nursing Administration, 25*(7/8), 68-92.

and provides a multitude of services. For example, entrepreneurs serve as consultants for risk management or provide direct client services, such as nurse practitioners, or produce and market a product, such as uniforms or software. For the past several years the *Journal of Nursing Administration* has published an annual list of consultants and *Perspectives in Psychiatric Care* has published a comparable list for nurse therapists in private practice. The *Journal of Nursing Administration's* 1995 *Directory of Consultants* lists consultants and the services they provide. The box above lists examples of the variety of services provided.

In addition to the services noted in the box, nurses have created companies that provide air ambulance service, home health care, temporary staffing, uniforms and client hospital gowns, pediatric surgical preparation kits, educational toys, corporate employee health programs, child care, elder care, editorial services, injury prevention, and emergency management training. Other nurse-run businesses provide direct client services, such as chronic pain management, breastfeeding counseling, health teaching, enterostomal therapy, family therapy, parenting classes, and home adaption for patients with neurological disabilities.

To determine the characteristics, work style, benefits, and problems of entrepreneurs, we surveyed a convenience sample of 22 nurse entrepreneurs; the return rate was 85%, ($n = 19$). A listing of the respondents appears in Table 7-1.

WHAT ARE THE CHARACTERISTICS OF SUCCESSFUL ENTREPRENEURS?

Not everyone wants to be an entrepreneur, and not everyone who attempts self-employment will be successful. In 1985, the Center for Entrepreneurial Management surveyed its 2,500 members in an attempt to develop a profile of an entrepreneur. The box on page 48 presents characteristics found to be present in the entrepreneurs surveyed. Examine the list in the box, and check those characteristics that best describe you. How many characteristics of a successful entrepreneur do you have?

Drucker (1985), "Entrepreneurs always search for change, respond to it, and exploit it as an opportunity" (p. 21). In our survey, several entrepreneurs emphasized the need to have good interpersonal skills (Dolan, Fishman, Gostel, Puetz). Hall Johnson emphasized good listening skills as a method to generate marketable ideas. Burgess wrote that one had to be "open to changing as the market requires and to look down the road as to what is changing and developing a response, while focusing on what needs to be done now." Meredith wrote "willingness to step out of established norms."

The majority of the respondents said that entrepreneurs should be creative, humorous, flexible, and enthusiastic. Alfaro-LeFevre expanded on the above by adding curiosity, humility, and persistence. When faced with problems or failure, one needs the ability to face rejection and stand back (Milazzo) and to have "thick skin" (Porter-O'Grady). Manthey emphasized that one needs a "strong desire to keep moving forward in personal growth and willingness to change." All respondents agreed that an entrepreneur must be a self-starter, self-disciplined, "driven," and have a great deal of energy. Carroll-Johnson described the need to have the willingness to invest money in anticipation of long-term gains. Jansen wrote that one needed bravery to give up the familiar financial security. In response to the question "What are the forces that led you to start your own business?" two respondents

Table 7-1 Survey Respondents

Roberta Abruzzese Consultant RELSA Garden City, NY	Suzanne Hall Johnson Director Hall Johnson Communication, Inc. Lakewood, CO
Rosalinda Alfaro-LeFevre President N.D.N.P. Consultants Malvern, PA	Marie Manthey President Creative Nursing Management, Inc. Minneapolis, MN
Christine Bolwell Owner Diskovery Saratoga, CA	Amy Meredith President The North American Center for Injury Medford, NJ
Connie Burgess President Connie Burgess & Associates Long Beach, CA	Vicki L. Milazzo President Medical-Legal Consulting Institute, Inc. Houston, TX
Rose Mary Carroll-Johnson Editor Nursing Diagnosis, Oncology Nursing Forum Valencia, CA	Tim Porter-O'Grady Senior Partner, CEO Tim Porter-O'Grady Inc. Atlanta, GA
Mariam B. Dolan President Heritage Home Health Bristol, NH	Belinda E. Puetz President, CEO Belinda E. Puetz & Associates, Inc. Pensacola, FL
Dorothy J. Fishman President Fishman Associates Farmington, CN	Roxane Spitzer-Lehmann President S/L Associates San Diego, CA
Roberta Gostel President Healthcare Multimedia Design Richmond, VA	Ann VanSlyck President VanSlyck & Associates, Inc. Phoenix, AZ
Elise T. Gropper President Gropper & Associates Inc. Miami Beach, FL	Sylvia Weber Psychiatric Nurse Clinical Specialist Counseling & Mental Health Services Cranston, RI
Sandra Jansen President Birth Plus Los Angeles, CA	

reported termination from their positions, and two reported unsatisfactory work situations. Since the profile mentioned earlier listed termination from position or resignation from an unsatisfactory position as characteristics of entrepreneurs, it would be interesting to ask those surveyed, "Were you happy in your position before starting your business?"

When asked, "What is the best aspect of being self-employed?" several respondents cited being their own boss, enjoying the freedom, and reaping the benefits of their hard work. Manthey replied, "Being able to stretch yourself as far as you can go without hitting a wall put up by someone else." Weber wrote, "I can be as creative as I want without needing to get everything I do approved by

CHARACTERISTICS OF SUCCESSFUL ENTREPRENEURS

- Have been fired from a job
- One or both parents were self-employed
- Had a business, e.g., babysitting, yard work, baking before the age of 20
- Is the oldest child in the family
- Has a bachelor's or master's degree
- Wanted to start a business to work primarily for him- or herself
- Tends to fall in love too quickly with new ideas
- Very organized
- Extroverted
- Enjoys people

From (1985). *The Entrepreneur's Quiz*, by J. Mancuso, New York: Center for Entrepreneurial Management.

a board, boss, etc." Carroll-Johnson liked the flexibility to be able to take a few hours during the day to work at her child's school. Bolwell said that the best aspect of being self-employed was also the most difficult, that is, "having the ability to self-determine goals and approaches to achieving those goals." One of this chapter's authors (Carpenito) likes the freedom to choose her direction and focus but suffers from taking on too many projects. Spitzer-Lehmann enjoys assisting many organizations and the freedom from politics.

WHAT ARE THE CHALLENGES?

Most entrepreneurs will agree that those not self-employed usually view entrepreneurs as having a great deal of freedom to decide if they want to work today and, if so, when and at what. Others have an impression that self-employed persons work fewer hours than their company-employed counterparts. Respondents to our survey reported working a range of 4 to 18 hours a day, with only one reporting 4 hours. Nine of the 15 reported usually working 6 days per week. Weekends were viewed as very productive because of fewer interruptions, e.g., telephone, staff.

When asked, "How many vacation days did you have last year?" one respondent said none and one reported 1 day. Of the 14 remaining, 8 took 2 weeks, 3 took 4 weeks, 1 took 6 weeks, and 1 vacationed 2 months. Milazzo wrote, "The real challenge is not to let your business pervade your personal life." Most entrepreneurs report difficulty turning off their creative thinking when they walk out of their office. Carpenito found initially that an office in her home made her home no longer a place of respite.

In addition to days worked, entrepreneurs often do not count the time involved in traveling. For example, if a person travels for work for 1 week, travel time takes Sunday and Friday evenings; thus two of the three weekend evenings are gone.

Inherent in every business are the activities, personnel, equipment, and supplies necessary to accomplish the business goals. When employed by someone else, most nurses are concerned primarily with their work activities. They utilize personnel, supplies, and equipment but may not be aware of their cost. Several respondents said that they had anticipated big expenses for copiers, computers, and fax machines but were surprised at the "little things" required to set up an office, such as paper products, postage, phone calls, and office supplies. In addition, they were surprised about the cost of taxes, legal fees, professional services (printing, editing), unemployment compensation, health insurance, airfares, and marketing. What previously were called benefits, i.e., sick time, vacation, health insurance, are now a business expense. No income is earned when you are on vacation.

The question "What is the downside about being self-employed?" evoked some interesting responses. One respondent described the impositions made on her time by phone calls or requests by friends and relatives for rides to appointments because "she is always available and not really working." Gropper responded "Being able to accept rejection when contracts do not come through."

Fear of financial failure, an uneven income, and the uncertainty of one's income year to year was cited by most respondents. One respondent said, "You can't pass the buck," while another reported the difficulty of letting go at the end of the day. Four respondents reported the "loneliness" of being self-employed, the isolation from colleagues, and the lack of office atmosphere.

The statement, "Describe one business experience which was a nightmare," yielded descriptions of several situations that future entrepreneurs will probably experience. One respondent replied, "When faced with the first cancellation of a seminar, I immediately concluded my venture was a total failure, when in fact I had been canceled because the RNs went on strike." Another described consulting at a hospital that had just recently been unionized so that, "When I showed up I was everybody's bait; nothing was going to change them. Everything I did was sabotaged." Another respondent wrote, "In the past when I have met with CFOs or CEOs and another person is present who is not a nurse, they automatically turn to the other person as if I couldn't possibly understand the 'business issues' because I am a nurse." One respondent reported that when she decided to start her business, her director of nursing wrote her a letter warning her that she would fail, "as most nurses do."

STARTING YOUR OWN BUSINESS

In a review of the literature on risk taking as a crucial component of entrepreneurship, Herron and Herron (1991) concluded that although early management studies seemed to support that belief, more recent studies "hold that risk-taking propensity is not a distinguishing characteristic of entrepreneurs" (p. 310). Herron and Herron (1991) state that "the empirical management literature strongly suggests that need for achievement is crucial to the decision to become an entrepreneur" (p. 310).

Nevertheless, there are many risks with which to be dealt. There are financial risks. (Can I derive sufficient income from the enterprise? Will I be able to sustain the services I provide? Will my practice be successful? Will it grow?) There are the psychological risks as well. (Do I see myself as an independent practitioner? Will I be able to work on an individual basis versus as part of a team? Will I succeed? Can I do it?)

One of the best ways to find the answers to these questions is to do your homework. For example, ask yourself why you want to start your own business. Are your answers realistic? Like any working position, being an entrepreneur has many rewards, but it also involves hard work and long hours; it can bring moments of great elation offset by despair. In short, it is not a panacea to all problems in other work areas. It does, however, provide an opportunity for creativity and an internal locus of control over one's work.

Once you are clear as to why you want to be an entrepreneur, you need to go through some other checklists (see the box on this page). The next step is to write a business plan. The actual writing of the plan is very important because it forces you to focus on your goals, objectives, and means of achieving them. Like any good plan or budget your business plan will be a guide. It is important that it be flexible to allow you to take advantage of unforeseen opportunities, which always appear.

Many books, software, and articles are readily available to help you write a business plan. For example, there are combination software and book packages that instruct you on how to write a business plan and provide a template for creating the plan, e.g., Business Plan Writer (Graphic Software Inc.), Business Plan Tool Kit (Business Essentials Library). At a minimum, the plan should include the purpose of your business, your specific goals and objectives, a definition of your products/services, a financial forecast of proposed expenditures and income for the first 6 months (in detail) and for the first 3 years (in less detail), and initial funding resources. It also needs to include your plans for initial funding resources. One respondent was surprised at her personal living expenses rather than her business expenses when she had to budget.

A crucial part of any business plan is the marketing component. In our experience, this is the most difficult aspect for nurses. Going from the position of an employee—where the direct marketing is done by others—to an entrepreneurial status—where the individual must do his or her own marketing—is difficult. This transition is a little like going to a non-English–speaking country without an interpreter armed with only a few words of the new language.

A marketing plan is essential unless, of course, you are one of those fortunate few who have people sitting on their doorstep begging to buy their services. If so, lucky you. Otherwise, consider these questions:

- How will you tell your target market about your business?

PLANNING AND EVALUATING ECONOMIC OPPORTUNITY

What services/products will you provide?

Will they be the same as others now available?

- How will yours differ?
- What is your rationale for choosing them?
- Will you start with one service/product or several?
- What are your qualifications to provide these services or produce the product?
- Are your services something that people need? or want? or both?

Who is your target market?

Hospitals? Schools? Individuals? Organizations?
Why should they buy from you?

- You're a nice person and you deserve a chance.
- You're just starting out and need a break.
- You have a sound product.
- You have a service not available elsewhere.

Who are your competitors and what are they selling?
How will these services/products generate income for you?

- Why do you think people will buy what you are selling?
- Who and what are your competitors, and how will you differentiate yourself from them?
- What are the features of your services/products and what benefits will they provide?
- What will you charge?

Students often ask how a person comes up with new ideas. The question recalls to us a friend who was an art director in an ad agency. She always said, "The more creative you are, the more creative you become." That is how you come up with new ideas. They emerge. You are automatically on alert to new ways of doing things, of looking for an unmet need. Then you check it out, ask questions, weigh the risks and opportunity, and make plans. Finally, Meredith advises to "gain all the information possible about your area of interest and that it takes time to establish a reputation."

SUMMARY

For would-be entrepreneurs, Alfaro-LeFevre advises to "have a clear vision of what you want to do" and "to look at false starts as stepping stones to getting there rather than signs to give up." Several respondents (Abruzzese, Puetz, Manthey, Burgess, VanSlyck) advise neophyte entrepreneurs to have the financial resources to make it through the hard times of the first year or two. VanSlyck also advises to hire talented staff. Burgess suggests that you know your product well, know how you are going to sell it, and expand slowly. Weber advises to set a plan with target dates and then to triple the timeline on the dates.

Because entrepreneurs are responsible for their successes and failures, Gostel recommends that you learn as much as you can about yourself before starting your own business. What is your work style? What are your peak- and low-energy periods during the day? Plan activities according to energy levels, e.g., answer mail during low-energy periods. Porter-O'Grady responded with, "Stick it out through the tough first two years," and "the client always comes first." And Milazzo poignantly advises to "go for your dream and be sure you can pursue something you are genuinely passionate about. Money should not be your motivation!"

Meredith advises nurses contemplating self-employment, "Don't be afraid to set standards and to stick to them, never be so anxious for a contract that you are willing to compromise what you know is right." Finally, as expressed by Burgess, "It is mine. The autonomy, the accountability, the decisions, the relationships with clients are all up to me. So the good decisions as well as the poor ones are my responsibility. I am responsible for my successes. It constantly stretches my creativity."

REFERENCES

Aydelotte, M., Hardy, M., & Hope, K. (1988). *Nurses in private practice: Characteristics, organizational arrangements, and reimbursement policy.* Kansas City, MO: American Nurses Foundation.

Directory of Consultants. (1995). *Journal of Nursing Administration, 25* (7/8), 68-92.

Drucker, P.F. (1985). *Innovation and entrepreneurship.* New York: Harper & Row.

Herron, D., & Herron, L. (1991). Entrepreneurial nursing as a conceptual basis for in-hospital nursing practice models. *Nursing Economic$, 9,* 310-316.

Keough, J. (1977). Guest editorial. *Journal of Continuing Education, 11*(3), 4.

Mancuso, J. (1985). *The entrepreneur's quiz.* New York: Center for Entrepreneurial Management.

Shoultz, J., Hatcher, P., & Hurrell, M. (1992). Growing edges of a new paradigm: The future of nursing in the health of the nation. *Nursing Outlook, 40,* 57-61.

Webster's New Collegiate Dictionary. (1993). Springfield, MA: G&C Merriam, Webster Inc.

Nurse informaticists

Who are they, what do they do, and what challenges do they face?

MARY N. McALINDON

Technology and information overwhelm us! We find computers in use at the bank, the grocery checkout, in our cars, on our telephones, and in almost every other aspect of our lives. The purpose of this technology is to gather data and provide information. This allows businesses to become more efficient and effective in providing their services. Information technology involves the use of computer hardware and software to process data and information in order to solve problems. The business of health care also benefits from the use of information technology.

Nurse informaticists are specialists in managing health care information and technology. Information is the communication or reception of knowledge. Since earliest times, nurses have collected, processed, and communicated information. Technology is a scientific method of achieving a practical purpose. When personal computers were introduced in health care in the 1970s, nurses began to use this technology to assist with communication. Today we combine computer science and information science to manage and process data, information, and knowledge to support the practice of nursing in all settings.

HISTORY OF NURSING INFORMATICS

Nurses comprise the largest segment of health care professionals. Many nurses with advanced knowledge and education are in specialized practice. In January 1992, the American Nurses Association (ANA) Congress of Nursing Practice designated informatics as a nursing specialty. The ANA Council on Computerized Applications in Nursing (CCAN) was thus authorized in 1992 to develop the scope of practice and standards for the new specialty. The Congress also requested a definition of the nursing informatics specialist. By 1994, the ANA Task Force on the Scope of Nursing Practice for Nursing Informatics published *The Scope of Practice for Nursing Informatics* (1994), followed by the *Standards of Practice for Nursing Informatics* in 1995.

Graves and Corcoran (1989) defined nursing informatics as the combination of computer science, information science, and nursing science to support the delivery of patient care. The ANA Task Force defined nursing informatics as

> the specialty that integrates nursing science, computer science, and information science in identifying, collecting, processing and managing data and information to support nursing practice, administration, education, research, and the expansion of nursing knowledge. It supports the practice of all nursing specialties in all sites and settings of care whether at the basic or advanced practice level. (*The Scope*, 1994, p. 3)

Nursing informatics is considered part of the field of medical informatics. Hannah, Ball, and Edwards (1994) defined medical informatics as "the field that concerns itself with the cognitive information processing and communication tasks of medical practice, education, and research, including information science and the technology to support these tasks" (p. 4). The American Medical Informatics Association (AMIA) is composed of 12 working groups including several that are not necessarily "medical." These groups include Dental Informatics, Hospital/Medical Information Systems, Nursing Informatics, and Prevention and Health Evaluation Informatics. The premise is that the term *medical informatics* refers to all health care professions and includes those information technologies that are concerned with the patient care decision-making process performed by health care practitioners. Many nurses, however, would like to see the term "medical" broadened to "health care" or be omitted altogether.

Nursing informatics is a practice discipline and the

term itself refers to the use of information technologies that focus on the recipient of care. In 1988, Peterson and Gerden-Jelger described three levels of competency for nursing informatics: a user level, a developer level, and an expert level. The user has the ability to use the information system, the developer has the ability to participate in development, and the expert is able to direct development and implementation and to serve as a consultant, evaluator, or researcher.

These competencies were intended for the four major roles in nursing: the nurse practitioner, administrator, educator, and researcher. *Competency* is defined as having sufficient knowledge, judgment, skill, or strength. Informatics practice assumes a degree of excellence in nursing practice as well as competency in informatics.

The core phenomena of nursing informatics consists of all data, information, and knowledge involved in the patient care process. McAlindon (1995) provides the following illustration: data, information, and knowledge constitute three aspects of a concept generally called "information." Data are discrete entities that describe or measure something without interpreting it. The number 30 has no meaning without interpretation. Information consists of interpreted, organized, or structured data. The number 30 interpreted as milliliters or as a length of time in minutes or hours has meaning. Knowledge refers to information that is combined or synthesized so that interrelationships are identified. For example, the number 30, when included in the statement "all patients with indwelling catheters longer than 30 days developed infections" becomes knowledge, something that is known (p. 228).

Nurse informaticists understand the progression from data to information to knowledge and the use of computers and programs to process data and information. They assess information needs, analyze requirements, design solutions, and develop, modify, and implement whatever technology will solve the identified problem (*Standards of Practice,* 1995, p. 3). They analyze and maintain information-handling technologies so that patient care data can be entered once and stored in a central repository called a database for access by all health care team members.

All health care professions interact, share the same mission, have access to the same published knowledge, and to some degree overlap. Nursing informatics applications are designed to serve nurses, but they do not exist alone and the informaticist assumes an important role in ensuring that nursing's data and knowledge are structured so that they are accepted and acceptable to the larger health care community.

The ANA's *Standards of Practice for Nursing Informatics* (1995) describes a generalist level of practice. At this level, the informatics nurse has a bachelor of science in nursing degree and additional informatics knowledge and experience. The informatics nurse specialist has a master of science degree in nursing and has taken graduate level informatics courses. Other nursing specialties focus on the substance of information and use informatics methods and tools to advance their understanding of patient care information.

ORGANIZATIONS SUPPORTING INFORMATICS

Four organizations have supported nursing informaticists: the ANA Council for Computer Applications in Nursing (CCAN), the National League for Nursing (NLN) Council for Nursing Informatics, the AMIA Nursing Informatics Working Group, and the Healthcare Information and Management Systems Society (HIMSS). The ANA CCAN was organized in 1986 and was combined with the Council for Nursing Administration in 1994 to become the Council for Nursing Service and Informatics. This council has been renamed the Council for Nursing Systems and Administration. The NLN Council for Nursing Informatics was formed in 1987 and had 389 members in 1994. The ANA serves the interests of nurses in practice and administration, while the NLN is more oriented to nurses in education and research. The AMIA Nursing Informatics Working Group was formed in 1982 and had 229 members in 1994. Each of these organizations believes that information and technology should be diffused throughout the organization. CCAN and Council for Nursing Informatics present the latest in technology during the biennial meetings of the ANA and the NLN. The ANA has software exchange sessions in which software developers can demonstrate their wares to those attending the convention. The Nursing Informatics Working Group of AMIA promotes nursing informatics during the AMIA fall and spring meetings. The fall meeting has come to be called the Symposium for Computer Applications in Medical Care. The International Medical Informatics Association has had an international meeting every 3 years since 1974. This meeting, called MEDINFO, provides an opportunity to learn about informatics and technology in other countries and to meet and network with other informaticists. MEDINFO will take place again in 1998. Nurses who are new to informatics are encouraged to attend these meetings to learn about the latest technologies and to network with others in the field. All of these organizations have their own publications, but the official

Table 8-1 Comparison of annual dues charged by nursing/informatics organizations

American Nurses Association	$297.00
National League for Nursing	$110.00
American Medical Informatics Association	$175.00
Healthcare Information and Management Systems Society	$105.00

journal of nursing informatics is *Computers in Nursing,* which has been published since 1984. Another useful journal is *Healthcare Informatics.*

The HIMSS meeting is the largest and provides an opportunity to hear from informatics experts in all professions and fields such as medical, nursing, engineering, and computer science. It also has the largest vendor display of any of the meetings mentioned. Table 8-1 provides a comparison of the dues charged by these organizations.

TITLES, ROLES, AND CHARACTERISTICS OF THE NURSE INFORMATICIST

There are titles, roles, and personal characteristics that describe the nurse informaticist. Many nurses working in this field have created their own positions, titles, and job descriptions as the informatics role in nursing has evolved.

Some of the position titles include consultant in nursing, systems analyst, systems nurse, project manager, systems coordinator, nurse analyst, nursing informatics coordinator, nursing information specialist, and director of informatics. The position title often depends on whether the nurse informaticist is working for nursing, information services, or a vendor.

New roles are evolving for informaticists; hospitals are hiring nurse consultants to help in the design and implementation of hospital and nursing information systems. Nurse educators are using computers to manage the educational environment and to develop computer-assisted instruction. Vendors are hiring nurses to develop applications that will be useful for patient care and to market these products to the health care industry. Nurses are needed to develop theory and methods of inquiry, collaborate in the development of manual and computerized information systems, and to teach nurses, nursing students, and others about the effective and ethical uses of information technology in nursing practice. Consultation with administrators, nurse practitioners, educators, researchers, and vendors as well as collaboration with other health informatics specialists and professional groups is important. Roles for the nursing informaticist can involve all phases of the life cycle of patient care information systems: design, development, selection, testing, implementation, user education and support, system maintenance, evaluation, and enhancement.

Personal characteristics of the nursing informaticist include flexibility, humor, high tolerance for meticulous work, computer literacy, knowledge of hardware, software, and database management, and good verbal, written, and communication skills. He or she must also be intelligent, inquisitive, diplomatic, eager to learn, and able to balance technology with human needs. Informaticists are energetic, creative self-starters. Diplomacy is a critical characteristic for the building of bridges and coalitions.

WHAT DO NURSE INFORMATICISTS DO?

Nursing informatics is the management of patient care–related systems, but nurses in administration, education, and research working in diverse fields may also be informaticists if what they do involves information handling, communication, and transformation rather than patient care, administration, education, or research (*The Scope,* 1994, p. 7). The box below lists some of the tasks found in the job descriptions of nurse informaticists.

In addition, the informatics nurse specialist must be able to (a) analyze and evaluate information requirements; (b) design and implement applications to solve patient care problems; (c) determine the appropriateness, effectiveness, and impact of the technology for the situa-

SOME RESPONSIBILITIES OF THE NURSE INFORMATICIST

- Systems analysis and design (reengineering if necessary)
- Development of data dictionaries and naming conventions
- Evaluation and testing of applications for patient care
- Configuration of hardware and software
- Translating the language of nursing to engineers and system designers and vice versa
- Using applications software and computer networks
- Installing and maintaining hardware and software
- Programming in one or more computer languages
- Skill in integrating two or more computer systems
- Coordinating projects of various sizes involving diverse team members

tion; and (d) analyze ethical issues concerned with safety and privacy.

Nurses in practice

Nurse informaticists are concerned with information management for all roles in nursing, but are particularly concerned with the information and technology in support of patient care. Nurse-users of information collect data as part of their patient care activities, interpret it, and make decisions based on their interpretations. Nurses in practice deliver and manage patient care through continuous communication with patients, families, other professionals, and staff. They add observations to the patient record to communicate with other health care providers. They monitor instruments that provide current information about patients. They perform tests and review the results of tests performed by others. All of these are examples of giving and receiving data, information, and knowledge.

According to McAlindon (1995), as nurses advance from novice to expert practitioner, interpretations of the data become intuitive and automatic, based on previous experience. When the information gained from previously cared for patients is combined or synthesized so that new interrelationships are identified, nurses gain new knowledge. At this point they begin to think of other uses of data and information for improving patient care.

The progression from data to information to knowledge occurs quickly in practice as data are interpreted and compared with previous information about the patient to provide knowledge. Much of this value is lost, however, because the data are not stored where others might retrieve and use them to synthesize new knowledge. It is the role of the nurse informaticist to examine what it is that nurses do in the care of patients from a technology perspective and to find ways to improve this process. An informaticist can help with the process of restructuring the health care delivery system because of the ability to collect, aggregate, organize, and re-present information in a way that is useful. For example, as shown in Fig. 8-1 the nurse informaticist and nursing staff will review the components of work on the left of the chart, filter the data through the questions in the center column, and make the decisions found in the right column. If client requirements are duplicated, eliminate them. If they are necessary (required), decide whether they should be modified, automated, or continued as is. This type of exercise will serve as a needs analysis for designing a system that will assist with data and information capture and communication.

Once the need or problem is identified, the informaticist will proceed to help with systems design. What is the system to do? Who will enter the data? Who will use the data? What will it look like? Where will it be stored? Is the system built to stand alone or to be networked or integrated with other systems? Does the information remain in the hospital or extend beyond it? Once the design is completed the informaticist will coordinate the building of the database, the testing processes, the choice and placement of the hardware devices, education of the staff, and implementation. Following implementation, staff support and issue resolution are essential for continued system success.

Working with others

Nurse administrators use information technology for quality management, personnel files, communication networks, budgeting and payroll, summary reports, and forecasting and planning. Nurse informaticists provide assistance in the choice of systems (hardware and software), as well as education, installation, and support.

Informaticists help *nurse educators* integrate information technology into the curriculum. For instance, interactive video assignments may be used to augment other types of instruction. Educators need to understand and teach the aspects of information science so that students will understand that they must look at what they do and try to find more effective and efficient ways of using information technology to improve patient outcomes. Students also need to learn how to use computers for bibliographic retrieval, word processing, database management, and spreadsheets.

An informaticist might assist the *nurse researcher* in the selection and purchase of hardware and software for bibliographic retrieval, statistical analysis, and word processing. In addition, informatics researchers are needed to (a) build and analyze databases of clinical information; (b) determine how nurses use data, information, and knowledge to provide patient care; (c) develop and test patient care decision support systems; (d) develop nurse workstations to provide patient care information linked to an integrated system; and (e) evaluate the effect of information systems on patient care.

WHAT CHALLENGES DO NURSE INFORMATICISTS FACE?

As professionals, nurse informaticists have an obligation to keep abreast of evolving patient care practice and information technologies. This is not easy because the amount

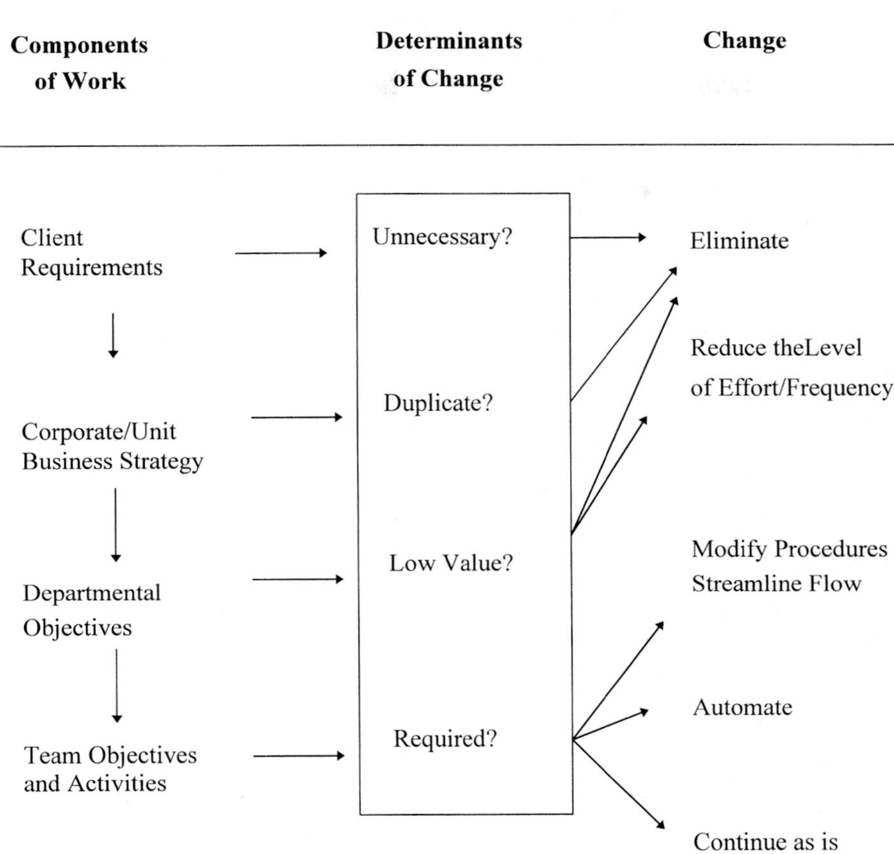

Fig. 8–1. Analysis of current work in preparation for automation.

of health care information available doubles every 2 years and hardware and software applications are outdated by the time they are purchased. Specialization within the field of informatics is necessary because development experts, installation experts, hardware and software experts, and reengineering experts will be needed.

Credentialing may become important as informatics gains recognition as a specialty in nursing. However, there are many nurses working with information and technology who are self-taught from the early days of computers. They may have degrees in computer science or engineering. If they do not have a bachelor's or a master's degree in nursing they are currently not qualified to take the ANA credentialing exam to become certified informatics nurses. Will this result in a "closed shop" of a chosen few? How valuable will certification be if many of the "experts" are excluded?

As departmental barriers in health care are disappearing, health care providers are contributing to a single patient chart. Many health care providers in an institution are involved in patient care, while nurse informaticists work with personnel in all other departments. Because their work crosses interdepartmental boundaries, many institutions are moving these nurses to the information services department. This provides the advantage of having experienced nurses who know what nurses need communicate with programmers so that usable programs will be written for all to use. It also presents the disadvantage of the informaticist being perceived by the nursing staff as "one of them" instead of "one of us." In addition, it becomes difficult to stay in touch with what is happening in the nursing department and the latest developments in patient care.

As the continuum of care moves to the community

(homes, clinics, streets, churches) the nurse's worksite also moves. Patient care information will be necessary in these environments. The informaticist will have to be prepared to support nurses and other health care providers in these settings.

Privacy, security, and confidentiality are important issues for the profession and the public. The question of protecting the public while granting access to information is being discussed, regulated, and challenged. Informaticists will have to understand and defend both sides of the issue.

Educators, administrators, and researchers must be aware of the latest technologies as they are preparing those entering the profession. This becomes a challenge for the informaticists working in these settings because these professionals must be prepared in time to teach students. Another difficulty occurs when students are in clinical settings with different information systems. Instructors and students need to be kept informed in these situations so that patient care is not compromised.

Informatics is the newest specialty in nursing and nurse informaticists have unlimited opportunities in health care as managers of information and technology. As roles and opportunities emerge, the challenge for the profession is to assist others to provide the care that gives life, health, and death their meanings in a technological organization that strives for efficiency and cost-effectiveness. Can we do it? We think so!

If you are an expert nurse who enjoys working with others, and you have a vision beyond "how we've always done it," and an insatiable curiosity about how and when and why not, and the patience to design and build and test and teach and support again and again, and you are flexible, fun, energetic, communicative, eager and bright —you too can be a nurse informaticist!

REFERENCES

Graves, J.R., & Corcoran, S. (1989). The study of nursing informatics. *Image 21*(4), 227-231.

Hannah, K.J., Ball, M.J., & Edwards, M.J. (Eds.). (1994). *Introduction to nursing informatics.* New York: Springer Verlag.

McAlindon, M.N. (1995). In Yoder-Wise, P. (Ed.). *Leading and managing in nursing* (pp. 227-249). St. Louis: Mosby.

Peterson, H.E., & Gerden-Jelger, U. (1988). *Preparing nurses for using information systems: Recommended informatics competencies.* New York: National League for Nursing.

Standards of practice for nursing informatics. (1995). Washington, DC: American Nurses Publishing.

The scope of practice for nursing informatics. (1994). Washington, DC: American Nurses Publishing.

International nursing leaders past and present

VERNA HUFFMAN SPLANE, RICHARD SPLANE

This chapter is about international nursing leaders that we either encountered or learned about as we proceeded with a study on a particular type of nursing leadership—that associated with the position of chief nursing officers (CNOs) in national ministries of health (Splane & Splane, 1994). We set out in 1985 to explore what we were to call the CNO Movement and, to gather the data for our joint study, we traveled to more than 50 countries and interviewed over 90 CNOs, past and present, as well as other nursing leaders and authorities in the associated human services.

Although the study started out as an inquiry about present-day nursing leaders, our growing fascination with the present-day CNO Movement in its entirety caused us to search out its origins and to discover the preconditions to its development. The hunt for the roots of the CNO Movement further served to arouse our interest not only about nursing leaders whose working lives were wholly or largely within their native land, but increasingly about those whose careers had led them to serve internationally and, in most instances, to establish international linkages and networks that were to be of great importance to their own countries and to nursing throughout the world. Our interest then extended from asking *who* the influential international nurses were, to enquiring about the challenges they faced and how, in meeting them, their influence extended in many directions and to many entities including the CNO Movement.

In reflecting on our experiences and our associated studies and enquiries we were able to link international nursing with identifiable movements, organizations, influences, and individuals that were connected with international nursing leadership in two ways: exemplifying it in at least some part of their endeavors and bringing it into being in the pursuit of their health-related objectives. Principally among them were the Nightingale influence, the International Council of Nurses (ICN), the International Red Cross, the World Health Organization (WHO), and the CNO Movement. This chapter is largely a discussion of these entities with special attention directed to nursing leadership that would have bearing on public policy as it relates to health and to the socioeconomic and political milieu that sets the parameters of health policy and thus of the work of many of those engaged in the health field.

The question of how deeply into history our enquiries should take us led to a decision to reach back to at least as far as what Bullough, Bullough, and Stanton (1990) have called "the Nightingale Era," 1850 to 1910.

THE NIGHTINGALE INFLUENCE ON INTERNATIONAL NURSING LEADERS

In exploring the story of the Nightingale influence on international nursing and on the CNO Movement we must begin in 1854 when the telegraphed reports to the *London Times* on the scandalous treatment of the wounded and dying in the Crimea and in the Scutari barracks brought Florence Nightingale from genteel obscurity onto the world stage, where her Crimean and post-Crimean achievements would keep her throughout her lifetime.

Florence Nightingale's standing as an international nursing leader is unchallengeable, even if her self-imposed immobility kept her in one part of the world for half of her unceasingly creative career. Her influence during that part of her life was largely based on what she wrote, to whom she wrote, and to whom she granted audience. Nonetheless, the breadth of her contacts and networks was global. Many were within the British Empire, then at its zenith, and a goodly number centered on India, the jewel in the imperial crown, to which no Viceroy departed London without consulting Miss Nightingale (Strachey, 1966). Her network spread beyond the Empire, however, reaching parts of the Orient, all of Europe, the

Middle East, Australasia, and the Americas, where she was greatly revered, sometimes to the point of idolatry. In addition, of some importance in the present context was Florence Nightingale's practice of identifying leadership potential in young nurses and dispatching them, somewhat imperiously at times, to numerous locations where leadership was acutely needed.

To ask what challenges Florence Nightingale faced and what she did about them is to call for yet another two-volume biography. In the simplest terms, she was challenged by every contemporary obstacle to human health and well-being, and what she did was attack them systematically and unrelentingly, believing that "never to know that you are beaten is the way to victory" (Cook, 1913). Poor and nonexistent nursing were obstacles to human well-being and Nightingale was convinced she had a mission to confront these obstacles and overcome them, and from that conviction emerged the genesis of modern nursing. Nursing, however, was not her central interest, nor was a voluntary hospital, like St. Thomas', representative of the means she employed to promote her main objectives. Described as "nursing's most astute political operator" (Cox, 1989, p. 18), she focused rather on legislatures and the public service. More specifically, she channeled her energies and skills toward the British Parliament and on those who would carry out the laws it enacted: the civil and military bureaucracy. It was thus mainly to public policy that she looked for the attainment of her broad range of social goals.

Table 9-1 Presidents of the International Council of Nurses

Name	Country	Years
Ethel Gordon Bedford Fenwick	United Kingdom	1900-1904
Susan McGahey	Australia	1904-1909
Agnes Karll	Germany	1909-1912
Annie Goodrich	United States	1912-1915
Henny Tscherning	Denmark	1915-1922
Sophie Mannerheim	Finland	1922-1925
Nina Gage	China	1925-1929
Leonie Chaptal	France	1929-1933
Alicia Lloyd Still	United Kingdom	1933-1937
Effie Taylor	United States	1937-1947
Gerda Hojer	Sweden	1947-1953
Marie Bihet	Belgium	1953-1957
Agnes Ohlson	United States	1957-1961
Alice Clamageran	France	1961-1965
Alice Girard	Canada	1965-1969
Margarethe Kruse	Denmark	1969-1973
Dorothy Cornelius	United States	1973-1977
Olive Anstey	Australia	1977-1981
E. Muringo Kiereini	Kenya	1981-1985
Nelly Garzon	Colombia	1985-1989
Mo Im Kim	Korea	1989-1993
Margretta Styles	United States	1993-1997

From Annual Reports, ICN.

THE INTERNATIONAL COUNCIL OF NURSES AND INTERNATIONAL NURSING LEADERS

The ICN stands first in any assessment of international nursing leadership. It was founded in 1899 by a small group of international nursing leaders. Among them were Ethel Bedford Fenwick of Great Britain, Lavinia Lloyd Dock of the United States, Agnes Karll of Germany, Charlotte Gordon Norrie of Denmark, Mary Agnes Snively of Canada, and Grace Neill of New Zealand. Each played historically important roles in nursing in their own countries, but it is the part they played in the birth and early nurture of the ICN that doubly ensures their place in nursing history.

The ICN justifiably describes itself as the first international professional organization to be established in the health field. It could take no less pride in surviving through the early decades of the 20th century, through the depression of the 1930s, and through a second world war. Its membership has consisted of national nursing organizations and, by requiring diverse nursing organizations in a given country to form a single unified national association, ICN has greatly strengthened organized nursing. The number of national nursing organizations grew from 7 in 1910 and 43 in 1940, to 112 in 1995. In almost all respects, including that of international nursing leadership, ICN and the national organizations were interdependent. It was from the national organizations that ICN's leadership was inevitably drawn; it was the ICN that provided international leadership challenges and opportunities.

The most visible and important leadership positions are those of the president and executive director of the ICN whose names and dates of service are presented in Tables 9-1 and 9-2. Between 1900 and 1995, there were 22 presidents who served 4-year terms. Over the same span of 95 years ICN was served by 12 executive directors. The first was Lavinia Dock, who carried the role as a volunteer; the second was Christiane Reimann of Denmark, who bequeathed from her estate the resources for the prestigious award in her name given quadrennially to a nursing leader who has made a pre-eminent contribution to global health and nursing.

Table 9-2 Executive directors of the International Council of Nurses*

Name	Country	Years
Lavinia Dock	United States	1900-1902
Christianne Reimann	Denmark	1922-1934
Anna Schwarzenberg	Austria	1934-1947
Daisy Bridges	United Kingdom	1948-1961
Helen Nussbaum	Switzerland	1961-1967
Sheila Quinn	United Kingdom	1967-1970
Adele Herwitz	United States	1970-1976
Barbara Fawkes	United Kingdom	1977-1978
Winnifred Logan	United Kingdom	1979-1981
Constance Holleran	United States	1981-1995
Judith Aulton	Canada	1996-

**Note.* The title of executive director has changed a number of times and has included executive secretary and general secretary as well as executive director.
From Annual Reports, ICN.

Constance Holleran of the United States was the Executive Director from 1981–1995, and has provided exceptionally creative leadership through a turbulent period. She brought to the position a wealth of experience in working with governments and a clear understanding of the vital importance of a collaborative relationship between nursing organizations and governments at every level. Accordingly, she has given a high priority to working closely with WHO, with which ICN enjoys consultative status. During the annual meetings of the World Health Assembly (WHA), Constance Holleran and her staff honor the CNOs and other nursing leaders who have been included in their respective country's official delegation.

The ICN brings nurses to the international stage in numerous ways including committees, commissions, task forces, and consultancies. Of special note is the policy-making body, the Council of National Representatives (CNR), which is composed of presidents of the national nurses associations, and the Professional Services Committee, which recommends direction on professional issues referred to it by the board of directors.

The quadrennial election of the board of directors gives national associations—the ultimate power base of the CNR—the opportunity and responsibility to nominate and elect nursing leaders who have made strong contributions in their own countries and who often have had significant international experience. With the election of Trevor Clay of the United Kingdom as a Vice President of the board in 1981 the precedent was established for the election of male nurses to the board. His outstanding leadership and, later, that of the second male nurse, Robert Tiffany, also from the United Kingdom, added a valued dimension to the deliberations of the Board.[a] With the election of Maximo Gonzales Jurado of Spain as a vice president at the Madrid Congress in 1993, a pattern of male nursing leaders participating at the highest level in the affairs of ICN seemed firmly established.

Individual nurses within the national nursing organizations in membership in the ICN number more than 1.5 million. They are encouraged to recognize that they are part of nursing worldwide and can aspire to become international nursing leaders or, more modestly but no less vitally, play a part in the governance of their global association. Large numbers of nurses, often exceeding 10,000, attend the Council's quadrennial congresses, where existing and potential international nursing leaders are able to experience the strength of their global association and forge international networks.

THE RED CROSS AND INTERNATIONAL NURSING LEADERS

Among the countless benefits that have flowed from the International Red Cross are the development of high standards of nursing and nursing leadership (Yule, 1983). The ideas and convictions that brought the Red Cross into existence in the 1860s were those of Swiss author, Henry Dunant, who credited Florence Nightingale with inspiring his endeavors. However, it was the battlefield experiences of the American Civil War and of the Franco-Prussian War of 1870-1871 that brought to the forefront most emphatically the need for professional nursing training. In response, the Red Cross played the leadership role in the movement to establish nursing training schools of high standards.

By World War I (1914-1918), nurses from Red Cross nursing schools provided a corps of nurses, on both sides of the conflict, whose record as qualified nurses and trainers of volunteer auxiliaries was beyond praise. It served to guarantee nurses a significant role in the historic Red Cross Conference held in Cannes, France in 1919. Nursing was superbly represented at the Conference by nursing leaders from France, Italy, Great Britain, and the United States. The American nurses were Carrie Hall, who had been the Chief Nurse of the American Red Cross, Julia Stimson, Director of the Army Nurse Corps,

[a]The death of these two outstanding international nursing leaders, Robert Tiffany in 1993 and Trevor Clay in 1994, constituted a loss that extended beyond national and professional boundaries.

Table 9-3 Nursing directors/advisers, League of Red Cross Societies, 1919-1986

Name	Country	Years
Alice Louise Florence Fitzgerald	United States	1919-1921
Katherine Olmstead	United States	1921-1926
Maynard Linden Carter	Great Britain	1927-1938
Yvonne Hentsch	Switzerland	1939-1971
Barbara Yule	Great Britain	1971-1975
Margaret Robinson	Great Britain	1975-1986

and Lillian Wald, renowned for her forthright stands on controversial social issues, her contributions as a leader in public health nursing, and founder of the Henry Street Settlement and the Visiting Nurse Service of New York.

The League of Red Cross Societies (LORCS) was the major outcome of the conference, bringing together in membership the national Red Cross Societies of the world. A second important outcome was the establishment in LORCS of a nursing division, with Alice Louise Fitzgerald of the United States as its first director.

The League, based in Geneva, undertook a range of health and social service endeavors, one of which was to extend the promotion of the establishment of Red Cross schools of nursing with high standards of nursing education that became models for other schools to emulate.

The nursing component in LORCS was greatly strengthened by a Nursing Advisory Committee composed of the CNOs (directors, advisers) of the national Red Cross Societies who met on a regular basis with the international director of nursing.

The most dramatic nursing initiative of LORCS was the sponsoring and support of Bedford College from its founding in 1921 to 1934. This postbasic school for nursing education in public health, administration, and teaching, centrally based in London, brought nurses from every continent for a year's training to prepare them for leadership positions in their own countries. Over the whole period of its operation—1921 to 1939—Bedford College served some 400 students from 46 countries. The graduates of the program formed an association—the Old Internationals—a networking group that underlined the importance of the program in promoting formal and informal linkages for the sharing of ideas, for international friendship and understanding, and for exchanging visits to each other's national programs.

Table 9-3 lists the directors/advisers of nursing of the LORCS from 1919 to 1986. Their contributions to the range of nursing endeavors to which they provided leadership merits separate and extended examination supplementing the study by Barbara Yule (1983) on the impact of Red Cross nursing on health care written in 1983.

THE WORLD HEALTH ORGANIZATION AND INTERNATIONAL NURSING LEADERS

The establishment of WHO as one of the United Nation's major specialized agencies was of monumental importance to nursing. WHO's mandate, as formulated in 1948, was to promote the attainment of the highest possible level of health by all peoples, with health defined as "a state of complete physical, mental and social well-being and not merely the absence of disease or infirmity" (WHO, 1948, p. 4). Those guidelines were in harmony with the expressed ideals of nursing, and nurses welcomed the advent of the new international body.

A variety of factors contributed to a good beginning for nursing in the life of WHO:

- The high status of nursing because of the praiseworthy contributions it had made in World War II and in rehabilitation agencies in the following years
- The strong interest and support evinced in the formation of the organization by nursing leaders, two of whom, Effie Taylor and Virginia Arnold, were able to influence the formulation of its policies while it was still in its interim stage (before it had moved from New York to its permanent home in Geneva)
- The American delegation to the first WHA of WHO had within it Lucile Petry Leone who, as the first woman and first nurse to address the WHA, made the case for the immediate appointment of senior nurses to the nascent WHO Secretariat (Splane & Splane, 1994)
- The availability of highly qualified nurses to fill the position of chief nurse in the Geneva Headquarters; to head the nursing programs in the six regional offices located in Washington, D.C., Copenhagen, Alexandria, Brazzaville, New Delhi, and Manila, and to provide nurses for subregional and country appointments and expert consultancies throughout the Organization.

A full account of the achievements of the nurses in WHO in both the developed and developing world during that initial period would support the view that in the first quarter century after the founding of WHO, nursing throughout the world, and especially in the developing world, was transformed and that WHO played the major role in that remarkable transformation. Contributing to the strong performance of nursing within WHO was the support nursing was given to convene five high-profile expert committees together with a prestigious multidisci-

Table 9-4 Senior nurses in the World Health Organization Headquarters, Geneva

Name	Country	Years
Olive Baggallay, Chief Nurse	United Kingdom	1949-1954
Lyle Creelman, Nursing Consultant	Canada	1949-1954
Lyle Creelman, Chief Nurse	Canada	1954-1968
Lilian Turnbull, Chief Nurse	Canada	1968-1975
Amelia Maglacas, Chief Scientist for Nursing (*de facto* Chief Nurse)	Philippines	1976-1989
Miriam Hirschfeld, Chief Scientist for Nursing (*de facto* Chief Nurse)	Israel	1989-

plinary meeting on nursing within the WHA in 1957. The reports of the expert committees of those early years provided authoritative guidelines for nursing: The first and second reports dealt largely with problems of nursing education, the third largely with nursing administration, the fourth with public health, the fifth again with education—basic, postbasic, postgraduate, and continuing—relating its analysis to quality in nursing and nursing research (Splane & Splane, 1994).

Much of the credit for the strong performance of WHO nursing can be attributed to the quality of leadership provided by its first three CNOs, listed with their successors in Table 9-4. The exemplary record of the work they directed from the headquarters nursing unit makes it difficult to account for the damaging blow to the nursing program that occurred in 1973—the elimination of the CNO position in WHO's Geneva headquarters and the relegation of the nursing unit into the functional programs of the Secretariat (Splane & Splane, 1994).

Progress in gradually rebuilding the influence of nursing within WHO, despite the termination of the CNO position at WHO headquarters, is associated with the one new nursing position established at Geneva after the abolition of the unit. The position, ultimately designated as chief scientist for nursing, was established in 1976 and was held for 14 years by Amelia Mangay Maglacas, a nursing leader from the Philippines who brought extensive international experience in administration and research to the formidable task of renewal. She was assisted in this by the worldwide reaction of the nursing profession to the loss of the CNO position and by the advent of primary health care—the strategy proposed in 1978 in the historical Declaration of Alma Ata for the achievement of "health for all by the year 2000." Among the health professions it was nurses and their leaders who emerged on the world stage as the major group promoting the goals and implementing the practices of primary health care.

When this was finally recognized, Dr. Halfdan Mahler, the Director General of WHO, took a number of measures to rectify the damage of the 1973 decision and to promote leadership in nursing. In a paper, *Nurses lead the way*, published by WHO in 1985, he referred to nurses as "a powerhouse for change," and called for the "optimal use of nurses in program planning and evaluation and in senior management, policy development and decision making" (Mahler, 1986, pp. 28–29). He also gave support to another initiative proposed by Amelia Maglacas in concert with the regional nurse advisers, namely the founding of a Global Network of Collaborating Centers for International Nursing Development.

These nursing initiatives have been carried forward from 1989 with the appointment of Miriam Hirschfeld, an Austrian-born Israeli nursing leader with a strong background in nursing education and research. The scope for renewed nursing leadership in WHO headquarters was immeasurably enlarged in 1992 by the passage in the Forty-Fifth WHA Resolution, WHA 45.5, calling for the strengthening of nursing and midwifery worldwide (WHO, 1992). It provided for a global advisory group (GAG), advisory to the director general with Miriam Hirschfeld as Secretary. GAG is multidisciplinary, with the majority of its 12 members being outstanding international nursing leaders from different specialties and different countries. Among its members Hiroko Minami of Japan and Yvonne Moores of the United Kingdom have chaired the group's meetings, sharing attendance with Mo Im Kim of Korea, Muringo Kiereini of Kenya, Julia Plotnik of the United States, and Judith Shamian of Canada (WHO, 1993). In its advisory capacity to the director general, GAG provides one of the most encouraging aspects of world leadership for global health and nursing. With strong support from the group, Miriam Hirschfeld has been able, despite financial limitations, to carry out *inter alia* two significant events: in 1993, a WHO Study Group on *Nursing Beyond the Year 2000* (WHO, 1994), and in 1995, an Expert Committee on Nursing Practice (M.J. Hirschfeld, personal communication, 1995).

THE CHIEF NURSING OFFICER MOVEMENT AND INTERNATIONAL NURSING LEADERS

Although our study had CNOs in *national* settings at its core, it also revealed that the functions of the CNO extend beyond national borders. The CNO position, indeed, is described as the focal point in the ministry with respect to both "domestic and international nursing issues" and the incumbent CNO is identified as "representing the Ministry at regional and global meetings and conferences in which nursing issues are involved" (Splane & Splane, 1994, p. 27).

Scores of examples can be cited of CNOs who have become international nursing leaders. Some have already been mentioned: Grace Neill (CNO from 1895 to 1901), Lucile Petry Leone (CNO from 1948 to 1966), and Nita Barrow of Barbados (CNO in Jamaica from 1955 to 1964). Many others are noteworthy: Eli Magnussen (CNO in Denmark from 1950 to 1971), who carried senior consultancies for WHO (and could be seen as exemplifying the qualities of other early international leaders of the Nordic countries; Sophie Mannerheim, Venny Snellman, Ingrid Hamelin, and Toini Noussianen of Finland; Emmy Rapp, Kersten Nordendahl, and Majsa Andrell of Sweden); Kofoworola Pratt (CNO in Nigeria from 1965 to 1971) and Muringo Kiereini (CNO in Kenya from 1968 to 1985), two nurses whose influence has extended throughout Africa and beyond; Tehmina Adranvala (CNO in India from 1948 to 1966), who carried numerous international assignments and, as in the case of a number of CNOs, was a founding member and president of her country's nursing association; Rukhmini Charan Shrestha (CNO in Nepal from 1984 to 1991), who demonstrated what nursing leadership can achieve in a country with very limited resources; Clara Sovenji (CNO in Hungary since 1985), who provides exemplary nursing leadership in eastern Europe in ideologically turbulent times; Sophia Kyriakidou (CNO in Cyprus since 1994), who has brought to international assignments her experience in the cultural and political milieu of the Eastern Mediterranean; Faye Abdellah (CNO in the United States from 1970 to 1989), whose leadership in developing the field of nursing research gave an added dimension to her work for WHO and especially for its work in the Americas; and Julia Plotnik (CNO in the United States since 1992), whose leadership qualities have been brought to bear on the important work of WHO's Global Advisory Group on Nursing and on Midwifery. Meriting special mention are the succession of CNOs in the United Kingdom from 1941 to the present, all of whom represented their country in numerous international undertakings including the WHA of WHO in almost every year since 1948. The more recent examples are Anne Poole (CNO from 1981 to 1992), organizer and chair of the meeting of Commonwealth Chief Nursing Officers and Professional Associations in Malta in 1992, and Yvonne Moores (CNO since 1992), serving in 1994 as chair of WHO's Global Advisory Group.

Table 9-5 Chief nursing officers serving on the board of the International Council of Nurses

Name	Country	Years
Mary Lambie	New Zealand	1947-1951
Tehmina Adranvala	India	1961-1965
Majsa Andrell	Sweden	1961-1965
Kofoworola Pratt	Nigeria	1965-1969
Jadwiga Izycka	Poland	1969-1977
Docia Kissieh	Ghana	1973-1977
Verna Huffman Splane	Canada	1973-1981
Muringo Kiereini[a]	Kenya	1977-1985
Annanna Cherian	India	1977-1981
Jean Grayson	Trinidad & Tobago	1985-1993
Merel Hansen	Jamaica	1987-1993

[a]President 1981-1985.

Some of those mentioned above are included in the list of CNOs who are serving or have served on ICN's board of directors, as shown in Table 9-5.

COLLABORATIVE WORK OF INTERNATIONAL NURSING LEADERS

Although the foregoing set out to discuss international nursing leadership under discrete headings, it is apparent that the parameters were permeable and that collaboration has been common among nursing leaders from all the identified areas. Many additional examples could be cited of CNOs working for a given objective with nursing leaders from WHO and ICN. Perhaps the most dramatic was the collaboration that brought about the passage of the WHO Resolution 45.5 of the WHA in 1992. Destined to greatly strengthen the capacity of Miriam Hirschfeld, the WHO's *de facto* CNO, and the Geneva nursing unit, it was achieved as a result of a key meeting of Constance Holleran with WHO's Executive Committee (Holleran, 1992), the work of many CNOs in securing support for the resolution among the member countries, and the crucial intervention in the concluding session debating the WHA resolution by the highly experienced CNO from the United Kingdom, Dame Anne Poole (Splane & Splane, 1994).

This example, selected from many, of the collaboration of international nursing leaders, indicates that the nursing profession is carrying forward, toward the end of the

20th century, the legacy of strong and effective commitment to the fields of health and nursing handed down by the founders of ICN at the end of the last century.

OTHER AREAS OF NURSING LEADERSHIP

The approach to international nursing leadership taken in this chapter has remained largely within the sociopolitical channel outlined at the outset. That the field of international nursing and the corps of international nursing leaders extends far more broadly is acknowledged. International nursing leaders come from national and subnational nursing associations, from universities, institutes, WHO collaborating centers, nursing associations organized along the lines of religious faith, and other types of professional groupings, including the Sigma Theta Tau International Honour Society of Nursing. Their work extends to international conferences, workshops, bilateral and multilateral undertakings, and specialist nursing groups. They are at the foreground as well in other undertakings that clearly involve public policy: the unending and vital question of the regulation of nurses and the complex issues of defining and monitoring nursing standards to deal with the increasing cross-border mobility of nurses.

A CLOSING COMMENT

It is encouraging to know that international nursing leadership has flourished to the point that a single chapter can touch on only one of its numerous aspects.

REFERENCES

Bullough, V., Bullough, B., & Stanton, M. (Eds). (1990). *Florence Nightingale and her era: A collection of new scholarship.* New York: Garland.

Cook, E. (1913). *The life of Florence Nightingale* (Vols. I & II). London: MacMillan.

Cox, C. (1989). *Forging nursing's future: A socio-political perspective.* Paper presented at the 19th Quadrennial Congress of the International Council of Nurses, Seoul, South Korea, 1989, (p. 18). Geneva: International Council of Nurses.

Holleran, C. (1992). ICN Statement to the WHO Executive Board 22 January 1992. *International Nursing Review, 39, 2, 36.* Geneva: International Council of Nurses.

Mahler, H. (1985, July). Nurses lead the way. *World Health.* (pp. 28–29). Geneva: World Health Organization.

Splane, R.B., & Splane, V.H. (1994). *Chief nursing officers in national ministries of health: Focal points for nursing leadership* (pp. 27-28, 119-139). San Francisco: University of California, San Francisco.

Strachey, L. (1966). *Eminent Victorians.* London: Harcourt Brace Jovanovich.

World Health Organization. (1948). *Official document 13. First Word Health Assembly.* Geneva: Author.

World Health Organization. (1992). *Resolution WHA 45.5: Strengthening nursing and midwifery in support of strategies for health for all.* Geneva: Author.

World Health Organization. (1993). *Report of the second meeting, Geneva 8 to 10, November 1993. Global Advisory Group on Nursing and Midwifery.* Geneva: Author.

World Health Organization. (1994). Nursing beyond the year 2000. *Report of WHO Study Group.* Geneva: Author.

Yule, B.M.G. (1983). *Red Cross nursing: Impact on health care* (pp. 1-123). Geneva: International Red Cross.

Section Two

CHANGING INFORMATION

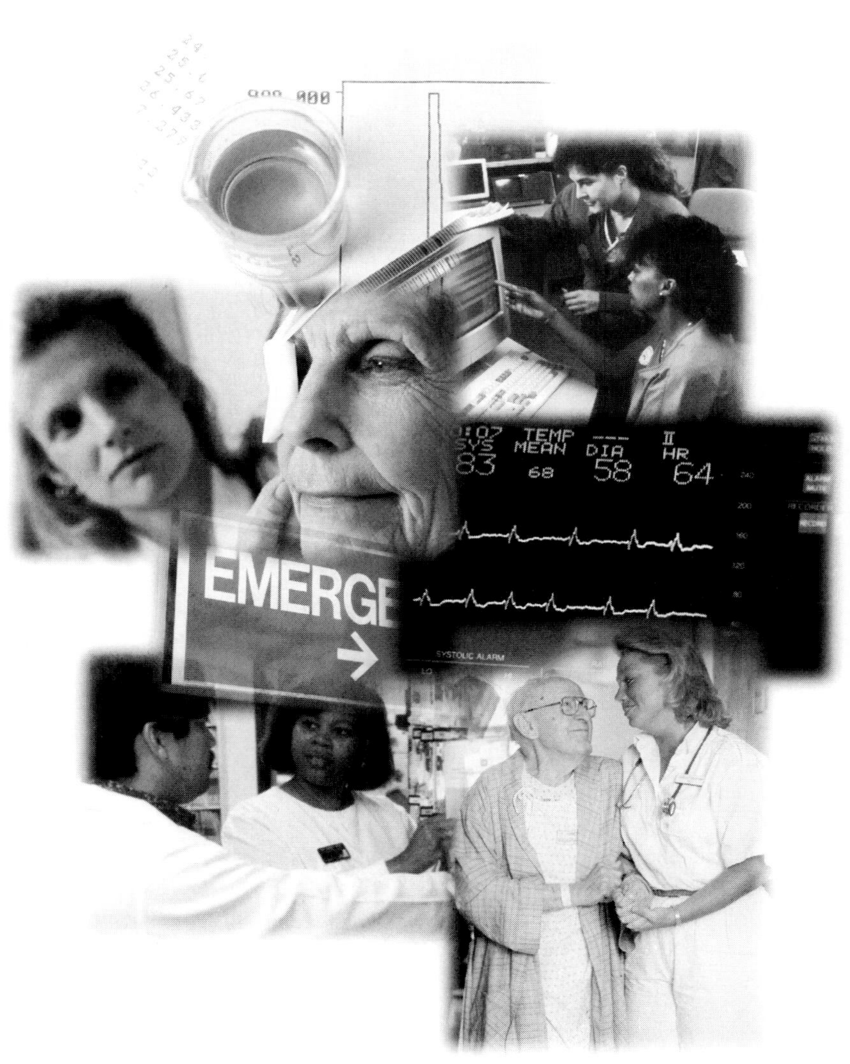

Data, information, knowledge

JOANNE COMI McCLOSKEY, HELEN KENNEDY GRACE

In order for nursing to advance as a scientific discipline we must generate data about patient encounters and the various systems of health care delivery. These data can then be organized in ways that yield information, which can then be explored, and tested either to confirm what we know or to reveal new knowledge. The links between practice, research, and theory are data links, and our science is only as good as our data and what we do with it. This section explores some of the new advances in this area of information management.

The first chapter in this section is a well-reasoned and thought-provoking debate about the relationships among nursing theory, nursing research, and nursing practice. After defining the terms, Blegen and Tripp-Reimer discuss the advantages and disadvantages of three positions. First, nursing theory, research, and practice should be kept as separate categories; second, the three categories should be connected; and third, the categories should be separate with bridges between them. They indicate their choice of the third position with middle range theory providing the connecting bridges. This position is now a real possibility due to the development of taxonomies of diagnoses, interventions, and outcomes, which provide the "skeletal framework for nursing knowledge." This very clear overview of the relationships among theory, research, and practice should provide good debate and discussion among all those interested in knowledge generation and use.

The first viewpoint chapter, by Henry and Costantino, provides a thorough overview of the challenges related to transforming nursing data into knowledge. The authors begin by addressing the question of why traditional automated nursing information systems have not fostered the development of nursing knowledge, citing the lack of standardized nursing vocabularies and classifications as a major handicap. They overview six classification systems and conclude that these systems are essential in order to transform our current record systems into ones that will foster the development of nursing knowledge. The role of informatics in fostering knowledge development in nursing is reviewed through the system design framework of the National Commission on Nursing Implementation Project. The framework's four types of information system processes (data acquisition, storage, transformation, and presentation) are reviewed with examples from the literature. This chapter illustrates the central role of the computer in building nursing science.

The key to nursing knowledge is good data about nursing practice. Nursing practice data are generated through a reasoning process usually referred to in nursing as the nursing process. In their chapter, Pesut, Herman, and Fowler propose an alternative to the nursing process called the OPT model of clinical reasoning (Outcome state, Present state, and Testing or comparing the present situation to the desirable outcome state). The juxtaposition of the current state with the desired state is, they assert, the essential element of clinical reasoning. Clinical reasoning in nursing is critical thinking embedded in practice. Clinical decision making is defined as the selection of interventions to achieve the desired outcome state. The authors argue that clinical reasoning that focuses on outcomes should replace clinical reasoning that focuses on problems. They say that nurses consider problems, solutions, and outcomes concurrently and that a new model is needed to illustrate this. The authors wish to stimulate debate and invite your comments and dialogue. This is a controversial but timely proposal that warrants consideration and discussion.

Health care providers generate a good deal of data that must be organized and managed in order to provide useful information. A major tool for managing data is benchmarking, which is explained in the chapter by Smeltzer, Leighty, and Williams-Brinkley. Benchmarking is the continuous process of comparing measures of services and practices against excellent competitors in order to improve practice in the organization. The authors discuss three types of benchmarking: internal, competitive, and functional. They also overview the four phases of the benchmarking process: planning, analysis, integration, and action. While performance measures (e.g., length of stay, total, expense, number of patient days) are the indicators that most hospitals typically benchmark against other hospitals, these authors believe that hospitals also need to benchmark against health maintenance organizations to compare patient care processes (e.g., treatments and medications administered, surgeries performed, and room maintenance services) as well as performance indicators. Process benchmarking can be very valuable in indicating the strategies that will achieve superior performance. As more regional and national databases become available, the tool of benchmarking will be used increasingly by managers to make decisions about cost and quality changes in their organizations. This chapter is a good overview of how the use of data can help organizations to improve their services continually.

More and more, communication of data and information is via the Internet. The chapter by Sparks overviews the Internet and some of the issues related to its use in nursing. Use of the Internet began with the U.S. military but has expanded rapidly to include research and education institutions and commercial organizations as well as individual subscribers. While usage is expanding rapidly, there are compatibility problems and a lack of standardization that make it difficult and costly to use. Sparks says that the nursing profession currently makes little use of the Internet and generally lacks appreciation of its benefits and applicability to the work of nursing. While more nurses are joining LISTSERVs, few post messages regularly. According to Sparks there is a tremendous need for research in telenursing and a need for more nurses prepared to teach others about the Internet. She makes a good case that this is an opportune time for more standardization of technical features and functions. Standardization would help new users overcome the effort required to become Internet literate. This chapter is an excellent overview of a tool that is changing the way information is shared and one that has great potential for nursing education and care delivery.

Nursing care delivery should be enhanced based on new knowledge discovered through research, but is it? The chapter by Titler examines research utilization, or the process of using research findings as a basis for practice. Titler begins her chapter with a brief history of research utilization. She overviews the steps of research utilization through a model that indicates when a problem needs research conduction versus the development of an intervention to change practice. Titler says that the conduct of research and research utilization are distinct yet complementary. Research is often not used by practitioners because of several barriers, which Titler discusses in four categories: organizational and professional, the nurses themselves, the nature of the innovation, and dissemination. In each category, strategies to overcome the barriers are discussed and then highlighted in a helpful table. Titler concludes her chapter with some suggestions on how to streamline research utilization activities. She believes that research utilization is a necessity for professional nursing practice, but for it to survive in the managed care environment it must be streamlined.

The international chapter of this section by Clark of England overviews the work by the International Council of Nursing to develop an International Classification for Nursing Practice. This is an effort to establish a common language about nursing practice that can be used worldwide in the areas of nursing diagnoses, interventions, and outcomes. Clark does an excellent job of overviewing the need that nurses around the globe share for a common language for data collection. While nurses in the United States were the first to recognize the need and to begin the work, there has been considerable work recently in Europe as well as in several other countries. Clark overviews the benefits for a worldwide nursing classification and discusses some of the limitations. More than anything, she stresses that we must value this kind of work. The challenges are enormous, she says, but the work is essential.

While nursing has made tremendous progress in the area of information management, we still have much work to do. Some of the challenges include better preparation of nurses with computer skills, the need to teach clinical decision-making skills in a more systematic way, the need for widespread use of standardized languages, and integration of nursing data in state and national databases. While we will continue to conduct and value single research studies that collect small samples of data, we must also begin to collect data in standardized forms on the computer for each patient encounter. These data can be aggregated across units and facilities and connected with other data to build large samples that can be used for sophisticated data analysis. Practitioners and researchers must work together to generate and analyze the data and then to improve practice based on what we learn. This is the computer age—let's be sure we are a part of it.

Nursing theory, nursing research, and nursing practice: Connected or separate?

MARY A. BLEGEN, TONI TRIPP-REIMER

Nursing knowledge is often discussed in three categories: practice knowledge, knowledge based in research or science, and theoretical knowledge. Dividing knowledge in this manner reflects and reinforces the idea and the actuality that the three categories of knowledge related to nursing are separate and distinct and are regarded as unrelated except that nursing claims each of them. Nursing scholars have acknowledged this separation in their calls to end it (Benoliel, 1977; Conant, 1967; Fawcett, 1978a; Fawcett & Downs, 1992; Jacobs & Huether, 1978; Walker, 1973).

Nursing practice is the "diagnosis and treatment of human responses to actual and potential health problems" (ANA, 1980). The knowledge nurses use while engaging in practice comes from many sources and is learned initially in the courses taken during undergraduate education. These courses are carefully selected from all disciplines—biophysical sciences, social sciences, humanities, and finally nursing science. The courses in nursing science present both knowledge based in other disciplines and knowledge generated by nurses. This nursing knowledge tends to be practical and is applied as soon as possible in a clinical setting. Nurse educators have worked diligently to present knowledge based in research and organized around a conceptual framework or nursing theory. Articles in nursing education encourage faculty to include nursing research and to use nursing theories. Again, these exhortations emphasize the existing separateness of practice, research, and theory.

Nursing research is the conduct of systematic studies to generate new knowledge or confirm existing knowledge. The fact that nursing research may not be informed by theory and is seldom applied in nursing practice has been lamented for some time. In the previous edition of this book, Weiler, Buckwalter, and Titler (1994) describe this state of affairs very well. They optimistically conclude, in agreement with other recent articles, that nurses are increasing their application of research in practice (Baessler et al., 1994; Coyle & Sokop, 1990; Pettengill, Gillies, & Clark, 1994). The idea of applying knowledge from research in practice implies the crossing of a boundary. This boundary is composed in part of difficulties finding, reading, understanding, and preparing the research for application. Another part of the boundary between research and practice is the different orientations of nurses who conduct research and those who care for patients directly. The orientation of nurse researchers leads them to increase the validity of the general knowledge produced by their studies by removing or controlling the influence of unique individual characteristics of each patient or subject and setting. Nurses oriented to practice must focus on those individual unique characteristics to provide care that truly meets each patient's needs. These different perspectives and tools continue to keep knowledge from research separate from knowledge used in practice until a nurse takes pieces of the knowledge from one arena and uses it in the other.

Nursing theory, on the other hand, is often portrayed as connected to neither practice nor research. Two reviews of research articles conducted to identify the nursing theory underpinning the research found that few of the studies were related to nursing theory. Silva (1986) found that 53 of the 62 research articles she reviewed were not tied to nursing theory. Moody et al. (1988) found that only 3% of clinical research articles actually tested nursing theory. Some of the inattention to theory-testing research comes from the researchers themselves; however, it is increasingly recognized that the older "grand" theories of nursing's recent past are not testable (Acton, Irvin, & Hopkins, 1991).

Many conceptual models emerged in the late 1960s to early 1980s as efforts to define the discipline and foster curricular reform. Although these models were historically essential in nursing's articulation of its identity, they evolved parallel to, rather than interwoven with, research (Blegen & Tripp-Reimer, 1994). These models were statements of nursing philosophy and ideology but did not present knowledge that could be applied directly in practice. They were separate from the world of nursing practice and were neither developed from research nor tested through research. Nursing theory as a type of knowledge in that era was often considered by both practitioners and researchers to be too abstract to be useful. As others have noted, nurses seemed to believe that, in order to be theory, the knowledge needed to be obscure and lack immediate use and meaning (Levine, 1995). Therefore, theory was relegated to a place separate from other types of nursing knowledge. When the grand theories of this era were used, they were most often superimposed on educational, clinical, and research environments with little regard to the fit. While the models are still selected by schools and hospitals as organizing frameworks, they do not drive practice, nor do they serve as frameworks for significant research programs.

In the 1980s, following Ura and Torres' (1975) National League for Nursing survey of curricular commonalities in baccalaureate schools of nursing, nursing scholars identified four common constructs (man-human, health, society-environment, and nursing) and declared that the metaparadigm of nursing had been established (Fawcett, 1978b; Flaskerud & Halloran, 1980; Newman, 1984). Scholars gratefully accepted this paradigm for nursing, in large part because perspectives in the philosophy of science had made achievement of disciplinary status contingent on having a paradigm. However, as Downs admonished, "To say that the metaparadigm of nursing is person, environment, health and nursing is to say virtually nothing at all" (Downs, 1988, p. 20). At its best, the metaparadigm of four central concepts provided a rationale and mechanism for the discipline to move beyond the conceptual models. Even after the identification of nursing's paradigm, nurse practitioners and researchers continued for the most part to ignore nursing theory in their work.

This chapter addresses several questions regarding the categories of nursing knowledge. Are the three categories still separate and, if so, is that situation inevitable? What are the advantages of keeping these categories separate? What are the advantages of connecting them? Can the three categories be separate and still useful? To stimulate debate, we present three positions: keep the categories separate, closely connect them, or keep them separate but structure the knowledge with built-in bridges.

POSITION ONE: THREE SEPARATE CATEGORIES

Each category of nursing knowledge will develop most fruitfully when tended carefully with full focus on one primary category. Nurses with interests and skills in each of the three areas have different perspectives. Nursing practice focuses on specific unique patients with immediate needs in concrete situations. Researchers, however, must carefully control the unique features to produce findings that can be applied across settings as well as to individual patients. Theorists focus on general abstract knowledge that may or may not be directly applicable in practice or tested in research at any given time. Their job is to develop the metanarrative of nursing; to articulate the patterns of knowledge, naming, defining, and relating concepts and patterns; to sketch boldly the phenomena of nursing and nursing care; and to clarify how nursing is a unique discipline (Reed, 1995).

Most nurse theorists, researchers, and practitioners currently have highly developed skills in only one of these areas, and knowledge in each category is developing well. Continuing in this manner will produce the knowledge needed and will use the currently developed skills and abilities efficiently.

If the categories of knowledge are kept separate, we must continue to develop the mechanisms to carry nursing theory both to practitioners to inform their practice and to researchers to guide their work. That is, a boundary-spanning role must be developed for persons who move and translate knowledge from the theoretical category to practitioners and researchers. Initially, nurse educators would fill this boundary-spanning role by organizing the knowledge learned by beginning students around nursing theories and capturing the knowledge available from existing research and using it to support nursing practice knowledge. After nurses complete their basic education, they must then rely on boundary-spanning activities in the form of continuing education or publications for practicing nurses. These publications would provide practitioners with nursing theory and current research findings. Useful research results must be translated into interventions and imported to practice by way of boundary-spanning persons or publications. Several publications have recently made valuable contributions in this area, e.g., *Applied Nursing Research, Nursing Scan in Administration,* and specialty journals that bring research to the practicing nurse.

Research utilization methods have been developed by nurses over the last two decades to provide this boundary-spanning role (Burns & Grove, 1993). While this type of activity is greatly needed by many applied professions, nurses are unique in constructing these methods in great detail. The profession has responded eagerly to this approach. Research utilization projects, often conducted by groups of staff nurses with advice and consultation from nurse research experts, have developed intervention protocols successfully for use in practice (Titler et al., 1994). The research utilization process is an example of successful boundary spanning across the knowledge categories of research and practice.

To reach across the categories of theory and research, boundary-spanning persons will need to identify theoretical developments that need testing and form research questions that need study. Research findings that inform theory development must be communicated back to the theoreticians. Practice problems without current solutions, or with questionable current solutions, must be identified and delivered to researchers for study. Researchers generally take on the role of boundary spanners themselves. That is, they have attempted to frame their research with theory and to derive research questions from practice. As previously noted, however, this has not been totally successful.

Keeping the categories of knowledge separate would allow the continuation of the present pattern of development, with which nursing has made great strides. Theoreticians focus on development of broad abstract statements of what nursing is and does, while researchers discover and develop knowledge from nursing's specific perspective. To facilitate fruition of each category separately and to use this knowledge in practice, boundary-spanning persons are needed to package and deliver knowledge from nurse theorists to researchers and practitioners and back. Basic and continuing nursing education, research utilization, and specialized publications have all functioned to span the boundary between research and practice. To continue to enhance progress in this mode, we must find better ways to span the boundaries between theory and practice and theory and research. These persons would also promote cross-fertilization use and stimulate the use of knowledge and promote development in concert with the needs of nurses in clinical practice.

POSITION TWO: CATEGORIES CLOSELY CONNECTED

The professional discipline of nursing must have a body of knowledge that is unique, coherent, and as seamless as possible. There must be one unified body of knowledge that belongs to nursing. This knowledge must be organized by theoretically identified concepts, patterns, and relationships; the statements of this knowledge must be generated from and tested by systematic research; and knowledge needs must be identified in practice and generated knowledge applied immediately to practice. Anything less than full connectedness will continue the current pattern of separateness and the ongoing necessity for the special roles of boundary spanners.

Models for accomplishing this connectedness have been described. The ideal model brings together academic researchers, nurse theorists, and practicing nurses to identify knowledge needs, to carry out basic research projects, and to bring research findings systematically into nursing practice. Three subtypes can be identified. The first is the researcher-practitioner collaboration. Two examples of this model come from northern California and involve collaboration among several health care agencies and nurse research experts (Chenitz, Sater, Davies, & Friesen, 1990; Rizzuto & Mitchell, 1988). Another example comes from the Midwest and describes a collaborative research project that began as a utilization project, became a research conduct project due to lack of adequate base for interventions, and concluded as the results of the research were used and evaluated in practice (Blegen & Goode, 1994).

The second type of collaboration is the theorist-practitioner model. Examples of this kind of collaboration are found in discussions of implementation of the conceptual models. The language and focus of a conceptual model is instituted in the nursing documentation and organization of a hospital or other patient care facility. Unfortunately, it is difficult to analyze the success of these efforts. How can we determine whether implementing model A or model B in a hospital leads to better outcomes? Real world problems are too complex to conclude unequivocally that the model implemented resulted in the changes specified.

The third type of collaboration is the researcher-theorist group, which most often evolves from an exploratory qualitative approach to research—the grounded theory approach. Yet another suggestion for increasing the connectedness of the production and use of knowledge is offered by Boyd (1993). The nursing practice research method features the relationship between the nurse researcher-as-clinician and the patient. The research process is a collaboration between nurse and patient; it is therapeutic to the patient and leads to development of the nurse. It can be questioned whether the knowledge produced by these efforts is generalizable beyond the setting and patients involved in the project. Even researchers from the perceived view call for the creation of knowledge that can be used by all nurses, i.e., knowledge that is generalizable (Schumacher & Gortner, 1992). The greater the need for knowledge that is generally useful by all nurses, the less this approach will be satisfactory.

There are no examples of models combining all three knowledge areas. While needed—and this need is often discussed in published literature—no working models have been described. One recently suggested approach may be able to facilitate this. Theories can be "tested" using means other than traditional empirical research methods. Silva and Sorrell (1992) suggested that there are four approaches to testing theory: verification through correspondence with empirical research, testing to verify through critical reasoning, testing through verification of personal experiences, and verification through assessment of problem-solving effectiveness. If a theory were tested with all these approaches, it will clearly increase the connectedness between practice, theory, and research. However, theory testing using any one of these four methods also involves advanced skills that many practicing nurses either do not have or have little time to use. If the theories being tested with personal experience or problem-solving effectiveness were closer to practice and more narrow in scope than the grand theories, the possibility of practicing nurses carrying out these tests is more likely than if the theories were conceptual models or grand theories.

While collaboration is generally to be recommended and is essential if we set out to develop one coherent, seamless body of knowledge, there are limitations to the extent of collaboration that can actually take place. It is difficult to cross the differing perspectives of the persons involved. Practitioners focus on individual and unique patients; researchers focus on systematically collecting knowledge that transcends the individual subjects from whom they collect data; and theorists focus on general and abstract concepts and the relationships among them. A great deal of time and effort must be expended to ensure good communication among collaborators.

This highly connected approach to nursing knowledge would put to rest the problem of separated areas of knowledge; however, working in teams that draw persons from multiple settings consumes a great deal of time and other resources. If an approach to nursing knowledge creation and use that produced a coherent, seamless body of knowledge were developed, the boundary-spanning activities encompassed by research utilization would no longer be needed. This would allow some resources to become available for use in the collaboration needed for success of the connected approach. At this point in time, the actual success of this model is questionable.

POSITION THREE: STRONG CONNECTIONS BETWEEN SEPARATE CATEGORIES

Nursing knowledge must be separated by type of knowledge (action-oriented specific practice applications, controlled systematic and narrow research findings, and abstract and general theory) and by the perspectives of the nurses associated with each category. The development and use of nursing knowledge are facilitated by keeping these separate and allowing clear and concentrated application of the different approaches used for each type. However, we need stronger connections than are presently provided by the boundary-spanning activities discussed in position one. These connections should be structural and intrinsic to the knowledge itself rather than dependent on boundary spanners. If the knowledge developed was closer to practice, amenable to research testing, and built around structures intrinsic to the discipline of nursing, we would then have the best of all worlds—separateness for development and connectedness to practice.

The best solution for keeping the three separate categories more closely connected is to use middle-range theory as the connecting point. Middle-range theory, when developed from research and thoughtful consideration of practice and tested by other research projects, does represent the most valid and useful type of knowledge available in nursing and other disciplines (Lenz, Suppe, Gift, Pugh, & Milligan, 1995).

Middle-range theory provides the means of articulating general knowledge, confirmed by the specific results of research projects, to nurses in clinical practice. When middle-range theory is used to guide research and knowledge development, the theorist and researcher are either the same person or two persons focusing on the same carefully delineated topic. The scope of knowledge within the topic area is more narrow than the grand theories and the metaparadigm concepts. This restriction of scope allows for far more precision and depth than the grand theories and conceptual models have allowed. This precise, in-depth and focused knowledge can then be used to inform and guide practice in specific and useful ways.

Theories of the middle range were first suggested by the sociologist Merton. The discipline of sociology also initially developed large theories attempting to differentiate sociology from other disciplines and to explain all of social phenomena with one effort. Merton (1967) responded by suggesting middle-range theories and differentiating them from the grand theories. Middle-range theory can be used to guide empirical inquiry because it lies between the minor working hypotheses that evolve in abundance during day-to-day practice and the all-inclusive systematic efforts to develop one unified theory that would explain all behavior. It is intermediate to the general theories, which are too remote from specific classes of behavior to account for what is observed, and to those detailed orderly descriptions of particulars that are not generalized at all. Middle-range theory, according to Merton, involves abstractions, but they are close enough to observed data to be expressed in propositions that permit testing with systematic research.

Merton has suggested that the search for the perfect grand theory led to a multiplicity of philosophical systems in sociology and, further, to the formation of schools, each with its own cluster of masters and disciples. Nursing perhaps has fallen to a similar fate. That is, we became differentiated from other disciplines but also became internally differentiated not in terms of specialization, as in other sciences, but in terms of schools of philosophy, held to be mutually exclusive and largely at odds. It is time to refocus from discussing these larger philosophical systems to producing knowledge that explains patient-related phenomena and helps in the choice and evaluation of interventions.

Merton further described the middle-range orientation as one that involves the specification of ignorance. Rather than pretend to have knowledge when it is, in fact, absent, the work on middle-range theories expressly recognizes what must yet be learned in order to lay the foundation for more knowledge. It does not begin with the task of providing theoretical solutions to all the urgent practical problems of the day, but addresses itself to those problems that might now be clarified in the light of available knowledge and to the identification of problems about which we know very little.

Our major task is to develop middle-range theory for the general advancement of nursing knowledge and to provide closer connections among theory, research, and practice. A large part of what is now described as theory consists of general orientations toward the discipline, suggesting types of variables that theories must take into account, rather than clearly formulated, verifiable statements of relationships between specified variables. We have many concepts but few supported propositions relating them—many points of view but few confirmed theories. It is time to move on.

To make use of the knowledge provided by middle-range theories, practicing nurses would need some grasp of research methods but they would not have to read and critique directly the often complex reports of research methods and findings. In addition, practicing nurses would not have to attempt to apply the global, highly abstract grand theories to everyday practice. Middle-range theories, developed and tested by research, would contain much more specific descriptions of human responses to illness and the nursing interventions applicable to these responses. Although understanding the theory and deriving specific nursing actions would be necessary, these activities would not be as daunting with theories developed in the middle range as they are with the grand theories.

Some boundary-spanning activities would still be needed. While the knowledge articulated with middle-range theories is much closer to practice, it still must be found and critiqued. Nurse educators and research utilization projects could provide this necessary assistance. Their job would be much easier with theory in the middle range that been tested systematically by researchers. Knowledge built in this way is more easily synthesized: the cumulation of knowledge across individual studies occurs as part of the process of conducting research and testing a theory. Persons actively engaged in research utilization could provide an additional service by formally feeding back to researchers the evaluation of utilization projects. This would provide a test of pragmatic usefulness for the knowledge.

Recent developments in nursing knowledge could provide other strong bridges connecting the three categories of nursing knowledge. In the last decade more of the theoretical work has been in the middle range. Some of these middle-range theories, however, were drawn from other disciplines and did not cohere naturally within the practice discipline of nursing. While these theories were used to support nursing research, they did not fit as well within the practice arena. Recent developments in nursing knowledge structures may be able to ground these theories within the discipline.

Developments in the structure of nursing knowledge, (the taxonomies for nursing diagnoses, interventions and outcomes) hold great promise for capturing the middle-range theories within a thorough and extensive framework of nursing knowledge. The Iowa Intervention Project has advanced even beyond the taxonomy of interventions and has identified a three-dimensional structure underlying these interventions (Tripp-Reimer, Woodworth, McCloskey, & Bulechek, 1996). Classes of interventions were characterized along four factors that were then related to the dimensions. The dimensions indicated principle elements describing patient needs and setting characteristics that nurses use in selecting the interventions, and four factors characterized the interventions available. Combined, these produce three descriptive categories. The first dimension nurses might use in selecting interventions is the *intensity of care* dimension; and the groups of interventions range along two bipolar factors—healthy self-care to provider illness care and continuous routine care to sporadic emergency care. The second dimension describing intervention selection is *focus of care* and the interventions range from individual independent to system collaborative. The third dimension is *complexity of care* and includes two groups of interventions—continuous routine to sporadic emergency and high-priority difficult to low-priority easy. These three dimensions and the factors within them could serve as the framework for guiding development of middle-range theories describing nurses' decision making in the selection of interventions.

The taxonomies of nursing diagnoses, interventions, and outcomes will provide a full skeletal framework for nursing knowledge. This skeleton could then be filled in with middle-range theories, the impetus and context for which would be clear. Theories would suggest explanations and predictions of relationships between diagnoses of actual or potential health problems, nursing interventions chosen to deal with these problems, and the patients' eventual outcomes. Each theoretical linkage would need to be tested in systematic research studies. The theories and the framework itself would be modified as this research progressed.

To bring about the close connections among theory, research, and practice using middle-range theories, nurses from each perspective must understand and appreciate the uniqueness of each perspective and the need to communicate across all perspectives. Researchers must accept the responsibility of truly testing the middle-range theories. That is, not only must their research be guided by the theory, but their results must be used explicitly to develop and modify the theory further. In addition, the researchers must ensure that the theory is described comprehensively and is useful to practitioners. Nurse theorists must work to develop theories that are testable by researchers and can be applied by practitioners. This knowledge, confirmed by research, could be incorporated into educational programs. Nurse educators must have a continually updated grasp of current research and the state of the knowledge pertaining to these middle-range theories.

Even with well-grounded theories in the middle range, nurses may still need assistance in applying the knowledge in practice. As other disciplines have found, the time lapse from discovery of knowledge to full application is often quite long. This assistance may not need to be as extensive and formal as the current research utilization process is. If research specifically tested middle-range theories and if the process of replication and extension is followed systematically, the knowledge will cumulate naturally and findings should be directly applicable in practice. This would make the job of research utilization much easier. Furthermore, if these middle-range theories are organized around knowledge structures as closely tied to practice as the taxonomies currently under construction, and if they are indexed using the standardized languages, they will be readily found and immediately pertinent.

Nurse educators and nurses involved in research utilization projects are important to the goal of incorporating nursing knowledge produced by theory building and testing in practice. However, nurses in practice must accept the primary ongoing responsibility of seeking out the most current developments in a theory and either applying it in practice or communicating to the researchers and theorists the reasons why it cannot be applied. Nurses in clinical practice must continue to provide the final test of the theories and the frameworks that organize these theories.

CONCLUSION

We presented three positions in answering the opening questions. First, the three categories of nursing knowledge should be kept separate to facilitate full development of each unique type; and boundary-spanning activities must be enhanced to ensure that the knowledge developed in each area is communicated to nurses working in the other areas, particularly nursing practice. In the second position, we argued that the three categories must be closely connected in order to have a body of knowledge that is coherent and seamless. To achieve this goal, new methods of conceptualizing, testing, and applying knowledge must be developed. Third, while nursing knowledge must be separated for the full focused development of each category, the connections between the categories must be strengthened by building bridges within the structure of the knowledge itself. These bridging structures are middle-range theory and the taxonomies of nursing knowledge currently under construction.

This third position was built on the recognition that the perspectives of theoreticians, researchers, and practitioners are different, and these differences are strengths that should be used well. This position also recognizes that the three categories must be closely connected and suggests both structural connections and continued use of boundary-spanning activities. Nursing theory, nursing research, and nursing practice would then be both separate and connected.

REFERENCES

Acton, G.J., Irvin, B.L., & Hopkins, B.A. (1991). Theory-testing research: Building the science. *Advances in Nursing Science, 14*(1), 52-61.

American Nurses Association. 1980. *Nursing: A social policy statement.* (p. 9). Kansas City, MO: ANA.

Baessler, C.A., Blumberg, M., Cunningham, J.S., Curran, J.A., Fennessey, A.G., Jacobs, J.M., McGrath, P., Perrong, M.T., & Wolf, Z.R. (1994). Medical surgical nurses' utilization of research methods and products. *Medical Surgical Nursing, 3*(2), 113-121.

Blegen, M.A., & Tripp-Reimer, R. (1994). The nursing theory-nursing research connection. In J. McCloskey & H.K. Grace (Eds.), *Current issues in nursing* (4th ed., pp. 87-91). St. Louis: Mosby.

Blegen, M.A., & Goode, C. (1994). Interactive process of conducting and utilizing research in nursing service administration. *Journal of Nursing Administration, 24*(9), 24-28.

Benoliel, J.Q. (1977). The interaction between theory and research. *Nursing Outlook, 25*(2), 108-113.

Boyd, C.O. (1993). Toward a nursing practice research method. *Advances in Nursing Science, 16*(2), 9-25.

Burns, N., & Grove, S.K. (1993). *The practice of nursing research: Conduct, critique, & utilization* (2nd ed.). Philadelphia: Saunders.

Chenitz, W.C., Sater, B., Davies, H., & Friesen, L. (1990). Developing collaborative research between clinical agencies: A consortium approach. *Applied Nursing Research, 3*(3), 90-97.

Conant, L.H. (1967). Closing the practice-theory gap. *Nursing Outlook, 15*(11), 37-39.

Coyle, L.A., & Sokop, A.G. (1990). Innovation adoption behavior among nurses. *Nursing Research, 39,* 176-180.

Downs, F. (1988). Doctoral education: Our claims to the future. *Nursing Outlook, 36*(1), 18-20.

Fawcett, J. (1978a). The relationship between theory and research: A double helix. *Advances in Nursing Science, 1*(1), 49-62.

Fawcett, J. (1978b). The "what" of theory development. In *Theory development: The what, why, how* (pp. 17-33)? New York: National League for Nursing.

Fawcett, J., & Downs, F.S. (1992). *The relationship of theory and research* (2nd ed.). Philadelphia: F.A. Davis.

Flaskerud, J.H., & Halloran, E.J. (1980). Areas of agreement in nursing theory development. *Advances in Nursing Science, 31*(1), 1-7.

Jacobs, M.K., & Huether, S.E. (1978). Nursing science: The theory-practice linkage. *Advances in Nursing Science, 1*(1), 63-73.

Lenz, E.R., Suppe, F., Gift, A.G., Pugh, L.C., & Milligan, R.A. (1995). Collaborative development of middle-range nursing theories: Toward a theory of unpleasant symptoms. *Advances in Nursing Science, 17*(3), 1-13.

Levine, M.E. (1995). The rhetoric of nursing theory. *Image: Journal of Nursing Scholarship, 27*(1), 11-14.

Merton, R.K. (1967). *On theoretical sociology.* New York: Free Press.

Moody, L.E., Wilson, M.E., Smyth, K., Schwartz, R., Tittle, M., & Von-Cott, M.L. (1988). Analysis of a decade of nursing practice research: 1977-1986. *Nursing Research, 37*(6), 374-379.

Newman, M.A. (1984). The continuing revolution: A history of nursing science. In N.L. Chaska (Ed.), *The nursing profession: A time to speak.* New York: McGraw-Hill.

Pettengill, M.M., Gillies, D.A., & Clark, C.C. (1994). Factors encouraging and discouraging the use of nursing research findings. *Image: Journal of Nursing Scholarship, 26*(2), 143-147.

Reed, P.G. (1995). A treatise on nursing knowledge development for the 21st century: Beyond postmodernism. *Advances in Nursing Science, 17*(3), 70-84.

Rizzuto, C., & Mitchell, M. (1988). Research in service settings: part I. Consortium project outcomes. *Journal of Nursing Administration, 18*(2), 32-37.

Schumacher, K.L., & Gortner, S.R. (1992). (Mis)conception and reconceptions about traditional science. *Advances in Nurse Science, 14*(4), 1-11.

Silva, M.C. (1986). Research testing nursing theories. *Advances in Nursing Science, 9*(1), 1-11.

Silva, M.C., & Sorrell, J.M. (1992). Testing of nursing theory: Critique and philosophical expansion. *Advances in Nursing Science, 14*(4), 12-23.

Titler, M.G., Kleiber, C., Steelman, V., Goode, C., Rakel, B., Barry-Walker, J., Small, S., & Buckwalter, K. (1994). Infusing research into practice to promote quality care. *Nursing Research, 43*(5), 307-313.

Tripp-Reimer, T., Woodworth, G., McCloskey, J.C., & Bulechek, G. (1996). The dimensional structure of nursing interventions. *Nursing Research, 45,* 10-17.

Walker, L.O. (1973, March). *Theory, practice, and research in perspective.* Paper presented at the American Nurses Association Ninth Nursing Research Conference, San Antonio, TX.

Weiler, K., Buckwalter, K.C., & Titler, M.G. (1994). Is nursing research used in practice? In J. McCloskey & H.K. Grace (Eds.), *Current issues in nursing* (4th ed., pp 61-75). St. Louis: Mosby.

Yura, H., & Torres, G. (1975). Today's conceptual framework within baccalaureate nursing programs. In G. Torres & H. Yura (Eds.), *Faculty-curriculum development. Part III: Conceptual framework—Its meaning and function.* (pp 17-25). New York: National League for Nursing.

Classification systems and integrated information systems: Building blocks for transforming data into nursing knowledge

SUZANNE BAKKEN HENRY, MORI COSTANTINO

The premises of this chapter are two. First, nursing theory, nursing research, and nursing practice must be related integrally in order to foster the development of nursing knowledge. Second, building blocks for the development of nursing knowledge include classification systems for patient problems, nursing interventions, and nursing-sensitive patient outcomes as well as integrated information systems to support the acquisition, storage, transformation, and presentation of data relevant to nursing. The discussion supporting these premises is organized around three questions:

- Why have traditional automated nursing systems not fostered the development of nursing knowledge?
- What is the role of classification systems in linking nursing theory, nursing research, and nursing practice?
- How can classification systems and integrated information systems foster the development of nursing knowledge?

WHY HAVE TRADITIONAL AUTOMATED NURSING SYSTEMS NOT FOSTERED THE DEVELOPMENT OF NURSING KNOWLEDGE?

Although various types of automated nursing systems have been in place for several decades, these systems have, for the most part, failed to foster the development of nursing knowledge. Several reasons can be posited for this void, including the traditional role of the nursing record as a transaction log rather than an evolving repository of nursing knowledge related to patient care; entry of abstract data requiring duplicate entry and having limited use, rather than atomic-level, patient-specific data; lack of standardized schemata for coding and classification of health care data; and application-specific rather than integrated information systems.

The nursing record as a transaction log

In his discussion of a framework for the transition from nursing records to a nursing information system, Turley (1992) notes that storage of the transaction log (what the nurse does when) is not likely to add to the understanding of the patient's condition and problems. He states,

> Alone, transaction logs do not reflect the evolvement of patient status, condition resolution, or expected long-term outcomes. All those lost data represent the forfeiture of documented nursing knowledge and will critically affect the development of decision support components of any nursing information system. (Turley, 1992, p. 178)

This thought is consistent with the recommendation by the Institute of Medicine (Dick & Steen, 1991) report on the computer-based patient record (CPR), which identified the documentation of the logical bases for all diagnoses or conclusions and the clinical rationale for decisions about the management of the patient's care as an essential attribute of CPR systems. In addition, these attributes are critical to knowledge development in health care.

Limited use and re-use of data

Until recently there has been limited use and re-use of data entered into computer-based systems. Multiple health care providers were faced with entering the same piece of patient information. Current development efforts are aimed at the collection of atomic-level, patient-specific data that can then be transformed using informa-

USERS	DATA/INFORMATION	SCOPE
World health officials Policy makers Researchers Lawmakers	General health status and health-related needs of individual nations	WORLDWIDE DATA
	ABSTRACTED. SUMMARIZED. AGGREGATED	
Policy makers Lawmakers Researchers Insurers	Trends in incidence, prevalence, outcomes, and costs by region, by diagnosis, by type of agency	NATIONWIDE DATA
	ABSTRACTED. SUMMARIZED. AGGREGATED	
Analysts Researchers Quality management Public health officials	Comparisons of treatments, outcomes, and costs by locality and by agency Incidence and prevalence of diagnosis by region	COMMUNITY/REGION-WIDE DATA
	ABSTRACTED. SUMMARIZED. AGGREGATED	
Administrators Researchers Accreditors Quality managers	Costs of care by category of patient Number of patients admitted with specific diagnosis Volume of tests, procedures, and interventions Outcomes for patients grouped by diagnosis	AGENCY-WIDE DATA
	ABSTRACTED. SUMMARIZED. AGGREGATED	
Care givers Agency departments Insurers QA personnel	Atomic level patient-specific data e.g., assessments, diagnostic test results, diagnoses, interventions, procedures, hours of care, outcomes Used to provide most appropriate care	INDIVIDUAL PATIENT DATA

Fig. 11-1. Examples of uses of atomic-level patient data collected once, used many times.

tion system processes. Figure 11-1 illustrates the manner in which data collected at the point of care can be aggregated for numerous purposes including quality assurance, research, and health care policy development (Zielstorff et al., 1993).

Lack of standardized vocabularies and classification systems

Standardized vocabularies and classification systems are a prerequisite for computer-based systems including databases, knowledge bases, patient records, and expert systems. In addition, a standardized clinical vocabulary is a key attribute of the CPR: it is required for the inclusion of nursing-related data elements in databases used for health care financing and policy development, and for facilitating clinical and outcomes research (Clark & Lang, 1992; Dick & Steen, 1991; Lange & Jacox, 1993).

There is currently no internationally accepted, standardized clinical language or classification system for nursing practice (Clark & Lang, 1992; Henry, Holzemer, Reilly, & Campbell, 1994). However, nursing diagnoses/patient problems, nursing interventions, and nursing-sensitive patient outcomes are widely acknowledged as essential elements of such a language. While developers of individual taxonomies or classification systems, such as the North American Nursing Diagnosis Association (NANDA) taxonomy (NANDA, 1994) and the Nursing Interventions Classification (McCloskey & Bulechek, 1996) continue to expand and refine their systems, efforts by the American Nurses Association (ANA; McCormick et al., 1994), the European Union (Mortensen et al., 1994), and the International Council of Nursing (Clark & Lang, 1992) are focused on the establishment of a unified system to describe nursing diagnoses/patient problems, nursing interventions, and patient outcomes.

While the interest in developing standardized nursing

vocabularies and classification schemata has been great, several authors have identified perceived barriers to the development of the universe of relevant nursing data, including the whole-person perspective of nursing; multiple conceptual frameworks guiding nursing practice; identification of the data elements in a nursing minimum data set; differentiation between nursing diagnoses and other problems of interest to nursing; defining the data elements required to capture different nursing diagnostic or classification systems, interventions, and outcomes; and the lack of a uniform coding format for nursing diagnoses (Clark & Lang, 1992; Ozbolt, Abraham, & Schultz, 1990; Simpson & Waite, 1989). Today, however, it may be possible to build this universe inductively through the classification of nursing concepts based on clinical data.

Challenge of information systems integration

Systems integration is still a major challenge in most health care organizations, thereby limiting the potential of information systems to influence the quality of nursing practice and also providing a barrier to nursing knowledge development. Stand-alone, application-specific information systems constrain the relationships that can be examined among various types of data as well as the transformation processes applied to the data.

Great strides made during the last decade have the potential to decrease the technological barriers to using information systems as a facilitator of knowledge development. Future efforts must include enhanced understandings of human-computer interaction and clinical decision making.

WHAT IS THE ROLE OF CLASSIFICATION SYSTEMS IN LINKING NURSING THEORY, NURSING RESEARCH, AND NURSING PRACTICE?

The language of nursing

The National Institute of Nursing Research Priority Expert Panel on Nursing Informatics (1993) defined nursing language as

> . . . the universe of written terms and their definitions comprising nomenclature or thesauri that are used for purposes such as indexing, sorting, retrieving, and classifying varied nursing data in clinical records, in information systems (for care documentation and/or management), and in literature and research reports. . . . Determining the way that nursing data are represented in automated systems is tantamount to defining a language for nursing. (p. 31)

Development of classification systems for nursing concepts

Since the late 1970s, NANDA Taxonomy I has been the predominant, although not universal, classification system for nursing diagnoses (NANDA, 1994; Ozbolt et al., 1990). The design and testing of a nursing minimum data set, led by Werley, has provided the framework for research on additional standardized vocabularies for nursing (Werley, Devine, & Zorn, 1988). The development of classification schemata is the focus of several recently completed or ongoing nursing research projects including the Iowa Intervention Project (McCloskey & Bulechek, 1992, 1996), the Georgetown Home Health Care Project (Saba, 1992a), the Omaha Community Health System (Martin & Scheet, 1992), the Nursing Intervention Lexicon and Taxonomy (Grobe, 1991, 1992), and the development of standardized terminology and codes for nursing diagnoses/patient problems, patient care activities, and expected patient outcomes by Ozbolt, Fruchtnicht, and Hayden (1994). Investigators (Griffith & Robinson, 1992, 1993; Henry, Holzemer, Reilly, & Campbell, 1994) have also demonstrated the feasibility of using terminologies not specifically designed for nursing such as the Physicians' Current Procedural Terminology (CPT) codes (American Medical Association, 1993) and Systematized Nomenclature of Human and Veterinary Medicine International (SNOMED) (Côté, Rothwell, Palotay, & Beckett, 1993) to represent some types of nursing concepts.

Evaluation criteria for a classification system to support nursing theory, nursing research, and nursing practice

Standardized vocabularies or classification schemata vary in purpose, scope, structure, and the level of granularity (abstract vs. atomic) of the data elements (Ozbolt & Graves, 1993). While a gold standard has not been identified, a number of authors have proposed evaluation criteria for a classification system designed to support clinical practice. These criteria are equally relevant for systems that will also support nursing theory development and testing as well as nursing research. The authors and the resulting criteria represent a variety of perspectives. Cimino (1989) identified nine criteria for a multipurpose controlled vocabulary for clinical information systems. These criteria were aimed at increasing the sensitivity and specificity of information retrieval queries. Clark and Lang (1992) described criteria from the perspective of the development of the International Classification of Nursing Practice. McCloskey and Bulechek (1995, 1996) generated criteria specifically for the evaluation of the taxo-

Table 11-1 Evaluation criteria for classification systems to support nursing practice

Criteria	Examples
Domain completeness	The classification system must include all the terms necessary to describe the domain (Cimino, 1989; Clark & Lang, 1992).
Conceptual clarity and coherence	The classification system should be consistent with a clearly defined conceptual framework, but not dependent on a particular theory or model of nursing (Clark & Lang, 1992; McCloskey & Bulechek, 1996). Other criteria related to conceptual clarity and coherence include: (a) clear, understandable definitions (McCloskey & Bulechek, 1996); (b) only one way to express each concept (nonredundancy) (Cimino, 1989); (c) terms should refer to only one concept (unambiguous) (Cimino, 1989); and (d) all terms within a category are members of the same class (homogeneity) (McCloskey & Bulechek, 1996).
Data structures and relationships among terms	The relationships among terms should be explicit (Cimino, 1989). For instance, in the Nursing Interventious Classification (Iowa Intervention Project, 1996) Bowel Incontinence Care is an Elimination Management intervention, a statement of EXPLICIT Relationship. Other types of explicit relationships among terms include EQUIVALENT-TO, PART-OF, and ASSOCIATED-WITH.
Clinical concept capture	Classification systems for clinical practice should be clinically expressive, i.e., include the types of natural language terms used to describe patient problems and health care interventions in the medical record (Campbell & Musen, 1992; Chute et al., 1992). To do this, the classification system should include modifiers such as those related to time and severity.
Utility	Three criteria related to utility of a classification system were described in the context of the International Classification of Nursing Practice. First, the system is ". . . simple enough to be seen by the ordinary practitioner of nursing as a meaningful description of practice and a useful means of structuring practice" (Clark & Lang, 1992, p. 111). Second, the classification system is complementary with the family of disease and health-related classification systems. Third, the classification system is based on a central core that can be updated through a continual process of development and refinement.

nomic structure of the Nursing Interventions Classification (NIC). Several authors have focused on criteria related to the clinical expressiveness of classification systems (Campbell & Musen, 1992; Chute, Atkin, & Ihrke, 1992). These evaluation criteria fall into five broad areas: domain completeness; conceptual clarity and coherence; data structures and relationships among terms; clinical concept capture; and utility. The criteria are defined in Table 11-1.

Overview of classification systems for representation of nursing concepts

Six classification systems were selected for review in this chapter. The four nursing classification systems are those officially recognized by the ANA Database Steering Committee (McCormick et al., 1994): NANDA, NIC, Georgetown Home Health Care Classification, and Omaha Community Health System. In addition, two more general health care classification systems with demonstrated potential for some nursing concept representation are included: SNOMED International and CPT. The six systems are discussed in the following section and summarized in Table 11-2.

North American Nursing Diagnosis Association Taxonomy 1. The NANDA Taxonomy 1 is a classification of nursing diagnoses by human response patterns (NANDA, 1994). Related factors and defining characteristics are included for each diagnosis. This classification system continues to be refined by the ongoing research and development efforts of NANDA (McFarland & McFarlane, 1993; NANDA, 1994). Five specific issues are being addressed: levels of abstractions of the diagnoses; placement of wellness-related diagnoses; methods for testing the taxonomic structure and classification schema; use of the structure in practice; and revision or deletion of diagnoses that do not meet the criteria specified in NANDA's definition of nursing diagnoses (McFarland & McFarlane, 1993).

Nursing Interventions Classification. The NIC (McCloskey & Bulechek, 1992, 1996) is a categorization

Table 11-2 Comparison of standardized classification schemata with data elements relevant to nursing

Scheme/Author	Major focus	Contents
Home Health Care Classification System (Saba 1992a, 1992b)	Home health care	147 diagnoses, 20 home health care components, 166 interventions, discharge status
NANDA Taxonomy 1 (NANDA, 1994)	Nursing diagnoses	128 diagnoses
Nursing Interventions Classification (Iowa Intervention Project, 1993, McCloskey & Bulechek, 1996)	Nursing interventions	6 domains, 27 classes, 433 interventions, related nursing activities
Omaha Community Health System (Martin & Scheet, 1992)	Community health	40 client problems, 62 targets of interventions, 4 intervention categories, 3 outcome measures
Physicians' Current Procedural Terminology (American Medical Association, 1993)	Physician procedures and services	Evaluation and management, anesthesiology, surgery, radiology, pathology and laboratory, medicine
SNOMED International (Côté et al., 1993)	Human and veterinary medicine	NANDA diagnoses, nursing procedures; signs, symptoms; medical diagnoses; changes found in cells, tissues, and organs; bacteria and viruses; occupations, devices, and activities associated with disease; general modifiers

Note. NANDA = North American Nursing Diagnosis Association.

of both direct and indirect care activities performed by nurses. Each intervention consists of a label describing the concept, the definition of the concept, and a set of related activities or actions. The three-tiered taxonomy contains six domains (physiological-basic, physiological-complex, behavioral, safety, family, and health system), 27 classes, 433 interventions, and related nursing activities for each intervention (Iowa Intervention Project, 1993, 1995; McCloskey & Bulechek, 1996).

The NIC was developed using an inductive approach. Interventions were initially collected from the nursing literature and three nursing information systems. The iterative definition of intervention labels and classification of activities into interventions included content analysis by the experts on the research team and clinical nurse specialists. Refinement of the intervention list and activities was accomplished by a two-round Delphi questionnaire and focus groups. The taxonomic structure was constructed using cluster analysis, and was judged to be adequate on five criteria by 121 experts in nursing theory. A series of three validation surveys by individual nurses and special organizations provided support for the domain completeness of NIC. NIC is being implemented in the nursing information systems of five field sites (McCloskey & Bulechek, 1996) and other agencies.

Home Health Care Classification System. The Home Health Care Classification System (Saba 1992a, 1992b) includes 20 home health care components, 147 nursing diagnoses (NANDA-plus additional homecare diagnoses), 166 nursing interventions within four classes of nursing interventions (assess, care, teach, and manage), and discharge status (improved, stabilized, or deteriorated). Examples of home health care components are activity, self-care, health behavior, and metabolic.

The Home Health Care Classification System was developed using an inductive approach to examine the Medicare patient records of a national sample of 646 home health agencies. Each agency abstracted 5 to 50 records providing a total of 8,961 cases for the analysis. The coding schema was generated from two open-ended questions used to collect nursing diagnoses or patient problems, or both, and nursing services. The first 1,000 cases were used to create the coding schema, which was tested interactively and refined and then used to code the two questions for the remaining cases. A total of 40,361 nursing diagnoses/patient problems and 80,283 nursing services were collected. The system is being tested currently in a number of settings including university medical centers (Ozbolt, Fruchnicht, & Hayden, 1994) and psychiatric home care settings (Parlocha, 1995).

Omaha Community Health System. The Omaha Community Health System (Martin & Scheet, 1992; Martin, Scheet, & Stegman, 1993) consists of standardized schemata of nursing diagnoses, interventions, and ratings of outcomes for patient problems. The problem classification schema includes 40 client problems or nursing diagnoses, two sets of modifiers, and clusters of signs and symptoms. The intervention schema is a taxonomy of four intervention categories and 62 targets or objects of the nursing interventions. In the outcomes schema, client progress in relation to specific problems is rated on the dimensions of knowledge, behavior, and status.

The Omaha Community Health System problem schema was developed using an inductive approach on empirical chart data of 338 families. Field testing in four agencies provided evidence for the domain completeness, interrater reliability, and test-retest reliability of the classification schemata (Martin & Scheet, 1992). The intervention schema was created using data from 275 charts, which were sorted into seven categories that had been identified in the literature and by consultants to the project. The seven categories were reduced eventually to four and the schema was further refined following completion of a pilot study. The Omaha system has been implemented widely in the community health setting.

SNOMED International. SNOMED International (Côté et al., 1993) is a compilation of nomenclatures that classifies patient findings into eleven modules or taxonomies: (1) *topography,* i.e., anatomic terms (12,385 records); (2) *morphology,* i.e., changes found in cells, tissues, and organs (4,991 records); (3) *living organisms,* i.e., bacteria and viruses (24,265 records); (4) *chemicals, drugs, and biological products,* i.e., drugs, chemicals, and plant products (14,075 records); (5) *function,* i.e., signs and symptoms (16,352 records); (6) *occupation,* i.e., terms to describe occupations (1,886 records); (7) *diagnosis,* i.e., diagnostic terms used in clinical medicine (23,623 records); (8) *procedure,* i.e., administrative, therapeutic, and diagnostic procedures (27,033 records); (9) *physical agents, forces, and activities,* i.e., devices and activities commonly associated with disease (1,355 records); (10) *social context,* i.e., social conditions and relationships of importance in medicine (433 records); and (11) *general,* i.e., syntactic linkages and qualifiers (1,176 records). NANDA diagnoses are included in SNOMED International in the function module and a limited number of nursing procedures are included in the procedure module. Other nomenclatures in SNOMED include the International Classification of Diseases, 9th Rev., Clinical Modification (ICD-9-CM), Diagnostic and Statistical Manual of Mental Disorders, 3rd ed., Revised DSM-III-R, International Standard Classification of Occupations, and the CPT. Plans are in place for the addition of the NIC, Omaha, and Home Health Care systems into SNOMED International. The feasibility of using SNOMED to represent some types of nursing concepts has been demonstrated by Henry, Holzemer, Reilly, and Campbell (1994), who reported that nurses frequently describe patient problems in terms of signs, symptoms, and medical diagnoses as well as nursing diagnoses and demonstrated the ability of SNOMED to represent those categories of terms.

Physicians' Current Procedural Terminology. Griffith and Robinson (1992, 1993) conducted two surveys focused on the degree to which physicians' CPT-coded services were provided by nurses in a variety of nursing specialties. These studies provided evidence that nurses do perform a limited number of interventions that can be represented using the CPT codes. A recent study by Henry, Holzemer, Reilly, Miller, and Randell (1995) demonstrated the superiority of NIC to CPT in representing nursing interventions for hospitalized patients with AIDS.

Several conclusions can be posited from the state of knowledge related to development of standardized vocabularies and classification systems for patient problems, nursing interventions, and nursing-sensitive patient outcomes. First, the existing nursing classification systems are not yet domain-complete for the domain of nursing. Second, some types of data used by nurses, e.g., patient assessment data, can be represented adequately with terms from nonnursing classification systems such as the symptom codes in SNOMED International. Third, nursing-specific schemata for the classification of nursing interventions are essential to the development of nursing knowledge. Last, the representation of nursing-sensitive patient outcomes in classification systems is less well developed than is the case for patient problems and nursing interventions. Classification systems are essential in the transition from automation of current nursing record systems to the development of nursing information systems that will foster the development of nursing knowledge and exploit the linkages among nursing theory, nursing research, and nursing practice. Specific strategies are discussed in the next section within the framework of information system processes.

HOW CAN CLASSIFICATION SYSTEMS AND INTEGRATED INFORMATION SYSTEMS FOSTER THE DEVELOPMENT OF NURSING KNOWLEDGE?

Framework for design characteristics for nursing information systems

"Nursing informatics is a combination of computer science, information science, and nursing science designed to assist in the management and processing of nursing data, information, and knowledge to support the practice of nursing and the delivery of nursing care" (Graves &

Corcoran, 1989, p. 3). The phenomena of interest in nursing informatics are nursing data, nursing information, and nursing knowledge. Nursing informatics involves the rules and processes that relate to symbolic representations of nursing phenomena.

The role of nursing informatics in fostering knowledge development in nursing will be reviewed using the framework for design characteristics of a nursing information system provided by the National Commission on Nursing Implementation Project (NCNIP) Task Force on Nursing Information Systems (Zielstorff et al., 1993). The framework includes three categories of information required to support professional nursing practice. *Patient-specific data* are data about a particular patient and may be acquired from a variety of data sources. *Agency-specific data* are those data relevant to the specific organization under whose auspices the health care is provided. *Domain information and knowledge* are specific to the discipline of nursing or to other related health care disciplines. The NCNIP framework also delineates four types of information system processes that relate to the three categories of information. *Data acquisition* is the set of methods by which data become available to the information system, e.g., from data entry by the nurse or from a medical device. *Data storage* includes the methods, programs, and structures used to organize data for subsequent use (i.e., type of database and indexes to search the database). *Data transformation* or processing comprises the methods by which stored data or information is "acted upon" according to the needs of the end user (i.e., calculations, search for matches with system rules). *Presentation* encompasses the forms in which information is delivered to the end user after processing (i.e., charts, graphs, multimedia).

While the NCNIP framework identifies the design characteristics of a nursing information system, it does not convey the dynamic relationship of data, the transformations across data types, and the process of knowledge development from data. Figure 11-2 operationalizes the NCNIP framework by illustrating the integration and transformation of patient-specific data, agency-specific data, and domain-specific information and knowledge using the clinical example of pressure ulcer management. As the figure shows, domain-specific knowledge (practice guidelines) is applied to patient-specific assessment data resulting in the generation of a "pressure ulcer risk score." The level of pressure ulcer risk score triggers agency-specific policies and protocols, e.g., ordering the appropriate type of mattress suitable to the level of risk. Multiple use of the data is illustrated by multiple presentation formats such as a patient education plan and critical path. The individual-level data can then be aggregated and transformed both to refine agency-specific needs and to add to the body of domain information and knowledge related to pressure ulcer management, e.g., does care given in compliance with the practice guidelines affect patient outcomes?

Transforming data into nursing knowledge through information system processes

Data acquisition. Regardless of the category of information (patient-specific, agency-specific, or domain-specific), the three major strategies for acquiring nursing data for storing, processing, and presenting in an information system are data entry by a member of the health care team or the patient, transfer of data from a medical device to an information system, and sharing of data among computer-based systems.

Patient-specific data such as patient assessments and history collected by the provider at the point of care can be entered into the information system via a number of interface devices such as the keyboard, trackball, mouse, touch screen, or light pen. While not yet widely implemented, pen-based and voice-recognition interfaces are being studied by a number of investigators (Dick & Steen, 1991; Gillis, Booth, Graves, Fehlauer, & Soller, 1994). Although strides are being made in the development of clinical work stations, for the near future, dictation and transcription by clerical or data entry personnel may continue as a predominant method of data entry for admission history and physical examination in some institutions.

Assessment data related to defining characteristics for nursing diagnoses can also be acquired from medical devices such as monitors, ventilators, intravenous pumps, urimeters, and pulse oximeters (East, Young, & Gardner, 1992; Shabot, 1994). For example, increased values for intracranial pressure are a defining characteristic for the NANDA diagnosis of *decreased adaptive capacity: intracranial.* The acquisition of these types of data has been hampered by the lack of a standard for electronic data exchange between the devices and the information system necessitating custom programming (Shabot, 1994). However, a recent effort by the Institute of Electrical and Electronic Engineers, entitled the Medical Information Bus Standard, is aimed at "the development of a hardware and software communication standard that would allow 'plug and play' connection of medical devices to data monitoring and data management systems" and thus enhance

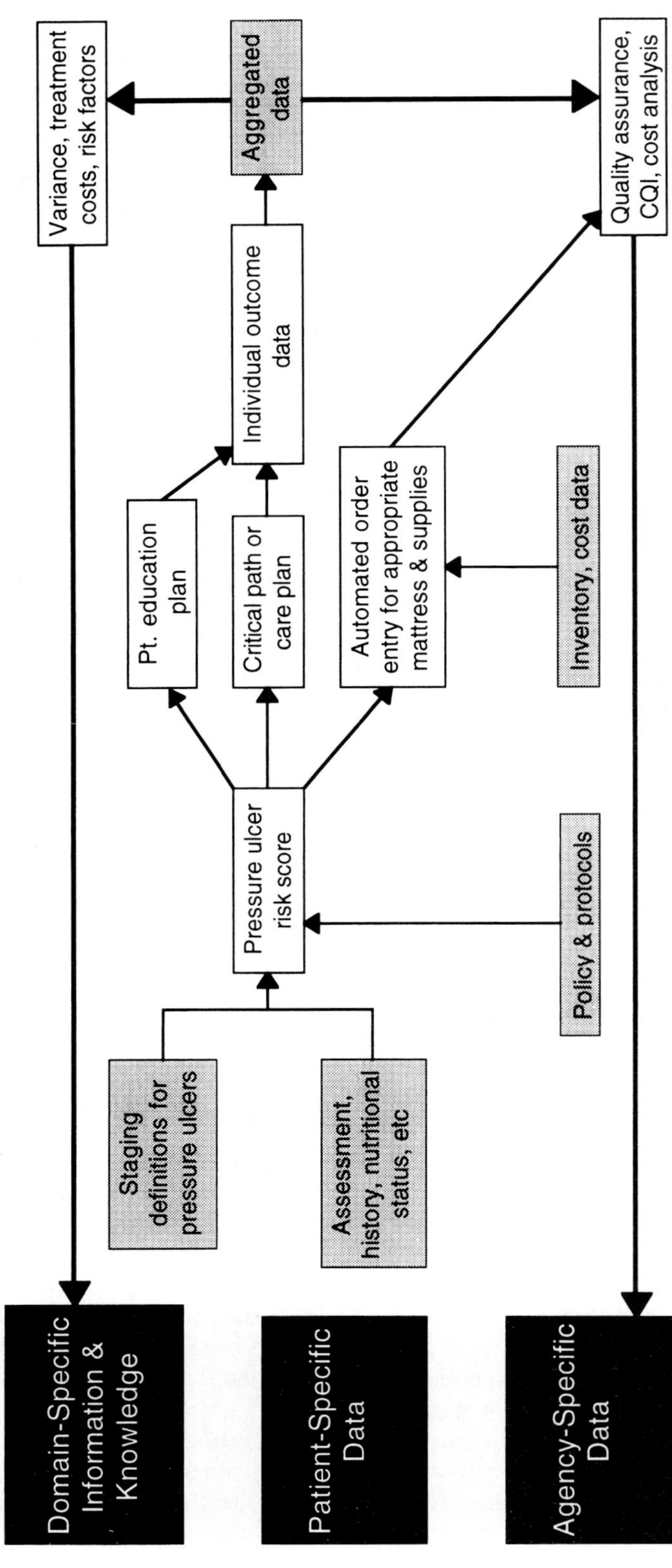

Fig. 11-2. An illustration of the dynamic relationships among the types of data and the iterative data transformation process in the management of pressure ulcers.

electronic data exchange (Shabot, 1994, p. 109). This proposal is currently under review for adoption as a standard.

Petrucci and Canfield (1992) advocate the shift from care planning systems, which do not communicate with other parts of a patient care system, to "intelligent" automated care planning libraries. For example, sources of knowledge in the care planning library may include agency-specific nursing care plans, standards of care, clinical practice guidelines, and critical paths. In this model, the care planning library, and medical record, administrative, and clinical databases would be searched for influences that could potentially affect the care plan's success including patient and provider preferences. The care plan database would also have the potential to learn and be modified by patient data. This type of "intelligent" care planning library has not yet been implemented in nursing, but has had some success in medicine.

Domain information and knowledge are acquired frequently through access with external databases and knowledge bases, and for the most part, are not integrated into "point of care" information systems. Such linkages, however, have been identified as an essential attribute of the evolving computer-based patient record (Dick & Steen, 1991). An example related to nursing is that of the Research and Application of Research in Nursing (RARIN) project (Bostrom & Wise, 1995). In this project, research articles from bibliographic databases were abstracted and entered into a customized software program on the experimental nursing units. Selection of topics was based on the nursing diagnoses from the nursing care plans and from a survey of staff. Although there were no significant differences in research innovations between the control and experimental units, the system was used by "opinion" leaders on the unit.

Data storage. The principles for storage of data, information, and knowledge, whether patient-specific, agency-specific, or domain-specific are the same. Independent of the type of acquisition strategy, the majority of data should be stored using widely accepted classification systems, data dictionaries, and lexicons to enhance single-entry, multiple use; and stored contents should be indexed extensively to facilitate retrieval, review, and update.

While standardized vocabularies and classification systems do not yet exist for all data relevant to nursing practice, the standardization is essential for comparative studies across organizations, communities, countries, or regions. In addition, storage in a standardized format and extensive indexing of nursing data will facilitate the development and sharing of computer-based interventions such as knowledge-based clinical decision support systems. These strategies must be complemented by electronic data interchange standards and standardized instruments to measure health care outcomes.

Data transformation. Data transformation is the major type of information process related to the development of nursing knowledge. In the following section, three specific examples are provided in the areas of validation of nursing diagnoses; machine learning using inductive algorithms; and linking patient problems, nursing interventions, and nursing-sensitive patient outcomes.

Validation of nursing diagnoses and defining characteristics. Databases containing nursing diagnoses and predicted defining characteristics as well as other patient characteristics have the potential to serve as the infrastructure for large-scale validation studies for nursing diagnoses (Brennan & Romano, 1987; Chang, 1993). Chang reviewed the applicability of Bayes' theorem in linking defining characteristics with nursing diagnoses and stated that it is clinically useful to know the conditional probability of the presence of a diagnosis given the presence of a particular characteristic (positive predictive power) or the conditional probability of the absence of a diagnosis given the absence of the defining characteristic (negative predictive power). For instance, in her sample of 414 client assessments using the Computer Aided Research In Nursing database, Chang found a 76% positive predictive power for the presence of the defining characteristic of a problem with moving body parts and the diagnosis of *self-care deficit*.

Rios, Delaney, Kruckeberg, Chung, and Mehmert (1991) used a measure of sensitivity (proportion of subjects with the defining characteristics for a given diagnosis among the total number of subjects with the diagnosis) to examine the validity of the defining characteristics of four nursing diagnoses related to alterations in fluid volume: *fluid volume, excess; fluid volume, active loss; fluid volume, loss secondary to regulatory mechanism;* and *fluid volume, potential deficit.* In addition to validating predicted defining characteristics, the study also identified never-documented defining characteristics.

Inductive algorithms. Several authors have identified the potential for the use of inductive algorithms to discover nursing knowledge from nursing data in large databases (Abraham, Fitzpatrick, & Jewell, 1986; Jones, 1991). A number of investigators have also demonstrated the ability of inductive algorithms such as SuperExpert, Learning from Examples using Rough Sets, C4 Extension of Concept Learning System, and Classification and Regression Trees to generate production rules or decision trees that could serve as an alternative, complementary mechanism for other approaches to knowledge acquisition for expert system development (Jones, 1991; Henry, 1995; Henry, Holzemer, & Gennari, 1994; Woolery & Grzymala-Busse, 1994). For example, an appropriate inductive algorithm could generate production rules based on the relationship between the data elements of defining characteristics and nursing diagnoses. These relationships could then be refined by a panel of nurse experts before being used in the knowledge base for an expert system. This type of approach has the potential to significantly decrease the amount of data to be examined by the experts.

Linking patient problems, nursing interventions, and nursing-sensitive outcomes of care. Several studies have demonstrated the increase in capture of data related to patient problems and nursing interventions with structured manual (Ehnfors, 1994) and computer-based approaches (Prophet, 1994) to care documentation. Large nursing databases built on these types of data are needed to examine the relationships between the processes and outcomes of care for care delivery, for building the base of nursing knowledge, and for health policy decision making at the local, national, and international levels (Zielstorff et al., 1993). While these databases do not exist currently, several investigators are focused on the development of outcomes infrastructures. Ozbolt et al. are developing a clinical database for nursing research in collaboration with the University Hospital Consortium (Ozbolt & Graves, 1993; Ozbolt et al., 1994). Nursing-specific information to be added to the demographic and medical information includes nursing diagnoses/patient problems, patient outcomes, patient care activities, principal nursing care unit, other nursing care units, patient's average nursing acuity score, and average staffing level on unit during a patient's hospitalization. Lush (1994) has described the plans for incorporation of a 14-item outcome measure based on the Quality Audit Marker (Holzemer, Henry, Stewart, & Janson-Bjerklie, 1993) across the continuum of care in a large health maintenance organization. The resultant three-dimensional (self-care, health care engagement, mental and social well-being) outcome measure will be linked with nursing acuity data and traditional outcome data such as length of stay, complication rate, and cost as well as patient problems and nursing interventions. A research team at Iowa is developing the Nursing Outcomes Classification (NOC)—patient outcomes sensitive to nursing treatments (Johnson & Maas, 1995). Each outcome consists of a label name, a definition, and a set of indicators.

Data presentation. Transformed patient-specific data can be presented in a variety of ways. Numeric data may best be presented as charts or graphs in order to examine trends while the compilation of potential nursing diagnoses generated from patient assessment data may best lend itself to an alphanumeric list format or categorization by human response pattern.

Different types of data lend themselves to a variety of presentation formats. Common among all, however, is the need for presentation at the point of care. Alerts, reminders, and other types of notifications are a type of presentation format integrated with the clinical information system, e.g., notification of the bedside nurse as she or he collects assessment data that the patient is eligible for a particular practice guideline or standard of care within the institution. For example, if the nurse activates the diagnosis of *pain,* the clinical information system could generate a reminder if the patient is eligible for the Agency for Health Care Policy and Research Acute Pain Management Guideline (Acute Pain Management Guideline Panel, 1992) and then provide electronic access to the guideline. In another example, Blaufuss and Tinker (1988) described the implementation of a computer-based falls alert in the HELP system. Using the alert designed by expert clinicians, the decision logic within the system is applied to current and past information to identify a patient at high risk for falling. The user is then guided by the system during the selection of appropriate interventions.

Document-handling technologies such as hypertext are suited to the presentation of data such as policy and procedures related to a particular diagnosis. If the nursing diagnosis of *impaired skin integrity* is activated, appropriate policies and procedures could be browsed using hypertext links. Whereas hypertext is appropriate to textual information, multimedia technology is useful to document procedures. In addition, the use of multimedia technology to visualize the steps of a particular procedure has the potential to decrease the variation in the application of the procedure. Zielstorff et al. (1994) implemented an on-line system in the critical care unit for providing computer-based access to synthesized expert knowledge in the area of troubleshooting pulmonary artery catheter wave forms. Additional implementations are planned in the areas of prevention and management of pressure ulcers and in the management of patients on ventilators. Another potential use of multimedia technology is in the presentation of defining characteristics. The defining characteristics of *altered oral mucous membrane,* which include leukoplakia, hyperemia, and hemorrhagic gingivitis, could be presented appropriately and effectively using video. Audio may be the most effective format for presenting the defining characteristics of *impaired verbal communication* as well as for tracking changes in the status of that nursing diagnosis over time.

Figure 11-2 and the discussion that follows highlight the dynamic nature of the integration and transformation of patient-specific data, agency-specific data, and domain-specific information and knowledge. Refinement of such models has the potential to generate additional design characteristics for information systems that will facilitate the development of nursing knowledge.

CONCLUSIONS

This chapter has described the essential role of classification systems and integrated information systems as building blocks for the development of nursing knowledge. The manner in which these building blocks can facilitate the interrelationships among nursing theory, nursing research, and nursing practice has also been posited. This was done by answering three questions:

- Why have traditional automated nursing systems not fostered the development of nursing knowledge?
- What is the role of classification systems in linking nursing theory, nursing research, and nursing practice?
- How can classification systems and integrated information systems foster the development of nursing knowledge?

However, answers to these questions suggest only a beginning understanding of the relationships among classification systems, integrated information systems, and nursing knowledge. Once the technological building blocks are in place, new types of questions will evolve. For example:

- Is knowledge only created in our heads or is the process of transformation of data, and its reiteration in many forms, a new way of developing nursing knowledge?
- Will integrated information systems help delineate a distinct nursing knowledge or will they blur the distinctions between the areas of knowledge and practice of different disciplines?
- How will nursing skills and competencies change as nurses evolve to the role of knowledgeworker as envisioned by Ozbolt and Graves (1993)? Who will the expert be?

REFERENCES

Abraham, I.L., Fitzpatrick, J.J., & Jewell, J.A. (1986). The artificial intelligence in nursing project: Developing advanced technology for expert care. In K.J. Hannah, M. Reimer, W.C. Mills, & S. Letourneau (Eds.), *Clinical judgment and decision making: The future with nursing diagnosis* (pp. 468-470).

American Medical Association (1993). *Physicians' current procedural terminology.* Chicago: Author.

Blaufuss, J., & Tinker, A. (1988). Computerized falls alert: A new solution to an old problem. *Proceedings of the Symposium for Computer Applications in Medical Care* (pp. 69-73). Los Alamitos, CA: IEEE Computer Society Press.

Bostrom, J., & Wise, L. (1995). The RARIN project: What we learned. *Communicating Nursing Research, 28,* 83.

Brennan, P.F., & Romano, C.A. (1987). Computers and nursing diagnoses: Issues in implementation. *Nursing Clinics of North America, 22,* 935-941.

Campbell, K.E., & Musen, M.A. (1992). Representation of clinical data using SNOMED III and conceptual graphs. In M. Frisse (Ed.), *Proceedings of the Sixteenth Annual Symposium on Computer Applications in Medical Care* (pp. 380-384). New York: McGraw-Hill.

Chang, B.L. (1993). CARIN system: Database for Bayes' theorem applications. *Western Journal of Nursing Research, 15,* 644-648.

Chute, C.G., Atkin, G.E., & Ihrke, D.M. (1992). An empirical evaluation of concept capture. In K.C. Lun, P. DeGoulet, & T.E. Piemme (Eds.), *MedInfo92* (pp. 1469-1474). Geneva: North-Holland.

Cimino, J.J., Hripsak, G., Johnson, S.B., & Clayton, P.D. (1989). Designing an introspective, multipurpose, controlled medical vocabulary. In L. Kingsland (Ed.), *Proceedings of the Thirteenth Annual Symposium on Computer Applications in Medical Care* (pp. 513-518). Los Alamitos, CA: IEEE Computer Society Press.

Clark, J., & Lang, N.M. (1992). Nursing's next advance: An international classification for nursing practice. *International Nursing Review, 39,* 109-112.

Côté, R.A., Rothwell, D.J., Palotay, J.L., & Beckett, R.S. (1993). *SNOMED International.* Northfield, IL: College of American Pathologists.

Dick, R.S., & Steen, E.B. (1991). *The computer-based patient record: An essential technology for health care.* Washington, DC: National Academy Press.

Ehnfors, M. (1994). Nursing information in patient records towards uniform key words for documentation of nursing practice. In S.J. Grobe & E.S.P. Pluyter-Wenting (Eds.), *Nursing informatics: An international overview for nursing in a technological era* (pp. 643-647). Amsterdam: Elsevier.

East, T.D., Young, W.H., & Gardner, R.M. (1992). Digital electronic communication between ICU ventilators and computers and printers. *Respiratory Care, 37,* 1113-1123.

Gillis, P.A., Booth, H., Graves, J.R., Fehlauer, C.S., & Soller, J. (1994). Translating traditional system development principles into process for designing clinical information systems. *International Journal of Technology Assessment in Healthcare, 10,* 235-248.

Graves, J.R., & Corcoran, S. (1989). The study of nursing informatics. *Image: Journal of Nursing Scholarship, 21,* 227-231.

Griffith, H.M., & Robinson, K.R. (1992). Survey of the degree to which critical care nurses are performing Current Procedural Terminology-coded services. *American Journal of Critical Care, 1,* 91-98.

Griffith, H.M., & Robinson, K.R. (1993). Current Procedural Terminology (CPT) coded services provided by nurse specialists. *Image: Journal of Nursing Scholarship, 25,* 178-186.

Grobe, S.J. (1991). Nursing intervention lexicon and taxonomy: Methodological aspects. In E.J.S. Hovenga, K.J. Hannah, K.A. McCormick, & J.S. Ronald (Eds.), *Nursing Informatics 91: Proceedings of the Fourth International Conference on Nursing Use of Computers and Information Science* (pp. 126-131). Berlin: Springer-Verlag.

Grobe, S.J. (1992). Nursing intervention lexicon and taxonomy: Preliminary categorization. In K.C. Lun, P. Degoulet, T.E. Piemme, & O. Rienhoff (Eds.), *MedInfo92* (pp. 981-986). Geneva: North-Holland.

Henry, S.B. (1995). An inductive algorithm approach to knowledge acquisition for expert system development: A pilot study. *Computers in Nursing, 13,* 226-232.

Henry, S.B., Holzemer, W.L., & Gennari, J. (1994). A computer-based approach to knowledge acquisition for expert system development. In S.J. Grobe & E.S.P. Pluyter-Wenting (Eds.), *Nursing informatics: An international overview for nursing in a technological era* (pp. 321-325). Amsterdam: Elsevier.

Henry, S.B., Holzemer, W.L., Reilly, C.A., & Campbell, K.E. (1994). Terms used by nurses to describe patient problems: Can SNOMED III represent nursing concepts in the patient record? *Journal of the American Medical Informatics Association, 1,* 61-74.

Henry, S.B., Holzemer, W.L., Reilly, C.A., Miller, T.J., & Randell, C. (1995). A comparison of Nursing Interventions Classification and Current Procedural Terminology codes for representing nursing interventions in HIV disease. In R.A. Greenes, H.E. Petersen, & D.J. Protti (Eds.), *Proceedings of MedInfo 95* (pp. 131-135). Edmonton, Alberta: Healthcare Computing and Communications Canada, Inc.

Holzemer, W.L., Henry, S.B., Stewart, A., & Janson-Bjerklie, S. (1993). The HIV quality audit marker (HIV-QAM): An outcome measure of hospitalized AIDS patients. *Quality of Life Research, 2,* 99-107.

Iowa Intervention Project (1993). The NIC taxonomy structure. *Image: Journal of Nursing Scholarship, 25,* 187-192.

Iowa Intervention Project (1995). Validation and coding of the NIC taxonomy structure. *Image: Journal of Nursing Scholarship, 27,* 43-49.

Johnson, M. & Maas, M. (1995). Classification of nursing-sensitive patient outcomes. In *Nursing Data Systems: The Emerging Framework.* (pp. 177–183). Washington, DC: American Nurses Association.

Jones, B.T. (1991). Building nursing expert systems using automated rule induction. *Computers in Nursing, 9,* 52-60.

Lange, L.L., & Jacox, A. (1993). Using large data bases in nursing and health policy research. *Journal of Professional Nursing, 9,* 204-211.

Lush, M. (1994). Developing an infrastructure for outcomes analysis with a nursing utilization database in a health maintenance organization. *Proceedings of the 1994 Spring Congress of the American Medical Informatics Association,* Rockville, MD: American Medical Informatics Association.

Martin, K.S., & Scheet, N.J. (1992). *The Omaha System: Applications for community health nursing.* Philadelphia: Saunders.

Martin, K.S., Scheet, N.J., & Stegman, M.R. (1993). Home health clients: Characteristics, outcomes of care, and nursing interventions. *American Journal of Public Health, 83(12),* 1730-1734.

McCloskey, J.C., & Bulechek, G.M. (Eds.). (1992). *Nursing interventions classification* (NIC). St. Louis: Mosby.

McCloskey, J.C., & Bulechek, G.M. (Eds.). (1996). *Nursing interventions classification* (NIC). St. Louis: Mosby.

McCloskey, J.C., & Bulechek, G.M. (1995). Construction and validation of a taxonomy of nursing interventions. In R.A. Greenes, H.E. Petersen, & D.J. Protti (Eds.), *Proceedings of MedInfo 95* (pp. 140-143). Edmonton, Alberta: Healthcare Computing and Communications Canada, Inc.

McCormick, K.A., Lang, N., Zielstorff, R., Milholland, D.K., Saba, V., & Jacox, A. (1994). Toward standard classification schemes for nursing language: Recommendations of the American Nurses Association Steering Committee on Databases to Support Clinical Nursing Practice. *Journal of the American Medical Informatics Association, 1,* 421-427.

McFarland, G.K., & McFarlane, E.A. (1993). *Nursing diagnosis & intervention* (2nd ed.). St. Louis: Mosby.

Mortensen, R., Mantas, J., Manuela, M., Sermeus, W., Nielsen, G.H., & McAvinue, E. (1994). Telematics for health care in the European Union. In S.J. Grobe & E.S.P. Pluyter-Wenting (Eds.), *Nursing informatics: An international overview for nursing in a technological era* (pp. 750-752). Amsterdam: Elsevier.

NANDA. (1994). NANDA nursing diagnoses: Definitions and classification 1995-1996. Philadelphia: Author.

NINR Priority Expert Panel on Nursing Informatics. (1993). *Nursing informatics: Enhancing patient care.* (Publication No. 93-2419). Bethesda, MD: U.S. Department of Health and Human Services, U.S. Public Health Service, National Institutes of Health.

Ozbolt, J.G., Abraham, I.L., & Schultz, S. (1990). Nursing information systems. In E.H. Shortliffe & L.E. Perreault (Eds.), *Medical informatics: Computer applications in health care* (pp. 244-272). Menlo Park, CA: Addison Wesley.

Ozbolt, J.G., Fruchnicht, J.N., & Hayden, J.R. (1994). Toward data standards for clinical nursing information. *Journal of the American Medical Informatics Association, 1,* 175-185.

Ozbolt, J., & Graves, J. (1993). Clinical nursing informatics: developing tools for knowledgeworkers. *Nursing Clinics of North America, 28*(2), 407-425.

Parlocha, P.K. (1995). *Defining a critical path for psychiatric home care patients with a diagnosis of major depressive disorder.* Doctoral Dissertation. University of California, San Francisco.

Petrucci, K., & Canfield, K. (1992). Improving automated care planning with plan libraries: A future use of technology in nursing. *Nursing Economic$, 10,* 297-301.

Prophet, C.M. (1994). Nurses' orders in manual and computerized systems. In S.J. Grobe & E.S.P. Pluyter-Wenting (Eds.), *Nursing informatics: An international overview for nursing in a technological era* (pp. 286-289). Amsterdam: Elsevier.

Rios, H., Delaney, C., Kruckeberg, T., Chung, Y., & Mehmert, P.A. (1991). Validation of defining characteristics of four nursing diagnoses using a computerized data base. *Journal of Professional Nursing, 7,* 293-299.

Saba, V.K. (1992a). The classification of home health care nursing: Diagnoses and interventions. *Caring Magazine, 11*(3), 50-56.

Saba, V.K. (1992b). Home health care classification. *Caring Magazine, 11*(4), 58-60.

Shabot, M.M. (1994). Standardized acquisition of bedside data: The IEEE P1074 medical information bus. In M.M. Shabot & R.M. Gardner (Eds.), *Decision support systems in critical care* (pp. 107-117). New York: Springer-Verlag.

Simpson, R.L., & Waite, R. (1989). NCNIP's system of the future: A call for accountability, revenue control, and national data sets. *Nursing Administration Quarterly, 14,* 72-77.

Turley, J.P. (1992). A framework for the transition from nursing records to a nursing information system. *Nursing Outlook, 40,* 177-181.

U.S. Department of Health and Human Services Acute Pain Management Guideline Panel (1992). *Acute pain management: Operative or medical procedures and trauma. Clinical practice guideline.* (AHCPR Publication No. 92-0047). Rockville, MD: Author.

Werley, H.H., Devine, E.C., & Zorn, C.R. (1988). *Nursing minimum data set data collection manual.* Milwaukee, WI: School of Nursing, University of Wisconsin.

Woolery, L., & Grzymala-Busse, J. (1994). Machine learning for an expert system to predict preterm birth risk. *Journal of the American Medical Informatics Association, 1,* 439-446.

Zielstorff, R.D., Barnett, G.O., Fitzmaurice, J.B., Oliver, D.E., Ford-Carleton, P., Thompson, B.T., Estey, G., Eccles, R., & Martin, M. (1994). A decision support system for troubleshooting pulmonary artery catheter waveforms. In S.J. Grobe & E.S.P. Pluyter-Wenting (Eds.), *Nursing informatics: An international overview for nursing in a technological era* (pp. 362-366). Amsterdam: Elsevier.

Zielstorff, R.D., Hudgings, C.I., & Grobe, S.J., and the National Commission on Nursing Implementation Project (NCNIP) Task Force on Nursing Information Systems (1993). *Next-generation nursing information systems: Essential characteristics for professional practice.* Washington, DC: American Nurses Publishing.

Toward a revolution in thinking: The OPT model of clinical reasoning

DANIEL J. PESUT, JOANNE HERMAN, LATRELL P. FOWLER

The traditional nursing process, based on a linear problem-solving model, is inadequate for nursing practice in the 21st century. We believe that adherence to the nursing process as the mode of practice impedes the acquisition of clinical reasoning skills. The ambiguity of today's nursing practice demands more complex thinking skills than the nursing process accommodates (Miller & Malcolm, 1990). Changes in the discipline of nursing and the health care system require nurses with expert outcome-oriented clinical reasoning skills. The current health care system demands accountability in minimizing client costs and maximizing care outcomes.

OUR VIEWPOINT

Current methods of organizing thinking in nursing depend on the nursing process. This method focuses on problems. Nursing care that is problem-focused is not necessarily outcome-specific. Our view is that nurses need to reason about client outcomes given present state information. Outcomes focus on an end result or desired state. Tests that provide evidence for achievement of desired outcomes are derived from clinical decisions and clinical judgments. Because of our research and academic and clinical experience, we have developed the Outcome-Present state-Test (OPT) model of clinical reasoning. In this model, problems are juxtaposed with outcomes. This juxtaposition is the essential element of clinical reasoning. We believe the OPT model deserves consideration as an alternative to the nursing process.

In this viewpoint chapter, we differentiate clinical reasoning from decision making and define clinical judgment. We describe the OPT model of clinical reasoning and discuss the cognitive operators and strategies that support the thinking activated by the model. We then illustrate the use of the model with an example. Finally, we share our opinions and discuss how this model moves beyond traditional use of the nursing process and represents the essential tension involved in clinical reasoning.

CRITICAL THINKING, CLINICAL DECISION MAKING, AND CLINICAL JUDGMENT

The traditional framework for thinking about clinical situations is the nursing process: assessment, diagnosis, planning, implementation, and evaluation. A variety of terms have been used to describe the thinking involved in nursing process. Hamers, Abu-Saad, and Halfens (1994) underscore the disparity and confusion in the nursing literature about terms and definitions used in clinical decision making. These terms include diagnostic reasoning, problem solving, critical thinking, decision making, and clinical reasoning. The outcomes of each of these thinking processes vary. Diagnoses come from diagnostic reasoning. Answers result from problem solving. Decision making yields approaches for care. Clinical judgments result from clinical reasoning (Fowler, 1994). Regardless of the disparity of terms used to describe clinical decision making, all of the thinking processes are based on a foundation of critical thinking.

Since the National League for Nursing (NLN) revised its criteria for evaluation of baccalaureate programs in nursing to include critical thinking, communication, and therapeutic interventions, there has been a flood of articles on critical thinking in nursing (NLN, 1992). Information about critical thinking has fueled debate about the viability of the nursing process. People are seeking ways to incorporate critical thinking into nursing curricula and nursing practice. Consequently, there is a demand for reassessment of the usefulness of the nursing process model

(Ford, & Profetto-McGrath, 1994: Frisch, 1994; Jones & Brown, 1993; McHugh, 1986; Radwin, 1995; Tanner, Benner, Chelsa, & Gordon, 1993).

In fact, evidence suggests that expert nurses do not use the nursing process (Brykczynski, 1991; Jones & Brown, 1993; Tschikota, 1993). Additional evidence supports the fact that nursing students do not gain skill in clinical reasoning during their educational program (Brooks & Shepherd, 1992; Kintgen-Andrews, 1991). As debates continue, authors (Katoaoka-Yahira & Saylor, 1994) propose critical thinking models for nursing education and not for guiding thinking in practice or patient care. Such models do not clarify the nursing process. Many proposed models focus more on the critical thinking attributes of the nurse rather than on the clinical reasoning process used to achieve patient outcomes.

Radwin (1995) criticizes the use of linear analytic models of thinking and argues for models that involve "knowing the patient" (p. 21). In our opinion, any model that fails to include the patient as a central focus fails to contribute something important to the discipline of nursing. If we continue to focus on the linear problem-solving nursing process and critical thinking skills of the nurse, we will maintain the status quo and fall into the trap of studying ourselves rather than clients within the context of our practice. There is a need to reconceptualize our thinking about clinical reasoning.

We concur with the Delphi Report (1990), which defines critical thinking as purposeful self-regulatory judgment that gives reasoned consideration to evidence, contexts, conceptualizations, methods, and criteria. Clinical reasoning in nursing is critical thinking embedded in practice (Fowler & Herman, 1995). Specifically, we define *clinical reasoning* as the concurrent, creative, critical thinking processes nurses use to juxtapose and test the match between a patient's present state and his or her desired outcome state. *Clinical decision making* is the process of selecting interventions from a repertoire of actions that facilitate the achievement of a desired outcome state. Clinical decision making supports clinical reasoning. We believe our definitions of clinical reasoning and clinical decision making describe more explicitly the critical thinking embedded in nursing practice.

Clinical reasoning that focuses on outcomes needs to replace clinical reasoning that focuses on problems. Holistic nursing care involves the juxtaposition of problem states and outcome states. As long as a problem-solving process is ascendent in nursing, we will not be able to move ahead with reflective judgment that contributes to quality patient care. These models of the past need to be replaced with outcome specification models (Pesut, 1989). We encourage a revolution in clinical thinking. However, such a revolution requires leadership and the development of models that move beyond rote application of the problem-oriented nursing process. We have developed an alternative model to nursing process, which we believe more accurately reflects the reality of thinking required in clinical practice.

REFLECTION: THINKING ABOUT THINKING

Think back to the last time you made clinical decisions about patients. Did you gather all the information about the patient, organize that information into a problem list, develop goals for the patient, select a group of interventions, implement the interventions, and evaluate their effectiveness? Did you organize your care around the problem or did you intervene to achieve an outcome? Were your actions really guided by the nursing process or did you use some other strategy to make decisions about what you would do? What was the nature of your purposeful self-regulatory judgments about this situation?

In our opinion, the nursing process today focuses on problems rather than on outcomes. We argue that experienced nurses do not use the nursing process. Our conjecture is that experienced nurses consider problems, solutions, and outcomes *concurrently*. It is a challenge to explain a process that occurs both concurrently and iteratively. Perhaps this is one reason why the nursing process has endured despite criticism. Following is a description of our model. Keep in mind that the process we describe is recursive rather than linear and occurs in the context of "knowing the patient."

THE OPT MODEL

Using the theory derivation method described by Walker and Avant (1995), the OPT model was derived from the work of Miller, Galanter, and Pribam (1960), Dilts, Epstein, and Dilts (1991), empirical evidence from research involving home health nurses (Fowler, 1994), and academic experience teaching clinical reasoning to generic and registered nurse completion students (Herman, Pesut, & Conard, 1994; Pesut & Herman, 1991, 1992). Clinical reasoning is a nonlinear iterative process as depicted in Figure 12-1.

Clinical reasoning is best represented by use of the OPT model (*O*utcome state of the client, *P*resent state of the client, and *T*esting for the match or mismatch of the two states). In the OPT model, reflection is a component

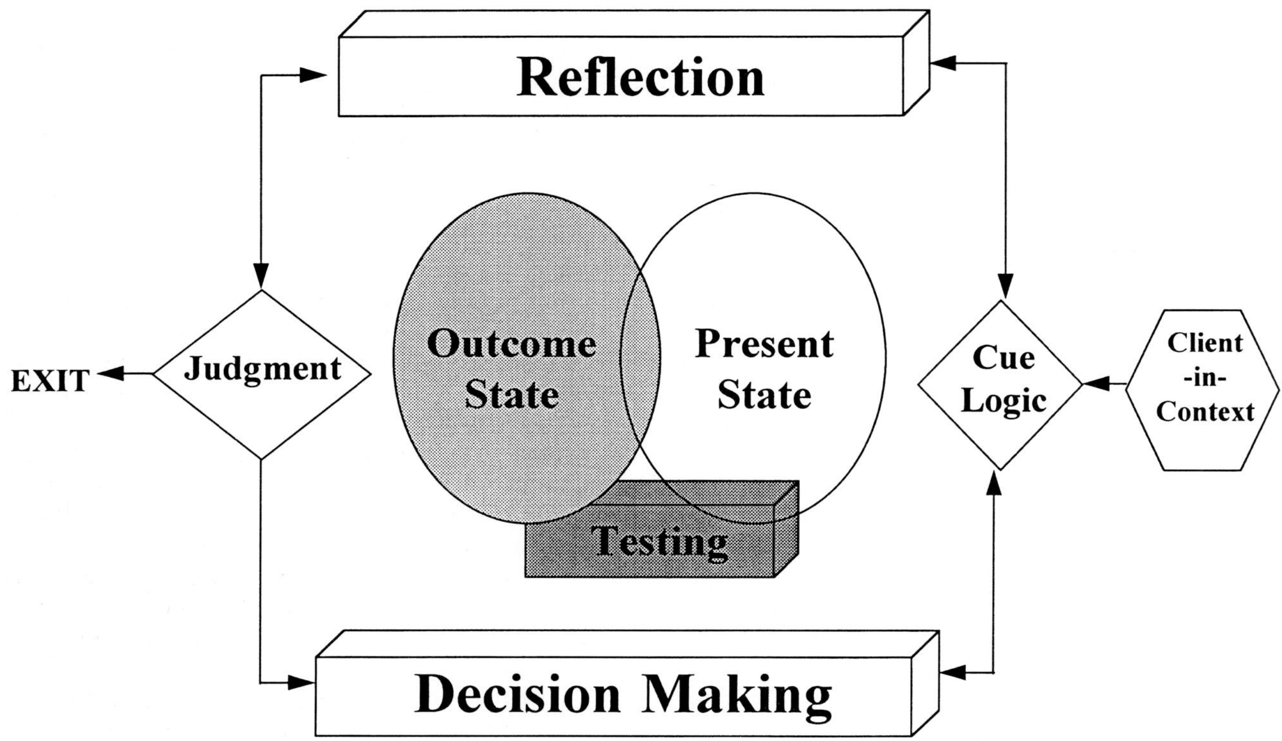

Fig. 12-1. The Outcome, Present state, Test (OPT) model of clinical reasoning. (© 1995 Pesut, Herman, Fowler)

of executive cognitive control processes and consists of self, task, and strategy knowledge as well as skills in monitoring, analyzing, predicting, planning, evaluating, and revising (Bruner, 1983; Flavell, 1979; Sternberg, 1988; Worrell, 1990). In our academic, clinical, and empirical experience, we have noted that nurses use a variety of means to juxtapose outcome and present state information about clients. Cue logic is one strategy nurses use to organize data about clients in context. Cue logic can be inductive, deductive, or a combination of induction and deduction that frames the test. In this model, test is a reflexive comparison of the client's outcome state to his or her present state. Clinical judgments are conclusions and decisions based on the test. Clinical decision making is the selection of nursing interventions that enhance clients' transitions from present states to desired outcome states. Clinical decisions are made in the context of nursing actions. If the match between present state and outcome state is unsatisfactory, reflection reactivates concurrent processing of available cues related to the client in context. Concurrent processing includes critical and creative decision making about interventions. Concurrent reflection and clinical decision making continue until there is a satisfactory test that supports a match between a client's present and desired outcome states. If a match exists, the nurse can exit this reasoning task.

The dynamics of the OPT model: cognitive operators

Clinical reasoning, decision making, and judgments are accomplished through the use of cognitive operators and strategies (Fonteyn, Kupiers, & Grobe, 1993; Fowler, 1994). Cognitive operators are reasoning processes that produce judgments about incoming information. Cognitive operators facilitate self-regulatory judgments. Clinical reasoning engages these operators as nurses use cognitive strategies to make clinical judgments. A closer analysis of clinical reasoning data reveals specific cognitive operators at work. Fowler (1994) developed definitions and descriptions of cognitive operators used by nurses. When asked to think aloud about client situations in a home health practice, nurses employed the following cognitive operators: (a) *describing*—presenting details of the representation of a situation; (b) *evaluating*—comparing the presence or absence of cues with some standard, prototype, or previous experience; (c) *explaining*—providing reasons or a rationale for a representation or an action; (d) *connecting*—considering possible relationships among cues or findings; (e) *planning*—formulating possible future actions; and (f) *judging*—formulating conclusions based on evaluation or contrast analysis (Fowler, 1994). As you reflect on your own clinical reasoning, which of these cognitive operators do you use most often and which are less familiar? In addition to cognitive operators, cognitive strategies support clinical reasoning.

The dynamics of the OPT model: cognitive strategies

Fowler (1994) defined cognitive strategies as heuristics that individuals naturally use to reduce cognitive strain when processing multiple cues. She identified and defined six cognitive strategies: (a) *induction*—reasoning from specific cues toward a general judgement; (b) *deduction*—reasoning from a general premise toward a conclusion; (c) *cue connection*—grouping two or more cues to form a pattern to guide inferencing; (d) *hypothesizing*—forming possible relationships among contrasting evidence; (e) *prototypical reasoning*—using past cases as reference points; and (f) *reflexive comparison*—making judgments about the state of a situation after gauging the presence or absence of some quality against a standard usually using the current case as a reference criterion (Fowler, 1994). The simultaneous use of operators with cognitive strategies provides a means to explain how nurses concurrently juxtapose present state information with desired outcomes and make clinical decisions that support nursing actions and clinical judgments.

Using the OPT model in practice

The OPT model relies on the use of cue logic, framing, and testing to juxtapose the client's outcome state with his or her present state. Clinical evidence about the client in context is processed according to the nurse's cue logic, which frames the test. Testing involves a comparison of the present situation to the desirable outcome state. Testing is accomplished through the use of prototypes or reflexive comparison (Fowler, 1994). Concurrent reflection and clinical decision making continue until there is a satisfactory test that supports a match between the client's present and outcome states. If a match exists, the nurse can exit this reasoning task. Consider the following client-in-context case example.

> Cora James is a 65-year-old grandmother living in substandard housing. She presents in the clinic with the following cues: progressive weight loss, productive cough, oral temperature 101°F, weight 106 lbs, extended family living in substandard housing, five young children at risk for infectious diseases, two child-bearing daughters and an alcoholic son living with her. Her records show that she is supposed to be receiving medication for tuberculosis. The nurse evaluates her clinical status and determines a plan of care for this family situation.

How would you approach this case using the nursing process? The nursing process is valuable in that it makes explicit the problem and the present situation. For example, one could focus on symptoms of pulmonary infection, possible noncompliance with the medication regimen, weight loss, family at risk for contacting and spreading tuberculosis, and questionable availability of resources.

Clinically, focusing on the present state or presenting problems does not provide direction for action. Once outcomes are specified, the path of action is clear and the tests of achievement are made explicit. Transforming problems into outcomes involves thinking beyond the present to the end results of action. This outcomes specification step is a missing link in the nursing process and a strength of the OPT model.

Consider use of the OPT model and monitor your thinking processes as you decide how to approach this situation. For example, the outcomes important in this case are that the infection is clear; that the patient is afebrile, taking medication as prescribed, and has adequate resources and transportation for follow-up; and that screening and treatment are provided for family members. Focusing on the outcome of taking medication as prescribed, the nurse juxtaposes the present state with outcome state and uses decision making to concurrently generate possible actions. For example, the nurse might determine that the client does not have resources to obtain the medication. The nurse could then implement a plan to obtain medication for the client using social service resources. Another possibility is that the client is unable to remember to take medication. The nurse could develop a plan for a family member to manage administration of the medication. Iteratively, the nurse uses mental prototypes and reflexive comparisons about past clients with successful outcomes to make judgments about what to do in the present situation to achieve the desired outcome.

The *test* will come later when the nurse compares the present state to desired outcome. Now the present state is that a family member obtained medication from social services and reported administering it as prescribed. The outcome of taking medication as prescribed has been achieved. The nurse can go on to another reasoning task.

Based on this example, the outcome, present state, and test were made explicit. Through the use of cognitive operators and strategies, reflection and clinical decision making continued until testing revealed a match and judgment was made that the desired outcome was achieved. The nurse chooses interventions to bring client and family from their present state to a healthier outcome state. Once judgments of the present state match closely the desired outcomes, the nurse exits.

SUMMARY

It is time to move beyond the nursing process. We believe the OPT model differs considerably from the nursing process. The model has several strengths. First, it is built on a foundation of reflective judgment and is derived from empirical data. Second, the OPT model is iterative and recursive, thus honoring the holistic nature of nursing. Third, the OPT model approaches patient situations in terms of cue logic and outcome specification. Fourth, the model identifies the cognitive operators and strategies involved in making clinical decisions and judgments. Finally, it is parsimonious and elegant.

We recognize that the OPT model needs further development. Education and documentation strategies need to be developed to support the model. We invite your comments and dialogue. The OPT model is one alternative to the nursing process. We believe it supports a revolution in clinical reasoning and will guide nurses' clinical reasoning into the 21st century.

REFERENCES

Brooks, K.L., & Shepherd, J.M. (1992). Professionalism versus general critical thinking abilities of senior nursing students in four types of nursing curricula. *Journal of Professional Nursing, 8*(2), 87-95.

Bruner, J. (1983). *In search of mind.* New York: Harper and Row.

Brykcynski, K. (1991). Judgement strategies for coping with ambiguous clinical situations encountered in primary family care. *Journal of the American Academy of Nurse Practitioners, 3,* 79-84.

Delphi Report—Critical thinking: A statement of expert consensus for purposes of educational assessment and instruction (1990). Research findings and recommendations prepared for the American Philosophical Association. Newark, DE. P. Facione, Project Director, ERIC Document No. ED 315-42.

Dilts, D.B., Epstein, T. A., & Dilts, D.W. (1991). *Tools for dreamers: Strategies for creativity and the structure of innovative operations.* Cupertino, CA: Meta Publications.

Flavell, J. (1979). Metacognitive and cognitive monitoring: A new era of cognitive-developmental inquiry. *American Psychologist, 34,* 906-911.

Fonteyn, M., Kupiers, B., & Grobe, S.J. (1993). A description of the use of think aloud method and protocol analysis. *Qualitative Health Research, 3*(4), 430-441.

Ford, J., & Profetto-McGrath, J. (1994). A model for critical thinking within the context of curriculum as praxis. *Journal of Nursing Education, 33*(8), 341-344.

Fowler, L.P. (1994). *Clinical reasoning of home health nurses: A verbal protocol analysis.* Unpublished doctoral dissertation, University of South Carolina, Columbia, SC.

Fowler, L., & Herman, J. (1995, June 24). *Using reflective verbalization as a strategy for promoting nurses' critical thinking.* Paper presented at University of New Hampshire Fifth Annual Institute on Critical Thinking, Durham, NH.

Frisch, N. (1994). The nursing process revisited [Editorial]. *Nursing Diagnosis, 5*(2), 51.

Hamers, J., Abu-Saad, H., & Halfens, R. (1994). Diagnostic process and decision-making in nursing: A literature review. *Journal of Professional Nursing, 10*(3), 154-163.

Herman, J., Pesut, D.J., & Conard, L. (1994). Using metacognitive skills: The quality audit. *Nursing Diagnosis, 5*(2), 56-64.

Jones, S.A., & Brown, L.N. (1993). Alternative views on defining critical thinking through the nursing process. *Holistic Nursing Practice, 7*(3), 71-75.

Katoaoka-Yahira, M., & Saylor, C. (1994). A critical thinking model for nursing judgement. *Journal of Nursing Education, 33*(8), 351-356.

Kintgen-Andrews, J. (1991). Critical thinking and nursing education: Perplexities and insights. *Journal of Nursing Education, 30*(4), 152-157.

McHugh, M. (1986). Nursing process: Musings on the method. *Holistic Nursing Practice, 1*(1), 21-28.

Miller, G., Galanter, E., & Pribam, K. (1960). *Plans and the structure of human behavior.* New York: Holt, Rinehart, and Winston.

Miller, M.A., & Malcolm, N.S. (1990). Critical thinking in the nursing curriculum. *Nursing and Health Care, 11*(2), 67-73.

National League for Nursing, Council for baccalaureate and higher degree programs. (1992). *Criteria for the evaluation of baccalaureate and higher degree programs in nursing* (6th Ed.). (NLN Publication #15-1252.) New York: Author.

Pesut, D.J. (1989). Aim vs blame: Using an outcome specification model. *Journal of Psychosocial Nursing and Mental Health Services, 27*(5), 26-30.

Pesut, D.J., & Herman, J.A. (1991). *Learning styles and teaching strategies: Creating a match.* Unpublished final report, University of South Carolina Office of the Provost, Columbia, SC.

Pesut, D.J., & Herman, J.A. (1992). Metacognitive skills in diagnostic reasoning. *Nursing Diagnosis, 3*(4), 148-154.

Radwin, L.E. (1995). Conceptualizations of decision-making in nursing: Analytic models and knowing the patient. *Nursing Diagnosis, 6*(1), 16-22.

Sternberg, R. (1988). *The triarchic mind.* New York: Viking Press.

Tanner, C.A., Benner, P., Chelsa, C., & Gordon, D. (1993). The phenomenology of knowing the patient. *Image, 25*(4), 273-280.

Tschikota, S. (1993). The clinical decision making processes of student nurses. *Journal of Nursing Education, 32*(9), 389-398.

Walker, L.O., & Avant, K.C. (1995). *Strategies for theory construction in nursing.* Norwalk, CT: Appleton and Lange.

Worrell, P. (1990). Metacognition: Implications for instruction in nursing education. *Journal of Nursing Education, 29,* 170-175.

Benchmarking: A tool for management decision making

CAROLYN HOPE SMELTZER, SCOTT LEIGHTY, RUTH WILLIAMS-BRINKLEY

The globalization of industries and the rapid advance of technology have resulted in a world in which change is a way of life. Corporations in many industries have responded to increasing competition by focusing an enormous amount of resources on change, through total quality management, reengineering, and other processes. Benchmarking is an important tool that has evolved over the past 15 years through the work of leading corporations that have continued the search for superior performance. With tremendous changes in the U.S. health care sector in this decade, benchmarking has become an essential source of information for managers in health care organizations as well.

HISTORY: SIGNIFICANCE OF CHANGE

Fundamental changes in the financing and delivery of health care have resulted from the rapid growth in health care expenditures. In 1980, national health expenditures represented 9.2% of the gross domestic product, while in 1994 it represented 15.8% (Standard & Poor, 1994). While medical price inflation slowed to 5.4% in 1993 from a peak of 9% in 1990, it still outpaced the general rate of inflation, which was 2.9% in 1993 (Standard & Poor, 1994). This tremendous growth in health care spending has been fueled by many factors, including an aging population, the proliferation of expensive medical technologies, and the expansion of publicly financed health insurance programs such as Medicare and Medicaid. The effects on private industry and government bodies have been significant: Major corporations complain that health care costs for employees and retirees hinder their ability to compete with foreign competition, while Congress debates sweeping changes in Medicare and Medicaid to eliminate in excess of $200 billion in spending by the year 2000 ("The State of Health Care in America," 1995). Meanwhile, employers have responded by embracing managed care programs in order to slow the growth of health care premiums. In fact, enrollment in health maintenance organizations (HMOs) had grown to 52.4 million members, or 20.3% of the population, by June 1994 (Marion Merrell Dow, 1994).

Increasing managed care penetration and decreasing reimbursement from government programs has had significant effects on health care providers. HMO inpatient utilization is less than two thirds the national average (Standard and Poor, 1994), which has contributed to a significant excess of available hospital beds. One result has been consolidation in the hospital industry, with the number of U.S. hospitals declining by 9% to 5,292 from 1982 to 1994. Meanwhile, home health care has become the fastest growing segment of the health care industry, with an estimated $40.1 billion in expenditures in 1994 ("The State of Health Care," 1995).

RESPONSE TO CHANGE

Why is the provider industry consolidating and reorganizing so rapidly? In order to maintain growth and profitability, a provider has three options: increase prices, increase volume, or decrease costs. In today's environment, in which customers have consolidated to increase their leverage, government has committed to reductions in health care spending, and a large percentage of the population is enrolled in managed care plans, health care providers cannot remain viable by relying on price and volume increases. They have quickly come to the realization that increased productivity, cost reduction, and the elimination of excess capacity must play a leading role.

Cost containment cannot alone explain the dramatic

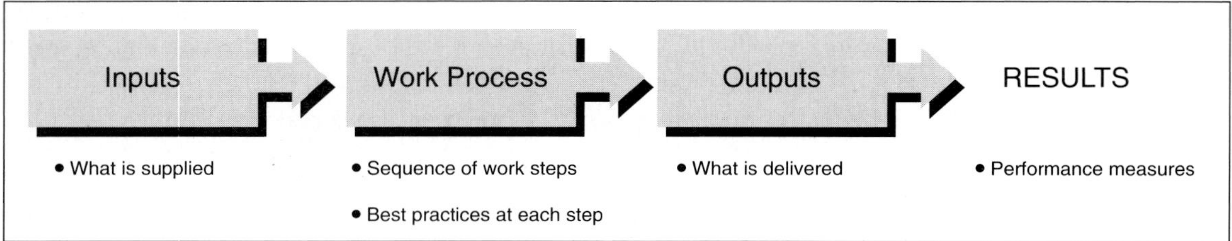

Fig. 13-1. The benchmarking process.

changes occurring in today's health care providers. Managed care customers press for reduced prices, yet demand that providers also compete on the basis of quality and service. Achieving an attractive blend of cost, quality, and service is driving significant changes in most health care organizations. Experience from other industries has shown that the most successful organizations have remained leaders through a continual process of changing and adapting to their environments. Expertise in benchmarking is one consistent feature of such leading organizations today. In order to meet the needs of today's health care customers, radical changes are being made by providers, and the current environment favors those organizations that seek superior performance and manage change effectively. As with leaders in other industries, successful health care organizations increasingly rely on benchmarking to maintain a competitive edge.

BENCHMARKING DEFINED

Benchmarking is a tool used for the achievement of superior performance through continuous improvement. Xerox Corporation, a leader in the field of benchmarking, has used the following definition: "Benchmarking is the continuous process of measuring products, services, and practices against the toughest competitors or those companies recognized as industry leaders" (Camp, 1989). Benchmarking involves establishing operating goals based on industry best-practice standards and adopting superior practices in order to improve one's own operations significantly.

WHAT TO BENCHMARK

It is common for line managers and administrators to view benchmarking only in terms of *performance measures,* and experience with a broad range of our clients has reflected this approach (Camp, 1995). Performance measures (*see* Results in Figure 13-1) offer a snapshot for managers to compare their results with others in the field. However, performance measures do not offer insight into *how* another organization has achieved superior results. Thus, managers are often left with the problem of explaining a "performance gap" that is identified through comparisons of performance measures without an understanding of the *processes* that achieved the superior results. Most experts now believe that the focus of benchmarking should be on business processes, because ultimately it will be the adoption of proven practices and technologies to one's internal operations that will result in increased value to one's customers. Performance measures are important, however, in identifying superior performers and in estimating the magnitude of improvement necessary once superior practices have been benchmarked.

Why do health care providers typically focus less on processes than on performance measures? Performance measures are generally inexpensive, readily available, and seemingly offer a quick answer to the question "How are we doing?" In addition, because providers for many years enjoyed consistent growth in the absence of serious pressures on operating margins and profitability, cost containment and productivity gains were less important than they are today. This resulted in a management orientation on budgets in which planning was done based on past performance, with allowances for inflation and growth. In an expanding market, an internal focus was effective because any necessary cost reductions were generally minor and were executed through the budget process. Fundamental changes in operating processes were rarely required. While suitable in its day, this approach is no longer desirable because of increased competitive pressures and a volatile health care marketplace. An external focus on customers, competitors, and industry best-practice organizations, including the continual search for superior practices, is now a key to industry leadership.

TYPES OF BENCHMARKING

There are several major categories of benchmarking from which to choose, including internal benchmarking, competitive benchmarking, and functional benchmarking. *Internal benchmarking* involves comparisons among similar operations within one's own organization. With the rapid consolidation of health care providers, especially hospitals, opportunities for benchmarking with members of a system or network are increasingly available. Our experience has also shown that pursuing internal benchmarking within a single hospital can also be valuable. A typical example would be a hospital that measures trends in certain performance measures, such as expense/adjusted discharge, over a period of 5 years. The advantage of this method is that the underlying practices that produce the best results over time should be known to the institution. The main disadvantage of this method is that, by definition, its focus is strictly internal.

The next level of analysis, *competitive benchmarking*, assumes an external focus on best-practice competitors. In the hospital industry, it is also common for institutions to include other hospitals that are not considered direct competitors due to geography; this follows from the extensive similarities found among most hospitals throughout the country. Panels of hospitals with similar sizes, services, and patient acuity can be compiled readily from various databases, facilitating comparisons of processes across institutions.

Competitive benchmarking has several advantages over internal benchmarking, the most important of which is that it capitalizes on the significant amount of information available on the processes employed by best-practice organizations that achieve superior levels of quality, service, or productivity. Another benefit is that competitive benchmarking requires an external focus, which reduces the organization's attention on itself and increases its attention on customers. Finally, this tool provides a means to gauge how key competitors fare versus various process and performance standards.

An example of competitive benchmarking with which we are familiar involves an acute-care hospital (hospital A) that was interested in making significant reductions in its budget without sacrificing quality or service. Having identified a nearby hospital (hospital B) that appeared to have much lower costs, the leadership from hospital A decided that further evaluation of hospital B's processes was desirable. Following a detailed examination, it was found that hospital B had succeeded in significantly standardizing and reducing the utilization of clinical resources, thereby gaining efficiencies and reducing costs. Hospital A is now in the process of adopting hospital B's clinical resource management practices.

Functional benchmarking compares the methods of one's organization with similar processes in other industries. It also offers the greatest potential rewards through the discovery of the best practices that industry has to offer. A classic example in health care is bar coding, which is used extensively to track the flow of patients and information, as well as to ensure accurate medical records. Bar coding originated in the grocery industry as a mechanism to improve distribution, inventory tracking, and customer check-out. Another example of functional benchmarking is the use of practices employed by auto racing pit-stop crews to evaluate operating room practices. When viewed from a process perspective, the objectives of pit crews and operating room teams are similar, including minimizing cycle times and effectively managing materials inventories.

These examples illustrate the importance of resisting the "not invented here" mentality that prevails in many organizations. An external focus combined with a process orientation provides avenues to performance improvement that would otherwise be unavailable to an organization.

BENCHMARKING PROCESS

The benchmarking process can be divided into four phases (see the box below), each of which consists of several steps. The *planning* phase involves three key steps: deciding what to benchmark, identifying whom to benchmark, and gathering data and observing best practices. In order to decide what to benchmark, it is important to have identified and prioritized key work processes. In our experience, the prioritization of processes is often enabled through the use of performance measures, which can help to identify areas of weakness. Identifying whom to benchmark will first require a decision as to the type of benchmarking to be done: internal, competitive, or func-

BENCHMARKING PROCESS

- Planning
- Analysis
- Integration
- Action

SAMPLE SCREENING CRITERIA

- <500 beds
- Provide cardiac surgery services
- At least level II trauma center
- Case Mix Index ≤ 1.6
- Recognized industry leaders
- Urban or suburban location

tional. Once this has been accomplished, it may be helpful to establish criteria in order to screen the pool of potential benchmark organizations. These criteria will vary and will be driven by the desired goals and the processes to be benchmarked. Possible criteria for a competitive benchmarking process involving a large acute-care hospital are outlined in the box above.

Gathering data involves a thorough review of relevant literature and on-line databases. In addition, industry associations and watchdog groups, securities analysts, consultants, suppliers, and the benchmark organization itself can serve as important sources of information on benchmark organizations. A number of benchmarking clearinghouses have also been developed in the past 5 years that provide a range of services and cover a wide range of industries.

The *analysis* phase consists of estimating the current performance gap and projecting future performance. Once benchmarking organizations have been identified and data collected, analysis will help to determine how much better their best practices are than the current internal practices. Further, these data should be used to project the magnitude of performance improvement that would result from the adoption of best practices, as well as the implications for the organization.

The *integration* phase of the benchmarking results involves extensive communication of the findings to all relevant constituencies in the organization. This is a critical step to maximize buy-in and commitment from others. In addition, the findings must be translated into operational statements that describe specifically how internal practices must change in order to adopt the characteristics of best-practice organizations.

Finally, the *action* phase involves the development of detailed implementation plans for the adoption of best practices, including monitoring results and communicating with key stakeholders on a consistent basis. Continual updating of benchmarks should also be done in order to keep pace with industry changes.

PERFORMANCE MEASURES

In our experience, most hospitals typically benchmark specific performance measures against other hospitals. The data needed to perform such comparisons are readily available from a number of vendors, consultants, and publicly available sources.

Performance measures can be oriented to costs, quality, or service. Historically, most benchmarking in hospitals has been done on the basis of productivity in an effort to monitor expenses. Regional and national databases to facilitate comparisons of quality and service have only recently become available; however, as the enrollment in HMOs grows and competition among health care providers intensifies, hospitals will be evaluated increasingly against these criteria.

Most performance measures that track productivity have an input and an output component. Typical inputs and outputs used in a hospital environment are provided in Table 13-1. These inputs and outputs can be combined in a variety of ways to create performance measures used by administrators and patient care executives. Examples include salary cost per full-time equivalent (FTE), worked hours per patient day, and total expense per discharge.

Performance measures are of great importance to leadership for at least two reasons. First, they provide a mechanism to evaluate the ongoing operations of an organization over time. For a manager with a broad scope of responsibility, performance measures are an efficient means for tracking performance at a macro level across functions. Performance measures also provide executives with the ability to compare their organizations against others in the industry. This type of competitive benchmarking is widespread, especially in an environment of increased competition. However, external benchmarking based solely on performance measures is not always straightforward and usually leaves important questions unanswered.

When comparing productivity measures across institutions, both external and internal consistency are of

Table 13-1 Common performance measures in acute care hospitals

Inputs	Outputs
• Average length of stay • Total worked hours • Total expense • Total salary cost • Total supply cost	• Full-time equivalent • Patient day • Discharge

great importance. From an external perspective, relevant comparisons require that both inputs and outputs be measured consistently in all institutions included in the benchmarking. One common issue involves the grouping of input data (e.g., salary dollars, worked hours, supply costs), which is often done by department. Due to organizational and operational differences between hospitals, the consistency of departmental groupings for inputs can vary significantly, thus affecting any resulting comparisons.

From an internal perspective, productivity measures should be consistent with the objectives of the organization and the needs of customers. For example, measuring productivity by tracking FTEs/patient day may not be consistent with the drivers of success in some markets. In markets with a high percentage of per-case reimbursement, the organization should be focused on providing the most cost-effective care per case. In such cases, discharges may be a more appropriate output unit than patient days. In markets in which per-diem reimbursement predominates, patient days may be an important indicator; however, expenses are likely to be more relevant than FTEs. Customers are less concerned with a hospital's number of FTEs than with its costs. Further, while FTEs are an indicator of costs, they can be misleading. In reengineering their patient care operations, some of our clients have reduced labor expenses significantly while increasing the number of FTEs. An increasing number of hospitals are now examining productivity on an expense per discharge basis for these reasons.

In summary, hospital-specific performance measures are an extremely important tool for managing day-to-day operations. They are also valuable in identifying suitable partners to benchmark in the hospital industry. However, performance measures do not provide information on *how* best-practice institutions achieve superior performance. In order to understand how superior results are achieved by others and how one's own organization can benefit from this knowledge, competitive and functional benchmarking must be done based on *processes.*

PATIENT CARE PROCESSES

Benchmarking processes provide insight into the practices of organizations that have achieved superior results and provide an excellent foundation for subsequent operations improvement and reengineering initiatives (Table 13-2). Our experience has shown that many hospitals desire to benchmark processes with other hospitals because of the similar nature of their operations. While perhaps limiting in terms of breakthrough potential, this type of benchmarking can offer significant potential yield along the dimensions of cost, quality, and service. One such process is the administration or provision of medications to patients. When examining the medication administration process, it is important to benchmark not only the cost of the medication itself, but also the steps involved from order inception (prescription) through procurement and administration or provision of the drug to the patient. This entire process most often occurs across at least two or more functional operating units within the organization (patient care unit and pharmacy); therefore, it is essential that each step be examined and improvements made to the *entire process,* rather than just to the steps that occur in either functional unit. The gains in cost, quality, and service to customers (patients and others) are usually more significant when the boundaries of the process are defined and the worksteps evaluated across functional groups.

While not yet used in many health care organizations, patient care executives have begun to recognize the value of process benchmarking within and across industries. As the health care market continues its pace of rapid change, process benchmarking will be an important tool

Table 13-2 Sample patient care processes

Illness management		
Diagnosis/treatment	**Operative procedures**	**Customer service**
Order entry	Preoperative preparation	Patient processing
Order processing	Surgery	admission
Scheduling	Postoperative care	discharge
Patient preparation	Follow-up clinic appointment	Room preparation/maintenance
Treatment/medication/procedure administration		Meal distribution
Test results reporting		Pastoral care
Documentation		Social work

to achieve superior performance and stay ahead of the competition.

SUMMARY

Benchmarking is one of the most important tools available to health care leadership to provide information for management decision making. As the environment in which health care organizations compete continues to evolve, they too must change. Further, one of the most effective methods to ensure successful organizational change is to learn from others who have addressed similar issues. Among the industry leaders, benchmarking is becoming part of the organizational culture to achieve superior long-term performance. It is an ongoing process—part of the continual search for excellence.

REFERENCES

Camp, R. (1989). *Benchmarking: The search for industry best practices that lead to superior performance.* White Plains, NY: Quality Resources.

Camp, R. (1995). *Business process benchmarking: Finding and implementing best practices.* Milwaukee, WI: ASQC Quality Press.

Marion Merrell Dow. (1994). *Managed care digest update edition.* Kansas, MO: Author.

Standard & Poor's health care products & services basic analysis (1994, October 6).

The state of health care in America, 1995. (1995). *Business and Health Magazine, 13*(3) (Suppl C).

The Internet and electronic information

SUSAN M. SPARKS

The Internet, a major component of the "information superhighway," offers nurses great opportunity for access to information and instruction, for delivery of nursing care, and for collaboration in the development of new nursing knowledge. This chapter discusses some of the technological and social issues related to nurses and their travels on the Internet, including some barriers to Internet use.

The Internet consists of a large number of smaller computer networks. In April 1995, it was estimated that 56,800 networks and 5 million host computers comprised the Internet. These networks and computers share data, information, computer programs, and various kinds of personal communication. Terminology related to the Internet is defined in the box on page 100.

Most of the Internet activity is generated in the United States. In April 1995, the United States accounted for an estimated 32,400 networks. Canada, the United Kingdom, and Australia also account for significant usage; and European, Asian, and Eastern European participation is increasing rapidly. Access to and use of the Internet in African, South and Central American, and Caribbean countries is growing, although more slowly than in other places. The total number of non-U.S. networks connected to the Internet was estimated to be 24,400 in April 1995.

In its earliest years, the Internet (then called ARPANet [Advanced Research Projects Administration Network]) was used for U.S. military and security projects. Later, with management by the National Science Foundation, research and educational institutions were granted access and Internet usage increased. In the late 1980s networks in other countries were allowed to link with the U.S. component of Internet. In the early 1990s, when commercial organizations and individual subscribers were allowed to participate, the amount of Internet activity burst, increasing far beyond the most educated projections. While research and educational institutions still account for the greatest number of Internet users, there has been a steady and huge increase in the number of commercial subscribers. Of the business enterprises on the Internet, an increasing number are charging for access and using what they consider to be secure communications to protect the passage of credit card and other private information. Individual subscriptions are also increasing rapidly. America Online added nearly a million subscribers during a 6-month period in 1994 alone. In January 1995, there were an estimated 6.3 million individual subscribers connected by CompuServe, America Online, and Prodigy.

Now not only is there more and more Internet traffic, but there are also growing kinds of electronic resources. To satisfy increasing appetites for features and functionality, new products are on numerous computer "drawing boards" and in development. The "stuff" of science fiction is becoming reality, or virtual reality. By the time this chapter is published it may even be becoming commonplace.

A technological advance called the World Wide Web (WWW, W3, or Web) was released in the fall of 1993. Web technology (a hypermedia, graphical interface to the Internet) brings together text, data, graphics, still and motion images, sound, live video and audio, executable computer programs, and hypermedia. Web technology now permits experimentation with the use of simultaneous multisite realtime multimedia conferencing, including live audio and video. While these technological advances allow us to do much now, they encourage the vision of the integration of media into one platform, bringing together the computer with broadcast, satellite, and cable television; telephone; realtime audio and video conferencing; and new kinds of applications, such as multisensory simulations of nursing situations and activities for learning and telenursing, and distance technology for remote nursing care delivery.

Fulfillment of this vision will require much technical

DEFINITION OF TERMS

ftp (file transfer protocol):	The standard by which a text or file containing executable computer programming is transferred from one computer to another.
gopher:	A hypertext, menu-driven computer interface that is easy to use. It requires that the user (client) and host (server) adhere to certain standards contained in special software (gopher client and gopher server).
LISTSERV:	A computer (server)-maintained electronic mailing system. LISTs are usually focused on specific interest areas. Messages sent to the LIST are distributed automatically to all members of the LIST.
telnet:	A communications session with a host computer, where the user is permitted use of the host's capabilities and files almost as though the host computer were under their control.

innovation and effort, such as developing efficient video and audio compression processes and increasing network bandwidth, both of which will enhance the efficiency of communications. Since the Internet is based on digital technology, the more digital infrastructure there is the easier it will be to facilitate one-platform integration. Already, all-digital telephones are becoming more commonplace. All-digital video production and editing have been widespread for several years now. "More and better" will happen because of the huge potential social and financial incentives involved.

As of now, some of the Internet-related technologies are rather "primitive," requiring much technical expertise to install on the computer and connect to the Internet. Compatibility problems and lack of standardization are major impediments. With more advanced technologies will come more problems for many future users. Many feel that waiting, rather than jumping in now, is appropriate given the difficulties and costs they perceive.

The foregoing are some major trends, visions, and impediments of Internet technologies and their applications. Next are some of the issues specific to nursing that significantly impede nursing's effective participation in these trends, potentially creating a mirage rather than actualizing a vision.

Among the issues of nursing, the Internet, and electronic information, perhaps the most important are the low level of the profession's participation in the use of these currently available resources and the lack of appreciation of the benefits and applicability of network technologies to the work of nursing. Potentially aggravating the situation may be a lack of appreciation of the importance of information in the delivery of nursing care.

Multiple interrelated factors are probably involved in this situation, including a history of nonapplication of instructional and information technologies in nursing; the rapid, but largely invisible to nurses, development of electronic networking technologies adequate for professional application; and insufficient appreciation of the need to become involved in the use and development of electronic resources to meet nurses' own professional needs.

Most nurses don't know how to begin using the Internet and its resources. They haven't been involved in the usual channels of distribution of information about the Internet, its resources, and its potentials. Even within educational and care institutions with Internet connectivity, nurses tend to be unaware of its availability to them. In the popular metaphor, these nurses don't know where their "on-ramp" to the information superhighway is. In addition, even if they do get onto the information superhighway, many do not know how to access or display the resources there for nurses. Nurses who have no roadmap or tour guide to the information superhighway are quite likely to miss their destinations.

Because most nurses have little training in electronic networking, computer, and information technologies, they tend to feel overwhelmed by the technology involved and somewhat embarrassed about not being Internet literate. These are powerful inhibitors to electronic networking. And while many recognize their personal discomfort, they tend to be uncertain as to what to do about it. As a result, many nurses stall before they even find the on-ramp.

Thus, it is not surprising that there is a lack of a critical mass of users among nurses. While there are some effective users and many nurses who say they want to be able to use Internet resources, too few have adequate experience and expertise to meet the needs of all the nurses who seem to want to take advantage of the technologies of the Internet (not to mention those who aren't even sure what the information superhighway is).

There has been a small cadre of nurses actively engaged in developing Internet-accessible resources for some time now. However, nurses with the expertise in informatics, computer science, or instructional technology needed to develop effective resources for nursing applications are scarce. Although integration of informatics content in undergraduate nursing programs is becoming more common, in 1995 there were only two graduate level nursing informatics educational programs in the United States, both of which were clinically oriented. A few nurses have studied medical or health care informatics and are working in nursing roles. Even more scarce are nurse experts in instructional/educational technology. There are less than 10 nurses who are adequately prepared in this important specialty field in the United States.

There has been a lack of professional leadership simply due to the small number of truly knowledgeable, credible Internet advocates within nursing. As a consequence, there has been a lack of strategic resource planning within nursing—including within educational and research institutions and professional organizations—for the education of members of the profession in the use and development of Internet-accessible resources. While nearly all the national nursing organizations have, since at least 1993, been considering developing electronic resources, only a handful have actually done so. Some of those that have provided electronic networking have not been Internet-accessible and, when they have been Internet-accessible, they have not offered full-service resources.

Thus, there is a "chicken-egg" phenomenon taking place. There aren't enough nurses traveling on the information superhighway, nor are there enough nurses sufficiently knowledgeable to teach large numbers of nurses how to find the on-ramp and where to go to visit important destinations. There aren't enough nurses developing great nursing destinations on the information superhighway. The nursing leadership hasn't paid much attention to the potentials of the information superhighway.

There are some hopeful signposts of nursing involvement on the information superhighway. Awareness of the Internet for sharing and exchange of information seems to be growing. Individuals are exchanging e-mail addresses and organizations are including them in the data they gather on members. Nursing listserver membership appears to be increasing. And the number of LISTSERVs for nurses also seems to be increasing. There are a few great telnet, gopher, ftp, and Web sites for nurses. However, real collaboration via electronic networking remains quite limited. Appendix 14-1 lists free Internet-accessible resources related to nursing.

There seems to be widespread reluctance to share nursing information, data, or an opinion. This observation is based on the fact that a large number of nurses belong to electronic resources but do not post messages. This reluctance, which may arise from privacy and proprietary concerns or differences in personal style, needs investigation.

The potential of the Internet to serve as a major new nursing care modality, through its resources, has had very limited consideration within nursing. There have been a few notable demonstration projects using telnet sessions on the Internet; however, because few nurses have seen them, future potentials are not even visible to most of the profession. Certainly, nurses who have not even seen well-developed sites on the Web are limited in what they can envision. The opportunity for telenursing, using telecommunications for nursing assessment/diagnosis and delivery of nursing care, will not materialize unless the leaders and the professional cadre begin to explore its potentials.

There is a tremendous need for research in telenursing. The study of what nursing activities are appropriate for this new modality and how to perform them is critical. Nurses need to devote their attention to the nursing aspects of the technology and not be diluted by tangential issues as they have in the past. Let the experts who are developing the systems for network secure access and privacy worry about those domains. Let nurses focus on nursing. After all, nurses wouldn't want experts outside of nursing to design nursing resources. Nurses should call on other experts when there is sufficient nursing information and prototype development to warrant concern with privacy and security.

In addition to collaboration with other nurse-technology specialists, collaboration with university-based medical or nursing informatics or computer science and telecommunications groups, the private sector, or elements of national, state, or local government might supply the needed expertise and resources, such as hardware or money. While there have been a few collaborations of major information system vendors and nurses, joint efforts in the areas of telecommunications and electronic networking have been much more rare. Collaborative efforts need to be stimulated. However, because of the limited market for nursing applications, it may be difficult to find private partners.

Nurses should plan to develop compelling demonstrations showing the value of Internet technology to the health of the nation and the world. Nurses must gather the data needed as convincing evidence. They should be prepared to educate the general public and policymakers about the nursing applications of Internet technologies. However, nurses who can barely perform their own literature searches on the Internet can hardly be expected to develop great demonstration projects or prototypes or to craft competitive proposals for research or demonstration projects.

In summary, there is a tremendous lack of knowledge about the Internet and its resources. There are few nurses prepared to teach others about it, and even fewer to develop Internet-accessible nursing resources. Any standardization of Internet-accessible nursing resources is probably accidental. There is an absence of strategic planning for the use and development of such resources within professional organizations and educational institutions. The nursing leadership, lacking the vision of the potential new nursing opportunities, has not advocated exploration and research of Internet technologies for the profession. Without having convincing, compelling demonstrations of Internet-accessible resources, grants and funding from private, commercial, and governmental sources are likely to remain limited or nonexistent.

The Internet itself could be a means of addressing many of the issues outlined here. It could serve as a forum to identify and discuss the elements of nursing resources that should be standardized; as the medium to help the nursing leadership develop a vision of the potentials of the Internet; and as the educational medium for use and development of Internet-accessible resources for nursing.

Standardization of technical features and services, without compromising purpose and creativity, has hardly even been discussed among those who manage the nursing resources on the Internet. For many nurses, each resource looks and feels like a unique technological barrier or challenge to master. One often hears determined comment about "learning" to use a networked resource such as, "I am going to try to learn AJN Network," or "I've got to learn how to do an ftp from the National Library of Medicine."

While some nursing resources are already available, there are many more in germination and many more not yet conceived. There may be no better time for the standardization of technical features and functionality. Standardization would help nurses by decreasing the sheer number of variables with which they must contend. Another outcome would be that the user and prospective developers would know what supporting viewer or helper applications and other operational software are required. New-user nurses could be assured of what software and special devices they need for a variety of Internet-accessible resources. There would be some assurance for developers that the nurse users could access and display their resource appropriately and that they themselves could also use the resources developed by others.

In addition, this could make user support much easier and less redundant. It might even be possible to develop one user support resource, linking to it from many nursing resources or mirroring it at a number of sites. Using the Internet, a nurse developer discussion forum could be developed to address standardization issues and also serve as information sharing and support for each other.

Nurse technologists could promote the visibility of Internet potentials through electronic publishing. Opportunities exist now for nurses to publish using Web technologies, creating exemplary hypermedia publications. Nurse experts should work in teams with nurse technologists to ensure the incorporation of appropriate hypermedia features and resources. These teams of nurses could develop outstanding peer-reviewed Web publications, which in turn could serve as a major platform to convince nursing leadership of the significance of the technology and its application to the scholarly work of nursing.

The Internet itself could serve as a medium for the gathering and distribution of expert knowledge in many content areas, not just for informatics or instructional/educational technology in nursing. The Internet can be used as a collaborative workspace both to share and exchange expert knowledge and to prepare and deliver hypermedia coursework, especially in the content areas of informatics and telecommunications and the Internet. Compelling demonstrations could be developed by experts who could participate wherever they are in the Internet-accessible world. The best, most current expertise could be brought to the learners, who also could be anywhere in the Internet-accessible world. Student assignments could involve international and multidisciplinary collaborative work either using the Internet or for Internet accessibility. The philosophy, logistics, and administration of such an informatics educational program would require a paradigm shift in nursing. However, paradigm shifts are difficult to engineer.

While the potential of the Internet for nursing is tremendous, our goals can only be actualized if nurses appreciate the value of information to the care of their patients, know enough about the Internet to effectively use and develop resources there, develop the vision of a new modality (telenursing) for actual care delivery, and then work to materialize that vision. Let's all get on the information superhighway, knowing where our own on-ramp is and being able to visit outstanding useful destinations, some of which were developed by and for nurses and their clients! Rev up your engines, nurses!

Appendix 14-1

The following is a selection of Internet-accessible resources related to nursing available at no charge as of August, 1996. They provide useful information for clinicians, researchers, administrators, and educators, as well as for patients and clients. In addition, many of them incorporate great applications of networking technologies. In the future, some of these sites will be viewed as pioneering efforts that laid the foundation for the much more advanced information superhighway destinations to come.

AJN WWW

This site includes the major journals of the AJN Company: *American Journal of Nursing, Maternal Child Nursing,* and *Nursing Research.* It provides hypermedia authoring capability.

http://www.ajn.org

Australian Electronic Journal of Nursing Education

An electronic publishing opportunity for rapid submission, review, approval, and electronic dissemination of peer-reviewed and non-peer-reviewed articles. Hypermedia authoring is possible.

http://www.csu.edu.au/faculty/health/nurshealth/aejne/aejnehp.htm

CancerNet

Everything professionals or patients would want to know about cancer, its treatment, studies that are completed, and those currently accruing patients. An electronic patient referral form is provided for rapid processing.

http://wwwicic.nci.nih.gov

Centers for Disease Control

This site is a rich source of information about all the Centers for Disease Control and Prevention's publications, including the *Morbidity and Mortality Weekly Report,* and surveillance activities, grants, and employment opportunities.

http://www.cdc.gov

GOLDFISH (Generation of Little Descriptions for Improving and Sustaining Health)

An experimental site being developed as a tool for (diabetic) patients to browse their own medical record with hyperlinks allowing users to access information on all aspects of diabetes.

http://www.gla.ac.uk/~ec19g/goldfish

HHS GrantsNet WWW

A "one-stop" source of information about grants and contract opportunities available at many, but not all, agencies within the U.S. Department of Health and Human Services.

http://www.os.dhhs.gov

The Interactive Patient

A hypermedia site for continuing medical education that requires a diagnosis and treatment plan based on the history, physical examination, and other diagnostic findings. An outstanding demonstration of great technology application.

http://musom.marshall.edu/medicus.htm

National Library of Medicine

Telnet to text.nlm.nih.gov (Health Service/Technology Assessment Texts, clinical practice guidelines)

ftp to nlmpubs.nlm.nih.gov

http://www.nlm.nih.gov

TraumaNET

Includes case histories and management techniques. Especially significant is the virtual surgery component of this excellent resource.

http://www.trauma.lsumc.edu/

Virtual Hospital

First of the well-developed resources for hypermedia in continuing medical education. There is information available for patients and all manner of health care professionals, including multimedia textbooks and testing.

http://indy.radiology.uiowa.edu/Welcome/Welcome.html

World Health Organization

Provides a profile of all the activities and programs of the World Health Organization.

http://www.who.ch

Research utilization: Necessity or luxury?

MARITA G. TITLER

Improvements in care delivery and patient outcomes are among the primary reasons for conducting nursing research, but this scientific knowledge must be translated into practice to be of value. Because patients who receive research-based interventions have better outcomes than those who do not, health care practices must be based on the best body of scientific knowledge available (Goode and Bulechek, 1992; Heater, Becker, & Olson, 1988; Iezzoni, 1994). However, as practice agencies respond to managed care markets by cutting costs, the viability of research utilization (RU) is questioned. Can RU be a reality in times of economic cutbacks? Can practice agencies afford the resources needed to support RU activities? How can the processes of RU be streamlined?

This chapter presents an overview of the history and process of RU, barriers to RU, strategies used to overcome these barriers, and future strategies to streamline RU. It seems that RU is a necessity for professional nursing practice and that the viability of RU is possible if the suggestions set forth herein are acted on.

HISTORY AND OVERVIEW OF RESEARCH UTILIZATION

Use of research in practice was not an issue for Nightingale, who used data to change practices that contributed to high mortality rates in hospitals and communities (Nightingale, 1858, 1863). "Indeed, nursing research and modern nursing were twin-born and their mother was the Lady of the Lamp, a term that aptly describes both aspects of her work" (Stewart, 1962, p. 5). In the early 1900s, few nurses built on the solid foundation of RU exemplified by Nightingale. Separation of the conduct and use of research is rooted in the 1930s and 1940s—a period in nursing when there were few educationally qualified nurse researchers, most nursing research was being done by nonnurses, and hospitals were being used as the primary setting for nursing education. During the mid-1900s, nurses were being prepared as researchers in fields other than nursing and most research focused on nurses rather than on patients (Titler, 1993). Today, more nurses are being prepared as researchers in nursing, and the scientific body of nursing knowledge is growing. It is now every nurse's responsibility to facilitate the use of that knowledge in practice.

Defined in various ways by experts, RU is essentially a process of using research findings as a basis for practice (Gift, 1994). RU can be undertaken from either an individual or organizational perspective and encompasses dissemination of new scientific knowledge, applying that knowledge in practice, and evaluating the impact on staff, patient outcomes, and cost/resource utilization (Goode & Bulechek, 1992; Stetler, Bautista, Vernale-Hannon, & Foster, 1995; Titler, Kleiber, et al., 1994).

Cronenwett (1995) describes two forms of RU: conceptual and decision driven. The purpose of conceptual RU is to influence thinking, not necessarily action. Exposure to new knowledge occurs but the new knowledge may not be used to change or guide practice. An integrative review of the literature, formulation of a new theory, or generating new hypotheses may be the result. This type of RU is referred to as "knowledge creep" or cognitive application and is most often used by individuals when they read and incorporate research into their critical thinking (Stetler, 1994; Weiss, 1980).

Decision-driven forms of RU are those we think of most often when discussing RU. Decision-driven RU encompasses application of scientific knowledge as part of a new practice protocol, policy, procedure, or intervention. In this process, a critical decision point is reached to change or not to change practice based on review and critique of the scientific knowledge. Examples of decision-driven models of RU are the Iowa model of research in practice (Figure 15-1), the Conduct and Utilization of Re-

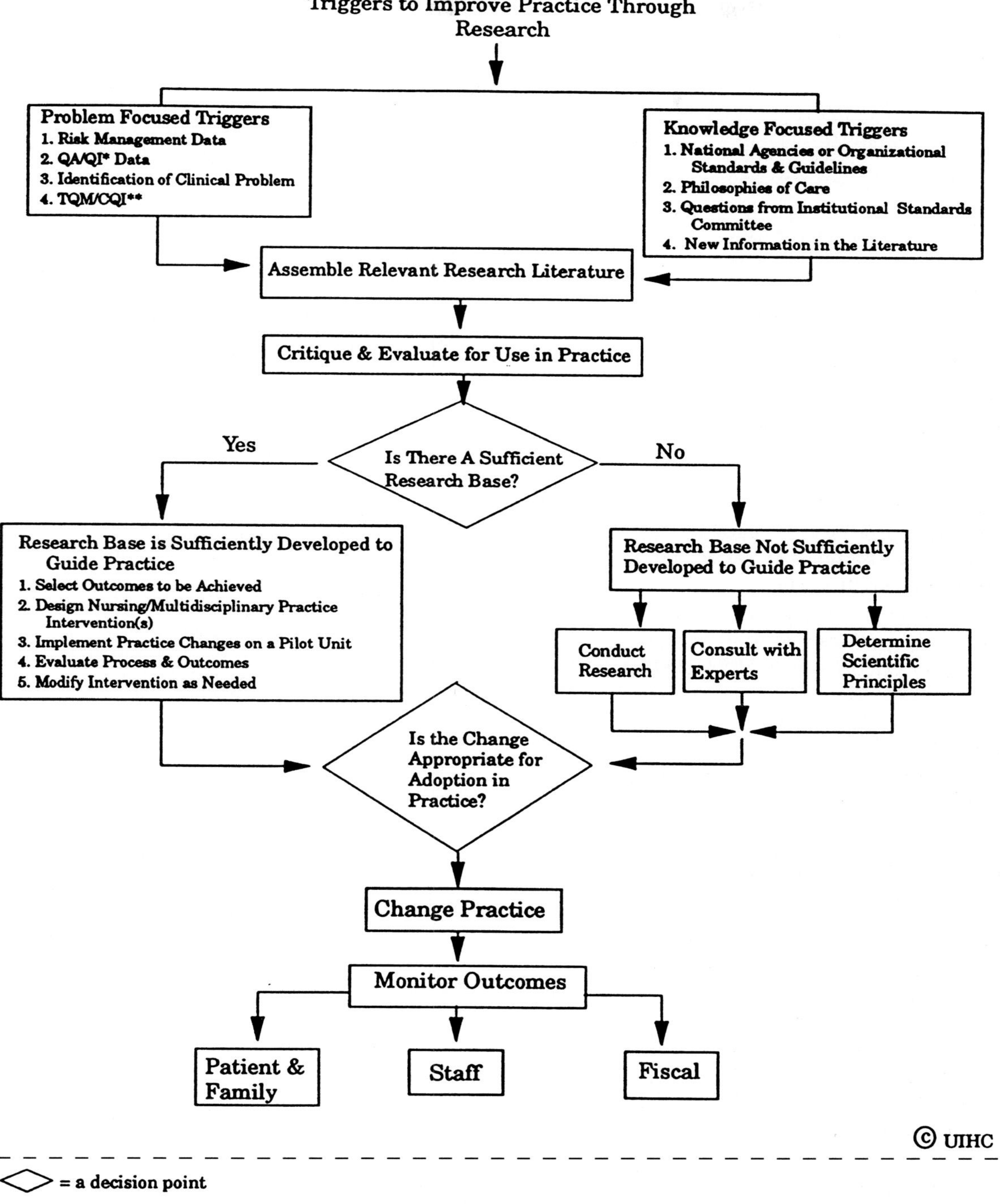

Fig. 15-1. The Iowa Model: Research based practice to promote quality care. (From Titler MG, Kleiber C, Steelman V, Goode C, Rakel B, Barry-Walker J, Small S, and Buckwalter K [1994]. Infusing research into practice to promote quality care. *Nursing Research,* 43(5), 307-313.)

search in Nursing project (Horsley, Crane, Crabtree & Wood, 1983), and the Stetler model (Horsley, Crane, Crabtree & Wood, 1983; Stetler, 1994; Titler, Kleiber, et al., 1994). It is the decision-driven form of RU that is the focus of this chapter.

In comparison with RU, the conduct of research is analysis of data collected from a homogeneous group of subjects that meet study inclusion and exclusion criteria for the purpose of answering specific research questions or testing specified hypotheses. Methods of research design and statistical analyses are guided by the state of the science in the area under investigation. Traditionally, conduct of research has included dissemination via research reports in journals and at scientific conferences. RU begins when nurses are exposed to this new knowledge.

The conduct of research and RU are distinct yet complementary interactive processes of learning and applying new knowledge. For example, one component of RU, as illustrated in the Iowa model, is determining whether there is enough scientific evidence on which to base practice. If there is not a sufficient scientific base for practice, a set of research questions is generated that could be addressed through the conduct of research.

Components of the RU process are reflected in the Iowa model and encompass the following: (a) acquisition, critique, and synthesis of studies in an area of interest that was generated by exposure to new knowledge (eg, Agency on Health Care Policy and Research [AHCPR] guidelines) or heightened awareness of a practice problem (e.g., quality improvement data); (b) deciding whether there is a sufficient research base to support or change current practice; (c) adopting the change in practice; (d) evaluating the impact of that change on patients and families, staff, and resource use; (e) refining the practice change based on evaluation data; and (f) incorporating and reflecting the research-based practices in the appropriate written documents such as policies, procedures, or practice standards (Goode, Butcher, et al., 1991; Horsley et al., 1983; Nolan, Larson, McGuire, Hill, & Haller, 1994; Titler, Kleiber, et al., 1994).

Incorporation of research findings into practice is a difficult and challenging process. Although we expect that nurses use research to guide practice, this is not always the case (American Nurses Association [ANA], 1991; Baessler, Blumberg, & Cunningham, 1994; Brett, 1987; Coyle & Sokop, 1990). Experts in the field of RU note that, in many ways, utilization presents more challenges to overcome than does the conduct of research (Prevost, 1994). Influencing the behavior of multiple caregivers to let go of ritual-based practices is not an easy task. Diffusion of an innovation, such as a set of research findings, is influenced by the nature of the innovation (the research findings) and the manner in which it is communicated (disseminated) to members (nurses) of a social system (institution, nursing profession) (Rogers, 1983). This framework is helpful for understanding the barriers to and strategies for facilitating RU activities within an institution and in the profession of nursing.

According to Funk, Tornquist, and Champagne (1995), findings regarding barriers to RU are quite stable across studies, across time, and among nurses in different roles. Limitations in the setting; research knowledge, skills, and attitudes of nurses; the manner in which the research is communicated; and the quality of the research itself have all been reported as interfering with using research to inform and guide nursing practice.

The remainder of this chapter addresses each of these areas in relation to barriers as well as current and future strategies to promote RU (Table 15-1). The chapter concludes with a description of what is needed to streamline RU if it is to survive in a managed care environment.

THE SOCIAL SYSTEM

Barriers

Organizational and professional barriers to RU have been described. Organizational characteristics reported as great or moderate barriers to RU include insufficient authority to change patient care procedures, insufficient time on the job to read and critique research and to implement new ideas, and little cooperation from physicians, administrators, or both, to implement change. What staff most frequently report as great or moderate barriers differs somewhat from those of administrators (Funk et al., 1995).

From a professional perspective, conduct of research has historically been viewed as the responsibility of academics in university settings. The majority of federal funds for nursing research have gone to colleges of nursing in university centers. Implicitly, a major priority of academic institutions is generation of new knowledge whereas the emphasis in practice agencies is the care of patients. These differing values have contributed to the gap between research and practice (Titler, 1993).

Current strategies of organizations

Several strategies to address these barriers are currently in use (Nolan et al., 1994). To maximize the benefits of RU, it is essential that RU be viewed and operationalized from an organizational perspective (Goode & Bulechek, 1992). Several characteristics are common in organizations with successful RU programs (Barnsteiner, Ford, & Howe, 1995; Butcher, 1995; Cole & Gawlinski, 1995; Cronenwett, 1995; Specht, Berquist, & Frantz, 1995; Stonestree & Lamb-Havard, 1994; Titler, Kleiber, et al., 1994; Titler, Moss, et al., 1994).

First, the value of research to the organization is explicitly stated in mission and governance statements, and reflected in job performance criteria, clinical ladders, and merit programs. Secondly, the units and institutional environments possess a culture of professional practice. Specifically, nurses are delivering quality care, participating in the resolution of practice issues, subscribing to professional journals, and participating in their professional and specialty associations (Titler, Goode, & Mathis, 1992). In addition, these organizations promote critical thinking, data-based decision making, questioning of current practices, and adoption of innovations. Thirdly, research objectives and how they support departmental and organizational objectives are articulated (Goode & Bulechek, 1992). Priorities for RU activities are delineated via strategic or operational plans. Being selective about the type and content of RU activities is more likely to result in success rather than being too broad in scope with frustration and perceived failure resulting (Kirchhoff & Titler, 1994).

Furthermore, the value of research is operationalized through joint appointments or hiring a full-time doctorally prepared nurse researcher; developing committee structures for research that involve nursing staff from all levels of the organization; and clearly delineating role responsibilities for RU activities.

Although role responsibilities vary somewhat among these institutions, commonalities exist. Staff nurses are essential to effective RU because they question current practice, identify practice areas that would benefit from examining research findings, and read research and ask "what does this mean for my practice?" They also champion the necessary research-based practice changes with their peers and participate in the critique and synthesis of studies (Titler, Kleiber, et al., 1994). Staff nurses who are effective in RU activities are often viewed as informal leaders; have clinical credibility with their peers; are enthusiastic, motivated, and willing to learn; follow through with commitments; and persevere in making the needed changes.

Advanced practice nurses (APNs) and other master's prepared nurses have the knowledge and skills to provide leadership for RU projects (Gawlinski & Henneman, 1994; O'Malley, 1994; Stetler et al., 1995). Role components of the APN include research. Specifically, APNs operationalize RU activities by leading others in organizing the acquisition and critique of studies, synthesizing findings, and determining what the synthesized findings mean for current practice. If a change in practice is warranted, they work with staff to develop and implement a plan for making and evaluating changes.

The roles of nurse executives and nurse managers are important to set the tone and expectations regarding research and practice (Kirchhoff & Titler, 1994). Responsibilities of nurse executives include articulation of research objectives, allocation of resources, ensuring that expectations regarding research are communicated to nursing staff at all levels of the organization, and making an organizational commitment to RU.

Nurse managers directly and indirectly contribute to the success or demise of RU. When selecting from several potential topics for RU projects, eliciting support and direction from nurse managers is an important step. Nurse managers have a responsibility at the unit(s) level similar to that of the nurse executive once the organization is committed to RU (Kirchhoff & Titler, 1994). They support the process by (a) having informal dialogue with staff and other health care professionals; (b) using RU job performance criteria in evaluation of staff; (c) supporting staff by arranging clinical release time; and (d) rewarding staff who participate by increasing salaries, supporting their attendance at local, regional, or national conferences, nominating them for local, regional, or national awards, and giving them positive written or verbal feedback. Nurse managers create a unit culture for staff to use research, think critically, and initiate questioning of current practices. They role model positive behaviors of RU by initiating journal clubs, participating in critiques of studies, posting selected research articles, assisting staff in troubleshooting problems that arise with implementing change, and encouraging their staff to inquire about practices via reviewing current research findings.

The role of the nurse scientist in clinical agencies is variable and influenced in part by the type of appointment. Hiring clinical nurse researchers into practice settings has enhanced RU activities (Kirchhoff, 1993). The nurse scientist provides consultation and direction for staff in learning the knowledge and skills for carrying out RU activities. Staff often need guidance in understanding statistics, learning how to put the findings from several studies together in a meaningful way for practice, deciding whether practice changes are warranted, and developing simple ways to evaluate the practice changes. Working with staff to encourage and support their efforts is an essential part of this role. Staff need mentoring in

Table 15-1 Barriers and facilitators of Research Utilization (RU) using Roger's (1983) framework

Areas of innovation diffusion	Barriers	Past and current strategies	Future strategies
	Characteristics of the social system		
Organizational	Lack of authority to change practice Insufficient time on the job Little cooperation from physicians or administrators	Organizational values for research incorporated into governance documents Value of research operationalized in job descriptions, merit programs, and committee structures Hiring a doctorally prepared nurse researcher in practice Allocation of human and monetary resources	Use of investigative teams Combining RU and QI activities into one committee Creating partnerships with organizations in the same geographic location Implementation across integrated delivery systems
Professional	Priorities of universities and practice differ Majority of federal research funds allocated to academic centers Historical perspective of research occurring in academic centers	Articulation of importance of RU in practice standards by professional associations and external accrediting agencies (e.g., JCAHO) Development and use of RU models	Increase funding for doctoral preparation Multisite RU projects Identification by specialty organizations of content areas ready for RU
	Members of the social system		
Knowledge and skills of nurses	Lack of awareness of research Isolated from knowledgeable colleagues Difficulty evaluating the quality of the research	Development and use of educational aides Federally funded RU projects (WICHEN, CURN, NCAST, OCRUN) RU conferences and preconferences	Incorporating journal clubs as a touching strategy in undergraduate programs Integrating RU skills into baccalaureate and graduate programs Requiring participation and/or leadership for RU projects as part of the educational experience
Attitudes	Feeling that research is not valued Not feeling rewarded for participation in RU	Administrative support for RU Reward system Feedback of data to illustrate how RU improves quality of care	Increase educational activities that socialize nurses into reading research Use of textbooks that have research-based interventions
	Nature of the innovation		
Quality of the research	Few replication studies	Emphasis placed on scientists building a program of research Increasing numbers of nurses prepared at the doctoral level in nursing Publication of integrative reviews and meta-analyses	More emphasis and value for replication studies More emphasis on development of midrange theories Devoted programs of research on the science of RU

Table 15-1—cont'd. Barriers and facilitators of Research Utilization (RU) using Roger's (1983) framework

Areas of innovation diffusion	Barriers	Past and current strategies	Future strategies
	Communication		
Dissemination of research findings to nurses in practice	Manner in which statistics are reported Relevant literature not compiled in one place Research reports written in research-ese, with implications for practice being unclear	Development of journals that emphasize application of findings Published summaries of research findings (*Annual Review of Nursing Research, On-line Journal of Knowledge Synthesis for Nursing*) Research columns in practice journals RU conferences Research conferences with a practice focus RARIN—Stanford University Hospital	Journal dedicated to report of RU projects More federal funding for national RU conferences Increase use of electronic superhighway to show RU protocols Central clearinghouse for dissemination of written research-based practices

Note: CURN = Conduct and Utilization of Research in Nursing; JCAHO = Joint Commission on Accreditation of Healthcare Organizations; NCAST = Nursing Child Assessment Satellite Training; OCRUN = Orange County Research Utilization in Nursing; QI = Quality Improvement; RARIN = Retrieval and Application of Research in Nursing.

this process and the nurse scientist should be providing this mentorship experience. Campbell and Chulay (1990) suggest targeting nurse managers and APNs for early involvement in initial research activities. By building on their enthusiasm and areas of interest, core leadership personnel will evolve to support and guide subsequent RU projects.

Developing an organizational culture that values RU is an ongoing process that requires the collective effort of nurses in all roles (Kirchhoff, 1991). It is important that small successes and the contribution of nursing research to improving the quality of care are acknowledged. The value of research-based practice to the organization is communicated to all staff through behaviors such as providing some clinical release time for participating in RU activities, instituting research recognition programs, and encouraging staff to attend and present at research conferences (Kirchhoff & Titler, 1994).

Allocation of resources for RU follows from the departmental objectives. Fixed expenses typically include research texts and journals, computer hardware, office space, and labor costs associated with budgeted staff positions. Variable costs include videotapes and other learning aides, computer software, posters for regional and national conferences, copying, and travel to research meetings. Additional resources to consider are library facilities, time for staff to participate in RU activities, and secretarial support (Kirchhoff & Titler, 1994).

The amount of fiscal dollars allocated for research depends on the size and scope of the objectives set forth by the nurse executive. Major impediments to effective RU include the lack of tangible resources such as time and money (Pettengill, Gillies, & Clark, 1994). Critical issues that must be addressed are the cost center (general nursing budget, quality improvement budget, independent cost center) for these activities and how resources are being allocated despite cost-containment efforts (Kirchhoff & Titler, 1994). Including research in the general nursing administrative budget provides more flexibility than establishing a separate cost center (Chance & Hinshaw, 1980).

Costs associated with supporting RU activities can be justified by illustrating the benefits of cost savings and improved quality of care derived from these activities (Titler et al., 1992). In addition, RU is some of the best continuous process improvement required by external crediting agencies. Furthermore, studies have demonstrated that research-based practices contribute to positive patient outcomes (Daly, Rudy, Thompson, & Happs, 1991; Fagin, 1990). Basing practice on research saves health care dollars (Goode, Lovett, Hayes, & Butcher, 1987; Goode, Butcher, et al., 1991; Goode, Titler et al., 1991).

Current strategies: A professional perspective

Several characteristics of the nursing profession enhance RU activities. Explicating the importance of research-based practice has been set forth by professional nursing associations as described elsewhere (Funk et al., 1995; Cronenwett, 1995; Kirchhoff & Titler, 1994; Nolan et al., 1994; Stonestreet & Lamb-Havard, 1994; Weiler, Buckwalter, & Titler, 1994). For example, ANA standards for nursing services and clinical practice delineate the expectation that research findings will be incorporated into practice. The American Association of Critical-Care Nurses, Sigma Theta Tau International, and the Association of Women's Health Obstetric and Neonatal Nurses all have initiatives targeting research-based practice such as regional and national RU conferences and awards, grant monies, and research priorities designated for RU. The accrediting standards for the Joint Commission on Accreditation of Healthcare Organizations expect that organizational policies, procedures, and practice standards be developed from current scientific knowledge.

Development and use of several RU models have also advanced the use of nursing research in practice (Nolan et al., 1994; White, Leske, & Pearcy, 1995) Some of these models focus on RU from an organizational perspective and others from the individual nurse perspective. All of these models have important similarities. They were developed as prescriptive models for RU. They conceptualize RU as a process with a discrete set of activities. They advocate an evaluation component. A variety of mechanisms are used to disseminate the research findings to the bedside (White et al., 1995). These developments in nursing are evidence that the profession has made a commitment to transfer the findings from a program of research into clinical practice standards.

Future strategies

In the future, continued attention is needed for increasing the number of doctorally prepared nurses, building focused programs of research that will result in findings for practice, developing research teams with members from academia and practice, and providing more forums for dialogue between researchers and clinicians. Investigative teams such as the Nursing Interventions Classification team (McCloskey & Bulechek, 1996) and the Family Intervention Research team (Johnson et al., 1993) illustrate the importance of collaboration in translating findings from a program of research into a practice setting.

As economic constraints continue in the health care setting, institutions may find it more efficient to combine RU and quality improvement (QI) activities and use RU projects as part of the QI program. Creating partnerships with nearby organizations to share integrative reviews, critiques, and research-based protocols would also save staff time (Titler et al., 1992).

Most RU programs have been instituted in acute care institutions of varying size. Administrators of the future will be challenged to determine what modifications are needed to support RU activities across an integrated delivery system as well as in other agencies such as long-term and home health care.

From a professional perspective, associations must continue to support innovative ways to stimulate nurses to look to research for practice improvements. Participation in multisite RU projects and provision of funding are important strategies for associations to continue. In addition, staff would benefit from speciality organizations identifying content areas that have a sufficient research base for practice, and appointing small groups from their membership to review, critique, synthesize, write, and update research-based protocols.

MEMBERS

Nurses comprise the members of the social system within which research findings are used. The knowledge, skills, and attitudes of these nurses vary, in part because of the varying educational credentials of nurses in the profession.

Barriers

Barriers most frequently reported by nurses as great or moderate obstacles to research use are the lack of awareness of research, being isolated from knowledgeable colleagues who would provide some dialogue and discussion about research, and not feeling capable of evaluating the quality of the research. Nurses complain about the lack of access to research and confusion that ensues when findings are different across studies.

Learning the art and science of critiquing research, synthesizing several critiques, and determining if there is enough research to change current practice are time-consuming but necessary endeavors. Skills of negotiation, influencing the behavior of others, educating others about research findings, being a change agent, and evaluating the change are also essential components of RU.

Current strategies

A variety of educational aides are available to teach nurses and students the knowledge and skills necessary for RU.

These include textbooks and study guides, an interactive computer program on critique of research, and videotapes on other components of the RU process (Burns & Grove, 1993; Goode, Butcher, et al., 1991; Mateo & Kirchhoff, 1991; Stetler et al., 1995; Tornquist, Funk, & Champagne, 1993).

Several broad-based, federally funded projects such as the Western Interstate Commission for Higher Education in Nursing regional program for nursing research development, and the Conduct and Utilization of Research in Nursing, Nursing Child Assessment Satellite Training, and Orange Country Research Utilization in Nursing Projects have focused on education, resulting in several RU teaching aides (Cronenwett, 1995; Horsley et al., 1983; Nolan et al., 1994; Rutledge & Donaldson, 1995; White et al., 1995). Preconferences to assist staff in learning how to do various components of RU are also used.

A majority of educational efforts to date have focused on increasing the knowledge and skill of staff in the practice setting. Although the majority of baccalaureate programs include content related to nursing research in their curricula, the knowledge and skills needed for RU receive little attention. "For the most part, education is lagging behind practice in its efforts to promote research utilization and research-based practice" (Crane, 1995, p. 570).

Future strategies

Crane (1995) describes the RU behaviors expected of baccalaureate, master's, and doctorally prepared nurses. Teaching strategies for each are described in Table 15-2. Nursing students need to be socialized into reading research, even if they can only make sense of the introduction and discussion section. Use of journal clubs is one teaching strategy to help students learn how to read and interpret research. Students' clinical conferences should include presentations of at least one scientific paper on a

Table 15-2 Research Utilization (RU) teaching strategies for Baccalaureate, Master's, and Doctoral students

	Baccalaureate	Master's	Doctoral
RU behaviors	Value of science-based practice How to access research reports How to read and critique research for use in practice How to use research methods to serve practice purposes Conceptual use of research findings in their practice	Evaluation of patient outcomes Use of electronic technology to access research and network with researchers and those doing RU Pilot testing of research-based interventions Advanced ability to critique research for scientific merit Synthesis of research critiques for application to practice Change strategies Decision-driven form of RU	Research training for conduct of research Increased value for replication studies Understanding of RU and innovation diffusion theory, nursing minimum data sets, nursing classifications (diagnoses, interventions, outcomes)
Teaching strategies	Assignments requiring use of electronic data bases such as CINAHL, MedLine Use of Internet to communicate with research about a practice issue Required research course, early in the program, that focuses on reading, critique, and cognitive use of research methods for practice Developing one written research based protocol	Written papers on critique and synthesis of research for use in practice Development and implementation of research-based protocols Selection of variables and methods to evaluate patient outcomes in their area of specialization Practicum on RU in a practice setting	Written paper on implementation and evaluation of an innovation Analysis of organizational variables that support RU Research residencies in RU Research practicums with investigative teams Dissertations on the science of RU or replication studies

Adapted from: Crane, J. (1995). The future of research utilization. *Nursing Clinics of North America, 30,* 565-577.

topic applicable to their patient population. Textbooks that incorporate research-based practices are needed for use in undergraduate curriculums.

Graduate students at the master's level would benefit from doing RU projects during their program of study. These could be incorporated into clinical course work or be a final project required for graduation. APNs have a major leadership role in RU efforts and must be taught how to lead staff in an RU project during their educational experience.

Graduate students, particularly at the doctoral level, benefit from working outside the classroom with investigative teams to learn first-hand how the theory of research is applied in day-to-day functioning. Doctoral students should have course work in RU and methods of evaluation, particularly if they plan to assume roles as directors of research in health care organizations (Crane, 1995).

NATURE OF THE INNOVATION

Barriers

The quality of the research is not reported frequently as a moderate or great barrier to RU as compared with communication, knowledge and skills, and organizational barriers (Funk et al., 1995; Pettengill et al., 1994). The most frequently reported barrier in this area is that research has not been replicated (Funk et al., 1995; Crane, 1995). Perhaps the reason that the quality of the research is perceived as less of a barrier is related to the emphasis placed on scientists building programs of research in specified areas, resulting in research findings that can be used in practice.

Current strategies

Nursing is accumulating a body of scientific knowledge in selected areas and beginning to build middle range theories that are applicable to practice (Blegen & Tripp-Reimer, 1994). Continuing emphasis on funded programs of research that tests middle range theories is essential if nursing is to have a scientific base to transfer to the practice setting.

As accumulation of research evidence continues to grow, more comprehensive integrated reviews and meta-analyses will be needed to summarize and understand these findings. A number of meta-analyses have been conducted on clinical problems relevant to nursing treatments (Burns & Grove, 1993, p. 696). This type of analysis is helpful for translation of findings into practice.

Future strategies

There is a greater need than ever for replication studies. Replication should be made more credible for dissertation work, particularly if it adds the missing link to a specific research base for practice (Crane, 1995). More middle range prescriptive theories are needed to guide practice and more emphasis should be placed on this component of scientific knowledge development in doctoral programs.

The science of RU is in its infancy (Nolan et al., 1994; Pettengill et al., 1994). The science of what makes some organizations centers of excellence in RU is minimal. We need to move beyond descriptive and educational studies on RU to demonstration and health services research projects that explicate and test the variables for successful RU programs.

DISSEMINATION/COMMUNICATION

Barriers

A major barrier to using research in practice is dissemination, i.e., how findings from research are communicated for use and application in the practice setting (Cronenwett, 1995; Funk et al., 1995; Pettengill et al., 1994). These dissemination barriers are related to and interact with characteristics of nurses who are trying to understand and use this information for their patients. These barriers include the manner in which statistics are reported, relevant literature not being complied in one place, and unclear implications for practice. The researchese used in oral and written research reports makes understanding research difficult for many nurses (Cronenwett, 1995).

Current strategies

Journals that emphasize reporting research in a manner that facilitates use in practice have been developed. These include *Applied Nursing Research, Clinical Nursing Research* and speciality journals such as *American Journal of Critical Care.* In addition, it is increasingly common to see research columns in practice journals such as *American Journal of Nursing, MedSurg Nursing,* and *Dimensions of Critical Care Nursing.* Summaries of research findings and guidelines for practice are available in Sigma Theta Tau International's electronic journal, *Online Journal of Knowledge Synthesis for Nursing,* as well as from the AHCPR. The *Annual Review of Nursing Research* publishes integrative research reviews that are helpful in understanding the state of the science in a particular area and components of the science that may be ready for practice (Cronenwett, 1995).

There is a paucity, however, of RU projects published in the nursing literature. Clinicians need to share their utilization experiences with others, i.e., what is learned when knowledge gained from a "controlled" setting is applied in a setting with a more heterogeneous population of patients using multiple caregivers. The formats of most journals do not lend themselves to reporting RU. Report of RU projects in a format designed for conduct is confusing, particularly for novices who are trying to distinguish between the conduct and utilization of research.

Research conferences traditionally have focused on scientific methods and data reporting with little mention of implications for practice. Experts in dissemination and RU have helped break this mold. Funk et al. (1995) at the University of North Carolina, Chapel Hill received federal funding to support conferences in which nurse researchers summarized their research. Clinicians were able to discuss the knowledge base for an area of practice with nurses currently doing the research. Conference proceedings were published and these books are major contributions to the literature in the field (Cronenwett, 1995; Nolan et al., 1994).

An annual conference entitled "Toward Research-Based Nursing Practice," sponsored by Dartmouth-Hitchcock Medical Center and St. Aslem College in New Hampshire, focuses on integrative research papers. Presenters describe a practice problem, integrate the findings of relevant research, and describe the meaning for practice. An annotated bibliography of the most relevant studies is also prepared and compiled in a syllabus for distribution to participants. The conference has been well attended with two thirds of the presenters from practice and one third from academia. This conference is exemplary of the type of conferences that help bridge the gap between conduct and utilization of nursing research (Cronenwett, 1995).

Lastly, the University of Iowa Hospitals and Clinics, in cooperation with the College of Nursing, hosts an annual RU conference that includes invited papers as well as a call for paper and poster presentations. Attendance at this conference ranges from 100 to 150 with representatives from throughout the United States and Canada. Similar RU conferences are sponsored by others. These types of conferences provide forums for nurses to exchange challenges encountered in changing practice and ideas for making RU a reality in their setting.

Mechanisms that increase nurses' access to research have also been trialed. The Retrieval and Application of Research in Nursing (RARIN) project at Stanford University Hospital provides nurses in their work areas with electronic linkages to locally and nationally maintained scientific information systems (Bostrom & Wise, 1994). Nurses are trained in database searching techniques. Significant mentoring is required to provide nurses with the expertise to use the literature once it is retrieved.

Future strategies

Much effort has gone into making research understandable for staff from a conference and written perspective. Few journals however, provide an avenue for reporting RU projects. A journal designed for nurses in practice that is dedicated to RU is needed. Articles could focus on the integrative review and research-based protocol, strategies used to change practice, and methods of evaluating implementation of the protocol.

More funding is needed for national conferences similar to those sponsored by the University of North Carolina, Chapel Hill. It is important that clinicians have an opportunity to discuss research with scientists, and that scientists learn how to present research in a way that is understandable for the clinician.

Finally, we need to make better use of the electronic "superhighway" to share research-based information and to minimize current duplicative efforts of critiquing and synthesizing research (Crane, 1995; Cronenwett, 1994). Standardization of the components and format for written research-based practice documents (e.g., protocols, policies, procedures) is necessary to promote similarity across practice settings. A central clearinghouse for dissemination of these written research-based practices would also be helpful (Crane, 1995; Cronenwett, 1995; Funk et al., 1995).

STREAMLINING RESEARCH UTILIZATION

As noted by Funk et al. (1995), cost efficiency is essential if RU is to survive. "We can no longer have nurses in practice settings throughout the nation duplicating the work of searching for the most up-to-date literature, evaluating it, synthesizing it, and drawing practice conclusions" (Funk et al., 1995, p. 403). Requesting time for nurses to participate in these RU activities may not be forthcoming. Research and practice expertise are both needed, however, to determine whether findings are ready for practice, to implement changes in practice, and to evaluate them.

In order for organizations to take full advantage of RU

EXAMPLES OF RESEARCH-BASED PRACTICES

- Facilitation of child visitation of a critically ill adult family member
- Family-centered critical care practice in the adult critical care unit
- Facilitation of sibling visitation of a critically ill neonate
- Endotracheal suctioning of the adult
- Endotracheal suctioning of children and neonates
- Latex allergy precautions
- Constipation management in the older adult
- Bathing persons with dementia
- Care of patients with Alzheimer's disease
- Music therapy
- Use of restraints
- Fall prevention
- Use of saline flush to maintain patency of peripheral intravenous locks
- Blood withdrawal from arterial lines in adults
- Intravenous tubing and peripheral site care in adults
- Prevention of deep venous thromboses
- Nasogastric and nasointestinal tube placement
- Vital signs monitoring for early detection and treatment of sepsis

projects undertaken at various sites throughout the country, a national center for RU is needed. This builds on the suggestion of others that speciality organizations take responsibility for the critique and synthesis component of RU, and make recommendations for practice (Funk et al., 1995; Crane, 1995; Cronenwett, 1995).

Many research-based protocols, however, are applicable across specialties (see Examples in the box). Thus, there would be an advantage to having research-based practice protocols centrally located, indexed, and updated via one center rather than by specialty associations. These organizations would need to facilitate the work by coordinating the identification of content and process experts in the field, disseminating the information to clinicians, and prioritizing content areas and research-based interventions essential for implementation.

Such a center would encompass a computerized database of research-based protocols that include the relevant policy and procedure, the population to which it applies, the quality improvement instruments that were used to evaluate it, a reference list, and helpful strategies for making the practice change (see the box on page 115). The names and types of institutions and contact persons where the practice change has been instituted would also be included. These prepackaged research-based protocols could also be available online through electronic communications such as the World Wide Web, Virtual Hospital System, or a list serve dedicated to RU.

The center would also serve as a network where health care personnel working on similar RU projects could identify one another, discuss issues encountered when instituting changes in practice, and link clinicians with researchers in the identified content area. For example, although it is clear that animal-assisted therapy is beneficial for patients, it is a challenge to implement this practice change in some agencies (Cole & Gawlinski, 1995).

Additional services the center could provide are (a) consultation with agencies that want to begin integrating research-based practice into the fiber of their institutions; (b) centralizing and cataloging educational aides on RU; (c) centralizing the tools and forms nurses have developed and used to help with various components of the RU process (e.g., critique forms, synthesis forms, selecting a topic form); (d) sponsoring "train the trainer" programs on RU via telnet to impart the knowledge and skills needed to make RU an integral part of the organization; and (e) assisting interested nurses in hosting regional or national conferences on RU.

The University of Iowa Hospitals and Clinics, in collaboration with the University of Iowa College of Nursing, is testing components of this national center through the Research Development and Dissemination Core of the Gerontology Nursing Intervention Research Center. Early lessons we have learned are that the prepackaged research-based protocols are highly valued by staff doing RU; limiting development of these protocols to gerontological topics may be premature because other interventions applicable to adults in general can also be used with the elderly; a training program for RU has general content applicable across specialties making it easy to modify the program by substituting examples with those from other specialties (e.g., critical care, pediatrics); and what we know about RU has been trialed in acute care agencies with minimal knowledge or experience about application to home health agencies, skilled nursing facilities, and long-term care. We have also learned that staff need guidance and clerical support for integrating the research-based practice changes into existing documents (e.g., standards, policies, procedures) in a manner that is easy for staff to tell what part is research-based.

SUMMARY

This chapter has provided an overview of RU, past and current strategies used to support RU, and changes to streamline RU activities. RU is a necessity for professional

COMPONENTS OF A WRITTEN RESEARCH-BASED PRACTICE STANDARD (Policy, Procedure, Protocol)

Purpose—A brief statement describing the patient care problem addressed (e.g., constipation) and the patient population to which it applies (e.g., hospitalized older adults [>60 years of age])
Example—An interdisciplinary protocol to prevent constipation in hospitalized older adults undergoing surgery

Definition of key terms—Operational definition(s) of major terms or concepts in the protocol; it is important that everyone knows the meaning of the concepts (e.g., peripheral locks; constipation; fall) central to the protocol, policy, or procedure
Example—Patients are considered constipated if the stool is hard and dry; if an impaction is palpable; if straining at stool is present; if abdominal distention/fullness is present; if rectal fullness is present; or there is absence of bowel movements beyond reported normal patterns of defecation.

Patients at risk—A brief statement or listing of patient populations that are most likely to benefit from this protocol; this can include a case definition, symptomatology, age/developmental level, and type of disease or condition
Example—Managing constipation
Elderly
Decreased mobility
Limited intake of fiber and/or fluids
Confusion

Assessment—Examples of patient and environmental assessments that indicate patients who are likely to benefit from use of the research-based practice
Example—For a constipation protocol, the following assessment criteria indicate patients at risk for developing constipation:
Age 70 or older
Hospitalized for 4 days
Restricted to bed rest
Nausea
Fluid intake of 800 ml/24 hr

Description of the practice—A description or step-by-step guideline on how to carry out the practice, indicating what part is research-based by referencing and footnoting the research reports. Algorithms, flow charts, and tables maybe helpful.
Example—To manage constipation for those at risk:
Maintain or increase fluid intake to 1.5 l/day.
High-fiber diet (25 to 50 g/day) when fluid intake is greater than 800 ml
Ambulate three times daily if not on bedrest.

Evaluation—A description of the process and outcome variables used to evaluate the change in practice. Inclusion of the tools used to measure these variables is helpful.
Example:
Outcome Variables—Through audit of patient records, incidence of constipation, impaction, and use of laxatives and enemas are noted. Patient interviews are used to evaluate whether bowel function is being maintained within normal limits.
Process Variables—Through use of a knowledge assessment test, nurses, physicians, and dietitians are queried regarding the various components of the constipation management protocol.

References—Bibliography of research reports used to develop the research-based practice.

nursing practice. Therefore, as the science of nursing continues to grow, it is imperative that the nursing profession respond by streamlining RU activities if it is to survive in managed care environments.

REFERENCES

American Nurses Association (1991). *Standards of clinical nursing practice.* Washington, DC: Author.

Baessler, C.A., Blumberg, M., & Cunningham, J.S. (1994). Medical-surgical nurses' utilization of research methods and products. *MedSurg Nursing, 3,* 113-121.

Barnsteiner, J.H., Ford, N., & Howe, C. (1995). Research utilization in a metropolitan children's hospital. *Nursing Clinics of North America, 30*(3), 447-455.

Blegen, M.A., & Tripp-Reimer, T. (1994). The nursing theory-nursing research connection. In J.C. McCloskey & H.K. Grace (Eds.), *Current issues in nursing* (4th ed., pp. 87-91). St. Louis: Mosby.

Bostrom, J., & Wise, L. (1994). Closing the gap between research and practice. *Journal of Nursing Administration, 24,* 22-27.

Brett, J.L. (1987). Use of nursing practice research findings. *Nursing Research, 36,* 344-349.

Burns, N., & Grove, S. (Eds.). (1993). *The practice of nursing research.* Philadelphia: Saunders.

Butcher, L. (1995). Research utilization in a small, rural, community hospital. *Nursing Clinics of North America, 30*(3), 439-446.

Campbell, G.M., & Chulay, M. (1990). Establishing a clinical nursing research program. In J.G. Spicer & M. Robinson (Eds.), *Managing the environment in the critical care setting* (pp. 52-60). Baltimore: Williams & Wilkins.

Chance, H.C., & Hinshaw, A.S. (1980). Strategies for initiating a research program. *Journal of Nursing Administration, 10*(3), 32-39.

Cole, K.M., & Gawlinski, A. (1995). Animal-assisted therapy in the intensive care unit. *Nursing Clinics of North America, 30*(3), 529-537.

Coyle, L.A., & Sokop, A.G. (1990). Innovation adoption behavior among nurses. *Nursing Research, 39,* 176-180.

Crane, J. (1995). The future of research utilization. *Nursing Clinics of North America, 30,* 565-577.

Cronenwett, L.R. (1995). Effective methods for disseminating research findings to nurses in practice. *Nursing Clinics of North America, 30*(3), 429-438.

Daly, B.J., Rudy, E.B., Thompson, K.S., & Happ, M.B. (1991). Development of a special care unit for chronically critically ill. *Heart & Lung, 20,* 45-51.

Fagin, C.M. (1990). Nursing's value proves itself. *American Journal of Nursing, 82,* 1844-1849.

Funk, S.G., Tornquist, E.M., & Champagne, M.T. (1995). Barriers and facilitators of research utilization: An integrative review. *Nursing Clinics of North America, 30*(3), 395-407.

Gawlinski, A., & Henneman, E.A. (1994). Research utilization in the critical care setting. In A. Gawlinski & L.S. Kern (Eds.), *The clinical nurse specialist role in critical care* (pp. 196-216). Philadelphia: Saunders.

Gift, A. (1994). Nursing research utilization. *Clinical Nurse Specialist, 8*(6), 306.

Goode, C.J. (1995). Evaluation of research-based nursing interventions. *Nursing Clinics of North America, 30*(3), 421-428.

Goode, C., & Bulecheck, G. (1992). Research utilization: An organization process that enhances quality of care. *Journal of Nursing Care Quality, Special Report,* 27-35.

Goode, C., Butcher, L., Cipperley, J., Ekstrom, J., Gosch, B., Hayes, J., Lovett, M., & Wellendorf, S. (1991). *Research utilization: A study guide.* Ida Grove, IA: Horn Video Productions.

Goode, C.J., Lovett, M.K., Hayes, J.E., & Butcher, L.A. (1987). Use of research based knowledge in clinical practice. *Journal of Nursing Administration, 17*(12), 11-18.

Goode, C.J., Titler, M., Rakel, B., Ones, D., Kleiber, C., Small, S., & Triolo, P. (1991). A meta-analysis of effects of heparin flush and saline flush: Quality and cost implications. *Nursing Research, 40,* 321-330.

Heater, B.S., Becker, A.M., & Olson, R.K. (1988). Nursing interventions and patient outcomes: A meta-analysis of studies. *Nursing Research, 37,* 303-307.

Horsley, J., Crane, J., Crabtree, M., & Wood, D. (1983). *Using research to improve nursing practice: A guide.* Philadelphia: Saunders.

Iezzoni, L.I. (Ed.). (1994). *Risk adjustment for measuring health care outcomes.* Ann Arbor, MI: Health Administration Press.

Johnson, S.K., Halm, M.A., Titler, M.G., Craft, M., Kleiber, C., Montgomery, L., Nicholson, A., Buckwalter, K., & Cram, E. (1993). Group functioning of a collaborative family research team. *Clinical Nurse Specialist Journal, 7*(4), 184-191.

Kirchhoff, K.T. (1993). The role of nurse researchers employed in clinical settings. *Annual Review of Nursing Research, 11,* 169-181.

Kirchhoff, K.T. (1991). Who is responsible for research utilization? *Heart and Lung, 20*(3), 308-309.

Kirchhoff, K.T., & Titler, M.G. (1994). Responsibilities of nurse executives in conducting and using research in the practice setting. In R. Spitzer-Lehmann (Ed.), *Nursing management desk reference* (pp. 606-628). Philadelphia: Saunders.

Mateo, M., & Kirchhoff, K.T. (Eds.). (1991). *Conducting and using nursing research in the clinical setting.* Baltimore: Williams & Wilkins.

McCloskey, J.C., & Bulechek, G.M. (1996). *Nursing Interventions Classification (NIC)* (2nd ed.). St. Louis: Mosby.

Nightingale, F. (1858). *Notes on matters affecting the health, efficiency, and hospital administration of the British Army.* London: Harrison & Sons.

Nightingale, F. (1863). *Observation on the evidence contained in the statistical reports submitted to her by the Royal Commission on the Sanitary State of the Army in India.* London: Edward Stanford.

Nolan, M., Larson, E., McGuire, D., Hill, M., & Haller, M. (1994). A review of approaches to integrating research and practice. *Applied Nursing Research, 7*(4), 199-207.

O'Malley, P.A. (1994). The role of the critical care clinical nurse specialist in critical care research. In A. Gawlinski, & L.S. Kern (Eds.), *The clinical nurse specialist role in critical care* (pp. 173-195). Philadelphia: Saunders.

Pettengill, M., Gillies, D., Clark, C. (1994). Factors encouraging and discouraging the use of nursing research. *Image, 26*(2), 143-147.

Prevost, S.S. (1994). Research-based practice in critical care. *AACN Clinical Issues in Critical Care Nursing, 5*(2), 101.

Rogers, E.M. (1983). *Diffusion of innovations.* New York: The Free Press.

Rutledge, D.N., & Donaldson, N.E. (1995). Building organizational capacity to engage in research utilization. *Journal of Nursing Administration, 25*(10), 12-16.

Specht, J.P., Bergquist, S., & Frantz, R.A. (1995). Adoption of a research-based practice for treatment of pressure ulcers. *Nursing Clinics of North America, 30*(3), 553-563.

Stewart, I.M. (1962). Remarks on research in nursing. *Nursing Research, 11,* 5-6.

Stetler, C., Bautista, C., Vernale-Hannon, C., & Foster, J. (1995). Enhancing research utilization by clinical nurse specialists. *Nursing Clinics of North America, 30*(3), 457-473.

Stetler, C.B. (1994). Refinement of the Stetler/Marram model for application of research findings to practice. *Nursing Outlook, 42,* 15-25.

Stonestreet, J., & Lamb-Havard, J. (1994). Organizational strategies to promote research-based practice. *AACN Clinical Issues in Critical Care Nursing, 5*(2), 133-146.

Titler, M.G. (1993). Critical analysis of research utilization (RU): An historical perspective. *American Journal of Critical Care, 2*(3), 264.

Titler, M.G., Moss, L., Greiner, J., Alpen, M., Jones, G., Olsen, K., Hauer, M., Phillips, C., & Megivern, K. (1994). Research utilization in critical care: An exemplar. *AACN Clinical Issues in Critical Care Nursing, 5*(2), 124-132.

Titler, M., Goode, C., & Mathis, S. (1992). Nursing research in times of economic cutbacks: Implications for nurse administrators. *Series on Nursing Administration, 4,* 167-182.

Titler, M., Kleiber, C., Steelman, V., Goode, C., Rakel, B., Barry-Walker, J., Small, S., & Buckwalter, K. (1994). Infusing research into practice to promote quality care. *Nursing Research, 43*(5), 307-313.

Tornquist, E.M., Funk, S.G., & Champagne, M.T. (1993). Advice on reading research: Overcoming the barriers. *Applied Nursing Research, 6,* 177-183.

Weiler, K., Buckwalter, K., & Titler, M. (1994). Debate: Is nursing research used in practice? In J. McCloskey & H. Grace (Eds.), *Current issues in nursing* (4th Ed., pp. 61-75). St. Louis: Mosby.

Weiss, C.H. (1980). Knowledge creep and decision accretion. *Knowledge: Creation, Diffusion, Utilization, 1,* 381-404.

White, J., Leske, J., & Pearcy, J. (1995). Models and processes of research utilization. *Nursing Clinics of North America, 30*(3), 409-415.

The international classification for nursing practice

JUNE CLARK

It is a cruel paradox that while we "know" that nursing is universal because the human needs that it exists to meet are universal, we have at present no empirical means of comparing nursing practice across countries, or even across clinical settings or client groups within a country. Is there such a thing as "nursing" that is the same whether it is being done by a nurse in a modern hospital in New York, in a mission hospital in Uganda, in a primary health care center in Finland, or in a clinic in the Amazon rain forest? The paradox is that until we have a language in which to ask and answer this question we cannot know; we can only believe. At present we do not have terms that are precisely defined or universally agreed on in any one language, let alone across languages, in which to express what Nightingale once called "the elements of nursing" (Nightingale, 1859), i.e., what nurses do, in response to what sorts of problems, with what sorts of effects. We cannot know the incidence or prevalence of the human responses to health problems that are the target of nursing actions; and we cannot describe, let alone measure, the effects of such actions because we do not have a shared meaning about what it is that we are trying to measure.

The problem is not new. Almost a century ago a nurse who attended one of the earliest meetings of the International Council of Nurses (ICN), held in 1909 in Paris, wrote,

> While attending a special meeting of the ICN in Paris, I was naturally at once struck by the fact . . . . that the methods and the ways of regarding nursing problems were . . . . as foreign to the various delegations as were the actual languages; and the thought occurred to me that . . . sooner or later we must put ourselves upon a common basis and work out what may be termed a "nursing esperanto" which would, in the course of time, give us a universal nursing language . . . . (Hampton-Robb, 1909)

In the 90 years that have passed since then, nursing has developed enormously, but the gap identified by Hampton-Robb has not yet been remedied.

Communicating among ourselves about nursing is, and always has been, important, but communicating with other people about nursing has acquired a new urgency in all countries as we are forced to recognize that the value of nursing can no longer be considered self-evident, but has to be made visible in the information systems that all countries are developing as part of their efforts to manage health care.

Examining the quality and effectiveness of nursing care requires linking nursing interventions to measurable improvements in people's health, i.e., linking interventions with nursing diagnoses and patient outcomes. This demands an infrastructure that consists of three elements: (a) standardized vocabularies that describe the elements of nursing; (b) computer-based methods for calculating clusters and correlations while controlling for the effects of such things as patient characteristics and comorbidities; and (c) integrated clinical information management systems in which data are not just collected, but are converted to information and fed back to the data collector and care provider to complete the cycle of assessment, planning, implementation, and evaluation. It is the first of these three requirements that is the focus of the International Classification for Nursing Practice (ICNP) project.

LANGUAGE AND CLASSIFICATION

The ICNP project is being undertaken by the ICN—an organization made up of national nurses' associations from well over a hundred countries across seven continents. Language in its everyday sense is a daily issue for such an organization: The ICN has three "official" languages in which all its work is conducted (English, French, and Spanish), but its members practice their nursing in literally hundreds of different languages and dialects.

Language can be a barrier to obtaining a shared meaning. Even within the English-speaking world different words describe the same things and the same words describe different things. English nurses constantly complain that they do not understand the language in which some American nursing textbooks are written, yet when English nurses work in the United States or American nurses work in the United Kingdom, it becomes clear that they are using much the same knowledge base to do many of the same things.

The problem does not lie only in making comparisons between countries, whether they use the same language or not. An even bigger issue in every country is that, "If we cannot name it, we cannot control it, finance it, teach it, research it, or put it into public policy" (Lang & Clark, 1991).

American nurses know that if they cannot name it, they cannot claim reimbursement for it. Even in countries where claiming reimbursement is not relevant because the health care system is different, the "invisibility" of nursing is a major problem. Experience in many countries has demonstrated the vulnerability to which this exposes nursing, especially in an environment in which there is competition for control of resources. How can one argue a case for more nurses or for a different kind of nurse, or even know how many nurses are needed, if there is no way of describing what nurses do in response to what kind of problems they face and with what results?

Terms or labels alone are not enough, however. It appears to be an intrinsic need of the human mind to organize information systematically by grouping data according to common features and distinguishing one group from another by their commonalities and differences. At an individual level, the process is frequently subconscious, and the criteria for the grouping are rarely made explicit. We use this mental process to make sense of the mass of data that continually bombards our senses, learning the "new" by contrasting and comparing it with the previously known, felt, or experienced. This is how babies learn, and children who are unable to manage the process become defined as having "learning difficulties." The process is, in effect, one of creating "categories" for classification.

This same process is also the basis of science, and recognition of its importance to the development of nursing science is also not new. In 1926, Harmer wrote,

> If nursing is ever to make even a remote claim to being a science, or even to being conducted on a scientific basis, it must be built up like all branches of science, that is by the most careful, unbiased observation and recording of often seemingly trivial details from which—by organising, classifying, analysing, selecting, drawing and testing conclusions—a body of knowledge or principles are finally evolved.

If the need was identified so long ago, why has it taken so long for us to respond? The linguistic problem should not be underestimated, but the real problems are conceptual and attitudinal. The conceptual problem has been the slow development of theoretical frameworks for nursing and the apparent resistance of practicing nurses to the relevance of theory to their practice. This attitudinal resistance leads many nurses to dismiss the intellectual activity of conceptualizing and categorizing what they do as "mere theorizing." The tragedy is that practicing nurses themselves fail to recognize the complexity of their practice and the intellectual processes that underpin it; they do not see any need to "fuss" about what Benner has called "the knowledge embedded in clinical practice" (Benner, 1984).

Until now. Where scientific imperatives failed, financial imperatives and technology are succeeding. Cost constraints and greater emphasis on the efficient (and therefore systematic) development of resources require sound information and management systems. The development of computers has leapt into the breach and spawned a whole new science (informatics) and new methods of communication. Computers work by sorting, classifying, and manipulating data items and, therefore, require clear rules for defining and categorizing data input.

In the excitement of the data processing, however, the significance of defining the data input may be overlooked. The invisibility of nursing in the policy and commercial aspects of health care has led to the assumption that medical nomenclature and classification systems such as the International Classification of Diseases (World Health Organization [WHO], 1992) are adequate for nursing or, worse, that some "common sense" or ad hoc system developed by the system vendors or information experts will do. Nursing must not leave the decision making about nursing's essential data to system vendors or other health care professionals. It is nursing's responsibility to define its own phenomena in ways that are consistent with its own purposes.

Nurses in the United States were the first to recognize the need and to begin the work. Werley began to develop the concept of the Nursing Minimum Data Set (NMDS) in the late 1960s (Werley and Lang, 1988). The work of the American Nurses Association (ANA) on the development of standards of practice during the 1970s identified the elements for a nursing practice classification in its delineation of "assessment factors, nursing diagnosis, interventions, and outcomes," (ANA, 1980) and these ideas were reinforced by their 1980 definition of nursing as "the diagnosis and treatment of human responses to actual or potential health problems" (ANA, 1980). One recommendation in this publication was the pursuit of a classification system for nursing and, in 1982 the ANA Cabinet on Nursing Practice appointed a steering committee on classifications of nursing practice phenomena. Meanwhile, the development of a classification of nursing diagnoses was being pursued through the North American Nursing Diagnosis Association (NANDA, 1994), and McCloskey and Bulechek began their work at Iowa on a classification of nursing interventions (1992, 1996). Werley and Zorn (1989) note that the work on NMDS spurred further elaboration of intervention classifications and the nursing diagnosis taxonomy and that similarly, continual testing and implementation of the NMDS are not possible without the development and refinement of the classification of nursing interventions. Many other American nurses are similarly working on a variety of projects, and the American literature is now considerable and rapidly expanding (Grobe, 1992; Martin and Scheet, 1992; Saba, 1992). Significantly, it was the American and the Canadian Nursing Associations that proposed the resolution to the ICN that led to the development of the ICNP project.

Developments in other countries began later, but have accelerated rapidly during the 1990s. In 1991 when we undertook our initial literature review and survey among our (then) 105-member nursing associations and the (then) 21 WHO Collaborating Centers for Nursing (Wake, Murphy, Affara, Clark, & Mortensen, 1993), we were able to identify some work in Australia and the beginnings of work in a few other countries, but not much, for example, in Europe. By 1994, classification activities were occurring all over Europe, and in 1995 a new organization—the Association for Common European Nursing Diagnoses, Interventions, and Outcomes (ACENDIO)—was launched. It is clear that the impetus for this development came from two sources: the accelerating concern in all countries with cost containment and resource management in health care, and the rapidly developing science and technology of informatics, which is providing the systems necessary to support these activities.

In Europe, driven no doubt by the imperatives of computerized information and management systems, several countries are developing minimum data sets for health care, but nursing has generally not been in the forefront of these initiatives, which are dominated overwhelmingly by medicine. The problems of Europe's linguistic variability are balanced by the political goals of standardization and harmonization within the European community that already includes 15 countries, soon to be joined by the remaining countries of Western Europe and soon, perhaps, the re-emerging countries of Eastern Europe.

Meanwhile, between 1976 and 1985, the WHO/Euro project, "People's Needs for Nursing Care," brought together nurses from Belgium, Czechoslovakia, Denmark, Finland, France, Greece, Norway, Poland, the United Kingdom, and Yugoslavia in an effort to standardize essential nursing data within the framework of the nursing process. This project was, however, pursued as part of the professional development of nursing and not as part of the development of computerized information system. As Mortensen (1991) has pointed out, European nurses (at least those in Denmark and the United Kingdom) seem to be divided into two groups: one interested in information technology but without any great interest in clinical nursing based on the concept of nursing diagnosis, and another actively interested in identifying nursing diagnoses in clinical practice but less interested in computers. This divide has to be overcome, and Mortensen's own work at the Danish Institute for Health and Nursing Research is designed to bring together the development of nursing diagnoses and the development of nursing informatics (Mortensen, 1992).

In all of these circumstances, the need for an ICNP is urgent. All around the world, we are faced with demands for information about health care and the development of systems for providing it, in which the largest component of health care—nursing—is at risk of being invisibly absorbed, its distinctive contribution unseen, undervalued, and sunk without trace.

THE HISTORY OF THE INTERNATIONAL CLASSIFICATION FOR NURSING PRACTICE

The ICNP project is the result of a resolution of the ICN's Council of National Representatives at its meeting in Seoul in 1989. Proposed and seconded by the ANA and the Canadian Nurses Association, the resolution asked that the ICN encourage member National Nursing Associations to become involved in developing classification systems for nursing care, nursing information management systems, and nursing data sets; to provide tools that nurses in all countries can use to identify nursing practice; and to describe nursing and its contributions to health.

The resolution was referred by the ICN Board of Directors to its Professional Services Committee, which appointed consultants first to study the feasibility of such a project and subsequently to take the work forward. The proposal was described in an article published by Clark and Lang in the *International Nursing Review* (1992). This document set out the shape of the project, in particular its goals and its criteria.

The specific objectives of the ICNP are:

- To establish a common language about nursing practice to improve communication among nurses and between nurses and other users of health information
- To describe the nursing care of people (individuals, families, and communities) in a variety of both institutional and noninstitutional settings
- To enable comparison of nursing data across clinical settings, client groups, and time
- To demonstrate or project trends in the provision of nursing care
- To enable the allocation of resources to patients according to their needs based on nursing diagnosis
- To stimulate nursing research
- To provide data about nursing practice to influence health policy decision making

To be useful and applicable to nurses in all countries, the ICNP must meet certain specified criteria. It must be:

- Broad enough to serve the multiple purposes required by different countries, and, as we now recognize, to serve the multiple purposes of information systems within countries
- Simple enough to be seen by the ordinary practitioner of nursing as a meaningful description of practice and a useful means of structuring practice
- Consistent with clearly defined conceptual frameworks but not dependent on a particular theoretical framework or model of nursing
- Based on a central core to which additions can be made through a continuing process of development and refinement
- Sensitive to cultural variability
- Reflective of the common value system of nursing across the world as expressed in the ICN Code for Nurses
- Usable in a complementary or integrated way with the family of disease- and health-related classification developed within WHO, the core of which is the ICD

A strategic plan that outlined the major goals and the means to their achievement was developed. The strategies on which the work is based are as follows:

- To develop an ICNP with specified process and product components
- To achieve recognition by the national and international nursing communities
- To ensure that the ICNP is compatible with and complementary to the WHO family of classifications and the work of other standardization groups such as the International Organization for Standardization and its related groups including the Comites European de Normalisation, and to secure inclusion of ICNP in relevant classifications
- To achieve utilization of ICNP by nurses at country level for the development of national databases
- To establish an international data set and a framework that incorporates the ICNP, the NMDS, a nursing resource data set, and regulatory data

These goals cannot be achieved by technical means alone, nor can they be achieved by the consultants or the ICN alone. They require the collaboration and commitment of many people in many organizations and many countries.

The ICN does not have a research team of the kind that has enabled so much work to be done in this field in the United States and some other countries, or indeed any personnel who can work full-time on the project. Since 1990 when the work began, however, a great deal has been achieved:

1. A literature search and three small surveys have been undertaken of member associations to identify classification systems either currently in use or being developed around the world (Wake et al., 1993).

2. In 1992, a Technical Advisory Group of nurses from six countries (Israel, Nepal, Chile, Kenya, Jamaica, and Japan) met in Geneva to test the feasibility and applicability of the work to date at global level. This is very important because one of our key challenges is to ensure that any system is applicable in all countries.

3. In 1993, a first draft list, derived from the literature, of terms that are currently used to describe nursing diagnoses, interventions, and outcomes was published (ICN, 1993). This initial list was recognized to be highly selective, biased by its over-reliance on English language sources, and certainly not comprehensive. For example, the UK Nursing Terms Project alone has already generated some 20,000 terms that are currently used by nurses in the United Kingdom (Casey, 1995). This list did not

incorporate any attempt at classification beyond alphabetical ordering under the three headings of diagnoses, interventions, and outcomes. The ICNP list, and the updating of the literature review, are being maintained by Wake at Marquette University in Wisconsin.

4. The ICN's 114 national nurses associations have been invited to submit new labels, using guidelines prepared by the consultants (ICN, 1994a).

5. As part of the commitment to collaborate with the WHO Department of Epidemiological and Health Statistical Services and the WHO Collaborating Centers for the Classification of Diseases, a review of ICD-10 and related classifications to identify labels that are relevant to nursing was undertaken, and a preliminary report of this work was included in an ICN Working Paper published in 1993 (ICN, 1993).

6. The Quadrennial Congress of the ICN held in Madrid in June 1993 included a plenary session, a special interest session, and a poster session about ICNP. All three were extremely well attended, demonstrating a quite overwhelming interest and enthusiasm for ICNP by nurses from many countries.

7. An Advisory Meeting on the Development of an Informational Tool to Support Community-Based and Primary Health Care Nursing Systems was held in Mexico in February 1994 (ICN, 1994b). This meeting brought together nurses from selected countries in Africa and North and South America to explore the potential of the ICNP for nursing in primary health care. This too is a major challenge because the ICN is totally committed to the development of primary health care, but unfortunately much of the work and many of the systems developed to date have been very oriented to acute and inpatient care. Another workshop, held in December 1995 in Taiwan, brought together nurses from nine Asian-Pacific countries.

8. During 1994 and 1995 the consultants and technical advisers worked on developing a taxonomic structure which enables existing terms and the new terms that are emerging from the work of nurses in many countries, to be classified within a logical framework. An Alpha Version, which contains a Classification of Nursing Phenomena (Diagnoses) and a Classification of Nursing Interventions is now available from ICN headquarters in Geneva. The first formal field testing is being undertaken in Europe in the TELENURSE project which is led by Dandi Mortensen of the Danish Institute of Health and Nursing Research.

SCOPE OF THE INTERNATIONAL CLASSIFICATION OF NURSING PRACTICE

The title ICNP is a kind of shorthand. The initials link the project to ICN, but the ICNP project involves more than a classification—it also involves developing a nomenclature, and, eventually, an internationally recognized nursing minimum data set. It will be both a new classification and a framework through which other nursing classifications can be cross-mapped.

The ICNP involves "naming, sorting, and linking phenomena that describe what nurses do, for what human conditions, and to produce what outcome" (ICN, 1991). This involves identifying and naming what Nightingale called the "elements of nursing" (Nightingale, 1859): nursing problems/diagnoses, nursing actions/interventions, and nursing outcomes. The structure of the task, showing how each stage leads on to the next, is shown in Figure 16-1.

Figure 16-1 shows how the practicing nurse finds words (terms) for the elements of his or her practice. When standardized among nurses, these words become a *nursing nomenclature.* This nomenclature can be sorted according to agreed upon principles to form a *classification.*

The nomenclature can be used in an NMDS, which is a minimum set of items with uniform definitions and categories concerning nursing. Many countries have already identified the need for collection, storage, and retrieval of nursing data, making it important to have a uniform nomenclature and classification of nursing practice so that meaningful and comparative data can be collected.

The data that are labelled according to a nursing nomenclature, structured into a nursing language, and classified by means of common features (an ICNP) can be collated for inclusion in an NMDS, which in turn can be fed back into nursing practice at the center of the spiral; and the continuous process of development, refinement and modification in response to external change begins again. But the most important thing to note is that the spiral begins and ends in nursing practice.

STRENGTHS AND WEAKNESSES, LIMITS AND OPPORTUNITIES

The ICNP project has been called "nursing's next advance" (ICN, 1991, unpublished data), but it is important also to recognize its limitations.

Firstly, the ICNP is not a panacea; it is merely a tool that nurses can use in whatever way they want to, and for

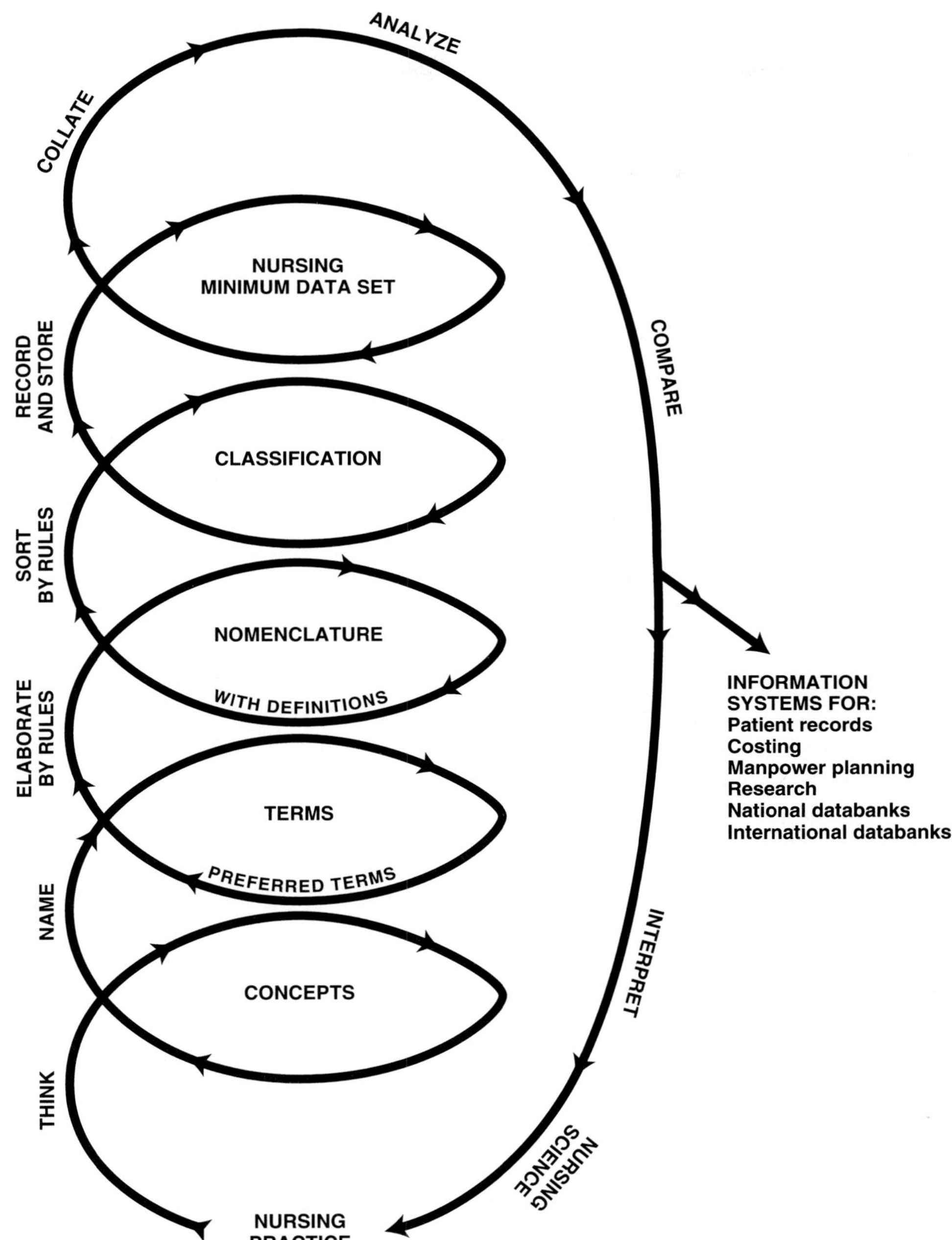

Fig. 16-1. Development of the ICNP.

whatever purposes. It will be of no use unless it is used, and just like any tool, we will have to learn how to use it well.

Secondly, it will only be as good a tool as we make it. For example, it will enable us to describe the full range of nursing practice only if it contains appropriate labels from all fields of nursing practice. Consequently, more work needs to be done in describing the nursing diagnoses and interventions used in community nursing and primary health care.

Thirdly, if we nurses do not value it, then nobody else will. There is a tendency, at least in the United Kingdom, to regard activities such as this as "mere theorizing"—as some kind of trivial intellectual game for academics that has no relevance to "real" nursing. This attitude is dangerous because it ignores the importance that computerized information, and therefore information systems, are beginning to have in all countries on the determination of nursing and health care, especially health care resources.

THE BENEFITS

If an ICNP were adopted on a worldwide basis and used to summarize data that were collected routinely and continuously, the benefits for nursing would be immense—for nursing practice, nursing administration and management, nursing research, nursing education, nursing policy, and health care policy.

For nursing practice an ICNP would:

- Provide a framework and a structure for nursing documentation that would encourage more precise and consistent documentation of nursing care and provide data to be used as a basis for individual clinical decision making
- Facilitate documentation (and therefore recognition) of those nursing actions that are not at present explicitly documented, recognized or, costed (e.g., those concerned with health promotion, identifying and utilizing people's own strengths and capabilities and coordinating care)
- Improve continuity of nursing care for patients who are transferred across settings by improving the quality of information about their nursing needs and previous nursing care
- Facilitate the collection and use of data for measuring and monitoring quality of care and for development of nursing practice standards and guidelines and quality assurance

For nursing administration/management an ICNP would:

- Facilitate the measurement of clinical nursing care for evaluation and other purposes
- Refine nursing resource allocation methodologies and improve the ability to estimate the need for nursing as a basis for planning, budgeting, and resource allocation
- Enable investigation of the cost-effectiveness of nursing by relating nursing interventions to outcomes
- Enable investigation of the effectiveness of differential staffing patterns relative to patient dependencies (acuity)
- Enable comparison of clinical nursing data and human resources data across units, regions, and countries
- Enable description and analysis of trends based on data about clinical nursing practice

For nursing research an ICNP would:

- Facilitate descriptive research on the kinds of problems that are the focus of nursing, and on the types of intervention nurses use to tackle them
- Stimulate and facilitate comparison of nursing diagnoses/problems across local, regional, national, and international settings
- Facilitate studies of the effectiveness of nursing treatments by relating nursing diagnoses, actions, and outcomes
- Permit the creation of a national and international database for development of nursing science, knowledge, and theory building

For nursing education an ICNP would:

- Provide a framework for curriculum planning and evaluation
- Provide a direct communication link between the curriculum and the practice arena
- Encourage research-based teaching by providing a similar communication link between curriculum and research data
- Encourage the integration of information management into basic, postbasic, and continuing education

For nursing policy an ICNP would:

- Make visible the full range of nursing practice including the nursing contribution to health promotion and prevention of illness
- Enable sound data instead of anecdotal information to serve as the basis for informed decision making and policy formulation

- Facilitate the definition of the evolving scope of practice for regulatory purposes
- Facilitate the definition of nursing roles for socioeconomic purposes

For health care policy an ICNP would:

- Identify the role of nurses in the multidisciplinary team and the contribution of nursing to multidisciplinary health care, especially in primary health care
- Provide nursing data comparable with and complementary to existing health care data
- Propose additional elements for epidemiological study
- Enable the inclusion of nursing data in cost-benefit ratios and quality assurance
- Enable the inclusion of nursing data in measurements of universal health status

CONCLUSION

The ICNP will be a useful tool to nursing in all countries and in many different ways. The challenges involved in its development are enormous, but it is fundamental to the continued development and recognition of nursing. It is the kind of project that never ends but for which the beginning is urgent: It is with justification that it has been called "nursing's next advance."

REFERENCES

American Nurses Association. (1980). *Nursing: A social policy statement.* Kansas City: MO: Author.

Benner, P. (1984). *From novice to expert: Excellence and power in clinical nursing.* Reading, MA: Addison-Wesley.

Casey, A. (1995). Standard terminology for nursing: Results of the Nursing, Midwifery and Health Visiting Terms Project. *Health Informatics, 1*, 41-43.

Clark, J., & Lang, N. (1992). Nursing's next advance: An International Classification for Nursing Practice. *International Nursing Review, 38*(4),109-112.

Grobe, S.J. (1992). Nursing lexicon and taxonomy: Preliminary categorization. In K.C. Lun, P. De Goulet, T.E. Plemme, & O. Reinhott (Eds.), *Med-Info'92: Proceedings of the 7th World Congress on Medical Informatics.* North Holland: Elsevier Science Publishers.

Hampton-Robb, I. (1909). *Report of the third regular meeting of the International Council of Nurses.* Geneva: International Council of Nurses.

Harmer, B. (1926). *Methods and principles of teaching the principles and practice of nursing.* New York: Macmillan.

International Council of Nurses. (1993). *Nursing's next advance: An international classification for nursing practice: Working papers.* Geneva: Author.

International Council of Nurses. (1994a). *Guidelines for submitting labels to the International Classification for Nursing Practice.* Geneva: Author.

International Council of Nurses. (1994b). *Report of an advisory meeting on the development of an information tool to support community-based and primary health care nursing systems.* Geneva: Author.

Lang, N., & Clark, J. (1991). Nursing's next advance: Development of an international classification for nursing practice: Final Proposal submitted to the Board of Directors. ICN (unpublished).

Martin, K.S., & Scheet, N.J. (1992). *The Omaha system: Applications for community health nursing.* Philadelphia: Lippincott.

McCloskey, J.C., & Bulechek, G.M. (Eds.). (1992). *Nursing interventions classification (NIC).* St. Louis: Mosby.

McCloskey, J.C., & Bulechek, G.M. (Eds.). (1996). *Nursing Interventions Classification (NIC)* (2nd ed.). St. Louis: Mosby.

Mortensen, R.A. (1991). *Experiences in health care data base development.* Paper presented to the WHO Workshop on Nursing Informatics in Washington, D.C., October 1991. Copenhagen: Danish Institute for Health and Nursing Research.

Mortensen, R.A. (1992). *Concerted action of nursing: European action on information requirements for nursing practice. European classification of nursing practice with regard to patient problems, nursing interventions, and patient outcomes, including educational measures.* Unpublished paper. Copenhagen: Danish Institute for Health and Nursing Research.

Nightingale, F. (1859). Notes on nursing.

North American Nursing Diagnosis Association. (1994). *Nursing diagnoses: Definitions and classifications.* Philadelphia: Author.

Saba, V.K. (1992). Diagnoses and interventions. *Caring, 11*(3), 50-57.

Wake, M., Murphy, M., Affara, F., Clark, J., & Mortensen, R. (1993). Toward an international classification for nursing practice: A pilot literature review and survey. *International Nursing Review, 40*(3), 77-80.

Werley, H.H., & Lang, N. (Eds.). (1988). Identification of the nursing minimum data set. New York: Springer.

Werley, H., Devine, E., Zorn, C., Ryan, P., & Westra, B. (1991). The nursing minimum data set: Abstraction tool for standardized comparable essential data. *American Journal of Public Health, 81*(4), 421-426.

WHO. (1992). *International statistical classification of diseases and related health problems: Tenth revision.* Geneva: Author.

Section Three

CHANGING EDUCATION

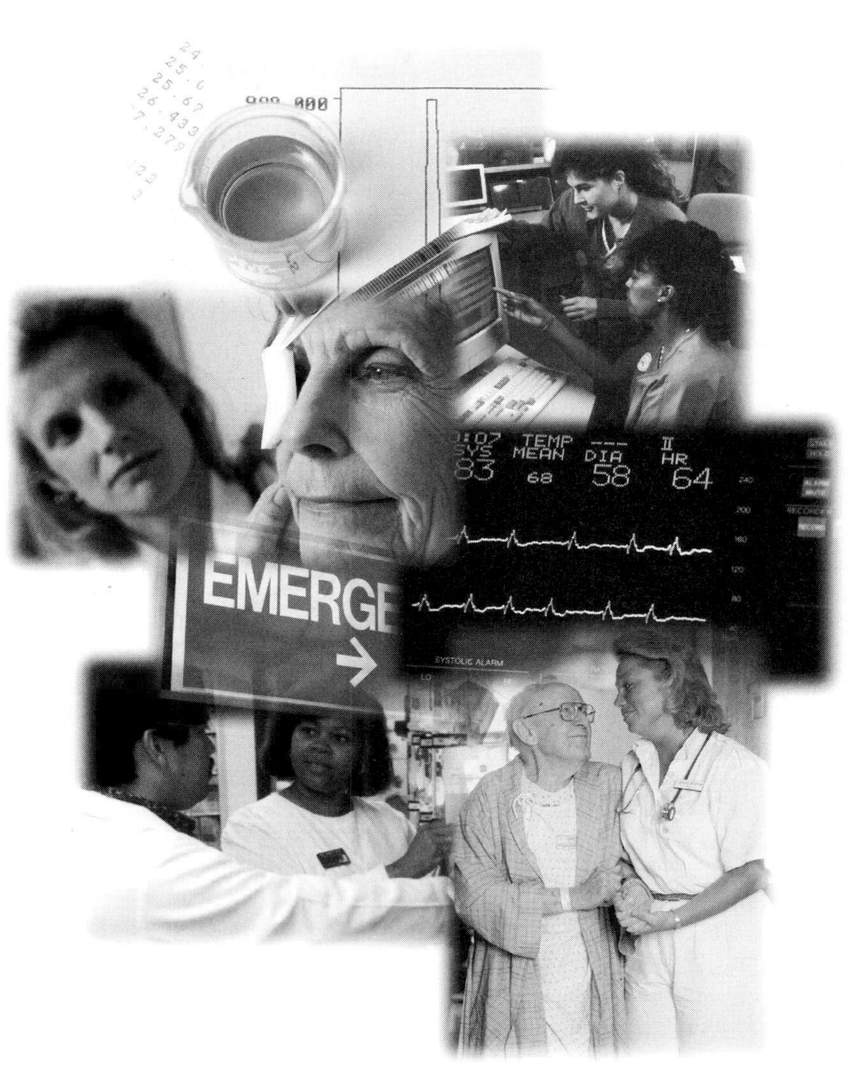

OVERVIEW

Nursing education in transition

JOANNE COMI McCLOSKEY, HELEN KENNEDY GRACE

As massive changes are occurring in the health care delivery system, nursing education faces challenges in preparing practitioners for the future. Over the past 50 years, much of the emphasis in nursing education has been on preparing nurses to practice in hospital settings. As hospitals have become increasingly specialized, nursing education has followed suit by preparing more and more nurse specialists. There are currently over 100 specialty groups within nursing, the majority of which are focused on in-hospital specialties. Changes in the health care system are moving now in the opposite direction—that of providing care in community and home settings to the degree possible. Patients who previously spent days in hospitals postoperatively now are sent home the day of surgery. There haven't been that many dramatic advances in the surgical procedures used, nor has the condition of patients changed appreciably; they are still as incapacitated as when they were placed in the hospital bed. It is now assumed, however, that patients can get well on their own. Even highly specialized care such as chemotherapy and other forms of infusion therapy is being provided in home settings. With the increased emphasis on keeping people healthy, a whole variety of new roles are opening for nurses. The challenge to nursing education is to make modifications that will prepare practitioners for the future rather than maintain the emphasis of the past. In this section a wide array of issues are addressed that challenge the very fundamentals of nursing education as we have known it.

In the opening debate chapter, Camilleri takes an historical look at nursing and nursing education and contrasts the conflicting perspectives of nursing as a craft versus as a profession. The context in which nursing has been practiced and in which nurses have been educated has valued nursing as a craft, while the development of nursing as a profession has posed a threat to those who have exerted control over the health care system. As we move to the 21st century, Camilleri identifies five major challenges to nursing education: change of the focus of care from hospitals to communities, the impact of the information superhighway, the ever-expanding role of technology, shrinking resources, and globalization with increased interdependency of communities all over the world. Meeting these challenges requires that we transform our thinking about nursing education to have much more of a career orientation, that we emphasize experiential learning in our curricula, that increased interdisciplinary collaboration be encouraged, and that we place emphasis on preserving resources and providing quality care.

Not only is the context of changing health care practices a challenge to nursing education, but the student body is also changing. Bednash, in the first issues paper in this section, points to the bifurcation of the student body with one part composed of students just out of high school, and the other composed of the growing group of adult learners returning to school to acquire new knowledge and skills. These two groups of students come from different experiential worlds and pose a challenge to nursing educators. Other challenges include the increased diversity of our population and the lag in the diversifying of students and faculty in nursing education. Nursing education increasingly must adjust to nontraditional students and modify teaching programs accordingly. Accelerated programs, allowing students additional time to complete degree study when needed, more attention to recruiting minority students, and addressing the special needs of a diverse student population are posed as some of the challenges.

Lacey advances the argument that one of the ways of meeting the challenges facing nursing education is by turning the focus to community health, thereby gaining understanding of the health issues confronting diverse communities. Pointing out that a large proportion of the health problems confronting us today are related to preventable diseases, nursing education should emphasize maintenance of health and the role of the family and the community rather than the treatment of illness in a hospital context. Lacey argues that communities and families provide a comprehensive matrix for teaching family dynamics and community health nursing practice, and that with this as a focal point nurses would be much better equipped to meet the challenges of the future. Using the example of her experience in establishing a health ambulatory clinic, a postdetoxification unit, and an infirmary in a homeless shelter, Lacey outlines the content of the nursing educational program that was developed in this setting. Contrasting paradigms are outlined that undergird traditional curricular constructs and the underpinning for the newly developed community-based curricula.

The nationwide Community College–Nursing Home Partnership project, headed by Waters, Tagliareni, Mengel, and Sherman, was successful in the transformation of associate degree nursing education to include an increased emphasis on gerontological nursing. This process of change is described, and it is proposed that associate degree nursing education build on these experiences to make further transformations from traditional hospital settings to the home and community. One of the major challenges in making these changes is the difficulty in dealing with the ambiguity of out of hospital settings. The future requires the acceptance of ambiguity in practice. Discovery learning and critical thinking will be essential in a community/neighborhood model of health care delivery.

Tracing the history and tradition of graduate education generally and nursing education specifically, Redman and Ketefian argue for diversity in master's degree programs while also meeting the challenge of ensuring that the standards for graduate education are comparable. At the doctoral level, the preservation of scientific integrity is identified as a major concern. This poses a particular challenge given the shallow "pool" of doctorally prepared faculty and the demands placed on them. Postdoctoral training is proposed as one way of addressing this issue.

The next three issues chapters in this section address teaching approaches. Krichbaum, Lewis, and Duckett address the problem of teaching the essential skill of critical thinking. Noting that the focus on preparing nurses for practice in critical care settings does not encourage critical thinking, the authors argue that this is a major issue for nursing education to address. They provide a comprehensive overview of the field and then offer suggestions for clinical and classroom teaching strategies that would encourage critical thinking. The challenge is for faculty and students to work side by side in developing this essential skill.

While distance education has traditionally been considered as an approach to address the needs of students who live and want to learn at a distance from the university campus, Rothert, Talarczyk, and Awbrey argue that the experiences drawn from finding ways of addressing student needs at a distance can play a role in facilitating transformation of the university to meet the challenges of the future. The use of computers and interactive television requires faculty to adapt their traditional teaching roles to the new technology. A particular issue for nursing education is assuring the quality of clinical instruction available to students studying at a distance. Nursing education, with its history of addressing the needs of adult learners through distance education, is uniquely positioned to be a part of the solution as universities move into the new world of partnerships with communities in entering the 21st century.

The challenge of using technology in nursing education is addressed by Clark. Noting the cost of technology and the lag in the readiness to make adequate use of these technologies, Clark advocates specific attention to faculty preparation as a critical issue. Emphasis needs to change from traditional forms of instructional delivery to developing the software for using the technology effectively. The role of the teacher changes from delivering instruction to serving as a facilitator or resource person to the student.

In all of these transitions, nursing education is confronted increasingly by the need to justify what is sometimes perceived as the high cost of nursing education. Forni and Burns point to a number of indices indicating that the costs of nursing education are being scrutinized closely. There are only two ways to address this concern: increase revenue streams or decrease costs. Expansion of approaches to generate revenues and ways of achieving greater efficiencies in teaching approaches are proposed.

Finally, the challenges of addressing the needs of a global society are addressed by Fenton. As the United States becomes an increasingly diverse society nursing education is faced with the need for preparing students to understand the cultural contexts of their patients. We have much to learn from health care systems in developing countries. Fenton suggests that some of the answers to our current health care problems could be enlightened by looking at models of care in other countries. Faculty exchange and international student programs are described as one approach to building international links. She concludes that "international exchanges result in better understanding of the differences and similarities of nursing around the world, and, most important, build confidence that nurses can make a significant impact on the health of the people."

Clark, in her article on technology, draws on Charles Dickens' "it is the best of times, it is the worst of times." Never have the opportunities been greater for nursing education to take the lead in making the transformations to address the challenges of health care in the 21st century. The shift of care from hospital to community, the emphasis on an increasingly diverse population, the opportunity to use diverse teaching technologies to improve nursing education, and the importance of interdisciplinary collaboration are unique opportunities. Can nursing meet these challenges through adaptive behavior, or will we cling to the old ways and maintain the self-defeating attitudes that have constrained us? If we cling to the past it will indeed be the worst of times.

Nursing education for the 21st century: Old traditions and new challenges

DOROTHY D. CAMILLERI

To stimulate spirited, sometimes contentious discussion among nurses, one has only to gather a heterogeneous group of nurse educators or nurses in clinical practice and introduce the topic of how nurses should be educated. Whether it is focused on education for today or for the challenging century ahead, the discussion would be spirited. Our differences of opinion on this topic are both a strength and a weakness for the nursing profession, but are hardly surprising given the diversity of types of practice covered by the designation "nursing" and the different paths that are taken to become credentialed for that practice.

OUR DIVERSE PATHS: TO A GARDEN OR A WEED PATCH?

The focus of this chapter is on nursing and nursing education as they have developed in the United States. In the United States, nurses constitute the largest single division of health care providers, and as a division are themselves quite segmented. Over two million people hold the registered nurse (RN) license, the credential that legally qualifies a person for the practice of professional nursing. During the first half of this century, the overwhelming majority of people qualifying for licensure were graduates of 3-year hospital diploma programs. Patterns have changed markedly, and today the majority of people meeting requirements graduate from 2-year associate degree programs. A growing minority graduate from baccalaureate programs, and a sharply shrinking minority from 3-year hospital diploma programs. Of 88,149 students graduating from basic RN programs in 1993, just under 7,000 were diploma program graduates, under 57,000 were associate degree graduates, and over 24,000 were baccalaureate degree graduates (National League for Nursing, 1994a). Some of the baccalaureate graduates undoubtedly already had a diploma or associate degree, because an increasing number of such graduates do go on to earn baccalaureate degrees—many in nursing, but some in other fields. Workplace pressures for nurses to complete a baccalaureate or advanced degree are thought to account for the willingness of so many nurses to return to school (Berlin and Bednash, 1995).

To further complicate matters, an additional small group of people who already have nonnursing degrees before entering nursing are qualifying for RN licensure through generic master's programs, or even professional doctorate programs (Berlin and Bednash, 1995). Some of these programs provide specialty as well as basic preparation.

Adding to the complex picture of nursing and its educational patterns, there are nursing groups on both sides of the basic professional preparation already outlined. On one side, there are a host of professional nurses with advanced practice or specialty designations such as nurse midwives, nurse practitioners, nurse anesthetists, and clinical specialists. These roles are becoming more numerous, and have always entailed some specialized training for the nurse to be recognized publicly in the specialized role. In more recent years, a graduate degree (master's or doctoral) has become a common requirement, and nurses claiming such roles are expected to be certified by a professional nursing association.

On the other side of the professional RN roles are the licensed practical or vocational nurses, whose scope of practice is legally defined but more limited than that of the RN. In addition, in health care settings it is also typical to categorize all individuals in assistive roles as nursing staff. These individuals and their roles are quite variable, ranging from certified nurse's aides to unlicensed assistive workers. The common denominator in this particular group is that their work falls under the direction and supervision of professional nursing staff. It is possible for a patient in a health care setting with a varied staff to report having talked to a nurse, and mean anyone from a nurse's aide to an advanced practice nurse.

The picture just described is considered confusing by most, and does at times seem more like an untended weed patch than a garden. Many nurses are troubled by it. On the issue of the basic licensure for professional practice, for instance, many critics argue that the wide range of educational programs at different educational levels, all purporting to prepare for professional practice, simply defies credibility. How would it be possible for such very different programs to produce the same ends? Some critics contend that our discipline is undermined by the claims to professional practice by this wide array of programs. They believe that the profusion of educational backgrounds as well as different professional roles make it highly improbable that other professionals and the public would take us seriously.

Other commentators acknowledge inconsistencies in our educational arrangements but advise a more tolerant attitude about the matter. This group reminds us that the RN credential is a legality with limited meaning. It is a political matter of legislation in each of the 50 states, and should not be taken as evidence of equality among programs or of true professional practice. In other words, passing the examination and meeting other standards for licensure ensures a minimum standard of safe practice; it does not measure degrees of quality or discriminate between higher and lower levels of ability or professionalism.

On the balance, there seems to be little point in bemoaning our lack of one precise meaning for the term "nurse," or our profusion of titles and educational paths. This is not because there is no confusion; there *is* confusion. It is because they represent the reality of our development, the breadth of nursing roles, and the very different ways that nurses are contributing to our nation's health care enterprise. We would do better to consider the factors that account for how we have evolved in concert with social circumstances, and to profit from our past in order to maximize our ability to contribute in the future. There is no doubt that nursing roles and educational practices will continue to evolve, as will health care and society in general. In trying to choose wisely the best directions to take in nursing education during the next century, we would do well to identify some of the important traditions we have had and to examine the different ways in which nursing is connected to and influenced by the society in which it is developing. This type of assessment provides a vantage point for predicting the challenges that will shape both nursing education and health care in the years ahead.

This chapter forwards such assessment by first looking to our past practice to identify two of the most potent traditions or cultures that have flourished, showing their fit into the larger social context of the times, and then turning to some of the challenges that can be expected in the years ahead. Some ideas about the implications of these challenges are elaborated, with differing points of view presented on a number of unresolved topics. The discussion is limited to the time period of the development of modern nursing, roughly the post-Nightingale era. Although the focus of the chapter is on nursing in the United States, we trace our heritage to Nightingale, and so need to take into account the forerunning developments as they occurred in Great Britain during that period.

DISCORDANT TRADITIONS

Historically, the story of modern nursing is closely tied to the story of women, with some special subplots related to social class and economics, as well as to gender. Trends or themes at odds with one another could always be identified as the story played out in Great Britain and the United States, and the updated version of these opposing trends sometimes seems clearly responsible for our current differences of opinion on educational practice.

The experiment in Great Britain

Most of us are familiar in broad outline, if not in detail, with the Nightingale Fund Nursing School program for staffing a number of hospitals in Great Britain with nurses who were well trained in comparison with the prevailing standards of that day. Worthy of note was the social class of the recruits (genteel rather than low), their status in the hospital (pupils rather than domestics), and the focus of their loyalty and identification (to the Fund rather than the hospital). These women were an experimental group who would use the skills and habits acquired through Nightingale's regimented system of training to bring about a transformation in the nursing care of hospitalized patients. Both pupil and trained nurses were responsible to the Fund, and were assigned to hospitals by that body. The elements of this Nightingale training had been established some years earlier by Breay, who clearly thought of the training as entailing a whole set of new principles, requiring new institutional arrangements, and yielding a new occupational identity (Williams, 1980). (I'm sure we all recognize an early "professionalizer" at work!) The Nightingale Fund program, of course, reflected the same principles as had been established by Breay. Physicians and superintendents in charge of the hospitals were quite happy with the advent of training because they were pleased at the upgrading or improvement in both the characters of nurses and the skills they possessed. Although the training ushered in the separation of nursing work from domestic work, the physicians and superintendents did not realize the significance of the change, nor did they recognize it as fuel for the start of a new occupation, with the potential for upsetting the status quo.

Before long, however, discordant voices were heard from the superintendent/physician group, based on their disapproval of the pupil nurses being taught theory. A medical historian wrote, "As time passed on the training of probationers became more specialized; from clinical and practical it became to a greater extent theoretical . . . and a bad style of nurse has resulted from this false training" (Williams, 1980. p. 52). According to Williams, the physicians were willing to accept the "skilled profession" in terms of changes in the character of nurses, but rejected it in terms of changes in their status and work that did not stem directly from a medical view of what nursing should be. The viewpoint of those in charge of the hospital was that nursing required a docile discipline, a good heart and character, and capable, well-trained hands. In their view, it clearly did not call for anything like independent thought or problem solving.

Thus, opposing trends are to be found at this first strong push to modernize nursing, with a small group of visionary women attempting to upgrade the status of nurses and reform nursing health care for patients. The positions of the different stakeholders were based on advancing or protecting their particular interests; when opposition arises, it is typically an indication that the opposer believes his or her interests are at risk of harm as some other interest is advanced. The men in control of hospitals welcomed improvements in nursing up to the point where the nurses seemed to be growing into a body with an identity and function of its own, outside the sphere of control of either the physician or the superintendent.

Note that the nursing care of the day *was* in need of change. Most stakeholders were in agreement on that point, although it is easy to imagine that one of the most powerless stakeholders of all, the lower class women whose hospital positions were low status sinecures of little accountability or responsibility, may have had other ideas about the changes that were indicated. While the nursing professionalizers did not achieve all of their goals, the balance that was struck between improvements in the structure and function of nursing, without altogether capsizing the boat of conventional hospital control, allowed the course of modern nursing to unfold—never out of trouble, but unfold nonetheless. The dynamic of stakeholders advancing or protecting their own interests is most fundamental. It is as pervasive today among and within all groups as it was in Nightingale's time.

The subordinate status of women in the Victorian era and early 20th century undoubtedly contributed to these developments. Davies (1980) suggests that only such a subordinate group would accept the compromises that these nurse reformers did, and she points out that only very meager resources were ever allocated to the training of nurses, and that the reform movement resulted in a minimal amount of change in the status quo. The nurse leaders of the day had not expected miracles; however, they regarded their efforts as one strand in the progress and social change of the day—promoting the wider participation of all women in society. Many in the cadre of well-educated women of respectable social class who were involved in upgrading nursing in both Great Britain and the United States were suffragists or feminists. Improving the general social order by improving the status of women was an important goal for them. For instance, responding to criticisms about nurses being taught too much, Dock, a renowned American nursing leader and suffragist of her day, said, "the thing of real importance is not that nurses be taught less, but that all women be taught more" (Melosh, 1982, p. 76).

The American scene

American women of similar class and bent as their British sisters were greatly influenced by the Nightingale system, and this was reflected in early efforts at reform and upgrading for nursing in the United States. There was fertile ground for such upgrading, and the same conflicting themes that were apparent between the nurse reformers and the conventional sources of social control in Great Britain found expression here. In an insightful review essay on nursing history, James (1984) characterizes the social ideology held by the professionalizing segment of turn-of-the-century nurses as the progressive view, one reflecting great faith in the strengthening of democracy through the education and elevation of women. Educated women and nurses would be forces for social reform and world peace. This viewpoint, James claims, infuses the history texts written by Nutting and Dock that were used for students in hospital schools in the early decades of the century. The students were thereby exposed to a morally uplifting, optimistic view of the nature of nursing that was a marked contrast to the realities of their daily life.

The conditions for nurses at the time were far from ideal. There was an explosive growth in the hospital industry as all classes of people, not just the poor, began to turn to hospitals for illness care (Vogel, 1979). At the same time, social changes were propelling women into the workforce, although the working woman was not commonplace and work choices were few. A window of opportunity had opened, creating a joint niche for hospitals and women. Hospitals survived by opening their own nurse training programs as a means of staffing their institutions, and women improved their situations, acquiring a toehold on a better life through the training and discipline they acquired in these programs. Note that for many women the need to be self-supporting was their motivation, rather than the wish to improve society or upgrade the status of women.

Typically, the hospital training programs were very short on curriculum, very long on hours of unpaid labor benefitting the hospital, very strong on discipline and subservience to authority, and very weak on career security for the fledgling nurse. Thus the cadre of nursing reformers of the day were injecting a note of high morale and moral purpose into the bleak nursing landscape experienced by students and trained nurses alike. Training was an apprenticeship affair, with students carrying out the work of the hospital wards under supervision of more advanced students or the nursing superintendent. Graduates left the hospital for private duty practice. Although the pattern had many positive points, service demands always took precedence over educational needs. Stewart commented:

> The big question was not how much the probationer understood about her duties but how much she could get done in a ten hour day and how fast she could learn to take a full share of the work of the hospital ward. (quoted in Davies, 1980, p. 110)

The reformers concentrated on issues such as raising standards of recruitment, allowing time for classes, and improving and standardizing the curriculum for nursing. For them, better education was the key to better health care for society and an improved status for nurses. The reformers had taken on a formidable task. James (1984) describes one group of them as "ambitious nurses [who] earned bachelor's and master's degrees [at Teachers College, Columbia] and dedicated themselves to the Sisyphean labor of upgrading the hospital training schools" (p. 571).

Loyal and not-so-loyal opposition. Disagreement with their agenda for upgrading nursing came from hospital officials as well as the trained nurses themselves. Those in charge of hospitals regarded the student apprenticeship training with its emphasis on submission to institutional authority as ideal. It created a disciplined, if temporary, workforce, and as students graduated, new students replaced them. Because students received little, if any, stipend, they were a relatively inexpensive source of labor. Any move to reduce the amount of service provided by students or to loosen the reins of hospital authority was, of course, objectionable.

Objections within the ranks of nursing itself had different bases. While the reformers were concerned with issues like the heavy workloads of students, their overarching concern was with the dual matter of improving health care and upgrading nursing into professional status, with all that implies about a conceptual knowledge base, autonomy, independent judgment and professional regulation of members, and professional organizations to foster professional goals. They wanted nursing programs to be in educational institutions, and had some success in achieving that goal, although progress was very gradual until after the midpoint of the century. They wanted entering students to meet the same requirements that entering students in other programs of study were meeting. In other words, the seeds of a professional culture, first sown by Breay in Great Britain, were transplanted by this early 20th century cadre of nursing reformers in the United States. Since then, the culture of professionalism has sometimes waxed and sometimes waned, as it has been tempered by developments in the women's movement, society at large and health care, and by both support and opposition within the ranks of nurses. Professionalism is undoubtedly one of our strongest traditions.

Professionalism was not a welcome prospect to many rank and file or mainstream nurses who were developing their own strong tradition. This group was reasonably satisfied with the apprenticeship training they had acquired in hospital schools and with the work that they now performed. They worried about being left behind, should the upgrading of standards proceed as the nursing leadership wished. If academic degrees became a *sine qua non* for practice defined as professional, they faced the prospect of becoming second class professionals or of being eliminated entirely. This seemed quite unjust to many of these nurses who considered themselves very well prepared for the work of nursing.

In addition to the threat of lowered status, they had a somewhat different perspective about the work of nursing, frequently identified as the craft orientation. They took great pride in their craft, with its hands-on skills, shared standards of work and deportment, and esprit de corp of their group. They downplayed the conceptual or theoretical and focused on the immediate conditions in their work situations. To oversimplify the differences in outlook between professional culture and the craft culture of the rank and file or mainstream nurse, it can be said that the leaders and aspiring professionals "looked outward, beyond the work experience to its social context and implications. [They] ... sought to improve nurses' positions within the medical division of labor" (Melosh, 1982, p. 5). Nursing for this group had an important cognitive aspect to it: It was to be a field of study. The rank and file, on the other hand, were absorbed in the nature, pace, requirements, and rewards of daily work. They looked inward, focusing on the immediate situation. Their concerns were on the practical, such as the conditions of work and whether the nurse had sufficient control over how it was performed. Their culture, constructed from their accumulated experiences and understandings of the workplace, guided and interpreted the tasks and social relations of work. Of value was their apprenticeship tradition, careful craft methods, practical experience, and self-control. Melosh (1982) claims that the mainstream in nursing has always embraced the craft culture; professional ideology, though influential, was a definite minority view. Throughout every decade of this century both cultures have been very much in evidence, though the issues generating the most passion for each group have varied, depending on other contextual factors of the times. Having different values, the cultures have often taken divergent, rather than convergent paths. Professional culture, over the years, has downplayed the apprenticeship means of learning because it was tainted with authoritarianism and illegitimate free labor, and because of its neglect or even disparagement of anything conceptual. With their eyes on the broader picture, professionalizers frequently paid little attention to the actual workplace concerns and welfare of the nurse in the trenches. The craft culture for its part has tended to distrust the theoretical approach of the professionals, thinking of them as abandoning nursing skills, being too upwardly mobile and creating an elitist class system in nursing. In the craft view patient care deteriorates as nurses' education moves away from the bedside (Melosh, 1982). Feelings over specific proposals have run high over the years, as demonstrated by this sentence from a letter to a nursing journal, following the publication of the 1948 Brown report (which recommended a baccalaureate education for nurses): "It's not the university graduate who knows how to give a better back rub or how to administer to the patient's comfort in countless ways, but the nurse who has been trained for it and who does not feel too far superior to carry out the everyday tasks" (Melosh, 1982, p. 68).

Nursing voices as just one section of the orchestra. The two quite different cultures or ideologies by no means represent the entirety of the positions taken by nurses over the years. Frequently, however, positions taken in educational or practice policy contain at least some elements from one or the other. Neither do professional and craft cultures explain all of the practices that have been adopted in nursing education and practice over the years. While some nurses feel that the confusion in our definition of the professional and in our pathways to practice happens because we, as a group, cannot or will not make up our minds, the facts are more complicated. It is true that nursing speaks with a chorus rather than with a single voice (Reverby, 1979), but it is also true, to continue the analogy, that our chorus is only one section of the orchestra. The panoply of events and conditions as they unfold in society add their own particular tunes and influence the outcomes. Economic factors, for instance, are potent. They have certainly played a key role in determining where and what kind of educational programs are supported, as well as in determining the degree to which we have layers of lesser prepared as well as more elaborately prepared nursing personnel. Economic factors have always played a commanding role in nurse shortages and nurse oversupplies, as reflected in the availability of jobs and the kind of qualifications required for all types of nursing positions. It is noteworthy that the addition of lesser prepared people usually occurs at the time of shortages as a less expensive mechanism for increasing supply, and that this usually occurs over the objections of nurses with both professional and craft ideologies.

Political factors frequently interact with economics in societal decisions about nursing and nursing education, and the case of the associate degree nurse is a good example of the interplay. The position and educational program were created as a compromise that was to meet diverse goals for diverse groups. The severe post-World War II nursing shortage would be addressed because the program would attract previously untapped pools of potential recruits. These recruits would be among the influx of students entering the community college system, which was rapidly developing as a publicly supported means for extending educational opportunities to previously non-college-bound people. The control of the program (college, not hospital) and level of practitioner (technical, not professional) overcame objections among many professional culture nursing groups, although it left many questions unanswered for other groups. The compromise acknowledged the need for different levels of practice within nursing, and was part of a strategy that placed all education in educational institutions, and placed professional practice at the baccalaureate level. The technical nurse would be under the direction of the professional nurse, a matter that would require appropriate licensing arrangements to be made by each state's board of nursing (Lynaugh, 1995). These boards of nursing never did, however, create that distinction in licensing (a political move for sure) and neither did hospitals (most likely an economic move). Consequently, we have a single license for practice, with various paths to achieve it.

The influence of an interacting web of societal events on decisions about nursing would be difficult to overestimate. Starting with politics, consider the occurrence of wars and the impact of them on available manpower, the need for health services for civilian and military populations, and the reorganization of male and female roles. Consider also the impact of the change in social and political ideology in this country regarding entitlements of all to health care, and redressing the inequalities of treatment and entitlement based on race and ethnic issues, gender, or economics. These are just examples of factors that, while external to nursing, form a powerful context for influencing decisions that are made about nursing.

THE CHALLENGES AHEAD

Nursing has spawned both a strong craft culture and a strong professional culture. How will understanding these traditions help us to design education patterns and policies that will be equal to the challenges ahead? Our traditional cultures have programmed us with a readiness to respond or think in certain ways, without testing the waters anew each time we must act to determine what response would be a good fit for the particular situation. Nurses become steeped in these cultures through the educational paths they take, and through their workplace experiences. Knowledge of how those cultures evolved out of the interacting web of factors that generated them enables us to take a more objective stance about them. It helps to reduce their automatic hold on our values and decision making, thus freeing us from what sometimes is the tyranny of blind adherence—to either culture. For both cultures encapsulate important insights about how nursing does, or might, fit into the emerging world of work, of health care, and of gender, yet both can constrict one's ability to problem solve in the most comprehensive way taking contextual factors into account. The tendency is to think one already has the answer.

Perhaps the biggest challenge that we face as a group is applying very comprehensive and creative problem solving to the process of reforming and adjusting nursing education to thrive in the face of the ambiguities of the 21st century. This kind of problem solving will require us to transcend the limitations of both cultures as they initially evolved and are outlined here, and to adopt a more negotiable blend or synthesis of elements from both. With the hindsight we have gained from experience, we might insist on a culture that will allow us to be more deliberate and self conscious about our values and priorities, how we weigh options, and how we can address the needs of many rather than a few. The options chosen would have to meet the litmus test of improving nursing's ability to respond to society's emerging health care needs, if we are to garner widespread support and become potent players in health care. This may require us to change our vision of the appropriate structure for nursing, from time to time, as we keep pace with social change.

LANDSCAPE OF THE 21ST CENTURY

What will the new century be like? Without the benefit of a crystal ball, certainty is quite elusive. How many times in years past was it predicted that hospitals would always be the primary and most important locale for the practice of nursing? That prediction would not be made with much conviction today. But caution notwithstanding, most evidence points to a high probability of certain conditions as prevailing, and ubiquitous change is topmost on the list (National Academy of Science Committee on Science, Engineering, and Public Policy, 1995). In addition to constant change, the information superhighway will be immense, and knowledge itself will become one of the most important assets that an individual can offer in the workplace (Smith, 1995). Nurses will need to be versatile in using the highway, and knowledge will be a vital commodity for nursing personnel at all levels. An ever-expanding role for technology is to be expected, and a shift toward a global perspective will be required as the interdependency of all communities on the planet becomes increasingly apparent. Finally, because the amount of most resources in the world is finite and the demand for resources is high from all societal sectors, we can expect a smaller share of the total resources to be allocated for either education or health care in general. This means we must find ways of sharing resources, rather than simply competing with others for them. Doing more with less will become a familiar refrain to those who have not become acquainted with it already.

Meeting the challenges

Ideas about how to meet these challenges can come from external as well as internal sources. We can profit from the insights of others. For instance, the National Academy of Science committee dealing with education for engineers and scientists, in response to the increasing rates of change and technological development expected in the coming century, asserts that, "A world of work that has become more interdisciplinary, collaborative, and global requires that we produce young people who are more adaptable and flexible, as well as technically proficient" (National Academy of Science, 1995, p. 2). In the face of intense development and rapid obsolescence of technology, they advocate avoiding the temptation of a vocational approach to education (meaning graduate education) that results in narrowness and overspecialization. Following their path and extending the argument to include undergraduate education, one would argue in favor of a sound generalist emphasis in all we teach, with the thought that a knowledge of principles is transferable and will be needed by practitioners as they face a future that is relatively unknowable at the present time. But the workplace is not always happy with this solution, feeling, with considerable justification, that expertise and skill are the qualities needed, not naive principles. If predictions about the future are correct, however, the workplace will have to think very seriously about a continuous learning mechanism for all employees. The informal "picking it up in the workplace" will not suffice. With the obsolescence of technology and changes in treatment modalities, no one knows now what technology or other knowledge he or she will need to know in 5 or 10 years, and adaptable learners will fare better than nurses with proficiency in a current technique who cannot accommodate change.

Additional questions can be posed for the nursing community to answer that grow out of the need for nursing to rise to the broad challenges listed above. There may be many ways of meeting the challenges ahead, and particularly from an international perspective, care should be taken so that our answers fit the requirements of the specific local situations. The following provisional list is not intended to be either exhaustive or to contain what are necessarily the most important issues. All entries on this list do, however, have at least a tangential connection to the dominant cultures described in this chapter.

1. *How can we transform our thinking about the conceptual in general and education in particular so that career awareness and mobility are enhanced?* As a corollary, how can we give the same kind of attention to access to education that has been given to the general area of access to health care? Our success in addressing these issues will determine to a great extent what we will accomplish in accommodating wisely and well to change, in increasing cultural diversity within nursing, and in increasing our ability to care for diverse and global populations.

The idea of ever finishing one's education is passe, and had best be replaced by a career orientation at every level from nurse's aide to advanced practice nurse. This development poses a challenge to both cultures. The craft culture's emphasis on the practical needs to make some room for recognizing the conceptual, and such change *has* been taking place widely, with the rapid spread and obsolescence of specific technologies and rapidly evolving roles outside of acute care settings. What about less intense, long-term settings, and particularly, nursing personnel at the lower ranks? A career orientation calls for looking ahead, assessing opportunities and demands of the future, and making a conscious effort to prepare for that future. The professional culture so prominent in academia and the rigidities of the workplace have been charged with setting roadblocks that make the pursuit of education difficult. Innovative programs to overcome these roadblocks need to be encouraged and more widely adopted. Distance education is one such strategy; devising ways of validating experiential learning is another.

2. *How can we provide experiential learning in our educational programs?* There are many thorny issues related to

this question because it is (or is it?) a critically important aspect of learning at all levels of nursing from entering novices to the specialized roles of advance practice nurses. With the rapid obsolescence of knowledge, what should be the focus of experiential learning?

3. *How can we change the sex stereotyping of nursing?* While nursing was a decidedly female occupation in the early years of this century, do we want it to continue that way? Whereas some argue that we should emphasize the women's identification as a particular strength in being care providers for women and children, others assert that such an identification plays to a perceived secondary (as compared with men) power position, is quite limiting, and is becoming less descriptive of the discipline, in any event. The number of men in nursing is small but growing, judging from the trends in graduations of men from all basic RN programs. Graduation rates for men grew from 5.8% of all graduates in 1981 to 9.9% of all graduates in 1992, with the highest percentage (10.4%) graduating from baccalaureate programs (National League for Nursing, 1994b).

4. *What are some safe, productive strategies for sharing resources and increasing our interdisciplinary collaboration?* Collaboration and the sharing of resources (as for learning experiences) are advocated frequently as means of doing more with less (Cawley, 1993; National Academy of Science, 1995; Smith, 1995). This is not always simple, however, and not always considered wise. Although becoming interdisciplinary is one way to break down traditional barriers between disciplines and between professionals and communities, it can also result in establishing hegemony on the part of one or another more powerful group when the power relations are not equal. Therefore, careful attention to establishing rational bases of equality among partners in the new group norms is necessary to ensure full participation and true collaboration. This usually means relative equality of educational preparation of the collaborators, and accepting patients and communities as full participants in decision making.

One final related note on limited resources comes from Havighurst, who has long been a scholar of the health care marketplace. Havighurst (1994) points out that the dynamics of the deregulated marketplace have changed, with industry coming between health provider and patient to take on the role of purchaser of services. This shift, Havighurst notes, points to the direction that nonphysician providers must take to fully realize practice opportunities. Instead of looking to the courts for judicial relief for claims of unfair monopolistic practices, Havighurst asserts that the real test will be to demonstrate to the businesses buying health care services that you can produce the least costly services with the desired degree of effectiveness.

SUMMARY

The challenges ahead for nursing and nursing education are plentiful. While our course is far from clear, we have a wonderfully diverse supply of courses of action to pursue in meeting our challenges, and these will be tested in the decades ahead. We also have the will, optimism, and perseverance to succeed in our quest.

Because what nursing ought or needs to be is dependent on the health care arrangements that come about in concert with other societal trends, we cannot know today what the final shape of our nursing workforce will or ought to be. We cannot be certain how many levels of personnel are best, or how each one should be educated. Therefore, it is still difficult to tell the weeds from the flowers in our garden of nursing positions and educational paths, although we know we may discover quite a few weeds. In the final analysis, tolerating some weeds is better than losing precious flowers, and most new role developments in nursing stimulated strong objection at the outset. With that fact in mind, let us remain open to a diversity of ideas and strategies that will promote interaction with other stakeholders in health care to bring about a system that produces a high level of care most effectively.

REFERENCES

Berlin, L., & Bednash, G. (1995). *1994-1995 Enrollments and graduations in baccalaureate and graduate programs in nursing* (AACN Publication No. 94-95-1). Washington DC: American Association of Colleges of Nursing.

Cawley, J. (1993). Physician assistants in the health care workforce. In D.K. Clawson & M. Osterweis (Eds.), *The roles of physician assistants and nurse practitioners in primary care* (pp. 21-39). Washington, DC: Association of Academic Health Centers.

Davies, C. (1980). A constant casualty: Nurse education in Britain and the USA to 1939. In C. Davies (Ed.), *Rewriting nursing history* (pp. 102-122). Totowa, NJ: Barnes and Noble.

Havighurst, C. (1994). *Practice opportunities for allied health professionals in a deregulated health care industry.* Unpublished manuscript, Duke University, Durham, NC.

James, J.W. (1984). Writing and rewriting nursing history: A review essay. *Bulletin of the History of Medicine, 58,* 568-584.

Lynaugh, J. (1995). Nursing and the W.K. Kellogg Foundation. *Nursing in Health Care, 16*(4), 174-183.

Melosh, B. (1982). *"The physician's hand": Work culture and conflict in american nursing.* Philadelphia: Temple University Press.

National Academy of Science Committee on Science, Engineering, and Public Policy. (1995). *Reshaping the graduate education of scientists and engineers.* Washington, DC: National Academy Press.

National League for Nursing. (1994a). *Nursing datasource* (Vol. I) (Publication No. 19-2642). New York: National League for Nursing Press.

National League for Nursing. (1994b). *Nursing data review 1994* (Publication No. 19-2639). New York: National League for Nursing Press.

Reverby, S. (1979). The search for the hospital yardstick: Nursing and the rationalization of hospital work. In S. Reverby & D. Rosner (Eds.), *Health care in America: Essays in social history* (pp. 206-225). Philadelphia: Temple University Press.

Smith, G. (1995). Lessons learned: Challenges for the future. *Nursing in Health Care, 16*(4), 188-191.

Vogel, M. (1979). The transformation of the American hospital, 1850-1920. In S. Reverby & D. Rosner (Eds.), *Health care in America: essays in social history* (pp. 105-116). Philadelphia: Temple University Press.

Williams, K. (1980). From Sarah Gamp to Florence Nightingale: A critical study of hospital nursing systems from 1840 to 1897. In C. Davies (Ed.), *Rewriting nursing history* (pp. 41-75). Totowa, NJ: Barnes and Noble.

The changing pool of students*

GERALDINE POLLY BEDNASH

Students obtaining higher education are increasingly heterogeneous and represent a variety of goals, life experiences, learning needs, and constituencies. Two contrasting groups of students are represented in the population of individuals seeking higher education degrees as the end of the 20th century draws near—from freshman students immediately out of high school to adult learners returning to school to acquire new skills or knowledge. The latter group is increasingly a predominant force in American higher education. To focus on high school students allows only a narrow perspective of the full spectrum of individuals who should be assessed as future professional nurses. In addition, although the number of high school graduates is increasing, and will continue to increase for the remainder of the 20th century, these new graduates are not engaging in traditional post–high school college learning patterns. Instead, high school graduates and adult students alike are increasingly nontraditional learners.

Students in higher education also have decidedly different values for themselves and perceive their relationships with their learning environments more pragmatically. The youngest portion of the higher education student population, often termed "generation X," is beginning its entry into career development. This group has been shaped by a world of media productions, global politics and disasters, and domestic struggles. The older and more experienced component of the higher education population is returning to school for an education that can improve their employability, their earning potential, and possibly their career satisfaction. In both of these groups, a growing percentage of the students are members of racially and ethnically diverse populations, and this percentage is increasing rapidly.

*This paper was written by Dr. Bednash in her private capacity. No official support or endorsement by the American Association of Colleges of Nursing is intended or should be inferred.

The differences in these populations represent both enormous potential and serious challenges for nurses in the education and practice worlds of the profession. The potential is represented by the increasing diversity that provides new pools from which nursing can draw. The challenges are a result of the need to reformulate how we educate nurses for the future with a population of students who are nontraditional learners and enrollees.

DEMOGRAPHIC REALITIES AND CHALLENGES

After a number of years of decline, the number of students enrolled in and graduating from high school is experiencing a steady and marked increase that is projected to continue through the end of the 20th century (Dortch, 1995). The most dramatic changes in high school graduation will be seen in southern states such as Virginia (+34%), Florida (+56%), and Georgia (+29%) and in western states such as California (+47%), Nevada (+77%), Arizona (+47%), and Colorado (+32%) (Western Interstate Commission for Higher Education, 1993). These increases are projected to result in increased enrollments in higher education over the next decade. The National Center for Education Statistics (1994) projects that the number of individuals enrolled in higher education will increase by 7.2% from 1995 to 2005.

A second, more dramatic demographic change is also reshaping the face of the increasing numbers of college students—the growth in the number of individuals who are members of a racial or ethnic minority group. According to the U.S. Census Bureau, in 1990, almost 25% of the population was a member of a racial or ethnic minority group (Figure 18-1) (Day, 1993). In the past half-decade, that percentage has increased. In some areas of the country, the term "minority" may be a misnomer. Hodgkinson (1992) reports that in "26 cities in Califor-

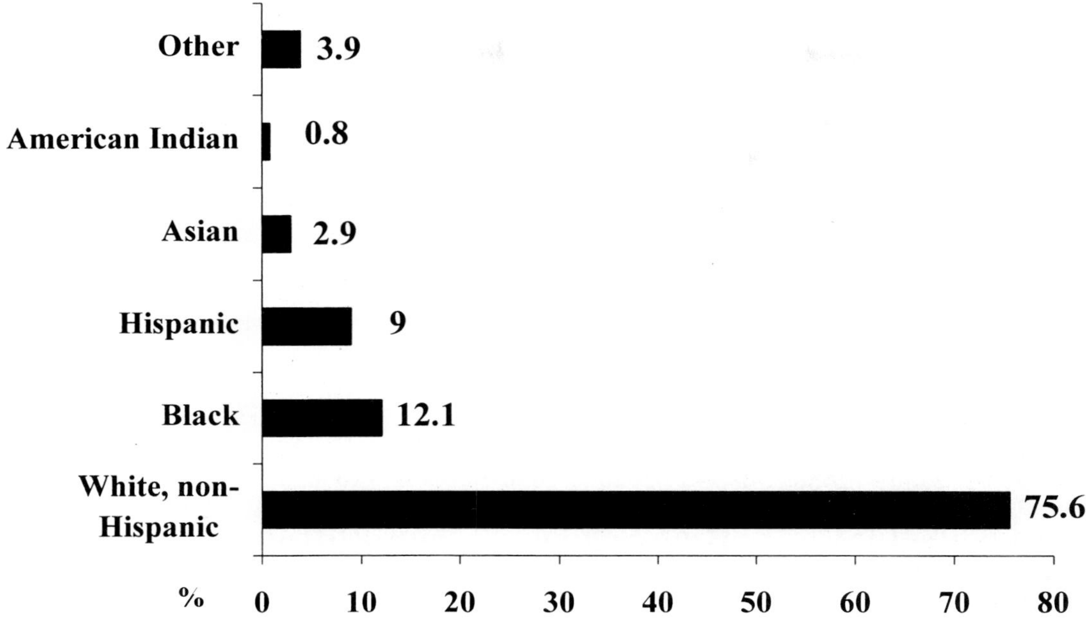

Fig. 18-1. Total population of the United States: 1990. (Source: *Women, Minorities, and Persons with Disabilities in Science and Engineering, 1994.*)
Notes: The 1990 population counts set forth herein are subject to possible correction for undercount or overcount. Percentages are based on unrounded numbers. Hispanics may be of any race. Because of rounding, percentages may not add to 100.

nia, no single racial or ethnic group made up a majority of the population" (p. 6).

The growth in ethnically and racially diverse populations is most dramatic in elementary and high school age populations. For example, in the elementary and secondary school systems in California, New Mexico, Hawaii, and the District of Columbia, over half of the population under the age of 18 are members of a racial or ethnic minority group. Claire Pelton, Director of Educational Services for the city of San Jose, California, reports that in the San Jose population of 30,000 elementary and secondary students 77 languages are spoken (personal communication, April 30, 1992) (Figure 18-2). These data suggest that the future composition of students in postsecondary programs will also have a much greater diversity.

Much of the growth in racial and ethnic diversity is a result of the surging growth in immigration to the United States. According to the U.S. Census Bureau, during the 1980s, almost 7 million legal immigrants entered the United States (Population-Environment Balance, 1992). An additional untold number of illegal immigrants have also entered the country, bringing demands for social, health, and educational services. This immigration boom, which is the largest in the history of the United States, has and will continue to create a dramatically different workforce. It will also bring a cultural richness and an enhanced level of strain to the higher education community.

The National Center for Education Statistics (NCES) of the U.S. Department of Education reports that black enrollments have risen recently to slightly higher percentages than those evidenced in the late 1970s. Moreover, Hispanic and Asian enrollments have seen consistent growth over the past two decades. From 1976 to 1992, minority students increased from 15% to 22% of the enrollments in the nation's colleges and universities (Smith et al., 1995). However, racial and ethnic minorities are still underrepresented in higher education. For instance, Hispanics, who represented 9% of the entire U.S. population in 1990, comprised only 5.5% of the student population in colleges and universities (Smith et al., 1995). In 1994, Hispanic enrollments had increased to 6%, but this minority group remains underrepresented in higher education (El-Khawas, 1995).

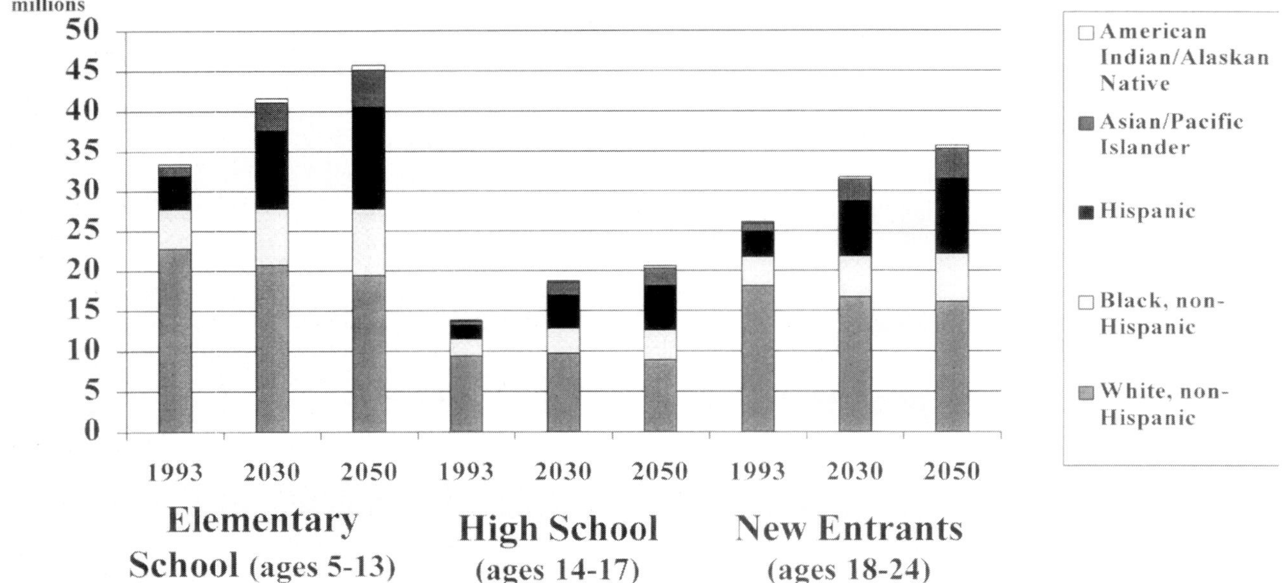

Fig. 18-2. Projections of the US population by selected age groups and race/ethnicity for 1993, 2030, and 2050. (Source: *Women, Minorities, and Persons with Disabilities in Science and Engineering, 1994.*)

Moreover, there is some evidence that students who are members of a racial and ethnic minority group are more likely to drop out of their education programs prior to completing the degree (National Science Foundation, 1994). Although no longitudinal analyses of minority student retention have been conducted, analysis of dropout rates indicates that minority students have higher attrition in the early years of baccalaureate education.

Minority students also have a greater potential to be nontraditional students. For instance, 50% of Hispanic students are enrolled on a part-time basis (NCES, 1994). Part-time students are not eligible for financial assistance, increasing their need to be employed. Further, blacks (59%) and Hispanics (34%) are more likely than whites (22%) to be from a family that is headed by a single parent—a factor that will often increase financial vulnerability and decrease the ability to complete studies. This creates an environment in which those students who are most likely to have their earning potential enhanced are least likely to be able to access or complete a higher education degree (National University Continuing Education Association [NUCEA], 1994).

NONTRADITIONAL EXPECTATIONS AND PATTERNS OF LEARNING

Nontraditional patterns of enrollment are not seen solely in minority student populations. The trend toward nontraditional patterns of learning began in the 1970s and has continued through the present with an end result that over three quarters of students of higher education are considered nontraditional learners. A report of the American Council on Education, titled *Financing Nontraditional Students,* analyzed the changes seen in postsecondary student populations as reported in the National Postsecondary Student Aid Study and in data reported to the NCES (Ross and Hampton, 1992). Ross and Hampton (1992) brought together diverse data sets to allow them, for the first time, to get an accurate total of the number of individuals who are now enrolled in postsecondary education programs—almost 18 million individuals—and to describe more fully this extremely large and diverse group.

Traditionally, a college student has been perceived to be immediately out of high school, in her or his late teens, financially dependent on parents or guardians, enrolled in a course of study full-time, and focusing full energies on the higher education experience. The reality, however, is quite different. Ross and Hampton (1992) were able to document that the traditional student is no longer the major force in higher education, but has instead been supplanted by a group of individuals who are older, studying part-time, working, and supporting families. Ross and Hampton (1992) define nontraditional students as those over the age of 22 who are no longer financially dependent on their parents or guardians, are most often enrolled on a part-time hourly basis, live off campus, have full-time or almost full-time employment, and have a greater likelihood of being a member of a racial or ethnic minority group.

Today, only one fourth of higher education students fit the earlier definition of "traditional students" (Levine, 1993). These students continue to be an important element of higher education today. However, nontraditional learning patterns considered in the past to be found predominantly in individuals returning to school after a career or child-raising experience are seen in students of all ages. More often, students are studying in nontraditional ways as they opt in and out of their education and explore life options, test new learning, and create a parallel life outside the higher education community.

This new reality has changed the nature of higher education dramatically and will likely continue to for the long-term future. Moreover, the clear domination of the nontraditional education patterns has created calls for new terms other than traditional or nontraditional to describe them.

Nontraditional students are also likely to view their education as they view other services, i.e., as a commodity that should be convenient, available at all times, and low in cost. Levine notes that students,

> Want a relationship with their college . . . like the one they already have with their banks, supermarkets, and the other organizations they patronize. They want the education to be nearby and to operate during convenient hours—preferably around the clock. They want easy, accessible parking, short lines, and polite and efficient personnel and services. (Levine, 1993, p. 4)

Levine further notes that today's students do not perceive the university environment as a multipurpose setting. Instead, they want education from their colleges and will seek their entertainment, sports, health, or counseling services elsewhere. Moreover, today's students are concerned about cost and quality and are seeking the highest-quality courses or curricula at the lowest possible costs. Data collected by the College Board (1988) indicate that adult students prefer classes that are held in the early morning (7 to 10 a.m.), or late evening (5 to 7 p.m.). Only 20% of adult students reported a willingness to take classes outside those time frames.

VALUE STRUCTURES AND CAREER GOALS

Clearly, the changing economic and social conditions in the United States today have created a surge in the number of individuals who are returning to college for a new career or reexamining college as an opportunity for enhancing their potential for economic security. Traditional patterns of education will not meet the needs of this new student majority. However, a focus on the utilitarian aspects of a higher education degree is not the sole concern of returning students. The freshman student entering college for the first time also reflects many of the same values for learning that are seen in their older student counterparts. Longitudinal analyses of the values and goals of entering college freshman have been conducted for over 20 years. In 1994, large percentages of American freshmen students entering college for the first time reported their most important reasons for entering college as the ability to get a good job (77.3%), the ability to make more money (72.4%), and the ability to learn more things that interested them (73%) (Astin, Korns, Sax, & Mahoney, 1994). These reasons reflect a pragmatic blend between individual learning and life skill goals.

This pragmatism is also reflected in the reported values of American freshmen, indicating that simple classifications of freshmen students as either conservatives or liberals are not possible. Over 80% of freshman in 1994 reported attendance at religious services, 73% reported that the courts had too much concern for the rights of criminals, and 80.6% felt that employers should have the right to test applicants or employees for drug use (Astin et al., 1994). Yet these students reported that the federal government should do more to control pollution (84%), that the government should have more control over handguns (79.9%), and that racial discrimination is still a problem in this country (82.9%).

NURSING STUDENTS: REFLECTIONS AND FAILURES

These data provide evidence that diversity is a part of the American mainstream, should be defined broadly, and must become a mainstay of nursing education in order to prepare an adequate number of highly skilled and capable nursing clinicians. The growing number of nontraditional students and the increasing racial and ethnic diversity of the U.S. population are the two student pool characteristics that will have the greatest impact on nursing education's ability to do that.

Nontraditional student trends have already affected nursing education. The average age of a graduate of an associate degree program in 1992 was 35.7, and the average age of graduates of baccalaureate nursing programs was 29.2 (Figure 18-3). Moreover, data from the American Association of Colleges of Nursing (AACN) study of the costs of a nursing education indicated that baccalaureate students took an average of 4.9 years to complete their degrees (Bednash, Redman, & Southers, 1989).

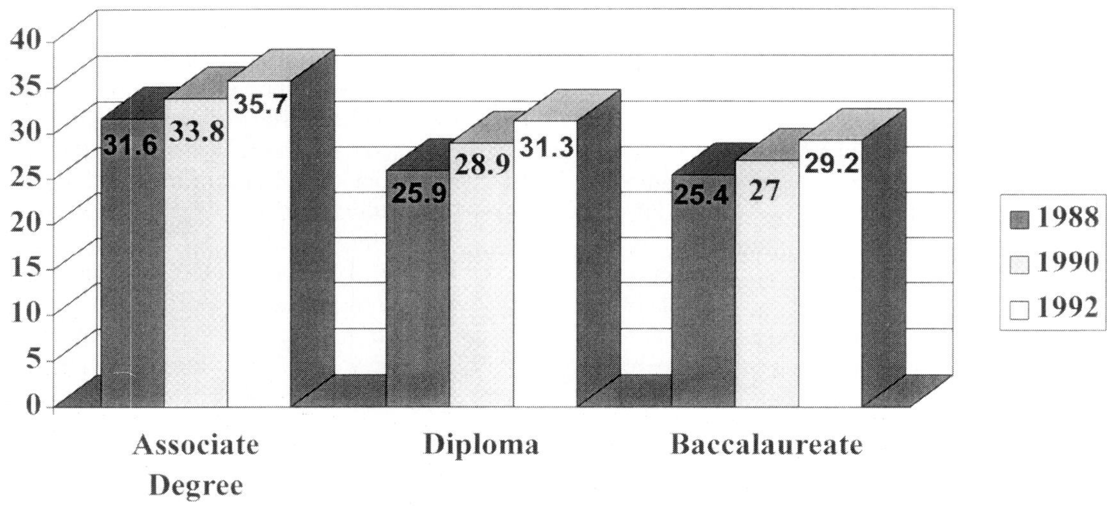

Fig. 18-3. Average age of newly licensed nurses by type of basic nursing education 1988-1992. (Source: Rosenfeld, *Profiles of the Newly Licensed Nurse,* NLN, 1994.)

These data suggest that nontraditional patterns of learning are a common part of nursing education.

Clearly, old ways of educating that require Monday through Friday, daytime class work will not meet the needs of the growing number of nontraditional students. In addition, if students are seeking the lowest-cost and highest-quality alternatives for their career goals, they are likely to vote with their feet as they select programs that provide alternative learning opportunities, creative scheduling, and learning that is real-world relevant. This shift in student populations has already changed dramatically the types of nursing programs that are being offered. Many nurse educators have responded to these changing realities with new programs for nonnurse students. These programs have seen marked growth in response to an older, nontraditional population of students. There has been dramatic growth in the new "accelerated" baccalaureate nursing programs, which were begun in the early 1990s as an option that allows individuals with baccalaureates in fields other than nursing to rapidly acquire the baccalaureate in nursing. In that short period, 59 programs have opened and another 5 are being planned (Berlin and Bednash, 1994).

These accelerated programs are an evolutionary variation on the generic master's programs for nonnurses that were incorporated with great controversy by Yale University. Yale's programs, designed to allow the individual with a baccalaureate degree in a field other than nursing to do entry level nursing studies at the master's level, were hotly debated as a workable model. Today, however, the number of generic master's in nursing programs is also increasing. A number of institutions other than Yale have begun these programs in response to a growing interest in nursing by nontraditional, older students with previous college education. In the academic year 1994-95, 14 of these generic master's programs existed and another 8 were in the planning stages (Berlin and Bednash, 1994).

Both the accelerated baccalaureate and the generic master's degree programs are clear indications that nursing education is evolving in response to new pools of students. Moreover, nurses returning to further their educations have also seen a number of options created for them to facilitate their pragmatic goals for efficient and cost-effective education. For instance, in 1994-95, 79 institutions offered programs for the registered nurse returning to school to acquire the master's degree without having to acquire the baccalaureate first. Another 22 such programs are in the planning stages. These variations are a beginning. However, other changes are vitally needed. The increasingly complex health care delivery system and the demands for more nurses with advanced clinical skills have caused an unprecedented growth in programs educating advanced practice nurses. The demand for master's educated and doctorally prepared nurses is projected to increase.

Unfortunately, many graduate programs in nursing require an entering student to have 1 or more years of experience prior to entering graduate studies. The requirement that a newly graduated nurse with a baccalaureate degree wait several years to begin advanced studies seriously elongates the time between entry into a generic nursing education program and availability to the health care system. As described earlier, the increase in the number of nontraditional students in nursing will greatly accelerate the aging of the nursing population. In 1992, less than 11% of all nurses were under the age of 30 (Moses, 1994). If graduates of nursing programs are finishing entry level studies at the ages listed previously, their career patterns will be affected by requirements that they step out of the educational arena for periods of time before progressing to graduate studies. Increasing the time required to complete graduate studies will truncate the number of years a nontraditional graduate will be able to practice as an advanced nurse clinician.

In addition, as was evident in the AACN study on nursing costs (Bednash et al., 1989), the majority of graduate students are employed an average of 32 hours per week during their studies, a factor that further lengthens the education experience and shortens the time the advanced nurse clinician is available to the health care system. Graduate students in general, including nursing students, are predominantly enrolled on a part-time basis (NUCEA, 1994). The goal of the educational system should be to facilitate progression to the highest level of practice with the fewest barriers.

The new realities of student pools also create a need to focus efforts on recruiting greater numbers of minority students. Although the percentage of nursing students who are members of a racial or ethnic minority group has increased in the last decade, these percentages still fall behind the total population representation. The most recent AACN report on enrollments and graduations in baccalaureate and graduate nursing education provides evidence that the greatest representation occurs at the undergraduate level (Tables 18-1 and 18-2). Minority enrollment at the graduate level continues to lag far behind as a result of the very small number of minority registered nurses (Figure 18-4).

The realities of the demographics of the future mandate greater attention to recruitment of larger numbers of minority students. Besides issues of equity and representativeness, the reality is that the student body of the 21st century is likely to be composed predominantly of minority students. In order to maintain a stable supply of nursing personnel, a consistent effort must be made to attract a diversity of students. In addition, Smith (1992) notes that by increasing the numbers of nurses and health professionals who are members of a minority group the professions also increase their ability to address the health care needs of diverse populations.

NEW DIRECTIONS FOR NEW ISSUES

In a recent policy discussion on human resources for health care, Bulger and Osterweis (1992) detail some of the dramatic changes that the system of health care delivery is undergoing. They note that, "[t]he number and kinds of health professionals society needs depends on the social choice we make in light of perceived threats to health, demographic shifts, technologic advances, costs, and the value that we place on health care" (p. 3).

In a world that is increasingly driven by concerns

Table 18-1 Type of program by race/ethnicity of students enrolled and number of nonresident alien students enrolled, Fall 1994

	Undergraduate			Graduate			Generic	
No. of schools reporting race/ethnicity	**Generic 412 (*n*[%])**	**RN 485**	**Total baccalaureate[a] 504**	**Master's 254**	**Doctoral 61**	**Post-doctoral 10**	**Generic master's 11**	**ND 3**
Asian	4,265 (4.5)	794 (2.2)	5,061 (3.9)	928 (3.1)	90 (3.1)	1 (3.6)	39 (4.8)	10 (3.2)
Black	8,527 (8.9)	3,078 (8.7)	11,620 (8.9)	1,859 (6.1)	155 (5.3)	1 (7.1)	25 (3.0)	16 (5.1)
American Indian or Alaskan native	564 (0.6)	187 (0.5)	751 (0.6)	130 (0.4)	9 (0.3)	0	4 (0.5)	2 (0.6)
Hispanic	3,461 (3.6)	1,022 (2.9)	4,487 (3.4)	768 (2.5)	47 (1.6)	1 (3.6)	27 (3.3)	1 (0.3)
White	76,770 (80.6)	29,112 (82.0)	105,920 (81.0)	25,530 (84.5)	2,456 (84.2)	23 (82.1)	703 (85.8)	284 (89.9)
Nonresident alien	377 (0.4)	193 (0.6)	570 (0.4)	353 (1.2)	123 (4.2)	1 (3.6)	5 (0.6)	2 (0.6)
Unknown	1,301 (1.4)	1,113 (3.1)	2,414 (1.8)	657 (2.2)	39 (1.3)	0	16 (2.0)	1 (0.3)
Total	95,265	35,499	130,823	30,225	2,919	28	819	316
Not reported	1,948	693	2,641	493	0	0	0	0

Note. RN = registered nurse.

[a]Two institutions that reported separate generic and RN baccalaureate race/ethnicity data are included in the total.

Table 18-2 Type of program by race/ethnicity of graduates and number of nonresident alien graduates, August 1, 1993 to July 31, 1994

	Undergraduate			Graduate		Generic	
No. of schools reporting race/ethnicity	**Generic 401**	**RN 482**	**Total baccalaureate[a] 496**	**Master's 249**	**Doctoral 61**	**General master's 11**	**ND 3**
Asian	911 (3.5)	222 (2.7)	1,134 (3.3)	183 (2.5)	3 (0.8)	12 (5.0)	0
Black	1,652 (6.4)	697 (8.3)	2,364 (6.9)	443 (6.0)	17 (4.7)	4 (1.7)	2 (7.7)
Native American	113 (0.5)	58 (0.7)	171 (0.5)	27 (0.4)	2 (0.5)	1 (0.4)	0
Hispanic	879 (3.4)	231 (2.8)	1,113 (3.3)	160 (2.2)	5 (1.4)	2 (0.8)	2 (7.7)
White	21,822 (84.8)	6,896 (82.3)	28,768 (84.1)	6,384 (86.4)	319 (87.4)	219 (92.1)	22 (84.6)
Nonresident alien	76 (0.3)	45 (0.5)	121 (0.4)	98 (1.3)	17 (4.7)	0	0
Unknown	284 (1.1)	230 (2.7)	516 (1.5)	90 (1.2)	2 (0.5)	0	0
Total	25,737	8,379	34,187	7,385	365	238	26
Not reported	471	600	1,030	268	0	0	0

Note. RN = registered nurse.
[a]Three institutions that reported combined generic and RN baccalaureate race/ethnicity data are included in the total.

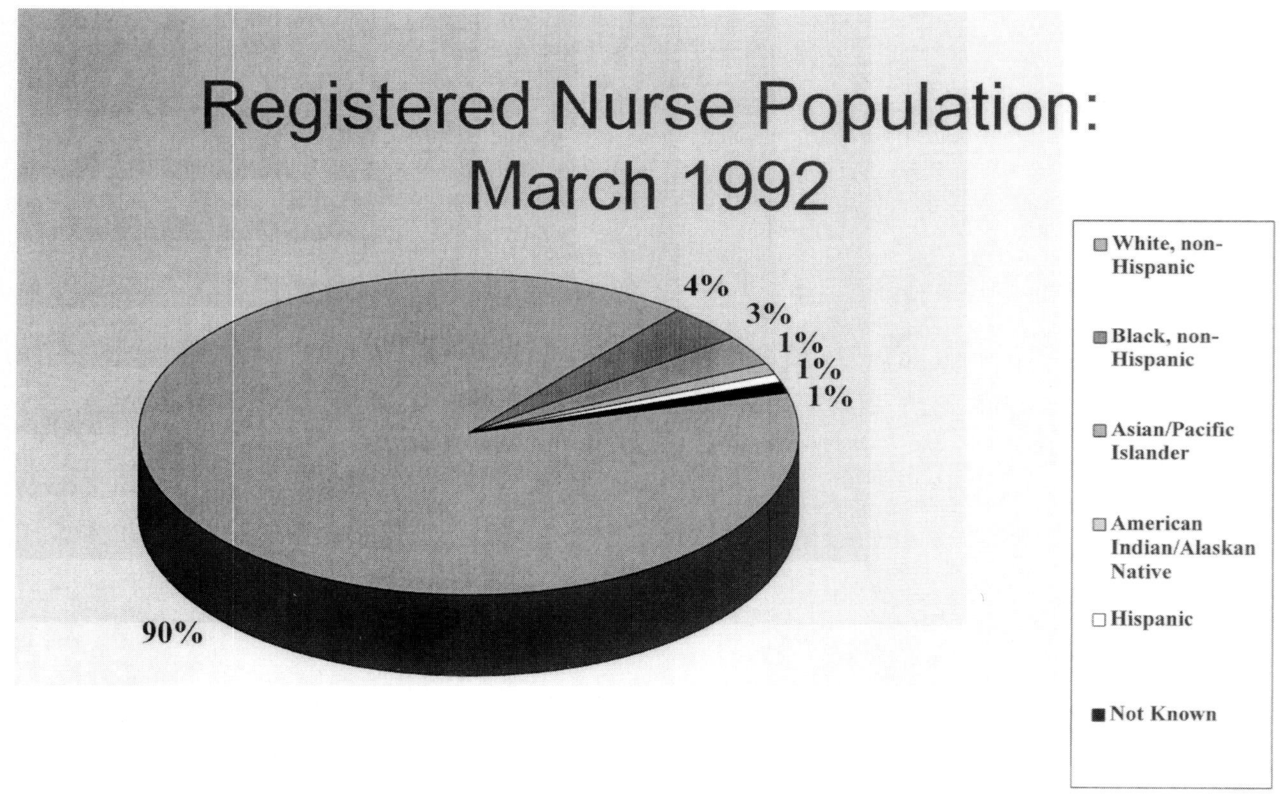

Fig. 18-4. Registered nurse population: March 1992. (Source: *The Registered Nurse Population 1992. Findings from The National Sample Survey of Registered Nurses, March 1992.* US Department of Health and Human Services.)

about the costs of health care, health care systems will need health professionals who are able to assess these changes and create a care ethos that is focused on the needs of the populations being served. Clearly, the nursing profession can only benefit from efforts to design programs that are creative, reflect the needs of the students being served, and create professionals who are reflective of the populations seeking health care. This outcome can not be achieved without attention to new student pools. Clearly, the nursing education community has made significant efforts to increase racial, ethnic, gender, and age diversity of nursing enrollments. Continued efforts are necessary, however. Particular attention must be paid to graduate enrollments and career mobility to improve diversity.

Detmer (1991) details the steps necessary to fulfill a vision of the future. First, realities must be understood clearly. Second, the goal or vision must be fully articulated. Finally, the infrastructure to achieve the vision must be put in place.

For nursing education, the reality is that new pools are and must continue to be tapped. The vision is to create a wealth of diversity in the nursing profession that is representative of social, economic, and cultural changes in the population at large. The infrastructure is only partially developed. The move to less traditional ways of becoming a professional nurse are a beginning. The challenge is to bring more diverse groups of individuals to these new options.

REFERENCES

Astin, A.W., Korns, W.S., Sax, L.J., & Mahoney, K.M. (1994). *The American freshman: National norms for fall 1994.* Los Angeles: Los Angeles Higher Education Research Institute, University of California, Los Angeles.

Berlin, L., & Bednash, G. (1994). *1994-1995 Enrollment and graduations in baccalaureate and graduate programs in nursing.* Washington, DC: American Association of Colleges of Nursing.

Bednash, G., Redman, B., & Southers, N. (1989). *The economic investment in nursing education: Student institutional, and clinical perspectives.* Washington, DC: American Association of Colleges of Nursing.

Bulger, R.J., & Osterweis, M. (1992). Human resources policy and academic health centers. In C.M. Evarts, P.P. Bosomworth, & M. Osterweis (Eds.) *Human resources for health: Defining the future* (pp. 1-12). Washington, DC: Association of Academic Health Centers.

Day, J.C. (1993). *Population projections of the United States, by age, sex, race, and Hispanic origin: 1993-2050.* (Bureau of the Census, Current Population Reports, P25-1104.) Washington, DC: U.S. Department of Commerce.

Detmer, D. (1991). Reducing the discontinuities between vision and practice. In C. Rich, A. Barbato, & J. Griffith (Eds.), *Vision: Leadership and values in academic health centers* (pp. 97-103). Washington, DC: Association of Academic Health Centers.

Dortch, S. (1995, May). Colleges come back. *American Demographics,* 4.

El-Khawas, E. (1995). *Campus trends: 1995.* Washington, DC: American Council on Education.

Hodgkinson, H. (1992). *A demographic look at tomorrow.* Washington, DC: Institute for Educational Leadership.

Levine, A. (1993). Editorial: Student expectations of college. *Change 25*(4), 8.

Moses, E. (1994). *The registered nurse population: Findings from the National Sample Survey of Registered Nurses, March 1992.* Washington, DC: U.S. Department of Health and Human Services.

National Center for Education Statistics. (1994). *Trends in minority enrollments in higher education, fall 1992.* (NCES 94-104.) Washington, DC: Author.

National Science Foundation. (1994). *Women, minorities, and persons with disabilities in science and engineering.* (NSF 94-333.) Washington, DC: Author.

National University Continuing Education Association (NUCEA). (1994). *Lifelong learning trends: A profile of continuing higher education.* Washington, DC: Author.

Population-environment balance. (1992, August). *Balance data,* Washington, DC.

Ross, L., & Hampton, D. (1992). How the nontraditional student finances her education. In J. Eaton (Ed.), *Financing nontraditional students: A seminar report* (pp. 7-32). Washington, DC: American Council on Education.

Smith, M. (1992). Health personnel in a diverse society. In C.M. Evarts, P.P. Bosomworth, & M. Osterweis (Eds.), *Human resources for health: Defining the future* (pp. 26-33). Washington, DC: Association of Academic Health Centers.

Smith, T.M., Perie, M., Alsalam, N., Mahney, R.P., Bae, Y., & Young, B.A. (1995). *The condition of education: 1995.* Washington, DC: National Center for Education Statistics, U.S. Department of Education, Office of Educational Research and Improvement.

The College Board. (1988). *How Americans in transition study for college credit.* New York: Author.

Western Interstate Commission for Higher Education. (1993). *High school graduates project by state, 1992-2009.* Boulder, CO: Author.

Advancing community based-community focused nursing education: Challenge for change

BERNADINE M. LACEY

Lillian Wald's founding vision of public health nurses in 1893 was one in which their services reflected the constantly changing needs of the people of those times, rather than a template of what a nurse should do (Salmon, 1993, p. 211).

In its initial stages, community health nursing provided health care to the poor and sick, and then later emerged as a force in augmenting preventive health care services to families within the community. Public health nurses struggled with problems of specialization and referral of patients to hospital settings. Essentially, community health nursing meant providing nursing care to the sick and health counseling and teaching for families under the sponsorship of governmental or voluntary health agencies.

As the growth of public health nursing practices took place, nurses recognized that their preparation in hospital schools was inadequate to provide the health care needed. Demands for advanced preparation in institutions of higher education were first met in 1910 by Columbia University, and the movement of nursing education programs into collegiate settings became a reality. Braving a resistance to change, courageous nursing leaders introduced concepts of family health care in the basic nursing curricula (Committee on Education of the National League for Nursing Education, 1919). Although the theoretical orientations were often lacking, the operational aspects, which gave recognition to the family as a unit of service and educational study, were identified as principles (Gardner, 1936).

Other mitigating factors against community health nursing education have focused around the reality that for the past century, nursing education and the practice of professional nursing was centered almost exclusively under the authority of physicians. Such care concentrated on providing curative measures within acute care hospital settings. The current revolution in health care requires an immediate change. Demographic changes as well as social and economic forces have focused increased attention on the dysfunctional health care system and a demand to improve the health of the entire community. The increasing attention given to the delivery of health services reflects many concerns about the manpower used to provide the necessary health care. There are advocates who suggest that emphasis on prevention, early diagnosis, and treatment of individuals is necessary to improve quality of life. For nursing education programs the need is to prepare nurses to meet the demands of diverse communities. In fact, the effectiveness of a nursing educational program may be judged best by the ability of its graduates to meet community needs. The curricula of nursing programs must reflect information relevant to the demographic shifts that concern health disparities among high-risk population groups as well as to the social and economic factors that have intensified concerns about the quality of life. Simply stated, nursing education programs must include curricula aimed at reducing the inequities in the delivery of health care to racial and ethnic minority populations who have increased exposure to air pollutants, hazardous waste, contaminated foods, violence, and sexually transmitted diseases.

EPIDEMIOLOGICAL CONCERNS RELATED TO COMMUNITY-BASED NURSING EDUCATION

Within the community each essential component of the health care system is affected by and has impact on the other components, and this ultimately determines the health care services and those persons served by the system. Using toxic waste as an example, among the relevant epidemiological findings are the following:

- Three out of five black communities have abandoned toxic waste sites in them.
- Sixty percent (15 million) of blacks live in communities with one or more abandoned toxic waste sites.
- Under the Comprehensive Environmental Response, Compensation, and Liability Act (generally known as Superfunds), cleanup programs for abandoned waste sites in minority areas take 20% longer to be placed on the national priority action list.
- Air-polluting facilities are not distributed evenly over the four regions of the country or between urban and rural areas. Almost half of nearly 300 major air-polluting facilities nationwide are in the southern United States, followed in order by the north central, western, and northeast regions.
- Native American lands have become prime targets for waste disposal proposals. More than three dozen reservations have been identified for waste dumps and for incinerators.
- In New York City, the most recent water treatment plant was built in the lowest socioeconomic neighborhood of Harlem. Although sewage treatment plants are important in the prevention of waterborne disease and in improving water quality, they may also be a source of exposure to toxic agents. Sewage sludge and waste water are very complex mixtures of heavy metals, persistent pesticides, and other organic compounds (Johnson & Coulberson, 1993).

In America at least 2.2 million people are victims of violent injury each year. In fact, our country ranks first among industrialized nations in violent death rates. More than 145,000 injury deaths occur each year and violence is now considered a leading health problem in the United States. Associated with acts of violence are the physical and psychosocial consequences that relate to the illnesses and disabilities of victims, their families, and their communities. The problems of violence require cooperation and integration across the health care, mental health, criminal justice, social services, and curricular components that address this problem.

Of equal concern for nursing community health education programs are the complex problems of communicable disease. Infectious diseases are now the third leading cause of death in the United States. These diseases require the practice of universal precautions and an urgent need for preventive educational content in promoting health.

Several initiatives have been made in promoting health. For example, a constructive effort to decrease the incidence of measles occurred on October 1, 1994, when the U.S. Department of Health and Human Services implemented a Vaccine for Children program. This program provides free vaccinations to children. One goal of the program is to increase vaccination levels for 2-year-old children to at least 90% by 1996. Comprehensive information concerning vaccination coverage for children in the United States can be found in the Centers for Disease Control and Prevention's October 7, 1994 report in *Morbidity and Mortality Weekly Report,* which is devoted to this important health promotion effort.

Despite these efforts, much remains to be done. Efforts to this point have been piecemeal and disconnected. The typical nursing curriculum may have a course in public health nursing, but usually it is more of an afterthought than an integrated part of the curriculum. Table 19-1 provides some evidence of the need to continue using more intensified methods of promoting health.

A COMMUNITY BASE FOR NURSING EDUCATION

Communities and families provide a comprehensive matrix for teaching family dynamics and community health nursing practice. A community-based nursing curriculum can provide the foundation for a thorough study of major family and community theories. This curriculum also provides opportunities for faculty and students to explore nursing interventions that consider the cultural, social, political, ethical, ecological, and economical factors affecting health. Students would be allowed to develop a reservoir of nursing approaches through the assimilation of the professional roles including providers of care and coordinators of care that are achieved through actual application within the community. Community health problems related to family disintegration, illegal drug use, violent crimes, and poverty highlight the need for community-based nursing education programs to be the primary focus for the future delivery of health care. In March 1995, the NLN endorsed community-based nursing practice as the ideal from which the nursing profession will evolve. Patricia Moccia, NLN's Chief Executive Officer, states,

Table 19-1 Cases of selected notifiable diseases in the United States

Communicable disease	Cumulative cases
Mumps	1,053
Malaria	777
Meningocaoccidal infections	1,990
Pertussis	2,528
Syphilis	16,105
Tuberculosis	15,800
Rabies, *animal*	4,723
AIDS	61,173
Gonorrhea	287,081
Lyme disease	8,252
Measles (rubeola)	832

Note. From Centers for Disease Control and Prevention, 1994 (October 7), *Morbidity and Mortality Weekly Report 43*, pp. 714-715.

> The future of health care delivery in America lies outside hospital complexes, in neighborhood based settings where collaborative relationships between individuals and health professionals can flourish. An individual's ability to become fully engaged in illness prevention and remain responsible for their health choices depends upon these strong community relationships. (Moccia, 1995, p. 1)

Moccia further contends that this is certainly a challenge to current models of health care delivery, although not in the sense of a declaration of war against the existing system. Rather, it is a challenge to the entire health care system to accept the necessary shift in focus toward a multidisciplinary, patient-centered health care system.

The NLN leadership notes that our health care system leaves large segments of our society with no access to health care, and the current biomedical view of health care overlooks the major societal conditions that lead to disease conditions, i.e., poverty, homelessness, and poor environmental conditions. Thus, the NLN endorses a focus on education for nurses that is committed to the social changes necessary for health promotion and disease prevention to combat illnesses.

Nursing centers, which are health promotion and disease prevention clinics for clients, are managed by nurses. These nursing centers take a futuristic approach, outlined in the NLN's Vision for Nursing Education, that endorses a nurse-centered transformation in health care delivery that is already happening in many communities across the nation. Nursing centers, such as that seen in Scottsdale's Community Health Services Clinic affiliated with Arizona State University, currently provide complete physical examinations that cost less than a third of what the average physician charges, and with greater client satisfaction.

Centers such as this tend to respond to a community's health care needs more accurately and humanely than hospital-based health centers, which are increasingly owned and operated by large for-profit corporations. Nursing educational programs exist in every neighborhood in this country and nursing centers should, likewise, be in these neighborhoods. Faculty and students have their roots in community settings, and nursing is well positioned to vitalize the mission of health care into our communities with the pride, purpose, and sense of responsibility we have always brought to acute hospital care.

A homeless project funded by the W.K. Kellogg Foundation in cooperation with Howard University's College of Nursing is another example of a nursing education project that focused on a nurse-managed clinic serving a high-risk population. Many of the individuals served were jobless, lacked the means to afford housing facilities, and had dysfunctional families and other social problems clearly linked to the health care problems of this population. While the homeless population has increased, the response of the health care delivery system to meet the needs of this population has lagged significantly. The W.K. Kellogg homeless project is used here to illustrate how a health care program was developed to be particularly sensitive to the health and social needs among the homeless population.

The origin of Howard University College of Nursing's response to health care for the homeless can be traced to the personal interest of one faculty member. In 1986, Lacey became associated with the Community for Creative Non-Violence (CCNV), which is one of the largest advocacy groups for the homeless. In this historically black university, with its mission of "social uplift," issues of homelessness were fully integrated into its nursing educational program and research activities. The history behind this initiative for integration, ways in which the model was implemented, and the constraints placed on the faculty members, are discussed briefly.

A federal appropriation, coupled with support from private foundations, provided the initial needed resources with which to transform a vacant federal building at 2nd and D Streets into a residential building with 1,400 beds and a health unit in the basement. Lacey was instrumental in the design of the health ambulatory clinic, a 24-bed postdetoxification unit, and a 32-bed infirmary.

With the funding from the W.K. Kellogg Foundation, the Howard University College of Nursing encouraged both undergraduate and graduate nursing students to take advantage of educational opportunities for health assessment, health education, referrals when indicated, and health promotion. Opportunities to enhance nursing clinical skills as well as to teach and learn case management, along with nursing administration, enabled nursing students to successfully accomplish course objectives within the curriculum. It was evident that innovation and critical thinking would unquestionably be required in addressing the complex problems imposed on the homeless population (Meleis, Isenberg, Koenner, Lacey, & Steven, 1995).

Although collaboration between the CCNV and the Howard University College of Nursing needed a period to cultivate and develop harmony of purpose and mission, a contract did emerge by which CCNV and Howard University could partner in the provision of health care to the homeless. A number of lessons were learned from these experiences that ultimately guided the project in modeling a concept of health care delivery for the homeless. Following is a summary of these lessons:

- An effective and accessible system of services for the homeless cannot be designed and implemented without the input, collaboration, and cooperation of the advocacy groups and homeless individuals.
- Trust is a basic requirement for collaboration, and develops over time.
- Myths, stereotypes, a false sense of dissonance, and "missionary zeal" must be replaced with respect, honesty, openness, and the right to self-determination.
- With understanding comes a recognition of what strengths, competencies, and potentials exist on both sides.
- Grassroots advocacy groups have a strong sense of what types of services are needed and wanted for their peers.
- Grassroots groups have opinions about how care can be delivered in culturally sensitive ways (the culture of poverty, rejection, and despair).
- Traditional nursing approaches can be modified to reflect the culture and environment in which services are needed.
- Students (undergraduate and graduate) can contribute to and benefit from nontraditional learning experiences through creative opportunities to problem solving.
- The greatest barriers to the effective delivery of services (fear, ignorance, and insensitivity) can be overcome by first recognizing that they exist.
- Academic institutions are inclined to engage in fairly detailed and logical theoretical determination of processes and models while grassroots groups tend to be action-oriented, practical, and driven by immediate outcomes.
- Mutual respect and interdependency, created out of learning to know each other, constitute the basis of a system of shared goals and responsibility (Lacey, 1994).

The W.K. Kellogg Homeless Project had profound impact on the undergraduate and graduate curricula of the College of Nursing at Howard University. The project was a catalyst for curriculum reform in the undergraduate program. Students were integrated into the setting from the start. During the first year of the project, student experiences were planned in a beginning level Fundamentals of Nursing course, followed by Health Assessment and Medical-Surgical Nursing. Later, Community-Mental Health Nursing along with Leadership and Management were added as courses that used the shelter for clinical experiences. These experiences had multiple benefits, one of the most important of which was to enhance opportunity for students to practice complex problem solving. In a setting in which minimum protocols existed and equipment and supplies were limited, students were forced to figure out what to do based on all their previous learning and by eliciting the knowledge and wisdom of the clients in collaborative problem solving. These experiences usually forced students to increase their awareness of community resources, the political system, and the need for interdisciplinary teams to address the concerns of patients.

These settings also provided faculty with the opportunity to expand problem solving readily as a teaching method. Hospital-based settings often impeded creative thinking and problem solving because pre-existing plans of care are often in place. Early experiences with the homeless caused faculty to become more willing to consider sites other than the hospital for clinical practice. Admittedly, faculty were reluctant to believe, initially, that students would find challenging and beneficial learning experiences within the shelter. Over time, many experiences were found to be superior—capable of supporting many clinical learning objectives and providing students with a more balanced nursing education.

Consequently, when the national debate on health care reform escalated to a level at which changes in nursing education were imperative to provide a properly trained nursing workforce, the College of Nursing was out front because of the positive, challenging, and beneficial experience gained over the first 2 to 3 years of the project.

Likewise, the graduate curriculum experienced some

changes and expanded direction, facilitated in part by the homeless project. The shelter provided an excellent setting for the preparation of nurse practitioners. Assessment skills, health education, diagnosis, and treatment skills can be practiced with various age groups including children, men, and women. The program made a decision to start a post-master's family nurse practitioner program with the shelter as a major practice site. The infirmary offered a rich learning environment for graduate students to meet the program objectives and to conduct research.

During the 4 years of project operations, 334 nursing students gained experience at the infirmary (Figure 19-1). Two hundred ninety-four (88%) were women and 40 (12%) were men; the median student age was 25 years, and the overwhelming majority were upper class students—freshmen, 5%; sophomores, 9%; juniors, 27%; seniors, 30%; and graduate students, 30%.

As the project developed and moved forward, the role of members of the homeless community also continued to expand. Specifically, homeless individuals from the CCNV community collaborated by assisting with admission and discharge planning; activities of daily living for infirmary clients; maintenance of a safe, clean, and comfortable respite environment; and the development of videos as health promotion messages.

Selected individuals of the CCNV community were also invited by the project director to participate as speakers on health care panels, specifically addressing issues of access to services for the underserved. The purpose of these appearances was to cultivate a sense of advocacy among the homeless for their own causes, to debunk some of the other popular stereotypical views of the homeless, and to give outsiders first-hand information on the cause of homelessness. The homeless, in turn, came to see the critical and crucial role of nursing in health care delivery.

Today's nurses, including nurse practitioners with advanced science degrees, are primary health care providers in widely varied communities, maintaining essential, personal services once provided by the family physician. The NLN's membership is ensuring that the community needs hold primary importance in planning for nursing's ever-expanding role in the health care system. Says Lindeman, past President of NLN's Board of Governors and Dean

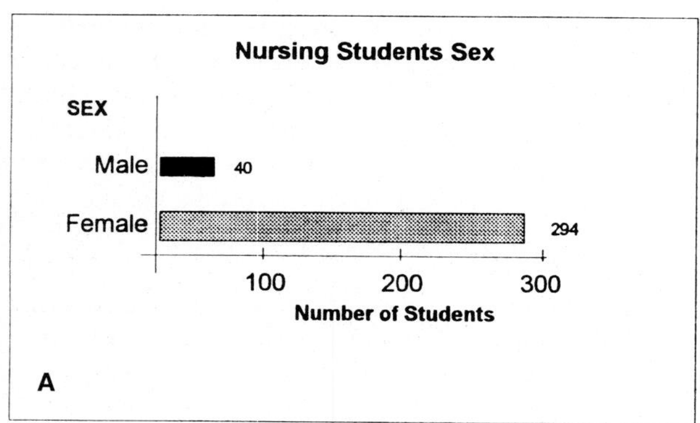

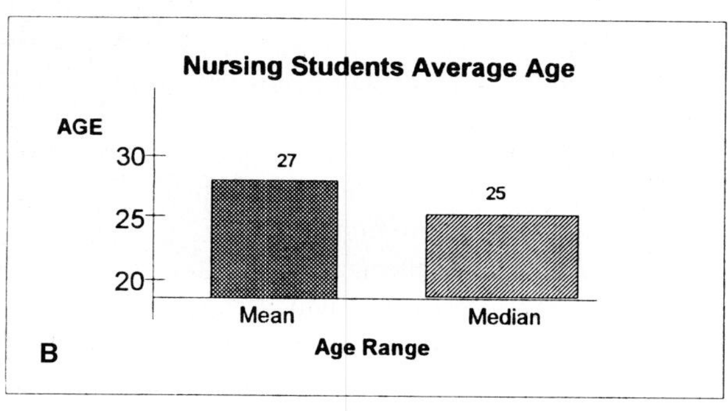

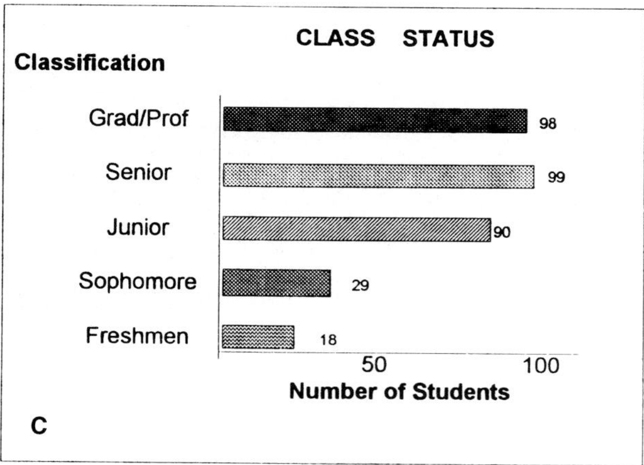

Fig. 19-1. Profile of 334 students participating in Howard University Homeless Project. **A**, by sex; **B**, by average age; **C**, by class status.

emeritus of the School of Nursing at Oregon Health Sciences Center, "Nurses' academic community, once the isolated domain of scholars, now includes practitioners, community and business leaders, and representatives of foundations, and public policy organizations as active partners in meeting its mission" (Lindeman, 1995, p. 8). Within this broadened context, nursing education has initiated a series of steps leading to fundamental reform.

Health care reform requires a restructuring of the health care delivery system into a community care network and with goals that are directed toward:

- Advancing patients and communities to the center of our attention
- Emphasizing prevention and minimizing illness and disability
- Making the health care system more user-friendly in order to improve the continuity and quality of health care services
- Realigning incentives that govern everyone's behavior in making decisions about the use of health care resources

Community health care networks must begin to share selected key characteristics such as

- A health focus on community
- A seamless continuum of care
- Management within fixed resources
- Community accountability ("Transforming Health Care Delivery," 1993)

It is very evident that the present and future paradigms for health care delivery will require that nurses perform more health promotion and wellness functions. In addition, the philosophy and conceptual framework that form the supporting matrix for designing nursing curriculum must reflect greater emphasis on community health promotion and practice to include practice in nursing centers. When and how these changes are made throughout the nursing profession constitutes a major challenge (Baldwin, 1995). As other options to expensive institutional care are sought and health care returns to the community, nursing will be returning to its roots in the public health design of community-based and community-focused care.

It is evident that old paradigms included ideas and methods thought to be effective in solving individual problems confronting nurses. As the health care focus has taken on a more dynamic and complex approach, many unsolved problems have been recognized. These unsolved problems have accumulated new ideas and approaches outside the old paradigms. As these new approaches develop, a new paradigm comes into place. Table 19-2 depicts a summary of the old and new paradigms of health. Both old and new curricular constructs

Table 19-2 Old and new paradigms of health

Old curricular constructs	Proposed and new curricular constructs
1. Hospital-focused health care of individuals to eliminate disease and repair of the diseased part is a primary concern of nursing.	1. There are demographic shifts that are population-based, with a focus on the concepts of equilibrium, interrelatedness of the universe, and an understanding of patterns. The focus is on *health promotion and disease prevention.*
2. Nursing professional is the authority. Nursing position with the client is in an advisory capacity.	2. Relationship-centered care in which the nurse is a partner with clients.
3. Nursing focus is on tasks, being efficient, and physician-dependent.	3. Human values and ethical principles are basic to holistic care using an interdisciplinary approach and fostering interdependence.
4. Mind-state of the individual is secondary to an organic illness.	4. Health and illness are expressions of life and the mind-state is co-equal in health promotion and illness prevention.
5. Health-care emphasis on cause-effect relationship in that negative is bad and positive is good.	5. Constant interchange between the environment and clients in which each influences the shaping of the environment and of the health of the client.
6. There is competition within the profession as well as with other disciplines.	6. Collaboration, cooperation, and mutual consensus in improving the health of the communities is the emphasis for nursing.
7. The individual is the focus and is viewed as a product with an illness.	7. Community-oriented nursing in assisting individuals, families, and communities to rebuild a sense of competence in their abilities to solve problems.

are presented, promoting a broader focus on health promotion and disease prevention.

Secretary of Health and Human Services, Shalala, made this statement concerning nurses as social leaders:

> A generation of nurses is being trained who will not only treat diseases of a society, they will understand intimately that their profession means a commitment to the social changes that are necessary for good health; personal and cultural. They will be not only staff nurses, nurse researchers, nurse administrators, nurse educators, and nurse practitioners, but nurse warriors (Shalala, 1993, p. 289).

The revolution has begun. May the nurse warriors presently engaged in this transformation persist and may future nurse warriors carry the changes forward.

REFERENCES

American Psychological Association. (1994). *Publication manual of the american psychological association* (4th ed.). Washington, DC: Author.

Baldwin, J. (1995). Are we implementing community health promotion in nursing? *Public Health Nursing, 12*(3), 159-164.

Carnegie, M.E. (1986). *The path we tread, blacks in nursing 1854-1984.* Philadelphia: Lippincott.

Centers for Disease Control and Prevention. (1994, October 7). *Morbidity and Mortality Weekly Report, 43*(39), 714-715.

Committee on Education of the National League for Nursing Education. (1919). *Standard curriculum for schools of nursing.* New York: National Nursing Association.

Gardner, M.S. (1936). *Public health nursing.* New York: Macmillan.

Grace, H.K. (1990, Spring/Summer). Building community: A conceptual perspective. *1, International Journal of the W.K. Kellogg Foundation.*

Green, A.H. (1995). Tennessee: A story of APN's and 16 months of managed care. *Nursing Policy Forum, 1*(4), 28-31.

Hanson, C. (1991). The 1990s and beyond: Determining the need for community health care nurses for rural populations. *The Journal of Rural Health,* 7 (1, Suppl).

Johnson, B., & Coulberson, S.L. (1993). Environmental epidemiologic issues and minority health. *Annals of Epidemiology, 3,* 175-179.

Lacey, B. (1994). *Howard University College of Nursing Final report to W.K. Kellogg Foundation.* Washington, DC: Howard University.

Lagermann, E.C. (1983). *Nursing history: New perspectives, new possibilities.* New York: Teachers College Press.

Lewis, J., & Farrell, M. (1995). Distance education: A strategy for leadership development. *Nursing and Health Care Perspectives on Community, 16*(4), 184-187.

Lindeman, C.A. (1995). Nursing education in changing times. *NLN Research and Policy Prism, 3*(1), 1-2, 8.

Moccia, P. (1995, March Press Release). League for nursing urges national focus on community-based health care. *National League for Nursing: Public information alliances.* p. 1.

Meleis, A.I., Isenberg, M., Koenner, J.E., Lacey, B., & Steven, P. (1995). *Diversity, marginalization, and culturally competent health care issues in knowledge development.* [Monograph]. Washington, DC: American Academy of Nursing.

National League for Nursing. *A vision for nursing education.* (1993). New York: Author.

Partnerships for Prevention. (1993). Prevention is the basis to health reform—A position paper. Unpublished manuscript, Washington, DC.

Salmon, M. (1993). Editorial: An open letter to public health nurses. *Public Health Nursing, 10,* 4.

Shalala, D. (1993). Nursing and society: The unfinished agenda for the 21st century. *Nursing and Health Care National League for Nursing, 14,* 6.

Smith, G. (1995). Lessons learned: Challenges for the future. *Nursing and Health Care: Perspectives on Community, 16*(4), 188-191.

Transforming health care delivery: Toward community care networks. (1993). [Booklet]. American Hospital Association: Chicago, IL.

Wald, L. (1915). *House on Henry Street.* New York: Holt.

CHAPTER 20

Clinical education in the nursing home becomes a step toward a community-based curriculum

VERLE WATERS, ELAINE TAGLIARENI, ANDREA MENGEL, SUSAN SHERMAN

In the previous edition of this text, strategies for change in nursing education used in the W.K. Kellogg–funded project, the Community College–Nursing Home Partnership: Improving Care Through Education, were described. That chapter noted different patterns of faculty development and faculty leadership emerging in six demonstration sites supported by the project, and provided speculation on the relationship between a given pattern and success in achieving curriculum change (Sherman & Waters, 1994).

Initiated in 1986, the Community College–Nursing Home Partnership: Improving Care Through Education project significantly increased curriculum emphasis on gerontologic nursing in associate degree education and fostered new clinical affiliations with nursing homes in more than a third of the nation's 850 associate degree nursing programs. Significant changes in curriculum design and development of innovative teaching strategies in nonacute care settings resulted from project activities. At least four assumptions or beliefs about conditions necessary to successfully bring about change emerged:

1. Change is more likely if the oligarchy advocates it. With this assumption in mind, six demonstration sites were selected. Each nursing program was accredited by the National League for Nursing and had a positive local reputation and a director who was seen as a national leader. Within the demonstration sites, the oligarchy principle argued for the recruitment of tenured, full-time, well-regarded faculty to coordinate project activities. However, not all six sites found it possible to place full-time faculty in project leadership positions.

2. Campaigns for change are made more effective by combining ideology and conceptual arguments with compelling demonstrations of how to do it. To achieve such campaigns, the project provided an "umbrella" structure identifying objectives and activities relating to a national perspective. A national advisory committee assisted in planning, analyzing, and synthesizing experiences from the six demonstrations. The six demonstration sites, on the other hand, built advisory committees that suited local needs and characteristics.

3. Change agents need support. For the period of the project, principals from all six sites met and worked together. At least two times per year, key people from each site gathered to collaborate, share, and plan. Faculty at each site received support from administration to redesign both classroom and clinical teaching learning models.

4. Systematic formative evaluation and feedback fosters successful change. An evaluation specialist assisted both the national project and each demonstration site to develop evaluation protocols and analyze data.

This paper offers a retrospective view of the project and describes how the lessons learned in the nursing home project provide a format and method for community college nursing faculty to continue curriculum change as nursing services move from the acute care hospital to the home and community settings.

In the years since its establishment in 1952, associate degree nursing education has demonstrated effectiveness in preparing significant numbers of nurses to meet the nursing needs of society. Located in community colleges—the segment of American higher education charged to offer curricula that respond to the community's needs—associate degree nursing programs emphasize the knowledge and job skills central to the practice of registered nursing and respond to the special needs of the local community. Until the last decade, the knowledge and skill areas were, in comparison with the present day, fairly easy to define: Because two thirds or more of registered nurses worked in acute hospitals, the faculty designed and implemented a curriculum based almost entirely on the practice of nursing within those hospitals.

The first major challenge to the acute hospital curriculum came with the recognition of changing demographics and the problems in providing health care to the elderly. The nursing home project, conceived and developed in the mid-1980s, responded to this challenge by demonstrating how care might be improved in nursing homes through staff development and affiliation with nursing students and how the curriculum might be changed substantially to prepare graduates for practice roles in both long-term and acute care organizations. By the time project funding ended in 1994, there were documented changes in the teaching of gerontology, and nursing homes had become a setting for clinical education in over 300 associate degree nursing programs (Hanson, 1995). By that time a sweeping change was occurring in the health care delivery system in the United States, and faculty were confronted with the realization that curriculum change responsive to the needs of the elderly was only a first step toward a major curriculum shift in both process and content. The curriculum that had based its definition of nursing on the role of nurses in the acute care hospital had suddenly become obsolete. In a remarkably short period of time, hospital stays decreased while care shifted to homes, ambulatory clinics, and nursing homes. Graduates of nursing programs confronted a diminished labor market for the registered nurse in acute care settings. These changes necessitated a shift in curriculum. The call to develop a community-focused curriculum posed an unnerving challenge to associate degree nursing faculty. For more than 40 years "community" had been the only clear-cut subject area difference between the associate and baccalaureate curricula. An unanticipated benefit of the Community College–Nursing Home Partnership project is that the change in thinking experienced by faculty groups provided the impetus for moving toward a community-focused program of study.

HELPING FACULTY DEVELOP A NEW PERSPECTIVE

In designing the Community College–Nursing Home project, project leaders were guided by the belief that faculty development is the gateway to curriculum change. Consequently the project plan called for early emphasis on faculty re-education (Hanson & Waters, 1991). An early lesson learned, as project activities got under way, was how deeply resistant some faculty were to the changes called for by the project. Project faculty were asked to agree to the clinical placement of senior students in nursing homes, a setting seen by most faculty as below par in standards of care and opportunities for student learning. These faculty, educated as and hired because they were acute care specialists, found conflict when asked to embrace long-term care nursing values. The emphasis on faculty development as an initial step in accomplishing the proposed changes in the curriculum allowed negative and skeptical attitudes to find expression and provided opportunities to address them. In retrospect, those who worked most closely with the project, when asked what they felt contributed to the success of the project, cited faculty development more than any other factor. Representative comments include the following:

- The focus on faculty development *first* gave faculty the confidence needed to move forward.
- The fact that the grant provided funds up front for educating faculty before they had to produce had a positive effect on students.
- Knowledge was the key factor; it was critical in helping us get over the hump.

Each of the six demonstration sites offered different approaches and activities for faculty development. One site scheduled periodic off-campus retreats for all faculty; another provided released time for a faculty member with a gerontological nursing background to share her knowledge with her peers; and another funded course attendance for faculty at a geriatric education center. Despite the wide range of differences in approach, there was agreement at the close of the project on the following guidelines for faculty development activities intended to facilitate educational change:

1. Involve all faculty in planning the faculty development activities.
2. Identify a "cheerleader" and give her or him time to coordinate planning; consult widely; recruit supporters; and find, photocopy, and distribute pertinent materials.
3. Provide constant, vigilant leadership, maintain the vision, keep people on target, encourage and validate success, and help faculty see value and purpose in their work.
4. As a leader, communicate the expectation that everyone will participate in some fashion.
5. Focus on those faculty members who are recognized

as informal leaders. Unless the oligarchy is supportive of, or open to, the intended changes, they are not likely to occur.

6. Bring out in the open as honest concerns what you know to be threatened self-interests: teaching favorite content, overwork, status associated with particular assignments, choice clinical settings, and so on.
7. Negotiate with people to take on a new assignment on a trial basis. Offer incentives and trade-offs. Make a genuine offer to discontinue if they wish after a trial period (Waters, 1995).

CLINICAL EDUCATION FOR COMMUNITY-BASED LEARNING

Clinical placement of students with geriatric populations was not new to nursing faculty; it had been (and is still) used for purposes of teaching nursing skills to beginning students. Such clinical placements call for working relationships between the college and the long-term care agency not unlike the relationships between college and hospital. In a clinical education pattern labelled "parallel play," the nursing faculty member arranged for a group of students to perform a set of nursing tasks selected by the teacher and carried out more or less independent of the work of nursing home staff. It became clear early in the project that its purposes required a very different pattern of college-agency relationships: In order to learn the role of the registered nurse in the long-term care setting and be prepared to assume such a role on graduation, senior students would need to become full participants in the daily care operations in the nursing home. Further, the project intention that nursing faculty would initiate and carry out staff development activities for nursing home staff required a new understanding of the ways in which the college and a clinical agency worked together.

A Delphi study done early in the project to determine essential factors in a community college–nursing home partnership confirmed the need for different college-agency relationships (Mengel, Simpson, Sherman, & Waters, 1990). This study showed that the basis for a solid partnership includes mutual respect and understanding, a commitment to high-quality education for students and high-quality service to patients, clear communication, and a collaborative approach to managing the partnership. Another finding was that both partners (the community college and the nursing home) wish to remain autonomous while collaborating on management of the partnership. However, one partner, most likely the community college, needs to assume responsibility for doing the majority of the work to maintain the partnership, because respondents felt that the benefits and responsibilities need not be equal.

These factors of a successful partnership seem applicable when developing collaborative relationships with agencies in the community. Like nursing homes, community agencies have a unique life of their own with respect to values, traditions, communication patterns, missions, constraints, and resources. Respecting this uniqueness is the first step for faculty trying to develop community-based clinical learning activities.

To flourish, partnerships must be negotiated and renegotiated as new needs arise. This is unlike the traditional relationships developed over the years between nursing programs and hospitals where a common language and set of expectations existed. In the community, nursing approaches to care delivery and nursing education outcomes are not necessarily known to personnel in community agencies. Attending to the needs and values that make each partner unique facilitates the collaborative process, and based on the Delphi analysis, ultimately results in richer clinical education experiences.

NEW FACULTY ROLES WHEN AMBIGUITY REPLACES CERTAINTY

Since the inception of associate degree nursing programs, faculty have enjoyed the privilege of a relatively clear definition of the role of the associate degree graduate and the benefit of relationships with hospitals that willingly provided direct feedback to the school about the fit between graduate's capabilities and the new employer's expectations. With the steady diffusion of jobs for new graduates—nursing homes, ambulatory clinics, and homes as well as acute care hospitals—uncertainty has grown about what exactly should be emphasized in the basic curriculum.

This sense of unrest, experienced by faculty involved in the Community College–Nursing Home Partnership project, occurred throughout the project. For faculty, movement out of the comfort zone of the acute care hospital, away from a cure-oriented, disease treatment model of curriculum design, resulted from project activities. That this movement was a significant shift for faculty cannot be overstated. Early in the project, faculty were asked to make a major paradigm shift, knowing that neither their education in a disease-focused, behavioristic curriculum nor their practice in an institution-based, acute care driven health care system had prepared them for this change. The resulting sense of ambivalence and uncertainty was inevitable.

Very quickly, project faculty recognized the need for

support as they moved into the new practice setting of the nursing home and designed new curriculum strategies. Faculty discovered that models for practice and teaching did not transfer intact from one setting to another. As faculty found themselves outside their comfort zones, specifically, outside the practice of teaching in an acute care environment, they began to realize that even as an expert teacher they temporarily experienced a novice role, creating what faculty termed the "expert teacher and expert practice dilemma" (Waters, 1991). The initial anxiety and ambivalence created by the transition to a new practice setting eventually led to new ways of thinking about curricula, about teaching, and about being with students. In fact, project faculty recognized the transforming nature of the transition experience and began to embrace, rather then resent, the novice role. They reached the conclusion that to be an effective change agent, to fully understand the environment and the culture of a new practice setting and take on new teacher roles, they must first become novices in the new setting. The term "expert novice" was coined to describe the transition process as faculty bring their expertise as teachers to an environment in which practice is new and where, at first, faculty are unaccustomed to procedures and ways of being with clients. Being an expert novice means being open to the differences in the practice setting in order to recognize opportunities for innovative nursing approaches to health care delivery. It means entering a new practice setting. It means being comfortable with ambiguity, recognizing that the acute-care, institution-focused curriculum, which seemed so clearly defined and universally understood, can no longer be the sole orientation of nursing education. Valuing the opportunity for new and different ways to be with students and patients when exposed to new environments of care became an essential posture to project faculty and may, in fact, have been the critical factor in project success. Understanding that the issue of ambiguity in practice is not solved through rigidity of curriculum design and accepting the role of the expert novice are essential leadership attributes to change nursing education effectively. This is a major lesson learned from the Community College–Nursing Home Partnership project.

There is a paradox, however. Nurses are magnetically attracted to certainty, to finding the right answer (Waters, 1995), and to following traditional and secure approaches to classroom and clinical learning. Yet the call to accept uncertainty and ambiguity in practice is now more imperative than ever.

> As American society becomes increasingly diverse and health care issues more complex, as the health care system moves swiftly and dramatically away from an acute care, disease-focused model, the traditional approaches to basic and continuing education come up short. Educational leadership today faces a daunting task: to facilitate the learning of unknown students who will care in the unknown tomorrows for unknown clients in unknown ways. It is time for fresh imaginings. (Waters, 1995, p. 75)

It is also a time to embrace ambiguity, not certainty, as an essential strategy to direct curriculum change.

NEW FACULTY ROLES WHEN A COLLABORATIVE TEACHING STYLE REPLACES TRADITIONAL MODELS

A struggle between ambiguity and certainty, between maintaining traditional approaches to teaching and embracing new, interactive methodologies is tellingly played out today in nursing education. Waters notes that "an earnest desire to graduate nurses who think critically and independently is often vitiated by teaching practices based on complying with authority and extolling factual knowledge" (1995, p. 75). Early in the Community College–Nursing Home Partnership project, faculty recognized the need to foster collaborative teaching approaches with students and to establish working partnerships with nurse colleagues in the nursing home. New patterns, traditions, and relationships among teachers, agency staff, and students emerged.

As faculty assumed the role of expert novice in the nursing home, they recognized the need to change the traditional faculty approach to clinical instruction, meeting clinical objectives "next to" rather than "with" their nurse colleagues in the practice setting (Tagliareni, Sherman, Waters, & Mengel, 1991). Throughout the years of the project, as faculty and staff became more comfortable with this collaborative model, one significant outcome evolved: The power relationship between faculty, staff, and students changed. Faculty no longer came to the setting with a pre-determined learning model for staff to follow and students to participate in—an approach that so often creates stressful environments that are oppressive for students, faculty, and staff. Faculty no longer fully directed the student's learning, but rather allowed time for students to challenge assumptions and be creative in personalizing care. Faculty learned that the relationship with staff often became the central factor in developing the learning environment, and that as staff assisted students in exploring a nursing model of care delivery, staff and students came to appreciate each other in new ways. These ongoing interactions led to a better understanding of the setting and the practice patterns within the setting, and subsequently to the establishment of new roles for students and new care-planning ideas for staff. Hopefully, a similar collaborative approach to staff in community settings will be achieved by nurse educators in the future.

Recognizing that the care-focused environment of the nursing home is characterized by ambiguity, personalized outcomes, and complexity of care planning, project faculty quickly rallied behind the notion that traditional teaching approaches did not foster collaboration and participatory nursing care delivery and that residents and clinical situations did not match the nice neat little boxes associated with traditional approaches to care planning. Project faculty were troubled by students who wrote elegant care plans but lacked the flexibility and creativity to respond rapidly to changing practice situations or, more importantly, the ability to personalize care planning within specific environments of care and to alter care plans based on context and personal meaning. Project faculty asked, How can we develop models of critical thinking that foster collaboration and help students attend to context?

At no time in nursing's history is this issue more salient than today, as nurse educators move to become faculty of the community (Moccia, 1993). The neat, behaviorist approach to care planning, which is rarely collaborative in nature, does not support thinking that is informed by reflection, collaboration, self-awareness, and understanding context.

To promote discovery learning, which is essential in a community-neighborhood model of health care delivery, nurse educators will need to reframe the way they teach students to think. Nursing faculty have relied on the nursing process and its five steps to foster comprehension and analysis. Problem solving or nursing process is a framework for solving problems; it may or may not have critical thinking as an element. In a community-based system, which involves a collaborative journey for nurses, the old models of teaching and thinking may be inadequate and may, in fact, inhibit critical thinking. This is a powerful lesson that emerged from the Community College–Nursing Home Partnership project.

SUMMARY

One purpose of nursing education is to serve society. Nursing education approaches the new millenium with challenges to adapt curricula to new care delivery systems, rapidly expanding technology, and dramatically different populations. Managing curriculum change is central in the worklife of every nurse educator.

Moving into the community is a new experience for most associate degree nursing programs. This move is appealing intuitively because most associate degree nursing programs are located in community colleges. Students come from the community and return to the community following graduation. Developing the potential in these connections seems to be a natural progression that will benefit both students and the community. Yet as this break with tradition occurs, resistance is natural. Faculty leading the way will need special skills to support other faculty, deal with ambiguity, and develop partnerships. Faculty will need to challenge each other to become expert-novices within their own neighborhoods and communities. As changes in health care delivery inform curriculum decisions and challenge the historic emphasis on the acute care setting as the primary focus of clinical learning, faculty will need to reframe their thinking about themselves as nurse educators, about students, and about health care for communities of people. They will need to move toward collaborative, interactive models of teaching-learning. Change in nursing education is often difficult to measure and accounting for why it was possible is considerably more difficult. Yet experiences associated with the W.K. Kellogg Community College–Nursing Home Partnership project have resulted in timely and successful ideas for changing nursing education—ideas that now serve as the catalyst for movement to a community-based associate degree nursing curriculum.

REFERENCES

Hanson, H.A. (1995). Evaluation highlights. In V. Waters. *The narrative enlarging: A biography of the community college-nursing home partnership project* (pp 101-108). New York: National League for Nursing.

Hanson, H.A., & Waters, V. (1991). The sequence of curriculum change in gerontology: Faculty first. *Nursing & Health Care, 12*(10), 516-519.

Mengel, A., Simpson, S., Sherman, S., & Waters, V. (1990, November). Essential factors in a Community College-Nursing Home Partnership. *Journal of Gerontologic Nursing, 16,* 26-31.

Moccia, P. (1993). Nursing education in the public trust: A faculty of the community: No unreal loyalties for us. *Nursing and Health Care, 14*(9), 472-474.

Sherman, S., & Waters, V. (1994). Community College-Nursing Home Partnership: Successful strategies for change in nursing education. In J. McCloskey & H.K. Grace (Eds.), *Current issues in nursing* (4th ed., pp 177-181). St. Louis: Mosby.

Tagliareni, E., Sherman, S., Waters, V., & Mengel, A. (1991). Participatory clinical education: Reconceptualizing the clinical learning environment. *Nursing and Health Care, 12*(5), 248-263.

Waters, V. (1991). *Teaching gerontology.* New York: National League for Nursing.

Waters, V. (1995). *The narrative enlarging: A biography of the community college-nursing home partnership project.* New York: National League for Nursing.

The changing face of graduate education

RICHARD W. REDMAN, SHAKÉ KETEFIAN

Rapid change characterizes today's society. Reform of the health care system has emerged at the forefront of public discourse and in recent political elections as a pressing domestic issue. The health professions both lead and follow changes in health care delivery. Rapid social and technological changes also present challenges in the education of health professionals. This is especially true in the graduate education of nurses.

A number of trends in society and health care have been identified that influence education for health professionals. These trends have been summarized by participants in the Future of the Health Professions Project of the Pew Charitable Trusts (O'Neil & Hare, 1990): the change in focus of health care from addressing individual needs in acute care settings to community and ambulatory settings concerned with broader populations and chronic conditions; the rising cost of health care, its impact on the economy, and its affordability; specialization in the professions while the need for primary care becomes greater; the need to incorporate quality measures into the assessment of clinical outcomes; a broader definition of health that transcends the traditional conception; changing expectations of "consumers," including patients and students; demographic trends in the population, including a rise in the number of elderly and minority groups; and expansion of knowledge.

These trends, and others unfolding with each passing day, demand a degree of unprecedented vigilance on the part of health professional schools if they are to prepare effective practitioners. This chapter aims to present selected issues and challenges in graduate education in nursing, including postdoctoral study from the perspective of current and evolving social, technological, professional, and clinical practice needs, and to suggest evolving trends in these areas.

To accomplish this aim, we begin with a historical overview of the development of graduate education in nursing. We then examine a number of critical issues in contemporary graduate nursing education at the master's, doctoral, and postdoctoral levels.

GRADUATE EDUCATION—HISTORICAL OVERVIEW

The original vision of the American graduate school was to train scholars for the transmission and creation of knowledge. The master's degree has been associated with pedagogy (Pelczar, Jr., 1980). First granted by Harvard University in 1642, the master's was a rigorous degree, involving 3 years of study beyond the bachelor's. This degree later diminished in importance, however. According to Pelczar, Jr., the University of Michigan is credited with reviving the master's degree. Adopted through regental action in 1858, achieving the master's degree involved a course of study and a thesis. This model was adopted by other institutions and variations of it were instituted throughout the country. The master's degree achieved its identity, as distinct from the doctoral degree, when offerings in education expanded, and institutions began admitting women to graduate study. The majority of the master's degrees were earned by public school teachers, a situation that continued through the late 1950s (Pelczar, Jr., 1980).

Graduate education received its impetus in 1867 with the opening of Johns Hopkins University, which was devoted exclusively to graduate study. The German model of education was adopted, emphasizing generation of new knowledge (Brodie, 1986). Following the German model, basic sciences gained ascendancy in the late 19th century, and the scientific model became the prototype for emerging disciplines. Thus was born the American Ph.D. degree, which was quickly adopted by major universities; the graduate school became the producer of the American scholar. The first part of the 20th century saw great expansion in graduate education and doctoral training. New knowledge generated gave rise to even more specialties and professional fields of study.

Rapid expansion in higher education occurred following the second World War. Many returning veterans sought undergraduate and graduate degrees. Government and foundations invested heavily in university research, students, and buildings (Brodie, 1986). Soviet scientific and space achievements in the late 1950s gave further impetus to graduate education. New national objectives were set for scientific training and fellowships were made available, although these fellowships tended to support doctoral rather than master's education (Pelczar, Jr., 1980).

Graduate education in nursing

Graduate education in nursing began at Teachers College, Columbia University in the early 1920s, and was designed to prepare educators and administrators. This model was used until 1954 when Rutgers University initiated a graduate program at the master's level to educate clinical nurse specialists in psychiatric nursing.

During the 1950s and 1960s the master's degree in nursing was viewed as a terminal degree (Jolly & Hart, 1987), and role preparation continued to be its focus. In the early 1970s clinical nurse specialist and nurse practitioner preparation emerged and continued to hold sway. By the late 1970s role preparation made a comeback. Such pendulum swings with regard to program focus and the development of new specialties and degrees reflected the discipline's readiness to evolve in response to changes in society and in nursing, and the need to incorporate the new knowledge that was becoming available at a rapid rate within nursing and related fields.

Forni (1987a) reported 11 master's degree titles being offered by nationally accredited master's programs in 1984. In 1983, Williamson's analysis of nationally accredited programs revealed 130 combinations of available areas of study from 109 accredited programs (Williamson, 1983). By 1986, Starck reported 247 different program titles and specialties being offered by 143 accredited master's programs (Starck, 1987).

Doctoral education in nursing was first initiated at Teachers College, Columbia University (1933) and at New York University (1934). These programs offered the doctor of education (Ed.D.) degree. In the next 25 years, only two more doctoral programs were established. Since then, the growth of doctoral programs has been exponential. At last count, 54 institutions were offering doctoral degrees. Grace (1978) and Murphy (1981) have described the development of doctoral programs in phases. Phase I included education *for* nurses for functional roles (inception to 1959); Phase II included education *for* nurses in a second discipline, referred to as nurse scientist training (1960 to 1969); and Phase III included education *in* and *of* nursing (1970 to present). Seven degree titles are currently offered, each claiming distinctive purposes and goals (Lash, 1987a, 1987b). The majority of the programs (72%) offer the Ph.D. degree, which is the research doctorate and has wide acceptance and recognition in higher education.

ISSUES IN GRADUATE EDUCATION

Graduate education in all disciplines has evolved to the present day in response to several driving forces. Graduate education parallels forces such as social values, priorities in the public sector, technological capabilities, knowledge development, maturity in the professions, and changing student demographics. These forces in turn shape curricular content, program requirements, and issues and challenges in higher education (Jolly & Hart, 1987).

For example, the rapid pace of change that is endemic in all types of industries has presented a number of challenges to graduate education. Workplace restructuring and reengineering of work processes have generally created such fundamental changes in the workplace that it becomes very challenging for colleges and universities to address knowledge and skills that will both be current when students enter practice and serve them throughout their careers. The balance between theory, technical skills, and application faces special challenges in contemporary graduate education.

The need for nursing research to address and inform pressing policy issues is also becoming increasingly apparent. Within the health care industry, the overriding concern today is on cost-effective interventions and programs that result in desired patient outcomes (Hegyvary, 1991; Jones, 1993). The need for health services research, with nurses as an integral part of the interdisciplinary research team, presents another set of challenges to graduate education. Learning the tools and methods of health services research and how to function as a contributing member of interdisciplinary research teams becomes as important during graduate education as acquisition of advanced clinical skills and knowledge.

The rapid social and technological changes taking place during the last 20 years in American society have also interacted with the evolution of professional nursing. During this time, there has been rapid growth in graduate nursing education. A number of issues have presented both challenges and opportunities for nursing education. While these issues vary somewhat depending on the level of graduate education, they present themes that are common to many professional disciplines.

Issues in master's education

At the master's degree level, the issues closely reflect the rapid changes in the profession and in clinical practice. In addition, they reflect the social, cultural, and technological transformations under way in society. Of a wide range of issues that could be examined, three critical ones have been selected to portray the types of challenges that master's education in nursing is facing today. They are meant to be illustrative rather than comprehensive.

Role of master's degree. The focus of master's degree education in many disciplines has evolved over time, reflecting both the maturity of higher education in the United States and changing social forces and values. Prior to 1900, the master's served primarily as a scholarly degree for college teachers. Between 1900 and 1945, the master's degree began to serve multiple purposes, ranging from being viewed as a terminal degree to a stepping stone to the doctorate. From 1945 to 1970, master's education underwent rapid expansion, diversification, and professionalization. Since 1970, change and innovation have been the hallmark of master's education. Rapid change in consumer demand has resulted in new formats such as external degree programs and interdisciplinary degrees (Conrad, Haworth, & Millar, 1993).

In many academic settings, particularly the research university, master's degree education has been assigned second-class citizenship. It is viewed primarily as a screening device or stepping-stone to the doctorate. In response to this designation, a study on master's education was commissioned by the Council of Graduate Schools to examine the role that master's degree education currently serves and the issues related to that role in American education. Data reveal that over 300,000 master's degrees are awarded annually in the United States, with 52% going to women and 12% to racial and ethnic minorities. Master's degrees comprise about one fourth of all academic degrees awarded. Nearly 85% are in professional fields. The overall conclusion of this study is that master's education has made a far greater impact than either doctoral or baccalaureate education in the lives of students and society. This impact is described as a "silent success" because of the major social benefits derived within various professions and across communities from master's-prepared individuals (Conrad et al., 1993).

Of particular interest in the Conrad et al. study is the typology of master's degree programs developed from their findings. Four major types of educational programs were described; these are presented in the box. Many of the issues in master's degree education in nursing parallel this typology.

One issue facing master's education is the type of educational program that will best address the pressing social and disciplinary issues that nursing faces. In graduate nursing programs, this issue is often described in terms of research versus professional degrees. In graduate programs in which the research doctorate is offered, the issue is particularly relevant. Whether one graduate program can offer two types of master's degrees, i.e., an ancillary and a career advancement or apprenticeship program, in a time of constrained resources is a dilemma that will be faced with increasing frequency. While it is clear that more than one type of master's degree is needed in nursing, it is not certain where these educational programs should be based.

Another issue deals with the rapid clinical specialization developing in nursing and the concomitant need for more apprentice-type programs where graduate students in nursing are involved with expert practitioners in clinical settings. This is an ongoing challenge for faculty, especially in university-based programs, who are pressed with

TYPOLOGY OF MASTER'S DEGREE PROGRAMS IN THE UNITED STATES*

Ancillary program: A stepping stone, screening device, and subordinate to the doctoral degree; learning takes place primarily through faculty-directed scholarly training; practical work experience is tacked on to degree requirements but not cherished

Career advancement program: Career-oriented training that provides terminal credential; heavy emphasis on preparing experts in a field with theory-to-practice focus

Apprenticeship program: Follows model used heavily in the biologic sciences with heavy emphasis on "doing" and strong foundation in theory; faculty serve as master practitioners who facilitate student apprenticeships into a profession

Community-centered program: A dialogical learning community wherein faculty and students are collegial participants; heavy emphasis on social stewardship and critically-informed thoughtful action.

*Adapted from: Conrad, C., Haworth, J., & Millar, S. (1993). *A silent success: Master's education in the U.S.* Baltimore, MD: Johns Hopkins University Press.

the need to maintain clinical proficiency along with demands for scholarly productivity. It also raises curricular issues concerning the balance between theory versus practice content at the master's degree level.

The rapid transformations taking place in master's degree education in general, and in nursing education in particular, will continue in these times of rapid social change. It is also clear that nursing is not the only academic discipline grappling with these issues.

Changing consumer demand. The graduate student population in nursing has undergone tremendous change. In fact, the typical graduate student is often characterized as nontraditional. The vast majority of nursing graduate students today are women with multiple professional and personal responsibilities. They are often full-time employees who are seeking part-time graduate study in programs that are flexible and designed to fit into their demanding schedules. Typically, students are not only placebound and unable to relocate to attend graduate school but also are dependent on the income that full-time employment provides. This transformation in graduate student demography has created several concerns in graduate nursing education.

One change, generated from student demand, has been in program structure and format. Several nontraditional approaches have been attempted that include a range of models from external degree programs to off-campus, satellite, outreach formats and include a blend of on-campus and off-campus offerings. Technological developments have enabled distance learning through video and electronic communications. Consortiums between existing programs also have been attempted. Several successful models for these new approaches exist (Holden-Lund, 1991, Reilly, 1990).

Many concerns have been generated by these nontraditional approaches to graduate education. When educational offerings are delivered off-campus, maintenance of program quality and integrity is always an issue. Another issue is the extent to which socialization toward role behaviors and values of the profession can occur when students are not in residence and do not have regular, ongoing interactions with nursing faculty. In addition, nonresidential students often have limited access to liberal arts course offerings and the wide range of learning resources available on campus. Program resources often are strained when both residential and nonresidential programs are offered within the same unit. Finally, the need for educating students in many advanced specialty practice areas must be balanced with the opportunities for learning experiences available off-campus.

We cannot anticipate that simply increasing the flexibility of educational programs will cause these barriers for those seeking graduate education in nursing to diminish sufficiently. It is clear that these issues will continue to challenge educational institutions and their faculty.

Curricular content and advanced practice roles. The rapid changes in undergraduate nursing education as well as in advanced practice roles have resulted in many challenges to the content in master's degree programs. The tensions between generalist versus specialist content and standardization versus diversity and flexibility have resulted in a wide variation among approaches. The diversity in master's education in nursing has been well documented and suggests there is a lack of consensus regarding the structure of master's degree programs. The content in many programs more typically reflects faculty philosophy than consensus within the discipline. In turn, this has resulted in role confusion across practice settings (Starck, 1987). The need for standardization in educational programs with a more uniform approach to preparation for advanced practice roles presents a major challenge to nursing education.

Given the agenda in the 1990s for reform in health care delivery, clinical practice in nursing has been changing rapidly, especially for nurses in advanced practice roles. Increased opportunities for advanced practice have become available across the entire continuum of care (Donley, 1995). Nurse practitioners typically practiced in primary care settings but now are used in acute care and even tertiary level settings (Keane & Richmond, 1993). In response to increased opportunities, there have been dramatic increases in graduate enrollments for a variety of advanced practice roles. Debate centers on the definitions and roles of advanced practice nurses and whether distinctions exist between clinical nurse specialist and nurse practitioner roles. There is a call for an alignment in graduate nursing education to prepare one educational product: the advanced practice nurse (Cronenwett, 1995; Watson, 1995). Yet consensus does not exist on the best approach for preparation of advanced practice nurses and the type of curricular content that is appropriate for specialization and practice.

In response to the rapid specialization in clinical practice, new issues have also arisen about certification and regulation. Various specialties within nursing are moving rapidly toward the requirement of advanced degrees for certification in a specialty. To date, certification has generally been on a voluntary basis and within the control of the profession. The lack of standardization of curriculum content takes on a new dimension in this realm. The National Council of State Boards of Nursing has proposed a second licensure for nurse practitioners to regulate through governmental authority the requirements for entry into advanced practice roles. This has resulted in extensive debate on the merits of certification versus licensure among professional nursing organizations (American Association of Colleges of Nursing [AACN], 1995; National Council of State Boards of Nursing, 1992).

As we rapidly move into a global community, program standardization becomes a challenge from another perspective. The need to consider standards beyond the United States must be dealt with as more international students seek education in American programs. Major variation exists in the health care and educational systems in the world community (Glittenberg, 1987).

The rapid changes that undergraduate nursing programs are experiencing also produce a problem of standardization. As these programs change to include content in areas such as conceptual models of nursing practice and research methodology, there is need for adjustment in graduate curricula. In addition, these changes affect the learning requirements of graduate students who have completed their undergraduate education at different points in time and at different institutions.

Another challenge relates to rapid scientific advances and technological changes and their impact on both process and content in graduate education. For example, the breakthroughs in genetics for both diagnosis and treatment of a wide range of conditions present both challenges and opportunities for nursing education and practice (McElhinney & Lajkowicz, 1994). Certainly information technology continues to change the way we carry out our personal and professional responsibilities. One result, however, has been ongoing debate about how it should be incorporated into graduate learning experiences. The same challenges exist with all the enabling technologies that are available in the patient care environment. It presents major challenges in terms of curriculum content, faculty proficiency, and program resources.

Issues in doctoral education

At the doctoral level, the issues reflect the evolving trends in society, the field as a whole, and especially the changes in the discipline and science of nursing. It is impossible to delineate an exhaustive list of issues in doctoral education. Those identified will give readers a sense of what doctoral programs and educators are grappling with, and hopefully stimulate them to explore this area further.

Conceptions of doctoral education. The broad goals of doctoral education are to prepare nurses who will expand the scientific knowledge base for the field through research and scholarly activities, and serve in leadership capacities in a variety of arenas within society and nursing (Crowley, 1977). There has been longstanding debate within nursing about the nature of each of the seven types of degree designations, and about which should be the standard or the ideal. On the one hand, the proponents of the professional doctorate (DNS/DNSc) have contended that as a practice discipline, all intellectual endeavors should be connected to the practice concerns of nursing. On the other hand, proponents of the PhD degree hold that the academic-research degree is needed to strengthen the scientific base of nursing (Lash, 1987a). Christman (1977) has advocated an even narrower conception, focusing on a clinical doctorate; Schlotfeldt (1966) and others hold that there is sufficient flexibility inherent in the nature of the Ph.D. to accommodate various types of pursuits; while Peplau (1966) has argued for the need for both professional and academic doctorates as being of value to the discipline. Many authors have reviewed and elaborated on these issues, and discussed the varying conceptions and justifications regarding doctoral preparation (Brodie, 1986; Forni, 1987b; Grace, 1978; Lash, 1987b; Meleis, 1988). (It should be noted here that the doctor of nursing (ND) degree is offered by three institutions, prepares individuals for basic practice in nursing, and represents neither an advanced nor an investigative degree.)

While these descriptions regarding differentiation of major degree types are ostensibly clear, in practice such differentiation is not clear in program goals or in program execution. Nor is there any evidence that prospective students make a deliberate choice of program on the basis of type of degree offered. Rather, it is the case that the more important elements in program differentiation have to do with the type of faculty expertise and their research, the nature of the substantive content being offered, and institutional support and resources available to the program, among others.

Substantive nursing knowledge. Historically, the majority of doctoral programs have focused on teaching "process" courses such as research methods, statistics, and theory development. More recently, a distinct move is evident toward focusing on substantive courses in the discipline of nursing. This movement has received impetus as a result of the efforts of groups such as the AACN and the National Forum on Doctoral Education in Nursing. It has been motivated by the expansion of the research base of nursing and the number of nurses engaged in knowledge generation. There is great variation across programs in the focus of nursing knowledge and phenomena being taught and investigated, and how that knowledge is organized (Ketefian, 1993). The consensus within the field at present is to endorse this diversity of theoretical and research approaches, because it is deemed premature at this juncture to dictate a uniform approach. It is felt that such diversity makes for richness and enhances the discipline.

In view of the rapidly diversifying population in the United States and the globalization of many universities and many industries, doctoral educators need to ask themselves what the impact of these societal changes are for what they teach. Ketefian and Redman (1995) contend that US-developed nursing science does not possess global characteristics, and in the main, international nursing issues and global content do not feature significantly in doctoral curricula. They have invited examination of these issues and have proposed recommendations for addressing them at the national and individual program levels.

For some time there has been a sense of disquiet on the part of some nurse educators that while we do a good job in socializing doctoral students for careers in research and scholarship, we do not pay sufficient attention to providing experiences that will prepare students for faculty positions, for institutional citizenship, and for overall professional service activities. Ketefian (1991) reports on national data in which the majority of students (93%) are pleased with the emphasis on research preparation in their programs, but 50% to 51% of the surveyed students would like more emphasis on preparing them for teaching and other roles. Ketefian describes ways of developing experiences and involving students in activities that would be broadening and would not require adding courses or deflecting emphasis from research or scholar preparation.

Scientific integrity. The recent spate of media cases involving various forms of scientific misconduct threatens to undermine the credibility of the scientific community at large. These cases also highlight an important oversight in the training process of scholars. Various governmental agencies have established offices and panels to deal with allegations of misconduct. Mostly, this development is the result of an inability or unwillingness of institutions themselves to set appropriate standards and monitor the integrity of science on their campuses.

In a recent survey of doctoral programs, Lenz and Ketefian (1995) and Ketefian and Lenz (1995) sought to determine current approaches to the teaching of scientific integrity and the issues encountered there. The extent and scope of instruction were highly variable, and the respondents themselves judged these to be inadequate. The role of senior faculty in mentoring junior colleagues and doctoral students was highlighted. Professional society and institutional level mechanisms were identified as means through which positive behaviors in the conduct of science could be promoted.

Disciplines vary in the ways in which they socialize their scholars in matters of scientific integrity. At present, nursing does not have its own guidelines about research integrity. The result is a situation whereby doctoral mentors aim to socialize their own students according to the tenets of their particular discipline and according to the tenets of their own best judgment. It is typically the case that doctoral program faculties include individuals with doctorates from many disciplines, each bringing different norms and expectations on matters of scientific integrity. In order to rectify this rather chaotic situation it is imperative for nursing to develop its own guidelines and set forth disciplinary norms related to scientific integrity. Research universities need to develop their own standards as well and have monitoring mechanisms in place. The Midwest Nursing Research Society (MNRS), a regional organization, has now developed its own guidelines and is in the process of promulgating it to the MNRS members (MNRS, 1996).

Accreditation. Following extensive discussions within nursing, it is now the case that doctoral programs are not accredited by the National League for Nursing (NLN), the specialized accrediting agency for baccalaureate and master's degree programs, or any other agency. It is the contention that such accreditation is not necessary, because quality monitoring is provided by the parent institution (Spero, 1987). The AACN (1987) has developed quality indicators in order to provide guidance with regard to various indicators of quality and program functioning. These indicators have been used widely by programs themselves; however, there are no data available at present to suggest the extent to which institutions do in fact monitor quality, whether they do this for the Ph.D. degree—which is typically administered under the aegis of the "graduate school"—or for the professional degree, and what type of variations might exist across institutions in this regard.

Students. Who are the students in doctoral study, and what is their composition? Currently, 10.8% of doctoral students are members of underrepresented minority groups (AACN, 1994); these are broken down as follows: 2.5% Asian, 6.1% black, 0.6% American Indian or Alaskan native, 1.6% Hispanic (AACN, 1994). These same groups comprised 10% of graduations (AACN, 1994, p. 26). The current climate in higher education unequivocally emphasizes diversity in its broader meaning. The population trends are changing and it is expected that the proportion of previously underrepresented minority groups will be high in the 21st century. Efforts to recruit a diverse student body need to be stepped up by doctoral programs. With regard to the matter of intellectual diversity, it is now the case that nonnurse potential applicants are not eligible for admission into nursing doctoral programs. While many nurses hold doctoral degrees in another discipline and are making important contributions both to nursing and those disciplines, nursing excludes nonnurses from becoming scholars of nursing. Inclusion of such individuals could imbue nursing with fresh perspective and enrich the field.

Another concern with regard to students is their age at entry to doctoral study and their age at graduation. The average number of years for doctoral study is 5 (Ketefian, 1991); many programs report the majority of their students as graduating between their late thirties and late forties. At this point in their careers, these individuals have families and many other obligations that detract from their ability to pursue doctoral study full-time, and this limits the length of the contribution they are able to make to the field after graduation.

Faculty. The majority of doctorally prepared nurses are employed in colleges and universities as faculty and academic administrators, and a small percentage are engaged in health care institutions, government agencies, and other enterprises. According to AACN data, in 1978, AACN member schools reported 15% of their faculties as having doctoral preparation (944 faculty); by 1991-92, the figure had risen to 48% (3690 faculty). Despite this growth, which has paralleled the growth in doctoral programs, the demand appears to be rising faster than the supply, with some schools reporting an inability to locate individuals to fill vacant faculty positions (AACN, 1992). Faculty salaries are not competitive with those within the service sector. This is a concern within the field; were this trend to continue, some educators fear that prospective students may not be motivated to seek doctoral degrees or will choose employment in settings other than higher education.

Another concern with regard to faculty is that a large majority are in their forties and fifties and are expected to retire within 8 to 15 years; this could leave a sudden vacuum in the ranks of senior faculty unless steps are taken to groom a new generation of young scholars to take their places. However, the impact of lifting the retirement age is not known at this time. How many people will choose to continue working indefinitely, and how many will retire at the "usual" time still remains to be seen. However, it is critical that the future be planned in a systematic way to avoid surprises.

POSTDOCTORAL TRAINING

Postdoctoral training is relatively recent within nursing. As nursing science has developed and the number of nurse scholars has increased, efforts to develop postdoctoral opportunities for nurses and in nursing have been stepped up. Historically, small numbers of nurses have sought postdoctoral training in a variety of disciplines, arranged through individual initiative. The impetus for postdoctoral training came following the establishment of the National Institute of Nursing Research (NINR; formerly the National Center for Nursing Research) within the National Institutes of Health in 1985. The purpose of postdoctoral training is "to provide time, space, an intellectual and colleague support system, as well as a safe, risk-taking environment for becoming an independent researcher" (Hinshaw, 1991, p. 83); this level of training is intended to enable nurses to "position ourselves so that we can shape the cutting edge of science" (Hinshaw, 1991, p. 82).

Under the aegis of the NINR, a career trajectory has been developed whereby scientific development is viewed as a lifetime commitment; under Institute programs opportunities are provided for nurse scholars to pursue postdoctoral training at different career phases. This conception is unique in nursing and is designed to be responsive to the unique career patterns of nurses and the needs of the discipline for science development. In most disciplines the typical pattern is for an individual to move into a postdoctoral fellowship immediately following the completion of the doctorate.

This level of study is now recommended more and more for individuals who expect to pursue research and teaching careers in research universities. Only a small number of nurses currently pursue postdoctoral training, mostly due to limited funding opportunities. Thirteen institutions currently offer postdoctoral training under funding from the NINR, the agency responsible for a large portion of funding for postdoctoral training; in addition, nine fellowships are individually funded through the NINR. Other sources of funding are available, or have become available from time to time from the National Science Foundation, the Robert Wood Johnson Foundation, the American Nurses' Association Minority Fellowship Program, and the W.K. Kellogg Foundation. A few drug companies, in collaboration with research universities, have made postdoctoral training opportunities available to nurses in areas of special concern to the company and the institution.

It is interesting to note that while many doctoral students express the interest and desire to pursue postdoctoral training (61%), only 5% of recent alumni in the same national survey have had postdoctoral training (Ketefian, 1991). This suggests that faculty need to take an active role in guiding students to this level of study, and for the field to expand the available opportunities. A broader policy consideration for academic institutions is to consider ways in which the age at which individuals embark on and complete doctoral study can be lowered, so that young scholars can focus on such training before they are burdened with a variety of family responsibilities.

It is expected that postdoctoral training will be a more common feature in the training of nurse scholars in the years to come.

CONCLUDING REMARKS

Graduate education in nursing at this moment is like a kaleidoscope, and is in a dynamic state of change. To what extent can graduate education in nursing be standardized? What are the tensions between standardization and flexibility? The NLN sets standards for master's education and accreditation of these programs, and the AACN has quality indicators that guide doctoral programs. While quality monitoring is crucial, flexibility needs to be maintained in order to make these programs responsive to the needs of both the society and the students. Nursing has been criticized for developing an ethnocentric science that is applicable to white, middle-class populations. Meleis (1988) calls for nursing to develop a world view of phenomena so that an awareness of issues faced by minority groups and by other nations can be an integral part of its science and instruction. She recommends that this criterion become an indicator of quality of doctoral programs.

Within the past few years a number of new specialties have developed in nursing, such as space nursing, AIDS, and addictions. A constraint to be mentioned relates to the fiscal picture across the nation that has affected graduate education. Many institutions are cutting budgets and are emphasizing the concept of "innovation by substitution" rather than by addition. In the 1970s and 1980s programs expanded offerings without much concern for cost. Now they are being challenged to be responsive to consumer demands, of high quality, and cost efficient all at the same time. The total quality management approach is now on our campuses, and this continuous improvement perspective is challenging us all.

At the time of this writing there are no data about how nursing programs are dealing with the constraints imposed on them, and whether the addition of a new specialty means the elimination of defunct specialties or subspecialties. This is a matter of urgent concern for educational administrators, because they are accountable for balancing the budget and for delivering high-quality programs. The environment in which we find ourselves is dynamic and the challenges are many.

While it is impossible to say what graduate education will look like in the 21st century, one thing is certain: It will be different than what it is today. If the past is a prologue, we have reason to believe that it will be stronger for the challenges, and will be even more central to the health care delivery system of the 21st century than it is today.

REFERENCES

American Association of Colleges of Nursing. (1987). Indicators of quality in doctoral programs in nursing. *Journal of Professional Nursing, 3*(1), 72-74.

American Association of Colleges of Nursing. (1992, June). *AACN Issue Bulletin*, p. 3.

American Association of Colleges of Nursing. (1994). *1993-1994 enrollment and graduations in baccalaureate and graduate programs in nursing* (Publication No. 93-94-1). Washington, DC: Author.

American Association of Colleges of Nursing. (1995). *Position statement: Certification and regulation of advanced practice nurses.* Washington, DC: Author.

Brodie, B. (1986). Impact of doctoral programs on nursing education. *Journal of Professional Nursing, 2*(6), 350-357.

Christman, L. (1977). *Clinical doctorates—A means of increasing the clinical competence of nurses.* Unpublished manuscript.

Conrad, C., Haworth, J., & Millar, S. (1993). *A silent success: Master's education in the U.S.* Baltimore, MD: Johns Hopkins University Press.

Cronenwett, L. (1995). Molding the future of advanced practice nursing. *Nursing Outlook, 43*(3), 112-118.

Crowley, D.M. (1977). Theoretical and pragmatic issues related to the goals of doctoral education in nursing. *Proceedings of the First National Conference on Doctoral Education in Nursing* (pp. 25-29). Philadelphia, PA: The University of Pennsylvania School of Nursing.

Donley, R. (1995). Advanced practice nursing after health care reform. *Nursing Economic$, 13*(2), 84-88.

Forni, P.R. (1987a). Nursing's diverse master's programs: The state of the art. *Nursing and Health Care, 8*(2), 70-75.

Forni, P.R. (1987b). Models for doctoral programs: First professional degree or terminal degree? In Hart, S.E. (Ed.), *Issues in graduate nurs-*

ing education (Publication No. 18-2196, pp. 45-73). New York: National League for Nursing.

Glittenberg, J. (1987). The scope and trends of international nursing education. In Roode, J. (Ed.), *Changing patterns in nursing education* (Publication No. 14-2203, pp. 133-142). New York: National League for Nursing.

Grace, H. (1978). The development of doctoral education in nursing: An historical perspective. *Journal of Nursing Education, 17*(4), 17-27.

Hegyvary, S.T. (1991). Issues in outcomes research. *Journal of Nursing Quality Assurance, 5*(2), 1-6.

Hinshaw, A.S. (1991). The federal imperative in funding postdoctoral education: Indices of quality. *Proceedings for the 1991 Forum on Doctoral Education in Nursing. Postdoctoral education in nursing science: Purpose, process, outcome* (pp. 81-108). Amelia Island, FL: The University of Florida.

Holden-Lund, C. (1991). Consortium model for master's education in nursing. *Nurse Educator, 16*(5), 13-17.

Jolly, M.L., & Hart, S.E. (1987). Master's prepared nurses: Societal needs and educational realities. In Hart, S.E. (Ed.), *Issues in graduate nursing education* (Publication No. 18-2196, pp. 25-31). New York: National League for Nursing.

Jones, R. (1993). Outcomes analysis: Methods and issues. *Nursing Economic$, 11*(3), 145-152.

Keane, A., & Richmond, T. (1993). Tertiary nurse practitioners. *Image: Journal of Nursing Scholarship, 25*(4), 281-284.

Ketefian, S. (1991). Doctoral preparation for faculty roles: Expectations and realities. *The Journal of Professional Nursing, 7*(2), 105-111.

Ketefian, S. (1993). Essentials of doctoral education: Organization of program around knowledge areas. *Journal of Professional Nursing, 9*(5), 255-261.

Ketefian, S., & Redman, R. (1995). Nursing science within the global community. *Proceedings of the National Forum on Doctoral Education.* Ann Arbor, MI: The University of Michigan, School of Nursing.

Ketefian, S., & Lenz, E. (1995). Promoting scientific integrity in nursing research, part II: Strategies. *Journal of Professional Nursing, 11*(5), 263-269.

Lash, A.A. (1987a). The nature of the doctor of philosophy degree: Evolving conceptions. *Journal of Professional Nursing, 3*(2), 92-101.

Lash, A.A. (1987b). Rival conceptions in doctoral education in nursing and their outcomes: An update. *Journal of Nursing Education, 26*(6), 221-227.

Lenz, E., & Ketefian, S. (1995). Promoting scientific integrity in nursing research, Part I: Current approaches in doctoral programs. *Journal of Professional Nursing, 11*(4), 213-219.

McElhinney, T., & Lajkowicz, C. (1994). The new genetics & nursing education. *Nursing & Health Care, 15*(10), 528-531.

Meleis, A.I. (1988). Doctoral education in nursing: Its present and its future. *Journal of Professional Nursing, 4*(6), 436-446.

Midwest Nursing Research Society (1996). *Guidelines for scientific integrity.* Glenview, IL: Author.

Murphy, J.F. (1981). Doctoral education in, of, and for nursing: An historical analysis. *Nursing Outlook, 29*(11), 645-649.

National Council of State Boards of Nursing. (1992). *Position paper on the licensure of advanced nursing practice.* Revised March 5th. Chicago: Author.

O'Neil, E.H., & Hare, D.M. (Eds.). (1990). *Perspectives on the health professions.* Durham, NC: Duke University Press.

Pelczar, M.J., Jr. (1980). *The value and future of graduate education leading to a master's degree: A national perspective.* Washington, DC: American Association of Colleges of Nursing.

Peplau, H.E. (1966). Nursing's two routes to doctoral degrees. *Nursing Forum, 5*(2), 57-67.

Reilly, D.E. (1990). *Graduate professional education through outreach: A nursing case study* (Publication No. 15-2340). New York: National League for Nursing.

Schlotfeldt, R.M. (1966). Doctoral study in basic disciplines—A choice for nursing. *Nursing Forum, 5*(2), 68-74.

Spero, J.R. (1987). Specialized accreditation of doctoral programs in nursing: To be or not to be. In Hart, S.E. (Ed.), *Issues in graduate nursing education* (Publication No. 18-2196, pp. 75-88). New York: National League for Nursing.

Starck, P.L. (1987). The master's-prepared nurse in the marketplace: What do master's-prepared nurses do? What should they do? In Hart, S.E. (Ed.), *Issues in graduate nursing education* (Publication No. 18-2196, pp. 3-23). New York: National League for Nursing.

Watson, J. (1995). Advanced practice nursing . . . and what might be. *Nursing and Health Care, 16*(2), 78-83.

Williamson, J.A. (1983). Master's education: A need for nomenclature. *Image: The Journal of Nursing Scholarship, 15*(4), 99-101.

Critical thinking: What is it and how do we teach it?

KATHLEEN KRICHBAUM, MARSHA LEWIS, LAURA DUCKETT

I can't believe that I have finished a year and a half of my nursing program already. This clinical is pretty easy, much to my surprise. My instructor has given me a good assignment today, a patient with cirrhosis, a diagnosis I haven't seen before. I came yesterday and read his chart; it fit with the text I reviewed last night in order to fill out his care plan for today. All I have to do is follow the orders on the chart, make sure I can assist with that paracentesis as laid out in the procedure manual, and turn in my care plan to my instructor on Friday. It is boring filling in all those rows and columns on the care plan—it takes so much time, and it's all the same stuff that is in the standardized care plans on the unit. But, now that it's done, I am ready to take care of this patient. Thank goodness this instructor doesn't pressure me with questions about the rationale for my care plan. I had that content early in the program and I hardly remember any of it.

Although hypothetical, these reflections of a baccalaureate nursing student could represent the thoughts of any nursing student in any one of the over 400 baccalaureate programs in the United States. The case is intended to raise questions among all those involved in nursing education—nursing students, nurse educators, and nurse researchers—about the methods we use to stimulate students to think and learn and the reasons that underlie our choice of strategies. As a result of students completing the nursing program, nurse educators expect that graduates will have learned to behave as nurses; that is, graduates will be able to solve clinical problems, to make decisions for themselves, and to help patients make decisions that will affect their health. Further, we expect that graduates will provide high-quality, skilled care grounded in a sound knowledge of the science of nursing. These are lofty expectations, yet the educational requirements designed to help achieve these outcomes often consist of attendance at theory classes, usually lectures, and practice in a variety of acute care settings where learning is measured by the student's ability to complete a care plan (Tanner, 1987). In reality, nursing curricular plans do not vary notably across programs, nor does implementation of curricula.

It appears that a focus on mastery of skill and content has consumed us. Ford and Profetto-McGrath (1994) refer to this orientation to curriculum as "the curriculum as product" informed by an interest in the technical aspects of nursing. That is, we in nursing education have a fundamental interest in controlling the educational environment by teaching rule-following action based on empirically grounded laws (Grundy, 1989). Ford and Profetto-McGrath go on to describe the other emphasis in most nursing curricula—a practical interest in understanding the environment that is rooted in the importance of "meaning-making." Decisions can then be made about appropriate actions or doing what is right. The basis for action is consensus about rightness, a prescriptive approach. Much effort has been expended on teaching students the correct formula to use for every problem.

Paul (1985) frames this view of education another way. He describes the approach used in nursing programs as monological. In monological systems, one set of rules prevails. An example is the almost exclusive use of the acute care setting for student nursing practice, a "system that operates only on a medical model, with medical rules of evidence and diagnosis" (Bandman & Bandman, 1995, p. 5). Other critics of the emphasis on the technical, practical, and monological approach to nursing education include Diekelmann (1988), who has called for an end to the "behaviorist paradigm" that she says restricts, among other things, the student's creative thinking and autonomy. Moccia (1990) supports this move away from behaviorism as well, advocating that nursing education foster in faculty and students alike a sense of responsibility and accountability for educating nurses. Even Bevis, one of the originators of standardizing the curricula using a behaviorist framework, has advocated, along with Gould, examining current models for their usefulness in today's complex health care environment, referring to these prescriptive models as "dragons" (Gould & Bevis, 1990). The National League for Nursing (NLN, 1988) held a forum that served as a starting point for the re-examination of the ways nurse educators construct programs, the means by which they are delivered, and the values that underlie these choices. Participants recognized that among the probable effects of using the current curricular models was the alarming trend discovered in empirical studies investigating the development of critical thinking (CT) in nursing students—*no gain* in CT scores while in their nursing programs.

The notion that the curriculum could negatively affect the growth of CT is of major concern to both nurse educators and researchers, and stands in direct opposition to the values expressed in the NLN forum. Further, it reflects the growing national concern about education generally, that "the heart of education lies exactly where traditional advocates of a liberal education always said it was—in the processes of inquiry, learning and thinking rather than in the accumulation of disjointed skills and senescent information" (Facione, 1990b). This chapter addresses issues related to the ability of graduates of nursing programs to think critically, examining current knowledge about the nature of CT, concerns with assessment of CT, and strategies at both the instructional and curricular levels that have shown promise for improving CT abilities in college students.

THE NATURE OF CRITICAL THINKING

Critical thinking has been discussed in recent education literature as an underlying value and as an outcome of a liberal education. Glaser (1985) asserts that the ability to think critically is essential to being a fully functioning individual in our complex, modern society; it is fundamental to democracy. Kreisberg (1992) sees it as basic to effective participation in a person's social and political worlds. Defining CT has been problematic, however. Some have defined it as a set of skills, while others describe it as a process, and others as a combination of skills and dispositions or characteristics (Siegel, 1988).

In Siegel's (1988) synthesis of rationality, CT, and education, he presents a review of theories of CT. He describes the seminal work of Ennis (1962), who defined CT as "the correct assessing of statements" (p. 83). A person who is able to think critically, according to this definition, has the skills to evaluate statements properly; there is no mention of the actual use of those skills. As his work continued, however, Ennis (1985) developed a "skills plus tendencies" conceptualization that included the idea of the importance of characteristics a person must possess in order to use appropriate criteria to evaluate statements or behave as a critical thinker. The addition of dispositions or characteristics to his theory, although important, served to complicate the previous thinking about CT as the process of rational thinking (Siegel, 1988).

Some of the other major CT theorists in recent years include Blair (1985), Facione (1990a, 1990b), Kurfiss (1988), McPeck (1981), Norris (1985), Paul (1985), Seigel (1985), Watson and Glaser (1980), and Yinger (1980). Among those who view CT as a process are Yinger and Kurfiss. Yinger (1980) defines CT as a cognitive activity associated with the evaluation of products of thought. Kurfiss (1988) views it as an investigative process but focuses on the purpose or goal of that investigation, which is to explore a situation, phenomenon, question, or problem in order to arrive at a hypothesis or conclusion about it that synthesizes all available information and that can be justified. Blair (1985) is among the theorists who describe CT as more than a set of skills or simple linear process. He says that argumentation is at the center of CT, but that CT is much more. It is a set of mechanisms that can be applied regardless of the subject matter, that consists of a vocabulary that has general applicability from field to field, and that is built on certain habits of mind that can transfer from one subject to another. Watson and Glaser (1980) also believe that CT consists of more than a specific set of cognitive skills. Rather it is a composite of skills, knowledge, and attitudes. Attitudes of CT denote a frame of mind that recognizes the existence of problems. CT knowledge involves an understanding of the nature of making inferences and generalizations, and the skills of being able to weigh the logic and accuracy of evidence.

Paul (1982, 1983, 1985) states that CT has been defined both narrowly and in a larger sense. The narrow definition implies that CT is a set of cognitive skills that can be learned and practiced but remain external to the learner. In his broader definition, CT is integral to the learner; the ability to think critically serves as evidence of the "free, rational, autonomous mind" (1985). Norris (1985) has developed the concept of skills to include metacognition. He describes two levels of cognitive skill. Lower-level cognitive skills include skills applied directly to carrying out a task. Metacognitive skills are used to plan and monitor the progress of lower cognitive skills. Siegel (1988) built the "reasons conception" of CT in which he explored and defined the dispositions to CT. True critical thinkers are "appropriately moved by reasons" (p. 32). His focus has been on the importance of educational methods that develop CT.

Based on these theories and on the growing interest in educating for CT, the American Philosophical Association (APA) in 1987 recruited Peter Facione, a noted philosopher and writer in the area of CT, to make a systematic inquiry into the current state of CT and CT assessment. Facione convened a panel of 46 experts, including Norris, Ennis, and Paul, who developed a consensus statement intended to guide curriculum development, instruction, and assessment of CT. This definition of CT and the ideal critical thinker follows:

> We understand critical thinking to be purposeful, self-regulatory judgment which results in interpretation, analysis, evaluation, and inference as well as explanation of the evidential, conceptual, methodological, criteriological, or contextual considerations upon which that judgment was based. CT is essential as a tool of inquiry. CT is a pervasive and self-rectifying human phenomenon. The ideal critical thinker is habitually inquisitive, well-informed, honest in facing personal biases, prudent in making judgments, willing to consider, clear about issues, orderly in complex matters, diligent in seeking relevant information, reasonable in selection of criteria, focused in inquiry, and persistent in seeking results which are as precise as the subject and the circumstances of inquiry permit. (Facione, 1990b, p. 4)

This definition, like Paul's, and Watson and Glaser's, represents the current view of CT as more than the process of problem solving. It is also a combination of skills and dispositions that transfer from one context to another.

CRITICAL THINKING IN NURSING EDUCATION

In recent years, nurse educators and researchers alike have begun to question whether or not graduates of nursing programs are able to think critically, to make appropriate, knowledge-based clinical decisions, and to implement those judgments to improve patient care (Creighton, 1984; Jenkins, 1985; Kintgen-Andrews, 1991; Miller & Malcolm, 1990; Tanner, 1983). Subsequent questions have been raised about the nature of CT itself and about both the effectiveness of the curriculum and the ability of individual instructors to contribute to students' achievement in these areas. Results of the few empirical studies designed to describe the impact of the nursing program on CT have been mixed.

In reviews of the CT literature, Kintgen-Andrews (1991) and Miller and Malcolm (1990) reported the results of recent studies in nursing education that examined the effects of nursing curricula on CT. Of the longitudinal studies reviewed, four showed no significant gains in CT (Bauwens & Gerhard, 1987; Kintgen-Andrews, 1988; Richards, 1977; Sullivan, 1987), whereas three others reported significant gains (Berger, 1984; Fredrickson, 1979; Gross, Takazawa, & Rose, 1987). Students in these studies represented diploma, associate degree, baccalaureate, registered nurse degree completion, and master's programs. Cross-sectional studies also had conflicting results. Matthews and Gaul (1979) and Dungan (1986) found no differences in CT related to level of students, but Scoloveno (1981) and Pardue (1987) reported significant differences. At the University of Minnesota, faculty are conducting an ongoing outcomes-based evaluation of curriculum effectiveness for outcomes including CT. Although the design includes both cross-sectional and longitudinal data, preliminary findings in the first two classes given the Watson-Glaser Critical Thinking Appraisal (WGCTA) showed no significant gain in CT scores (Krichbaum, Duckett, Miller, Ryden, & Wainwright, 1994). These studies have raised concerns about CT abilities of nursing students.

There are issues related to the conduct of the studies that should be considered as well. The sole use of cross-sectional designs is not recommended for studies of curriculum effectiveness (Brophy & Good, 1986). Further, many of the earlier studies are difficult to compare because of varying sampling techniques and research methodologies. In addition, all previous investigators studying nursing students used the WGCTA to assess CT. Other measures are now available. Despite the methodological flaws, the message conveyed by previous investigators is that we need to continue to examine the nature of critical thinking and what we are doing in nursing education to foster its development.

In a survey of nursing school administrators, researchers found that in most nursing education settings, CT is defined as linear problem solving (Jones & Brown, 1991), and the chief means used for problem solving is the nursing process. More recently, nurse researchers have focused on the development of clinical reasoning skills in nursing students and practicing nurses (Corcoran & Tanner, 1988; Corcoran-Perry & Narayan, 1995a, 1995b). Clinical reasoning, also called decision making or clinical judgment, is similar to but not synonymous with CT. Clinical reasoning has been defined as "the thinking and decision-making processes that are integral to clinical practice" (Higgs & Jones, 1995, p. xiv). Much of the effort at investigating clinical reasoning in nurses has helped to clarify the need to educate nurses in CT. It has further pointed out the lack of common understanding among educators and researchers in nursing relative to CT. The fact that the NLN has adopted the APA consensus definition of CT is a promising beginning. Knowing and understanding the nature of CT must necessarily precede any change in teaching strategies or curricula.

ASSESSMENT OF CRITICAL THINKING

Reasons to assess critical thinking

There are several compelling reasons why nursing educators should grapple with the problem of assessing CT. First, one of the hallmarks of a professional discipline is that there is a unique body of knowledge and ongoing knowledge development (Donaldson & Crowley, 1978; Johnson, 1974). Knowledge development requires both the constant critical review of existing knowledge and active engagement in the research process and other forms of scholarly inquiry (Fawcett, 1978). Intellectual curiosity and CT are essential to knowledge development. Second, professional practice, in contrast to the work of a technician, requires one to evaluate situations and apply knowledge from the discipline and related disciplines in each unique clinical situation that arises. Even when there are general guidelines that apply to certain types of patients, a professional must assess the particular person, group, or community and make judgments about how to modify guidelines to fit a particular situation. Third, because of the importance of CT to the discipline of nursing, nurse educators must attempt to develop it in their students. Without assessment of CT there is no way to determine the success or failure of nursing curricula, as implemented by nursing faculty, in developing CT in students. The fact that the NLN (1993) now includes CT as one of its criteria for accreditation is a reflection of these three reasons.

Methods used to assess critical thinking

Standardized tests. When researchers and educators think about assessing CT, they usually think about administering a standardized test to all students in a class or a program. A particular group may be assessed once, yielding cross-sectional data, or on two or more occasions (e.g., at program entry and exit), yielding longitudinal data.

The standardized tests that cover more than one aspect of CT skills and are suitable for college students are the (a) California Critical Thinking Skills Test (CCTST), (b) Cornell Critical Thinking Test-Level Z, (c) Ennis-Weir Critical Thinking Essay Test, (d) New Jersey Test of Reasoning Skills, and (e) WGCTA. With the exception of Ennis-Weir, all of these tests are multiple choice and machine-scored. More detailed information about these commercially available tests can be found in Ennis (1993) and Norris and Ennis (1989, pp. 54-100).

Based on a review of published nursing articles, it appears that the WGCTA (Watson & Glaser, 1980) has been used most frequently in nursing education settings. This 80-item test includes five sections (inference, recognition of assumptions, deduction, interpretation, and evaluation of arguments), each of which has 16 items.

Recently, nursing educators have started to use the newer CCTST (Facione, 1990a) and the companion test of CT dispositions, The California Critical Thinking Disposition Inventory (CCTDI) (Facione, N.C., Facione, & Sanchez, 1994; Facione, P.A., Facione, & Sanchez, 1994). The CCTST includes 34 multiple-choice items from which six scores are derived, a total score and scores for analysis, evaluation, and inference, inductive reasoning and deductive reasoning. All 34 items, divided into three clusters derived by expert concensus (Facione, 1990b), comprise the first three subscales. Thirty of the items, divided into two clusters based on traditional conceptualizations, comprise the last two subscales (Facione & Facione, 1993).

There are two forms of the CCTST, A and B, which Facione and Facione (1993) claim are conceptually and statistically equivalent based on data from testing the same 90 undergraduates with both forms. However, Jacobs (1995) administered Form A to one randomly selected group of 684 freshmen and Form B to a different group of 692 randomly selected freshmen and his results caused him to question the equivalency of the two forms. Internal consistency reliability of the CCTST is reported to be .70 for Form A and .71 for form B using the Kuder Richardson-20 formula (Facione & Facione, 1993, p. 12). Reliability coefficients for the five subscale scores are not reported in the test manual.

The CCTDI includes 75 items that are rated on 6-point scales with "agree strongly" and "disagree strongly" as anchors. The conceptual development of the CCTDI began in 1991 and was guided by expert conceptualization of

CT (Facione, 1990b). The CCTDI includes seven subscales: truth-seeking, open-mindedness, analyticity, systematicity, self-confidence, inquisitiveness, and maturity. Internal consistencies (Cronbach's alphas) of the seven CCTDI subscales ranged from .71 to .80 for the initial sample tested and from .60 to .78 for two additional samples. Cronbach's alpha for the total score was .91 for the initial sample and .90 for the later samples (Facione, P.A. et al., 1994).

Teacher-made tests. Given the increasing attention to developing CT in nursing students, it seems likely that there will be greater interest in developing classroom tests that assess students' CT in specific courses and content areas. Examples of open-ended tests and scoring guides used to assess students' CT related to selected content covered in an ethics multicourse sequential learning curriculum can be found in Duckett, Waithe, Rowan, Schmitz, and Ryden (1993). Several helpful sources are available for nurse educators who wish to create valid CT tests for either programmatic or classroom assessment (Ennis, 1993; Norris, 1988, 1989; Norris & Ennis, 1989).

Tasks to be undertaken before assessing critical thinking

Decide the specific purpose of the assessment. Different tests are appropriate for different purposes. Unless reasons for assessment of CT have been clearly conceived and articulated, it will be difficult to choose or create the best possible assessment instrument. Purposes of CT assessment and problems to consider are presented in the box.

Determine which tests are most suitable to the purpose of assessment. There are three major steps to take in attempting to match purpose and instrument if a commercially available test is to be used. First, obtain information about the test and its reliability and validity from the test publisher. Such information is usually summarized in the test manual (e.g., Facione & Facione, 1993). Second, do a literature review to determine what studies have been published involving the use of the particular instrument; find out what writers other than the test authors have to say about it (e.g., Frisby, 1992; Jacobs, 1995). Third, take each test being considered and score it yourself because there is no better way to get a picture of the content validity of the test in light of its intended purpose (Ennis, 1993).

Determine which of the tests that seem suitable to the purpose are feasible. Not all tests of CT will be feasible in all situations in which they are suitable. For example, one might decide that the Ennis-Weir Critical Thinking Essay Test (Ennis & Weir, 1985) is the best match with the purpose of the intended assessment, but that it will not be feasible to score the essay test. An essay test is typically more time-consuming to score and requires trained and certified scorers. The time and money investment will be higher than with a test that can be scored by machine (Ennis, 1993).

POSSIBLE PURPOSES OF CRITICAL THINKING (CT) ASSESSMENT AND PROBLEMS TO CONSIDER

Purposes of CT assessment

Diagnosing students' levels of CT
Giving students feedback about their CT
Attempting to motivate students to be better critical thinkers
Providing feedback to teachers about their efforts to help students develop CT skills
Doing research about questions involving CT
Providing help in making admissions decisions (a "high stakes" purpose)
Holding schools accountable for students' CT (a "high stakes" purpose)

Problems to consider

Most CT tests, especially those easiest to use, are not comprehensive.
Using the same form of test for pre- and posttesting may influence posttest results, but different forms are actually different tests.
Test makers and test takers may have different background beliefs and assumptions that affect test validity.
When a pre- and posttest are given without using a control group, other factors besides instruction may influence results.
Developing CT skills takes time; significant changes may be expected too quickly.
High-stakes purposes may interfere with test validity.
Results may be compared with norms and attributed to instruction when there are other possible explanations.
Scarce resources may lead to compromises that affect test validity.

Note. Adapted from "Critical Thinking Assessment," by R.H. Ennis, 1993, *Theory into Practice,* 32, 180-181.

Issues to be considered before assessing critical thinking

State of the art of critical thinking assessment and implications. From the evidence that has been accumulated to date, it appears justifiable to use the standardized tests of CT skills and the one published test of CT dispositions for purposes that are not in the "high stakes" categories. Use of standardized CT tests for high-stakes purposes (e.g., data for admissions decisions) is problematic for at least two reasons: The tests are not secure and are not comprehensive enough to be valid for high-stakes uses (Ennis, 1993). Ennis (1993) not only pointed out some of the shortcomings of multiple-choice CT tests, but also acknowledged their advantages. Norris (1988, 1989, 1992) and Ennis (1993) have described very specific ways of improving multiple-choice tests of CT. Subject-specific standardized tests of CT are needed, but have not been developed yet (Ennis, 1993).

Measuring critical thinking versus measuring verbal intelligence. Exactly what standardized tests of CT measure has been questioned. Do these tests serve as another measure of intelligence, a fairly stable trait, or do they measure specific CT skills that can be improved by educational interventions? Jacobs (1995) has claimed that the CCTST scores largely reflect the type of verbal intelligence measured by the Scholastic Aptitude Test, a claim that has been made about the Cornell CT tests as well (Hughes, 1992). If this claim is completely true, nurse educators should not expect to see improvements in CT scores when students are tested at entry and exit from a nursing program. Clearly, more research is needed both to evaluate evidence that might support or refute convergent validity of measures of CT skills and dispositions and to determine time frames necessary to effect change in critical thinking.

Obtaining valid student responses. Students may not produce results that are valid if the test and test situation are not suitable. Unless students are motivated to do their best on the CT test being used, their measured score may not be a reflection of their true score. Because faculty at the University of Minnesota School of Nursing had a strong hunch that the timing of the testing, the amount of time allocated for testing, and the content and length (80 items) of the WGCTA were causing students to fail to do their best on the exit tests, several modifications in the testing process were implemented. Changes included switching to the shorter CCTST (34 items) for classes entering in or after 1993 and adding the CCTDI in 1994. In addition, students now take their exit tests earlier during the last quarter before their minds are completely focused on graduation and job interviews. Until student data from the WGCTA and the two California tests are analyzed and compared, it is impossible to make a judgment about which approach to testing CT provides the most valid and useful results.

TEACHING STRATEGIES

The student in the case study presented at the beginning of the chapter sees her patient care assignment from a monological point of view, i.e., identifying one perspective—that of filling in the care plan and following the doctor's orders. Nurse educators and researchers have found little evidence to support the view that the nursing process is the most important approach to clinical reasoning, that care plans reflect that process, or that care plans reflect actual clinical performance (Diekelmann, 1988; Ford & Profetto-McGrath, 1994; Gould & Bevis, 1990; Tanner, 1986, 1987, 1993). How could the student's clinical instructor provide opportunities for students to view the client situation from multilogical perspectives and thus facilitate the development of CT skills? The literature on teaching CT and clinical reasoning and our many years of teaching experience suggest a number of strategies that could encourage the development of the cognitive skills identified in the APA definition of CT.

Clinical teaching strategies

The literature in nursing and medicine provides a number of strategies for teaching clinical reasoning or clinical decision making, including iterative hypothesis testing (Kassirer, 1983), paradigm cases (Benner, 1984; Benner & Tanner, 1987; Corcoran-Perry & Narayan, 1995b), reflection-about-action (Corcoran-Perry & Narayan, 1995a; Schon, 1987), and analogies, decision analysis, and thinking aloud (Corcoran & Tanner, 1988; Corcoran-Perry & Narayan, 1995a, 1995b). Following is a description of how a clinical instructor might incorporate two of these strategies during clinical conferences.

Iterative hypothesis testing. Kassirer (1983) proposed a method for teaching diagnostic reasoning that could be adapted to the student case study. Iterative hypothesis testing provides students with the opportunity to practice diagnostic reasoning in the safe environment of the clinical conference. The instructor asks the student who is assigned to the client with cirrhosis to present this client situation in clinical conference. However, instead of the student essentially verbalizing the care plan, the instructor interrupts after the student gives the basic demographic information and reason for hospitalization. The instructor then explains iterative hypothesis testing to the group, and the student acts as the repository of information about the client while the other students and the instructor ask questions. This strategy requires the students to ask questions to gather data, provide a rationale for why they asked the questions, explain what hypotheses (inferences) they had in mind when asking the questions, and, when the information is provided, interpret the new information and explain how it influences their hypotheses. The instructor guides the process by role modeling diagnostic reasoning and offering feedback. Although this strategy focuses on diagnostic reasoning, it can be broadened to encompass the planning process for intervening in the client situation. The strengths of this strategy are explication of details of the diagnostic process, active participation of students, instant feedback, and the opportunity to engage in clinical problem solving as it is done in practice (Kassirer, 1983).

Paradigm cases. A paradigm case may be used to help the student think critically about the client situation and the care provided (Benner, 1983; Corcoran-Perry & Narayan, 1995b). Even the novice nurse has stories to tell about client experiences that are salient and transform the student's view of nursing in some way. The student is asked to write down the client situation and describe the meaning derived from it. By sharing the case with peers during a clinical conference, the student has the opportunity to analyze the situation, interpret its meaning, evaluate personal responses, and make inferences. This inductive method of thinking helps both the student and his or her peers to gain new knowledge and insights from the paradigm case.

Classroom strategies

Strategies designed to foster CT skills come from a variety of disciplines and include structured controversy (Johnson & Johnson, 1979, 1988), problem-based learning (Krichbaum, 1995; Woods, 1994), role modeling (Brookfield, 1987; Ruggiero, 1988); critical questioning (Brookfield, 1987), and role playing (Brookfield, 1987; Ryden, McCarthy, Lewis, & Sherman, 1991). Structured controversy and problem-based learning are described next in relation to the case study.

Structured controversy. The notion of cooperative learning has been refined by Johnson and Johnson (1978, 1989, 1991) at the University of Minnesota. One strategy that reflects this type of learning is structured controversy (Duckett et al., 1993; Johnson, Johnson, & Smith, 1986, 1991; Pederson, Duckett, Ryden, & Maruyama, 1990). The clinical instructor might engage students in structured controversy to elucidate the issues surrounding the possibility of a liver transplant for the client with cirrhosis. Structured controversy differs from debate (Johnson & Johnson, 1985) in that in a debate students choose or are given a perspective to argue, construct logical arguments, and defend a proposition from one perspective. Structured controversy offers students the opportunity to view an issue multilogically as they construct arguments for one side of an issue but then also are expected to take on the opposite perspective. For example, one pair in a group of four students might present reasons for using taxpayer money to fund a liver transplant for a client with cirrhosis secondary to chronic alcoholism, while the other pair would present reasons for not doing so. The two pairs would then change sides and argue from the opposite perspectives. The students then would analyze the arguments made from both perspectives, offer counter-arguments, determine strengths and weaknesses of the counter-arguments, and reach a conclusion about what should be done.

Problem-based learning. The problem-based learning approach developed at McMaster University (Woods, 1994) facilitates the development of CT skills by requiring students to (1) explore the problem, create hypotheses, and identify issues; (2) identify what is already known and what still must be known to solve the problem; (3) prioritize learning needs, set learning goals and objectives, and allocate resources; (4) share new knowledge effectively; (5) apply knowledge to solving the problem; and (6) evaluate the process. Unlike subject-based learning that assumes students know very little and proceeds to lay out the information in a preselected sequence, problem-based learning uses a problem situation to drive the learning activities. Problem-based learning requires students to be active, self-directed learners. Although many disciplines at McMaster University have developed whole curricula around the problem-based approach, the teaching strategy can be useful as one method in a teacher's repertoire. The clinical instructor of the student in the case study might pose a problem about the client with cirrhosis and ask the clinical group to search for information and formulate a solution together.

Strategies across the curriculum

Writing across the curriculum. Although writing assignments have been a pervasive element in nursing curricula, the focus on developing thinking skills through writing is more recent. Because writing skills are essentially thinking skills, writing fosters higher levels of cognitive development (Lashley & Wittstedt, 1993). However, for a writing assignment to facilitate CT skill development, the instructor must require that students go beyond description and engage in analysis, interpretation, evaluation, inference, or explanation. Examples of written assignments that may promote CT skills include process recordings, journals, portfolios, research proposals and reports, writing for publication (Lashley & Wittstadt,

1993; Ruggiero, 1988), and analysis papers (White, Beardslee, Peters, & Supples, 1990).

Process recording. Process recordings have been used for many years in nursing education to help students analyze their interpersonal communication skills and develop a better understanding of client situations. At the University of Minnesota, process recording is used in an interpersonal communications course, with the student choosing a client from the practicum for the assignment.

For example, the student in the case study might be instructed to write a verbatim account of an interaction with the client, including nonverbal behavior. The major emphasis in the process recording lies in the analysis of the client and nurse communication. The student would then address a series of questions meant to probe beyond the spoken words and nonverbal behavior. Some of the prompts would include providing a rationale for your responses (including references); describing how your feelings and needs may have influenced the interaction; writing alternative responses to improve your communication based on the analysis; identifying client strengths and patterns of behavior; making inferences from the data regarding client's behavior; and describing how the context of the situation influenced both your and the client's responses. The outcomes from this assignment would include identifying biases and how they affect the interaction, realizing the complexity of human behavior and the importance of looking beyond the surface, making inferences that encompass the context, and interpreting the impact of the student's own communication on the interaction.

Multicourse sequential learning. Faculty at the University of Minnesota (Ryden, Duckett, Crisham, Caplan, & Schmitz, 1989) have developed a model, MCSL ("muscle"), that "weaves an identifiable strand of content throughout a curriculum by including the content in a vertical course, with units embedded in existing courses across various levels of a program" (Duckett et al., 1993, p. viii). Using the MCSL approach, content is carefully sequenced from course to course in the various levels of the program, and teaching strategies are employed to develop CT skills systematically.

Educational climate

Although the literature describes many discrete teaching strategies for facilitating the development of CT, several authors present a more general view for teaching CT. Some authors focus on classroom climate, instructor attitude, and role; while others present a new instructional or curricular paradigm.

Classroom climate. Brookfield (1987) and Meyers (1986) suggest that fostering CT involves "helping learners to acquire new perceptual frameworks and structures of understanding" (Brookfield, 1987, p. 82). They describe a reflective or connected classroom as one in which class begins with a problem or controversy. Periods of creative silence are encouraged for pondering new perspectives. The environment of the classroom is open and safe for risk taking; seating is in a circle to facilitate small group discussion, and classes last at least 2 hours to provide time for processing. An example of using a reflective classroom to teach leadership and management to baccalaureate nursing students was described by Krichbaum (1993, 1995).

Clinical climate. The idea of a reflective practicum was introduced by Schön (1987). In the reflective practicum, students learn by doing in an environment that represents the world of practice; novices learn from experts through reflection-in-action and reflection-about-action. The teacher in the reflective practicum acts as a coach and engages in dialogue with the student. In this dialogue messages are conveyed both verbally and through performance, both by the student and the coach. The student attempts to perform what is being learned. The coach provides advice, criticism, explanations, and descriptions to the student and role models the expert's own performance to the student. Schön (1987) describes the ideal dialogue as "reciprocal reflection-in-action" (p. 163).

Curricular climate. Diekelmann (1988) proposes a paradigm shift away from the technical models to an emancipatory model, curriculum as dialogue and meaning. As described in the model, dialogue "is a joint reflection on a phenomenon; it is a deepening of experience for all participants; it is talking, generating questions, and possibly interpretations" (p. 145). Dialogue involves teachers, practitioners, and students engaging in enlightened debate about issues, viewing problems from different perspectives, and achieving solutions together. This curricular model emphasizes respect, openness, responsibility, and willingness to learn.

Another paradigm shift is proposed by Ford and Profetto-McGrath (1994). They advocate a shift from the narrow technical and practical perspectives of the past to one that is grounded in an emancipatory interest. Curriculum developed in an emancipatory interest is defined as *curriculum as praxis* (Ford & Profetto-McGrath, 1994). Praxis is a form of action informed by reflection; and reflection is, in turn, informed by action. Curriculum as praxis is based on an "interest in emancipation and empowerment to engage in autonomous action arising out of authentic, critical insights into the social construction of human society" (Grundy, 1989, p. 19). Grundy attributes the foundations of curriculum as praxis to Habermas (1972) and Friere (1972).

Curriculum as praxis seeks to develop critical consciousness and freedom from tradition in the learner. A paradigm shift such as this requires that faculty and students define nursing education and its outcomes differently. It requires a different conceptualization of CT, beyond linear problem solving toward viewing it as an interactive, dynamic process that challenges the status quo. Until now, nursing education has been invested in developing and maintaining the status quo. The rightness of action and rule orientation must give way to a mutual exploration by faculty and students of presenting patterns of information. These patterns then serve as the basis for dialogue about what is true and what constitutes knowledge. Developing this type of knowledge necessitates the active involvement of the learner with the information—a new way of learning for both students and faculty.

THE FUTURE OF CRITICAL THINKING DEVELOPMENT IN NURSING EDUCATION

As the discipline of nursing continues to change, define its role in health care, and create nursing knowledge, there is an urgent need to accept CT as an outcome of highest value for nursing education and for practice. As educators, we must learn to facilitate its development. The list of potential teaching strategies to develop CT in students continues to grow. As it does, a number of questions and issues arise regarding the use of these teaching strategies and the responses of the recipients. Do the teaching strategies produce the desired outcomes in students and in clients? What are the desired outcomes? How can a strategy be used most effectively? Is there a hierarchy of teaching strategies that requires careful sequencing throughout the curriculum? How much of a strategy is sufficient to effect change and how much is too much? How do teachers help students to value and actively engage in these strategies? Little research has been conducted in past years that addresses these questions. In this era of diminished resources, knowledge explosion, and the changing health care scene, it is essential that educators develop effective strategies to help students learn to think critically.

In order to do this, educators first must be willing to accept responsibility for failing to stimulate sufficiently the development of CT in students, i.e., to recognize the existence of the problem. This may require a shift in the values of nursing faculty. Second, administrators must be committed to supporting faculty in revising curriculum and learning teaching strategies that foster CT. Third, faculty and students need to be prepared to deal with the discomfort inherent in changing from methods that are comfortable to new strategies that may seem unfamiliar and awkward at first.

Many current nursing educators experienced some teaching strategies as students that encouraged CT and others that seemed to hinder it. As educators we tend to pass that same legacy on to our students unless we learn more about CT and work hard to gain skill in teaching strategies that foster CT. Do we want our students to be copying information from textbook care plans onto a care plan for their patient and memorizing notes from lectures? Or will we hold them accountable for identifying and clarifying problems, deciding what they need to know, going on scholarly quests for valuable, relevant information, weighing evidence, and making discerning judgments? When you need the services of a nurse, what do you want that nurse to be able to do? If we want graduates of nursing programs to think critically, to solve problems, and to decide with clients on the best course of action, we must be willing to give up old ways and to risk working alongside students and colleagues to develop CT dispositions and skills.

REFERENCES

Bandman, E., & Bandman, B. (1995). *Critical thinking in nursing.* Norwalk, CT: Appleton & Lange.

Bauwens, E.E., & Gerhard, C.G. (1987). The use of the Watson Glaser Critical Thinking Appraisal to predict success in a baccalaureate nursing program. *Journal of Nursing Education, 26,* 278-281.

Benner, P. (1984). *From novice to expert: Excellence and power in clinical nursing practice.* Menlo Park, CA: Adison-Wesley.

Benner, P., & Tanner, C. (1987). Clinical judgment: How expert nurses use intuition. *American Journal of Nursing, 87,* 23-31.

Berger, M.C. (1984). Critical thinking ability and nursing students. *Journal of Nursing Education, 23,* 306-308.

Blair, J.A. (1985). Some challenges for critical thinking. In J. Hoagland (Ed.), *Conference on critical thinking: Christopher Newport College.* Newport News, VA: Christopher Newport College Press.

Brookfield, S. (1987). *Developing critical thinkers.* San Francisco, CA: Jossey-Bass Publishers.

Brooks, K., & Shepherd, J. (1990). The relationship between clinical decision-making skills in nursing and general critical thinking abilities of senior nursing students in four types of nursing programs. *Journal of Nursing Education, 29*(9), 391-99.

Brophy, J., & Good, T.L. (1986). Teaching behavior and student achievement. In M.C. Wittrock (Ed.), *Third handbook of research on teaching.* New York: MacMillan.

Corcoran, S., & Tanner, C. (1988). Implications of clinical judgment research for teaching. In National League for Nursing (Ed.), *Curriculum revolution: Mandate for change* (NLN Publication No. 15-2224, pp. 159-176). New York: National League for Nursing.

Corcoran-Perry, S., & Narayan, S. (1995a). Teaching clinical reasoning to nurses in clinical education. In J. Higgs & M. Jones (Eds.), *Clinical reasoning in the health professions* (pp. 258-268). Oxford: Butterworth Heinemann Ltd.

Corcoran-Perry, S., & Narayan, S. (1995b). Clinical decision making. In M. Snyder & M. Mirr (Eds.), *Advanced practice nursing: A guide to professional development* (pp. 69-91). New York: Springer Publishing Company.

Creighton, H. (1984, May). Nursing judgment. *Nursing Management, 15*(60), 62-63.

Diekelmann, N. (1988). Curriculum revolution: A theoretical and philosophical mandate for change. In *Curriculum revolution: Mandate for change* (NLN Publication No. 15-2224, pp. 137-157). New York: National League for Nursing.

Donaldson, S.K., & Crowley, D.M. (1978). The discipline of nursing. *Nursing Outlook, 26*(2), 113-120.

Duckett, L., Waithe, M.E., Rowan, M., Schmitz, K., & Ryden, M.B. (1993). *MCSL building: Developing a strong ethics curriculum in nursing using Multi-Course Sequential Learning* (2nd ed., pp. F5-F15, F20-F29, S23-S39). Minneapolis, MN: University of Minnesota School of Nursing.

Dungan, J.M. (1986, November). *Relationship of critical thinking and nursing process utilization.* Paper presented at the University of Minnesota School of Nursing Research Conference, Minneapolis, MN.

Ennis, R.H. (1962). A concept of critical thinking. *Harvard Educational Review, 32*(1), 81-111.

Ennis, R.H. (1985). A logical basis for measuring critical thinking skills. *Educational Leadership, 43,* 44-48.

Ennis, R.H. (1993). Critical thinking assessment. *Theory into Practice, 32*(3), 180-186.

Ennis, R.H., & Weir, E. (1985). *The Ennis-Weir Critical Thinking Essay Test.* Pacific Grove, CA: Midwest Publications.

Facione, N.C., Facione, P.A., & Sanchez, C. (1994). Critical thinking disposition as a measure of competent clinical judgment: The development of the California Critical Thinking Disposition Inventory. *Journal of Nursing Education, 33*(8), 345-350.

Facione, P.A. (1990a). *The California Critical Thinking Skills Test.* Millbrae, CA: The California Academic Press.

Facione, P.A. (1990b). Executive summary—critical thinking: A statement of expert consensus for purposes of educational assessment and instruction. Millbrae, CA: The California Academic Press. [The complete Delphi report, including appendices, is available from The California Academic Press and as ERIC Doc. No. ED 315-423, P. Facione, Principal Investigator.]

Facione, P.A., & Facione, N.C. (1993). *Test manual: The California Critical Thinking Skills Test, Form A and Form B.* Millbrae, CA: The California Academic Press.

Facione, P.A., Facione, N.C., & Sanchez, C.A. (1994). *The California Critical Thinking Disposition Inventory: Test manual.* Millbrae, CA: The California Academic Press.

Fawcett, J. (1978). The relationship between theory and research: A double helix. *Advances in Nursing Science, 1*(1), 49-62.

Ford, J., & Profetto-McGrath, J. (1994). A model for critical thinking within the context of curriculum as praxis. *Journal of Nursing Education, 33*(8), 341-44.

Frederickson, K. (1979, March). Critical thinking ability and academic achievement. *Journal, New York State Nurses Association, 10,* 41-44.

Friere, P. (1972). *Pedagogy of the oppressed.* Harmondsworth: Penguin.

Frisby, C.L. (1992). Construct validity and psychometric properties of the Cornell Critical Thinking Test (Level Z): A contrasted groups analysis. *Psychological Reports, 71,* 291-303.

Glaser, E. (1985, Winter). Critical thinking: Educating for responsible citizenship in a democracy. *Phi Kappa Phi Journal, 65,* 24-7.

Gould, J., & Bevis, E. (1990). Here there be dragons. *Nursing & Health Care, 13*(3), 126-133.

Gross, Y.T., Takazawa, E.S., & Rose, C.L. (1987). Critical thinking and nursing education. *Journal of Nursing Education, 26,* 317-323.

Grundy, S. (1989). *Curriculum: Product or praxis.* Philadelphia: Falmer Press.

Habermas, J. (1972). *Knowledge and human interests.* (J. Shapiro, Trans.). Boston: Beacon Press.

Higgs, J., & Jones, M. (Eds.). (1995). *Clinical reasoning in the health professions.* Oxford: Butterworth Heinemann Ltd.

Hughes, J.N. (1992). Review of the Cornell critical thinking tests. In J.J. Kramer & J.C. Conoley (Eds.), *Eleventh mental measurements yearbook* (pp. 242-243). Lincoln, NE: University of Nebraska, Buros Institute of Mental Measurements.

Jacobs, S.S. (1995). Technical characteristics and some correlates of the California Critical Thinking Skills Test, Forms A and B. *Research in Higher Education, 36*(1), 89-108.

Jenkins, H. (1985, June). Improving clinical decision-making in nursing. *Journal of Nursing Education, 24,* 242-3.

Johnson, D.E. (1974). Development of theory: A requisite for nursing as a primary health profession. *Nursing Research, 23*(5), 372-377.

Johnson, D.W., & Johnson, R. (1978). Cooperative, competitive, and individualistic learning. *Journal of Research and Development in Education, 12,* 3-15.

Johnson, D.W., & Johnson, R. (1979). Conflict in the classroom: Controversy and learning. *Review of Educational Research, 49,* 51-70.

Johnson, D.W., & Johnson, R. (1985). Classroom conflict: Controversy vs. debate in learning groups. *American Educational Research Journal, 22,* 337-256.

Johnson, D.W., & Johnson, R. (1988). Critical thinking through structured controversy. *Educational Leadership, 45*(8), 58-64.

Johnson, D.W., & Johnson, R. (1989). *Cooperation and competition: Theory and research.* Edina, MN: Interaction Book Company.

Johnson, D.W., & Johnson, R. (1991). *Learning together and alone: Cooperative, competitive, and individualistic learning.* Englewood Cliffs, NJ: Prentice-Hall.

Johnson, D.W., Johnson, R., & Smith, K. (1986). Academic conflict among students: Controversy and learning. In R. Feldman (Ed.), *Social psychological applications to education.* New York: Cambridge University Press.

Johnson, D.W., Johnson, R., & Smith, K. (1991). *Active learning: Cooperation in the college classroom* (pp. 7:1-7:26). Edina, MN: Interaction Book Company.

Jones, J.A., & Brown, L.N. (1991). Critical thinking: Impact on nursing education. *Journal of Advanced Nursing, 16,* 529-33.

Kassirer, J. (1983). Sounding board: Teaching clinical medicine by iterative hypothesis testing. *New England Journal of Medicine, 309,* 921-923.

Kintgen-Andrews, J. (1988). Development of critical thinking: Career ladder P.N. and A.D. nursing students, pre-health science freshmen, generic baccalaureate sophomore nursing students. *Resources in Education, 24*(1). (ERIC Document No. 297 153).

Kintgen-Andrews, J. (1991). Critical thinking and nursing education: Perplexities and insights. *Journal of Nursing Education, 30*(4), 152-157.

Kreisberg, S. (1992). *Transforming power, domination, empowerment and education*. New York: State University of New York Press.

Krichbaum, K. (1993, April). Empowering nursing students for leadership. *Learning Resources Journal*, 11-14.

Krichbaum, K. (1995). *Strategies for developing critical thinking skills in nursing students*. Unpublished manuscript.

Krichbaum, K., Duckett, L., Miller, M., Ryden, M. & Wainwright, H. (1994). *A report on the effectiveness of the baccalaureate curriculum for helping students in nursing achieve program objectives*. Unpublished report to the faculty of the University of Minnesota School of Nursing.

Kurfiss, J. (1988). *Critical thinking: Theory, research, practice, and possibilities*. (ASHE-ERIC Higher Education Report No. 2.) Washington, DC: Association for the Study of Higher Education.

Lashley, & Wittstedt. (1993). Writing across the curriculum: An integrated curricular approach to developing critical thinking through writing. *Journal of Nursing Education, 32*(9), 422-424.

Matthews, C.A., & Gaul, A.L. (1979). Nursing diagnosis from the perspective of concept attainment. *Advances in Nursing Science, 2*(1), 17-26.

McPeck, J.E. (1981). *Critical thinking in education*. New York: St. Martin's Press.

Meyers, C. (1986). *Teaching students to think critically: A guide for faculty in all disciplines*. San Francisco: Jossey-Bass.

Miller, M., & Malcolm, N. (1990). Critical thinking in the nursing curriculum. *Nursing & Health Care, 11*(2), 67-73.

Moccia, P. (1990). No sire, it's a revolution. *Journal of Nursing Education, 29*, 307-11.

National League for Nursing. (1988). *Curriculum revolution: Mandate for change* (NLN Publication No. 15-2224). New York: Author.

National League for Nursing (1993). *NLN criteria for the evaluation of baccalaureate and higher degree programs in nursing*. New York: Author.

Norris, S.P. (1985, May). Synthesis of research on critical thinking. *Educational Leadership, 42*, 40-46.

Norris, S.P. (1988). Controlling for background beliefs when developing multiple-choice critical thinking tests. *Educational Measurement: Issues and Practice, 7*(3), 5-11.

Norris, S.P. (1989). Can we test validly for critical thinking? *Educational Researcher, 18*(9), 21-26.

Norris, S.P. (1992). A demonstration of the use of verbal reports of thinking in multiple-choice critical thinking test design. *The Alberta Journal of Educational Research, 38*(3), 155-176.

Norris, S.P., & Ennis, R.H. (1989). *Evaluating critical thinking*. Pacific Grove, CA: Midwest Publications.

Pardue, F. (1987). Decision-making skills and critical thinking ability among associate degree, diploma, baccalaureate, and master's prepared nurses. *Journal of Nursing Education, 26*, 354-361.

Paul, R.W. (1982). Teaching critical thinking in the 'strong' sense: A focus on self-deception, coordinating views and a dialectical mode of analysis. *Informal Logic Newsletter, 4*(2), 2-7.

Paul, R.W. (1983). An agenda item for the informal logic/critical thinking movement. *Informal Logic Newsletter, 5*(2), 23-4.

Paul, R.W. (1985). The critical thinking movement. *National Forum, 65*(1), 32.

Pederson, C., Duckett, L., Ryden, M., & Maruyama, G. (1990). Using structured controversy to promote ethical decision making. *Journal of Nursing Education, 29*(4), 150-157.

Richards, M.A. (1977). One integrated curriculum: An empirical evaluation. *Nursing Research, 26*(2), 90-5.

Ruggiero, V. (1988). *Teaching thinking across the curriculum*. New York: Harper & Row.

Ryden, M., Duckett, L., Crisham, P., Caplan, A., & Schmitz, K. (1989). Multi-course sequential learning as a model for content integration: Ethics as a prototype. *Journal of Nursing Education, 28*(3), 102-106.

Ryden, M., McCarthy, P., Lewis, M., & Sherman, C. (1991). A behavioral comparison of helping styles of nursing students, psychotherapists, crisis interveners, and untrained individuals. *Archives of Psychiatric Nursing, 5*(3), 185-188.

Schön, D. (1987). *Educating the reflective practitioner.* San Francisco: Jossey-Bass.

Scoloveno, M. (1981). Problem solving ability of nursing students in three program types. (Doctoral dissertation, Rutgers University, 1981). *Dissertation Abstracts International, 41*, 1396B.

Siegel, H. (1985). Educating reason: Critical thinking, informal logic and the philosophy of education. *Informal Logic, 7*(2), 69-81.

Siegel, H. (1988). *Educating reason*. New York: Routledge.

Sullivan, E. (1987, March/April). Critical thinking, creativity, clinical performance, and achievement in RN students. *Nurse educator, 12*, 12-16.

Tanner, C.A. (1983). Research on clinical judgment. In W.L. Holzemer (Ed.), *Review of research in nursing education*. New Jersey: Slack.

Tanner, C. (1986). The nursing care plan as a teaching method: Reason or ritual? *Nurse Educator, 11*(4), 8-9.

Tanner, C. (1987). Teaching clinical judgment. *Annual Review of Nursing Research, 5*, 153-173.

Tanner, C. (1993). More thinking about critical thinking and clinical decision making (Editorial). *Journal of Nursing Education, 32*(9), 387.

Watson, G., & Glaser, E.M. (1980). *Watson-Glaser Critical Thinking Appraisal*. San Antonio, TX: The Psychological Corporation.

White, N., Beardlsee, N., Peters, D., & Supples, J. (1990). Promoting critical thinking skills. *Nurse Educator, 15*(5), 16-19.

Woods, D. (1994). *Problem-based learning: How to gain the most from PBL*. Waterdown, Ontario: McMaster University.

Yinger, R.J. (1980). Can we really teach them to think? In R.E. Young (Ed.), *Fostering critical thinking. New directions for teaching and learning*. No. 3. San Francisco: Jossey-Bass.

Distance learning: An integral part of transforming the university and nursing education

MARILYN L. ROTHERT, GERALDINE J. TALARCZYK, SUSAN M. AWBREY

Distance education has traditionally been considered an educational model to address the needs of students who live and want to learn at some distance from the main university campus. Lewis and Farrell (1995) identify the underlying philosophy of distance learning to include

> the belief that when students have access to a program of planned instruction where the course materials are systematically designed and provide direction to additional resources, students can proceed in a self-directed manner and be successful in meeting the specified outcomes for each course. (p. 185)

The literature on distance education has focused primarily on the learner's experience, technological capability, and teaching strategies for adult learners.

The underlying premise of this chapter is that distance learning not only impacts the learner and the teacher, but is an integral part of the transformation of the university and redefinition of outreach with direct implications for nursing education. An understanding of the transformation is an essential base from which to envision the future role of distance education for nursing.

REDEFINING THE UNIVERSITY

As we enter the 21st century, we might pause to reflect on what universities of the future may look like. Will the new age of universities see only incremental change and adherence to traditional patterns or will we see radical changes based on new ways of organizing and involving the learner? The role distance learning plays in the future will depend on how far universities are willing to go in transforming themselves to meet the needs of society. In today's world of rapid change the public is grappling with complex ideas and problems in the economy, in society, and in their personal lives. As a diverse citizenry struggles to address complex dilemmas, more and more demands are being placed on universities to contribute to the solutions. Clearly society intentionally and unintentionally is challenging universities to actively alter the way they do business.

As demands on universities increase it is likely that the academy will evolve in new and dramatic ways. One scenario suggests that universities may no longer serve a narrow geographic area or even a nation but will draw from a worldwide clientele (Duderstadt, 1994). Universities may become virtual institutions that exist as technological links between students, faculty, learning resources, and the community—institutions that are re-formed to provide multidimensional connections across disciplines, cultural boundaries, and barriers to the broader society. Assisted by digital convergence, these learning institutions could disseminate knowledge in multiple forms over worldwide networks providing access to audiences unheard of in the past. A glimpse of such a vision of higher education can be found in the use of distance education, which began with the University of South Africa in 1951 and was followed by Open University in the United Kingdom. Lewis and Farrell (1995) indicate that the number of open universities around the world has grown to nearly 30. Open universities do not offer traditional, on-campus programs, but exist solely for the purpose of distance education.

This scenario opens possibilities for an "extended university" that moves beyond geographic boundaries, time frames, and formats (Lynton and Elman, 1987). However, the university must become more than a mere "knowledge server" or storehouse of information accessible on the World Wide Web. To remain relevant universities must form interactive human connections with the communities they serve. Universities must learn, teach, and apply knowledge as well as discover it. Knowledge does not move only from the locus of research to the place of application. There must be two-way interaction so that as the knowledge resources of the university extend to communities, changing their capacity and enabling their future, the expectations and environment of the community reflect back to the university, refining its teaching and research and influencing the definition of its mission, the roles of its faculty, and the expectations of its management. This is the "new" aspect of distance education that challenges our thinking and the very organization of universities.

It is not merely the technological infrastructure that must be transformed to create an institution of higher learning that is responsive and relevant to societal needs, but the vision of what an institution of higher education does, whom it serves, and the norms by which it operates must also be transformed. Our vocabulary, policies, and traditional understanding of higher education must evolve. Historically, the university was considered a place, in fact *the* geographical location, where research, teaching, and service take place, thereby creating the environment necessary for learning. The students were expected to share common characteristics in background, experience, and age. Teaching and learning, research, and service in sites away from the university campus were external to the central mission and the central site of the university. Students who were not of standard age, experience, or background were considered "nontraditional" students. This view influenced not only our vocabulary but also the policies and procedures of the academy including the matriculation and graduation processes for students and the reward processes for faculty. The residency requirement for students exemplifies a remnant from the time when the campus was considered the best and only place for true learning and scholarship. Reluctance to involve junior faculty in community-based scholarship prior to tenure is another vestige of the historical definition of scholarship. In a world linked by technology and celebration of diversity, these notions are not only outdated, but can become barriers to achieving the goals of higher education, currently defined as the generation, dissemination, and application of knowledge. Distance learning must be understood as part of a movement to the new paradigm of higher education, developing the capacity of the academy to meet these goals.

Senge (1990) has defined the notion of a "learning organization" as one that is able to deal with the problems and opportunities of today and invest in its capacity to embrace tomorrow, an organization prepared for change and able to succeed in a dynamic environment. Taking Senge's advice, what can be done today to build toward tomorrow and position the university for the future?

UNIVERSITY OUTREACH

One resource that can play a key role in the university's transformation of educational delivery and its quest to form linkages with the community is university outreach. As the "wall" between the university and the world begins to soften, outreach can act as an experimental laboratory for developing the future and a mechanism for initiating changes that foster new ways of thinking about how we implement our mission.

Outreach has been defined as "a form of scholarship that cuts across teaching, research, and service. It involves generating, transmitting, applying, and preserving knowledge for the direct benefit of external audiences in ways that are consistent with university and unit missions" (The Provost's Committee on University Outreach, 1993, p. 1). Using this definition, outreach is considered to be rooted in scholarship. Outreach crosscuts the university mission, sometimes generating knowledge (e.g., applied clinical research), sometimes transmitting knowledge (e.g., continuing professional education), sometimes applying knowledge (e.g., providing technical assistance), and sometimes preserving knowledge (e.g., creating electronically accessible databases). The goal of outreach is to bring the knowledge resources of the university to diverse audiences for the direct benefit of those audiences. To play a pivotal role in the transformation of the university, outreach must become a central function and integral part of the institution and an integral form of scholarship within the university.

Technological advances have provided the mechanism for the university to expand its campus to a broad geographical location. Technology enables the student 200 miles from campus to be fully qualified, working on a master's degree in nursing, strongly networked to faculty and support services such as the library. Technology links students in two or more sites, creating a "classroom" in which students separated by distance simultaneously gain classroom knowledge and share personal experiences, thus learning from one another. Students from the original campus as well as those in the community campus are in local clinical learning experiences and doing research, which is frequently focused on locally identified issues. Teaching, learning, and scholarship are occurring across sites, with distance learning expanding the boundaries of the traditional university.

Business and industry are using new management techniques focused on productivity and outcomes to create a more effective and efficient organization (Covey, 1989; Drucker, 1993; Senge, 1990; Walton, 1986). Many of these strategies value the concept of teamwork and desire to build an environment with systems supporting individuals functioning at an optimal level. With the expanded partnering between university and community, and strengthening of the ties between universities and industry, both universities and industries are now being expected to "re-engineer" their systems. This is an example of the two-way characteristic of distance learning. While the knowledge resources of the university are extended to communities, changing their capacity and enabling their future, the expectations and environment of the community reflect back to the university, impacting and influencing the definition of its mission, the roles of its faculty, and the expectations of its management. This reciprocity demonstrates that distance learning is that which links two sites separated by geographical distance. It does not assume that the teaching originates from one site and the learning takes place at the other.

Walshok (1995) has noted that it is rare to find research universities that include connections to off-campus publics as important components of central planning activities. Most frequently, nonfaculty expertise and support are usually sought only after faculty have determined what they want and need, and then they are usually sought for the purposes of gaining political or financial support for a new agenda. Walshok notes that change will require a cultural shift to bring a wider circle of perspectives and intellectual competencies to the discussion of institutional priorities and commitments. Distance learning can either act as a catalyst for change within the university, helping it to transform into an institution that is more integrated in its mission and connected to the society it serves, or it can become one more ancillary activity split off from the central core of university activities.

IMPLICATIONS FOR NURSING

The changing concept of the university to include distance education as an integral part of the total functioning requires the individuals and systems involved to change. The very definition of who is involved denotes change. Community-based faculty, students, partners, and systems bring a new dimension to nursing education. Faculty and administrators will have to work together to facilitate faculty and student success in distance learning (Willis, 1994). Organizational systems will require greater flexibility to respond to new instructional delivery systems as well as to changing characteristics and needs of both students and faculty.

We are moving into a new generation distance education model that uses a combination of print, videotape, audiotape, fax, computers and interactive television. Further, faculty involved in teaching are no longer in one site, creating the need for collaborative efforts across distances. This new model requires campus-based faculty to become oriented to the community and its culture as well as to new colleagues; it requires community-based faculty to become oriented to the university systems and to new colleagues. Faculty who are involved in the pioneering efforts in this distance education generation will need a strong support system. Not only are faculty needing to learn a new educational process but they are simultaneously adapting to a changing educational system as the university moves toward a transformation. Collaborative peer support groups for problem solving and sharing of ideas are important to relieve the insecurity faculty may feel and to avoid individual isolation. Ongoing training and support are important for faculty at all sites. An integrated approach would include one-on-one learning opportunities, workshops, and self-paced learning modules. The use of outside and local expertise provides both an opportunity to incorporate new ideas and ongoing support. Willis (1994) states that as distance education moves to the incorporation of new technologies such as computers and interactive television faculty will need assistance to (a) look at the course in a new way to adapt traditionally delivered courses for effective distance delivery; (b) shift from the role of content provider to content facilitator in which the backgrounds and accomplishments of the learners are drawn on to enhance individual and group learning; (c) gain comfort and proficiency in using technology as the primary teacher-student link; (d) learn to teach effectively without the visual control provided by direct eye contact; and (e) develop an understanding and appreciation for the distant students' lifestyle.

With distance education the role of the student is also affected. With the classroom expanded to include students in multiple sites learning simultaneously, the challenge is to create an environment in which the students learn from one another as well as from the faculty, enriched by the diversity rather than burdened by the challenge. This requires students to redefine their "classmates" to include those they know only through technology. To accomplish this goal, students must be oriented early to the redefinition of the university and the boundaries of the college campus. Greater responsibility for independent learning is also required. The passive learner attitude of, "I paid my tuition, now here I sit, so tell me everything you know about the subject," will no longer be appropriate to facilitate learning. In addition to an early orientation to the new academic philosophy, it is necessary for students to have an opportunity to become familiar with the use of new technologies used in instructional delivery in order to interact fully with the content, the instructor, and other learners (Hillman, Willis, & Gunawardena, 1994). While distance learning may require rapid learning of new technologies, familiarity with technology is also necessary for their professional responsibilities. Students at distant sites who are concentrated in a geographical area or who have access to computer communication with each other will find that their interaction is a source of learning opportunities, and these students often become a more cohesive group than main campus students in similar programs.

It is critical that the goals and expectations for distance education be related to the mission of the unit and clearly understood by administrators and faculty. It has not yet been demonstrated that distance education can reduce costs or serve greater numbers of students with the same funds. Threlkeld and Brzoska (1994) state that "there is little evidence in the United States that distance education reduces costs over traditional instruction. There is some evidence that cost-effectiveness can be demonstrated, if one examines cost over a period of time" (p. 62). This, however, is dependent on media costs, the costs of program development and maintenance, and long-term student and instructional support.

Administrators and faculty must work together to incorporate distance education into the institutional reward system, which includes promotion and tenure, and into the tripartite mission of research, teaching, and service (Billings et al., 1994; Caffarella, Duning, & Patrick, 1992; Willis, 1994). Developing or adapting instruction for distance education requires time and effort. Issues to be considered include instructional workload, which is related to students at multiple sites, simulcasting instruction to multiple sites, and administrative meeting time. As for on-campus instruction, student and faculty issues include the use of compressed time frames for courses, weekend instruction, and evening course hours. Provision must also be made to provide support staff, hardware, software, and services needed to carry out distance education to maintain quality and faculty support.

Distance education fosters collaboration, requiring coordination with multiple university units and community resources. For example, it is critical that distant learners have access to library materials. To accomplish this goal, systems and arrangements must be developed by the university library, the local community college, the local health care agencies, and the nursing academic unit offering the course.

Research has demonstrated that there is no significant difference between the level of achievement of distance learners and those in traditional classrooms (Billings and Bachmeier, 1994; Threlkeld and Brzoska, 1994). In nursing these studies have been done predominantly with nonclinical courses and baccalaureate completion registered nurse and master's students. Although there is some evidence that socialization into new roles can be achieved with distance education (Cragg, 1991; Lenburg, 1990), further study needs to be done for registered nursing students in this area.

Providing distant students with quality clinical instruction is another issue that requires further attention (Henry & Ensunsa, 1991; Rosenlieb, 1993). The common method is to use community-based practicing nurses as preceptors or instructors. This challenges the campus faculty to address creatively issues of orientation of distant faculty to course and academic requirements, and development of distant faculty in relation to teaching skills. It is essential that distant faculty become part of the academic unit to which they are volunteering their services or by which they are employed. With increased distance education the meaning of "faculty" may be redefined as increased interdependence occurs between the academic community and the greater communities of which it is a part.

In the United States distance education for both degree granting and continuing education programs is leading us to increased cooperation and collaboration for resource sharing at local, state, and regional levels. This will result in an examination of state policies regarding recognition of academic programs, review of programs for duplication and cost-effectiveness, and incentives for collaboration rather than competitiveness. Because distance education at the university level is available in many countries throughout the world, it seems that in the near future as technologies are developed further and the costs for using these technologies decrease there will be global distance education. While this will solve the problem of travel and relocation and will enhance information exchange and learning, it will provide another set of challenges related to policies, laws, cultures, and customs (Brown & Brown, 1994; Thach & Murphy, 1994).

Distance learning as a part of continuing professional education for practicing nurses is a growing area of university programming. As the university strengthens its linkage to the community, a natural outcome is the community-based educational offering to upgrade clinical skills. With the advances of technology, the expertise of a community practitioner can be linked with that of a faculty member to demonstrate the partnership between theory and practice.

In summary, distance learning is closely linked to the transformation of universities and redefinition of their mission. Stronger linkage with communities will stimulate reciprocal relationships and bring about university and community change. University outreach will continue to move from a position of isolation in mission and operation to an integral part of the scholarship of the institution. Nursing will be challenged to position itself as part of the solution to the changes facing universities. Distance learning will assist nursing to build on a history of community partnership in education and service to enhance capacity and quality in nursing education.

REFERENCES

Billings, D., Durham, J., Finke, L., Boland, D., Smith, S., & Manz, B. (1994). Faculty perceptions of teaching on television: one school's experience. *Journal of Professional Nursing, 10*(5), 307-312.

Billings, D.M., & Bachmeier, B. (1994). Teaching and learning at a distance: a review of the nursing literature. In L.R. Allen (Ed.), *Review of research in nursing education* (Vol. VI, pp. 1-32). New York: National League for Nursing.

Brown, F.B., & Brown, Y. (1994). Distance education around the world. In B. Willis (Ed.), *Distance education: Strategies and tools* (pp. 3-39). Englewood Cliffs, NJ: Educational Technology Publications.

Caffarella, R.S., Duning, B., & Patrick, S. (1992). Delivering off-campus instruction: changing roles and responsibilities of professors in higher education. *Continuing Higher Education Review, 56*(3), 155-167.

Covey, S.R. (1989). *The seven habits of highly effective people.* New York: Simon & Schuster.

Cragg, C.E. (1991). Professional resocialization of post-RN baccalaureate students by distance education. *Journal of Nursing Education, 30*(6), 256-260.

Drucker, P.F. (1993). *Managing for the future.* New York: Truman Talley Books/Plume.

Duderstadt, J.J. (1994). *The challenge for the 1990s: Transforming the university.* [Speech.] The University of Michigan, 1994.

Henry, S.B., & Ensunsa, K. (1991). Preceptorship in nursing service and education. In P.A. Baj & G.M. Clayton (Eds.), *Review of research in nursing education* (Vol. IV, pp. 51-72). New York: National League for Nursing.

Hillman, D.C., Willis, D.K., & Gunawardena, C.N. (1994). Learner-interface interaction in distance education: An extension of contemporary models and strategies for practitioners. *The American Journal of Distance Education, 8*(2), 30-42.

Lenburg, C.B. (1990). Do external degree programs really work? *Nursing Outlook, 38*(5), 234-238.

Lewis, J.M., & Farrell, M. (1995). Distance education: A strategy for leadership development. *N&HC: Perspectives on Community, 16*(4), 184-187.

Lynton, E., & Elman, S. (1987). *New priorities for the university: Meeting society's needs for applied knowledge and competent individuals.* San Francisco: Jossey Bass.

The Provost's Committee on University Outreach. (1993). *University outreach at Michigan State University: Extending knowledge to serve society.* East Lansing, MI: Michigan State University.

Rosenlieb, C.O. (1993). A profile of preceptorships in baccalaureate degree nursing programs for registered nurses. In N.L. Diekelmann & M.L. Rather (Eds.), *Transforming RN education: Dialogue and debate* (pp. 256-272). New York: National League for Nursing.

Senge, P.M. (1990). *The fifth discipline: The art & practice of the learning organization.* New York: Currency Doubleday.

Thach, L., & Murphy, K.L. (1994). Collaboration in distance education: From local to international perspectives. *The American Journal of Distance Education, 8*(3), 5-21.

Threlkeld, R., & Brzoska, K. (1994). Research in distance education. In B. Willis (Ed.), *Distance education: Strategies and tools* (pp. 41-66). Englewood Cliffs, NJ: Educational Technology Publications.

Walshok, M.L. (1995). *Knowledge without boundaries.* San Francisco: Jossey-Bass Publishers.

Walton, M. (1986). *The Deming management method.* New York: Putnam Publishing Group.

Willis, B. (1994). Enhancing faculty effectiveness in distance education. In B. Willis (Ed.), *Distance education: Strategies and tools* (pp. 277-290). Englewood Cliffs, NJ: Educational Technology Publications.

New teaching strategies and technologies

CHARLENE E. CLARK

To paraphrase Charles Dickens, "It is the best of times, it is the worst of times." Those words apply appropriately to contemporary teaching methods in schools of nursing and apply formidably to the future of nursing education as one projects the potentials and possibilities of the 21st century. Technological opportunities are currently presented to educators that combine a number of strategies and methodologies that have never before been available to faculty. However, the multiplicity of these options frequently are neither used by nor made accessible to the "grass roots" faculty, due at least in part to limited institutional financial resources, lack of advanced training or education of nursing faculty and administrators, or a combination of both. While instructional delivery systems have become more and more sophisticated in the last several years, their effective use, in many instances, has been restricted.

To understand the contemporary status of teaching technologies it would be helpful for the reader to review a brief historical perspective of the relative speed of media advancement in this century. Audiovisual instruction, which combined audio onto motion film, became available in the late 1920s. While use of this technology advanced slowly in the public education sector, military and business applications expanded as interest and application in using the new media began to flourish. Development and use of the overhead projector emerged toward the end of World War II, yet Heinich, Molenda, and Russell (1993) indicate that it is still proclaimed to be the most widely used single piece of audiovisual educational hardware (p. 23). In the 1950s, educators began to identify the importance of television as an instructional strategy, and research studies initiated in those years substantiated its efficacy. Use of this technology at all levels of the educational process continues to be documented in the literature, and nursing has recognized its potential for content delivery on site as well as for off-campus learners (Clark, 1989).

Theories of communication and human learning have been studied throughout the 20th century by educators, psychologists, sociologists, and other research scientists. Of major midcentury interest were the first efforts of programmed instruction, which had been developed in the early 1950s based on previous studies by Skinner. Although programmed instruction is rarely used at any level in today's educational system, the pedagogical basis it provided led the way for many of the self-directed applications incorporated into courses during the last two decades. Development and use of computer-assisted instruction (CAI), modules and packets, and interactive laser discs (ILD) have emerged from the theoretical research initiated during this earlier era. Use of interactive technologies including CAI and ILD in nursing education was begun in the mid-1980s and continues to gain momentum as educators become more sophisticated in planning its effective integration into curricula.

STRATEGIES AND TECHNOLOGIES

As nursing moves into the 21st century there are many instructional options potentially available for use in the classroom, in the home for patient teaching, and in acute or tertiary care centers. Two salient factors that may impede access to these resources include the cost of the technology and readiness of administrators and educators to utilize the strategies and technologies.

Cost factors

Learning laboratories have a significant place in schools of nursing as well as in health care centers. These areas provide students and professional employees opportunities to acquire new knowledge without the risk of error that could lead to patient injury or reprisal from teachers or supervisors. Students, functioning at a pace most conducive to their personal learning styles, thus challenge faculty to create and efficiently utilize a variety of educational materials.

The expenditure at the outset of developing a computer laboratory or an audiovisual laboratory for learners' independent use outside classroom hours can be significant. Therefore, prior to embarking on major expenditures to support such areas, nurse educators first must decide whether the technology supports the mission and goals of the program. Is the initial cost of equipment and software a sound investment for current learners as well as for those who will enroll in the program in the near future? Are there adequate technical support staff to assist students as they pursue literacy with the technology? Are personnel knowledgeable and available to provide hardware maintenance to ensure the learner's time is not wasted in troubleshooting bothersome equipment?

Previewing and acquisitioning newly produced computer and audiovisual software is critical to ensure that students are afforded the opportunity to work with materials that reflect current trends and contemporary standards of practice. Educators must take the time to search software catalogs and attend media showcase events to identify those programs that will offer learners the best possible educational experience. Software that provides interactivity, i.e., CAI and ILD, is encouraged because it promotes active participation, critical thinking, and problem-solving skills. Such activity denies passivity in student learning and furthers their understanding and long-term retention of principles and concepts.

Cost related to equipping and staffing a practice (or skills) laboratory is also very important to those responsible for allocating budgetary resources. Support for practicing psychomotor nursing skills is highly expensive, particularly if simulations using contemporary patient care equipment is a goal. Unless the student has the opportunity to use equipment and supplies that provide near-reality experience, it will have little meaning in the transfer of knowledge. Therefore, despite the cost, educators must ensure that simulations and practice laboratory experiences have as much realism as possible. Preceptors who are nonfaculty registered nurses staffing the laboratory are essential to reinforce learning and assist students in the hands-on applications of content studied through videotapes, texts, journals, CAI, and ILD. The salaries for these critical support positions is another cost consideration.

Readiness factor

A second major factor that may impede utilization of new technologies and related teaching strategies is a lack of readiness of either administrators or faculty (or both) to embody these pedagogically sound methods. Such reticence can be the result of fear of being replaced by the technology or fear of the technology itself. Reflection based on such questions as "Can the computer do what the teacher once did?", "Can I break the equipment?", or "How will the students think of me if I do break it or have difficulty using it?" complicate the educator's acceptance of technology. In addition, because many of today's technologies evolved after a large number of those faculty who are currently teaching completed their own education, they have neither seen the technologies modeled nor had relevant theoretical background preparing them for its use. One or more of these issues frequently places constraints on the desire to risk innovation in the classroom or in assigning outside-classroom work.

Another concern expressed by some teachers is that students will not learn unless the information is heard from the expert, i.e., the teacher. Faculty have failed to allow themselves the pleasure of shifting from the role of content giver to that of facilitator or resource person. Educational and nursing research documents that adult learners, a category in which nursing students are considered, will rise to the expectations of the teacher. Those expectations developed as clearly stated course objectives and programmatic outcomes set the plan for student progress. Once learners understand the criteria for successful completion of the program of study, they usually will complete the required and self-directed work.

Faculty and administrators will continue to be faced with their readiness to divert scarce budgetary resources toward meeting technologic needs. Such funding decisions, as mentioned earlier, should be based on the academic goals of the institution and department. Faculty also must "buy into" the benefits of new technology lest the electronics be purchased and remain unused. Well-planned training or inservice programs are of key importance in assisting faculty to develop their personal skill levels in using the technologies and in having a knowledge base on which to apply their use pedagogically.

In an effort to assist faculty and administrators to become more familiar with the potential for effective use of new technology, continuing education programs are offered by many universities and other entities that endeavor to stimulate innovative thinking in course delivery. While campus workshop efforts are extremely helpful and easily accessed, other sources are also available for nurse educators. For example, the National Institutes of Health, with special funding assistance from the Division of Nursing, Health, and Human Services, offered a series of workshops for nursing leaders in continuing education and staff development. Experts from the Lister Hill Center's Learning Center for Technology and the American

Journal of Nursing Company led the workshop with assistance for hands-on application from nurse facilitators selected from across the country who might later serve as resource people in dispersed geographic areas after participants returned to their homes and workplaces. Technology available for use in a "wet" carrel, an electronically equipped learning station, offered participants hands-on experience. ILD with various levels of interactivity, CAI, and CD-ROM software programs were demonstrated and used during the workshops. In addition, exposure to electronic computer networking quickly convinced participants that they, too, could implement this as a usable, efficient communication and information-gathering resource.

The Fuld Institute for Technology in Nursing Education and other somewhat more commercial vendors regularly offer programs throughout the country in the use of electronic technology. These workshops all contribute in preparing faculty and administrators toward becoming more familiar with the plethora of technologies available to them. Fears of being replaced by the technology are decreased as professionals are led to see more clearly the value of becoming less resistant to change, and of working *with* the technology to provide better student learning experiences. Such preparation encourages use of efficient, high-quality teaching aids and enhances the educator's readiness to implement use of these strategies.

COMPUTERS

While CAI has been in use for the last decade, computer conferencing has only recently gained momentum as universities increasingly seek efficient alternative ways to provide distance education to learners who are restricted to acquiring advanced degrees while remaining within the geographical area in which they live and work. Computer conferencing provides students and teachers a mechanism by which they can interact with one another without regard to time or place. It is defined by Halstead, Hayes, Reising, and Billings (1995) as using "the computer to establish a network on a mainframe or file server in which an unlimited number of individuals can communicate with each other using personal computers linked by a local or wide area network or modem" (p. 56). This technology is one example of providing connectivity between faculty and all students regardless of their learning site. A question posed by the teacher is responded to by all class members who will each have the opportunity to read their peers' answers. Dialogue across the miles is thus facilitated as learners acknowledge and reply to one anothers' comments at times convenient for them.

The use of computers to manage nursing education records or health care delivery records is an essential resource in today's educational infrastructure. Efficiency in gathering pertinent data related to student learning styles and past educational performance is imperative for the faculty member as he or she prepares to use various learning strategies. Similarly, relevant patient data is essential for the nurse to efficiently plan care for an individual or group. Doorley, Renner, and Corron (1994) have indicated that opportunities for students to have connectivity within their school to an actual hospital information system have "enhanced student motivation, professional socialization, the ability to understand the 'whole clinical picture,' and decreased [their] fear of computer technology" (p. 160). Such alliances between medical centers and colleges of nursing clearly lead the way for elevating student learning in the information age of the 21st century.

INTERACTIVE LASER DISC

Interactive laser discs and CD-ROM have provided opportunities for learner interactivity with the medium, thus increasing the potential for effective student assignments requiring skills of critical thinking and problem solving. Because most nursing students could be considered adult learners based on the usual age of those registered, it can be assumed that these enrollees bring with them to the school of nursing program a number of years of life experiences. Interactive technologies provide a mechanism and the potential for students to incorporate their previous cognition into their current learning activity. In addition, the student remains actively engaged in the learning process.

Effective use of interactive media places expectations on the teacher to serve as a facilitator or resource person. An understanding of the pedagogical advantages and disadvantages of the use of these technologies will be imperative for the faculty member to ensure that assignments are appropriate for meeting course objectives or outcome goals. Consideration should be given to using ILD or CD-ROM for exposure to new material, remediation, and "trigger" points for theory or course discussion. Faculty must have a comfortable working knowledge of the medium so they can assign the programs effectively or utilize them efficiently within a class session.

MULTIMEDIA

Educators recognize that there is increased student retention of content when more than one physiologic sense is stimulated. In the early years of audiovisual instruction, the combination of audio and motion film was the first step toward stimulating multiple senses in the learner. In the 1990s we find that the possibilities have increased considerably. Multimedia technology, in basic terms, refers to the use of more than a single medium. Presentations considered to be multimedia frequently involve computer and projected video or other motion imaging, slides, or audio. Such programs can be purchased commercially and used in their entirety, can be repurposed for use other than that for which they were initially intended, or authored as original programs. Since commercially developed programs may have an initially higher cost for purchase, they should be evaluated critically for content, organization, presentation style, and "fit" with course objectives. Conversely, to author one's own multimedia courseware can rarely be done with a high degree of sophistication unless a design team is available to do specific areas of the production. While the content is developed by the faculty member(s), the programming and visual and audio segments are best presented by those professionals who have expertise in these areas and are able to pull together the entire package. Dependent on institutional support or the financial resources available for this type of undertaking, it is frequently more expeditious to purchase commercially prepared multimedia courseware. Regardless of the origination of the software, "health care educators will need to incorporate multimedia training techniques as part of a multi-dimensional educational process" (Gleydura, Michelman, & Wilson, 1995, p. 169).

Although multimedia programs are usually considered to be a part of a formalized setting, such options also can be assigned as an effective "outside the classroom" curricular experience. Audiovisual laboratories equipped to provide multimedia services furnish an enriched instructional facility. Education and health care institutions should consider the benefits of having a well-planned and adequately supplied centralized location for the learner to view materials and interact with media designed for that purpose.

VIRTUAL REALITY

Within an early decade of the 21st century it is realistic to expect that nursing education will incorporate virtual reality experiences into undergraduate and graduate curricula. Such opportunities will allow students to actually practice psychomotor nursing skills on a simulator using the exact motor movements they would in the clinical setting. These scenarios will provide learners with the stimulation of conversation with the client in a replicated environment like that in which an actual clinical interaction would take place. Student recall in addition to responses to verbal and nonverbal cues will be incorporated into the learning experience.

Another form of "virtual learning" is already commonplace in higher education in the form of distance education. Colleges and universities have identified that providing education to learners who live and work in areas distant from the home campus can be an effective method of meeting educational needs in rural populations. Strategies that include interactive teleconferencing, satellite, audioconferencing, and computer conferencing are being implemented increasingly into nursing curricula throughout the country. Teaching in the "virtual university" will require modifications in the institution's infrastructure. Adjustments to traditional teaching methodologies and materials must be well planned by faculty as they prepare to offer distant didactic courses through one or more of the various technologies (Clark, 1993).

SUMMARY

To discuss new technologies and strategies one must both reflect on the past and consider futuristic opportunities. To relate technology to pedagogy one can simultaneously be alarmist and utopian. Never before have nurse educators faced such technological challenges—some of which have been and will continue to be a basis for restructuring colleges of nursing and the health care workplace. The new focus on student learning options and new approaches to communication among scholars can only serve to stimulate our creative abilities and endeavors. We must rise to the challenges presented in an effort to ensure that the best of times, indeed, can be the best of times!

REFERENCES

Clark, C.E. (1989). Telecourses for nursing staff development. *Journal of Nursing Staff Development, 5*(3), 107-109.

Clark, C.E. (1993). Beam me up, nurse! Educational technology supports distance education. *Nurse Educator, 18*(2), 18-22.

Doorley, J., Renner, A., & Corron, J. (1994). Creating care plans via modems: Using a hospital information system in nursing education. *Computers in Nursing, 12*(3), 160-163.

Gleydura, A., Michelman, J., & Wilson, C. (1995). Multimedia training in nursing education. *Computers in Nursing, 13*(4), 169-175.

Halstead, J., Hayes, R., Reising, D., & Billings, D. (1995). Nursing student information network: Fostering collegial communications using a computer conference. *Computers in Nursing, 13*(2), 55-59.

Heinich, R., Molenda, M., & Russell, J. (1993). *Instructional media and the new technologies of instruction* (4th ed.). New York: Macmillan.

Decreasing nursing education costs: Where is the bottom line?

PATRICIA R. FORNI, PAULETTE BURNS

Higher education is not experiencing the levels of funding achieved in past decades, nor will it in the foreseeable future. This forecast includes nursing education, which will continue to be faced with fluctuating enrollments and decreasing sources of revenue. Budgetary adjustments will have to be made if nursing is to meet its educational goals. The fact is that 33 states experienced budget cuts in higher education in fiscal year 1992 and 42 states cut budgets in fiscal year 1993. Given the federal budget deficit, little help can be expected from the federal government. Pressures from state legislators and higher education coordinating agencies for cost-effectiveness and accountability continue to mount.

Faculty productivity is being scrutinized in many states as a natural consequence of tightening resources. Former vice president of the education commission of the states Patrick M. Cullan, speaking on this issue, says, "Higher education is not going to be exempt from the economic, technological, and demographic pressures that are causing every type of institution we have to reconsider how to organize itself to get the job done" (Jacobson, 1992, p. A16). Nor is it any wonder that policymakers and taxpayers expect a reasonable return on their investment dollar when one considers that a sizable portion of state budgets go to higher education. Over $38 billion was spent in fiscal year 1991 for public colleges and universities according to Research Associates of Washington (Layzell, 1992, p. 82).

Faculty workload and productivity is only one facet of accountability that is being examined. Educational institutions across the nation are being asked to demonstrate "outcomes" as a requirement for academic accreditation as well as for funding allocations from legislatures and governments. Departments, schools, and colleges, by discipline, are being judged on aspects such as numbers of students, numbers of graduates, student credit hour production, faculty:student ratios, and funded research dollars per square foot of space. These challenges are being brought to bear while maintaining the quality of programs without regard to the resources needed and justified by tradition.

Academic programs are being called on increasingly to demonstrate innovative ways to achieve their goals within budget limitations. As a first step the educational program must decide how a budget reduction will be absorbed in relation to the three university missions of teaching, research, and service. The goals for productivity among the three missions must be determined as well. For example, faculty teaching workloads could be increased to allow fewer faculty to teach the same number of students. In this example, however, faculty research and service activities would of necessity be reduced in order to accommodate greater teaching loads. This issue is especially important to nursing because many schools are at a critical point in building research programs.

There are at least two strategies for addressing the challenge of shrinking budgets: increase revenue streams from other sources and/or decrease expenditures. These strategies must be considered in tandem with assumptions and goals about productivity and outcomes of the educational unit. For example, does a budget reduction mean decreased enrollment or could the status quo be maintained by doing the same with less?

For discussion purposes, we have made the following assumptions about the higher education funding picture:

1. For the foreseeable future, allocations of state and federal funds for higher education will not see great increases and, in fact, may be reduced.
2. Accountability for the use of public funds for educa-

tion will take on paramount importance in the public view.

3. The trend toward privatization of public-supported institutions of higher education will continue.
4. Higher education institutions will be forced to adopt new ways of achieving budgetary resources.
5. Part of the costs for higher education will be passed on to students through higher tuition and fees.
6. Demographic changes in society will have significant consequences for higher education.
7. Issues of program quality will have to be addressed in the face of shrinking budgetary resources.
8. Educational institutions or programs that fail to respond to the above-identified changes will be forced either to close or to reduce operations significantly.
9. The present focus on outcomes as a measure of productivity and quality will continue to be important for program funding.

Insofar as the strategies and assumptions discussed in this chapter are drawn from the public sector, they also apply to private institutions of higher education and may be considered for their use as well.

Nursing educators must address how they will meet these challenges if program viability is to be maintained. There is a general perception among some university administrators that nursing programs are expensive compared with programs in other academic disciplines. However, in a study of three baccalaureate nursing programs Melvin (1988) found that program costs were lower than the average instructional expenditures for full-time-equivalent (FTE) students in the respective universities. In a Canadian study, Roberts (1989) found that the cost of obtaining a baccalaureate degree in nursing was not significantly different from the mean cost of obtaining an honors arts degree and was below the cost of obtaining an honors science degree. In 1986 the American Association of Colleges of Nursing (AACN) undertook a study of the costs of generic baccalaureate nursing education. According to Kummer, Bednash, and Redman (1987) the study found that the three most important groups of variables in constructing costs were as follows: "1) faculty size and instructional costs including teaching load, salaries, and benefits; 2) student enrollment and curriculum patterns including student attrition; and 3) other institutional costs including support staff costs, direct instructional costs for nonnursing courses taken by nursing students, and indirect costs" (Kummer et al., 1987, p. 182).

The questions on the minds of educators and administrators are, Can nursing decrease the institutional costs of nursing education? If so, how and where is the bottom line? These questions will be explored under the two strategies of increasing revenues and decreasing expenditures.

INCREASING REVENUES

Given the first assumption stated above, any increase in revenues will likely not come from tax-supported sources. What, then, are the possible sources of revenue streams for nursing education? Sources of revenue include those external to the nursing unit and those that can be generated within the nursing unit. External sources include private foundations, individual donors including alumni and friends, Medicare pass-through funds, special arrangements with hospitals and health care agencies, and extramural grants and contracts. Internal sources of revenue include student tuition and fees, faculty practice, continuing education offerings, royalties, inventions, service contracts, and nurse-managed clinics and community nursing centers. Figure 25-1 suggests sources of revenue streams.

External sources of revenue

A number of large private foundations such as the W.K. Kellogg, Robert Wood Johnson, and Helene Fuld foundations typically fund programs of interest to nursing. Additionally, there are numerous small foundations that have funds for nursing education. Library resources containing data on funding priorities, amounts, application deadlines, and proposal formats can be consulted for more information. One such source is *The Foundation Directory* (1994), edited by Feczko, which provides authoritative sources of information on private philanthropic giving in each state.

Another revenue stream consists of monies and gifts from donors such as alumni, friends of nursing, and corporations. Many nursing education programs have not developed this source to its fullest potential. As part of their education, nursing students should be socialized that annual giving is a professional responsibility of alumni. Special fundraising events such as banquets, galas, and athletic events serve as revenue streams that can tap into donors other than alumni and gross considerable returns. Gifts such as bequests of property should not be overlooked as sources of revenue.

The phenomenon of privatization of public institutions is on the rise. Privatization refers to the fact that public-supported institutions are increasingly turning to private

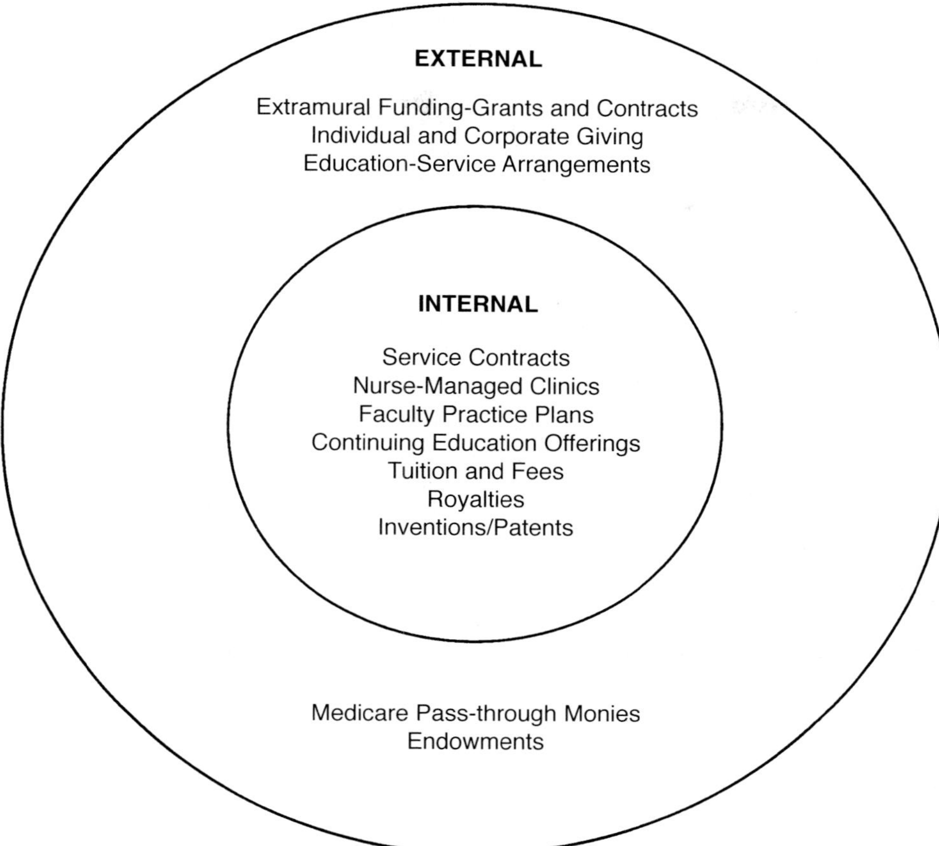

Fig. 25-1. Sources of revenue streams.

donors, money-making enterprises, and tuition for support as state allocations continue to shrink (Blumenstyk, 1992).

Medicare pass-through monies are available to some nursing programs through their affiliating hospitals. This money is derived from Medicare funds ". . . for those portions of direct education costs that reflect the average Medicare patient population of hospital services" (Frank, 1990). Funds are allocated to hospitals and are used to help defray the costs of educating health professionals. According to a study by Aiken and Gwyther (1995), Medicare pass-through monies represent the single largest source of federal funding for nursing. However, the majority of funds ($114 million or 66%) went to support diploma programs. Moreover, 48% of these funds went to just three states (Pennsylvania, New Jersey, and Ohio).

Education-service arrangements provide links between nursing programs and hospitals or other service agencies for purposes of funding faculty or staff positions, e.g., to provide clinical supervision of students, for academic advisement, or for other academic needs. Joint appointments are an example of such arrangements. The University of Oklahoma College of Nursing had such an arrangement with its University-affiliated hospital to fund an academic counselor's position and for clinical supervision of two groups of undergraduate students.

Endowments are sources of money from generous benefactors that are set up in perpetuity. Income from endowments is derived from the interest earnings on the principal. Endowed monies usually are earmarked for purposes specified by the donors. Some states have matching fund programs whereby private donations are matched with state funds. Endowed chairs in nursing are on the increase. According to data on institutional resources and budgets (AACN, 1991), 57 schools of nursing reported endowed chairs, ranging from one to six, with a range of monies from $10,000 to $2,137,225.

Endowments, while providing additional support, do not provide predictable funding because interest income fluctuates with the economy.

Extramural funding through research and training grants and contracts is another source of revenue. This funding can provide both direct and indirect cost recovery funds. Direct costs are those associated with the conduct of the grant or contract such as salaries, equipment, travel, and supplies. Indirect costs are administrative costs and are figured as a percentage of the direct costs. These monies are intended for use to support grant activities. For example, indirect cost recovery monies may be allocated throughout the institution to extend support of other research efforts in order to generate more funds. These monies may be used for secretarial assistance, research assistants, purchase of equipment, and other support of further research efforts.

Internal sources of revenue

The sources of revenue streams discussed so far have been external to the institution and the nursing unit. What revenue streams can the nursing unit generate?

Tuition is the major source of revenue for educational institutions: more students mean more tuition. Nationwide, there is a growing dependence on tuition as a major source of income. Yet in most state institutions, tuition covers only a portion of total costs for in-state students. In 1960 tuition accounted for 17.7% of the total cost of instruction and support, and this rose to 24.8% in 1990 (Blumenstyk, 1992). In general, tax-supported institutions are formula-funded, which is tied to student enrollments in terms of FTEs and student credit hours produced. Unlike most other academic disciplines, but like many health profession disciplines, nursing is limited in the number of students it can enroll, primarily because of the required student:faculty ratios for clinical experiences and the availability of clinical sites for practicums. Over time, enrollments in nursing programs have vacillated from extreme declines experienced in the mid-1980s to record highs experienced in the early 1990s. Billingsly (1991) reported that some colleges have assessed students in the health professions additional costs and concludes that this may be a future trend for nursing.

Student fees serve as another source of revenue to support operating budgets. Schools have implemented fees for various program components such as computer use, nursing skills laboratory, program application, and equipment.

Traditionally, medical schools have relied on income from faculty practice plans to support large portions of their budgets, whereas nursing has relied primarily on allocations from the parent institution for budget support. In the future, nursing faculty practice plans may be looked on as a major source of income for the nursing unit. In the Houston Linkage Model at the University of Texas School of Nursing, Houston, faculty practice occurs on a contractual basis (Starck, Walker, & Bohannan, 1991). In a personal communication in June 1995, Dean Patricia Starck reported, "Faculty practice including revenues from the nurse run clinic and a satellite is generating around $1,000,000 per year. There has been a shift from hospital-based practice to ambulatory/community care." The AACN (1991) reports that 53 schools have written practice plans.

Continuing education offerings, if managed carefully, may provide another source of income to nursing programs. Many continuing education programs are self-supporting and realize profits. Contracting with large organizations, for example, to provide learning packages for employees is a revenue source because many service agencies are decreasing their in-house staff development programs. In states where continuing education in nursing is mandatory, universities have a potential earning opportunity.

Royalties from publications, production of computer software programs, videos, and packaged learning materials developed by faculties could also serve as a revenue source for the nursing unit. Patents for inventions are another source of revenue. However, they are subject to the rules and regulations of the governing institution and revenues derived from this source may have to be shared.

Nurse-managed clinics operated on a fee-for-service or capitated basis are growing in numbers. Under managed care arrangements a fixed amount of reimbursement is allocated to the provider on a per-member (capitated) basis. The potential for income generation from nurse-managed clinics is on the increase. This is in part a function of reimbursement for nursing services being available from third-party payers including Medicare and Medicaid. According to the AACN (1991), nurse clinics and centers were operant in 76 schools of nursing with sources of support from internal schools of nursing funds, fees for service, grants, free space, and others. Increasing revenue streams is in consonance with Hegevary's (1992) ideas for diversifying schools' funding to survive economic slumps. An additional resource on nursing centers is a National League for Nursing publication of the proceedings of the Seventh National Conference on Nursing Centers (Murphy, 1995).

Service contracts are arrangements for specific services

such as provision of health assessments for employees of private corporations, health assessments for HeadStart or day care for children and mental health services. These types of services, which focus on prevention, are increasingly in demand as the nation moves toward managed care and monies for illness care are limited.

REDUCING EXPENDITURES

Expenditures are a function of many factors including mission and goals, type and size of the parent institution, nursing organizational structure and curriculum organization, and number and level of programs offered by the academic unit. The box lists suggested sources of cost savings.

Nursing units that exist in large research institutions have different expectations for scholarship than those located in small liberal arts colleges. Accordingly, the costs for meeting their respective missions and goals are different. In institutions where the major focus is on teaching, the costs of operating the nursing program are generally less.

Organizational structure

The organizational structure of the academic unit determines how many administrative and support staff are required to carry out the functions of the program. As a general rule, the more complex the structure, the more costly it is to run. Reductions can be achieved by simplifying the structure and reducing administrative and staff positions. How much administrative time is allocated to carry out the mission of the academic unit? Can responsibilities be consolidated? Does the nurse administrator have instructional as well as administrative responsibilities?

Consortial arrangements whereby several institutions join forces to offer a degree program have been developed in some states. These arrangements are cost-effective in that they avoid duplication of programs and conserve state resources. The University Center at Tulsa is such an arrangement. The University Center at Tulsa is a consortium of four state universities offering unduplicated undergraduate and graduate programs. The University of Oklahoma College of Nursing is designated to offer the master's degree in nursing at this site.

If the nursing unit has a continuing education program or nurse-managed center, are they self-supporting or do they require funding from the nursing budget? How are the faculty organized? How many committees are there, what is their membership requirement, and what is the frequency of meetings? Faculty time (as spent in committee meetings) is a valuable resource. A school could calculate the number of hours spent in meetings, place a dollar figure on this use of time, and then ask the question, does the outcome justify the cost? All of these questions have bearing on costs associated with organizational structure.

SOURCES OF COST SAVINGS

- Organizational structure
- Curriculum organization
- Student body size/characteristics
- Faculty/staff size/characteristics
- Workload policy
- Material resources
- Instructional costs
- Staffing practices
- Teaching methodologies

Curriculum organization

Curriculum organization, including length of the nursing major, the number and type of specialties available, and levels of programs affects costs in many ways. The lengthier the program, the more costly it is in terms of personnel requirements. The more career tracks offered within a program level, the more costly the program is to run. For example, the master's curriculum at the University of Oklahoma College of Nursing requires 38 to 48 semester credit hours, but a total of 134 credit hours are required for the five specialty areas and four role preparation areas. Master's programs in the United States offer from 1 to 24 specialty areas and from 1 to 19 functional role areas (Burns et al., 1993). The more specialty tracks that are offered, the smaller the class size is per course. Small classes are expensive. Costs are also related to the levels of the programs offered. Master's and doctoral programs, requiring low student:faculty ratios with doctorally prepared faculty, are more costly than undergraduate programs. Thesis and dissertation guidance is labor-intensive for faculty and thus incurs costs. It would be interesting to compare thesis versus nonthesis costs in master's curricula.

Frequency of course offerings is another cost consideration. Low-enrollment master's courses could be scheduled less frequently, e.g., every other year, to provide for a larger enrollment and to free faculty for other activities. Multiple teaching and clinical sites also require additional resources.

Teaching methodologies can have a great impact on the budget. A plethora of nursing electives with low enrollments is a luxury most programs can no longer afford. Team teaching whereby a number of faculty sit in on all classes of one course is expensive and outdated. The least expensive method that provides the most credit hours is when one professor lectures to a large class. Expensive methodologies are those requiring special equipment and low enrollments, thus increasing faculty requirements.

Distance learning is a means to increase enrollment and tap into populations that would otherwise not be reached. Distance learning technology requires costs up front for purchase of equipment, faculty development, and support services but eventually results in increased revenues from tuition and fees.

Class size and mix are important cost factors. Class size may be increased by offering courses that are open to enrollment by nonmajors. Some nursing programs have developed nursing courses that are required of nonnursing majors. This strategy would be a consideration for increasing student credit hours, which are in turn tied to formula-funded budgets. On the other hand, costs can be reduced by limiting class size and downsizing programs.

Another cost consideration in undergraduate education is student mix with regard to generic vs. registered nurse students. In general, it is less costly to educate registered nurses because they do not require as extensive skills laboratory instruction as do generic students. Moreover, clinical supervision of registered nurses is not as labor-intensive in most clinical areas. At the graduate level nurse practitioner programs are more expensive to operate because they require more resources in terms of equipment and personnel.

Student:faculty ratios are cited as the most costly component of nursing education. According to the 1974 Institute of Medicine study on education costs in the health professions, student:faculty ratios were found to be the major source of variation in baccalaureate nursing program costs. Higher costs were associated with lower student:faculty ratios (Melvin, 1988). Because of the nature of the nursing discipline, requiring close supervision of students in the clinical setting, this ratio cannot be increased significantly without jeopardizing safety and quality. Furthermore, boards of nursing in each state generally specify a maximum number of students per faculty member.

Another emerging consideration in the supervision of undergraduate students is related to changes in the health care delivery system, i.e., the dramatic reduction in acute care beds resulting in shrinking clinical sites for student learning. It has yet to be resolved how the supervision of students in nonacute care settings such as homes, clinics, and schools will be managed and how it will be funded. For example, the current model of having one faculty member supervise 8 to 12 students in one place at one time will no longer apply.

The ratio of laboratory to credit hours is another cost factor. The more contact hours faculty spend in clinical laboratory, the more costly it will be. A related factor is the number and ratio of clinical credits required in the curriculum. Using a 1:3 ratio, a course with 4 hours of clinical credit would require 12 contact hours of supervision per week per academic term, whereas using a 1:4 ratio, a course with 4 hours of clinical credit would require 16 contact hours per week per academic term. In the future, a more efficient method of achieving clinical learning objectives may be through clinical simulations using advanced technology. The concept of "virtual reality" is another strategy that may help to reduce faculty workload strain with regard to helping students meet clinical objectives. It is predicted that ". . . there will be virtual hospital units, nursing homes, communities, patients, and families" (Anonymous, 1991).

Insofar as students require remediation, cost factors increase because of the faculty time involved in helping students. However, student retention and graduation rates are extremely important in an era in which outcome measures are being used to evaluate program effectiveness and determine funding.

Personnel costs

The largest cost category in any educational budget is personnel. Dienemann (1983) suggested options for reducing faculty workload: changing class size, supplementing full-time faculty with other types of personnel, and changing classes from one location to another. Cost variables include number of faculty, faculty rank mix, faculty tenure mix, faculty turnover and longevity, and length of contracts. Faculty salaries are related to all of these variables. One can assume that tenured faculty at the higher ranks who have the longest time in service will usually be paid the most. Mix refers to the proportion of individuals in each category so that a large proportion of professors would cost more as would a large proportion of tenured faculty. High faculty turnover is expensive because replacement is costly. Faculty contracts may vary from 9 to 12 months and costs vary proportionately. The same applies to full-time vs. part-time employees not only in relation to salaries but also to the fringe benefits covered.

Cost is also related to the number and type of staff required to meet program goals. The practice of using graduate teaching assistants is cost-effective because it frees higher paid faculty for other activities. How much of the academic support services does nursing provide for its programs? If the nursing unit has responsibility for recruitment, advisement, and financial aid, for example, then the costs will be greater than for programs in which this is handled centrally.

Faculty requirements (numbers) are closely tied to workload. When faculty carry heavy teaching loads, fewer faculty are required for instruction. Workload policies should permit attainment of the mission and goals of the nursing unit as well as the requirements for faculty promotion and tenure. To illustrate, in a 36 credit hour master's curriculum with one specialty track using a teaching workload of 6 credit hours per semester for graduate faculty, six faculty would be required. Using a workload of 9 credit hours, four faculty would be required. Assuming faculty were at the associate professor rank at salaries of $48,000, the cost savings in the latter example would be $96,000.

The use of part-time faculty to provide clinical supervision of students is also cost-effective. In many situations, staff nurses serve as mentors or preceptors at no cost to the academic unit. The benefits to service agencies when staff nurses serve as mentors or preceptors need to be taken into account when negotiating these arrangements. Studies reported by Hawken and Hillestad (1987) and Starck and Williams (1988) conclude that service agencies gain tangible resources through these collaborations.

Other cost factors

A number of expense categories can be manipulated to reduce costs. These include instructional materials, computer hardware and software, library, laboratory, research, equipment, supplies, communications, travel, printing, renovation, and repair.

Factors external to the institution that affect costs are accreditation and requirements imposed by state boards of nursing under the rules and regulations of nursing practice acts.

Other considerations

"It takes money to make money" may be a cliché but it is true. In order to generate revenue it is sometimes necessary to spend money up front. For example, student recruitment is a necessary first step in attracting students to an institution for purposes of increasing enrollment. Costs associated with recruitment include travel, development of brochures or other promotional materials, personnel time, and communication costs. Fund raising can be profitable but requires similar resources in terms of personnel, communications, and public relations activities. Grantsmanship is a labor-intensive endeavor with associated costs, but the payoff in terms of funded grants or contracts is well worth the effort.

Demographic changes will have important effects on higher education in the following ways. The average age of students in nursing is increasing. Registered nurses and licensed practical nurses are returning to school in increasing numbers to attain higher degrees. These factors are forcing nursing programs to develop innovative means for these nontraditional students to meet their educational goals such as weekend and evening classes, accelerated tracks, and tracks for second-career students.

Moreover, funding is affected in another way in that older taxpayers are exhibiting reluctance to support a system of education that competes with dollars for health care, a matter of more immediate concern to them (Yudof, 1992, p. A48). Nursing educators should not lose sight of the fact that investors in higher education (taxpayers) want an accounting of the returns on their investments and want to know that their tax dollars are being used in the most efficient manner possible. In the future accountability for faculty time and effort will be scrutinized more closely. Productivity will be measured in outcomes such as graduation rates, student credit hours produced, and funded research dollars. Geitgey (1982) urges nursing educators to become more involved in politics and public policy formation in order to influence state and federal funding decisions.

Any discussion of cost cutting should take into consideration quality issues. It is incumbent on the individual institution to determine which cost-effective measures can be undertaken without compromising the educational outcomes of the program. In this chapter, we have demonstrated that there are sources of revenue streams for nursing education programs to pursue and there are cost-savings measures that can be employed. Nursing can respond creatively to the budgetary challenges of the future through implementation of innovative strategies and ideas.

The bottom line is that nursing must become more proactive in generating new revenue streams, more efficient in containing costs, and more diligent in achieving quality. A further consideration and one that is paramount in the context of costs of nursing education has to do with the number and level of nursing programs that are needed to meet current and future health care needs. We believe that the number of baccalaureate and advanced practice nursing programs needs to be *increased* while the number of associate degree and diploma programs needs to be *decreased.* This position is based on the facts that (a) the setting for health care delivery is shifting from institutions to the community; (b) emphasis is being placed increasingly on health promotion and disease prevention; (c) primary care is expanding; and (d) reengineering of organizations and systems is occurring. All of these changes require nurses educated at baccalaureate and higher levels.

REFERENCES

Aiken, L.H., & Gwyther, M.E. (1995). Medicare funding of nurse education. *Journal of the American Medical Association, 273*(19), 1528-1532.

American Association of Colleges of Nursing. (1991). *Institutional resources and budgets.* Washington, DC: Author.

Anonymous. (1991). Virtual reality: A technology in nursing education's future. *Nursing Educators Microworld, 5*(3), 17, 19.

Billingsley, M. (Winter, 1991). Hard times all around. *Nursing Connections, 4*(4), 13-14.

Blumenstyk, G. (1992, May 13). College officials and policy experts ponder implications of 'privatizing' state colleges. *Chronicle of Higher Education,* A25-27.

Burns, P.G., Nishikawa, H.A., Weatherby, F., Forni, P.R., Moran, M., Baker, C.M., Booton, D.A., & Allen, M.E. (1993). Master's degree nursing education: State-of-the-art. *Journal of Professional Nursing, 9*(5), 267-277.

Dienemann, J. (1983). Reducing nursing faculty workloads without increasing costs. *Image: The Journal of Nursing Scholarship, 15*(4), 111-114.

Feczko, M. (Ed.). (1994). *The foundation directory* (16th ed.). New York: The Foundation Center.

Frank, K.M. (1990). Funding for nursing education: Passthrough or pass over? *Nursing Economics, 8*(3), 132.

Geitgey, D. (1982). Financing nursing education: A public perspective. In *Economics of higher education in nursing* (pp. 13-14). Washington, DC: American Association of Colleges of Nursing.

Hawken, P.L., & Hillestad, E.A. (1987). Weighing the costs and benefits of student education to service agencies. *Nursing & Health Care, 8*(4), 223-227.

Hegevary, S.T. (1992). Funding of schools of nursing. *Journal of Professional Nursing, 8*(3), 142.

Hines, R. (1992). State higher education appropriations: A retrospective of fiscal year 1993. *Grapevine, 34*(384), 3137.

Jacobson, R.L. (1992, April 15). Colleges face new pressure to increase faculty productivity. *The Chronicle of Higher Education,* A1, 16-18.

Kummer, K., Bednash, G., & Redman, B.K. (1987). Cost model for baccalaureate nursing education. *Journal of Professional Nursing, 3*(3), 176-189.

Layzell, D.T. (1992, February 19). Tight budgets demand studies of faculty productivity. *The Chronicle of Higher Education,* B2-3.

Melvin, N. (1988). A method for the comparative analysis of the instructional costs of three baccalaureate nursing programs. *Journal of Professional Nursing, 4*(4), 249-261.

Murphy, B. (Ed.). (1995). *Nursing centers: The time is now.* New York: National League for Nursing.

Roberts, P.M. (1989). An estimate of the cost of educating a BN graduate and graduates of other disciplines at a Canadian university: A case study. *Journal of Nursing Education, 28*(3), 140-143.

Starck, P.L., Walker, G.C., & Bohannan, P.A. (1991). Nursing faculty practice in the Houston linkage model: Administrative and faculty perspectives. *Nurse Educator, 16*(5), 23-28.

Starck, P.L., & Williams, W.E. (1988). What does nursing education cost? Turning the question around. *Journal of Professional Nursing, 4*(1), 38-44.

Yudof, M.G. (1992, May 13). The burgeoning privatization of state universities. *The Chronicle of Higher Education,* A48.

Development of models of international exchange to upgrade nursing education

MARY V. FENTON

WHY INTERNATIONAL EXCHANGE?

International exchange is becoming a reality for many schools and colleges of nursing that would not have considered it as part of their scope 5 or 10 years ago. Rapid changes in our world are not only facilitating more international exchange but demanding it. Barriers have fallen and borders have changed almost overnight, and many countries, including the United States, are placing a greater priority on nursing as an underutilized health care resource. Because of more international conferences and the availability of international travel, nurses from all over the world are meeting colleagues in other countries and discovering that nursing speaks a common language regardless of the country, native language, or culture. This has led to increased interest in learning about other countries' health care systems and nursing education programs. Many of the foreign nursing students who came to the United States for nursing master's and doctoral degrees in the 1970s, 1980s, and 1990s have returned to their countries to provide nursing leadership. Thus, the development of an exchange program with a foreign university or ministry of health is often facilitated by an initial contact with a nurse administrator or faculty member who has studied in the United States.

Many pressing reasons exist for international exchange in nursing education. First, the increase in immigration and travel has greatly increased the ethnic diversity of our population, and U.S. nurses are providing care for patients with a wide variety of customs, beliefs, and health practices. This diversity often leads to frustration and values conflicts. There is a tremendous need for students and nurses to have multicultural experiences, which can be provided through international exchange programs. Second, the last decade has brought about an explosion of knowledge in the biomedical sciences. Today's nurses and nursing students all over the world face a far more complex environment requiring advanced clinical skills in both acute and primary care settings. Third, in many countries, both developing and developed, people still do not have access to basic health care including disease prevention and health promotion. International exchange can address this problem directly by making possible the sharing of models and concepts for the development and implementation of community-based primary health programs.

The impact of a global economy

The international trend toward a global economy is also influencing nursing education and practice. The North American Free Trade Agreement (NAFTA) and the European Common Market are increasing not only the exchange of products but also the exchange of workers and cultures. A global economy promotes common goods and services and shared occupational hazards and concerns as well as more similar day-to-day experiences and health practices for those affected by the agreements (Naisbit & Aburdene, 1990). Nurses outside the United States are already responding to these changes. For example, because of the existing regional markets, regional nursing associations, such as the Asociacion Latinoamericana de Escuelas y Facultades de Enfermeria (ALADEFE), i.e., the Association of Latin American Schools and Nursing Faculties, the Federacion Panamericana de Enfermeras (FEPEN), i.e., the Federation of Panamerican Nurses, and the Fundacion Ibero-americana de Enfermeria (FIDE) have been created. ALADEFE is using the existing market regions in the Americas to create chapters and has named them according to geographic regions: Andean Market, Central American Market, South Market, Caribbean Market, and NAFTA Region. FIDE includes ALADEFE and

FEPEN from South America and Concejo de Enfermeria de España (Spain) from the European community. The purpose of these groups is to foster nursing collaboration among the countries, cultures, and institutions involved through networking.

The implications of a global economy on nursing are great. The global economy has increased the availability of electronic communication both with and within less developed countries. Unfortunately, in order to take advantage of electronic communication, nurses from less developed countries still may need to travel long distances to attain training or information that is not yet available through computer-based systems. Access to electronic communication enables nurses in less developed countries to gain information to respond to changes in health needs. Life expectancy has increased, resulting in the increased incidence of chronic diseases and disabilities, which are becoming more of a major concern for health professionals. New discoveries in the biomedical field are leading to new techniques for diagnosis and treatment of old and new diseases. Environmental pollution and occupational hazards resulting from deregulation of environmental protection acts in some countries provide new health risk factors. Ethical considerations are increasing in importance as genetic researchers find more ways to prevent or treat diseases. Availability of the latest information empowers nurses to assume more responsibilities such as translating scientific information into lay terminology for the populations they serve.

The continuing need for international exchange

Access to basic health care has become an even bigger issue at both the consumer and political levels in the United States. For example, the United States no longer ranks at the top for common health statistics such as infant mortality. In 1918, with an infant mortality rate of 77 per 1000 live births, the United States ranked 6th in the world for the lowest death rates (Mason, 1991). By 1993, the infant mortality rate had been reduced to 8.3 per 1000—a vast improvement, but a rate that now places the United States 22nd in international rankings (Wegman, 1994). This may be more of a reflection of our increased ability to save sick babies than to produce healthy ones (Mason, 1991). The overall infant mortality rate, too, is misleading if specific ethnic minorities are studied. Black infants, for example, are twice as likely as white infants to be born preterm, to be of low birth weight, and to die at birth (Behrman, 1995). These statistics become even more significant if we accept Assistant Secretary for Health Mason's assertion that "a nation's infant mortality rate is a measure of its success in combating poverty, ignorance, and disease" (Mason, 1991, p. 475).

Mason's assertion raises the question of why the United States, with its vast resources and health care expenditures, has health indices worse than many developing countries. One answer can be found by looking at the deteriorating infrastructure of our health care system. For the past 10 to 15 years, many basic public health disease prevention and health promotion programs have been cut at the federal, state, and local levels and literally made unavailable to much of the population. This policy was carried out in the United States at the same time that many developing countries were developing programs that focused less on high technology and more on the provision of basic primary health care to the population. These programs had to be cost-effective because of the lack of available resources. Therefore, you will find developing countries with immunization rates for children that exceed that of the United States. For example, in the United States as of 1991, state vaccination rates for children 1 to 4 years of age for measles, rubella, diphtheria, polio, and mumps ranged from 58.9% to 64.9%, although technically speaking, 90% of all children "have access" to immunization (National Center for Health Statistics, 1992). Some individual cities and large urban areas had even much lower rates. In Houston, for example, the rate of immunization in 1991 for 1- to 4-year-old children was an alarming 11%, and while in 1995 the rate has increased to 64% for school-age children, for the most part immunization of toddlers is difficult to track (SoRelle, 1995). Even with increased emphasis on immunization, reported cases of measles alone have more than doubled since 1970 (National Center for Health Statistics, 1992). Therefore, both developing and developed countries have much to learn from each other about health care and the education of health professionals.

Efforts at health care reform in the United States in 1994 brought primary health care into the discussions of health care providers, educators, and policymakers. The collapse of health care reform led to a highly competitive managed care system based on rationing care, insuring the healthy, and discouraging those more likely to be ill—the poor—from using the system. The United States has gone from being the world model for public health policy and structure in the early and mid-20th century to one of "disarray" that must be redefined and restructured if we are to assume that a healthy population will move into the 21st century. A focus on primary health care is critical to addressing problems here in the United States and worldwide. Alternative models of health care with appropriate technology are needed to demonstrate that in many situations more can be done with less.

THE ROLE OF NURSING AND HIGHER EDUCATION

With the U.S. system of health care no longer affordable or accessible to many segments of the population, nurses functioning in both traditional and advanced practice roles are being utilized in more and more diverse ways. They cost less than physicians and can perform a wider range of responsibilities appropriate to meet primary care needs. Thus, nurses prepared for advanced clinical nursing roles are in higher demand than ever before, and many legal barriers to advanced nursing practice from the past are disappearing primarily because of economic reasons. The situation is right for nurses to move toward more active participation in shaping a system that will be effective in meeting the needs of the population. This fact, however, is not enough on which to base a newer, better, more efficient system. Serious deficiencies and the focus of our delivery system are difficult issues for a country that has always considered its health care system as the "biggest and best."

Since the end of World War II, world politics and health care have undergone a radical transformation, and the late 1980s and 1990s will be remembered as a time when whole nations and people demanded rapid change. One of the most difficult aspects of rapid evolution is general confusion as to which direction to go and who should lead. Backman, as early as 1983, asserts in *Approaches to International Education* that if Americans are to be able to understand and cope with the changing environment, "the higher education community should—in fact, must—take the lead in developing international education programs" (Backman, p. XIV, 1984). However, in the United States as elsewhere, funding is scarce for development and sustenance of such programs, and the bulk of the burden for development and implementation of programs will fall directly to institutional leaders and participating faculty (Backman, 1984). If we are going to utilize some of the successful experiences of our colleagues in other countries in developing cost-effective and accessible systems of health care to restructure our own system, there will be a need to research, evaluate, present, and publish these ideas and systems in order to promote change. Higher education institutions, including schools of nursing, are logical choices because these educational programs will produce the health care leaders of tomorrow, and they must be prepared to understand health care as it relates to people all over the world.

In summary, as we near the century mark, we have as a nation reached a crisis in health care. It has become unaffordable, and while managed care promises to decrease costs, the verdict is out as to whether it will provide adequate access to quality care. Having fallen behind in meeting many basic health needs of the population, we are increasingly forced to look internationally for health care models. Nurses have a vital role to play in primary health care in both developing and developed countries. International exchange is a viable method of increasing our knowledge and ability to meet the needs of our population, and to educate nurses prepared to deal with life and nursing practice in the future.

DEVELOPMENT OF MODELS OF INTERNATIONAL EXCHANGE

There are a wide range of models of international exchange in schools of nursing today. These may range from individual efforts by faculty and largely informal contacts with individuals overseas to more highly formalized models with university agreements and contracts spelling out specific objectives and even including international exchange as a mission of the school. Activities may include faculty exchange or consultation, project and research collaboration on common problems, joint publications, sharing of ideas and resources, student exchange and sharing of courses, materials, and resources from both institutions.

Many issues are encountered in the development and implementation of an international educational exchange program. Some key questions include: How does a school of nursing committed to development of an international educational exchange program identify resources for funding and planning and use them most efficiently? How can the use of scarce resources for international exchange be justified? Is it possible to work within the existing academic system? How do faculty and students become involved and committed to such a program? Should the program stand alone in the nursing school or be integrated into the overall university program if one exists? How should institutional goals and objectives be designed? How could a program be designed to meet the needs of the institution, faculty, administration, and students? (Backman, 1984). In addition to these general questions, schools of nursing have additional concerns. First, this is a time of diminishing budget support for higher education and a time of competition for available funds. Finding funding is often difficult and may require creative financing ideas. Second, nursing is a discipline that requires complex licensing and registration procedures in order for graduates to practice; therefore, to bring foreign students and visitors to the United States to gain educational and clinical experience often requires special policies and in some states may be considered illegal unless the person is licensed in the United States.

In order to deal with these issues, great commitment on the part of faculty and nursing school deans is required. Numerous models have been developed and implemented for international exchange in schools of nursing with various degrees of success. The most important concept is that the model be feasible, for no two institutions or schools will or should have identical programs, if only because no two institutions can or will have the same needs or populations. Some schools have been able to integrate international health concepts into their programs and activities, while others have treated it as a separate entity.

International faculty exchange

An international faculty exchange program between schools of nursing is a two-way street. Although the transfer of high-tech acute care knowledge may be seen as flowing primarily one way from the United States, the transfer of knowledge about using less invasive, less expensive, and less intense methods may be flowing primarily in the opposite direction. It is often surprising to U.S. nurses to discover that many less technological methods obtain equivalent results when compared with outcomes of health care in the U.S. Therefore, visits and discussions with colleagues from other countries often stimulate thinking about more creative and less expensive ways to provide health care.

Faculty often return from an international consulting visit with more questions about the U.S. health care system. They often become more politically astute about the role of women in society and the role of nursing in health care and come to the realization that until those inequities are addressed, "health for all" will probably only remain a slogan and unattainable goal. Faculty are exposed to a wealth of information relating to health such as World Health Organization (WHO) programs and publications, and by incorporating this information into their curricula, are able to create a more common language for working with schools in other countries. Because of the more centralized government-controlled systems of health care in countries other than the United States, nurses from other countries have been more exposed to WHO's goals, policies, and information than have U.S. nurses.

U.S. faculty also come face-to-face with the influence that nursing in this country has had on nursing education abroad. Because the United States has often taken the lead in development and innovation of nursing education, many countries have adopted U.S. curriculum models that may or may not have relevance for nursing in other countries. One may also see either outdated or even brand new equipment and technology sitting in classrooms with no one trained to use it, no repair or parts available, or in the case of computers, no software to run on it or no printer. The problems of exporting inappropriate technology without knowing the setting or needs of the country or situation become evident. As a result, faculty begin to question the appropriateness of their own curriculum and teaching methodologies not only for the United States, but for other countries as well.

One example of this is the export of U.S. nursing theory as the basis for conceptualization of nursing school curricula and research. In most cases, U.S. nursing theorists did not expect their theories to be used as the basis for developing curricula. However, during the 1970s and early 1980s many schools of nursing in the United States adopted developing nursing theories as the basis for their curricula. This use of theory sometimes resulted in disjointed, awkward, and confusing curriculum design that was difficult to transfer into learning experiences for students. When international graduate students and visiting faculty returned from U.S. schools to their countries, they attempted to use the theories, often with similar results. The result was that in many cases the new curriculum stayed on the shelf and was only shown to visiting dignitaries, and the old curriculum continued to be taught.

Research is another area in which international collaboration attempts have been made with various results. Long travel distances between collaborators, difficulties in both technical communication and communication related to language, cultural differences in understanding the research problem and design, and funding are just some of the issues that must be addressed if a successful project is to result. Having experienced the above problems in various attempts to initiate international research projects, the University of Texas Medical Branch School (UTMB) of Nursing through its WHO Collaborating Center for Nursing Development in Primary Health Care designed a primary care research program for nurses from Central and South American countries. Nurses are selected by their governments or universities to come to

Texas for a 5-week intensive course conducted in Spanish that is designed to assist them in developing research plans and proposals to address pressing health needs in their home countries. The emphasis is on identifying resources in their own countries to support the project as well as to identify technologically appropriate ways to communicate internationally to access needed information and assistance continuously as they develop and implement the project on their return.

This program has expanded with the participation of the UTMB Department of Family Medicine to include a family medicine physician as part of the team because it is obvious that no serious changes will occur in health care systems unless both medicine and nursing are involved and have similar goals. There is no one source of funding for this program. Funding comes from a variety of sources including the universities and governments involved, and the Pan American Health Organization (the WHO Regional Office for the Americas), which provides consultants during the programs. In addition, the UTMB School of Nursing donated time from many professionals and individuals who are interested in the program. All classes are either held in Spanish or with an interpreter and electronic translation equipment. This research course has responded not only to a need for more research development in Latin America but also to needs for culturally tailored information. Research education programs of this type are a valuable step in addressing many of the recent global transitions and their epidemiological fallout.

International exchange programs that concentrate on evaluation of the relevance and application of theory, research, and clinical practice to a country's needs could be very valuable if efforts are made to avoid the transfer of inappropriate technology and ideas. The term *cultural paternalism,* for example, was coined to refer to instances in which consultants from well-developed countries offer inappropriate counsel given the available financial, human, and infrastructural resources of their host country (Beunza, Boulton, Ferguson, & Serrano, 1994). Care must be devoted to determination of the participating countries' values, needs, and resources, particularly when disparities exist between and among the cultures involved. The exposure to other countries' primary health care models and projects has influenced the development of both inner city and rural models in this country by U.S. nursing faculty and students, demonstrating the leadership role of nursing in providing primary health care. The testing of U.S. nursing theories for relevance in other cultures and countries could also be a valuable step for developing more universal nursing theory related to health and response to disease.

International students

In 1994, 449,749 foreign students were enrolled in U.S. colleges and universities, the largest foreign population of students in the world (Davis, 1994). Many of these students are sponsored by their governments or home institutions in hopes that the education they gain will provide them with the professional, social, and personal skills required to play meaningful leadership roles in their societies. Many of these programs are successful, but when they are not, it is often due to students' difficulty in adaptation to U.S. culture (Gay, Edgil, & Stullenbarger, 1993; Lee, Abd-Ella, & Burks, 1981). To counter this problem, educational exchanges must be planned carefully. The first step after committing to develop an international exchange program is to assess the needs of the students, faculty, school, and institution and to identify the available resources.

Providing an international exchange program for students can range from accepting foreign students into the program, to taking and accepting students on exchange visits either for short or long periods of time, to arranging for preceptorships for students in other countries. All of these experiences will broaden and enrich the knowledge and understanding of students from all countries. For example, in collaboration with faculty from the University of Nuevo Leon School of Nursing in Monterrey, Mexico, the UTMB School of Nursing conducted a community health elective for undergraduate students in Mexico. The program consisted of intensive preparation classes including information on culture, customs, and simple Spanish phrases before leaving the United States, and then classes and community health clinical experiences with faculty and students from Nuevo Leon. The majority of students who took the elective were RN-BSN students, most of whom had considerable nursing experience in the United States. For many of them, it was not only an experience in culture shock but also a turning point in their careers. They came home convinced that they could do a better job of providing health care, even with fewer resources. They also had a better appreciation of the origins and experiences of many of their patients from Mexico and the border areas of Texas. They were proud of their ability to cope with all the situations they encountered, although at the time they were not sure they would be able to do so. If you asked them today what was one of the most significant learning experiences they had while earning their BSN, they would all say their elective in Mexico. The fact is that even though faculty may try to create experiences to challenge students and to make them critically evaluate our health care system, an international experience makes that happen.

Most schools of nursing have students enrolled who are not necessarily classified as international students because they are U.S. citizens but may be first- or second-generation Americans who are still highly influenced by their family and country of origin. These students provide a wonderful resource for any international exchange program because not only are they interested in meeting people from their own countries and others but their knowledge of other customs and cultures as well as that of the United States is invaluable. In addition, there are students who either have an interest or have traveled or lived in other countries who are interested in interacting with international visitors or working or international projects. Recognizing this, the UTMB School of Nursing organized a student association to give students a means of participating in the school's international activities. The organization is called the Student Ambassadors for International Nursing. Students who participate receive an orientation and volunteer to assist in a variety of activities. Many of these activities are social in nature and enjoyed by both visitors and students alike. Many of the students already speak Spanish as a first or second language so they are of great assistance to our visitors from Central and South America. The students gain insight into the nature of international collaboration as well as knowledge of health care problems and issues around the world.

An international exchange program brings a nursing school faculty and students face to face with the policies of the U.S. government. For many faculty and students, it is often the first time they have been exposed to any viewpoint other than that of the United States. In many cases the experience is positive, but in other situations it may be negative. It often results in the development of more political awareness and interest in the U.S. role in world politics both nationally and internationally. For example, faculty and students have become aware that the United States does not discourage U.S. companies from aggressively developing new markets for cigarettes in developing countries in which the principal targets are young people and women. This has happened concurrently with the outlawing of most cigarette advertising in the United States and more stringent control over second-hand smoke. A second example is the U.S. policy that allows the exportation of pesticides that have been banned in the United States because of their harmful effects on the people and environment. Awareness of such policies can raise faculty and students' awareness of the connection between politics, economics, and health care policy in their own communities and states.

Funding of international exchange

Over the last 30 years, many state and private universities have implemented international education programs with the assistance of the federal government and private foundations such as Carnegie, Kellogg, Rockefeller, and, prior to 1970, the Ford Foundation (Backman, 1984). The emphasis on international affairs in the 1940s resulted in the development of international assistance programs in the early 1950s, particularly through the Federal Operations Administration, which awarded contracts to several large universities to develop and implement programs. After 1960, the United States Agency for International Development continued this unique role (Backman, 1984).

However, many successful international programs are not the result of large grants from private foundations and U.S. governmental agencies. Many programs are supported on an individual project-by-project plan by the schools themselves. For example, a successful short-term faculty exchange program can be conducted by simple agreements between the two schools involved. In many situations, the institution sending the faculty member continues to pay his or her salary and also for airfare and travel expenses while the host school provides housing and transportation. The faculty member is responsible for paying for food and incidentals. This does not put a great drain on either institution to find large amounts of new money and yet can result in a very successful exchange. Longer term exchange programs may require the assistance of private foundations and government agencies. Another way to fund a successful program is to write grants jointly to fund programs that benefit both schools. This can be especially effective when U.S. schools can provide technical and writing assistance for international schools applying to U.S. foundations.

SUMMARY

In summary, the effect of international exchange on schools of nursing both in the United States and other countries is just beginning to be realized. International exchange programs have exposed students and faculty to other cultures' beliefs and health care models. They are having a major impact on developing a more culturally sensitive approach to health care around the world. Although in the beginning there was more of a one-way exchange, with the United States exporting ideas and technology, this is beginning to change as we become more exposed to different ways of providing health care developed in other countries and as we learn to do more with less. International exchange is contributing to the development of more relevant nursing curricula and research as we search for better ways to meet the health care needs of our societies. It also contributes to better educated nurses who are more willing to participate in the development of health policy for their communities, states, and countries due to their increased awareness of the effect of policy on health care. International exchanges also result in better understanding of the differences and similarities of nursing around the world and, most importantly, build confidence that nurses can make a significant impact on the health of the people.

REFERENCES

Backman, E.L. (Ed.). (1984). *Approaches to international education.* New York: American Council on Education/MacMillan.

Behrman, R.E. (Ed.). (1995). Low birth weight: Analysis and recommendations. In *The future of children.* Los Altos, CA: The Center for the Future of Children, The David and Lucille Packard Foundation.

Beunza, I., Boulton, N., Ferguson, C., & Serrano, R. (1994). Diversity and commonality in international nursing. *International Nursing Review, 41*(2), 47-56.

Davis, T. (1994). *Open doors, 1993-94.* New York: Institute of International Education.

Gay, J.T., Edgil, A.E., & Stullenbarger, E.N. (1993). Graduate education for nursing students who have English as a second language. *Journal of Professional Nursing, 9*(2), 104-109.

Lee, M.Y., Abd-Ella, M., & Burks, L.A. (1981). In S.C. Dunnett (Ed.), *Needs of foreign students from developing nations at U.S. colleges and universities.* Washington DC: National Association for Foreign Student Affairs.

Mason, J.O. (1991). Today's challenges to the Public Health Service and to the nation. *Public Health Reports, 106*(5), 473-477.

Naisbit, J., & Aburdene, P. (1990). *Ten new directions for the 1990's: Megatrends 2000.* New York: William Morrow and Company.

National Center for Health Statistics. (1992). *Prevention profile. Health, United States, 1991.* Hyattsville, MD: Public Health Service.

SoRelle, R. (1995, August 26). A successful shot in the arm. *Houston Chronicle,* pp. 1A, 18A.

Wegman, M. (1994). Annual summary of vital statistics—1993. *Pediatrics, 94*(6), 792-803.

Section Four

CHANGING PRACTICE

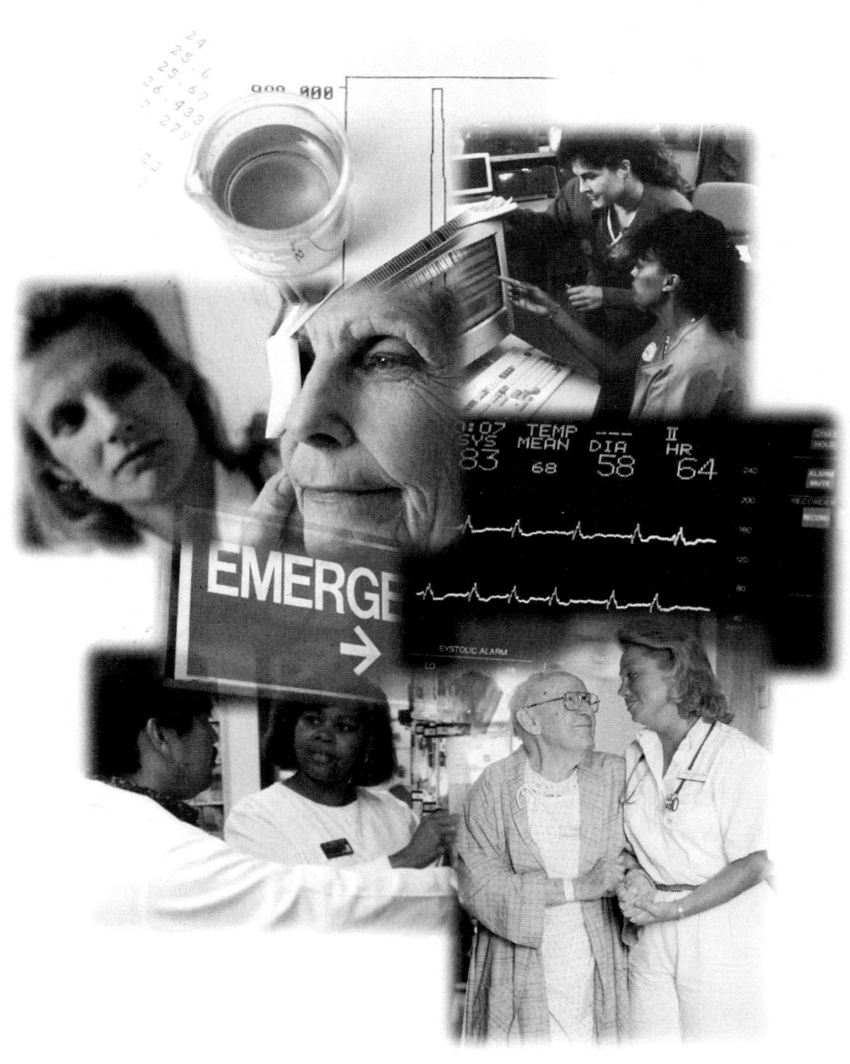

OVERVIEW

A nurse is not a nurse is not a nurse

JOANNE COMI McCLOSKEY, HELEN KENNEDY GRACE

While we have always had a section on issues in nursing practice in this book, this is the first time that the changes and issues in practice are presented by specialty area. While all nurses share certain perspectives and experiences, the chapters in this section reflect that nurses working in different specialties have a wide range of skills and are faced with different issues. Communicating these differences with each other helps us all to understand the vast profession that we share. Space limitations prevent us from including all of the specialties; we have selected for inclusion those areas of practice that reflect the majority of nurses and may be of most interest to nursing students.

The debate chapter by Joel is about home care and turf battles that are developing as this arena of care delivery assumes more importance. Joel begins by relating the history of home care in the United States. While nursing has traditionally dominated the home care scene things are changing. Consumers of home care want more say, and physicians and other providers are now competing with nurses to offer services. The definition and even the label of home care are being challenged by new consumer groups such as the disabled. Joel addresses many questions: To what extent should providers and consumers be able to exercise choice in the selection of a setting for care? Does the consumer have the right to choose home care regardless of cost, or only as the least costly option? Joel frames the debate statement as to whether the recipients of in-home services should have increased autonomy and responsibility in making decisions about their care. On the pro side is a strong consumer lobby complicated by the need to make policy decisions about reimbursement. On the con side are the opinions of providers, especially physicians who are returning to home care driven by economics and need and the issues related to supervision of assistive personnel. This debate is only beginning. Joel's chapter helps us to understand the current situation as the issues continue to emerge and take shape.

The viewpoint chapters are in alphabetical order by specialty, with the first being that of ambulatory nursing. According to Androwich and Haas, by the year 2000 approximately 700,000 nurses will be employed in some type of ambulatory care setting. Despite the growing workforce, the role of these nurses remains undefined. What exactly is ambulatory nursing and what do ambulatory nurses do? A definition is difficult because of the multiple settings in which these nurses practice, including outpatient departments, physician offices and group practices, health maintenance organizations, and nurse-managed centers. Furthermore, each setting may have a different model or philosophy of health care. The authors discuss several issues related to ambulatory care: the diversity of practice settings, inadequate documentation, educational preparation, the use of unlicensed assistants, the rapid pace of care, preparation for telephone communication, and the difficulty of maintaining a common culture across various settings. Despite the issues, they believe that there are a number of opportunities and many rewards for nurses in this specialty.

As health care moves rapidly into the community, nurses working in this setting face multiple challenges. Gutt begins her chapter with a brief overview of population trends that are changing the role of community nurses. She then discusses the need and ways for community health nurses to be more active in health care policy making. She says that "community health nurses need to become more aware of the sociopolitical realities of their world and develop a positive group self-esteem and the political skills necessary to bring about change proactively in the health care system." Nurses in the community must address difficult decisions relevant to quality and sustenance of life as well as affordability and rationing of equipment related to such decisions. A clear personal value system is needed. This chapter is a strong statement about why nurses must take a proactive visible role in community advocacy. Well-educated nurses working in partnership with consumers and other providers are needed as health care evolves into the community setting.

The specialty of emergency nursing is discussed by Rice and Smith. The issues for nurses in this specialty include working with unlicensed caregivers, increasing exposure to unknown infectious diseases, increasing patient acuity, the addition of observation units, the high risk of violence, the movement to contracted services, and the need for data management skills. The authors also overview the numerous credentials and certifications these nurses are required to have, the use of advance practice nurses in the emergency room, and the opportunities for expanded roles. Legislative changes frequently impact the role and responsibilities of the emergency room nurse. The authors conclude with an overview of the role of the Emergency Nurses Association in the popular television show "ER." Despite the many changes and challenges facing nurses in this specialty, it remains a preferred field of work for many.

Some specialties focus on setting, others on the age of the population. While the elderly population is growing, the number of nurses specializing in gerontology remains small. In their chapter, Zwygart-Stauffacher and Rantz provide an overview of the issues related to the care of our aging population. Increasingly, the elderly are using services across the continuum of care, and new roles for care givers are emerging as a result. The authors point out that within the new reimbursement systems, gerontological nurses must often assume tough gatekeeping functions about what services will be provided. They discuss the role of the gerontological clinical nurse specialist compared with that of the gerontological nurse practitioner. Qualifications of faculty, adequacy of associate degree programs to prepare nurses to work in nursing homes, and the need for specialty gerontological content in master's practitioner programs are discussed. In this chapter the authors wrestle with many of the issues related to this specialty that will be helpful to others working in the area.

Medical-surgical nurses have typically cared for adult patients in hospitals. These patients are now older, sicker, and require treatments that use more acute care technology. As hospitals downsize and close, jobs for medical-surgical nurses are disproportionately affected. Fetter and Grindel overview the many challenges facing medical-surgical nurses, including the need to retool with skills and knowledge in health promotion and disease prevention, the need to measure the outcomes of their interventions, and the need to include family teaching as part of an expanded role. The authors acknowledge the difficulties facing nurses in this specialty but believe that the health care system of the future requires more generalists and that these nurses can capitalize on their generalist preparation. They raise important questions: Is medical-surgical nursing bound to the hospital setting? How does medical-surgical nursing differ from critical care and home care nursing? They challenge medical-surgical nurses to be positive about the changes and to recognize their high level of expertise in adult health and create opportunities to use their expertise in all settings.

At the other end of the age continuum Kurtt and Budreau describe the challenges facing pediatric nurses. These challenges are caused by the use of sophisticated technology and by changes in the social fabric of society. Pediatric nursing work in hospitals is increasingly more high-tech and fast-paced, and children receiving home health care require more intense nursing care. As technology and treatment become more complex, pediatric nurses need more ethical knowledge and family counseling skills. The authors discuss several problems including infant mortality and low birth weight, inadequate immunization coverage, and poor access to health care for a large number of children not covered by insurance. Poverty and violence affect a large number of children and cause many complicated problems for pediatric nurses. Kurtt and Budreau urge pediatric nurses to be advocates for children, to design new patient care delivery models that bridge gaps, and to open neighborhood and school-based health clinics.

Brooten begins her chapter on issues in perinatal nursing by listing several, including in vitro fertilization, access problems, and a high low-birth-weight rate compared with that in other countries. She focuses the chapter, however, on the problems resulting from earlier hospital discharge of mothers and newborns. Length of hospital stay for having a baby has declined dramatically since the 1950s, so much so that a few states have now passed legislation to incorporate a minimum stay. Brooten overviews the advantages and disadvantages of early discharge. Early discharge often requires follow-up home care but budget restrictions have eliminated these services for many groups. Brooten describes in some detail the model of transitional care provided by advance practice nurses at the University of Pennsylvania. This model and others are challenged by issues of maintaining continuity between the hospital and home, knowing the most cost-effective provider, and determining the type and length of services. Brooten raises several questions that demonstrate the need for more information. This is a thoughtful analysis of a timely and important issue.

Perioperative nursing, a specialty that is currently under siege, is the topic of the next chapter. Steelman gives a fascinating explanation of the current situation in which registered nurses working in operating rooms are increasingly being replaced by unlicensed assistants due to economic pressure. In 1994 the Joint Commission on Accreditation of Health Care Organizations changed its standard to allow increased use of lesser prepared assistants. Steelman overviews both external and internal factors contributing to the reduction of registered nurses in the operating room. Internal factors include the focus on technical practice, segregation from mainstream nursing, lack of a tool to predict patient needs for intraoperative nursing care, and a history of catering to surgeon preference. According to Steelman, the drastic reductions in nursing personnel in some operating rooms are dangerous and unnecessary. She proposes instead the reduction of expenses through standardization of expensive supplies, implants, and instruments, combined with some use of assistants for nonnursing functions. She also discusses what the specialty is doing to build a more supportive foundation. Hers is an interesting, hard-hitting chapter.

Psychiatric nursing is the subject of the next chapter by Stuart, who begins by listing several areas of vulnerability that nurses in this specialty face. Stuart believes that psychiatric nurses may become extinct and replaced by others unless they can expand their roles and present a case for why their skills are needed. She overviews the changes that have occurred in five areas: role, activities, models of care, treatment settings, and outcome data. She first reviews the history of psychiatric nursing and how the role has evolved since the emergence of the specialty in the 1950s. Next she lists psychiatric practice activities in three groups: direct care, communication, and management. She says that communication and management activities need to be better integrated in the current role of the psychiatric nurse. In the area of model of care she outlines four stages of treatment and gives the goal, assessment, intervention, and outcome for each. This is a very helpful model because hospital length of stay continues to decline and much of psychiatric treatment is now given in community-based settings. She then discusses the expansion of mental health treatment settings and the challenges and opportunities provided by the change. Finally, she urges psychiatric nurses to articulate the nature of their care and collect data on the outcomes that they achieve. This is an informative chapter about a specialty that is undergoing a number of changes and is being challenged to respond.

The international chapter in this section addresses primary health care in developing countries, specifically South Africa. Robertson describes a very sobering and challenging situation as South Africa experiences a massive movement of people into major cities with resulting overcrowding, crime, and illness. The challenges to health care workers in these situations are many and include the threat of safety. Unfortunately, the promotion of primary health care has had limited success as providers and the public cling to the curative mindset of the medical model and traditional ways of working. Implementation of primary health care has also suffered from poor management skills. Delivery of primary care by nurses has received mixed reviews from community members. Despite the many problems, however, Robertson believes that primary health care still has much potential. She discusses four steps that nurses must take to make a difference: develop a vision; value diversity; create community partnerships; and engage in learning. Robertson also lists the new skills and changes in educational curricula that need to take place. While the focus of the chapter is on attempts to make a transition to primary health care in South Africa, the chapter's content and the author's experience are relevant and helpful to nurses everywhere.

As the chapters in this section demonstrate, nurses in all specialties are challenged to keep up with many health care system changes. As we attempt to streamline our care to save unnecessary steps and cost, we must also continue to provide enough time to attend to the tasks of caring for people. Nurses need to be vocal about the services that must be retained to ensure safety and quality. We also need to help others see that nurses are not interchangeable. The nursing profession is large and composed of a vast array of individuals with differing skills and knowledge. We need to acknowledge our similarities and differences as we move forward amid the turmoil of overwhelming change.

Moving the care site from hospital to home: Whose turf?

LUCILLE A. JOEL

Many view the growth of the home health care market in recent years as a direct response to the more prudent use of inpatient settings, most notably hospitals and to a lesser extent nursing homes. This is only one aspect of a multidimensional scene. The explosive demand for community services, and for the home as a major community setting for care, is closely related to changing American demographics (i.e., the increasing elderly population), a declining presence of family caregivers, expanding public entitlement benefits for community and home care, technological refinements that allow more sophisticated treatment in the nonhospital environment, and economic pressures to limit the use of costly inpatient facilities (Silverman, 1990). This analysis conveys the picture of two distinct home care markets—the patient following an acute illness and the frail, disabled, and chronically ill. This distinction will grow in importance as our discussion continues.

A very clear sequence of events over the past 30 years has shaped modern home care and generated the dilemmas we face today. Titles 18 and 19 of the Social Security Act created Medicare and Medicaid. It was within those entitlements that home care was recognized as reimbursable, although not at first mandatory. Subsequent legislation in 1971 made home health services mandatory as a covered benefit under these programs, and service was expanded to the disabled in 1972 and to patients with end-stage renal disease in 1978. Elimination of the prior hospitalization requirement and a more flexible redefinition of the term "homebound" followed over time, and brought home care into its own. The Medicare hospital prospective pricing system and diagnosis-related groups (DRGs) of 1982 heightened the utilization of a segment of the industry—home care—that had already begun to experience significant growth (Estes et al., 1993). Incentives were offered to hospitals to decrease the length of stay for their patients. Referral to home care was the natural consequence.

A few statistics demonstrate the profound effect of public policy. Table 27-1 shows that no proprietary (for-profit) agencies existed in 1967 that were Medicare-certified, and 3,730 existed in 1995, with the most significant growth occurring between 1980 and 1985, from 186 to 1,943 proprietary agencies. The dramatic growth of for-profit agencies ended the historic dominance of the field by visiting nurse associations and nonprofit and governmental agencies (Estes, 1993). This transition was bound to impact the home care industry as a business, if not as a professional service (if the two can be separated). In many ways, home care may have been the precursor to the current shift toward privatization in all sectors of health care. The entire home care industry has become very dependent on government dollars. By 1992, almost 75% of home care was funded publicly (Burner et al., 1992), and 74% of the recipients of care in 1993 and 1994 were 65 years of age or older (Marion Merrell Dow, 1995). Nonprofit and hospital-based agencies were the most dependent on government reimbursement (80%), with nonprofit organizations operating in deficit. In contrast, for-profit organizations derived only 55% of revenues from public funding and ran at a profit (Marion Merrell Dow, 1993, 1995). This is not to cast dispersion; the lower reimbursement levels from public programs and the need for clients who can pay out of pocket or have richer insurance benefits is just good business.

Whether expansion of the home care market is a response to the declining use of hospitals or is due primarily to other factors, it is a trend that seems irreversible. From 1980 to 1990, there was a decline from 1,163 to 709.5 annual hospital days per 1,000 population

Table 27-1 Number of medicare-certified home care agencies, by Auspice, 1967–1995

	Freestanding agencies						Facility-based agencies			
Year	**VNA**	**COMB**	**PUB**	**PROP**	**PNP**	**OTH**	**HOSP**	**REHAB**	**SNF**	**TOTAL**
1967	549	93	939	0	0	39	133	0	0	1,753
1975	525	46	1,228	47	0	109	273	9	5	2,242
1980	515	63	1,260	186	484	40	359	8	9	2,924
1985	514	59	1,205	1,943	832	4	1,277	20	129	5,983
1986	510	62	1,192	1,915	826	4	1,341	17	117	5,984
1987	500	61	1,172	1,882	803	1	1,382	14	108	5,923
1988	496	55	1,073	1,846	766	1	1,439	12	97	5,785
1989	491	51	1,011	1,818	727	1	1,465	10	102	5,676
1990	474	47	985	1,884	710	0	1,486	8	101	5,695
1991	476	41	941	1,970	701	0	1,537	9	105	5,780
1992	530	52	1,083	1,962	637	28	1,623	3	86	6,004
1993	594	46	1,196	2,146	558	41	1,809	1	106	6,497
1994	586	45	1,146	2,892	597	48	2,081	3	123	7,521
1995	579	38	1,161	3,730	667	59	2,357	3	153	8,747

Reproduced by permission of the National Association for Home Care, from *Basic Statistics About Home Care 1995*; Data from HCFA Office of Survey and Certification.

Note. COMB = Combination agencies are combined government and voluntary agencies, and are sometimes included with counts for visiting nurse associations.

HOSP = Hospital-based agencies are operating units or departments of a hospital. Agencies that have working arrangements with a hospital, or perhaps are even owned by a hospital but operated as separate entities, are classified as freestanding agencies under one of the categories listed above.

OTH = Other freestanding agencies are agencies that do not fit one of the categories for freestanding agencies listed above.

PNP = Private nonprofit agencies are freestanding and privately developed, governed, and owned home care agencies.

PROP = Proprietary agencies are freestanding, for-profit home care agencies.

PUB = Public agencies are government agencies operated by a state, county, city, or other unit of local governemnt having a major responsibility for preventing disease and for community health education.

REHAB = Agencies based in rehabilitation facilities.

SNF = Agencies based in skilled nursing facilities.

VNA = Visiting nurse associations are freestanding, voluntary, nonprofit organizations governed by a board of directors and usually financed by tax-deductible contributions as well as by earnings.

(Mezey & Lawrence, 1995). By 1993, utilization rates for hospitals in association with health maintenance organizations (HMOs) were about 335 hospital days per 1,000 members (Marion Merrell Dow, 1995). American Hospital Association data indicate that there were 892,126 community hospital beds in September 1994 compared with 918,786 beds the previous year (American Hospital Association, 1995). If this trend continues, an additional 54% of current beds could close over time (Immigration Nursing Relief Advisory Committee, 1995). It seems useful to project using the HMO or managed care standard, given the domination of the health care market by these programs. Since there is no reduction in the volume nor complexity of health care problems of the American public in sight, the future seems to hold even greater challenges for the management of both health and illness.

It is logical to predict using the HMO or managed care standard, given the domination of the health care industry by these programs. As hospitals decline in use, community and home care will grow proportionately.

This shift in the dominant venue for health care places in question the roles and relationships that were assumed in a medicalized inpatient environment. Turf battles are inevitable as we either settle into new patterns of authority and accountability or reestablish those from other times and places. There will be questions about who has the right to authorize services; where the quality controls are, if indeed quality can be defined or is even an issue; and who is responsible for the practice of nonprofessionals who have proliferated more than any other category of caregiver in home care?

Nursing has long dominated the home care scene. The roots of many of our most illustrious leaders can be traced to home care. This has often been touted as the setting that provides the best showcase for our practice, promising autonomy, equality, respect. The pioneering home care agencies were nurse-managed and nurse-controlled and built on a social model that ranged far beyond the diagnosis and treatment of illness. As the treatment of complex disease in the post-acutely ill moves into the community and the home, will this tradition continue? Should it? This is part of the debate, but it is only tangential.

The wild card in this equation is the consumer. Consumerism has taken on a new militancy. The recipients of care have become uncomfortable deferring to professionals. The common practice of "protecting the public from themselves" is eroding as consumers gain increasing direct access to diagnostic and therapeutic products (Joel, 1995a). Additionally, consumer satisfaction and dissatisfaction as expressed to insurers, particularly in managed care plans, are a driving determinant in who does what and which providers and facilities will be included in a network. The good will of plan members is necessary if they are to continue their subscription.

CIRCUMSCRIBING THE DEBATE

The meaning of home care seems obvious, but has been challenged by many advocates of a more contemporary view. A broad concept of home care was included in the long-term care entitlements proposed to Congress by President Clinton in 1993 (Kane & Wilson, 1993). Recommendations supported increased flexibility in the form of personal assistance for persons with functional impairment where they live, where they recreate, where they work, and where they do business. The intent was to normalize life through personal assistance suited to the needs and preferences of the individual (Kane & Wilson, 1993). The extreme application of this philosophy proposes to extend it to nursing homes by separating personal care and nursing services from nontherapeutic and hotel services so the client or his or her agent (usually the family) may choose what suits them best, thereby controlling resources, which is the ultimate weapon. It suffices to know that this broader vision of home care and in-home services exists, has been proposed for public policy, and enjoys growing support.

Inevitably there are a number of issues folded into the debate. Following are only some of these issues:

- What are the appropriate criteria for maintaining a patient in the home, putting aside economic motivation?
- To what extent should providers and consumers be able to exercise choice in the selection of a setting for care?
- How appropriate is the medical model to the home care population?
- How much direct consumer access to providers and services should exist?
- What is the extent of services that should be reimbursed in favor of maintaining a person in the home?
- If home care is a cost-efficient proxy for the hospital or nursing home, how is the break-even point identified and what happens once it is reached?
- Does the consumer have the right to choose home care regardless of cost, or only as the least costly option?
- Who is responsible for the supervision of volunteers in the home, including family members if they undertake medical or nursing activities?
- When is the registered nurse personally accountable for the service rendered, and when and for what is the system accountable?
- Should family members be supervised or are they the supervisors?
- To what extent can activities be delegated?
- Should volunteer and family caregivers receive reimbursement either through dollars paid or tax credits allowed?
- When and to what extent do nurses supervise home care workers?

THE CONTEXT OF CARE IN THE 1990S

Senge (1990) tells us that wisdom lies in tracing the patterns of social trends so that we may position ourselves strategically to create our own preferred future. This statement is not an oxymoron; rather it is a truth that is so basic as to be frightening. Trends are set in motion by a society and are undebatable (assuming they are interpreted correctly), yet they are broad enough that stewards of the society can be creative in their response. The challenge is to rise above self-interest, the temptation to protect our field of work, and our natural caution about change. Once we have faced our own biases, the world looks more logical, if not more acceptable.

The American public is intrigued by high technology, specialization, and the myths of freedom of choice and fierce individualism. Deriving from these origins, many would define our ethic toward health care as a basic package of services for everyone, but the guarantee that those who have the resources can obtain more for themselves and their own. In contrast, countries with more socialized systems would say it is the greatest good for the most people. This contrast may answer many questions about why we act as we do.

Many among us expect health to be an individual responsibility. Because most of us suffer a small amount of serious illnesses in our lives, this makes good sense. On the other hand, the progress of medical science has created a cohort of the frail and vulnerable for whom health care takes on a new meaning. The frail elderly, those who are disabled or chronically ill, persons with AIDS, and low-birth-weight babies are all among those whose health becomes a public concern and can create serious liabilities if they are ignored. Homelessness, poverty, the absence of family, and environmental pollution are all by-products of industrial progress, further complicating the picture and generating more need for personal health services.

The financial burden of health care has become substantial for Americans as they continue the search for efficiencies that will allow them to honor a commitment to the needy yet maintain some control over the total number of dollars spent. Americans are neither proud nor complacent about the fact that 14% of the population has no guaranteed access to health care and an equal number have inadequate provisions.

The search to produce access has begged the question of a defined standard in health care but has focused on the irrational cost. Hospitals have been targeted as a major offender, given their association with high technology and aggressive and defensive diagnostics and therapeutics. Rather than searching for programmatic options that promise a better use of resources, the years since 1982 have held a flurry of public policy activity with the obvious goal of preserving the status quo in the health care industry to whatever extent possible. These antics included reducing reimbursement for services to the poor so that few providers would care for them, increasing the cost-sharing and deductible requirements for the elderly under Medicare, and cross-subsidizing the cost of public entitlement programs through private sector payers. During this same period, several generations of statistical equations were developed: DRGs, common procedural technologies (CPTs), resource based relative value scales (RBRVSs), resource utilization groups (RUGs), minimum data set (MDS), minimum data set, version 2 (MDS2), and minimum data set-plus (MDS+) with the ultimate purpose of reducing the cost of services; each has been gamed creatively by the industry. We continue to pursue technical solutions to political problems. The most hopeful programmatic or infrastructure redesigns began to surface from the private sector: the expansion of community and home care services, the use of primary care providers as gatekeepers to the system challenged to refocus on disease prevention and health promotion, and seamless programs that provide access for individuals to all services through a single point of entry.

The declining use of hospitals has been sensationalized by the press and fueled by some provider groups with cries of "quicker and sicker" discharge. A more productive response has been to create support for periods of recuperation and rehabilitation in the home and community. Within an environment of limited resources, this requires getting the proper services to those who need them, no more and no less. The Health Security Act of 1993 (finally defeated in the early fall of 1994) recommended demonstration grants to make clearer distinctions between levels of care: intensivist, critical, acute, subacute, skilled, intermediate, custodial, ambulatory, nursing home, and home care. There was also the call for funding of assisted living programs with a broad range of in-home services that are currently nonreimbursable. Although largely doomed from the outset because of its political naivete (Joel, 1995b), this bill introduced a social model to the public conscience that cannot be ignored.

ISSUES OF CONTROL

As the home and community become the prevailing sites for care, the control of the medical establishment (including nurses) declines. Some may say that consumer demand for more control was a major catalyst in this reformation rather than its by-product. Consumer allegations of forced dependence on entering the health care system and frequent distrust of provider professionals should have been an anticipated consequence of specialization and high technology. Without adequate attention to the human relationships between provider and patient, the vulnerable easily come to feel victimized. This distrust and the search for cost efficiency have contributed to the growth of managed care plans in which decisions are made (hypothetically) on objective criteria, and primary care providers or case managers are, or could be, the essential ingredient to make the system work to the advantage of the consumer.

The position of the consumer is further strengthened by the growing trend to have public entitlement recipients (Medicare, Medicaid, Champus) use their resources to "buy" into a managed care plan of their choice. Currently, this ability to choose is compromised when managed care plans are designed specifically for the poor, and choice is often limited to providers and facilities that can not attract a middle class or private payer client base.

Discussion inevitably leads to issues inherent in the

idea of "turf," which is so central to our debate. A medicalized system has concentrated services in settings where the balance of power weighs in the direction of the industry and provider professionals. Public dissatisfaction with this paradigm was slow in coming but long in building. The issue is who defines the nature and context of services. The thrust of the Agency for Health Policy and Research, the Patients' Bill of Rights and the Final Directives requirements, are examples of public policy intended to guarantee the ability of consumers to make their own informed choices. Home care has always been distinguished by consumer domination and the absence of medical control. The migration toward home care is motivated primarily by cost, but what home care has been and the prevailing public sentiments will play a major role in any emerging paradigm.

The frail and the chronically ill have been the major recipients of home care, and they have frequently been poor. Today they are joined by those recuperating patients who may be in a position to demand more and different services, having access to more personal resources such as private insurance and workplace benefits. There is also the addition of younger disabled persons who object to both the terms "home" and "care" because of the connotations that have become associated with them in this society (Asch, 1993). They prefer to reserve the term "care" for relationships of intimacy and affection, and note that assistive services should not be limited to the home in the usual sense of the word. Rather, services that allow patients to maintain a home in the community should help them to live and flourish wherever that home might be. Rather than promoting a "caring in place" philosophy, services should follow patients from the home to places where they can be productive, recreate, socialize, or do business. Advocates of the disabled, this often younger and more militant constituency, contend that the recipients of services should be able to select those in an assistive relationship and decide whether family is an option. This is contrary to the traditional view, which bases the authorization of services on the potential for rehabilitation or the need for skilled nursing. The expanded definition of "homebound" was a breakthrough, but rigid interpretations still exist. More latitude has been observed in state-funded or Medicaid waiver programs in which personal assistance and functional impairment are the priorities. This has been the response in programs created to substitute for nursing home placement rather than hospital confinement.

The ability of home care personnel to provide some rather technically complex care and the frequency and immediacy of supervision, if any, are very controversial. Many arguments for the increased use of nonprofessional personnel hinge on the ability of the disabled to direct their own care, thereby maintaining control. Other controversy focuses on the delegation of specific activities by the professional, notably the nurse. In Oregon, nonnurses may perform nursing functions if they have been taught by a nurse on a patient-specific and procedure-specific basis.

THE DEBATE

Any pro or con position must consider the attitudes and values of the 1990s, the trends that have already been put into motion, and the continued stewardship, on their own terms, of the professions to the public. It is hardly debatable that we are migrating toward new settings for care and that new models will be needed that are more harmonious with those settings. *The recipient of in-home services should have increased autonomy, flexibility, and commensurate responsibility in making determinations about their care.*

Pro

The medical model is increasingly inconsistent with the restructuring delivery system. Primary health care, integrated systems of care, and community-based services all begin to move us toward a new paradigm that values self-care, personal responsibility, prudence in resource use, and increased responsibility for the common good. The frail elderly, a major market for in-home services, are more concerned with functionality and their perceptions of their own health than they are with illness. Illness only becomes a priority when it gets in the way of living. Managed care plans, in either their broadest or more restrictive forms, value consumer satisfaction above most other indicators of success. The Clinton administration's 1993 report on health care reform recommended eligibility for assisted living and home health services based on measurable functional impairments as opposed to medically defined problems and a shift to personal, client-directed care with the standard being that the persons providing service be selected, trained (to the degree possible), supervised, and evaluated by the recipient. Although enabling legislation failed, support for such models of home care remains strong and its advocates are dedicated (Estes, 1993).

Realistically, a fence may have to be put around the liberties and choices allowed within the context of home care, especially where public dollars are used. One approach is a cap on the total amount of funding available in a preestablished period. Caution would have to be taken that the spirit of flexibility and choice is not violated by inadequate funding. Withholding funding is a common back-door strategy to reach one's goal without the unpleasant policy decisions that would be required with a more forthright approach. Examples abound, but two examples in health care should be very familiar. Few, if any, restrictions are placed on the services provided to Medicaid recipients, but the fees are so low that few providers accept these patients. If dollars are limited, priorities should be established. Defining a basic benefit package or directing dollars to specific clinical situations is politically risky, but the state of Oregon did it in 1993. Similar manipulation plagues the abortion issue. The procedure is legal, but the poor are denied the public dollars to access it.

The tough policy decisions to allow the consumer to retain maximum control will be slow in coming. The first challenge requires the honesty to separate the control and funding aspects. Although only a finite number of dollars may be available to an individual, allowing decisions about the use of those dollars could honor the spirit of consumer choice. Supporting flexibility may lead to some creative options. Pooling resources in a setting such as a group residential home may bring more services and consequently more freedom (Mollica et al., 1992); for the more acutely ill or those recovering from acute illness, fluid movement between levels of care including (but not limited to) the home, all within a predetermined spending cap, may help. Good experience can be derived from true hospice programs. Any of these decisions are most comfortably made if they are supported by case management, at best independent case management. A case manager engaged by the payer could be plagued by conflict of interest, i.e., the need to hold a job versus advocate for the client. The ability to exercise personal choice in the selection of benefits and to convert resources within reasonable limits should do much to temper the adversarial attitude that often characterizes those with long-term needs and ends in litigation.

Con

Consumer militancy and the growing political influence of both elderly and younger disabled persons has led to a gradual restructuring of home care in order to distance it from the mainstream of health care in this country, broaden the definitions of home care and in-home assistance, and increase the consumer's right to engage and dismiss services.

A first wave of consumerism pre-dated the dramatic onslaught of acute and subacute clinical situations into the home (mostly from 1982 and the advent of DRGs). With the appearance of this new clinical population in the home, there is new justification for medicalization. Physicians who once abandoned home practice are returning to that setting, some out of economic motivation and others as a response to consumer need. The federal government has just approved Medicare reimbursement to physicians for their supervision of the medical regimen in home care, based on the observation that much of home care has become so medically dependent that close supervision is not only justified but also necessary.

Putting aside the very apparent medical needs in home care, there remain the chronically ill, frail, and disabled. These populations have traditionally used significant amounts of nonprofessional and assistive services in the home. Surveys indicate that home health agencies rely on part-time, temporary workers and have been assigning heavier caseloads resulting in alienation of the workforce. In keeping with job dissatisfaction, high turnover among home health aides was common and often led to a lack of reliability and consistency of services. Observable quality of care problems follow, such as incomplete work, inadequate skills even for simple ministrations, failure to carry out specific orders, client injury or abuse, exploitation of the client, theft, and absenteeism (Eustis et al., 1993). Given these indicators and the basic vulnerability of many home care recipients, the justification for closer professional control builds.

Despite the outcry for consumer empowerment, the American public has always found comfort in the medical establishment and the assurance that professionals will act in their best interests. There is clear distinction in home care between those situations in which medical necessity drives the use of resources and situations in which functional ability and basic services to compensate for functional deficits are the primary need. It was just such a distinction that differentiated Medicare and Medicaid (i.e., episodic versus continuing care). Whether these distinctions should be perpetuated and how they should be reflected, if at all, in the process of authorizing services for the public are serious questions, more rooted in philosophy than financial expedience. Quick answers are in order as the country moves toward merging these systems.

IN CONCLUSION

The dispute over turf ownership in home care or any other sector of health care pits the consumer against the government bureaucracy and their agents, the industry, and the professions. Over time home care and in-home services have moved to a functional/social model that is more suitable to the needs of some, while a growing constituency of the post-acutely ill have a real need for continuing medical expertise in the home and are confronted with decisions beyond the capability of most lay people. The challenge will be to see the distinctions and accommodate them. These were the original observations on the needs of the Medicare and Medicaid populations. There may be something we can learn from past experience—the successes as well as the blunders.

REFERENCES

American Hospital Association. (1995). *Hospital statistics*. Chicago: Author.

Asch, A. (1993). Abused or neglected clients—or abusive or neglectful service systems? In R.A. Kana & A.L. Caplan (Eds.), *Ethical conflict in the management of home care: The case manager's dilemma*. New York: Springer.

Burner, S.T., Waldo, D.R., & McKusick, D.R. (1992). National health expenditures projections through 2030. *Health Care Financing Review, 14*(1), 1-29.

Estes, C.L. (1993). *The restructuring of home care*. Conference on the future of home care and community based care. New York: Harriman.

Estes, C.L., Swan, J.H., & Associates. (1993). *The long term care crisis: Elders trapped in the no-care zone*. Thousand Oaks, CA: Sage.

Eustis, N., Kane, R., & Fischer, L. (1993). Home care quality and the home care worker: Beyond quality assurance as usual. *The Gerontologist, 33*(1), 64-73.

Immigration Nursing Relief Advisory Committee. (1995, March). *Report to the Secretary of Labor on the Immigration Nursing Relief Act of 1989*. Washington, DC: Author.

Joel, L.A. (1995a). Expanding paradigms of self-care. *American Journal of Nursing, 95*(8), 7.

Joel, L.A. (1995b). Health care reform: Getting it right this time. *American Journal of Nursing, 95*(1), 7.

Kane, R.A., & Wilson, K.B. (1993). *Assisted living in the United States: A new paradigm for residential care for the frail elderly*. Washington: American Association of Retired Persons.

Marion Merrell Dow. (1993). *Managed care digest: Long term care edition*. Kansas City, MO: Author.

Marion Merrell Dow. (1995). *Managed care digest series, institutional digest*. Kansas City, MO: Author.

Mezey, A.P., & Lawrence, R.S. (1995). Ambulatory care. In A.R. Kovner (Ed.), *Health care delivery in the United States*. New York: Springer.

Mollica, R.L., Ladd, S., Dietsche, K.B., & Ryther, B.S. (1992). *Building assisted living for the elderly into public long-term care policy: A guide for states*. Portland, ME: Center for Vulnerable Populations, National Academy for State Health Policy.

Senge, P. (1990). *The fifth discipline*. New York: Doubleday.

Silverman, H. (1990). Use of Medicare-covered home health agency services. *Health Care Financing Review, 12*(2), 113-126.

Ambulatory care nursing: Concerns and challenges

IDA M. ANDROWICH, SHEILA A. HAAS

Ambulatory care nursing offers numerous opportunities for nurses to practice in a variety of roles. It is predicted that by the year 2000 ambulatory (outpatient) services will account for nearly half of most hospitals' net revenue and that over 700,000 nurses are expected to be employed in some type of ambulatory care setting (Curran, 1992). Given the size, growth, and importance of the field, defining the practice would appear straightforward. Yet Stavins (1993) claims that the most difficult challenge facing ambulatory nursing is "defining our role" (p. 67). This chapter focuses on the definitional aspects of the ambulatory care nursing role and identities and discusses several of the issues facing nurses in this practice field.

DEFINING AMBULATORY CARE NURSING

Verran is credited with an early interest in the delineation and definition of ambulatory care nursing. In her seminal study (1981) she used a Delphi methodology and ambulatory nurses' expert opinions to delineate seven "responsibility areas" in the ambulatory nurse role. Other researchers have continued this effort (Haas & Hackbarth, 1995a; Hackbarth, Haas, Kavanagh, & Vlasses, 1995; Hastings & Muir-Nash, 1989; Hooks, Dewitz-Arnold, & Westbrook, 1980; Joseph, 1990; Parrinello & Witzel, 1990; Pinkney-Atkinson & Robertson, 1993).

In the American Academy of Ambulatory Care Nursing's (AAACN) "Administration and Practice Standards" (1993), ambulatory care nursing is operationally defined as ". . . nursing practice in an ambulatory care setting. Nursing care provided to patients with institutional episodes of care of less than 24 hours" (p. 19). This definition delineates nursing practice by the environment in which the nurse practices and by the amount of time the nurse spends with a patient, but is not useful in capturing essential characteristics and role elements.

This need to depict ambulatory nursing as it is today for practicing nurses, other health care providers, policy makers, and the public led the American Nurses Association (ANA) and the AAACN to establish a joint Task Force charged with writing a monograph on ambulatory care nursing. As part of this charge, the Task Force is developing a conceptual definition of ambulatory care nursing. In the absence of a rich and recent literature base from which to cull the universal characteristics of ambulatory care nursing, members of the Task Force were asked to assemble focus groups in their ambulatory care organizations. Each focus group responded to the question, "What are the universal characteristics of ambulatory care nursing?" (ANA/AAACN Task Force, 1995). Commonly occurring themes in the reports assisted the Task Force in the evolution of a conceptual definition of ambulatory care nursing.

Using the ANA's Social Policy Statement (1995) as a foundation, the Task Force developed the following definition: Ambulatory care nursing is the diagnosis and treatment of actual and potential health problems in patients who are home-based and engage predominantly in self-care or care provided by family members or significant others, but who come to health care environments in need of assessment, advice, counsel, monitoring, teaching, treatment, evaluation, and care coordination.

The AAACN is

> the association of professional nurses who identify ambulatory care nursing as essential to the continuum of high quality, cost-effective patient care. The goals of the AAACN are to shape professional practice and the environment, build collaborative relationships, and provide innovative thinking and vision in ambulatory care. (AAACN, 1993, p. 5)

The AAACN was established in 1978 by a group of nursing directors and supervisors in ambulatory care who recognized the need for well-prepared nurse administrators in the expanding arena of ambulatory care. Originally named the American Academy of Ambulatory Nursing Administration, the name was changed to AAACN in 1993 to reflect the organization's commitment to development of all nurses working in ambulatory care. As part of this commitment, the AAACN publishes and updates standards for ambulatory care nursing.

The third edition of the "Ambulatory Care Nursing Administration and Practice Standards" (1993, p. 6) reflects five core ambulatory care nursing values:

- Shared responsibility among patients, families, and other members of the health care team in all phases of the episode of care
- Education to enable patients and families to understand and make informed decisions
- Continuity of care
- Excellence in care that balances patient needs, cost-effectiveness, and appropriate resource utilization
- The opportunity to serve as patient advocate

The nine "Ambulatory Care Nursing Administration and Practice Standards" (1993) are designed to "promote effective management of increasingly complex ambulatory care nursing roles and responsibilities in a changing health care environment which requires not only expanded clinical and administrative skills but methods to evaluate the quality, appropriateness and effectiveness of services" (p. 4). The standards are designed to be used in conjunction with specialty practice nursing organization standards such as those promulgated by the ANA. They address issues such as the structure and organization of ambulatory care nursing, staffing, competency of nursing staff, nursing practice, continuity of care, ethics and patient rights, environment, research, and quality management. Each standard includes a rationale and criteria by which "to measure nursing's contribution" (p. 4). The AAACN standards are presented as recommendations and are intended to be adapted to fit many diverse ambulatory care settings. Because ambulatory care practice is continually expanding and changing, the AAACN is committed to revising, updating, and promulgating its standards.

CURRENT ISSUES IN AMBULATORY CARE NURSING

Along with the need for definitional clarity, there are also several issues relating to the ambulatory care environment. These include (1) the diversity of practice in ambulatory care settings, including the use of varied conceptual models of health; (2) inadequate documentation of nursing practice leading to limited understanding of ambulatory nursing practice; (3) the limited number of nurses with baccalaureate or advanced academic preparation; (4) the increased need for delegation and supervision of unlicensed assistive personnel; (5) the rapid pace of ambulatory patient encounters; (6) the expectations placed on the nurse related to telephone communication; and (7) the need to negotiate within multiple organizational cultures.

Diversity in practice

There is marked diversity in the types of settings where ambulatory care is delivered. Among the major private sector ambulatory care settings are university hospital outpatient departments, community hospital outpatient departments, physician group practices, health maintenance organizations (HMOs), physicians' offices, and nurse-managed centers. Ambulatory care settings that are funded publicly include community health clinics, Indian Health Service, and Community and Migrant Worker Health Centers. Within each of these distinct settings, the philosophy of care and the model of care delivery may have a different model of health as a foundation.

It is not surprising that the medical model is frequently the driving force in physician group practices and even in university hospital ambulatory care and community hospital ambulatory care settings. However, it is somewhat surprising that this model predominates in many HMOs (Haas, Hackbarth, Kavanagh, & Vlasses, 1995). By definition, HMOs should be more focused on health promotion and disease prevention.

Diversity in the types of settings, models of health, and consequent models of health care delivery is an issue for nursing when nurses who work in a setting find that they have difficulties working under the prevailing model and philosophy. Furthermore, they may have difficulty identifying this lack of congruence in values as the root of the problem. They will say, "I want to have time to do health promotion with my clients, yet I have so much paperwork and clerical work that I just can't get to it"; or "I want to work with the vast array of patient/family problems, but all I have time for is their physical ailments"; or "I want to work as a colleague with the physicians and really get into health promotion." Operative in each of these situations is a clinical model of health driving the practice model. Consequently, the scheduling of patient visits and the provider's time is dictated by this view of health.

Solutions to this issue involve educating nurses about the many and various types of ambulatory care settings, educating nurses and physicians about multiple models of health with their practice implications, and enhancing the care provider's ability to diagnose operative models of health in different settings. The optimal outcome would be health care professionals who will choose a practice setting for employment where there is a good fit between their professional goals and the mission, philosophy, model of health, and care delivery model of the organization. If there is not a good fit, at least the professional enters the organization with an understanding and awareness of the model currently operating and, if needed, the wherewithal to initiate change.

Inadequate documentation of practice

The nature of ambulatory practice, with its relatively rapid pace for patient encounters, high patient volume, and scheduled time constraints does not contribute to comprehensive documentation of nursing care. Use of the nursing minimum data set (NMDS) (Werley & Lang, 1988) in ambulatory practice is limited (Androwich & Stoupa, 1994). With no paper or electronic documentation trail, justifying the value of nursing is problematic and the care rendered by nurses becomes invisible. At a research conference held by the AAACN (Androwich & Phillips, 1992) several documentation concerns were identified, including limited use of the elements of the NMDS in practice settings, documentation systems designed primarily for physicians, no classification scheme for interventions or outcomes, and limited use of the problem list. When nursing interventions are documented, the assessment data leading to the individual nursing judgement is omitted, and any link to patient outcome is unknown. In addition, there are no generally accepted methods of measuring productivity, nursing intensity, or patient acuity in the ambulatory setting, nor have we defined the concept of *episode of care* in a manner that could link visits within an episode of care to determine the effectiveness of specific interventions in achieving outcomes. Documentation needs to be captured in an automated patient record system in order to link encounters in a meaningful, retrievable manner.

In 1992 the Iowa Nursing Interventions Classification (NIC) was published (McCloskey & Bulechek, 1992). In order to prepare to implement the NIC in an ambulatory field test site an assessment survey asking about the interventions used in practice was distributed to professional nursing staff ($N = 197$) at that site. This survey was modelled after a similar national survey employed by the Iowa Research Team (Bulechek, McCloskey, Denehey, & Titler, 1994) that was designed to elicit the frequency of use of each of the 336 nursing interventions in the taxonomy. Respondents were asked to identify the frequency of use of each of the interventions based on a 5-point Likert scale, ranging from "rarely or never" to "many times a day."

Table 28-1 Frequency of use of the top 30 Nursing Interventions Classifications interventions ($n = 126$)

	Rating (%)	
	Rarely or never	**Many times daily**
Active Listening Intervention	10.32	76.19
Vital Signs Monitoring	15.32	60.48
Infection Control	17.60	57.60
Body Mechanics Promotion	30.16	50.79
Emotional Support	17.46	47.62
Health Screening	24.59	42.62
Specimen Management	22.40	41.60
Teaching: Prescribed Medication	16.80	40.80
Communication Enhancement	16.80	39.20
Infection Protection	27.64	39.02
Medication Management	19.05	38.89
Presence	18.40	38.40
Teaching: Disease Process	18.55	37.10
Humor	24.00	36.80
Touch	28.00	36.80
Teaching: Individual	24.19	36.29
Teaching: Procedure/Treatment	21.77	33.06
Medication Administration	33.60	32.00
Medication Administration: Parenteral	31.75	31.75
Energy Management	38.40	31.20
Technology Management	41.13	29.84
Preparatory Sensory Information	30.08	28.46
Environmental Management: Safety	32.26	28.23
Fall Prevention	36.80	26.40
Anxiety Reduction	24.80	25.60
Risk Identification	36.00	25.60
Medication Administration: Oral	34.40	25.60
Decision-making Support	20.63	25.40
Transport	41.13	25.00
Environmental Management: Comfort	39.20	24.00

The response rate for the ambulatory survey was 64%, yielding 126 completed surveys from each of 12 service areas in the outpatient center. Table 28-1 lists the top 30 interventions by frequency of use in ambulatory care across all 12 settings. Interestingly, the intervention "Active Listening" was the top intervention in both this survey and in the Iowa survey, which queried nurses in all specialty areas.

The responses from the nursing specialty areas ($N = 277$) (Bulechek, McCloskey, Titler, & Denehey, 1994) were drawn from member nursing organizations in the ANA's Nursing Organization Liaison Forum. Ambulatory nurses used a number of these top 30 interventions "many times daily" in higher percentages than the mean "many times daily" use response percentages of overall nursing in the Iowa study. When the top 30 interventions identified by the ambulatory nurses in the Androwich (1994) study are compared with the frequency of use of the same interventions in the Bulechek et al. (1994) overall nursing study, some interesting dimensions are evident about the ambulatory nursing role. The interventions that are more frequently used in ambulatory care include "Body Mechanics Promotion" (51% vs. 45%), "Health Screening" (43% vs. 23%), "Teaching: Prescribed Medication" (41% vs. 35%), "Teaching: Disease Process" (37% vs. 35%), "Humor" (37% vs. 30%), "Teaching: Individual" (36% vs. 31%), "Teaching: Procedure/Treatment" (33% vs. 22%), "Preparatory Sensory Information" (28% vs. 24%), and "Risk Identification" (26% vs. 23%).

Interventions with more than 10% greater "many times daily" use frequency in the Bulechek et al. (1994) overall nursing study than in the ambulatory care nursing study include "Vital Signs Monitoring" (71% overall vs. 60% ambulatory care), "Emotional Support" (63% vs. 48%), "Communication Enhancement" (49% vs. 39%), "Presence" (53% vs. 38%), "Touch" (57% vs. 37%), "Medication Administration" (65% vs. 32%), "Medication Administration: Parenteral" (59% vs. 32%), "Energy Management" (43% vs. 31%), "Technology Management" (48% vs. 30%), "Environmental Management: Safety" (39% vs. 28%), "Fall Prevention" (39% vs. 26%), "Medication Administration: Oral" (58% vs. 26%), and "Environmental Management: Comfort" (35% vs. 24%).

In the multispecialty setting that was used for this study, *all* of the 336 interventions were identified as being used. This provides evidence of the practice diversity that is inherent in most ambulatory settings with several different service areas. Of the 6 domains of interventions identified in the taxonomy (McCloskey & Bulechek, 1992), 5 were reflected in the top 30 interventions, with the "Behavioral" (n = 12) and "Safety" (n = 7) domains drawing the largest number. The domain "Family" was not represented in the top 30, although it was present in the top 20 interventions in the maternal and child health service areas. This absence of interventions from the family domain is interesting given that families are specifically mentioned in two (shared responsibility for care and education) of the five ambulatory care nursing administrative and practice standards (AAACN, 1993).

The use of standardized language systems such as NIC for interventions is an important step toward implementing an NMDS in ambulatory care and will allow collection and aggregation of data across ambulatory care sites.

Another major issue with documentation involves the inability to link visits into meaningful units where goals are set over varying time periods. For example, many of the nursing interventions that are identified for a pregnant woman occur over the duration of the pregnancy and into the postpartum period. When the single visit is documented, but not linked to related visits, there is an inability to demonstrate an effective outcome related to nursing care. As we move to increasingly automated documentation in ambulatory care, we will need to determine the best method to conceptually examine and capture an entire episode of care.

Educational preparation

Significant numbers of nurses currently working in ambulatory care have many years of nursing and ambulatory care experience, but many also have less than baccalaureate preparation as their highest level of nursing education (Hackbarth et al., 1995). With expansion of ambulatory nursing roles, there are increasing expectations that ambulatory nurses coordinate care within the health care network and the community. Yet nurses without baccalaureate preparation have not had formal coursework or clinical experiences with community health nursing. Adding to this problem is the fact that significant numbers of currently practicing ambulatory care nurses do not belong to any professional nursing organizations (Haas & Hackbarth, 1995a). Therefore, continuing education through programs, newsletters, and collegial information sharing is less available to ambulatory nurses who are not members of professional organizations.

The issue of basic nursing preparation and continuing education for nurses practicing ambulatory care presents a challenge. Creative mechanisms are needed to provide incentives for nurses to enhance their formal educational preparation and to keep current with regional and national practice issues and trends. Clinical ladders or professional nursing advancement programs offer mechanisms that provide both incentives and rewards for nurses who seek educational opportunities to enhance their practice. The need for more nurses with baccalaureate degrees working in ambulatory care organizations has been identified, yet there is currently no way to provide entre to employment of these new graduates into ambulatory care.

Ambulatory care organizations might be more willing to hire new nurse graduates if they were educated to practice in ambulatory care. For example, bachelor of nursing students should have parallel ambulatory care clinical experiences. Students should spend as much time caring for pediatric, obstetric, mental health, and elderly clients in ambulatory settings as they do in hospital settings.

Delegation and supervision

Nonlicensed assistive workers have traditionally been used in ambulatory care settings. As in inpatient settings, there is a push in ambulatory care to maximize the use of assistive personnel. There is even a movement to remove all professional nurses from some ambulatory care organizations, based on the misinformed assumption that "nursing care" in ambulatory settings is strictly technical care and can be provided by technicians at a lower cost.

There are patient care delivery roles for both assistive personnel and professional nurses in ambulatory care. Assistive personnel should be performing lower level nursing activities that do not require discretionary judgment or critical thinking. Nurses working in ambulatory care want to delegate many activities that fall under the dimensions of enabling operations and technical procedures (Haas & Hackbarth, 1995a). Activities in these dimensions are listed in Table 28-2. Delegation of these dimensions would allow the professional nurse time for higher level activities in dimensions such as teaching, care coordination, and community outreach. Nurses working in ambulatory care also need time to both delegate and supervise assistive personnel. There is currently no empirical data that give direction as to the optimal number of assistive personnel that one nurse can supervise in the ambulatory setting. In addition, because many nurses grew up under primary nursing in hospitals they have little experience with delegation and supervision of assistive workers, and many have mistaken notions about how assistive workers are "working on their license." Consequently, they are reluctant to delegate to them for fear of what may happen not only to the patient but also to their license and livelihood.

As more assistive workers are incorporated in delivery models in ambulatory care organizations, nurses will need to be educated regarding delegation and supervision, and evaluation studies will be necessary to identify optimal staffing ratios including optimal spans of control. There is also a need for nursing intensity indices and systems in ambulatory care so that client demands for nursing care can be tracked and appropriate staffing can be planned and budgeted (Haas & Hackbarth, 1995b; Hastings, 1992; Verran, 1986). Caveats to consider regarding assistive workers are that assistive workers are more costly than professional nurses when there is insufficient work to occupy their time for an entire shift. When assistive workers are in a delivery model a significant portion of professional nursing time will be consumed in delegation and supervision; thus when the bulk of the care needs are at a higher level, it may be more cost-effective to hire a nurse who can perform all aspects of care and who does not require supervision. For example, there will be more activities that can be assigned to assistive workers in high-volume clinics such as general surgery or ophthalmology and perhaps less work for assistive workers in an oncology clinic where chemotherapy is being given and emotional support, care planning, and education needs are many.

Rapid pace of care

The high volume of patients with whom the nurse must interact affords a limited time for each individual patient. This means that the nurse must make rapid assessments, plan nursing care, and execute that plan in quick order. This leads to a continuing tension between the available time in an encounter and the ideal time needed for a complete nursing assessment. It is difficult for the nurse to be the patient's advocate if there is no time to spend in understanding what the patient's needs are.

Continuity of care (i.e., the extent to which the same provider is seen during a sequence of encounters) has been given attention with physician providers as a determinant of quality of primary care (Spooner, 1994). If we believe that nursing care can impact patient outcomes in ambulatory practice then it is necessary to develop models of care delivery to ensure continuity of the nurse provider.

Nurses in ambulatory care settings are often used primarily to leverage the physician's practice, and little value is placed on the dimensions of the nursing role or the nursing interventions themselves. There are a number of differentiated nursing practice models that can be used to address this (Hermann, 1993). In the model described by Hermann, nursing practice is diversified to incorporate registered nurses with differing educational preparation and practice experience. There are three levels of nursing: the staff registered nurse (usually associate-degree- or diploma-prepared), who typically supervises unlicensed personnel, provides basic triage patient education, and administers medications; the level II registered nurse (with a bachelor's degree in nursing), who functions with a broader yet still limited scope; and the clinical nurse specialist-nurse practitioner (master's prepared), who functions independently.

Another solution to the limited time a nurse can spend

Table 28-2 Dimensions of the future staff nurse role

Nine core dimensions of the future staff nurse clinical practice role and three core dimensions of the future quality improvement/research role in ambulatory care.

Factor	Dimension
Clinical practice role	
Factor I	*Enabling operations*: Order supplies, locate records, set up room, search for space/equipment, schedule appointments, transport clients, witness consent forms, maintain traffic flow, and enter data in computer
Factor II	*Technical procedures*: Assist with procedures, prepare client for procedures, chaperone during procedures, inform client about treatment, administer oral and intramuscular medications, measure vital signs, and collect specimens
Factor III	*Nursing process*: Develop nursing care plan, use nursing diagnosis, and conduct exit interview
Factor IV	*Telephone communication*: Telephone triage, call pharmacy with prescription, and call client with test results
Factor V	*Advocacy*: Make clients aware of rights, promote positive public relations, act as a client advocate, and triage client to appropriate provider
Factor VI	*Client teaching*: Assess client learning needs, instruct client on medical/nursing regimen, instruct client on home and self-care, and evaluate client care outcomes
Factor VII	*High-technology procedures*: Administer blood/blood products, perform complex treatments, and monitor clients before and after procedures
Factor VIII	*Care coordination*: Long-term supportive relationship, act as a resource person, coordinate client care, assess needs and initiate referrals, and instruct on health promotion
Factor IX	*Expert practice/community outreach*: Expertise in advanced nursing practice, function as advanced nurse resource, design and present in-service education, serve as preceptor for students, independently provide primary care, organize and conduct group teaching, participate in community outreach, follow up clients in the home
	Reliability alpha = .9098
Quality improvement/research role	
Factor I	*Quality improvement*: Implement professional standards, participate in preparation of quality improvement plan, collect and analyze quality improvement data, use quality improvement plan in practice, participate in interdisciplinary quality improvement teams, develop expected client outcomes, and utilize a client classification system
Factor II	*Research*: Facilitate nursing research, participate in research of others, follow guidelines to protect human subjects, serve on research review board, identify researchable questions, evaluate nursing research findings, and conduct own nursing research
Factor III	*Continuing education*: Participate in on-site and off-site continuing education

in a patient encounter is to develop an ambulatory care exit interview (K. Phillips, personal communication, 1994). Here the nurse has the opportunity to go over the visit with the patient, assessing learning needs and correcting any misapprehensions the patient may have with respect to future therapeutic plans, medications, or educational needs.

Phone communication

The phone communication dimension (Haas & Hackbarth, 1995a; Hackbarth et al., 1995) of the ambulatory nurse role is an aspect that is unique to ambulatory nursing practice. It is also a role dimension about which ambulatory nurses have concerns, some of which are related to the amount of education they receive regarding phone communication, particularly phone triage and phone advice, both of which have a high-liability risk potential. Assessment of the client over the phone requires a high level of assessment, including the ability to identify nuances in each situation, well-developed communication and decision-making skills, and proficiency in documentation. Nurses in ambulatory settings need to collaborate with physicians and other members of the health care team in establishing protocols that include health promotion and disease prevention as well as treatments for symptoms. Finally, nurses need to be educated that all phone communication must be documented appropriately.

Promulgation of organizational culture across settings in a network

As more acquisitions and mergers occur, health care networks will encompass multiple health care organizations and agencies. There will conceivably be networks that include several different types of ambulatory care agencies. For example, an academic health center may have in its network one or more HMOs, a university hospital outpatient center, a community hospital outpatient center, and two or more physician group practices. Ambulatory patients will move between these settings. Patients may receive primary care in an HMO or physician group practice or the community hospital outpatient center and then be referred to the university hospital outpatient center for consultation with specialists. Referrals may be made from the university hospital outpatient center back to the original primary care referral source. Ambulatory care nurses working in each of these agencies will need not only excellent negotiation skills, but they will also need to be expert at assessing the cultures in each of the agencies with which they interact. A "seamless system of care" demands that each agency's culture and requisite practices not impede a patient's progress. At this point in time, we are but neophytes in understanding organization culture. The survival of evolving health care networks will depend on management and blending of multiple organizational cultures.

CONCLUSION

Although concerns and challenges abound in the rapidly evolving world of ambulatory care nursing, they also provide multiple opportunities for nurses. Experienced ambulatory care nurses say that they would work in no other field of nursing. The opportunities to provide primary health care and build long-term relationships with patients, families, and health care colleagues are but a few of the rewards of working in ambulatory care nursing.

REFERENCES

American Academy of Ambulatory Care Nursing Standards Revision Task Force. (1993). *Ambulatory care nursing administration and practice standards.* Pitman, NJ: Janetti.

ANA & AAACN Task Force, in process. *Ambulatory care nursing (Monograph).* Washington, DC: ANA.

ANA. (1995). *Social policy statement.* Washington, DC: Author.

Androwich, I. (1994). Use of the Iowa Nursing Interventions Classification (NIC) in Ambulatory Settings. Paper presented at the American Academy of Ambulatory Care Nursing Annual Meeting. San Diego, CA.

Androwich, I., & Phillips, K. (Eds.). (1992). *The use of the minimum data set in ambulatory nursing.* American Academy of Ambulatory Nursing Administration. Pitman, NJ: Janetti.

Androwich, I., & Stoupa, R. (1994). Count what counts: The nurse manager's role in automating data. *Seminars for Nurse Managers, 2*(2), 85-91.

Bulechek, G.M., McCloskey, J.C., Titler, M.G., & Denehey, J.A. (1994). Report on the NIC project: Nursing interventions used in practice. *American Journal of Nursing, 94*(10), 59-62.

Curran, C. (1992). An interview with Mary Ann Moore. *Nursing Economics, 10*(2), 87-93.

Haas, S., Hackbarth, D., Kavanagh, J., & Vlasses, F. (1995). Dimensions of the staff nurse role in ambulatory care: Part II. Comparison of role dimensions in four ambulatory settings. *Nursing Economics, 13*(3), 152-165.

Haas, S., & Hackbarth, D. (1995a). Dimensions of the staff nurse role in ambulatory care: Part III. *Using research data to design new models of nursing care delivery. Nursing Economics, 13*(3), 230-241.

Haas, S., & Hackbarth, D. (1995b). Dimensions of the staff nurse role in ambulatory care: Part IV. *Nursing Economics,* 13(5), 285-294.

Hackbarth, D., Haas, S., Kavanagh, J., & Vlasses, F. (1995). Dimensions of the staff nurse role in ambulatory care: Part I—Methodology and analysis of data on current staff nurse practice. *Nursing Economics, 13*(2), 89-98.

Hastings, C. (1992). Classification issues in ambulatory care nursing. *Journal of Ambulatory Care Management, 10*(3), 50-64.

Hastings, C., & Muir-Nash, J. (1989). Validation of a taxonomy of ambulatory nursing practice. *Nursing Economics, 7,* 142-149.

Hermann, C.E. (1993). Diversified nursing practice in ambulatory care. *Nursing Economics, 11*(3), 176-177.

Hooks, M., Dewitz-Arnold, D., & Westbrook, L. (1980). The role of the professional nurse in the ambulatory care setting. *Nursing Administration Quarterly, 4*(4), 12-17.

Joseph, A. (1990). Ambulatory care: An objective assessment. *Journal of Nursing Administration, 20*(11), 18-24.

McCloskey, J.C., & Bulechek, G.M. (Eds.). (1992). *Nursing interventions classification.* St. Louis: Mosby.

Parrinello, K., & Witzel, P. (1990). Analysis of ambulatory nursing practice. *Nursing Economics, 8,* 322-328.

Pinkney-Atkinson, V., & Robertson, B. (1993). Ambulatory nursing: The handmaiden/specialist dichotomy, *Journal of Nursing Administration, 23*(9), 50-57.

Spooner, S.A. (1994). Incorporating temporal and clinical reasoning in a new measure of continuity of care. *Proceedings of the 18th Annual Symposium on Computer Applications in Medical Care,* 716-721.

Stavins, M. (1993). Ambulatory nursing: Facing the future. *Journal of Ambulatory Care Management, 16*(4), 67-71.

Verran, J. (1981). Delineation of ambulatory care nursing practice. *Journal of Ambulatory Care Management, 4*(2), 1-13.

Verran, J.A. (1986). Patient classification in ambulatory care. *Nursing economics, 4*(5), 347-251.

Werley, H.H., & Lang, N.M. (Eds.). (1988). *Identification of the nursing minimum data set.* New York: Springer.

Recent changes and current issues in community nursing

CAROLE A. GUTT

In an effort to stop lives from being ruined by preventable diseases, nurses need to be given greater recognition as being paramount to the quality of America's health care. Each, as a valued provider, makes daily differences in the lives of individuals and communities. (Clinton, 1993, p. 186)

Historically, nurses have been in the vanguard as champions and leaders for health in their dealings with individuals, families, and communities. The challenges of the 21st century are many and community health nursing is faced with many complex issues. As the nation struggles to address community health needs, nursing *must* move to the forefront as a resource for quality health care delivery.

Nursing's Agenda for Health Care Reform (American Nurses Association [ANA], 1991) calls for a clearly defined health care package for all U.S. citizenry through a meshing of both private and public funding sectors. Health promotion and disease prevention must be stressed with community settings serving as sites for primary health care services. Indeed, from its inception, nursing has provided community care in the domains of public health, occupational health, school health, and home care—all key sites for health care in the new millennium (de Tornyay, 1993).

In the United States in 1990, 12% of the gross national product (approximately $671 billion) was allocated to health care expenditures (Levit, Lazenby, Cowan, & Letsch, 1991). Quality health care and reduced health care costs both in the home and in community-based settings has been validated as being assisted by nursing's unique body of knowledge and services (Aiken & Fagin, 1992; Avorn, Everitt, & Baker, 1991; Evans, Strumpf, & Williams, 1991; Etheridge & Lamb, 1989). It is important to note that the system is being changed by strong forces exerting influence on the marketplace. These forces in turn must cause nursing as a profession to review its caring ethic within the perspectives of political empowerment, managed care, innovative sites for practice, and advanced roles for its community health practitioners. Community health nursing will be called on increasingly to assess the population it serves, to determine the areas of greatest need, to implement cost-effective collaborative interventions in conventional and futuristic community-based settings, and to evaluate future markets and trends as well as the quality outcomes of services provided.

POPULATION TRENDS

Community health nursing in the late 1990s and into the next century will assess the health care needs of an increasingly diverse population with continually changing needs. The U.S. Senate Special Committee on Aging (1988) projects that by the year 2020, 17% of the population will be comprised of persons over the age of 65 years. Working families can neither provide the physical care needed for the elderly in the home nor meet their special developmental needs. In addition, we will also see a much more culturally diverse population, with women and minorities representing two thirds of the workforce by the year 2000 (Nelton, 1988). One third of the country's total population will be comprised of minorities by the end of the 1990s (Hudson Institute, 1987). Mason, McEachen, and Kovner (1993) project that the effects of this in terms of both our clients and personnel must be taken into consideration in the formulation of policy and delivery of health care. Illiteracy, unemployment, poverty, homelessness, substance abuse, the return of infectious diseases (including tuberculosis), chronic illness, women's health, violence, teen pregnancy, sexually transmitted diseases, HIV/AIDS, and well child care can be seen as a web with demands and changes in each layer causing a ripple effect of the needs in other areas. For example, a Canadian study on 12 self-reported indices of health status found that the unemployed reported more stress, depression, disability days, health problems, and hospitalizations, lower activity levels, and fewer physician contacts. When one considers that the number of unemployed persons at the time of the study was approximately 3 million, the obvious effects on health care costs are significant. Unemployment is also linked to crime, abuse, and myriad other social problems (Jin, Shah, & Svoboda, 1994). Certainly community health nursing alone cannot rectify all of these rampant social ills, but it does possess the expertise and power to assist all of its publics in a healthy, quality life from birth to death.

EMPOWERMENT

Political empowerment is needed to facilitate movement of community health nurses to a proactive role in policy making for health care initiatives and reform. Empowerment as defined by Mason, Backer, and Georges (1991, p. 73) is "the enabling of individuals and groups to participate in actions and decision-making within a context that supports an equitable distribution of power." Community health nurses need to become more aware of the sociopolitical realities of their world and develop a positive group self-esteem and the political skills necessary to bring about change proactively in the health care system. Nursing as a profession, and particularly those nurses practicing in the community, need to begin to relate their work issues to those of the broader social environment. Seeking change in the legislative and executive government branches is suggested by Kjervik (1996) as a prime vehicle for community health nurses to become empowered and engender policy change. This involves becoming familiar with the law-making process at all levels of government. Public health laws have direct bearing on the areas previously mentioned such as the abuse of vulnerable populations, communicable diseases, and disease prevention, all of which are focal to community health nursing's domain of practice (Northrup & Kelly, 1987). Empowerment involves anticipatory planning and lobbying to visualize problem areas rather than being forced as a profession to react to crisis situations created by forces external to nursing.

POLITICAL AND POLICY CHANGE

Batra (1996) sees nurses as the fulcrum for grassroots sociopolitical change in their communities because of their majority position as providers of primary care and their role as gatekeepers of access, cost, and quality of care. Kjervik (1996) stresses that community health nurses must take an aggressive, and if necessary, confrontational stand with the power structure as lobbyists in Congress, expert consultants in legislative hearings, expert witnesses in courtroom settings, and participants in health care agencies' processes for rule making. Rudimentary decisions made in client screenings and referral to social and health care services are examples of individual nurses and agencies determining allocation of health care resources in the gatekeeper role.

Vance (1993) suggests that nurses utilize the three *C*s of political influence: communication, collectivity, and collegiality. Political skills are communication skills, according to Vance, and include the entire range of verbal and behavioral interpersonal communication activity. Collaboration with other nurses, professionals, consumers, and community groups provides for more effectiveness in politics and policy development. Creating change can only occur through caring and sharing of mutual convictions and values with both lay groups and professional associates.

Nurses possess or can learn the basic skills of politics (Leavitt & Barry, 1993). Through education and practice, nurses have developed the repertoire of communication skills and knowledge of the health care system that is needed to be "movers" in health care policy reform. Collegiality encompasses mentoring and role modeling. Mentors can provide guidance, advice, expertise, and inroads to opportunity for policy change. Internships and fellowships can provide positive learning and exploratory opportunities for nurses moving into political/policy arenas. Specific knowledge and information can be sought through graduate education and continuing education programs. When choosing a graduate program or registered nurse/bachelor's of science in nursing program, applicants need to verify that courses are offered in health policy and political action and ensure that the faculty have expertise in these areas.

Workshops and conferences offer opportunities to develop political sensitivity and skills. The ANA, the National League for Nursing, state nurses associations, and other providers of continuing education programs are resources for a variety of educational programs and active involvement in policy and political issues related to health. Informal learning, on the other hand, involves personal involvement and can include organizing experiences such as fundraisers or community awareness campaigns on a health-related issue. Nurse lobbyists, collective bargaining activities, and shared governance participation are all examples of hands-on experiences (Leavitt & Barry, 1993).

Basic skills in politics must be accompanied by a working knowledge of policy process if nurses are to be effective in the political arena. Policy process develops a working program for a policy that starts at the problem level and can be approached through an interactive model or a more pragmatic approach such as Anderson's sequential model (Anderson, 1990). Anderson's model has five sequential steps starting with policy agenda setting, which is the identification of a policy problem and refinement of that problem to a policy issue. The next stage is policy formulation, in which the type of policy options to be developed are addressed. Policy adoption involves getting input from all stakeholders, budget development, and funding processes. Policy implementation charges the executive or regulatory body for the program to develop the guidelines and regulations necessary for the program to function. The last phase is the policy evaluation stage to assess how the program has met its goals and objectives and whether it should be continued in total, modified, or restructured based on a changing societal need (Hanley, 1993).

Nurses can play a key role in policy analysis because they are primary stakeholders in the health care system. Policy analysis moves beyond the process to examine the causes and results of government action or lack of it. Policy issue papers identify underlying issues, give structure to the problem, collate agreements for and against the issue, and outline strategies to move the issue through the policy cycle (Hanley, 1993).

Nursing can no longer function in isolation. Empowerment can be given new meaning and integrity for nursing by expanding leadership and role modeling for policy action in health care. Figure 29-1 depicts the role and functions leading to empowerment for nurses.

ADVOCACY

Quality of life and advocacy issues are and will continue to be crucial to the practice of community health nursing in the future. Client advocacy, client rights, and accountability are contained within the basic tenets of community health standards published by the ANA ("Standards of Community Health Nursing Practice," 1986).

With the advent of formal efforts to implement cost-control policies in health care delivery, clients are being discharged to their homes more rapidly than in the past, often while still acutely ill, and are requiring high-technology care previously given in hospitals. Hyperalimentation, tracheotomy care, chemotherapy, and ventilators are now commonplace in the home settings where community health nurses practice. Nurses are called on to deal with affordability and rationing of equipment and to evaluate the impact of this care on the client and his or her family. Nurses must also enable families in the difficult judgements relevant to quality of life. Do Not Resuscitate orders, health care proxies, living wills, and durable power of attorney are areas with which the public feels uncomfortable and is lacking in knowledge. Community health nurses are often sought for expert information, evaluation of resources, and support when these very difficult choices must be made.

Nurses dealing with these sensitive, value-laden topics must be very aware of their own moral philosophies as well as of the basic principles contained in theoretical orientations such as deontology, teleology, virtue ethics, and care-based ethics. Respect for clients' autonomy, beneficence, and maleficence have been incorporated into a model by Cameron (1993) that asks nurses to consider their intent in a given situation in the framework of the relevant ethical principles balanced against the consumers' wants and needs. Conflicts in any of these spheres must be addressed with clients and their support systems before decisions are finalized.

Nurses often feel at a loss when it is suggested that they need to work openly and advocate with community forces to bring about policy change and empowerment. The first step according to Lacey and Atwell (1993) is to recognize that a problem exists and then accept the challenge to work on solutions. Networking is imperative and must include the publics to be served as active participants in the decision-making process. Public policymakers must then be approached for their support as well as that of other professional and activist groups. Advocacy for community-client groups demands sincerity, credibility, working with people in the community at the grassroots level, suggesting alternative and concrete solutions, and maintaining a high level of enthusiasm. Dealing with politicians, lawmakers, and elected officials requires using appropriate means of "leverage" while distancing oneself from involvement in internal politics. Support personnel are excellent "helpmates" if approached in an open and respectful manner. Knowledge of the organizational structure and departmental functions of any organization approached speeds up contacts and eliminates wasted ef-

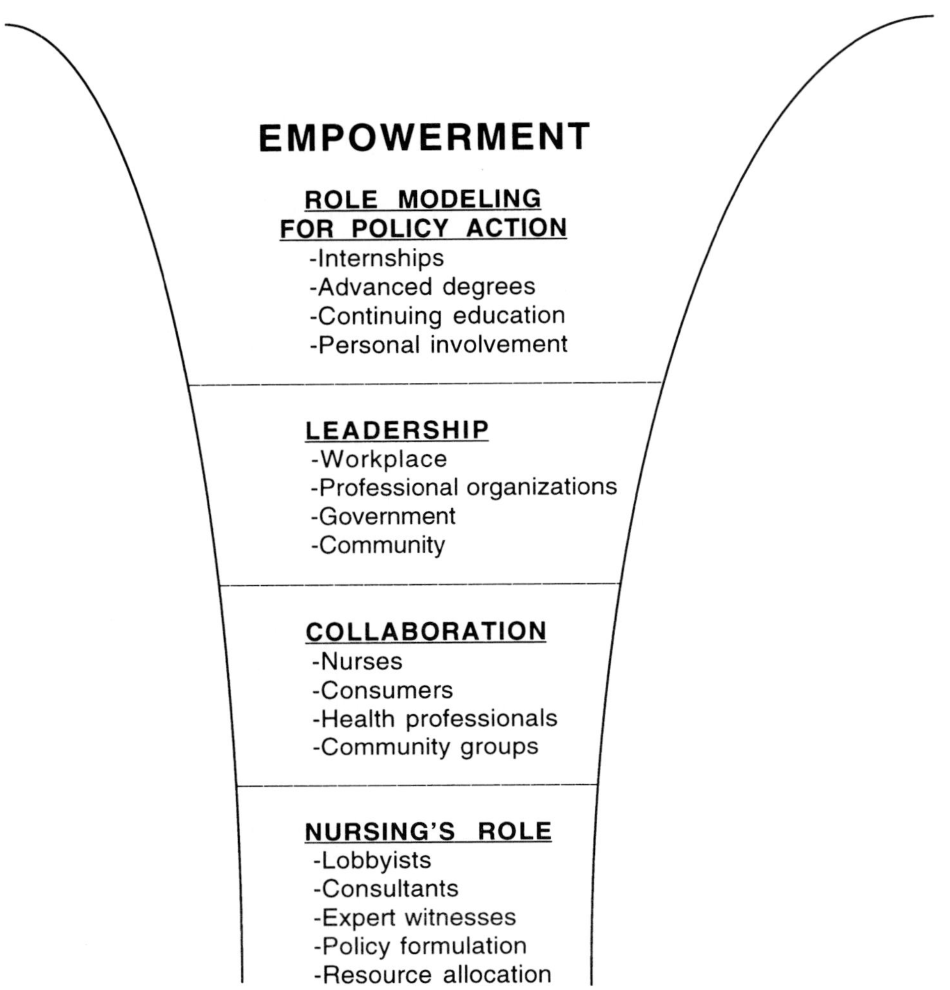

Fig. 29-1. The road to empowerment.

forts and stalemating. It is most crucial to keep all levels of the advocacy group informed and up to date to avoid closing them out and losing their participation and input. This method was used successfully by Lacey and Atwell (1993) to initiate an infirmary for homeless men in Washington, D.C. in 1986. Nurses can and *must* begin to take a more proactive, visible role in community advocacy and break from the restricted roles of the past.

FUTURE PRACTICE AND TRENDS

The year 2000 will witness drastic changes in the roles of nurses and the settings in which they practice. Community and ambulatory settings will come to the forefront as sites of care as hospital downsizing continues throughout the late 1990s. Cost containment will be a more pressing issue than ever before. Primary care, prevention, community-based practices, managed care, and collaborative provider partnerships are the wave of the future. As consumers of health care, clients will need to be empowered and knowledgeable participants in their health care.

Primary care, which involves basic health care with an emphasis on prevention, health assessment, diagnosis, and management of common acute and chronic illnesses, is the most reasonable means of guaranteeing affordability, access, and quality of care (Lancaster & Lancaster, 1993). This can be facilitated by increased use of midlevel providers (advanced practice nurses) such as clinical

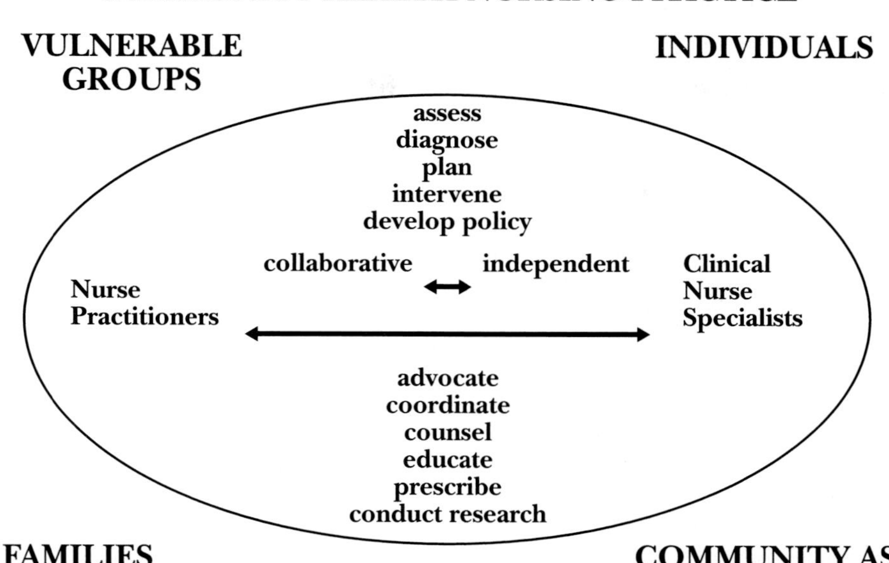

Fig. 29-2. Scope of practice and roles of community health nurses.

nurse specialists and nurse practitioners. Nurse practitioners are trained specifically to focus on health problems of individuals and families, to obtain histories and perform physical examinations including diagnostic tests, to diagnose and treat common health problems, to monitor chronic diseases, to prescribe or recommend prescriptive drugs and treatments, and to provide prenatal services, family planning, and well child services. Health maintenance care and health and lifestyle education and counseling are part of their role. The nurse practitioner works as part of the interdisciplinary health services team (Lancaster & Lancaster, 1993). McGarth (1990) has stated that the use of nurse practitioners is cost-effective and provides comparable care to that provided by physicians. Cost savings annually have been estimated between $6.4 and $8.75 billion (Nichols, 1992).

Community health clinical nurse specialists function in roles of administration, clinical practice, consultation, education, and research (Sparacino, Cooper, & Minarik, 1990, "Standards," 1986). The community health nurse synthesizes nursing practice and public health practice and applies the synthesis to promoting and preserving the health of populations (American Nurses Credentialing Center, 1993). Promotion of the health of the community is the primary objective of the community health clinical nurse specialist (Kupina, 1995).

Specialists in community health nursing are educated at the master's or doctoral level and have in-depth knowledge in the areas of sociopolitical theory, health policy, ethical and legal issues, health care delivery system economics and politics, quality assurance and change, and empowerment theory (ANA, 1986).

The community health clinical nurse specialist implements community programs to achieve health goals, collaborates with other community and professional factions to develop resources and implement such programs, maintains a channel of information to the community regarding its health status and resources, conducts and reviews research to evaluate outcomes, and has an active role in health and social policy. Individual, family, and community levels fall within their scope of practice (ANA, 1986).

Settings for advanced nursing practice in the future will include home care, ambulatory care, health promotion and disease prevention programs, nurse-managed clinics or nursing centers, private practice, and parish settings. Jenkins and Sullivan-Marx (1994) see nurse practitioners as key figures in case management in primary care settings. Coordination of a clinical database and follow-up is orchestrated by a health care provider who could be either a nurse practitioner or clinical nurse specialist. Case management roles encompass interviewing skills, negotiation ability, communication skills, and problem-solving skills (Mullahy, 1995). University–clinical agency partnerships are now being seen as venues to expand case management services into communities. Successful projects carried out through a collaborative effort between the School of Nursing at San Francisco State University and local health care agencies was successful in establishing a new patient care delivery system in a hospital, a school-based health center for high-risk adolescents, case management services for high-risk pregnant women, and a comprehensive perinatal care program. Faculty and students bring in-depth knowledge of grants, research, and evaluative techniques along with clinical expertise and program development skills. Health agencies bring current knowledge of changes and trends in health care and nursing practice, which in turn can be used to update and revise curricula. Certainly, the benefits to the populations served are the most positive outcome of the joint venture (Haw & Ferretti, 1995).

INTERDISCIPLINARY COLLABORATION

As community health nurses move into new settings and roles, perspectives and the practice of nursing are changing (Fig. 29-2). Figure 29-2 presents the scope of practice and roles of community health nurses. Interdisciplinary collaboration, which includes the consumer as a key player, is vital to a cost-effective, quality system of health care delivery. "The development of coordinated, efficient and effective services through the unique contributions of allied health, medicine, nursing, pharmacy and other health professionals is needed for patients who have increasingly sophisticated health care needs" (de Tornyay, 1993). For change to occur in the health care system, "nurses must develop support bases that cut across disciplines" (Mason et al., 1993). Creative problem solving can best be achieved through interdisciplinary alliances and coalitions with other health professionals with resultant quality care for the community.

REFERENCES

Aiken, L.H., & Fagin, C.M. (1992). *Charting nursing's future: Agenda for the 1990's.* Philadelphia: Lippincott.

American Nurses Association. (1991). *Nursing's agenda for health care reform.* Kansas City, MO: Author.

American Nurses Association. (1986). *The role of the clinical nurse specialist.* Kansas City, MO: Author.

American Nurses Credentialing Center. (1993). *American Nurses Credentialing Center certification catalog.* Washington, DC: Author.

Anderson, J.E. (1990). *Public policymaking.* Boston: Houghton Mifflin.

Avorn, J., Everitt, D.E., & Baker, M.W. (1991). The neglected medical history and therapeutic choices for abdominal pain: A nationwide study of 799 physicians and nurses. *Archives of Internal Medicine, 151*(4), 694-698.

Batra, C. (1996, in press). Professional issues. In J. Cookfair (Ed.), *Nursing process and practice in the community* (pp. 681-703). St. Louis: Mosby.

Cameron, M.E. (1993). *Living with AIDS: Experiencing ethical problems.* Newbury Park, CA: Sage Publications.

Clinton, H.R. (1993). Nurses in the front lines. *Nursing & Health Care, 14*(6), 286-288.

de Tornyay, R. (1993). Education: Staying on track. *Nursing & Health Care, 14*(6), 302-306.

Etheridge, P., & Lamb, G.S. (1989). Professional nursing care management improves quality, access and costs. *Nursing Management, 20*(3), 33.

Evans, L., Strumpf, N., & Williams, C. (1991). Redefining a standard of care for frail older people: Alternatives to reduce routine physical restraint. In P. Katz, R. Kane, & M. Mezey (Eds.), *Advances in long term care* (vol. 1, pp. 81-108). New York: Springer.

Hanley, B.E. (1993). Policy development and analysis. In D. Mason, S. Talbott, & J. Leavitt (Eds.), *Policy and politics for nurses* (pp. 71-87). Philadelphia: Saunders.

Haw, M.A., & Ferretti, C. (1995). University-clinical agency partnerships: Cost-effective opportunities to expand case management services and measure outcomes. *The Journal of Care Management, 1*(1), 10-36.

Hudson Institute. (1987). *Workforce 2000.* Washington, DC: U.S. Department of Labor.

Jenkins, M.L., & Sullivan-Marx, E.M. (1994). Nurse practitioners and community health nurses: Clinical partnerships and future visions. *Nursing Clinics of North America, 29*(3), 459-470.

Jin, R., Shah, C., & Svoboda, T. (1994). The health impact of unemployment: A review and application of research evidence. *Registered Nurse, 6*(6), 10-13.

Kjervik, D.K. (1996). Legal and ethical issues. In J. Cookfair (Ed.), *Nursing process and practice in the community* (pp. 663-680). St. Louis: Mosby.

Kupina, P. (1995). Community health CNSs and health care in the year 2000. *Clinical Nurse Specialist, 9*(4), 188-198.

Lacey, B.M., & Atwell, W.M. (1993). Working with the community for change. In D. Mason, S. Talbott, & J. Leavitt (Eds.), *Policy and politics for nurses* (pp. 622-635). Philadelphia: Saunders.

Lancaster, J., & Lancaster, W. (1993). Nurse practioners: Health care providers whose time has come. *Family & Community Health, 16*(2), 1-8.

Leavitt, J.K., & Barry, C.T. (1993). Learning the ropes. In D. Mason, S. Talbott, & J. Leavitt (Eds.), *Policy and politics for nurses* (pp. 47-61). Philadelphia: Saunders.

Levit, K.R., Lazenby, H.C., Cowan, C.A., & Letsch, S.W. (1991). National health expenditures, 1990. *Health Care Financing Review, 13*(1), 29-45.

Mason, D.J., Backer, B.A., & Georges, C.A. (1991). Toward a feminist model for the political empowerment of nurses. *Image, 23*(2), 72-77.

Mason, D.J., McEachen, I., & Kovner, C.T. (1993). Contemporary issues in the workplace. In D. Mason, S. Talbott, & J. Leavitt (Eds.), *Policy and politics for nurses* (pp. 223-240). Philadelphia: Saunders.

McGarth, S. (1990). The cost effectiveness of nurse practitioners. *Nurse Practitioner, 1*(5), 40-42.

Mullahy, C.M. (1995). The case manager is the catalytic collaborator in managed care. *The Journal of Care Management, 1*(1), 7-10.

Nelton, S. (1988, July). Meet your new workforce. *Nation's Business,* 12-17.

Nichols, L.M. (1992). Estimating the cost of underusing advanced practice nurses. *Nursing Economics, 10*(5), 343-351.

Northrup, C.E., & Kelly, M.E. (1987). *Legal issues in nursing.* St. Louis: Mosby.

Sparacino, P., Cooper, D.M., & Minarik, P.A. (1990). *The clinical nurse specialist.* Norwalk, CT: Appleton & Lange.

Standards of community health nursing practice (1986). Kansas City, MO: American Nurses Association.

U.S. Senate Special Committee on Aging. (1988). *Aging America: Trends and projections* Government Document Y3.F31/15:2AG4/2/987-881089. Washington, DC: U.S. Department of Health and Human Services.

Vance, C. (1993). Politics: A humanistic process. In D. Mason, S. Talbott, & J. Leavitt (Eds.), *Policy and politics for nurses* (pp. 104-117). Philadelphia: Saunders.

Recent changes and current issues in emergency nursing

MARILYN RICE, DEBORAH S. SMITH

The professional association for emergency nurses, the Emergency Nurses Association (ENA), was chartered in 1970 as a result of the efforts of two nurses, Dorr from Buffalo, New York, and Kelleher from Downey, California. Originally called the Emergency Department Nurses Association, ENA now boasts over 24,000 members representing every state in the United States as well as 22 other countries. While the ENA represents a significant number of emergency nurses, the number of nurses practicing in emergency care settings in the United States is estimated at 70,000. This number is changing with the work redesign that is occurring across the country.

PRACTICE ISSUES

The changes occurring in health care in recent years have impacted the professional practice of emergency nursing. Many of these changes are exciting and provide new and unique opportunities for the emergency nurse, including role expansion beyond the primary role of direct caregiver to include collaborative practice with other disciplines, the facilitation and coordination of care utilizing assistive personnel, and involvement in aspects of management, education, and research (ENA, 1994b).

Nonlicensed caregivers in the emergency care setting

Emergency care settings have not been left out of the reengineering and restructuring efforts that are occurring throughout the health care industry. The use of nonlicensed personnel to assist emergency nurses in the delivery of patient care began in the 1950s (Curry, 1992). The number of nonlicensed personnel grew steadily in the 1980s as hospitals attempted to meet the increasing demand for nursing services. Today, the title of nonlicensed provider may be emergency department technician, orderly, patient care technician, care partner, or patient care assistant.

The use of nonlicensed personnel was originally task-oriented, including duties such as patient transport, stocking rooms, and making beds. The statement by the American Hospital Association (1991), which reported that hospitals that successfully implement "nurse extenders" could save as much as 60% of the cost of a nurse's salary, reflects the rationale of many health care institutions in allowing the registered nurse (RN) increased responsibility for professional nursing practice and decreasing their use as "universal worker bees" (Evans, 1991).

In attempting to decrease cost and maintain a high level of care, the skills and training of nonlicensed caregivers in the emergency care setting must be evaluated continually. Nonlicensed personnel frequently focus on fulfilling defined tasks and require more structure and supervision than do professional staff members (Beardsley & Hatler, 1994). A position paper by the ENA in 1993 states that the scope of practice, role, and lines of accountability for the non–registered nurse (RN) caregiver in the emergency department has not been clearly delineated or well defined, contributing to a fragmented approach to patient care and infringement on nursing's scope of practice and the potential for compromise of quality patient care (ENA, 1993).

As change occurs in all aspects of health care, emergency nurses cannot be immune to changes in their practice. The use of non-RN caregivers in the emergency setting can work, but only if these caregivers are under the direct supervision of the emergency nurse. Essential skills for the emergency nurse include effective delegation and follow-up. Tasks, such as taking vital signs, wound preparation and dressings, and patient transport can be delegated to non-RN practitioners who have received adequate orientation and skill validation. The RN, utilizing the nursing process, can use assistive personnel effectively as an adjunct in providing care to their patients.

Triage

One of the highest-level skills associated with the critical judgement of the emergency nurse is that of triage. Surprisingly, there continue to be emergency services that do not have any type of nurse triage system yet established. The need for well-educated, highly skilled triage nurses is key to the success of any triage program. A recent survey revealed that in only 59.4% of hospitals is triage performed by an RN (Purnell, 1993).

Triage includes not only the prioritization of care with the emergency department, but also the initial physical assessment and provision of emergency interventions. When a triage system is functioning most effectively, patient satisfaction is increased and total length of stay can be decreased (Geraci & Geraci, 1994). The triage nurse is facing increasing challenges with the expansion of managed care plans. The Consolidated Omnibus Budget Reconciliation Act (COBRA) legislation (discussed later in this chapter), patient rights, and reimbursement issues may all be at odds.

Changing patient populations

Infectious disease. Emergency care practitioners are perhaps the most susceptible of all health care providers to exposure to unknown infectious diseases. With the increased incidence of tuberculosis, the emergency nurse must be attuned to identifying the prevailing signs and symptoms from the initial presentation of the patient at the triage desk in order to protect caregivers from unforeseen exposure.

Unlike hospitalized patients, who may already be under isolation precautions, patients presenting the emergency department may not have any idea that they are infected with a communicable disease. With the rising incidence of tuberculosis and HIV, it is essential that emergency personnel receive continuing education regarding disease transmission, treatment, and protective measures (ENA, 1994c). Facility design of emergency care areas must include sufficient and strategically located negative pressure rooms. The necessary protective equipment must be present in sufficient quantities to meet patient volume and staffing demands.

Increasing acuity. In the last few decades emergency rooms have evolved into emergency departments, with state-of-the-art high-technology equipment and a growing acutely ill patient population being cared for in them. In some institutions a shortage of critical care beds or critical care nurses has caused the emergency department to hold acutely ill patients for longer periods of time, providing ongoing evaluation and treatment.

Care of patients with invasive monitoring, balloon pumps, and intracranial pressure monitoring is just one of many critical care skills that are frequently required of emergency nurses today. These patients may receive 1:1 or 2:1 nursing care in an intensive care unit, and staffing in the emergency department needs to be adjusted to meet the care needs of these acutely ill patients.

Early hospital discharges. As hospitals are decreasing the length of stay, recently discharged patients are returning to the emergency department with continuing symptoms and problems. Surgical procedures that previously required an overnight stay are being done on an outpatient basis. Postprocedure complications are being seen in the emergency department during evening and night hours. As the number of outpatient procedures and surgeries increases, the numbers of these patients can be expected to increase. This includes problems arising from mothers and babies discharged with the obstetrical short-stay programs being promoted nationwide.

Observation units

Observation units are springing up in hospitals across the country as a result of the need to provide longer periods of patient treatment for those who do not meet the sometimes stringent admission criteria imposed by payers. These may be handled as inpatient units but are being seen more frequently as an emergency department service.

When an observation unit is part of the emergency department, the nurse manager needs to be involved integrally in the development of the admission and discharge criteria, staffing patterns, and other operational issues relative to the unit (ENA, 1994a). Although certain advantages may exist in having an emergency department–based observation unit, the drawbacks may outweigh the benefits.

The patient care delivered in an observation unit more closely reflects the type of care delivered in a typical medical-surgical setting as opposed to the emergency department. Although the emergency department staff often enjoy the opportunity to spend more time with patients and their families, they may become frustrated with the constant changing of their roles. The flexibility of staffing, touted as an advantage, may not be the best way to meet the needs of the patients in the emergency department's observation unit. When deluged with high patient volumes or acuity, staff may be pulled from the observation unit to meet the immediate, staffing needs of the emergency department, leaving less than optimal staff in the observation unit. Staffing the unit with a nonemergency nurse would reduce the flexibility in crossing back and forth between the acute care and observation areas.

Credentials

One of the realities of emergency nursing is that an unusually high number of credentials and certifications are required by nurses practicing in the specialty (see Table 30-1). In addition to basic life support, advanced cardiac life support is the standard for any emergency nurse in this specialty practice setting (ENA, 1994a). The trauma nursing core course is the recommended minimal trauma nursing education standard (ENA, 1995d). For emergency departments caring for pediatric patients, pediatric advanced life support and an emergency nursing pediatrics course are recommended. In hospitals with prehospital care involvement, the mobile intensive care nurse credential may be required.

Certification in the specialty of emergency nursing is granted by the Board of Certification for Emergency Nursing. First established in 1980, the certified emergency nurse (CEN) credential is currently held by almost 23,000 practitioners in the United States and Canada. Prerequisites for the examination are 2 years of experience in emergency nursing care. The CEN's purpose is to validate the specialized body of knowledge that is unique to emergency nursing. Evaluation of this knowledge at the competency level by the CEN examination contributes to the quality of care by validating that a defined body of emergency nursing knowledge has been demonstrated. The CEN is gaining greater recognition internationally, with the first CEN examinations being offered internationally in 1995 in Australia and New Zealand. For emergency nurses in the specialty of flight nursing, the certified flight registered nurse (CFRN) examination has been available since 1993.

Advanced practice nurses

The role of the advanced practice nurse, particularly that of the nurse practitioner, is gaining momentum throughout the various emergency care settings. During the 1970s emergency nurse practitioner programs arose with roles more similar to those of a physician's assistant. Graduate level preparation was not a requirement. It is estimated that approximately 200 emergency nurses completed such programs before this type of federally funded program was discontinued in the early 1980s.

Table 30-1 Credentials for emergency nurses

Credential	Description	Offered By
BLS	Basic life support	American Heart Association
ACLS	Advanced cardiac life support	American Heart Association
TNCC	Trauma nursing core course	Emergency Nurses Association
ENPC	Emergency nursing pediatric course	Emergency Nurses Association
PALS	Pediatric advanced life support	American Heart Association
MICN	Mobile intensive care nurse	State or local regulations
CEN	Certified emergency nurse	Board of Certification for Emergency Nursing
CFRN	Certified flight registered nurse	Board of Certification for Emergency Nursing

With the increase of alternative care settings has also come an increase in the use of the nurse practitioner in the emergency care setting. It is currently estimated that only 1% of all nurse practitioners (approximately 320) are practicing in emergency department settings (Curry, 1994). New programs are being developed to meet the increased demand. In 1994, the first students were selected to begin studies in the newly established emergency nurse practitioner program at the University of Texas Houston Health Science Center School of Nursing. Upon graduation, the emergency nurse practitioners will be prepared to care for emergent, urgent, and nonurgent patient populations in a busy hospital emergency department, flight program, urgent care setting, or rural, underserved emergency department setting.

The Board of Certification for Emergency Nursing is currently looking at issues and exploring the potential for a certification for emergency services advanced practice nurses. For ENPs to practice to their fullest potential, autonomous practice and third-party reimbursement must become more prevalent.

Changing practice settings

No longer is the practice of emergency nursing limited to the hospital emergency department. With the movement to improve access to care and to provide customer-friendly, convenient care, there has been an increase in the development of urgent care settings, either community-based or within the walls of the hospital.

Although a separate specialty represented by the National Flight Nurses Association, the roots of flight nursing are firmly planted in emergency nursing. Many flight programs require nurses to have previous emergency care experience. Poison control nurses similarly have an emergency nursing background.

The practice of the emergency nurse in the prehospital care setting has been a source of continuing debate. Just as nurses are concerned about the infringement of prehospital care providers (emergency medical technicians) on their scope of practice within the hospital, emergency medical technicians in several states have effectively blocked the nurse from practicing in the prehospital setting. These are issues that must be dealt with at the state nurse practice act level.

As hospitals develop innovative programs to generate new revenues, the development of occupational health clinics offers expanded practice opportunities for emergency nurses. Similarly, walk-in clinics for nonacute treatment and procedures are becoming more common (Bailey, 1991).

Even within the traditional hospital setting, new roles and responsibilities are available for the emergency nurse. The emergency services case manager is a relatively recent role, often limited to larger, tertiary care centers to help coordinate the services of the many departments and agencies involved in meeting the needs of the emergency patient. As the development of critical paths and practice guidelines for the emergency department becomes more widespread, it is anticipated that the number of emergency service case managers will increase. Emergency nurses will, in general, serve as the overall coordinators of patient care.

LEGISLATIVE ISSUES

COBRA

Enacted in 1985, COBRA was a response by Congress to the mounting concerns of denial of care and inappropriate patient transfers. The COBRA legislation, revised several times since its initial passage, requires that hospitals receiving Medicare funds provide a medical screening examination to determine whether an emergency condition exists to all patients presenting to a hospital for care. Such a condition, if found, requires the hospital to provide immediate and stabilizing care prior to considering a transfer. These provisions also include patients in active labor (Southard, 1989).

The increased prevalence of managed care plans throughout the country, many of which require precertification for emergency treatment, presents a dilemma for emergency departments. Patients may not be questioned about financial considerations prior to being screened for an emergency medical condition. Therefore, many emergency departments have adopted the position of triaging and providing treatment to all presenting patients, and then obtaining financial information following treatment (Hulen & Beeler, 1995). Patients then may be "stuck with the bill" if the managed care plan will not authorize the emergency department treatment. The ethics presented by this situation have caused emergency nurses and physicians to work with their legislators to develop solutions.

Access to care

In July 1995, a bill entitled Access to Emergency Medical Services Act of 1995 was introduced to Congress. This legislative initiative, developed in cooperation with the American College of Emergency Physicians and supported in concept by the ENA Board of Directors, establishes a uniform "prudent layperson" definition of an emergency medical condition and enacts it for all health plans, including Medicare and Medicaid (ENA, 1995a). Passage of the bill would end a traditional practice by many managed care plans to retrospectively deny coverage for the provision of legitimate emergency health care services and establishes other important standards for managed care plans as they relate to emergency health care services. At time of this writing, the bill is still in committee.

Trauma

Issues related to trauma include the incidence of the disease and the systems in place to care for its victims. With the increase in domestic violence and other violent crimes, emergency nurses must not only keep their clinical skills relative to trauma fine-tuned, but must also work with their respective governmental agencies and legislators to promote prevention and enforcement.

Continued funding for trauma centers and trauma patient care is also an issue for education of the public and legislators. Reimbursement by insurance companies for trauma-related incidents and government funding of trauma centers is the responsibility of all care providers. Personnel in trauma care must manage their programs in an "extremely cost effective, efficient, quality program . . . and be willing to speak to the legislature or the insurance companies when proposals come forward that could eventually diminish the effectiveness of the trauma system" (Southard, 1994, p. 423).

Legislative agendas

Issues that remain a high priority to emergency nursing practice include those related to the scope of nursing practice, the welfare of emergency care workers, bans on the sale of assault weapons, the prevention of domestic violence and the treatment of its victims, support for vehicle passenger safety measures, monitoring child health issues, and legislation that addresses other means of injury prevention, trauma care, and emergency care.

MANAGEMENT ISSUES

As organizations become flatter, the emergency service managers may find themselves accountable for a broader scope of responsibility. With decentralization, many of the layers of management are being eliminated, thus empowering the emergency services staff with previous managerial responsibilities such as scheduling, quality improvement, practice issues, and others. The previous nurse manager role is broadening to include responsibilities reflecting the entire scope of emergency care and often more than one department. The traditional role of the manager is becoming that of a facilitator, adviser, and coach. A variety of management changes are being seen in that emergency departments may not have a manager, or the manager may not be a nurse. The emergency department nurse manager must interface not only with all hospital departments, but also with agencies and services within the community (Bailey, 1991).

Contract management

Over 50% of the approximately 5,200 hospital emergency departments in this country have contracted to manage their services (Greene, 1994). Similar to the rest of the health care industry, contract management companies are engaged in a flurry of mergers and acquisitions. In the future, it will become more common for emergency physician contract groups to provide emergency settings not only with physician staff, but also with all caregivers including nurses. Leasing the emergency department entirely, including the facility and human resources, is a business venture clearly on the horizon (Lorenz, 1994).

Physician practice management companies provide capital, managed care expertise, and information systems and achieve economies of scale in return for a percentage of revenues or a management fee. Some hospitals are entering into joint ventures with these companies to ensure a piece of the capitation dollar or a steady referral stream (Jaklevik, 1995). The emergency nursing manager may be an employee of one of these companies, or, as a hospital employee, may be closely involved with working with a contract management company in the provision of emergency health care services. Nurse entrepreneurs may find opportunities by venturing within these groups and perhaps nurse-owned and -managed practice management companies will become a reality in the not too distant future.

Managed care

Managed care is no longer limited to the East and West Coasts of the United States. With the market-driven health care reform initiatives taking place across the country, emergency nurse managers must position the services of their departments to compete in this arena. Even Medicare reimbursement, which has remained fee-for-service, is not far from changing to a prospective payment system.

It is believed that health care reform and its ensuing and often tumultuous changes are the biggest challenges faced by emergency nurses today (Lee, 1994). The emergency department is often the only location where some patients can receive the care they need. If a family is without insurance coverage or does not have access to a primary care physician, the emergency department, open 24 hours a day, 365 days a year, is available to them. This presents funding issues for the departments as well. In some areas, emergency departments are establishing primary health care clinics just to meet this demand (Lee, 1994).

Utilization review, new product and service development, managed care contracting, and innovative pricing strategies are just a few of the elements the nurse manager must include in any plans to compete in a managed care marketplace (Donker, 1992). Even in communities where managed care has had little impact, these strategies can be used to help provide the delivery of cost-efficient emergency health care.

Informatics

The expression, "We're drowning in information but starved for knowledge," represents the need for improved automation of emergency department data (Maclean, 1995). The efficient processing of this data into systems useful in the management of emergency services is in its infancy. The increased data management capabilities in emergency services has expanded to include complex registration capabilities; automated triage; patient flow monitoring; clinical uses including reference information retrieval, automated diagnoses based on symptoms, and other data; drug dosage calculations; patient history profiles; medical record management, including system-driven and voice-activated report dictation; trauma registries, point-of-service billing; hospital-to-hospital linkages; and automated patient discharge instructions (Matson, 1992). Until recently, computerization and informatics development within the typical emergency department was limited to registration and order-entry/ results-reporting capabilities. With the explosion in computer-based technology, patient assessment and treatment information, on-line consultation via teleconferencing, and voice recognition documentation are becoming realities. Paperless patient information systems in the many facets of emergency care are the goal. Emergency nursing practice must evolve to include competency with the information systems available in the practice setting. Emergency nurse managers must develop the skills and comfort with data management, utilizing databases and spread sheets as aides to their management tasks.

OTHER ISSUES

Violence in the emergency care setting

A 1994 ENA survey of 4,600 emergency department nurse managers (response of greater than 1,400) revealed that violence is a frequent, if not daily, occurrence in many emergency departments (ENA, 1995c). Emergency personnel are exposed to high levels of violence on a regular basis (see Table 30-2 for findings).

Violence in the emergency care setting can be precipitated by a number of factors, including emergency department overcrowding, easy hospital access through the emergency department, the families and friends of patients in a crisis situation, long wait times, and the availability of controlled substances and other drugs. A study performed by the California Emergency Nurses Association (Keep & Glibert, 1992) of five metropolitan areas revealed that 58% of 103 hospitals surveyed reported injuries by staff members, visitors, or patients as a result of violence. The most common weapons used were guns and knives.

Table 30-2 Violence in the emergency care setting: results of survey

Question	Response (%)
Staff exposed to verbal abuse more than 20 times per year	97
Staff exposed to physical assault without weapons 1 to 5 times per year	87
Staff exposed to physical violence with weapons 1 to 5 times per year	24
Physical injuries to staff	67
Minor	96
Resulting in lost work time	18

Note. From "Emergency Nurses Association Violence in the Emergency Care Setting Survey Results," Emergency Nurses Association, 1995, Park Ridge, IL, Author. Reprinted with permission.

Information from the ENA survey is being used extensively for legislative action at state levels to protect health care workers from violence. Additionally, education of staff relative to recognition of hostile situations and the skills with which to handle them, the use of trained security personnel, and environmental controls that serve as a deterrent against violence are being promoted.

Media representation of emergency nursing

With the highest-rated television show in 1995 being NBC's "ER," emergency nurses have had the unique opportunity to help shape and significantly impact the image portrayed of the profession and specialty to the general public. Taking the positive position to work with the producers, writers, publicists, and others from Warner Brothers and NBC to develop an authentic and accurate portrayal of emergency nursing and emergency department operations, emergency nurses from across the country have been interviewed by telephone, in person, and in focus groups for story ideas and opinions by the shows screenwriters. Members of the cast portraying nurses attended the ENA 1994 and 1995 annual meetings to meet and network with practicing emergency nurses from various practice settings and to learn about the complex realities of emergency care in this country.

Following the pilot episode in which the nurse manager attempts suicide via a drug overdose, the portrayal of emergency nursing has improved to the point at which the show received a Special Board Recognition Award from the ENA in 1995. The award acknowledges the program's positive effect on the public perceptions of emergency nursing, recognizing that there is a degree of artistic license taken with the presentation of an ongoing dramatic series.

On a weekly basis, "ER" reinforces strong favorable impressions of emergency nursing to millions of viewers. The number of student nurses aspiring to the emergency nursing specialty has been no doubt influenced by the show. Actors and representatives of the program have also helped promote nursing benefits, such as the Violence Benefit in June 1995 held by the American Nurses Foundation in Washington, D.C. Emergency nurses have learned that a powerful message of education and prevention can be sent out to the public through programs such as this. The 1995 ENA theme of "Know us before you need us" was demonstrated throughout nursing's involvement with the media and can be enhanced and built upon in the future.

REFERENCES

American Hospital Association. (1991, November 23). *Hospitals cut cost, relieve nurse shortage with nurse extenders* [News release]. Chicago: Author.

Bailey, M.M. (1991, September). What the future holds for E.D. nursing. *Nursing 91*(3), 84-89.

Beardsley, S., & Hatler, C. (1994). Nonlicensed, multiskilled workers in the emergency department: One hospital's experience. *Journal of Emergency Nursing, 20*(5), 377-382.

Curry, J.L. (1992). Oil on troubled waters: Unlicensed assistive personnel in the emergency department. *Journal of Emergency Nursing, 18*(5), 428-431.

Curry, J.L. (1994). Nurse practitioners in the emergency department: Current issues. *Journal of Emergency Nursing, 20*(3), 207-212.

Donker, R.B. (1992). Managed care. In T.A. Matson & P. McNamara (Eds.), *The hospital emergency department: A guide to operational excellence* (pp. 115-124). Chicago: American Hospital Publishing, Inc.

Emergency Nurses Association. (1993). *ENA position statement on the use of non-registered nurse (non-RN) care givers in emergency care.* Park Ridge, IL: Author.

Emergency Nurses Association. (1994a). *Emergency nursing core curriculum.* Philadelphia: Saunders.

Emergency Nurses Association. (1994b). *ENA position statement on the role of the emergency nurse in clinical practice settings.* Park Ridge, IL: Author.

Emergency Nurses Association. (1994c). *ENA position statement on tuberculosis exposure in the emergency department.* Park Ridge, IL: Author.

Emergency Nurses Association. (1995a, July 27). *Federal legislative report.* Park Ridge, IL: Author.

Emergency Nurses Association. (1995b). *ENA position statement on observation/holding areas.* Park Ridge, IL: Author.

Emergency Nurses Association. (1995c). *ENA position statement on violence in the emergency care setting.* Park Ridge, IL: Author.

Emergency Nurses Association. (1995d). *ENA position statement on minimal trauma nursing education recommendations.* Park Ridge, IL: Author.

Evans, S.A. (1991). Delegation: What do we fear? [Editorial]. *Heart Lung, 20,* 17A-20A.

Geraci, E.B., & Geraci, T.A. (1994). An observational study of the emergency triage nursing role in a managed care facility. *Journal of Emergency Nursing, 20*(3), 189-194.

Greene, J. (1994, January 31). Contracts are catching on. *Modern Healthcare,* 29-34.

Hulen, K.D., & Beeler, L.M. (1995). TennCare: The impact of state health care reform on emergency patients and caregivers. *Journal of Emergency Nursing, 21*(4), 282-286.

Jaklevik, M.C. (1995, August 14). Doc practice management set to explode. *Modern Healthcare,* 26-31.

Keep, N., & Glibert, P. (1992). California Emergency Nurses Association informal survey of violence in California emergency departments. *Journal of Emergency Nursing, 18*(5), 433-439.

Lee, M. (1994). Emergency nursing at the crossroads. *American Journal of Nursing, 93,* 65-66.

Lorenz, S.D. (1994, October 1). The changing face of emergency services. Paper presented at the Emergency Nurses Association Annual Meeting.

Maclean, S.L. (1995). The ENA national emergency department database. *ENA Management Update, 2*(3), 5.

Matson, T.A. (1992). Information systems. In T.A. Matson & P. McNamara (Eds.), *The hospital emergency department: A guide to operational excellence* (pp. 115-124). Chicago: American Hospital Publishing, Inc.

Purnell, L. (1993). A survey of the qualifications, special training, and levels of personnel working in emergency department triage. *Journal of Nursing Staff Development, 9*(5), 223-226.

Southard, P. (1989). COBRA legislation: complying with ED provisions. *Journal of Emergency Nursing, 15*(1), 23-25.

Southard, P. (1994). Trauma in a reformed health care environment. *Journal of Emergency Nursing, 20*(5), 422-423.

Recent changes and current issues in gerontological nursing

MARY ZWYGART-STAUFFACHER, MARILYN J. RANTZ

We have been hearing for the past 30 years about the projected explosion in the number of older adults in the United States. That time is now, and the elderly population projections for the 21st century are staggering. Cost implications for caring for the elderly are equally staggering. Costs are associated not only with vast increases in numbers of elderly but also with the complexity of the multiple chronic diseases and acute exacerbations that occur in this population. While people over the age of 65 years comprise approximately 12% of the population they account for more than one third of the country's personal health care expenditures (U.S. Senate Special Committee on Aging, 1991). As the older population grows, so will their use of health care services. In 1990, about 1.5 million impaired people over the age of 65 used some type of community service at least once. By the year 2020, 2.4 million impaired older people will use community services (U.S. Senate Special Committee on Aging, 1991). To understand the scope of the costs of these services, in 1992 more than $60 billion was spent on long-term care and home and community care for the elderly (Cohen, Kumar, McGuire, & Wallack, 1992). Acute care and physician services push this amount to over $160 billion for those over 65 years of age (U.S. Senate Special Committee on Aging, 1991). Considering the costs and needs for services for older people today and in the future, we must ask whether we have the nursing workforce to address the needs of gerontological clients, whether today's workforce can adjust to work effectively in our changing delivery systems, and how we can better prepare the gerontological nursing workforce of tomorrow. These are major issues confronting gerontological nursing today.

CHANGING DELIVERY SYSTEMS

Older adults are using services across the continuum of health care, and they no longer depend on hospitalizations coupled with ongoing supervision from their primary care physician to manage their chronic conditions. Older adults are using a multitude of community-based home care and social services, subacute care, and long-term care services delivered in multiple sites (Vladeck, Miller, & Clauser, 1993). New roles are emerging as nurses assist seniors to manage the continuum of care. The nurse becomes the person who helps them manage those uncertain waters as they try to use services from various settings across multiple agencies funded from a variety of sources. New nursing roles are not without dilemmas. Gerontological nurses must now make decisions that are not only client-focused but also economical. Seldom before have nurses played such integral roles in the allocation of resources. Nurses in the past cared for seniors without concern for cost implications. Today, as nurses assume case management or care coordination roles, cost must be considered. Nurses must make tough decisions about the allocation of resources for their clients. It is a new era for gerontological nurses. We must be aware of what services cost and help seniors make wise cost-effective choices while ensuring that they receive the service they need.

As seniors use a variety of services across the continuum of care, funding of services via managed care contracts becomes a tremendous challenge for gerontological nurses. When funded via managed care contracts, services must be provided within a capitated budget. This means that there is a set fee for *all* services that people will use, and nurses must assume gatekeeping functions and make tough decisions about which types of services seniors will receive. Capitation is very different than the fee-for-service approach in which costs of services are totaled and billed at the end. As managed care is fully implemented for Medicare recipients, limits on acute care utilization and hospitalization will become very apparent. No longer will seniors with multiple chronic illnesses utilize multiple hospitalizations primarily for the management of their illnesses. As much as possible, they will be managed on an outpatient basis; and some tough decisions will have to be made about when to stop treatment. Subsequently, the elderly who will be seen in the acute care setting will have the most complex problems, with multiple-system disorders or illnesses requiring a tremendous depth and breadth of knowledge for care. The nurse in the community will be part of a health care team that will be making some tough decisions not to hospitalize some very sick people with complex illnesses and allow them to die at home, in a nursing home, or in a subacute unit.

ADVANCED PRACTICE NURSE IN GERONTOLOGICAL NURSING

With the evolution of managed care and complex care delivery systems the gerontological nurse prepared at the graduate level is being viewed as the appropriate provider or coordinator of care services. Therefore, an increase in the number of individuals prepared with graduate degrees in gerontological nursing is required. Historically, the advanced practice gerontological nurse is master's prepared with a clinical specialization in gerontological nursing.

In the 1970s there were few programs at the master's level preparing gerontological nurse practitioners; this specialty was not embraced by the nursing community until the mid- to late 1980s. There are now two advanced clinical practice roles in which gerontological specialization developed: the gerontological clinical nurse specialist and the gerontological nurse practitioner. Yet even with the expansion of two graduate preparation options the number of individuals prepared with gerontological nursing specialization has not been realized. For instance, in 1993 the number of certified gerontological nurse practitioners was 1,570 (American Nurses Credentialing Center [ANCC], 1994), while the number of pediatric nurse practitioners was in excess of 4,500 (National Certification Board of Pediatric Nurse Practitioners and Nurses; personal communication, 1995).

There is support in the literature that these two roles (clinical specialist and nurse practitioner) will merge into that of a single advanced practice gerontological nurse in the near future (Fulmer & Mezey 1994). Although there are similarities between the two roles, there are also differences that have had little discussion within all of the nursing communities (Page & Arena, 1994). At issue is whether one individual can be prepared who can integrate the competencies of both of these roles when very minimal research has been conducted to compare them (Fenton & Brykczynski, 1993). These roles have traditionally been setting-specific with the nurse practitioner as the provider of ambulatory and primary care services and the clinical nurse specialist providing services to special patient populations in long-term and acute care settings and staff education or development. If a blending of these roles can occur the resulting issue becomes whether we can prepare clinically competent people in a role who can successfully meet the demands of the role expectations across settings. Nurse practitioners have been prepared with a variety of primary care skills that have been targeted specifically to develop skills to direct primary care of older adults. That has not been the case for clinical nurse specialists, who have received information and education targeted to managing nursing problems older adults present, not assuming responsibility for directing with the client the management of his or her health alteration. These are two very distinct role functions.

Historically, the individuals who have merged these role functions have done so with a clinical nurse specialist master's degree followed with a postmaster's specialization for nurse practitioner. How to configure both the merged curriculum and the specialized focus is at issue. Another key issue is whether family nurse practitioners or adult nurse practitioners will be viewed as having the knowledge and experience necessary to work with the elderly in their health care management. Technically, individuals prepared as family or adult nurse practitioners were allowed to sit for the ANCC certification as gerontological nurse practitioners. Beginning in 1996, the ANCC is allowing only individuals who have been prepared in a gerontological nurse practitioner program to sit for the examination. No longer will cross-over from family and adult to gerontological nursing be allowed. Given the complexity of both the gerontological clients themselves and the knowledge base required for managing the role functions of the gerontological nurse practitioner successfully, it is clear that formal education needs to be the foundation for certification and clinical practice.

An additional issue related to preparing individuals at the advanced practice level is the need to restructure curricula in academic institutions in light of cost containment. There is a growing trend to minimize specialization content in an effort to try to include more students in all courses. These cost-containment efforts are very likely to impact specialized courses, such as gerontological courses. It is likely that these efforts will delete those courses as options for students because it is more costly and time-consuming to arrange both specialized didactic and clinical components. It is presumed by some that one can obtain the knowledge that is necessary for delivering gerontological care simply by completing clinical practicums with older adults without specialized didactic content within the graduate program. This is a disturbing trend.

Assuming that broad didactic courses such as a general primary care management course applied across the life span and clinical experience with older people are adequate for preparation as an advanced practice gerontological nurse is a disservice to both students *and* clients. Students need both didactic and well-planned clinical experiences with theoretical content specific to the gerontological population. Courses should be available for further specialization. Haight and Stewart (1994) describe geropsychiatric specialty courses for graduate nursing education. In light of the scope of clinical problems and the frequency with which nurses are confronted with mental health and behavior problems of older adults, such specialty courses are very appropriate and needed. Students also need an understanding of cost of care delivery. We can no longer afford to teach students how that care should be delivered without an understanding of what that care will cost.

Aside from the content issues of what should be taught, qualifications of the faculty are at issue. A report of the planning committee for the White House Conference on Aging reveals that an alarming 40% of the nursing faculty now teaching in graduate-level gerontological nursing programs have *no* formal gerontological preparation. Three fourths (77%) of all clinical preceptors and instructors in all nursing programs have no formal preparation for working with the elderly (Dye, 1992). How can gerontological advanced practice nurses be prepared by faculty without gerontological preparation?

UNDERGRADUATE NURSING EDUCATION

Based on our experience, we concur from with Fulmer and Mezey (1994) that traditionally basic nursing programs have included very little geriatric nursing content and that most faculty lack preparation in geriatric nursing. If they do have course work in geriatric nursing, the faculty lack the preparation to be qualified to teach those courses. Yurchuck and Brower (1994) report that only 12% of undergraduate faculty have specific gerontological preparation. When one considers the approach to undergraduate nursing education, it is clear that nurse educators would not be put in the position of teaching pediatric or obstetric nursing without preparation in those fields. Why have we allowed nurse educators to teach gerontological nursing with neither a knowledge base nor a practice base for their instruction? Because of the sheer numbers of older adults using the health care delivery system and the complexity of the clinical problems they present, it is imperative that faculty be prepared both clinically and theoretically to teach these courses. Bahr (1994) said it so well:

> What's wrong? Despite the amount of money made available for post-doctoral study, few faculty are taking advantage of the opportunity to upgrade their knowledge in gerontological nursing. I would hazard a guess that the attitude problems of students not wishing to choose gerontological nursing as a career starts with the faculty who also have an attitude problem. To be based in reality means that all of us are on the continuum of aging. All persons will get old unless a traumatic event occurs that ends life much earlier. What are faculty afraid of that they shy away from content and clinical experience that evolves around the care of the aged? (p. 38)

Issues surrounding undergraduate nursing education must include grappling with the problem of associate degree education. Most of the registered nurses working in nursing homes are prepared at the associate degree level. Many associate degree curricula do include content concerning gerontological nursing; however, most do *not* contain a specialized gerontological nursing course.

The Institute of Medicine Committee on Nursing Home Regulations (1986) has recommended that

> Nursing homes should place their highest priority on recruitment, retention, and support of adequate numbers of professional nurses who are trained in gerontology and geriatrics to insure an adequate number and appropriate mix of professional and non-professional nursing personnel to meet the needs of all types of residents in each facility. (p. 103)

However, many nursing homes have received waivers from even OBRA's minimal increases in staffing standards (Francese & Mohler, 1994). These homes claim that shortages of registered nurses and inadequate reimbursement to pay their salaries are the reasons they cannot meet the staffing standards. Nursing must become involved to correct these delivery system problems.

Additionally, nursing must deal with the issue of how much preparation a student can receive in a 2-year program to be able to deal with complex problems of the

TABLE OF CONTENTS OF JOURNALS REVIEWED FROM 1992 TO 1995

Journal of Gerontological Nursing
Geriatric Nursing
The Gerontologist
Journal of the American Geriatrics Society
Journal of Gerontology
Journal of Long-Term Care Administration
Image: The Journal of Nursing Scholarship
Nursing Research
Research in Nursing and Health
Nursing Outlook

TRENDS IN THE GERONTOLOGICAL LITERATURE IDENTIFIED BETWEEN 1992 AND 1995

Clinical issues

Reminiscence
Restraints
  Problems associated with
  Efforts to reduce usage
Disruptive or aggressive behavior
  Nursing strategies to manage
Wandering behavior
Functional status
  Maintaining functional abilities
  Measuring functional status
  Using functional status to predict illness
Activities of daily living
Elderly response to hospitalization
Use of life-sustaining or life-saving procedures
Tube feedings
  Positive and negative aspects of use
  Ethical dilemmas of use
Relocation stress
Urinary incontinence
Failure to thrive
Substance abuse
Depression
Alzheimer's disease
Elder abuse
Wellness promotion

elderly in nursing homes and other settings. However, it must be acknowledged that one of the major providers of nursing services in nursing homes are licensed practical nurses prepared with even less formal education.

Home care is an exploding source of services for the elderly. Most nurses working in the home care arena are prepared at the associate degree level. Traditionally, public health or community-based services were to be provided by baccalaureate-prepared nurses, but this is no longer the case. We have nurses going into homes—a most challenging environment to care for people with complex clinical problems—with minimal formal nursing education. At some point nursing must address this issue and establish the baseline for professional gerontological nursing and general nursing practice at the baccalaureate level. Education aside, nursing assistants and homemakers with little or no formal nursing preparation are delivering many in-home services to seniors.

CURRENT CLINICAL AND SYSTEMS ISSUES

To identify current trends in clinical and systems issues of gerontological nursing discussed in the gerontological literature, the tables of contents of 10 journals (see box for list) for the years 1992 through 1995 were analyzed using qualitative methods. The trends identified are listed in the two boxes above. When one compares the trends in the gerontological nursing literature from 1992 to 1995 with those identified from a 1980 to 1990 literature review for a report to the Institute of Medicine (Lang, Kraegel, Rantz, & Krejci, 1990), some new issues have surfaced. These include the emergence of dementia special care and subacute units. Controversy surrounds these special care programs and units. Some see them as options for long-term care agencies to improve their financial position, while others are concerned about whether the agencies can provide the level of clinical expertise that these more acutely ill elderly need. The minimum data set (MDS) assessment instrument mandated for use in all nursing homes in 1990 is a new issue. Controversy surrounds the MDS instrument and the data collected from it. Some are concerned about pursuing research activities using MDS data, raising concerns about validity and reliability. Others are concerned about how regulators will interpret aggregated assessment information from MDS data, how payment mechanisms may be designed using the data, and how comparisons will be made across agencies.

There is a marked increase in the number of studies related to advanced directives and the use of life-sustaining procedures. It may be that the Patient Self-

TRENDS IN THE GERONTOLOGICAL LITERATURE IDENTIFIED BETWEEN 1992 AND 1995

Systems issues

Dementia special care units
- Resource use
- Regulation of
- Effectiveness of

Subacute units
Discharge from acute care settings
Family caregiving
- Collaboration between facilities and families
- Stress associated with

Community-based services
- Continuum of care
- Financing
- Gaps in home health coverage

Life-care community developments
Advance directives and self-determination
Delaying nursing home placement
Financing long-term care
Staffing issues in nursing homes
- Use of nurse practitioners and clinical nurse specialists
- Retention of staff and training issues

Minimum data set for nursing homes
- Validation of/and research using

Health care reform
Financing acute care

Determination Act of 1991 is raising these issues for discussion or perhaps the public debate surrounding health care reform and the costs of services is bringing these issues forward. Elder abuse in the current survey is more clearly represented in the gerontological nursing literature. It is likely that this is related to increased public and professional awareness of the problem and attention by nurse researchers.

The developments of community-based services across the continuum of care and of life-care communities for older adults are also recent phenomena in the nursing literature. These services are considered by many to be significant trends for the future of gerontological care delivery. Other trends for the future identified in the literature are delivery of acute care services in long-term care facilities and an increased emphasis on research about care delivery and care needs of older adults. These trends could hold much promise for improving the quality of care and quality of life of long-term care residents.

WHERE GERONTOLOGICAL NURSING NEEDS TO GO . . . NEXT

With the complexity and diversity of clinical problems it is clear that gerontological nursing education must be enhanced so that nurses working with older adults are educationally prepared to deal with this patient population. Additionally, nurses must be prepared to deal with the complex systems issues that permeate the complicated delivery systems that older persons must traverse. Gerontological nursing education must prepare professionals to not only deal with these complex issues, but to shape the future of care delivery for older adults.

We must have nurse researchers who have gerontological nursing experience to guide research that is relevant and clearly addresses the issues of health care for older adults. Gerontological nurse researchers who are grounded in clinical experience with older adults can direct relevant research that truly adds to improving the quality of care that older adults receive or improve the education that nurses receive for gerontological nursing. Additionally, nurse researchers who are out of touch with the realities of clinical service systems are not prepared to ask relevant questions that will make significant differences for older adults. With diminishing research dollars and increased competition for resources for research activity, the true relevance of the topic under investigation and the impact it will have on clinical practice and patient outcomes must be clear. Researchers who are formally educated and experienced in the care of the elderly are crucial to the future of gerontological nursing.

It is important that we recruit individuals into gerontological nursing practice who have a true commitment to the elderly and to the services they need. Gerontological services are in a growing market with expanding opportunities. As with any expanding market, it is not always clear whether people are motivated to choose gerontological nursing because they are truly interested in caring for older adults or whether job and economic security are the prime motivators. This motivation can clearly affect the outcome of care and the individualization of the care provision.

Nurses who are committed to gerontology need to embrace this time of health care reform and configure systems of care, determine what appropriate care outcomes will be, and pursue building those service delivery systems. It is time for gerontological nurses to design the future, not be reactive to someone else's designs. It is time for gerontological nurses to designate what the critical outcomes of gerontological nursing should be and design a path to achieve those outcomes. "In view of the projections of dramatically increasing elders in the next century, gerontological nursing will hold a critical position in the health of the nation and the world" (Southern Council on Collegiate Education for Nursing, 1995, p. 6).

REFERENCES

American Nurses Credentialing Center. (1994). *Credentialing catalog.* Kansas City, MO: American Nurses Association.

Bahr, R.T. (1994). Response to "Issues facing faculty in long-term care." In E.L. Middy (Ed.), *Mechanisms of quality in long-term care: Education* (pp. 37-41). New York: National League for Nursing.

Cohen, M.A., Kumar, N., McGuire, T., & Wallack, S.S. (1992). Financing long-term care: A practical mix of public and private. *Journal of Health Politics, Policy, and Law, 17*(3), 403-423.

Dye, C.A. (1992). *Education and training.* In the Report of the White House Conference on Aging Planning Committee. Washington, DC.

Fenton, M., & Brykczynski, K. (1993). Qualitative distinctions and similarities in practice of clinical nurse specialist and nurse practitioners. *Journal of Professional Nursing, 9*(6), 313-326.

Francese, T., & Mohler, M. (1994). Long-term care nurse staffing requirements: Has OBRA really helped? *Geriatric Nursing, 15*(3), 139-141.

Fulmer, T., & Mezey, M. (1994). Contemporary geriatric nursing. In W.R. Hazzard, E.L. Berman, J.P. Blass, W.H. Ettinger, & J.B. Halter (Eds.), *Principles of geriatric medicine and gerontology* (3rd ed., pp. 249-258). New York: McGraw-Hill.

Haight, B.K., & Stuart, G. (1994). Answering need: Gero psychiatric nursing course development. *The Journal of Gerontological Nursing, 209*(12), 12-18.

Institute of Medicine Committee on Nursing Home Regulations. (1986). *Improving the quality of care in nursing homes.* Washington, DC: National Academy Press.

Lang, N.M., Kraegel, J.M., Rantz, M.J., & Krejci, J.W. (1990). *Quality of care for older people in America.* Kansas City, MO: American Nurses Association.

Page, N., & Arena, D. (1994). Rethinking the merger of the clinical nurse specialist and the nurse practitioner. *Image: The Journal of Nursing Scholarship, 26*(4), 315-318.

Personal communication. (1995). National Certification Board of Pediatric Nurse Practitioners and Nurses.

National League for Nursing. (1991). *Gerontology in the nursing curriculum.* New York: Author.

Southern Council on Collegiate Education for Nursing. (1995). Gerontological nursing issues and demands beyond the year 2005. *Journal of Gerontological Nursing, 21*(6), 6-9.

U.S. Senate Special Committee on Aging. (1991). *Aging America: Trends and projections.* (DHHS Publication No. (FCoA) 91-28001). Washington, DC: U.S. Government Printing Office.

Vladeck, B.C., Miller, N.A., & Clauser, S.V. (1993). The changing face of long-term care. *Health Care Financing Review, 14*(4), 5-23.

Yurchuck, E., & Brower, H. (1994). Faculty preparation for gerontological nursing. *The Journal of Gerontological Nursing, 20*(1), 17-24.

Recent changes and current issues in medical-surgical nursing practice

MARILYN S. FETTER, CECELIA GATSON GRINDEL

The goal of medical-surgical nursing is to maintain, promote, and restore the health of adult clients. According to the American Nurses Association (ANA) scope of practice statement for the specialty, medical-surgical nurses use the nursing process to care for adults with known or potential physiologic alterations, trauma, or disability (ANA Division of Medical-Surgical Nursing Practice, 1980). Traditionally, the majority of medical-surgical nurses have worked in hospitals, while others are employed in private practice, outpatient, and long-term care settings (Brozenec, Levitt, & Poyss, 1994). Currently, health care delivery is undergoing sweeping reforms that are effecting unparalleled change, uncertainty, and challenges within medical-surgical nursing. Changes in patient problems and populations, technological advances, nursing departments and models of care delivery, hospitals and health systems, reimbursement for care, and the locus and focus of health care itself are prompting medical-surgical nurses to restructure their work. The future of medical-surgical nursing will be determined by how the specialty faces several key clinical and professional issues. Future challenges include incorporating outcomes management into the nursing process, enhancing professional accountability; retooling clinicians to function with clinical, technological, and organizational changes; incorporating a prevention, family-centered orientation to care; redefining and strengthening specialty identity; and developing education and practice models to facilitate the relationships among the many nurses and associates caring for adults.

RECENT CHANGES

Changing patient populations

Due to demographic and other factors, the conditions of medical-surgical patients are increasingly complex. Improved standards of living and health care have resulted in a significant increase in the elderly population. According to the U.S. Bureau of Census (1992), there were 20 million Americans 65 years of age and older in 1970. By 1995, this figure had grown to 33.6 million, and by the year 2010 it is expected to exceed 40 million and will represent more than 13% of the total population. The old-old, persons 85 years and older, are the fastest-growing segment of the elderly population and are expected to number 4.6 million by the end of the decade. Most older adults remain in the community, with only 1.3% of persons 65 to 74 years of age and 6% of older adults between the ages of 75 and 84 placed in long-term care (American Association of Retired Persons, 1993). While persons 65 and older can presently expect to live 16.4 more years, they average 12 additional years of healthy life before experiencing significant morbidity (National Center for Health Statistics, 1992). Despite their relative independence, older adults frequently have one or more significant chronic health problems such as cardiovascular disease, pulmonary disorders, diabetes mellitus, incontinence, visual and hearing impairments, and dementia, all of which can limit functional abilities and quality of life. Thus, when older adults are acutely ill, their multiple health problems challenge the treatment team. These patients often receive numerous medications, recover more slowly from operative procedures and other treatments, and require more assistance from nursing staff.

All hospitalized patients, not only those who are elderly, have more complex care needs as a result of the use of advanced technologies and changing reimbursement patterns for health care. Because of reimbursement-dictated shortened lengths of stay, patients are being moved through the system more quickly. Those who 5 years ago would have been hospitalized in intensive care are now the norm on general medical-surgical units (Russell, 1995). Many operative procedures, such as cataract and orthopedic surgery, cholecystectomy, and angiography, once requiring inpatient care, are now regularly performed with minimal or no hospitalization. Therefore, the remaining surgical patients are more acutely ill and likely to have experienced complications or other serious health problems. Central lines, invasive hemodynamic monitoring, ventilators, and the use of medications and treatments requiring vigilant patient monitoring are commonplace on general units. Managed care, with its focus on reducing overall cost, has forced shorter lengths of stay. Hence, overall unit acuity levels have risen sharply and are projected to increase to even higher levels as managed care and market forces continue to influence patient length of stay. Patients with more complex problems require nurses to engage in a higher degree of care coordination and collaboration with numerous physician specialists and other providers. The discharge of patients to home, rehabilitation, and subacute settings has intensified the demand for patient and family teaching and support, discharge planning, and case management. The work of the medical-surgical nurse has increased and is evolving.

Health care system changes

Managed care and other health care reforms have brought about enormous changes in the ways hospitals, many now functioning as integrated health systems, are structured, organized, and managed (Sovie, 1995). Medical-surgical nurses are experiencing these changes first-hand. Capitation, shortened lengths of stay, stricter controls on tests and procedures, and lowered reimbursements, along with industry over-capacity, have combined to reduce hospital revenues. In order to maintain fiscal controls, hospitals across the country are evaluating all programs and services to determine their effect on the bottom line. Hospitals are aligning into cooperatives to increase their bargaining power with third-party payers and are restructuring care delivery systems (Kerfoot, 1994). Nursing departments, and medical-surgical units in particular, have been subjected to intense scrutiny in terms of budget, organization, and outcomes. Hospital administrators and health systems consultants are recommending streamlining of the nursing service organizational table. In many hospitals, nurse manager, clinical nurse specialist, and staff development-clinical educator positions have been combined or eliminated. The administrative span of control has increased, with nurse managers now taking responsibility for two or more units.

Patient care delivery is being redesigned in order to enhance efficiency, reduce costs, and, as some experts and hospital administrators contend, improve quality and patient satisfaction (Bostrom & Zimmerman, 1993). Called "patient-focused care" in some institutions, these redesign efforts involve bringing services to the patient's bedside and using nonnurse technicians to provide some patient care tasks (Fritz & Cheeseman, 1994). In these systems, the role of the medical-surgical nurse shifts from that of direct caregiver to care coordinator and supervisor. Patient care associates or nursing assistants are being trained to deliver many of the services previously performed by primary care nurses (Hines, Smeltzer, & Galletti, 1994). However, the roles, skills, and training of these workers vary widely among institutions, as was found in a recent survey of 234 institutions employing unlicensed assistive personnel (UAP) (Barter, McLaughlin, & Thomas, 1994). Because the performance and liabilities of these assistants have not been well articulated or evaluated, many nurses have legal and ethical concerns about the delegation of previously considered "nursing responsibilities" to UAP. This lack of data, coupled with the reduced demand for nurses that such a system entails, has resulted in considerable anger and frustration in many institutions. Because these changes are occurring simultaneously with significant reductions in administrative support and resources, morale among many medical-surgical nurses is poor. Medical-surgical nurses are worried about the quality of patient care, patient safety, legal accountability issues, and personal employment options.

Changes in the locus and goals of care

Capitation, the philosophical and economic underpinning of managed care, is based on the principle that keeping people well is more cost-effective than treating them once they become ill; providers receive a set fee per year whether clients are sick or well (Enthoven, 1993). Because managed care pays an increasingly larger percentage of the nation's medical bills, maximizing the cost-effectiveness of services and providers is paramount. Shifting the locus of care to less expensive settings such as community centers, subacute units, and the home is a top priority. The diminishing role of the hospital to caring for only the most acutely ill patients has seriously affected employment patterns and the role of medical-surgical nurses. It is estimated that as many as one third of the nation's hospitals may close by the year 2000 (Sovie, 1995), and these closures will affect medical-surgical nurses disproportionately. While some experts contend that increased opportunities in community settings will be created, especially if a national health plan is enacted that includes universal coverage (Buerhaus, 1994), there is no guarantee that professional nurses at the generalist level will be placed in some or all of these new positions. Tighter cost controls by Medicare, Medicaid, and other payers will also retard expanded nursing employment opportunities in home care. There is the potential for an undetermined number of medical-surgical nurses, including those currently employed in ambulatory settings, to be displaced by nurse practitioners, physician assistants, and even UAP. While opportunities in home health and community nursing are rapidly becoming available, they will not exceed the number of positions lost. Further, these opportunities are not necessarily attractive or available to hospital-based medical-surgical nurses. Many diploma- and associate-degree-prepared nurses have had minimal or no didactic and clinical preparation in community settings. Nurses who have worked for years on general medical-surgical units feel comfortable in these environments and look on a transition to the community with fear and trepidation, even though many who do make the move report enjoying the increased autonomy and independence. Little is known regarding the educational, training, and supervisory needs of nurses and nurse associates making transitions from hospital to subacute and community settings.

In addition to providing services more economically in the community, managed care has redirected health care goals to promoting health, preventing disease, and limiting disability. Medical-surgical nurses in outpatient and ambulatory settings can easily incorporate these aims into their practice, although allocating adequate time and identifying effective methods is increasingly challenging. Home health nurses, many of whom are essentially performing medical-surgical nursing in the home, have always relied heavily on patient and family teaching regarding health behaviors, symptom management, and preserving quality of life. However, cost containment and the threat of reduced Medicare and other third-party reimbursements have placed pressure on these nurses to enhance productivity by shortening visit time and increasing the number of visits made per day. Further, because home health agencies receive payment based on meeting the identified individual patient's needs, medical-surgical nurses risk charge disallowal if they deviate from the individual plan of care to address other family health care needs. These nurses report instances of a double-bind, in which the identified problem that provides the rationale for the visit is the least of the family's problems in terms of health status. Hence, prevention and promotion efforts can be constrained under current care delivery structures.

The shift from a disease to prevention orientation is difficult for many hospital-based nurses. Conceptually and practically, they are relatively unfamiliar with models of prevention and promotion. Further, they feel overloaded by the existing care demands of their patients and report not having sufficient time to take on added responsibilities. Perceptions that they lack the training, tools, and feedback required to provide effective health promotion education are common. For example, in the case of cardiovascular disease, the number one cause of adult deaths in the United States, several of the major risk factors associated with heart attack and stroke are modifiable. Smoking cessation, moderate or lower alcohol consumption, a diet low in saturated fats and cholesterol, and regular physical activity can reduce morbidity and mortality in patients with cardiovascular disease (U.S. Public Health Service, 1991). However, many nurses believe that it is virtually impossible to change the lifelong behaviors of poorly motivated, elderly, culturally and ethnically different, or chronically ill clients. This is problematic because many patients who receive intensive cardiac intervention can reduce their risk of premature mortality and future morbidity by modifying their behavior (Dracup, Baker, & Dunbar, 1994). In the case of cancer, the number two national killer, avoiding tobacco, alcohol, and other known carcinogens are the only known, successful primary prevention activities. Secondary prevention efforts center around promoting awareness, surveillance, and early treatment. Implementing effective strategies to encourage these behaviors is a national priority, but significant research is needed to direct cost-effective, culturally competent approaches (McGinnis & Lee, 1995). Of particular concern to medical-surgical nurses is the timing of these interventions, because most acutely ill hospitalized patients may be unwilling or unable to attend to more general health promotion messages. Once these patients improve, they are quickly discharged and the "teachable moment" can be lost. For nurses uncomfortable with these interventions, these perceptions become a convenient rationale for avoiding prevention efforts.

Numerous changes are affecting the specialty. Medical-surgical patients are older, sicker, and have more complex problems. Highly sophisticated technologies are employed to save lives and return patients quickly to the community. Patients are discharged more quickly, units have higher acuity levels, and hospitals are restructuring to stay competitive. The very nature of the work of medical-surgical nurses is changing. In hospitals, they are providing less direct care, supervising UAP and other care associates, collaborating with increased numbers of physician specialists and other professionals, and coordinating more aspects of the treatment plan. As an increasing percentage of care is delivered in nonhospital settings and as numerous other personnel, including nonprofessionals, join the care team, traditional medical-surgical nurses are questioning their identity and role. Clearly the challenge for medical-surgical nurses is to prepare themselves to fit into the changing health care environment. Key to success in moving into the future are role clarification and specialty identification; professional development; outcomes measurement; and the development of creative practice and education models.

STRATEGIES TO MEET THE FUTURE

Role clarification/specialty identity

With the reality of downsizing, cost-containment, and new models for the delivery of patient care, medical-surgical nurses are experiencing unparalled job insecurity. Positions for medical-surgical nurses in acute care settings will decrease until hospitals stabilize patient care capacity and models for the delivery of patient care services. As the use of UAP increases, nurses who are stretched to the maximum caring for acutely ill patients feel threatened with job loss. Many see no future outside the walls of the hospital. Others are focused inward, mourning the loss of the health care environment of the past.

These changes prompt reconsideration of the role of the medical-surgical nurse. Is medical-surgical nursing bound to the hospital setting or does it revolve around adults, sick or well, requiring nursing care? As patient care increases in complexity and acuity, what are the distinctions between medical-surgical and critical care nursing? What expertise can the medical-surgical nurse offer to patients in community-based settings such as home care? Categorizing home health nursing is also difficult: Is it medical-surgical nursing or critical care? More fundamentally, what is the nursing role?

Recognition of the expertise they have to offer is key if medical-surgical nurses are to market themselves confidently in new practice environments. Nurses in this specialty are experts in patient assessment, patient/family teaching, broad-based clinical knowledge, and technical skills. Medical-surgical nurses are specialists in managing the care of the adult patient. For decades nursing curricula have taught nursing students to care for the patient across the continuum. Granted, the focus has been on the acute care setting; but these nurses have the foundation for professional growth in the areas of prevention and health maintenance. The challenge for medical-surgical nurses is to recognize their high level of expertise in adult health and look for opportunities to use this expertise in other practice settings. While the 1980s was the era of nursing specialization, the 1990s and beyond will see the rise of the expert generalists—clinicians who provide comprehensive patient care services in a wide variety of settings.

Professional development

As medical-surgical nurses seek opportunities to use their expertise in new roles, they must prepare themselves for changing roles and responsibilities. Developing a "retooling plan" is the first step in this process. A retooling plan involves identifying the knowledge and skills needed for new work roles and devising an action plan to accomplish these goals. Regardless of role or setting, a strong orientation to disease prevention, health promotion, and health maintenance forms the necessary foundation for future practice. For example, the nurse teaching the newly diagnosed Type I diabetic will not only teach the client and caregiver about diet, exercise, and medication, but will also emphasize the beneficial effects of smoking cessation for overall health status. Understanding the interrelationships of patient needs and outcomes, resource utilization and reimbursement for services as patients flow through wall-less health care systems is another critical informational need for the medical-surgical nurse. Enhanced knowledge and skills in managing the patient care needs across the care continuum, with an emphasis on health promotion and disease prevention, are imperative to the specialty's survival.

Political and economic realities will affect medical-surgical nurses as they attempt to retool for the future. Local, state, and national politics are influencing nursing employment opportunities and educational requirements. With the pace of national health care reform slowed, many states are proceeding with their own initiatives. In most instances, these efforts feature a reliance on nurses in advanced practice roles to deliver primary care to substantial segments of the population. Educational requirements, licensure and certification standards, supervision, and specific practice roles and responsibilities are evolving on a state-by-state basis. Consequently, there is a need for national professional and specialty organizations to facilitate the development of uniform practice standards. Without this standardization, job and geographic mobility are threatened, and individual states have the opportunity to diminish the nursing role. Creative medical-surgical nurses will use this time of change to identify opportunities to develop innovative nursing roles that fulfill previously unmet health care needs in their communities.

Economic changes have also affected nurses' professional development. In the past, nursing budgets often included money for professional nurse staff development. This luxury is no longer available. Nurses must now take responsibility for and invest in their own futures (Kerfoot, 1994). Hospitals and clinical agencies will continue to provide a minimum level of continuing education to ensure that nurses are competent to provide patient care. However, to expand their expertise and to obtain advanced training and higher degrees, medical-surgical nurses will need to make personal financial commitments. They must design their own retooling plans based on the consideration of numerous personal, professional, and political factors, and will need to work much harder to fund their career development.

Outcomes measurement

Historically the cost of nursing services was subsumed under the patient's room and board. It was assumed that the care nurses provided in implementing the physician's treatment plan was going to have a positive effect on patient outcomes. Of course, little or no energy went into demonstrating that this was indeed true. The focus in today's health care environment is on the delivery of high-quality care resulting in desired clinical outcomes at controlled costs (Sovie, 1994). Nurses must now demonstrate that the patient outcomes achieved are a direct result of their care, an unfamiliar orientation for most nurses. If patients got better and went home or died peacefully, it was assumed that all the interventions that nurses implemented helped achieve those goals. No longer can this assumption be made. Documentation in national health care databases will show that nursing interventions do make a difference.

The creation of a nursing minimum data set will provide structure for documentation of nursing diagnoses, interventions, and outcomes. In 1986, the ANA resolved to support the development of computerized nursing information systems in nursing services (ANA, 1986), and this initiative has been extremely productive. Systems that have been produced include the North American Nursing Diagnoses Association, the Nursing Interventions Classification, the Omaha System, and the Home Health Care Classification System, and a nursing-sensitive classification for patient outcomes is in development at the University of Iowa (Werley, Ryan, & Coenen, 1994). These classification systems require more uniform adoption as well as ongoing evaluation and refinement. The ANA and specialty organizations are collaborating to initiate or support programs to identify and refine data elements for data sets pertaining to nursing diagnosis, interventions, and outcomes. As a nursing minimum data set becomes part of national health care databases, documentation of the cost-effectiveness of nursing services is possible, which in turn allows for direct reimbursement.

Medical-surgical nurses must understand the goals and methods of improving and measuring patient outcomes. Valuing this initiative and supporting the implementation of the use of the nursing minimum data set nationwide is critical. Understanding the relationship of nursing diagnosis and interventions to patient outcomes is essential if medical-surgical nurses are to be at the table when health system strategic planning occurs. Nurses must be aware of outcome measurement issues, such as the types of patient outcomes that should be measured, the amount and type of nursing (or "nurse dose") needed to effect patient outcomes, the nurse dose needed in a given health care environment to demonstrate an effect, and the nurse dose needed for effects with differing patient groups (Brooten & Naylor, 1995).

The bottom line is that medical-surgical nurses must think evaluation. Staff nurses and nurses in advanced practice roles, by virtue of their ongoing assessment and treatment of patient care, are essential to both outcomes assessment and management (Titler & Reiter, 1994). As new caremaps, clinical protocols, procedures, and practice models are introduced, a plan for evaluating the effectiveness of these interventions must be in place. Data that are collected must be essential data that can show the effectiveness of the intervention because resources are not available to collect meaningless data. Cost data should also be included. These data must be examined to ensure that patient care services are effective and control costs; they also serve as the framework for enhancing practice when goals are not achieved. To make outcomes evaluation and management a reality, a global approach to outcomes measurement is suggested. Outcomes assessment must be integrated as a routine part of care and systems must be developed to score instruments, aggregate data and feed the data back to providers of care in a time-efficient manner (Titler & Reiter, 1994). A successful outcomes management initiative will address the selection of outcome domains and instruments and the development of an infrastructure to support data collection, analysis, and feedback of outcome data to providers of care (Titler & Reiter, 1994). Medical-surgical nurses are expected to be a part of the outcomes measurement process and must be prepared to do so.

Creative practice and educational models

Practice Models. As health care providers scramble to meet the cost-containment demands of the current health care environment, they are examining their services and the delivery of those services. In order to survive in this changing environment, providers are implementing new practice models that they hope will ensure quality patient care while saving health care dollars. Many institutions are expanding ambulatory care services, creating subacute facilities, developing hospital-based home care services, and redesigning inpatient services around the framework of patient-focused care. Many nursing staff feel these moves toward redesign are only financially based and that health care institutions are losing sight of quality patient care. If quality patient care is the expected outcome of redesign efforts, then it is clear that many nurses do not see that vision and probably have not been participants in redesign planning.

New practice models are most effective when all relevant stakeholders are included and the process is planned and evaluated. A plan that does not consider detail or one that does not get some "buy-in" from participants is likely to fail. Communication between administrators, nursing managers, and nursing staff is essential to obtain buy-in from staff; nurses who come to understand new systems will be more supportive. In addition, they are likely to suggest ways to ease the transition and enhance implementation. Furthermore, nurses are key elements to personalizing the new practice model to the patient population of the institution.

Medical-surgical nurses need to be open to change. Resistance to change itself can be very detrimental in the current environment. Rather than developing a mindset of negativism, nurses need to become active participants in decision making as plans unfold. Expanding their vision for the delivery of nursing care and using their knowledge of their patients' needs, these nurses can offer creative and insightful suggestions for care delivery. This input can "mold" the new patient care model into an efficient, effective system for the delivery of services.

Medical-surgical nurses have consistently included the family in the plan of the patient's care. Shortened hospital lengths of stay place a new emphasis on family-centered care. In the past, patients were discharged when they reached some level of self-care or independence, while patients today are discharged once it has been determined that they are stable. This situation places greater responsibility on the family for the patient's care. Family-centered education becomes an essential part of the patient's recovery. With less hospitalization time, the challenge to impart the necessary education to the patient and family is becoming increasingly overwhelming. Medical-surgical nurses have the expertise to develop innovative strategies that ensure patient care and safety.

New models for the delivery of services suggest novel dimensions for collaboration. Historically, nurses have viewed collaboration from the perspective of the nurse-physician relationship. Today's practice models suggest an expansion of that narrow perception of collaboration. Wall-less health care systems will broaden nurses' world view of resource utilization. The magnitude of the health care team will expand to include health care providers outside the walls of hospitals. Case managers, home care nurses, community social services, spiritual directors, financial consultants, patient education consultants, and others could be used to address the patient's and family's needs. Health care providers will tap into creative community networks to access needed resources. Using these community networks will provide a new challenge for medical-surgical nurses who are more accustomed to a one-step process of initiating a referral to the hospital's social services department.

Collaboration can only be as effective as the communication system in which it functions. Information systems that can link health care providers across the wall-less health care systems will offer efficient means of ensuring patient care without duplicating services. These information systems will not only facilitate communication among health care providers; they will record health care diagnoses, interventions, and outcomes into community, regional, and national databases. These data will be used to evaluate the effectiveness of patient care.

A wall-less hospital system suggests a need to ensure continuity of care because patient outcomes cannot be attained within the short time frame of hospitalization. Information systems can support this continuity of care, but they cannot guarantee it. Case management or some comparable process for managing and monitoring the patient's and family's progress along the health care continuum can ensure that quality health care is implemented and that the health status of the patient is maintained. The broad range of clinical expertise that medical-surgical nurses have makes them excellent candidates to assume roles as case managers. Critical to the success of such roles, however, will be the freedom to diagnose and manage all problems that affect the health of the family. To focus on one clinical problem without attention to the social system in which it occurs can limit the success of the treatment plan and the attainment of the expected patient outcomes. For example, educating the diabetic patient on insulin administration is ineffective if the patient cannot afford to purchase insulin and syringes. Instructing a patient on pharmaceutical management of hypertension is wasted if choices must be made between the purchases of groceries and the acquisition of the antihypertensive medication. If patient and family health outcomes are to be achieved, a more holistic approach to health maintenance and health promotion is necessary.

Educational Models. New educational models to prepare medical-surgical nurses for the practice environments of the future are needed. Increased emphasis on community-based practice is required as more nurses assume these practice roles. To date, only a few nursing programs report curriculum revisions emphasizing a community orientation. The practice roles for nurses in the 21st century demand an expansion of course content to include a broader perspective of resource identification and utilization, cost-benefits principles, access issues, and reimbursement concepts. Academic programs must change to be responsive to these educational needs for generic students. As well, there is an urgent need for quality registered nurse to bachelor's and master's of nursing programs that can help current practitioners retool for the future health care environment.

Changes in curricula should reflect the needs of professional nurses who seek to practice in new settings. A few research studies are under way to determine the needs of nurses who anticipate moving from acute care settings to home care or community-based practice. The results of these research projects can give direction to educational programs as nurses confirm what they do know and identify what they need to know. Add this information to what is expected of nurses working in community-based settings that focus on health promotion and maintenance and the framework for curriculum changes emerges.

Many colleges and universities have hastened to develop nurse practitioner programs to meet the predicted demand for such roles as the new health care system unfolds. Strong nurse practitioner programs that emphasize the nursing role are emerging, and nurses seeking graduate education are being encouraged to enter into them. What is unclear is the extent of the demand for such practitioners. State legislators and state boards of nursing are struggling to define the parameters of the role as it extends beyond the traditional boundaries of pediatric nurse practitioner and nurse midwife. Third-party payers are examining reimbursement for nurse practitioners for services rendered. Some physician groups oppose initiatives to expand the role of nurse practitioner, implying that quality patient care may be at stake. Finally, the failure of the 1994 Congress to legislate changes to the Medicaid and Medicare programs to emphasize health promotion and health maintenance hindered the expansion of nurse practitioner positions. Clearly, academic programs that include nurse practitioner programs would do well to monitor the development of this role as new delivery of care models emerge.

A large number of medical-surgical nurses will be seeking educational opportunities other than that of the nurse practitioner role. Creative continuing education programs that address key principles of health promotion, disease prevention, case management, cost-benefit analysis, outcomes measurement, resource utilization, and collaboration will be useful for nurses who are retooling. Again, these programs should recognize the clinical expertise and educational preparation of participants and plan programs that build on participants' knowledge base.

As medical-surgical nurses face numerous changes such as more complex patients and technologies, diminishing resources, and new practice roles and responsibilities, they are challenged to resolve several critical issues. First and foremost, they must view these changes with optimism rather than resistance. By conceptualizing what some might label a crisis as an opportunity, medical-surgical nurses can create future practice roles that are more consistent with the heart and soul of the specialty. Prerequisite to this evolution in practice is individual nurses accepting responsibility for their own professional development. The initiation of innovative, accessible educational programs to retool clinicians is essential. Further, health care organizations and nursing professionals must value and become facile with methods to measure and improve patient outcomes, in order to ensure that care redesign is driven by principles of sound patient management rather than simply short-term economic incentives. Medical-surgical nurses now have the charter to expand their focus to include health promotion initiatives and family-centered care as critical elements of their practice. In order to achieve these aims, medical-surgical nurses must reaffirm the specialty's identity as expert generalists caring for adults across the care continuum.

REFERENCES

American Association of Retired Persons (AARP). (1993). *A profile of older Americans.* Washington, DC: Author.

American Nurses Association. (1986). *Development of computerized nursing information systems in nursing services* (Resolution No. 24). Kansas City, MO: Author.

American Nurses Association Division of Medical-Surgical Nursing Practice. (1980). *Standards of medical-surgical nursing practice.* Kansas City, MO: Author.

Barter, M., McLaughlin, F., & Thomas, S. (1994). Use of unlicensed assistive personnel by hospitals. *Nursing Economics, 12,* 82-87.

Bostrom, J., & Zimmerman, J. (1993). Restructuring nursing for a competitive health care environment. *Nursing Economics, 12,* 35-41, 54.

Brooten, D., & Naylor, M. (1995). Nurses' effect on changing patient outcomes. *Image, 27,* 95-103.

Brozenec, S., Levitt, A., & Poyss, A. (1994). Introduction. *Core curriculum for medical-surgical nurses.* Pitman, NJ: A.J. Jannetti.

Buerhaus, P. (1994). Economics of managed competition and consequences to nurses. Part I. *Nursing Economic$, 12,* 10-17.

Dracup, K., Baker, D.W., & Dunbar, S.B. (1994). Management of heart failure: II. Counseling, education, and lifestyle. *Journal of the American Medical Association,* 272, 1442-1446.

Enthoven, A.C. (1993). The history and principles of managed competition. *Health Affairs, 12*(Suppl), 24-48.

Fritz, D., & Cheeseman, S. (1994). Blueprint for integrating nurse extenders in critical care. *Nursing Economic$, 12,* 327-331, 326.

Hines, P., Smeltzer, C., & Galletti, M. (1994). Work restructuring: The process of redefining roles of patient care givers. *Nursing Economic$, 12,* 346-350.

Kerfoot, K. (1994). Nurse managers, managed care, and the external, outward view: A critical success factor. *Nursing Economic$, 12,* 340-341.

McGinnis, J.M., & Lee, P.R. (1995). *Healthy people 2000 at mid decade. JAMA, 273,* 1123-1129.

National Center for Health Statistics. (1992). *Health United States 1991 and prevention profile.* Hyattsville, MD: U.S. Public Health Service.

Russell, S. (1995). Recognizing change. *MedSurg Nursing, 4,* 174.

Sovie, M. (1994). Nurse manager: A key role in clinical outcomes. *Nursing Management, 25,* 30-34.

Sovie, M. (1995). Tailoring hospitals for managed care and integrated health systems. *Nursing Economic$, 13,* 72-83.

Titler, M., & Reiter, R. (1994). Outcomes measurement in clinical practice. *MedSurg Nursing, 3,* 395-398, 420.

U.S. Public Health Service. (1991). *Healthy people 2000: National health promotion and disease prevention objectives.* Washington, DC: U.S. Dept. of Health and Human Services.

U.S. Bureau of Census. (1992). *Sixty-five plus in America.* Washington, DC: U.S. Government Printing Office.

Werley, H., Ryan, P., & Coenen, A. (1994). *A brief synopsis of the nursing minimum data sets (NMDS).* Washington, DC: American Nurses Association.

Recent changes and current issues in pediatric nursing

JODY L. KURTT, GINETTE BUDREAU

As the end of the 20th century approaches, it seems fitting to examine the changes that pediatric nurses have experienced in recent decades and the challenges we face. Pediatric nursing and the health of our nation's children have been dramatically affected during the past 2 decades by the unprecedented development of new technology and knowledge, the escalating cost of health care, and significant economic and societal trends, including changes in the traditional family structure, increasing poverty, homelessness, and violence among children, and the appearance of new and the reemergence of "old" infectious diseases.

NEW TECHNOLOGY AND KNOWLEDGE

Recent advances in technology and knowledge have transformed the U.S. health care system and significantly altered the character of child health care and pediatric nursing. The development of new and sophisticated screening methods, diagnostic tests, noninvasive monitoring techniques, interventions, and therapies has greatly improved the ability of health care providers to predict, prevent, diagnose, and treat many acute and chronic conditions (Smith, 1986). As a result, more children survive preterm birth, life-threatening illnesses and diseases, and severe trauma, so that the number of children with chronic illnesses, disabilities, and complex health care needs is increasing (Diamond, 1994).

The development of new knowledge has been due in part to the contributions of pediatric nurses. From the early work of Rubin (1963) describing maternal touch to the work of Hester (1979) and Eland (1985) over the past 20 years concerning assessment and management of children's pain and the more recent work of Kleiber and coworkers (Kleiber, Hanrahan, Fagan, & Zittergruen, 1993) on the use of heparin versus saline for peripheral intravenous locks, the research and expertise of pediatric nurses has significantly impacted children's health care in the hospital and community. Pediatric nursing has made great strides in providing care that is based in scientific principles and research and in establishing health care environments that are child-focused and family-centered.

COST OF HEALTH CARE

With advances in health care technology and treatment, health care costs in the United States have skyrocketed. By 1993, health care expenditures in the United States had risen to more than 14% of the gross national product—higher than any other nation in the world—and aggregate expenditures on health care for children nearly doubled between 1977 and 1987 (Center for the Future of Children, 1992, p. 10; Givens & Moore, 1994, p. 9).

While national efforts to reform health care and control costs have been unsuccessful, changes are occurring at the state and regional levels. Reimbursement structures are shifting from a fee-for-service–dominated system to a managed care, capitated system. This shift to a market-driven, managed care delivery system has had an impact on patient care. Hospital lengths of stay have shortened, resulting in earlier discharge of pediatric patients with ongoing health care needs. At the same time, utilization of outpatient visits and ambulatory surgery has risen so that children receiving home health care and day treatment services require more intense nursing care than ever before. In addition, capitated payment systems have stimulated a major paradigm shift in American health care, changing the focus from illness management to primary care and preventive services (Jackson, 1995; Kirby, 1995).

PEDIATRIC NURSING TODAY

New technology and the shift to managed care have had a significant impact on pediatric nurses. The hospital units that pediatric nurses work in today are high-technology and fast-paced. Neonatal nurses care for infants receiving high-frequency ventilation and nitric oxide who often weigh as little as 500 g. In the pediatric intensive care unit, nurses manage vasoactive drug therapy, hemodynamic monitoring, and at times even extracorpeal membrane oxygenation for children before and after cardiac surgery. Pediatric medical and surgical nurses are questioning long-standing practices and implementing research-based standards of care such as pain management protocols for children experiencing acute surgical or cancer pain (Schmidt, Eland, & Weiler, 1994; Schmidt, Holida, Kleiber, Petersen, & Phearman, 1994).

Hospital-based clinical nurse specialists are playing an increasingly important role in educating and assisting children and their families to manage chronic illness. They are adopting computer-assisted instruction as a tool to teach children to manage diseases such as diabetes at home (Engvall, 1994). A relatively new role for clinical nurse specialists as well as staff nurses in hospitals is that of case manager. As case managers, pediatric nurses are leading multidisciplinary teams in the development of critical paths to impact the cost and quality of care for their patients.

As the shift from inpatient to outpatient care escalates and the hospital is no longer the locus for health care services, pediatric nurses have had to refocus their roles as providers. Community-based pediatric nurses have traditionally specialized in health surveillance and promotion, teaching, counseling, and case management. Today, pediatric nurses are also managing home health care agencies that provide care to children with complex health care needs including ventilators, intravenous medications, and parenteral nutrition. With the increasing emphasis on primary care, pediatric nurse practitioners are experiencing myriad new opportunities as primary care providers.

It is clear that pediatric nurses in today's health care environment must possess a broad knowledge base and skill set. At the same time they are challenged to provide care that interfaces human caring with technology, ensuring that patient care is individualized, developmentally appropriate, and family-centered, yet efficient and effective. As technology and treatment options have become more complex and health care resources more limited, pediatric nurses have found it necessary to acquire knowledge of ethical principals and counseling skills to support families faced with difficult decisions.

The increasing cultural diversity and changing lifestyles in our nation have heightened the need for pediatric nurses to recognize and understand cultural variations, the context of the child within the family and community, and the impact these differences have on health beliefs and practices. As supporters of family-centered care, pediatric nurses have accepted responsibility to advocate for and empower children and families as "members" of the health care team.

In the new health care environment, nurses and other health care providers are being held accountable for reducing and controlling costs while maintaining or improving quality and outcomes. Pediatric nurses in all settings and roles are becoming more involved in multidisciplinary teams to evaluate and improve patient care. Experience and expertise in quality improvement, research, and research utilization is valued for staff nurses as well as advanced practice nurses and nurse managers. Strong leadership and communication skills are essential and acquisition of computer skills is becoming increasingly important for all pediatric nurses.

HEALTH STATUS OF U.S. CHILDREN

Despite significant advances in technology and knowledge and increased expenditures on health care, the United States has thus far been unsuccessful in providing access to nonfragmented, basic health care services for all its children. Several key indicators of children's health, including high infant mortality rates, lack of early prenatal care, high incidence of low birth weight, high levels of uninsuredness, and low immunization rates, warn that progress in improving children's health is suffering (Children's Defense Fund, 1994). In addition, the social conditions of changing families and increasing poverty and violence have put children at increased risk for health problems. The health status of children in the United States is not in line with our capabilities or expenditure levels (Center for the Future of Children, 1992).

Child health indicators

Infant mortality and low birth weight. While tremendous strides have been made in infant health during this century, there is still cause for concern. In 1992, the U.S. infant mortality rate of 8.5 deaths per 1,000 live births was higher than infant mortality rates in more than 20 other industrialized nations (Children's Defense Fund, 1994, p. 11; Givens & Moore, 1994, p. 10). Although rates in the United States have fallen significantly since 1960, improvement has slowed greatly since 1980 and has been primarily the result of improved technology for high-risk neonates, not improved primary and preventive care (Children's Defense Fund, 1994, p. 10; Givens & Moore, 1994, p. 10).

Our infant mortality rate is due largely to the nation's poor track record with early prenatal care and low-birth-weight infants (Children's Defense Fund, 1994). Birth weight is a key predictor of the health and survival of newborn infants. Despite two decades of new research, therapies, and technologies to prevent, identify, and treat preterm labor, there has been a consistent, slow increase in the number of low-birth-weight infants born in the United States (Givens & Moore, 1994, p. 11). In 1991, 7% of all American infants weighed less than 5.5 pounds when born, a condition placing them at greater risk of dying during their first year of life and of suffering from chronic health conditions and disabilities throughout life. In that same year, almost one of every four American babies was born to a woman who did not receive prenatal care during the first 3 months of her pregnancy. U.S. infants were less likely in 1991 than in 1980 to be born to mothers who received early prenatal care and were more likely to be born at a low birth weight (Children's Defense Fund, 1994, p. 10).

The risk of low birth weight and infant death in black infants is especially sobering. In 1991, almost 13.6% of black infants were born weighing less than 5.5 pounds, which is more than double the rate for white infants (Children's Defense Fund, 1994, p. 11). With an infant mortality rate of 16.8 per 1,000 live births in 1992, black infants were almost twice as likely as white infants to die within their first year of life (Givens & Moore, 1994, p. 10). These disparities among racial groups are likely related to sociocultural factors discouraging the use of preventive health care, the stresses of continued racism, and the effects of years of inequity among Americans with respect to income levels, family stability, education, nutrition, employment, and health care (Givens & Moore, 1994). If our nation is to lower its infant mortality rate substantially, these issues must be addressed.

Immunization rates. Childhood immunization rates are another key indicator of how well a nation is caring for its children. Since the 1960s when vaccines became widely available, many childhood communicable diseases and the associated risks of serious illness and death have been preventable through routine immunization. While most school-age children in the United States are fully immunized because it is required for entry to school, many younger children do not receive recommended immunization coverage. In 1992, only 55.3% of 2-year-olds and less than 40% of 2-year-olds living below the poverty line were fully immunized (Children's Defense Fund, 1994, p. 11).

The reasons for low immunization rates in children are not agreed on nationally and are most likely the result of multiple, complex, interacting factors, including inattention by the provider ("missed opportunities"), inadequate public education as to the seriousness of the diseases that immunizations prevent, and limited access to immunizations as a result of inconvenient clinic locations and hours, difficulty getting quick appointments, and the inability to pay.

The substandard immunization rate in the United States gained national recognition during the measles epidemic of 1989 to 1991, which resulted in 55,000 reported cases, over 100 deaths, and $20 million in hospital costs (Scudder, 1995). Most of the cases occurred in children under the age of 5 who were not immunized. Concern was further heightened in 1992 and 1993 by the increasing number of pertussis cases. President Clinton helped to bring the issue of low immunization rates to the forefront of the health care reform debate and increased public awareness. Soon after taking office he developed the Childhood Immunization Initiative, a national program of unprecedented scope to improve vaccination rates in preschool children, which eventually led to legislation under the Omnibus Reconciliation Act of 1993 (Scudder, 1995, p. 20-1, 26). Federal efforts at improving immunization rates have been supplemented by multiple private endeavors, most notably the "Every Child By Two" campaign organized by Rosalynn Carter and Betty Bumpers and joined by the American Nurses Association in 1992 (Scudder, 1995, p. 27).

Although the immunization rates of preschoolers in the United States appear to be improving, we must not be content. If we are to meet the "Healthy People 2000" goal of 90% immunization compliance (Igoe, 1990), nurses and other health care providers must support local, state, and national efforts that make immunizations a priority. Immunization is a low-cost, cost-saving measure that promotes and protects the future health of our children.

Access to health care services Both private and public health insurance play a crucial role in facilitating access to health care services and improving children's health. Health insurance is associated with increased use of prenatal care, improved pregnancy outcomes and infant health, and a positive impact on the entire spectrum of child health and developmental issues (Center for the Future of Children, 1992, p. 14). Uninsured children are less likely to have a consistent and comprehensive source of health care and be adequately immunized, have fewer physician visits for some acute illnesses, and are more likely to use costly emergency room and inpatient hospital care.

Despite the known benefits, in 1992 more than 8 million American children had no health insurance at all, and these numbers greatly underestimate the millions of other children who were uninsured at some time during the year or had insurance plans that failed to cover preventive care or preexisting conditions (Children's Defense Fund, 1994, p. 9; Center for the Future of Children, 1992, p. 14). For the past decade, the number of children covered by private health insurance has declined steadily. Only by expanding Medicaid coverage during the past decade has the United States prevented the number of uninsured children from increasing even more sharply. The percentage of children covered by Medicaid rose from 15.5% in 1988 to 21.4% in 1992 (Children's Defense Fund, 1994, p. 10).

Although Medicaid coverage has been expanded substantially, the protection it now provides helps primarily very young and very poor children. The income eligibility threshold significantly limits the relief that Medicaid can provide to children of the working poor and middle class. Furthermore, the slow phase-in of the eligibility expansion to children through age 18 leaves older children with little protection at this time (Cartland & Yudkowsky, 1993, p. 150).

Lack of private health insurance and ineligibility for Medicaid are not the only barriers that children face in gaining access to health care. Utilization, especially with regard to Medicaid, has been limited by complex programmatic and administrative issues and by low provider reimbursement rates, leading to low and declining participation in Medicaid by pediatricians. More recently, private insurers have increasingly tightened their programs to limit utilization and control costs.

Perhaps the most widespread obstacle to access of health care for children on Medicaid is the inadequate participation and distribution of providers. Although a generous supply of pediatricians has developed during the past decade, the number participating in Medicaid is low and their geographic distribution does not match that of U.S. children, especially poor children in urban and rural areas (Center for the Future of Children, 1992, p. 16-17).

Inadequate insurance coverage and limited access to care for pregnant women and children are important factors underlying the problems of low birth weight, infant mortality, low immunization rates, and other health problems in children. It is deplorable that the most expensive health care system in the world does not ensure even the most basic health care coverage for all of its children.

Societal effects

Changes in social conditions in our nation during the past three decades have dramatically affected the American family, children's health, and pediatric nursing practice.

Changing families. The children and families that pediatric nurses care for today are much different than those of a generation ago. The lives of most children and families have become significantly more complicated, busier, and riskier. Family life is increasingly challenged by the demands of parents' work, children's extracurricular activities, and the lure of interests and opportunities outside the family. The traditional structures, roles, and routines of families have been transformed and the economic stability of families has been threatened (Children's Defense Fund, 1994; National Commission on Children, 1991).

The rapidly rising divorce rate and increasing number of out-of-wedlock births, especially among teenagers, during the past 2 decades have increased the number of children living in single-parent families. In the United States in 1950 and 1970, 5% and 12% of children, respectively, lived with only one parent (National Commission on Children, 1991, p. 6; Spence, 1995, p. 10). Today, fully one fourth of the children in the United States live in single-parent homes.

One of the most dramatic social changes in the past 20 years has been the steady increase of mothers in the workforce. Between 1960 and 1994, the number of working mothers increased nearly fourfold, from 6.6 million to 24.2 million (Spence, 1995, p. 10). The long-term effects of this change on children's development is not yet clear.

Other societal factors that have significantly affected children, families, and pediatric nursing are the increasing levels of poverty and violence in our nation.

Poverty. Today, children are the poorest Americans (National Commission on Children, 1991, p. 7). It is troublesome that the number of children living in poverty in the United States continues to rise while the rate among other age groups has either remained relatively constant or decreased (Allen, 1994, p. 382). In 1993, 25% of all infants were born into families with incomes below the poverty line, more than in any year since 1964 (Givens & Moore, 1994, p. 13). More than 14 million children—one child in five—live in families with incomes below the federal poverty level (Allen, 1994, p. 382; Children's Defense Fund, 1994, p. x; Starfield, 1992, p. 32), and 5 million of these children are desperately poor, living in families with incomes at less than half the federal poverty level (National Commission on Children, 1991, p. 8). Millions more live in families that are barely above the poverty level (Allen, 1994, p. 82; Starfield, 1992, p. 32).

While the majority of poor children are white, poverty varies considerably by race and family composition. Minority children are much more likely to live in a poor family: About 44% of black children and 36% of Hispanic children are poor, compared with less than 15% of white children (Allen, 1994, p. 382). Children living with only their mothers are especially likely to be poor; more than 40% of single-parent families headed by a mother are poor, compared with only about 7% of two-parent families.

Poverty influences the health of children in many ways. Children living in poverty experience double the incidence of low birth weight and are at higher risk of neonatal and postneonatal mortality, receive delayed immunizations three times more frequently, experience tripled rates of lead poisoning, become ill more often and have more serious illnesses, and die three times more frequently from accidents and four times more frequently from diseases (Starfield, 1992, p. 33). Among the reasons for these risks are increased environmental exposures from poor housing and hazardous neighborhoods, inadequate nutrition, and limited access to health care. Poor children miss 40% more days of school as a result of illness and are at greater risk for academic failure (Igoe, 1995, p. 14; Starfield, 1992, p. 33). The health problems of poor children are of great concern not only because of the immediate consequences they pose to health, but also because of the compromising effect they have on future health and development and opportunities to succeed.

Injuries and violence. Injuries have been the leading cause of death and disability among children in the United States for more than four decades (Betz, 1993, p. 353; Center for the Future of Children, 1992, p. 9). However, the number of intentional violent injuries and deaths from homicides among children has been increasing in recent years (Center for the Future of Children, 1992, p. 9). Violence affecting children is now more visible throughout our nation. This problem is not confined to poor and minority youth. Rather, it crosses all socioeconomic boundaries and affects rural, suburban, and urban communities (Spivak, 1994, p. 577).

In 1992, 1.5 million violent crimes were committed against children, 23% more than in 1987 (Spence, 1995). Since 1988 more American children between the ages of 15 and 19 have died from gunshot wounds than from illnesses or other natural causes (Spence, 1995). In 1991, guns were the second leading cause of death after car accidents for all children 10 to 18 years of age and young adults (Children's Defense Fund, 1994, p. 64). Guns take their highest toll among young black males ages 15 to 24, in whom they are the leading cause of death.

While the number of children victimized by violence has soared, so has the number of teen offenders (Children's Defense Fund, 1994, p. xvi). Between 1988 and 1992, juvenile arrests for murder, robbery, and assault all increased by 50% (Spence, 1995, p. 10). The increased murder arrest rate is inextricably linked to guns—more than 80% of juvenile murders today involve firearms. Although our nation regulates the safety of many products including children's toys, blankets, and pajamas, it does not regulate the safety of a product that kills and injures thousands of children and adults each year. A new gun is produced every 10 seconds in America and is available to almost anybody who wants to own one, including children (Children's Defense Fund, 1994, p. xi).

The escalating violence against and by children is a cumulative manifestation of many serious and neglected societal ills, including epidemic child and family poverty, increasing economic inequality, racial intolerance, widespread drug and alcohol abuse, the disintegration of family and community values and supports that children need, and the pervasive violence in our popular culture (Children's Defense Fund, 1994, p. x). Images and models of violence surround us and are easily available to children: Children watch an average of 8,000 murders and 100,000 other violent acts on television before finishing elementary school. Experts link childhood violence to violence in the media, but also believe children would be less affected by media violence if families and communities provided proper guidance and support (Spence, 1995).

The epidemic of violence among our nation's young has created a new challenge for pediatric nurses, who are having to learn how to take care of the physiological and psychological needs of kids affected by violence.

CHALLENGES AND RECOMMENDATIONS

Children are our future

As we move into the 21st century, pediatric nurses must act collectively and in concert with other health care professionals and communities to improve the health status of our nation's children and their families. The economics of the health care market will continue to stretch our creativity and require us to develop new models of health care delivery that provide cost-effective, accessible, coordinated care across all settings.

It is imperative that our nation establish a comprehensive health care system for all children that ensures easy access to preventive services and primary care at a price society can afford (Center for the Future of Children, 1992, p. 22). As the state and federal governments move to make important policy decisions affecting children's health care, the involvement of pediatric nurses is important. Children have very little political clout and need pediatric nurses to advocate and speak for them. Through our own individual lobbying efforts and membership in professional organizations that support children, we must push for a national children's agenda and health policy legislation. While current reform efforts are proceeding incrementally at the state and federal levels, expansion of Medicaid programs is necessary to extend coverage to uninsured children, who are currently not eligible. In addition we must ensure that programs providing childhood nutrition (Women, Infants, and Children program, school and summer meal programs, food stamps) and opportunities for early learning and development (Head Start) are maintained and enhanced.

Delivery of care

As managed care and capitation forces health care organizations and providers to develop integrated delivery systems, pediatric nurses have the opportunity to design patient care delivery models that bridge the gaps across the entire spectrum of care. By being flexible and working across departmental and agency lines we can help to develop accessible, coordinated, nonfragmented systems that focus on wellness across the continuum, meet community-based needs, and demonstrate concern for cost-effective utilization (Kirby, 1995). These new models will take us steps beyond case management.

Primary care

It is glaringly evident that the our nation lacks a well-developed primary health care sector to complement our highly developed specialty services (Starfield, 1992, p. 37). Too many children, especially the poor and uninsured, experience fragmented services and episodic care. Until we can ensure access to efficient and effective primary care for all children in this country, we will be unable to improve the health status of our nation's children, especially those in high-risk groups. One group often overlooked is adolescents. Teenagers have the poorest health status and fastest rising death rates of any age group in the United States (Center for the Future of Children, 1992). However, because many adolescent health problems are related to high-risk behavior, this population often has problems accessing the health care it needs. Schools are an excellent but underutilized site for health promotion and the delivery of accessible, affordable, primary care. Alternative delivery models such as school-based clinics and neighborhood centers are being developed and should be encouraged. Advanced practice nurses are a valuable primary care resource and if utilized appropriately can expand assess to health care services for children and families.

Immunizations

As patient advocates and educators, pediatric nurses are in a logical position to assume leadership for promoting public awareness about the need to immunize infants and young children. Nurses can help define the problems of low immunization rates through practice and research and can promote legislation that offers a viable solution to this national health problem (Scudder, 1995). In our practice we must remove the barriers that families experience in getting immunizations for their young children and take advantage of every contact with a child to review immunization status and vaccinate as indicated. By networking with established immunization initiatives across the country and using research, pediatric nurses can provide the leadership needed to establish community-based programs that meet the immunization needs of local populations (Scudder, 1995).

Societal issues

Although the societal issues of poverty and violence are beyond the realm of health care alone, their negative effect on children's health and opportunities to succeed may be reduced by changes in the health care system and actions of pediatric nurses.

Pediatric nurses should take the opportunity to educate children and parents, health care professionals, and child care providers about violence in the media, child health issues associated with firearms, and how to childproof guns in the home. We must work with all factions to prevent guns from getting into the hands of kids and criminals, and support community-based programs that give children opportunities to have positive, supervised recreation and adult role models (Children's Defense Fund, 1994).

Nursing practice

The restructuring of health care has already significantly altered the role of pediatric nurses and many complex problems and challenges lay ahead. Feeg (1990, p. 77), editor of *Pediatric Nursing*, has encouraged us to meet these challenges with knowledge and enthusiasm. As we move into the 21st century we need to work collaboratively with multidisciplinary teams and communities to design accessible health care systems that are compatible with quality and cost indicators and responsive to children's needs (Kirby, 1995).

Pediatric nursing has made great strides in the past decade to develop standards of practice based on research and to infuse the elements of family-centered care into the health care environment. These efforts will continue to be critical in the years ahead. There will be an increasing need for research that demonstrates and evaluates the outcomes of our interventions and determines the effectiveness and costs of new patient care delivery models.

Children truly are our future and we must give new directed attention and societal commitment toward improving their health (Starfield, 1992, p. 38). We cannot afford not to care.

REFERENCES

Allen, C.E. (1994). Families in poverty. *Nursing Clinics in North America, 29*(3), 377-392.

Betz, C.L. (1993). Injury: Our children's greatest health problem. *Journal of Pediatric Nursing: Nursing Care of Children and Families, 8*(6), 353.

Cartland, J.D.C., & Yudkowsky, B.K. (1993, Spring). Datawatch. *Health Affairs*, 144-151.

Center for the Future of Children. (1992). Analysis. *The Future of Children, 2*(2), 7-24.

Children's Defense Fund. (1994). *The state of America's children yearbook.* Washington, DC: U.S. Government Printing Office.

Diamond, J. (1994). Family-centered care for children with chronic illnesses. *Journal of Pediatric Health Care, 8,* 196-197.

Eland, J.M. (1985). The child who is hurting. *Seminars in Oncology Nursing, 1*(2), 116-122.

Engvall, J.C. (1994). Tool chest: Use of computer-assisted instruction in diabetes education. *Diabetes Educator, 20*(5), 433-436.

Feeg, V.D. (1990). The future of pediatric nursing: Anticipating the health care needs of children. *Imprint, 37*(4), 70-77.

Givens, S.R., & Moore, M.L. (1994). Status report on maternal and child health indicators. *Journal of Perinatal and Neonatal Nursing, 9*(1), 8-18.

Hester, N. (1979). The preoperational child's reaction to immunization. *Nursing Research, 28*(4), 250-255.

Igoe, J.B. (1990). Healthy people 2000. *Pediatric Nursing, 16*(6), 584-586.

Igoe, J.B. (1995). School health . . . designing the policy environment though understanding. *Nursing Policy Forum, 1*(3), 12-36.

Jackson, P.L. (1995). Advanced practice nursing: Part 2. Opportunities and challenges for PNPs. *Pediatric Nursing, 21*(1), 43-46.

Kirby, A. (1995). Establishing a community health focus in perinatal nursing practice within a capitated environment. *Journal of Perinatal and Neonatal Nursing, 9*(1), 68-77.

Kleiber, C., Hanrahan, K., Fagan, C.L., & Zittergruen, M.A. (1993). Heparin vs. saline for peripheral IV locks in children. *Pediatric Nursing, 19*(4), 405-409.

National Commission on Children. (1991). *Beyond rhetoric a new American agenda for children and families.* Washington, DC: U.S. Government Printing Office.

Rubin, R. (1963). Maternal touch. *Nursing Outlook, 11,* 828-831.

Schmidt, K., Eland, J., & Weiler, K. (1994). Pediatric cancer pain management. *Journal of Pediatric Oncology Nursing, 11*(1), 4-12.

Schmidt, K., Holida, D., Kleiber, C., Petersen, M., & Phearman, L. (1994). Implementation of the AHCPR guidelines for children. *Journal of Nursing Care Quality, 8*(3), 68-74.

Scudder, L. (1995). Child immunization initiative: Politics and health policy in action. *Nursing Policy Forum, 1*(3), 20-29.

Smith, J.P. (1986). Nursing and health care in the twentieth century: Myth, reality, and dichotomy. *Journal of Advanced Nursing, 11,* 127-132.

Spence, A. (1995, August). Family instability leaves children vulnerable. *AAP News,* p. 10-11.

Spivak, H. (1994). Violence prevention: A call to action. *Pediatrics, 94*(4), 577-578.

Starfield, B. (1992). Child and adolescent health status measures. *The Future of Children, 2*(2), 25-39.

Recent changes and current issues in perinatal nursing

DOROTHY BROOTEN

Clinicians and practitioners providing perinatal care today are faced with issues involving in vitro fertilization, surrogate parenthood, continued high levels of adolescent pregnancy, a high low-birth-weight rate compared with other developed countries, continued problems with access to prenatal care, women receiving late or no prenatal care, and early hospital discharge of newly delivered mothers and their infants. Each of these issues holds important implications for nursing practice, the delivery of health care, ethics, the law, and public policy. Over the last several decades many studies and demonstration projects have focused on reducing adolescent pregnancy, the low-birth-weight rate, and the numbers of women receiving late or no prenatal care. The newer area of in vitro fertilization and surrogate parenting is replete with ethical, moral, legal, and public policy issues. However, the number of patients, families, and practitioners involved is far smaller than that of those affected by earlier hospital discharge of childbearing women and newborns. For this reason, this chapter focuses on early hospital discharge for mothers and newborns.

DISCHARGE TRENDS

Length of hospital stay for newly delivered women and their newborns and women hospitalized antenatally has changed dramatically over the last several decades. In the 1950s, the average length of stay for mother and baby was approximately 7 days. By 1982 and 1992, the average lengths of stay for women delivering vaginally were 2.9 days and 1.8 days, respectively (Commission on Professional and Hospital Activities, 1983, 1994). Some institutions have even mandated 6- to 8-hour lengths of stay. For women who deliver by cesarean, length of stay decreased from 6.1 days in 1982 to 4 days by 1992, and some providers are now advocating a 2-day length of stay for these patients (Strong, Brown, Brown, & Curry, 1993). The 1982 lengths of stay for normal-term and preterm infants were 3.7 days and over 40 days, respectively, compared with 1.7- and 18-day stays in 1992. Women previously hospitalized for problems and monitoring during pregnancy are now being maintained at home through the use of electronic monitoring and nurse home visits.

The driving force for this reduced length of hospital stay was largely a desire to control health care costs by federal and private insurers. Some consumers also voluntarily preferred an earlier hospital discharge. Arguments over the resulting costs and benefits of earlier discharge continue. Most recently Maryland and New Jersey enacted legislation requiring insurers to cover a minimum 48-hour length of stay for mothers and newborns following delivery and numerous states are following their lead. A 24-hour discharge is allowed if a home visit by nurses is supplemented by insurers (Begley, Springen, & Duigan-Cabrera, 1995).

ADVANTAGES AND DISADVANTAGES OF EARLY DISCHARGE

Potential advantages of early hospital discharge for newly delivered mothers and infants include returning them to the family sooner, decreasing exposure to nosocomial infections, decreasing the stress of a strange, often noisy environment with constant intrusions and unfamiliar routines and food, and reduced health care costs. Environmental assaults of excessive noise, constant bright lighting, and frequent, sometimes painful contact by nurses, physicians, and other providers on the hearing, sight, and responses of hospitalized preterm infants is well documented (Graven et al., 1992). The negative effects of decreased mobility and increased stress on women needing prolonged antenatal hospital bedrest

(Heaman, 1992; Maloni, 1994), and the difficulty of regulating blood sugar levels in pregnant hospitalized women with resulting altered activity and dietary intakes (York et al., in press), are also documented.

The most commonly cited disadvantage to early hospital discharge for mothers and babies is undetected complications. This potentially results in increased numbers of rehospitalizations and acute care visits to emergency rooms or physicians' offices (Brooten et al., 1995; Brown & York, in press; Jansson, 1985). Additional disadvantages include increased family stress, increased out-of-pocket expenses as the burden of care and costs shifts to families, fatigued mothers who assume household responsibilities prematurely, and less successful breastfeeding experience and duration (Brown & York, in press).

In an effort to maintain optimal outcomes for mothers and newborns while decreasing health care costs, a number of programs of early hospital discharge and home follow-up services have been developed, especially for high-risk, high-cost, high-volume patient groups (Brooten, et al., 1986, 1988, 1994; Dahlberg & Kaloroutis, 1994; Eaton, 1994; Goodwin, 1994; Heaman, Robinson, Thompson, & Heleva, 1994; Raff, 1986; York et al., in press). Such services are provided by community nurses, hospital-based home care services, home follow-up services provided by health maintenance organizations, and those services provided by contractual arrangements with entrepreneurial groups. Ideally, each program would include coordinated discharge planning, home follow-up visits by providers knowledgeable about care of the patient group they are serving, coordination of additional home services where needed, and planned health care follow-up.

HOME FOLLOW-UP SERVICES

Community nursing services

Community or public health nurses have historically provided home follow-up to preterm or high-risk infants and women with high-risk pregnancies or complicated postpartum courses. Their services are well known and accepted by the general public and health care providers. Nurses working within the community are also familiar with community resources, health care needs, values, and culture of the community residents. Unfortunately, over the past 10 to 15 years, budget reductions of community nursing services have all but eliminated home follow-up services to many perinatal and neonatal groups that were formerly served. Programs focused on prevention and well child care were curtailed to provide services to more acutely ill patients, mainly the elderly, who are now discharged earlier while they are still recovering. More recently, however, less stable, more acutely ill newborns and pregnant and newly delivered women were added to the caseloads of community nurses (National Association for Home Care, 1993).

Many community nursing services are currently challenged to update the specialty knowledge and skills of agency nurses with a generalist preparation; maintain continuity of patient care from the hospital to the home; and provide sufficient services to maintain good patient outcomes while insurers are reimbursing for fewer services (Brooten, 1995). To provide service to a more high-risk prenatal and neonatal group of patients, agencies have been providing continuing education for their nurses, using nurses with advanced practice skills (master's prepared clinical nurse specialists and nurse practitioners) as consultants for the agency or in agencies with sufficient caseloads, and hiring advanced practice nurses to provide direct care in the home. Attempts to improve continuity of care to high-risk groups has included predischarge hospital visits to patients by a community nurse and a community liaison nurse on site in the hospital. Some agencies now provide 24-hour nurse coverage 7 days a week and expanded use of ancillary personnel including homemaker–home health aids.

Hospital home care services and health maintenance organization follow-up services

As reimbursed length of stay for perinatal and neonatal patients decreases, hospitals' needs for improved discharge planning and postdischarge home care services for these groups increases. Documented discharge planning is mandatory for hospitals and many have hired discharge planners to facilitate earlier discharge. Some hospitals contract with community nursing services or independent home care agencies to provide home care services for their high-risk perinatal and neonatal patients. An increasing number are establishing their own home care services. In some instances this home care is provided by existing hospital nursing staff from the obstetrical and neonatal units where bed occupancy has decreased, thus reducing the nursing staff needed on the units. As Dahlberg and Kaloroutis (1994) note, one of the greatest advantages of a hospital-based program is the internal availability of knowledgeable and skilled nursing staff. They further note that physicians are more likely to refer patients to a program that is staffed with nurses they know and trust from the hospital setting. In others hospitals, home care services are provided by a nursing staff hired and managed by the hospital's home care department (Brooten, 1995).

Health maintenance organizations have a clear financial incentive for discharging perinatal and neonatal patients early and for preventing costly rehospitalizations. They have used case managers and nurses with specialty knowledge and skills to review patients' discharge and home care needs. Because realizing a profit is essential, their approach has been one of minimal hospital length of stay and postdischarge services. Home follow-up services provided vary in number of visits provided, type of nurse provider (nurse generalist or specialist), and length of follow-up. While more than the routine allowable number of home visits may be reimbursable for a patient, this must be negotiated between provider and insurer.

Entrepreneurial services

Over the past decade many entrepreneurial groups have established services to provide home care to perinatal and neonatal patients (Eaton, 1994). These groups usually are not involved in discharge planning but do provide home care services on a fee-for-service or contractual basis. The services provided may be determined by the company's medical advisory board or by the contracting agency and reviewed and approved by the company's medical advisory board. Nurses providing services may be full-time employees or temporary nursing staff who may or may not have specialty preparation and skills in caring for the patient groups they are following.

One service model established through research and demonstration

Research and demonstration projects have tested models of early hospital discharge and home care services over the past decade. In 1981, a model of transitional care provided by master's-prepared advanced practice nurse (APN) specialists (clinical nurse specialists and nurse practitioners) was established by Brooten et al. (1988). The model was designed to discharge patients early from the hospital by substituting a portion of hospital care with a comprehensive program of transitional home follow-up care by the nurse specialists. The model, consisting of both comprehensive discharge planning and home follow-up through the period of physiological stability or normally expected physiological recovery, examines patient outcomes and cost of care, and documents all nursing interventions.

Using the model, patients are discharged early provided they meet a standard set of criteria agreed on by the physician and nurse specialist that encompass physical, emotional, and informational patient readiness for discharge and a home environment that is supportive of convalescence. Discharge criteria include general physiological stability; the ability to assume self-care or a support person at home who is willing and able to assist in care; and a demonstrated knowledge of reportable signs and symptoms, temperature taking, activity limitations, dietary needs, and care specific to the patient population being discharged.

The APN specialist prepares the patient for discharge and coordinates discharge planning with the patient, physician, hospital nursing staff, and other health care personnel involved in the patient's care. The APN specialist also coordinates or performs patient teaching, helps establish a time frame for discharge, coordinates plans for medical follow-up, and makes referrals to community agencies when needed. When problems are encountered, the APN specialist consults with the physician and appropriate others to resolve the problem. If the difficulty cannot be resolved, and in the opinion of the APN specialist and physician the situation poses a significant threat to the patient's well-being, the patient is not discharged early (Brooten et al., 1988).

Following discharge the APN conducts a series of home visits and is frequently in touch with patients by telephone to monitor their physical, emotional, and functional status; provide direct care when necessary; assist in obtaining community resources or services; and provide teaching, counseling, and support during the period of convalescence.

The model, using randomized clinical trials, has been tested with several high-risk, high-volume, and/or high-cost perinatal/neonatal groups including very-low-birth-weight infants, women following unplanned cesarean birth, and women with high-risk pregnancies (e.g., women with diabetes and hypertension). Results using the model with very-low-birth-weight infants demonstrated that infants followed by an APN specialist could be discharged 11 days earlier than control infants with no increase in rehospitalizations or emergency visits and a 27% reduction in hospital charges (Brooten et al., 1986). Using the model with women following unplanned cesarean birth, women followed by an APN specialist were discharged 30.3 hours earlier, had significantly greater satisfaction with care, had significantly more infants immunized, and incurred 29% lower health care costs compared with women in the control group (Brooten et al., 1994). Women with high-risk pregnancies (diabetes and hypertension) who were followed antenatally by an APN specialist had fewer antenatal hospitalizations, gave birth to fewer very-low-birth-weight infants, and incurred almost 38% less in health care costs compared with the control group (York et al., in press).

Current research using the model focuses on substituting half of prenatal physician or clinic care for APN specialist care delivered in the home to women with high-risk pregnancies (i.e., diabetes, hypertension, preterm labor) (Brooten, 1991-1996; Stringer, Spatz, & Donahue, 1994). In addition, based on the results of more than a decade of testing and refining the model, a transitional care service for childbearing women and their newborns has been established by the University of Pennsylvania School of Nursing (M. Stringer, personal communication, August 30, 1995).

Other research and demonstration projects have examined the effects of nurse home follow-up on selected perinatal and neonatal outcomes. These programs, however, were not developed in response to earlier hospital discharge or to provide home care for vulnerable groups discharged earlier. The work of Olds et al. (1992) using nurse home visiting focused on improving pregnancy outcomes and reducing the number of low-birth-weight infants born to mothers in rural New York and urban Memphis. Barnard, Hammond, and Summer (1987) used nurse home visits to focus on improvement of parenting skills and child development with term and preterm newborns.

Current issues in earlier discharge and home follow-up care

All programs of early hospital discharge and home follow-up services are challenged by issues of how to maintain continuity of care between hospital and home, what type of provider is needed and most cost-effective for what patient group, what type and length of follow-up service is required to achieve optimal patient outcomes, and how to provide a level of reimbursable service that will maintain good patient outcomes.

Approaches to achieve continuity of care include using telephone contacts, home visits, or similar methods that provide patients with ongoing access to their care providers. Maintaining continuity is best achieved when the same provider or provider team is responsible for provision of care both in the hospital and at home. When different groups of providers are involved, attempts to maintain continuity of care have been somewhat successful using community liaison nurses who are hospital-based or who conduct predischarge hospital visits. Good communication between hospital and home care nurses is essential to avoid patients receiving conflicting information, which can erode both patient confidence and satisfaction with care (Brooten, 1995; Goodwin, 1994).

Data are now needed to match the most efficient, effective, and cost-effective type and level of nurse provider (e.g., nurse specialist, nurse generalist, registered nurse, APN) with specific patient groups. It is not clear, for example, which patient groups benefit most from the services of nurse generalists or nurse specialists, which groups require direct care from nurse specialists, and which would be best served by nurse generalists with consultation from nurse specialists. Data are also needed on the most effective mix of nurse services in combination with other types of health care personnel such as homemaker aides.

Data are also needed to determine the most effective and cost-efficient type and length of home care service. For some patient groups postdischarge telephone follow-up alone to provide support, counseling, and monitoring of a patient's condition may be sufficient. For high-risk groups, telephone follow-up in combination with home visits may be required to achieve similar good patient outcomes. Within each patient group, subgroups of patients such as those with morbidity, abusive situations, or overwhelming personal, social, or economic problems are already demonstrating that they require more nurse time to achieve the same health outcomes (Brooten et al., in press).

The most challenging situation now is how to achieve a match between patient need and reimbursable services. In some health care systems that mandate very short hospital stays the need for additional reimbursable hospital days or nurse home visits is being voiced clearly by consumers, providers, and politicians (Haddad, 1992). In other situations reimbursement is still allocated by days spent in the hospital and fees for services provided. Here provider and institutional incentives are clear and provide other sets of challenges. Very-low-birth-weight infants, for example, may be kept and discharged directly from neonatal intensive care units to maximize institutional reimbursement and perhaps provider fees. Such practices have the potential to increase parental stress and decrease confidence in parenting skills. For nurses, the challenge is to develop and implement the most effective and cost-efficient set of services acceptable and available to perinatal and neonatal patients who need them.

Implications for nursing education

Given the current changes in health care delivery for both perinatal and neonatal patients, what knowledge and skills are now required to care for patients who stay in the hospital for very brief periods? How can newly delivered women, for example, best be educated regarding their own physical and psychological condition or parenting skills given only brief encounters with a multitude of different health care providers? What is required to care for more acutely ill patients in their homes? What skills are needed to negotiate plans of care with family members when the provider is a guest in the home and removed from readily available consultants as in the hospital setting? What is required to keep mothers and neonates well, out of the hospital, and not using inappropriate visits to the doctor or emergency room? Finally, what is required to accomplish these goals within the broader system of health care services?

Interestingly, current changes in health care are reflective of those occurring in the corporate world. This includes the need for a changed workforce whose members are flexible and focused on thinking and problem solving rather than carrying out a set of discrete tasks. This is also true in nursing. To keep patients healthy or to return them to health after an illness episode requires knowledge of their health problem, thinking, problem solving, flexibility, and providers focused on improving health outcomes rather than on the conduct of discrete tasks.

For nurses providing care to high-risk populations in today's health care market, nurses must first and foremost possess depth of knowledge and exquisite clinical skills. Equally important, they must have the ability to plan for the care of patients over time and settings and possess the skills for negotiating the health, social, political, and reimbursement systems needed to support these patients. The level of clinical sophistication and system savvy that are required to meet the increasingly complex needs of this population in our changing health care market are the hallmarks of master's preparation in advanced nursing specialty practice.

REFERENCES

Barnard, K., Hammond, M., & Summer, G. (1987). Helping parents with preterm infants: field test of a protocol. *Early Childhood Development and Care, 27,* 255-290.

Begley, S., Springen, K., & Duigan-Cabrera, A. (1995, July 10). Deliver: Then depart. *Newsweek,* p. 62.

Brooten, D. (Principal investigator). *Nurse home care/high risk pregnant women: Outcomes and costs (1991-1996)* (NIH, R01-NR-02867). Bethesda, MD: National Institute for Nursing Research, National Institutes of Health.

Brooten, D. (1995). Perinatal care across the continuum: Early discharge and nursing home follow up. *The Journal of Perinatal and Neonatal Nursing, 9*(1), 38-44.

Brooten, D., Brown, L., Munro, B., York, R., Cohen, S., Roncoli, M., & Hollingsworth, A. (1988). Early discharge and specialist transitional care. *Image: The Journal of Nursing Scholarship, 20*(2), 64-68.

Brooten, D., Knapp, H., Borucki, L., Jacobsen, b., Finkler, S., Arnold, L., & Mennuti, M. (In press). Early hospital discharge and home care of women following unplanned cesarean birth: A report of nurse care time. *Journal of Obstetric, Gynecologic and Neonatal Nursing.*

Brooten, D., Kumar, S., Brown, L., Butts, P., Finkler, S., Bakewell-Sachs, S., Gibbons, A., & Delivoria-Papadapoulos, M. (1986). A randomized clinical trial of early hospital discharge and home follow-up of very-low-birth-weight infants. *New England Journal of Medicine, 315,* 934-939.

Brooten, D., Naylor, M., York, R., Brown, L., Roncoli, M., Hollingsworth, A., Cohen, S., Arnold, L., Finkler, S., Munro, B., & Jacobsen, B. (1995). Effects of nurse specialist transitional care on patient outcomes and costs: Results of five randomized trials. *The American Journal of Managed Care, 1*(1), 35-41.

Brooten, D., Roncoli, M., Finkler, S., Arnold, L., Cohen, A., & Mennuti, M. (1994). A randomized clinical trial of early hospital discharge and home followup of women having cesarean birth. *Obstetrics and Gynecology, 84,* 832-838.

Brown, L., & York, R. (In press). Early postpartum discharge. *Nursing Clinics of North America.*

Commission on Professional and Hospital Activities. (1983). *Length of stay by operation, United States, 1982.* Ann Arbor, MI: HCIA, Inc.

Commission on Professional and Hospital Activities. (1994). *Length of stay by diagnosis and operation, United States, 1994.* Ann Arbor, MI: HCIA, Inc.

Dahlberg, N., & Kaloroutis, M. (1994). Hospital based perinatal home care program. *Journal of Obstetric, Gynecologic and Neonatal Nursing, 23*(8), 682-686.

Eaton, D. (1994). Perinatal home care: One entrepreneur's experience. *Journal of Obstetric, Gynecologic and Neonatal Nursing, 23*(8), 726-730.

Goodwin, L. (1994). Essential program components for perinatal home care. *Journal of Obstetric, Gynecologic and Neonatal Nursing, 23*(8), 667-674.

Graven, S., Bowen, F., Brooten, D., Eaton, A., Graven, M., Hack, M., Hall, L., Hansen, N., Hurt, H., Kavalhuna, R., Little, G., Mahan, C., Morrow, G., Oehler, J., Poland, R., Ram, B., Sauve, R., Taylor, P., Ward, S., & Sommers, J. (1992). The high-risk infant environment: Part 1. *Journal of Perinatology, 12*(2), 164-172.

Haddad, A. (1992). Ethical problems in home health care. *Journal of Nursing Administration, 22*(3), 46-51.

Heaman, M. (1992). Stressful life events, social support, and mood disturbance in hospitalized and non-hospitalized women with pregnancy induced hypertension. *Canadian Journal of Nursing Research, 24,* 23-37.

Heaman, M., Robinson, M., Thompson, L., & Heleva, M. (1994). Patient satisfaction with an antepartum home care program. *Journal of Obstetric, Gynecologic and Neonatal Nursing, 23*(8), 707-713.

Jansson, P. (1985). Early postpartum discharge. *American Journal of Nursing, 95,* 547-550.

Maloni, J. (1994). Home care of the high risk pregnant woman requiring bed rest. *Journal of Obstetric, Gynecologic and Neonatal Nursing, 23*(8), 696-706.

National Association for Home Care. (1993). *Basic statistics about home care* (pp. 1-8). Washington, DC: Author.

Olds, D.L. (1992). Home visitation for pregnant women and parents of young children. *American Journal of Diseases of Childhood, 146,* 704-708.

Raff, B. (1986). The use of homemaker-home health aides perinatal care of high risk infants. *Journal of Obstetric, Gynecologic and Neonatal Nursing, 15*(2), 142-145.

Stringer, M., Spatz, D., & Donahue, D. (1994). Maternal/fetal assessment in the home setting: role of the advanced practice nurse. *Journal of Obstetric, Gynecologic and Neonatal Nursing, 23*(8), 720-705.

Strong, T., Brown, W., Brown, W., & Curry, C. (1993). Experience with early postcesarean hospital dismissal. *American Journal of Obstetrics and Gynecology, 169,* 116-119.

York, R., Brown, L., Samuels, P., Swank, A., Armstrong, C., & Robbins, D. (In press). A randomized clinical trial of early discharge and nurse specialist home follow up of high risk childbearing women.

Issues in perioperative nursing

VICTORIA M. STEELMAN

Recent economic pressure on hospitals has heavily impacted on perioperative nursing. Cost containment efforts initiated by hospital administrators and operating room directors have focused heavily on the cost of operating rooms, where immediate reductions can be made without time-consuming negotiations with surgeons. These rapid cuts have changed the meaning of "surgical knife" from "scalpel" to "staffing reductions in the operating room." Restructuring has involved replacement of many registered nurses (RNs) with unlicensed assistive personnel (UAP), including surgical technicians and multiskilled workers as well as lesser prepared licensed practical and vocational nurses. The resulting staffing mix varies greatly across settings. In many operating rooms, use of an RN in the role of scrub nurse is no longer viewed as cost-effective, and the ratio of RNs to technicians has been reduced to a reasonable 70:30 mix. However, some settings have moved to an even leaner skill mix (e.g., 50:50), with RNs absent during breaks and lunch. In other settings the changes have been even more critical: The circulator in the operating room is no longer an RN, but is an unlicensed assistant with one RN supervising many assistants in a number of operating rooms ("Use of Surgical," 1994). A 1994 survey of operating room managers found an increased use of technicians in 21% of hospitals. When technicians were circulating, 32% of hospitals reported an RN "immediately available" (not in the room), while others reported an RN scrubbed operating room monitoring the patient (Schrader, 1994). Anecdotal reports from perioperative nurses across the country indicate that this trend has become more common in 1995.

The pressure to restructure with fewer RNs has become a serious ethical dilemma for nursing administrators. In a recent survey of nurse executives, staffing level or skill mix was the issue identified that led most often to an ethical dilemma, and it was also the ethical decision encountered most often (Borawski, 1995). The impact of this dilemma has been felt in the operating room. Restructuring with fewer RNs and more UAP terrifies veteran perioperative nurses who vividly recall historical battles to keep professional nursing in the operating room. These nurses ask, How can this happen again? Yet, restructuring is equally frightening, if not more so, for junior nurses educated in an era of primary care. These nurses lack the delegation skills required to lead a team of unlicensed assistants, and feel cheated out of their collaborative relationships with peers. All share a genuine concern for the welfare of their patients, fear losing their jobs, and fear employer retaliation if they speak out about the resulting lowered quality of care. Their concerns were made public as perioperative nurses joined the American Nurses Association (ANA) and *Revolution* magazine cosponsored protest march in Washington, D.C., in March 1995. As veteran perioperative nurse Nancy Geisking, explains, "We needed to let the public know the qualifications of care providers as a result of downsizing and to protect RNs who blow the whistle. This downsizing must be done with safety of the patient in mind, not just the dollar" (Personal communication, August 30, 1995).

The public has heard the cries from nurses across the country about downsizing with inadequate staffing because serious hospital errors have reached the lay press. The now infamous University Community Hospital in Tampa, Florida was banned from doing surgery for 11 days while a series of errors, including amputation of the wrong foot, were investigated. The hospital was fined $341,000 by the state and lost $1 million in revenue as well as its accreditation status. Inadequate staffing and poorly trained technicians were identified by the Health Care Financing Administration as contributing to these errors ("1995 Top Ten," 1995; "Florida Hospital Cleared," 1995).

CONTRIBUTING FACTORS

A number of factors have contributed to the pressure for restructuring with unlicensed assistants replacing RNs in perioperative nursing. Some of these factors are external to the nursing specialty; others are internal. External factors include a rapid change in the health care economic environment, change in the standards of the Joint Commission for Accreditation of Health Care Organizations (JCAHO), and proposals in state legislatures to eliminate restrictions on delegation to unlicensed assistants.

The economic environment of health care has changed drastically during the 1990s. Reimbursement has changed from an almost exclusively fee-for-service system to a capitated payment system. In the past, the operating room was seen as a revenue generator. Under capitated systems, however, the operating room is considered a cost center, a necessary liability detracting from the bottom line. For-profit hospitals have flourished in this chaotic environment, equating low-cost health care with large profit margins. Businesses have demanded health care at a lower cost and have negotiated lean contracts with institutions offering "acceptable quality" at a lower rate. Administrators, anticipating steep competition for large corporate contracts, are considering all alternatives for rapid reduction of costs. The result has been the immediate implementation of extreme cost-cutting programs. Because a significant portion of a hospital expense budget is labor, restructuring the care delivery with increased use of unlicensed and lesser prepared personnel has become commonplace throughout the United States. In the operating room, rich with RNs, technicians offer an enticing, lower-cost alternative that can be implemented rapidly.

Responding to the changes in health care, the JCAHO has modified its standards to allow maximum flexibility in hospital staffing patterns. Historically, the JCAHO has supported the role of the RN as circulator in the operating room. However, in 1994 the standards covering the surgical and anesthesia services were revised and the wording in scoring guidelines changed to "other qualified personnel assisting in circulating are under the supervision of a qualified RN who is immediately available" (JCAHO, 1994, p. 10). "Immediately available" has been interpreted by some as an endorsement of the competency of technicians to circulate in the operating room with an RN elsewhere in the department. Against strong opposition by the Association of Operating Room Nurses (AORN), this wording remains in place in the 1995 standards (JCAHO, 1995). The JCAHO standard provides fuel for the ongoing debate over the legitimacy of the role of the RN in the operating room and provides a critical lack of support for directors faced with mandates of reducing labor costs.

The changes in the economics of health care have also been echoed in the state legislatures. On the West Coast, proposals have been put forth in legislatures to eliminate all restrictions on the amount of nursing practice that can be delegated to unlicensed assistants (Federici, 1995; "RNs, Patients Describe," 1995; "Title 22 Hearings," 1995). This raises serious questions about delegation of complex perioperative interventions to inadequately qualified persons. If passed, these proposals would permit hospitals to provide all intraoperative care by UAP.

In addition to factors outside of nursing, a number of factors within the specialty of perioperative nursing have also failed to support the role of professional nursing and have contributed to the current movement toward the use of unlicensed assistants. These include continued focus on technical practice, segregation from mainstream nursing, lack of a tool to predict patient needs for intraoperative nursing care, and a history of catering to surgeon preference.

Perioperative nursing has always focused heavily on technology. The amount and diversity of highly technical equipment in the operating room extends from complex positioning devices and monitoring equipment to fiber optics and lasers. Because troubleshooting technology poses more of a challenge to experienced perioperative nurses than changes in patient status, the focus is often on the surgical procedure and the technology rather than uniqueness of individual patient needs and risk factors. Advances in medical instrumentation have occurred so rapidly that almost continuous in-servicing is required to remain competent in the specialty. It is understandable that these nurses have developed a wide knowledge base about technical issues. However, they have also been resistant to using nursing terminology when describing their work. For example, care planning is usually done the working day before surgery, with the scheduled surgical procedure providing most of the information. Therefore, patient care is often planned without an assessment of the individual patient or review of the patient's record, and nursing diagnoses are not seen as valuable. This long standing technical focus is now endangering the existence of professional nurses in the operating room.

In addition to focusing on technology, perioperative nurses have traditionally emphasized the differences between their work and the work performed by other nurses. In doing so, they have segregated themselves from mainstream nursing. This segregation has been reinforced by the strength of the AORN. This organization has been very strong, and provides valuable services for its 47,000 members, including establishing standards for practice, coordinating legislative activities, providing continuing education, and, under the auspices of a certification board, credentialing nurses in the specialty. These services have met the needs of members to the extent that few belong to the ANA, and most do not understand the ANA's role or contributions to nursing, including the specialty of perioperative nursing. This segregation is no longer an asset to perioperative nurses. The differences, once hailed with pride, are now seen by outsiders as evidence that the work is not professional nursing, and can be performed by unlicensed assistants.

Another internal factor that is detrimental to perioperative nursing during this era of downsizing is the lack of a tool to predict staffing needs in an operating room accurately. Acuity systems to measure severity of illness are available. However, severity of illness neither predicts the need for intraoperative nursing care nor identifies the appropriate skill mix required in an operating room. For example, a critically ill patient undergoing a colon resection may require one RN and one technician during the procedure. However, additional personnel may be required for a variety of reasons, including increased risk associated with technology, the type of anesthesia administered, and the mental state of the patient. If blood loss is excessive, an additional RN may be required to check and administer blood. Intraoperative salvage of blood may require additional personnel to operate the equipment. These variables impact on the staffing requirements in an operating room, but are not identified on instruments used to measure patient acuity. In the absence of a tool to predict accurately the need for intraoperative nursing care, directors lack the foundation necessary to plan and support decisions about staffing and skill mix.

Another factor impacting on the movement to less costly personnel is a long history of catering to surgeons' preferences. Perioperative nurses have prided themselves in having the strong, collaborative relationships with surgeons that are required when working side by side during a surgical procedure. However, these relationships have been nurtured extensively by catering to surgeons' preferences, some of which are more costly than the alternatives. In the past, a hospital could pass along this added expense to the patient. Today, however, with the bulk of reimbursement based on capitation or a per-diem rate, the cost of every instrument, suture, supply, and implant is a direct loss to the hospital. For example, in one large, teaching hospital, over $1 million is tied up in maxillofacial implants marketed by five different vendors. Each type of implant requires a separate set of specialized instrumentation. Surgeons are unable to come to a consensus on standardization of the implants, even though no demonstrable differences in patient outcomes are available to justify their preferences. Sales representatives continue to foster cozy relationships with the surgeons by paying for dinners, trips to conferences, and other "perks," while the hospital continues to purchase all five brands based on surgeon preference. The same scenario has resulted in hospitals with millions of dollars tied up in other implant inventory (e.g., knee, hip, valve) which is sure to become obsolete in the near future. The problem with surgeon preferences extends beyond implants to many other surgical products (e.g., suture, gloves, drains) and expensive capital equipment (e.g., lasers, video equipment). Now, directors find themselves in the uncomfortable position of attempting to reverse this precedent and move toward standardization with less costly products. However, this change requires skills new to many directors and may negatively impact on relationships with surgeons. Depending on the setting, threats such as "I will take my business elsewhere" may override the director's incentive to reduce costs in this manner. An easier solution, not requiring collaboration with surgeons, is changing the skill mix in the operating room.

It is clear that sound financial management in the operating room setting is a required component of health care costs across the country. It is also clear that the foundation of perioperative nursing has some weaknesses that require attention. These limitations, not always seen by nurses within the specialty, are being scrutinized by others, including administrators looking for ways to reduce hospital costs.

BUILDING A SUPPORTIVE FOUNDATION

It would be short-sighted to deny that perioperative nursing is at great risk. However, there has been some progress toward building a foundation to support professional nursing in the operating room and providing directors with the guidance and tools necessary for reasonable, appropriate delegation of activities to assistants. One of these efforts has been the restructuring of the "Perioperative Care" class of the Nursing Interventions Classification. Many nursing interventions (e.g., laser precautions; positioning; intraoperative; and surgical precautions) have been added to this classification to reflect more comprehensively the work of perioperative nurses (Steelman, Bulechek, & McCloskey, 1994). The presence of these interventions in a classification describing all nursing activities assures perioperative nursing equal status with other specialties. Each intervention contains a list of activities, some of which can be delegated, but the accountability for the intervention remains with the RN. The AORN has begun initial work on identifying data elements (diagnoses, activities, outcomes) for perioperative nursing with the assurance that when completed, this work will be integrated into the standardized languages of mainstream nursing (Applegeet, Kleinbeck, & Sudduth, 1995). A team at Massachusetts General Hospital studied activities of perioperative nursing in that setting, and has developed a model identifying which activities can be delegated to unlicensed assistants (Coakley, 1995). Such research-based initiatives are necessary for the foundation of perioperative nursing and serve as building blocks to compare management interventions such as restructuring across settings.

Another significant movement is the development of the AORN Position Statement on Unlicensed Assistive Personnel (AORN, 1995). Concerns about restructuring resounded during the 1995 AORN House of Delegates, where this position statement was passionately debated and approved. The statement clearly articulates that "A 1:1 perioperative RN to patient ratio is required for each patient during operative and other invasive procedures" and the circulator in the operating room must be an RN. According to the AORN, unlicensed assistants may assist in the operating room with delegated activities, but the RN may not delegate assessment, diagnosis, outcome identification, planning, or evaluation. The AORN position statement reflects the national viewpoint of perioperative nursing and can be used to support appropriate restructuring in the operating room setting.

REDUCING EXPENSES IN THE OPERATING ROOM

Reducing an operating room expense budget first requires a close look at implants, supplies, and instruments. Standardization of these items offers an opportunity to save over a million dollars, without diminishing the quality of patient care. Instead of stocking an assortment of similar products, a hospital may identify specifications of an acceptable product and entertain bids from vendors meeting these specifications. In an exchange for a guarantee of 80% of the hospital's business related to that product type, a 10% to 40% reduction in the purchase price can be obtained ("Contracts with Vendors," 1994; "Cost Cutting Ideas," 1994; "Implant Prices," 1994; "Manager Cuts Inventory," 1994; "Orthopedic Implant Contract," 1995; Solovy, 1995). For example, standardization of orthopedic joint implants (e.g., hip, knee) can save hundreds of thousands of dollars on each type of implant. Utilizing consignment and "just in time" relationships with vendors eliminates the need for a multimillion dollar implant inventory that will likely be obsolete in the near future. Similar opportunities exist to reduce the cost of other supplies. For example, one medium-sized hospital saved $500,000 over 5 years by standardizing suture and stapling devices (G. VanMilligan, personal communication, August 31, 1995). In a large teaching hospital considering this change, a conservative estimate of savings is over $150,000 per year (M. Murphy, personal communication, September 6, 1995). Other high-volume products also lend themselves to cost savings without reducing quality. One large teaching hospital reported savings of $250,000 by standardizing to higher-quality surgical gloves (Patterson, 1995).

A close look at disposable instruments and supplies can also lead to cost savings. Reversing the trend toward disposable instruments can save large amounts of money. For example, by reverting to a reusable trocar, $378 can be saved on each laparoscopic cholecystectomy procedure (Fernsebner, 1995). A medium-sized hospital with an annual volume of 300 of these procedures can save $113,400 per year by this simple change. Similar savings may be realized with reusable surgical gowns.

Efficient instrument inventory management is another way of reducing costs in an operating room. An estimated 25% to 50% of instruments on the table during surgery are returned for decontamination postoperatively without ever being used. Technology is available to track individual instruments and provide the basis for redesigning sets based on the actual usage of these instruments. In a large teaching hospital, an estimated cost avoidance of over $200,000 in instrument purchases, repairs, and refurbishing may be realized, and the cost of labor associated with continual, unnecessary reprocessing can be decreased dramatically (M. Murphy, personal communication, September 6, 1995).

The volume of savings available through the efficient management of implants, supplies, and instruments is much greater than can be realized through replacement of RNs with unlicensed assistants in an operating room setting. Therefore, responsible financial management would indicate that the focus should clearly be in this direction first, where there is no negative impact on quality of patient care.

However, responsible perioperative management also requires evaluation of the use of human resources within the operating room. At times, the utilization of personnel can be maximized through restructuring and using unlicensed assistants to perform additional nonnursing functions. As with any management innovation, effective restructuring requires a systematic approach beginning with an assessment and ending with a comprehensive evaluation. The desired outcomes and any potential indirect effects should be identified in advance and should be an integral component of the restructuring plan. The evaluation should compare these patient, staff, and organizational variables before and after the change as well as an analysis of the cost of implementation (e.g., personnel time, training costs) (see the box below). The laws of physics also apply to restructuring: For every action, there is a reaction. The reaction may or may not be in the desired direction. For example, restructuring with a multiskilled worker to transport patients, restock supplies, and assemble supplies for a case cart may result in a reduction in labor costs, fewer preoperative delays, and decreased turnover time. However, this change could also result in dissatisfied employees, lowered productivity, and an increase in preoperative delays or increased turnover time. Identification of key variables to be measured before and after the change provides the manager with the means to evaluate comprehensively the true impact of the change. Although perioperative restructuring initiatives have been reported in the literature, none describe a comprehensive evaluation plan, and successes, when claimed, appear to be based on intuition alone.

EXAMPLES OF OUTCOME MEASURES

Patient Outcomes
Length of stay
Satisfaction
Readmissions
Surgical wound infections
Adverse outcomes
Cautery burns
Laser injuries
Skin breakdown
Waiting times
Staff Outcomes
Absenteeism
Competency level
Incorrect counts
Injuries
Laser safety compliance
Job performance
Medication errors
Productivity
Satisfaction
Turnover
Organizational Outcomes
Canceled procedures
Operating room utilization
Overtime paid
Use of agency personnel
Volume of procedures

SUMMARY

Economic pressure on hospitals has created a serious challenge for perioperative nursing. Directors across the country face administrative mandates for immediate reductions in expense budgets. Some efforts toward inventory control and standardization of implants and supplies have been undertaken. However, because these endeavors are time-consuming and may result in conflicts with surgeons, they have not been fully explored. A faster, easier approach to reducing expenses has been to focus on changing the skill mix of operating room staff. In some settings, this has resulted in reasonable restructuring, with additional nonnursing functions delegated to unlicensed assistants. However, in other settings, perioperative nursing care is being declared nonnursing, technical practice, and directors have indiscriminately replaced RNs with unlicensed assistants in the circulating role. This issue has risen to the forefront as potentially the most serious threat ever to face perioperative nursing. Efforts to contain hospital costs should be directed toward inventory management, where millions of dollars can be saved without impacting negatively on the quality of care. Nonnursing functions can and should be delegated to unlicensed assistants. In addition, restructuring of roles within the operating room should only be attempted with clearly identified goals and a comprehensive plan for evaluating the impact of the change on patient, staff, and organizational outcomes.

REFERENCES

AORN. (1995). A.O.R.N. position statement on unlicensed assistive personnel. *AORN Journal, 61*(6), 956-957.

Applegeet, C., Kleinbeck, & Sudduth, M. (1995, March). Perioperative data elements. Paper presented at the AORN Congress, Atlanta, GA.

Borawski, D. (1995). Ethical dilemmas for nurse administrators. *Journal of Nursing Administration, 25*(7/8), 60-66.

Coakley, E. (1995, September). A new model for perioperative nursing.

Paper presented at Managing Today's OR Suite conference, Washington, D.C.

Contracts with vendors. (1994). *OR Manager, 10*(6), 14.

Cost-cutting ideas. (1994). *OR Manager, 10*(1), 14.

Federici, N. (1995). Capitol chronicle . . . Nurse delegation. *Washington Nurse, 23*(1), 4.

Fernsebner, B. (1995). Disposables make differences in lap chole costs. *OR Manager, 11*(9), 13-14.

Florida hospital cleared to resume surgery. (1995). *OR Manager, 11*(6), 28.

Implant prices. (1994). *OR Manager, 10*(6), 15.

JCAHO. (1994). Operative and other invasive procedures. In *1994 Accreditation manual for hospitals: Scoring guidelines,* vol. 2, p. 10. Oakbrook Terrace, IL: JCAHO.

JCAHO (1995). Operative and other invasive procedures. In *1995 Accreditation manual for hospitals: Scoring guidelines,* vol. 2. Oakbrook Terrace, IL: JCAHO.

Manager cuts inventory. (1994). *OR Manager, 10*(4), 18.

1995 top ten myths on hospital and healthcare restructuring. (1995). *California Nurse, 91*(6), 8-9.

Orthopedic implant contract could save hospital 40%. (1995). *OR Manager, 11*(1), 12.

Patterson, P. (1995). Allergy issues complicate buying decisions for gloves. *OR Manager, 11*(6), 1, 8-14, 19.

RNs, patients describe care crisis to senate committee. (1995). *California Nurse, 91*(3), 3.

Shrader, E. (1994). Publisher's note. *OR Manager, 10*(10), 5.

Solovy, A. (1995). Hearts, knees, or hips: Where to focus savings efforts. *Materials Management, 4*(6), 74-78.

Steelman, V., Bulechek, G., & McCloskey, J. (1994). Toward a standardized language to describe perioperative nursing. *AORN Journal, 60*(5), 786-795.

Title 22 hearings: RNs urge DHS to protect patients. (1995). *California Nurse, 91*(3), 7.

Use of surgical techs upward trend in hospitals. (1994). *OR Manager, 10*(10), 8.

Recent changes and current issues in psychiatric nursing

GAIL W. STUART

The contemporary practice of psychiatric nursing is challenged both by issues internal to nursing and by changes in the external health care environment. Perhaps at no other time in their history have psychiatric nurses had to face the question of whether they are vulnerable to becoming extinct and replaced by others, or whether they are viewed as valuable, competent clinicians who can function in a world of changing mental health care needs, processes, and structures. The areas of vulnerability are many:

- Fewer nurses are attracted to the specialty of psychiatric nursing.
- The amount of content devoted to understanding psychiatric illnesses and to working with psychiatric patients in nursing educational programs has decreased steadily over the past decade and is almost nonexistent in some curricula.
- Graduate programs in nursing are moving away from the preparation of psychiatric clinical nurse specialists and toward that of nurse practitioners who have significantly less course work related to the diagnosis and treatment of psychiatric illnesses.
- Most psychiatric nurses work in inpatient psychiatric units, yet health care reform has stimulated the greater use of community health settings.
- The skills and expertise of psychiatric nurses are often poorly delineated and underused in mental health care systems.
- Psychiatric nurses are frequently viewed as expensive mental health care providers who can be replaced by two or more less costly personnel.
- There are increasing threats to nursing autonomy as state boards of nursing and other regulatory bodies restrict master's-prepared psychiatric nurses to practicing in the "extended" role, requiring the full supervision of physicians.
- There are relatively few outcome studies that document the nature, extent, and effectiveness of care delivered by psychiatric nurses.
- Psychiatric nurses continue to struggle to be perceived as revenue producers and to receive direct reimbursement from third-party payers for the services they provide.
- Role differentiation for psychiatric nurses based on education and experience is often lacking in the position descriptions, job responsibilities, and reward systems of the organizations in which they practice.

These issues must be addressed if psychiatric nursing is to continue to develop as a specialty area. Specifically, changes are occurring in five discrete areas of psychiatric nursing practice: role, activities, models of care, treatment settings, and outcome data. Each of these will be explored based on historical perspectives, recent developments, and future challenges in the field.

THE PSYCHIATRIC NURSING ROLE

The 1950s and 1960s are remembered fondly by psychiatric nurses because they mark the emergence of the identity of the specialty. It was an exciting and stimulating time; and the early psychiatric nursing leaders who contributed to this identity formation, Peplau (1952, 1962, 1978), Tudor (1952), Gregg (1954), and Mellow (1968), will forever remain larger than life for their early contributions to the emerging specialty area. The challenges they faced were to identify and describe the roles and functions for the psychiatric nursing specialty practice and to disseminate them widely within the broader community of nurses.

The challenges for psychiatric nurses in the 1970s and 1980s were somewhat different. During these years nurses worked to define the nature and focus of nursing as a practice discipline and examined aspects of both the art and the science of nursing. Psychiatric nurses worked parallel to the overall nursing profession and moved psychiatric nursing into the mainstream of nursing practice by helping to elaborate psychosocial concepts, thus further defining the caring and holistic dimensions of professional nursing practice.

Psychiatric nurses in the 1990s are faced with a new challenge—integrating the rapidly expanding bases of psychobiology, the neurosciences, and psychopharmacology into the holistic biopsychosocial practice of psychiatric nursing (Abraham, Fox, & Cohen, 1992; Babich & Tolbert, 1992; McEnany, 1991; Pothier, Stuart, Puskar, & Babich, 1990). Advances in understanding the interrelationships of biology, brain, behavior, emotion, and cognition offered new opportunities for psychiatric nurses (Laraia, 1995). In addition, the taxonomy used to categorize and diagnose mental illnesses was becoming increasingly precise and more interdisciplinary. A final issue to emerge was the importance of sociocultural factors in psychiatric care. Psychiatric nurses saw the need to become realigned with care and caring, which represent the art of psychiatric nursing and give balance to the science and high technology of current mental health care practices. These changes led to the 1994 revision of the *Standards of Psychiatric-Mental Health Clinical Nursing Practice* (American Nurses Association [ANA], 1994a) and the publication of *Psychopharmacology Guidelines for Psychiatric-Mental Health Nurses* (ANA, 1994b) in the same year.

The task for psychiatric nurses today and in the years ahead is to evolve beyond the formative work in the field and enact psychiatric nursing roles and functions based on current realities (Billings, 1993; Goering, 1993; Krauss, 1993; Schreter, 1993). For example, the nurse-patient relationship as first described by Peplau (1952) has grown in complexity from its original historical elements. It needs to be reconceptualized in a health care environment in which there is greater consumer responsibility and a broader context of clinician accountability. The concept of the nurse-patient relationship has thus evolved into that of the nurse-patient partnership, which incorporates new dimensions of the professional psychiatric nursing role (Fig. 36-1).

Enacting the nurse-patient partnership requires expanding the traditional roles of the nurse to include the elements of clinical competence across the continuum of care, patient-family advocacy, fiscal responsibility, interdisciplinary collaboration, social accountability, and legal-ethical obligations (Stuart, 1995a). No longer can psychiatric nurses focus exclusively on bedside care and the immediacy of patient needs. Rather, they must broaden the context of their care and the responsibility and understanding they bring to the caregiving situation (Mohr, 1995). Thus the current practice of psychiatric nursing requires greater sensitivity to the social environment and active advocacy for the diverse needs of patient and families of the mentally ill (Fisher, 1994). It also mandates thoughtful consideration of complex legal and ethical dilemmas that arise from a health care system that is embracing the efficiencies of managed care and often disadvantages and discriminates against those with psychiatric illness (McDaniel, 1992; Mechanic, 1994; Olsen, 1994; Scallet & Havel, 1994). New models of delivering mental health care require greater skill in interdisciplinary collaboration built on the psychiatric nurse's clinical competence and professional self-assertion (Merwin & Fox, 1992) and balanced by a clear understanding and respect

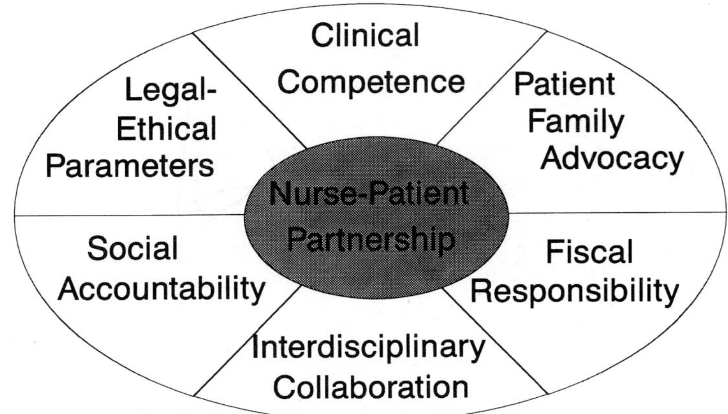

Fig. 36-1. Nurse-patient partnership.

for the cost indices and financial aspects of psychiatric care in general and psychiatric nursing care in particular (Baradell, 1994; Sharfstein, Stoline, & Goldman, 1993; Watson, Lower, Wells, Farrah, & Jarrell, 1991). Each of these elements must permeate to a greater degree the education, research, and clinical components of the current state of psychiatric nursing.

PSYCHIATRIC NURSING ACTIVITIES

There are three domains of contemporary psychiatric nursing practice—direct care, communication, and management activities. It is within these overlapping domains that the teaching, coordinating, delegating, and collaborating functions of the psychiatric nursing role are expressed. The communication and management domains of practice are often overlooked, minimized, or discounted in psychiatric nursing. However, these integrating activities are critically important and time-consuming aspects of the psychiatric nurse's role. They are also very valuable in a reformed health care system that places great emphasis on efficient patient assessment, triage, and management. Thus they are critical aspects of contemporary psychiatric nursing practice.

It is important for psychiatric nurses to be able to further delineate the various activities in which they engage within each of these domains. The box lists the range of specific activities that can be enacted by a psychiatric nurse in each area (Stuart, 1995a). While not all psychiatric nurses participate in all of these activities, they do reflect the current nature and scope of competent caring by psychiatric nurses. In addition, psychiatric nurses do the following:

- Make culturally sensitive biopsychosocial health assessments
- Design and implement treatment plans for patients and families with complex health problems and comorbid medical conditions
- Engage in case management activities, such as organizing, accessing, negotiating, coordinating, and integrating services and benefits for individuals and families
- Provide a "health care map" for individuals, families, and groups to guide them to community resources for mental health, including the most appropriate providers, agencies, technologies, and social systems
- Promote and maintain mental health and manage the effects of mental illness through teaching and counseling
- Provide care for the physically ill with psychological problems and the psychiatrically ill with physical problems
- Manage and coordinate systems of care integrating the needs of patients, families, staff, and regulators.

Finally, psychiatric nurses must be able to articulate both the general and the specific aspects of their practice to patients, families, other professionals, administrators, and legislators. When such skills and competencies are identified, psychiatric nurses will be able to ensure their appropriate role utilization, adequate compensation for the nursing care provided, and the most efficient use of scarce human resources in the delivery of quality mental health care.

A PSYCHIATRIC NURSING MODEL OF CARE

As a result of rising health care costs, changing reimbursement trends, and problems with accessibility of care, the model of care for psychiatric illness in this country has been reformulated. Just 10 years ago, the majority of psychiatric care was provided in hospital units where the average length of stay for acute inpatient treatment was about 25 days, as compared with 19 days in 1991 and 10 days in 1995. Not surprisingly, the majority of psychiatric nurses were employed by inpatient facilities. More recently, however, the average length of stay in many inpatient psychiatric settings is 7 days, and inpatient crisis stabilization programs may involve only a 2- or 3-day stay. These changes have stimulated reciprocal changes in the goals, assessments, interventions, and expected outcomes of psychiatric care. Mental health providers, including psychiatric nurses, have therefore reevaluated the models of care they use based on the patient's treatment stage, the treatment setting, and the available resources (Montgomery & Webster, 1993).

One current psychiatric nursing model of care identifies four treatment stages: crisis, acute care, maintenance, and health promotion (Stuart, 1995b). These stages reflect the range of the adaptive-maladaptive continuum of coping responses and suggest a distinct set of psychiatric nursing activities. For each stage, the psychiatric nurse identifies the treatment goal, focus of the nursing assessment, nature of the nursing interventions, and expected outcome of nursing care (Fig. 36-2).

In the *crisis stage* of treatment the nursing goal is stabilization of the patient; the nursing assessment focuses on risk factors that threaten the patient's health and wellbeing; the nursing intervention is directed toward managing the environment to provide safety; and the expected

PSYCHIATRIC NURSING ACTIVITIES

DIRECT CARE ACTIVITIES

- Advocacy
- Aftercare follow-up
- Behavioral treatments
- Case consultation
- Case management
- Cognitive treatments
- Community education
- Compliance counseling
- Crisis intervention
- Discharge planning
- Family interventions
- Group work
- Health promotion
- Health teaching
- High-risk assessment
- Home visits
- Individual counseling
- Intake screening and evaluation
- Medication administration
- Medication management
- Mental health promotion
- Milieu therapy
- Nutritional counseling
- Obtaining informed consent
- Parent education
- Patient triage
- Physical assessment
- Physiological treatments
- Play therapy
- Prescription of medications
- Providing environmental safety
- Psychosocial assessment
- Psychotherapy
- Relapse prevention
- Research implementation
- Self-care activities
- Social skills training
- Somatic treatments
- Stress management

COMMUNICATION ACTIVITIES

- Clinical case conferences
- Developing treatment plans
- Documentation of care
- Forensic testimony
- Interagency liaison
- Peer review
- Preparing reports
- Professional nurse networking
- Staff meetings
- Transcribing orders
- Treatment team meetings
- Verbal reports of care

MANAGEMENT ACTIVITIES

- Budgeting and resource allocation
- Clinical supervision
- Collaboration
- Committee participation
- Community action
- Consultation/liaison
- Contract negotiation
- Coordination of services
- Delegation of assignments
- Grant writing
- Marketing and public relations
- Mediation and conflict resolution
- Needs assessment and forecasting
- Organizational governance
- Outcomes management
- Performance evaluations
- Policy and procedure development
- Professional presentations
- Program evaluation
- Program planning
- Publications
- Quality improvement activities
- Recruitment and retention activities
- Regulatory agency activities
- Risk management
- Software development
- Staff scheduling
- Staff and student education
- Strategic planning
- Unit governance
- Utilization review

Note. From Stuart, G. (1995a). Roles and functions of psychiatric nurses: Competent caring. In G. Stuart & S. Sundeen (Eds.), *Principles and practice of psychiatric nursing* (5th ed., p. 12). St. Louis, MO: Mosby.

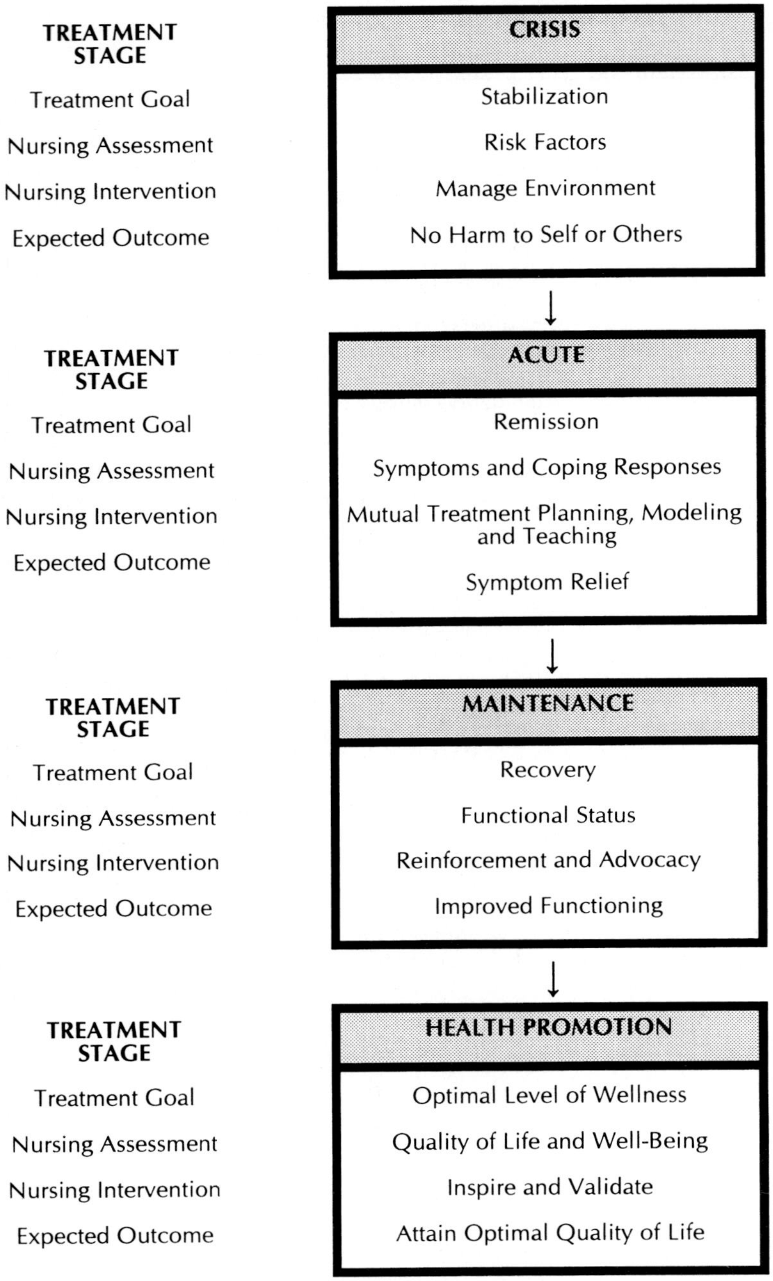

TREATMENT STAGE	CRISIS
Treatment Goal	Stabilization
Nursing Assessment	Risk Factors
Nursing Intervention	Manage Environment
Expected Outcome	No Harm to Self or Others

↓

TREATMENT STAGE	ACUTE
Treatment Goal	Remission
Nursing Assessment	Symptoms and Coping Responses
Nursing Intervention	Mutual Treatment Planning, Modeling and Teaching
Expected Outcome	Symptom Relief

↓

TREATMENT STAGE	MAINTENANCE
Treatment Goal	Recovery
Nursing Assessment	Functional Status
Nursing Intervention	Reinforcement and Advocacy
Expected Outcome	Improved Functioning

↓

TREATMENT STAGE	HEALTH PROMOTION
Treatment Goal	Optimal Level of Wellness
Nursing Assessment	Quality of Life and Well-Being
Nursing Intervention	Inspire and Validate
Expected Outcome	Attain Optimal Quality of Life

Fig. 36-2. Stages of psychiatric treatment.

outcome of nursing care is that no harm will come to the patient or others.

In the *acute stage* of treatment the nursing goal is for the patient's illness to be placed in remission; the nursing assessment is focused on the patient's symptoms and maladaptive coping responses; the nursing intervention is directed toward treatment planning with the patient as well as modeling and teaching adaptive responses; and the expected outcome of nursing care is symptom relief.

In the *maintenance stage* of treatment the nursing goal is the complete recovery of the patient; the nursing assessment is focused on the patient's functional status; the nursing intervention is directed toward reinforcing the patient's adaptive coping responses and patient advocacy; and the expected outcome of nursing care is improved patient functioning.

In the *health promotion stage* of treatment the nursing goal is for the patient to achieve the optimal level of wellness; the nursing assessment is focused on the patient's quality of life and well-being; the nursing intervention is directed toward inspiring and validating the patient; and the expected outcome of nursing care is that the patient will attain the optimal quality of life.

These treatment stages have often been overlooked in traditional psychiatric nursing practice that did not value or reimburse maintenance or health promotion activities. With health care reform and the emergence of managed mental health care, however, activities related to these stages are becoming essential aspects of the contemporary psychiatric nursing role.

This model of care also helps to determine how the psychiatric nurse functions in each setting. For example, in previous years most psychiatrically ill patients entered the psychiatric hospital in the acute treatment stage and were able to stay in the hospital until the goal of symptom remission was attained. This created the need for comprehensive treatment plans with long-term interventions for recovery. Today, however, the majority of patients are admitted to inpatient units in the crisis stage of treatment and have stabilization as their treatment goal, thus mandating very different nursing interventions and expected outcomes. The psychiatric care goals of symptom remission and recovery are now most often pursued in community-based settings, requiring new skills and competencies of psychiatric nurses.

PSYCHIATRIC NURSING TREATMENT SETTINGS

Traditional practice settings for psychiatric nurses have included psychiatric hospitals, community mental health centers, psychiatric units in general hospitals, residential treatment facilities, and private practice. With health care reform initiatives, however, alternative treatment settings throughout the continuum of mental health care are emerging for psychiatric nurses. Specifically, hospitals are being transformed into integrated clinical systems that provide inpatient care, partial hospitalization or day treatment, residential care, home care, and outpatient or ambulatory care (Fig. 36-3). Psychiatric nurses who continue to work within inpatient units have seen the goals, processes, and structures of care change drastically, reflecting the new models of psychiatric nursing care described above (Delaney, Ulsafer-Van Lanen, Pitula, & Johnson, 1995; McGihon, 1994; Queen, 1995). Nurses who staff inpatient units no longer have their responsibilities limited to activities delivered exclusively in the hospital setting. Rather, they are likely to be assigned flexibly on a daily basis to other settings in the continuum of mental health care based on fluctuating patient census and organizational need.

Current community-based treatment settings have expanded to include foster care or group homes, hospices, visiting nurse associations, emergency departments, nursing homes, shelters, primary care clinics, schools, prisons, industrial settings, homes, managed care facilities, and health maintenance organizations. This widened range of settings maximizes the psychiatric nurse's potential contribution to the delivery of mental health care (Carson, 1994; Haber & Billings, 1995; Mellon, 1994;

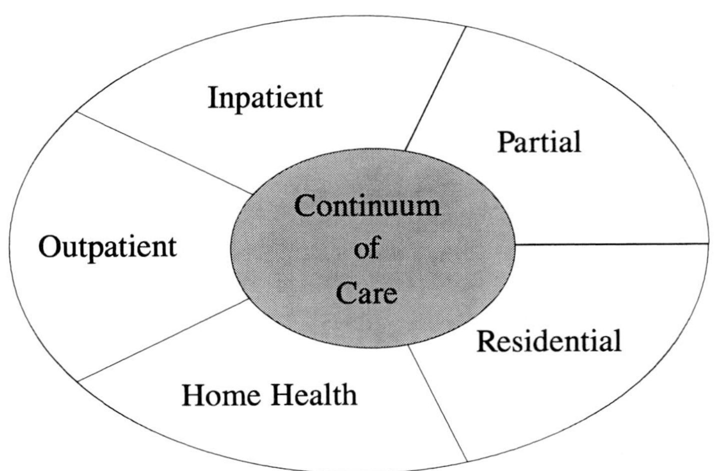

Fig. 36-3. Continuum of mental health care.

Mound, Gyulay, Khan, & Goering, 1991; Saur & Ford, 1995; Worley, 1995). The specific role the nurse assumes in any one of these psychiatric treatment settings, however, depends on a number of factors:

- Legal parameters of practice as defined by the state's nurse practice act
- Clinical competence of the nurse as a consequence of education, experience, and certification as either a generalist (C.) or certified specialist (C.S.) in psychiatric nursing
- Philosophy, mission, values, goals, and organizational structure of the treatment setting
- Needs of the consumers of mental health services
- Number of available staff and the services they are able to provide
- Consensus reached by the mental health care providers who work together regarding their respective roles, responsibilities, and accountabilities
- Resources and revenues available to offset the cost of care needed and provided

The new opportunities for psychiatric nursing practice that are emerging throughout the continuum of mental health care are very exciting for the specialty. They allow psychiatric nurses to demonstrate their flexibility, accountability, and self-direction as they move forward into these expanding areas of practice. They also require that psychiatric nurses be proactive in articulating their skills and activities and demonstrate their expertise in designing interventions, planning programs, implementing treatment strategies, managing staff, and collaborating with other health care providers in a variety of traditional and nontraditional treatment settings. Perhaps most important, the expansion of mental health treatment settings is providing psychiatric nurses with the opportunity to implement primary, secondary, and tertiary prevention functions from a holistic, biopsychosocial perspective, thus expanding their base of practice to better meet the mental health needs of individuals, families, groups, and communities.

PSYCHIATRIC NURSING OUTCOME DATA

The final area of current psychiatric nursing practice involves the identification, description, and measurement of data pertaining to the effectiveness of the care provided by psychiatric nurses. This is the greatest area of challenge for the specialty because psychiatric nursing is noticeably absent from the numerous published reviews of the value and effectiveness of the profession (Fagin, 1982a, 1982b, 1990), and the specialty has found it difficult to articulate the nature and outcomes of psychiatric nursing care (Merwin & Mauck, 1995). This has created problems in justifying the need for psychiatric nurses in various treatment settings and in giving psychiatric nurses the recognition and compensation they deserve based on their actual and potential contributions to the mental health delivery system.

Outcome data for psychiatric nurses can include health status, functional status, quality of life, presence or absence of illness, type of coping responses, and satisfaction with treatment. Outcome evaluation can focus on a psychiatric clinical condition, a nursing intervention, or the caregiving process. The outcomes that need continued examination by psychiatric nurses fall into four categories:

- Clinical outcomes—the patient's treatment response
- Functional outcomes—the maintenance or improvement in the patient's biopsychosocial functioning
- Perceptual outcomes—the patient's and family's satisfaction with the response to treatment, caregiving process, and health care providers
- Financial outcomes—costs and resources used to achieve the treatment response

Specific indicators related to each of these categories are presented in the box (Stuart, 1995a).

Outcome data documenting the quality, cost, and effectiveness of psychiatric nursing practice are perhaps the most important issue on the psychiatric nursing agenda. More work is needed in this area and studies must be able to stand up to the scientific review of the broader community of mental health professionals, regulators, and payers by being methodologically sound, empirically grounded, and replicated across the continuum of psychiatric treatment settings (Mirin & Namerow, 1991). The results of this work can then be used to provide a shared knowledge base, formulate practice guidelines, provide data on clinical course, and better manage mental health care and the way in which it is delivered in this country.

Finally, the need to focus on ways to critically evaluate the outcomes of psychiatric nursing practice is a task for each and every psychiatric nurse regardless of role, activity, model of care, or treatment setting. Psychiatric nurse clinicians, educators, administrators, and researchers all must assume responsibility for answering the question that is likely to determine the future of psychiatric nursing: What difference does psychiatric nurse caring make? Only a clear and credible answer to this question will position psychiatric nurses as central, visible, competent, in-

CATEGORIES OF OUTCOME INDICATORS

Clinical outcome indicators

- High-risk behaviors
- Symptomatology
- Coping responses
- Relapse
- Recurrence
- Readmission
- Number of treatment episodes
- Medical complications
- Incidence reports
- Mortality

Functional outcome indicators

- Functional status
- Social interaction
- Activities of daily living
- Occupational abilities
- Quality of life
- Family relationships
- Housing arrangement

Perceptual outcome indicators (patient-family satisfaction with)

- Outcomes
- Providers
- Delivery system
- Care received
- Organization
- Access and timeliness

Financial outcome indicators

- Cost per treatment episode
- Revenue per treatment episode
- Length of inpatient stay
- Use of health care resources
- Costs related to disability

Note. From Stuart, G. (1995a). Roles and functions of psychiatric nurses: Competent caring. In G. Stuart & S. Sundeen (Eds.), *Principles and practice of psychiatric nursing* (5th ed., p. 15). St. Louis, MO: Mosby.

terdependent, and collaborating professionals who have much to offer a reformed health care system.

REFERENCES

Abraham, I., Fox, J., & Cohen, B. (1992). Integrating the bio into the biopsychosocial: Understanding and treating biological phenomena in psychiatric-mental health nursing. *Archives of Psychiatric Nursing, 6,* 296.

American Nurses Association. (1994a). *A statement on psychiatric-mental health clinical nursing practice and standards of psychiatric-mental health nursing practice.* Washington, DC: Author.

American Nurses Association. (1994b). *Psychiatric Mental Health Nursing Psychopharmacology Project.* Washington, DC: Author.

Babich, K., & Tolbert, R. (1992). What is biological psychiatry? How will the trend toward biological psychiatry affect the future of the psychiatric mental health nurse? *Journal of Psychosocial Nursing and Mental Health Services, 30,* 33.

Baradell, J.G. (1994). Cost-effectiveness and quality of care provided by clinical nurse specialists. *Journal of Psychosocial Nursing, 32*(3), 21-24.

Billings, C. (1993). Psychiatric-mental health nursing professional progress notes. *Archives of Psychiatric Nursing, 2*(3), 174-181.

Carson, V.B. (1994). Doing psych but talking med-surg language. *Caring Magazine, 2,* 32-41.

Delaney, K., Ulsafer-Van Lanen, J., Pitula, C.R., & Johnson, M.E. (1995). Seven days and counting: How inpatient nurses might adjust their practice to brief hospitalization. *Journal of Psychosocial Nursing, 33*(8), 36-40.

Fagin, C.M. (1982a). Nursing as an alternative to high-cost care. *American Journal of Nursing, 82,* 56-60.

Fagin, C.M. (1982b). The economic value. *American Journal of Nursing, 82,* 1844-1849.

Fagin, C.M. (1990). Nursing's value proves itself. *American Journal of Nursing, 90,* 17-30.

Fisher, D.B. (1994). Health care reform based on an empowerment model of recovery by people with psychiatric disabilities. *Hospital and Community Psychiatry, 45*(9), 913-915.

Goering, P. (1993). Psychiatric nursing and the context of care. *New Directions for Mental Health Services, 58,* 3-12.

Gregg, D. (1954). The Psychiatric Nurse's Role. *American Journal of Nursing, 54,* 210-212.

Haber, J., & Billings, C. (1995). Primary mental health care: A model for psychiatric-mental health nursing. *Journal of the American Psychiatric Nurses Association, 1*(5), 154-163.

Krauss, J.B. (1993). A nursing perspective on mental health policy. *New Directions for Mental Health Services, 58,* 85-97.

Laraia, M. (1995). Biological context of psychiatric nursing care. In G. Stuart & S. Sundeen (Eds.), *Principles and practice of psychiatric nursing,* (5th ed., pp. 103-139). St. Louis, MO: Mosby.

McDaniel, C. (1992). Ethical issues in restructuring of psychiatric services. *Issues in Mental Health Nursing, 13,* 31-37.

McEnany, G. (1991). Psychobiology and psychiatric nursing: A philosophical matrix. *Archives of Psychiatric Nursing, 5,* 255.

McGihon, N.N. (1994). Health care reform: Clinical implications for inpatient psychiatric nursing. *Journal of Psychosocial Nursing, 32*(11), 31-33.

Mechanic, D. (1994). Integrating mental health into a general health care system. *Hospital and Community Psychiatry, 45*(9), 893-897.

Mellon, S.K. (1994). Mental health clinical nurse specialists in home care for the 90s. *Issues in Mental Health Nursing, 15,*(3), 229-237.

Mellow, J. (1968). Nursing therapy. *American Journal of Nursing, 68,* 2365.

Merwin, E., & Fox, J. (1992). Cost-effective integration of mental health professions. *Issues in Mental Health Nursing, 13,* 139.

Merwin, E., & Mauck, A. (1995). Psychiatric nursing outcome research: The state of the science. *Archives of Psychiatric Nursing, 9*(6), 311-331.

Mirin, S., & Namerow, M. (1991). Why study treatment outcome? *Hospital and Community Psychiatry, 42,* 1007.

Mohr, W.K. (1995). Multiple ideologies and their proposed roles in the outcomes of nurse practice settings: The for-profit psychiatric hospital scandal as a paradigm case. *Nursing Outlook, 13,*(4), 215-223.

Montgomery, C., & Webster, D.C. (1993). Caring and nursing's metaparadigm: Can they survive the era of managed care? *Perspectives in Psychiatric Care, 24*(4), 5028.

Mound, B., Gyulay, R., Khan, P., & Goering, P. (1991). The expanded role of nurse case managers. *Journal of Psychosocial Nursing, 29*(6), 18-22.

Olsen, D.P. (1994). The ethical considerations of managed care in mental health treatment. *Journal of Psychosocial Nursing, 32*(3), 25-28.

Peplau, H. (1952). *Interpersonal relations in nursing.* New York: GP Putnam's Sons.

Peplau, H. (1962). Interpersonal techniques: The crux of psychiatric nursing. *American Journal of Nursing, 63,* 53.

Peplau, H. (1978). Psychiatric nursing: Role of nurses and psychiatric nurses. *International Nursing Review, 25,* 41.

Pothier, P., Stuart, G., Puskar, K., & Babich, K. (1990). Dilemmas and directions for psychiatric nursing in the 1990s. *Archives of Psychiatric Nursing, 4,* 284.

Queen, V. (1995). Inpatient psychiatric nursing care. In G. Stuart & S. Sundeen (Eds.), *Principles and practice of psychiatric nursing* (5th ed., pp. 811-829). St. Louis, MO: Mosby.

Saur, C.D., & Ford, S.M. (1995). Quality, cost-effective psychiatric treatment: A CNS-MD collaborative practice model. *Archives of Psychiatric Nursing, 9*(6), 332-337.

Scallet, L.J., & Havel, J.T. (1994). Reflections on the mental health community's experience in the health care reform debate. *Hospital and Community Psychiatry, 45*(9), 888-892.

Sharfstein, S., Stoline, A., & Goldman, H. (1993). Psychiatric care and health insurance reform. *American Journal of Nursing, 150,* 7.

Schreter, R.K. (1993). Ten trends in managed care and their impact on the biopsychosocial model. *Hospital and Community Psychiatry, 44*(4), 325-327.

Stuart, G. (1995a). Roles and functions of psychiatric nurses: Competent caring. In G. Stuart & S. Sundeen (Eds.), *Principles and practice of psychiatric nursing* (5th ed., pp. 3-19). St. Louis, MO: Mosby.

Stuart, G. (1995b). A stress adaptation model of psychiatric nursing care. In G. Stuart & S. Sundeen (Eds.), *Principles and practice of psychiatric nursing* (5th ed., pp. 79-95). St. Louis, MO: Mosby.

Tudor, G. (1952). Sociopsychiatric nursing approach to intervention in a problem of mutual withdrawal on a mental hospital ward. *Psychiatry, 15,* 193.

Watson, P., Lower, M., Wells, S., Farrah, S., & Jarrell, C. (1991). Discovering what nurses do and what it costs. *Nurse Management, 22,* 38.

Worley, N. (1995). Community psychiatric nursing care. In G. Stuart & S. Sundeen (Eds.), *Principles and practice of psychiatric nursing* (5th ed., pp. 831-849). St. Louis, MO: Mosby.

Reflections on primary health care in developing countries

BARBARA ROBERTSON

For most developing countries the change from a traditional curative health care service to one based on a primary health care (PHC) approach continues to be long and difficult. This may be due in part to many health professionals viewing PHC as the solution for the provision of rural health services. This has resulted in PHC being perceived as an appropriate cost-effective service for the poor. Community members have also resisted nurse-run clinics by bypassing them to see a general practitioner or a doctor at the nearest hospital outpatient department. Quality PHC is not a cheap Third-World service. It consists of a wide variety of skilled health care workers who together provide care for individuals, families, and communities. The hallmark of such a service is universal access and quality care in a culturally sensitive and cost-effective manner.

Successfully implemented, a PHC program in any given region should be able to control such well-known diseases as tuberculosis, malaria, diarrhea and respiratory tract infections, which occur most often in developing countries. One needs to ask why the incidence of such illnesses has not been significantly limited. The following factors must be held responsible, at least in part, for such failure.

DOUBT AS TO THE EFFICACY OF PHC

Some who previously accepted PHC with its principles of accessibility, affordability, acceptability, accountability, and equity are now doubting the likely success of such a system. The demand for such a high degree of change to the health care system and commitment to working with communities whose involvement in the decision-making process in health care consumes large amounts of health worker time. Community members are likewise disillusioned at the reluctance of the health team to listen to their needs and provide more than institutional care.

THE MEDICAL MODEL RESULTING IN A CURATIVE MINDSET

The curative medical model has benefited enormously in recent decades from medical and technical advances in treating illnesses. This model favors an emphasis on curative medicine. It provides a quick-fix approach; and the physician's inability to correct a health problem is considered a failure. With their busy schedules in the institution, the health care team is unable even to be concerned about how their patients, still unable to manage on their own, will cope when discharged. They find it difficult to accept the more long-term goals of PHC. Nurses are unwilling to move from the hospital environment to a PHC clinic because they feel that their training has better prepared them for the more technical hospital environment. The frequently observed patronizing and arrogant attitude toward patients by physicians and nurses is interpreted by the community as wielding power over them. The "doctor knows best" attitude and the fact that community members do not appear to be welcome when they are requesting information on health issues leads community members to feel alienated in the health system. Even the normal birth process becomes abnormal and is treated in a culturally insensitive manner if deliveries are done in high-care units. Midwife obstetrics units are perceived as a problem especially in urban areas because there is a reluctance for doctors to provide the backup service required.

LACK OF EMPHASIS ON PHC IN URBAN AREAS

A World Health Organization (WHO) report (1992) on urbanization states that the urban crisis will affect all major cities in both the developed and the developing world. South African cities will not be an exception because they are already experiencing an influx of people from rural areas seeking employment and a better life. Immigrants, many of whom are illegal, also flock to the inner city. In South Africa the rapid political change has resulted in the massive migration of people into the major cities. Adequate infrastructure for such rapid growth cannot be provided. The increased population is mostly concentrated into the decaying inner-city apartment buildings and in informal settlements where people illegally construct temporary housing in parks, empty plots, or open land around the periphery of the cities.

This uncontrolled influx is destroying health, societal values, and human lives and contributes to illness, accidents, and crime. Streets abound with the homeless, the chronically sick, and poor and abandoned children. Accommodations are overcrowded and the owners of apartment blocks renege on the repair of electricity, water, and sewage systems. It is estimated that in a central area of Johannesburg, the largest city in South Africa, 60% of the population are young people under 30 years of age. Prostitutes and drug peddlers ply their trade in night clubs, escort agencies, and on the streets. Sexually transmitted diseases are common and the incidence of HIV infection (Coulson, 1994; Seager, 1994) is rising. Acculturation and the weakening of support systems result in the breakup of family life. Physical and sexual abuse, crime, violence, alcohol abuse, stress, and mental disorders become everyday occurrences, promoting insecurity, fear, and stress in vulnerable groups such as the elderly, who are afraid to venture into the streets. However, health is not a priority for many of these city dwellers, whose energies are concentrated on survival and job seeking.

This scenario sketches clearly the need for PHC services in inner-city communities. The health care workers in the area do render a service but experience many frustrations:

- Health services are currently divided into preventive/promotive and curative health services. This division makes it impossible for either group to handle health problems as a whole.
- Violence prevents clinics being from opening at times convenient to working people. Clinics are also targets of crime at night, thus preventing essential services like midwifery from being available to the community.
- Because of the high mobility of the population, the group being served is changing constantly. Maintaining contact and a satisfactory follow-up service for these patients, especially those with tuberculosis, is difficult.
- Secondary and tertiary health services are close at hand. Not only do they overshadow the PHC approach, but they also consume an ever-increasing amount of the budget. This further mitigates against providing a comprehensive PHC service.
- Because the major training universities and institutions are situated in these areas, as long as the curative medical model is promoted as the appropriate way to train health professionals, the struggle to provide adequate comprehensive health services will continue.

COMMUNITY PARTNERSHIP IN PRIMARY HEALTH CARE

Communities are divided in their opinions of the effectiveness of PHC. The medical model has led even the most remote communities to believe that the best service is provided by a medical doctor (a doctor trained in a medically approved Western facility) or in some instances by a traditional doctor (diviner, herbalist prophet, spiritual healer, or traditional birth attendant). A service in which the front-line health care worker is a nurse is often viewed by the community as inferior.

Many community members feel demotivated, powerless, and abused. They lack knowledge and have lost the hope of having their needs met. They are angry and blame the government for not delivering what it has promised. After a visit to the Cameroons and parts of the Congo, Robbins (1995), a health correspondent writing in a leading Johannesburg newspaper, states that comanagement and cofinancing of PHC is the only way to achieve real partnership with the community. Health care workers are reluctant to give up their power bases and control over the health services. They feel threatened because they still see community clinic services as their prerogative and are not willing to engage in action that will upset their status and privileges. It is regretful that they cannot see that an effective partnership will enhance rather than reduce their power base. Inner cities in particular are not homogeneous and lack leadership. Residents are either illegal or have moved in from overcrowded areas and are therefore hesitant to participate or volunteer for community activities. Farley (1993) elaborates on this, stating that the health cost of powerlessness among these people is interpersonal violence, dangerous housing, chronic disease, alcohol and drug abuse, and teenage pregnancy. Creating partnerships is a transformational process that will be long term, slow, and painful because it involves redistribution of power and changes in health workers' attitudes, beliefs, and perceptions.

POOR MANAGEMENT

Many of the PHC plans that are well researched and well developed seem to fall apart at the implementation phase because of a lack of management skills. The importation of overseas management models has not had the expected impact because these models have not taken into consideration whether the system fits the values, knowledge, and management needs of the country in which they are to be used. Skills are often taught in a didactic rather than experimental manner, and the nurse finds it difficult to put them into practice. Major problems in the management of PHC services were identified in a national workshop (Department of Health, 1995):

- Lack of strategic planning at the national level
- Inadequate training of health workers at all levels in leadership and management practice
- Maldistribution and misuse of resources, including wastage of money, ineffective use of human resources, and unrealistic goals and time frames
- Inaccessibility of information; low priority is given to the development of information systems, and a skills deficit exists in using and managing information
- Lack of ownership of service by the community; there is no strong link to ensure that the community is part of the decision-making process and that a common vision is shared
- A paternalistic attitude that provides for people rather than working with them
- Poor communication
- Lack of organizational, personnel, and budgeting skills
- Excessive paperwork
- Structures that are top down, with centralized decision making, which results in role-bound services that are inflexible and resistant to change
- Fragmentation of health services delivery
- Lack of a user-friendly records system
- Power struggle between different professionals with each one striving to retain its grip over their particular piece of health territory, resulting in the duplication of services and treatment overlap

THE EXTENDED ROLE OF THE NURSE—HOW FAR?

A PHC model needs to deal with both the psychosocial and physical aspects of health. The question is, how far should the nursing curriculum go in teaching aspects such as the environment, housing, water supplies, family disintegration, and lifestyle issues, among others, and how far should nurses be involved in them? Should nurses be a resource to link communities with the relevant departments that are able to provide these needs or should they be able to deal with them? What should nurses do if the relevant departments are unresponsive? What is really meant by the extended role of the nurse? If nurses expand their role are they legally covered by practice acts, and what aspects of the traditional nursing role can or would be lost? Do nurses remain nurses or should a new type of health worker be created who is neither a nurse, a doctor or a social worker? This issue is being debated by health planners in South Africa and poses a new threat to nurses. Another question being asked is whether nurses can share their decision-making role with the community and still be credible health workers. What if the community priorities are not realistic? Will both parties then become frustrated? How can traditional evaluation measures for workload productivity and quality care be used to evaluate the effectiveness of the service? Health professionals need to look critically at themselves, at the people they care for, and at the system of which they are a part. The free flow of information will help the parties to adapt continuously. The process must include appropriate research and should include both quantitative and qualitative studies to monitor and adapt what is largely a human interactive process in which teamwork skills are important.

RELUCTANCE OF NURSES TO BE INVOLVED IN POLITICAL ISSUES

Most nurses have felt that political involvement in health issues is the prerogative of others. From the beginning of their education nurses are socialized into believing that their chief task is patient care and that involvement in anything that could be perceived as being political (usually interpreted in the party political context) is unacceptable. Nurses in PHC will need to accept that their service is linked inextricably with power and politics (Walts, 1990). This includes negotiation with local, district, provincial, and national government. In addition, they will also act as resource people and advocates to redress the injustices of the past (e.g., inequitable resource allocation, lack of appropriate services, and devolution of power to community level). This will mean acquiring networking and lobbying skills.

TRADITIONAL WAYS OF WORKING

Existing clinic routines are rigid and usually divided into special sessions. Patients coming to a facility on the "wrong" day are given very cursory care and are asked to return when the particular service they need is next being offered. In urban settings nurses are reluctant to treat homeless children because they are unaccompanied by an adult and cannot give a permanent address. This may result in the children being sent away. The pattern of running clinics is based on the hospital's outpatient system and results in queues and long waits for community members. Most patients must be seen in the morning and are expected to arrive well before they will be seen. Health education talks are given before the commencement of a session and waiting patients must listen regardless of whether the subject is appropriate to their needs. Most staff members tend to go to tea and lunch at the same time, leaving gaps when no one is available to see patients. Nurses control the way they work and what they do. They have difficulty in acknowledging and accepting the fact that community members are able to understand health issues and gain knowledge to undertake tasks that have traditionally been the responsibility of nurses.

THE TRADITIONAL CURATIVE NURSING CURRICULUM

Health training institutions all have an uncomfortable feeling that they must change to ensure that health professionals are trained to be competent to function within the changing emphasis in health care delivery. Because change is a threatening issue the tendency is to cling to traditional ways of teaching. Lecturers are comfortable with it; it has worked well in the past; and in this time of change it is important that international credibility is not lost. Even for those who have taken the plunge to change it is not smooth sailing. Community-based education becomes a problem because there are no well-structured student programs available and clinic staff do not see a role for first-and second-year nurses in their services because they do not have sufficient nursing skills to be able to function in the clinic. Issues related to interdisciplinary teamwork and intersectoral cooperation need to be demonstrated and students need to be involved actively with the community in the sociopolitical process of improving health. There are risks related to change, and these are discussed in the sections that follow.

Professional risks

There is always a fear that standards will be lowered, and that the institution will loose its credibility and therefore its ability to recruit top-quality staff.

Program risks

Excellence seems to be measured by the number of publications from lecturers and the quality of their fundamental research. There is less concern for appropriate research that is performed to investigate community needs and for change in teaching approaches.

Organizational risks

Exposure of the students to communities is to risk credibility and to expose the organization to criticism. Extra expenses are incurred in transport cost and vehicles are in danger of being hijacked at gunpoint. Personal safety risks due to crime, robbery, and motor vehicle accidents are becoming a major problem for students going out into informal and inner-city areas (Showstack et al., 1992).

PROVIDING SOLUTIONS

It is still accepted that PHC has the potential to solve many of the problems in our health care system. For nurses in particular PHC poses both a challenge and a window of opportunity. If nurses are prepared to make the shift, there will be an opportunity for them to show that they can make a difference, be creative, and become the driving force in a health service. For this to happen four steps must be taken.

Developing vision and valuing diversity

Scripture says "where there is no vision the people perish." People work harder in a situation in which they understand the significance of their contribution and the goals and objectives of the overall service. When both health workers and community members achieve a common vision in which they create a sense of purpose and belief in the ability of PHC to satisfy the major needs of the community, PHC will be able to supersede the domi-

SUGGESTIONS FOR DEVELOPING A COMMON VISION

- Decide on what you want to create—a picture of what is to be achieved.
- Create a sense of excitement.
- Develop a personal vision and build on it.
- Sell the vision, and revise it on an ongoing basis.
- Obtain commitment from all players.
- Sustain the vision through sharing.
- Be prepared to take risks to make it happen.
- Identify the steps needed to fulfill the vision.
- Identify the core values because they will guide how you act.

From *The fifth discipline fieldbook: Strategies and tools for building a learning organisation* by P. Senge, C. Roberts, R.B. Ross, B.J. Smith and A. Kleiner, 1994. London: Nicholas Brealey. Adapted with permission.

HELPFUL HINTS FOR VALUING DIVERSITY

- Acknowledge differences.
- Know as much as possible about the cultures of your colleagues.
- Work in small groups and support each other, while knowing that you are part of a larger health team.
- Create your own identity as a group.
- Listen to each other.
- Promote mutual learning and development through open communication.
- Become involved in the change process.
- Develop a strong sense of membership and identity.

From "New futures, at whose cost" by E. Charles in R. Boot, J. Lawrence, and J. Morris, eds. 1994, *Managing the unknown by creating new futures*. London: McGraw-Hill; and Kendall F. "Diversity Issues in the workplace." In Griggs, L.B. and Luow, L.L. (eds.): Valuing Diversity: New Tools for a New Reality. New York: McGraw-Hill.

nation that the curative service has had. The box lists suggestions for developing such a common vision.

Valuing diversity

In a developing country it is not easy to have a homogeneous community with a single language. This difficulty poses a problem for the health worker because most people are more comfortable working in their own cultural or interest group. Working in a group outside of a person's own frequently leads to conflict situations and misleading perceptions, because only some aspects of what is really believed and felt surface. It is not our similarities that cause problems but our differences. Therefore, valuing diversity is at the heart of working relationships. It involves learning about yourself and other groups and accepting and appreciating the differences. People should be seen as equal but different. This is well explained in the African term *ubuntu,* which literally means "a man is a man." It can be further elaborated by the idiom "a person is a person through other people," which symbolizes collective solidarity. Mbigi and Maree (1995, p. 111) say "for the thumb to work efficiently it will need the collective operation of the fingers." These fingers embrace the concepts of respect, dignity, solidarity, compassion and survival. For PHC to be effective there should be a collective approach to planning and implementation that is based on the above concepts.

Community partnerships

Creating community partnerships is a process that is long-term, slow, and painful because it concerns the redistribution of power and the changing of health worker attitudes and perceptions. It is essential for community members and health workers to uncover differences, build bridges, and learn to understand each other. It can set in motion a process that is dynamic and continuing where people build one another up, seeking reconciliation and transformation. This teamwork or sharing process works well in typical South African community organizations called *Stokvels* (Chadford, 1995). These are highly successful credit unions in which people contribute money, draw from it on a rotational basis, or invest it and share the profits. They are rooted in African culture and have developed a highly successful way of conducting their affairs. The principles identified (see box) are understood and used by large numbers of community members and can well be incorporated into team-building in PHC.

Learning

Learning will need to take place on three fronts.

- *With the community.* The objective will be to empower the community to speak out and be involved in change because they have acquired the necessary knowledge and skills based on the principles of adult learning; sharing of experiences by the community members; active participation in small groups; and ongoing learning in which acquiring new knowledge and life skills are stressed. Building capacity in this way develops confidence and commitment and leads to action. Celebration when goals are reached further stimulates others to be involved in creating an environment for participatory involvement.

STOKVEL PRINCIPLES

Creation of a culture of learning, which is aimed at building the person, the group and the community
Inclusiveness, which creates a sense of belonging and provides common purpose, equal status, and a support group
Ubuntu, which includes showing respect for life and death for all people and promoting a sense of pride in self and others
Support based on reciprocity, which enables all members to benefit
Trust because of the insistence on transparency and a respect for all
Discipline through formal procedures, use of peer pressure, and speedy resolution of problems
Democratic governance based on transparency, consensus decision making, and conflict resolution through dialogue

• *Between health workers and community.* This involves the formation of appropriate attitudes and the acquisition of communication skills. These need to be based on agreed standards of conduct and ethics, mutual respect, and trust. Working together in small groups will assist in developing listening skills, provide practice in mutual decision making, and create opportunity to develop a respect for the cultural environment of both the community and the health workers.

• *With the health workers.* Deficits in knowledge and skills not acquired in basic education programs will need to be obtained through short courses, self-directed learning, or formal courses.

These courses will include PHC and management skills. *PHC skills* include the following:

- Diagnostic and treatment knowledge and skills for disease conditions prevalent in the district
- Situational analysis of community needs
- Investigation of a health problem
- Planning and implementation of health programmes
- Teaching of life skills, e.g., assertiveness, social adjustment, stress management
- Working within the legal requirements related to the use, prescription, and control of drugs

Management skills include the following:

- Leadership and team building
- Clinic organization and management, including budgeting

STEPS FOR NURSE EDUCATORS

- Introduce a community-based, problem-based approach to primary health care in all curricula.
- Encourage critical thinking and develop visionary leadership and creativity.
- Bring community members onto curricula committees and review student selection policies with them.
- Develop sites for community-based education and develop a cooperative model with the committees for joint teaching and involvement.
- Develop negotiating and networking skills.
- Encourage collaboration with nongovernmental organizations, traditional healers, and other community workers.
- Promote the development of women and prepare nurses to be active in policy making at the district, provincial, and national government levels.
- Promote research into community health issues and health administration.
- Encourage participation research with the community.
- Assist with the development of appropriate health information systems, quality assurance standards for primary health care, and evaluation systems.

- Health information systems
- Participatory research and evaluation
- Management skills to plan and manage a clinic using appropriate technology
- Proper use and control of essential drugs

In addition to postgraduate work there is a need to examine nursing curricula. More productive learning will take place with a community-based, problem-based curriculum that is modular and experiential. This is in line with the WHO (1994) report on nursing beyond the year 2000, which states,

> In planning nursing education, both the content and method should be considered. Countries may need to consider a variety of approaches—including problem-based learning, distance learning, self-directed learning, community-based education, continuing education credits and professional experience—in order to expand educational opportunities and career mobility. (p. 14)

A greater emphasis must be placed on subjects like epidemiology; knowledge of culture and cultural perspectives of illness; the impact of social and community influences on health, communication, team building, creative management, and risk taking; counselling skills; and cost-effectiveness of care.

IN CONCLUSION

Imagine a PHC center where community members are holding a health fair to celebrate the first anniversary of their partnership with the health team. A healthy lifestyle program has been completed that enabled community members to develop critical thinking, problem-solving, communication, and coping skills with township-living skills as well as specific health information on parenting, gardening, story-telling, self-defense, and budgeting. The community members are excited because they have been asked to run a similar program for one of the larger community churches. The nurses are equally excited as they share in the celebration. They fully acknowledge that they did not think it would be such hard work to assist in improving the health status of their community, nor did they anticipate how rewarding the result of their hard work would be. One was overheard to remark, "My involvement with the community this year has been the most exciting period in my nursing career. I have been enriched by the community, they have taught me more than I have taught them." In addition, the community members have begun to interact with local government. A major planning meeting will be held in the next month with the these authorities. It will address some of the sociopolitical issues worrying the community, the chief of which are safety and crime prevention. The community has prepared a memorandum for presentation to the meeting and has four major suggestions in which they feel they could assist the police in their task with very little financial outlay. They also have ideas on job creation that will assist in lowering crime. They have identified their spokeswoman and she has practiced her role. The nurses have chosen their representatives and they will support and facilitate discussion. Is this scenario myth or reality? I believe it can be more than an isolated happening!

REFERENCES

Chadford, K. (1995). *South African management principles within Stokvels: A case study.* Unpublished manuscript, Faculty of Management, University of the Witwatersrand, Johannesburg.

Charles, E. (1994). New futures, at whose cost. In R. Boot., J. Lawrence, & J. Morris (Eds.), *Managing the unknown by creating new futures* (p. 141). London: McGraw-Hill.

Coulson, N. (1994). A changing inner city, health workers respond: The Hillbrow PHC project. In *Critical Health, 46,* 39-46.

Department of Health. (1995). Report of the workshop on Human Resource Management. Pretoria: Author.

Farley, S. (1993). The community as partner in primary health care. *Nursing & Health Care, 14*(5) 244-245.

Kendall, F.E. (1995). Diversity issues in the workplace. In L.B. Griggs, & L.L. Louw (Eds.), *Valuing diversity: New tools for a new reality.* New York: McGraw-Hill.

Mbigi, L., & Maree, J. (1995). *Ubuntu: The spirit of African transformation management.* Randburg, Gauteng: Knowledge Resources.

Robbins, D. (1995, October 9). PHC must be a partnership. *Star Newspaper,* (p. 13).

Seager, J. (1994). Growing cities, new disease patterns: Urban health in the developing world. *Critical Health, 46,* 14-20.

Senge, P., Roberts, C., Ross, R.B., Smith, B.J., & Kleiner, A. (1994). *The fifth discipline fieldbook: Strategies and tools for building a learning organisation.* London: Nicolas Brealey.

Showstack, J., Fein, O., Ford, D., Kaufman, A., Cross, A., Madoff, M., Goldberg, H., O'Neil, E., Moore, G., Schroeder, S., Inui, T., & the Health of the Public Mission Statement Working Group. (1992). *Health of the public: The academic response. JAMA, 267*(18) 2497-2502.

Walts, R.J. (1990). Democratization of health care: Challenge for nursing. *Advances in Nursing Science, 12*(2), 37-46.

WHO Commission on Health and Environment. (1992). *Report of the panel on urbanisation.* Geneva: Author.

WHO. (1994). *Nursing beyond the year 2000. Report of a WHO study group* (p. 14). Technical Report series 842. Geneva: Author.

Section Five

QUALITY IMPROVEMENT

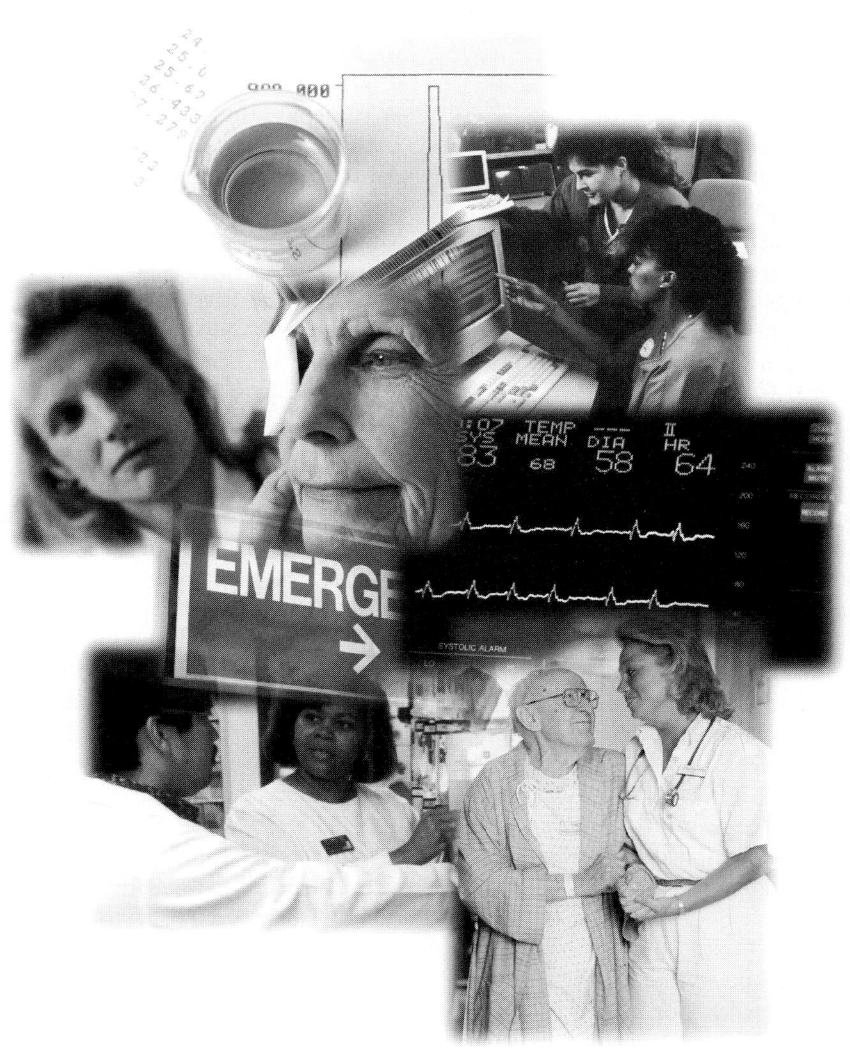

Preserving quality in an era of cost control

JOANNE COMI McCLOSKEY, HELEN KENNEDY GRACE

In this time of continual transition in health care with intense pressures to control costs, maintaining quality of care becomes a major concern. In the past, incentives have focused on doing more rather than less in a system in which payment was based on the services provided. Under managed care, however, the incentives have been reversed so that minimalist care could easily become the norm. Within a system in which funding is based on capitation and income to a practice is based on an average per enrolled member, the challenges to deliver care while making a profit are powerful. Costs can be controlled by reducing the numbers of laboratory tests and procedures, time spent talking to patients, and the amount of time spent in hospitals, and excluding from the system those with prior conditions that would necessitate costly care or underserved poor, and underrepresented groups in our society. These intense pressures to control costs create a unique opportunity structure for nursing. Nurses can play extremely important roles in managed care systems, bringing their unique skills to play as part of a cost-conscious, coordinated system. Nurses also play key roles in institutional settings, which are part of the fabric of health care. As part of these systems, with all the pressures to cut corners wherever possible, nurses have the important role of maintaining quality of care within the system. This is a particular challenge as increasing numbers of nonclinical administrators view health care purely from a business perspective. The challenge for nursing is to maintain its "rootedness" in clinical care while still serving as an effective spokesperson in the business aspects of health care. This section provides an interesting overview of the issues related to maintenance of standards at different points within the health care system.

In the opening debate chapter Vruwink and Mitchell pose the question of the potential for managed care to improve the quality of care for patients. The chapter opens by mapping out the complex terrain of managed care. Studies that have compared quality of care in both fee-for-service and managed care systems conclude that they are comparable. These studies, however, have used traditional measures of quality and have not tapped into some of the unique dimensions of managed care, such as preventive and primary care. The authors assess the potential role of accrediting agencies in establishing standards, and advocate that nursing take a leadership role in defining and assessing new quality of care measures. When these measures are clearer, quality of care issues can be addressed in greater depth. While quality of care for those who have managed to gain entry to managed care systems is one dimension, a larger question involves those who are denied access. What has happened to this population as the health care system has shifted?

The first issues chapter by Dean-Barr reviews the history of the development of standards and guidelines for nursing practice. While standards establish a broad direction for the overall practice of nursing, guidelines describe recommended courses of action to address specific problems. Dean-Barr advocates greater attention to the use of standards and guidelines to ensure quality of care. Nursing organizations working in collaboration with one another should be involved in the development of standards and guidelines to ensure quality of clinical practice.

While standards and guidelines provide a framework for evaluating quality, their implementation within the real world of practice may not be as positive as we had hoped. Quality patient care requires not only good nursing practice but also collaboration of caregivers in the process. The next three chapters in this section address multidisciplinary approaches to improvement of quality of care.

Clinical pathways, multidisciplinary plans for patient care that sequence interventions and clinical outcomes on a timeline, are advocated by Kyzer. Bringing together the multidisciplinary team to develop the clinical pathway and continually monitoring the progress of care are important parts of the process. Results from a cross-section of settings using the clinical pathways as a methodology indicate positive improvements in the quality of care provided.

In the business world, considerable attention has been paid to total quality management redesign, and more recently to the concept of reengineering. Triolo, Hendricks, and Duncan describe and contrast these approaches. Total quality management is an approach to improve practice (existing processes) continually, whereas reengineering involves "starting all over and reinventing the future." Contrasting these two approaches, Triolo and colleagues advocate the total quality management approach combined with some of the aspects of reengineering. The most important factor in this process is the people involved in improvement of the system in total quality management in contrast to the top-down approach of reengineering.

The next three issues chapters turn to the problems related to measurement of quality of care. Martin and Martin address some of the complexities in measuring quality of care and describe the implementation of the Omaha System to measure quality of care in community-practice systems. Use of this system provides a framework for orientation of new employees, improves client records, and enhances the development of information systems that allow for retrieval of information across cases within the organization. Most importantly, the use of the system allows for tracking of patient outcome data, providing a database for improved clinical practice and improved management.

Another way to address qualitative issues is to ensure that clinical practitioners are competent. One of the challenges in measuring clinical competence is assessing the ability of the individual to apply knowledge, skills, and judgment in the practice setting. Yocom provides a thorough overview of the underlying concerns and describes current approaches to measuring clinical competence. The use of new technologies offers the promise of being able to simulate clinical situations so that much more valid measures of clinical competence can be achieved.

Turning to the world of managed care, Stahl describes the various managed care arrangements available and the challenges to ensuring quality of care within the incentive frameworks of the various systems. While the parameters for quality of care have been defined by the National Committee on Quality Assurance and a tool has been developed, its application in measuring actual performance has been questioned. One area that is particularly problematic is the quality of subacute care. This is one of the areas in which the potential for cost savings is the greatest, but it is also the one in which abuses of quality of care may be most rampant. Strategies for improving quality of care in managed care systems are proposed.

In the final issues chapter, the focus moves to the international scene and the use of self-care as a model for improving health in Latin America. Lange and Jaimovich provide an overview of major health issues throughout the region. Engagement of individuals and their families in becoming active participants in health care has been demonstrated to be effective in improving the health of the community. Greater use of this model to guide practice and measure its effectiveness is advocated.

Ensuring quality of care for people requires a multifaceted approach. Professional associations have an important function in setting a framework of expectations. Engagement of those involved in the provision of care is essential in the practical application of this framework in the workplace. While the process of engagement of clinical staff in planning and implementing patient care is one thing, measurement of the impact of these approaches on outcomes of care is another. It is incumbent on the profession to continue to address the complexities of measurement so that the impact of quality of care can be addressed in the language of the marketplace—the cost-effectiveness of quality care. One of the most important facets of improved quality of care is the degree to which the patient and family are viewed as participants, rather than as recipients, of care. There is much to be learned from the Latin American experience that can be applied to the United States to ensure that all Americans have access to quality care at an affordable cost.

Improving quality of care: Can managed care make a difference?

MICHELLE VRUWINK, MARIA MITCHELL

Although efforts to achieve national health care reform have failed to date, a rapid and dramatic transformation of the nation's health care delivery system is under way. Managed care has been central to both the national health reform debate and the concomitant transformation of the health care system in the United States. Largely fueled by runaway inflation in the cost of traditional health care delivery, both the public and private sectors have firmly embraced managed care as a means to reform delivery and contain the costs of health care services. Managed care has clearly delivered on some of its promises, particularly in the area of cost containment. As more of our population enrolls in managed care organizations, however, what is the impact on the quality of health care? Can managed care provide a model of "doing more with less?" In this chapter, we examine the accomplishments of managed care to date and explore how the increasing competition in our health care market will foster the demand for continuous quality improvement.

WHAT IS MANAGED CARE?

The term *managed care* has come to represent a wide variety of health care financing and delivery structures. At its most basic level, managed care can be described as a model of health care delivery in which all of the health care needs of a patient are funneled through one party—generally referred to as the case or care manager or "gatekeeper." The goal of this model is to rationalize what has traditionally been a fragmented system of care delivery and financing, ensuring that patients receive coordinated and cost-effective health care and limiting the use of high-cost specialty and inpatient care.

There are many variations to this basic concept of managed care. Some of the most common types of managed care organizations include health maintenance organizations (HMOs), individual practice associations (IPAs), preferred provider organizations (PPOs), and the newer point-of-service (POS) plans. Each of these types is considered a "managed care organization" and is commonly used today. For clarification, we include brief descriptions of each.

Health maintenance organizations

An HMO is an organization that combines health care insurance and delivery, and there are several types. In the staff model the HMO employs physicians on a salaried basis who treat HMO members in central clinical facilities. In the group model a medical group practice contracts with the HMO to provide services, and in turn subcontracts with a group of physicians (either on a salaried, capitated, or fee-for-service basis). In the network model the HMO contracts with a number of independent group practices to provide medical services.

Individual practice associations

In a typical IPA, physicians maintain their own practices but associate with a central management organization to provide administrative services and function as the group's agent in negotiations. IPA physicians may be reimbursed on a fee-for-service basis or may be capitated for services.

Preferred provider organizations

Slightly more flexible provider organizations, PPOs include a group of physicians contracted to provide health care services to a discrete population, such as the employees of a large business, typically at a discounted rate. Insured members are then usually offered incentives, such as lower out-of-pocket costs, to use the "preferred" network of providers. However, members may choose to receive services outside this network.

Point-of-service plans

The POS plans offer the greatest flexibility to insured members. A POS plan is essentially a combination of traditional fee-for-service coverage, an HMO, and a PPO. Insured members select a primary care physician to serve as their care manager and receive referrals from this physician for specialty services. However, the member may choose to seek such services either from network providers or outside the network. Like the PPO, there are typically incentives for insured members to access care through network providers.

Managed care typically involves a different financing method than traditional fee-for-service health care. The most critical difference between managed and fee-for-service care is the concept of a prepaid fee per member per month—or capitation. In fee-for-service plans, a provider is reimbursed for each health service delivered to a patient, whereas in managed care, the managed care organization is prepaid a set fee to cover any and all health care services delivered to a particular individual in that month. This capitation significantly changes the incentives to deliver services. With fee-for-service plans, the incentive is to maximize payment by providing more care. In recent years, there has been increasing concern that this traditional model of care has led to an unnecessary, and sometimes harmful, overuse of care. With managed care, the capitated entity assumes the risk that the cost of care will not exceed their payment. This creates an incentive to monitor and limit the use of high-cost care.

Despite recent interest, managed care is not a new concept. An early form of managed care can be found in the late 1800s in arrangements between mining, lumber, and manufacturing companies and "town doctors" to provide health services for employees in exchange for a prepaid monthly fee. Managed care was not promoted widely until the early 1970s, when rapidly rising health care costs created a demand for reform. The term *health maintenance organization* was coined by Ellwood et al. at InterStudy, who recommended increased federal support for the concept and use of managed care in a position paper developed for President Nixon. The following year, federal legislation was passed to promote the development of HMOs. Prior to 1970, less than 2% of the insured population in the United States was enrolled in 50 HMO-like organizations. By 1989, 32.5 million people, or 13% of the insured population, were enrolled in HMOs (Shouldice, 1991).

The growth in managed care for Medicaid beneficiaries has also increased dramatically—nearly tripling in the past 2 years. In 1982, only six states had federally approved Medicaid managed care demonstration projects. Today, all but six states either have projects being implemented or are awaiting federal approval. In 1993 only 14% of all Medicaid beneficiaries were enrolled in managed care (Rowland, Rosenbaum, Simon, & Chait, 1995); by 1995 approximately 12 million people, or about 35% of Medicaid beneficiaries, were enrolled (Rachel Bloch, November 29, 1995). As federal efforts to reform Medicaid and Medicare move forward, this trend can be expected to accelerate. Managed care is truly becoming the mainstream model of health care.

QUALITY OF CARE IN MANAGED CARE

As our health care system shifts to managed care, it is important to assess what we have learned about the quality of managed care. As the Kaiser Commission found in their 1995 review on Medicaid and managed care, the literature reflects both the wide diversity of care delivery systems grouped under the term "managed care" and the mixed results that this model produces. We can capture this diversity by reviewing the findings of several recent studies.

Many of the studies published to date have focused on patient perceptions of health care as a measure of the quality of services delivered. Three of these surveys provide an interesting mix of findings. The first, conducted by the Health Institute at New England Medical Center in Boston and sponsored by Xerox Corporation, Digital Equipment Corporation, and GTE Corporation, found that managed care enrollees rated the performance of their plans higher than did fee-for-service enrollees (Winslow, 1994). The largest of its kind, this study was based on a detailed survey questionnaire administered to nearly 25,000 people. Specifically, the study found that 86% of the enrollees in managed care were satisfied with their health plans compared with 74% satisfaction with fee-for-service plans. The enrollees in managed care were also more likely to stay with their health plans during the open enrollment period (97%) than were members of fee-for-service plans (63%), most likely because of lower costs.

The second study, conducted by the Harvard School of Public Health and the Boston Globe, found that overall, Americans are satisfied with their health care (Blendon et al., 1994). This study also found no significant difference in satisfaction between managed care enrollees and members of traditional fee for service health plans. Conducted in September 1993, the survey asked 1,000 randomly selected adults to rank their health care plans on six factors: quality of primary care, ease of using primary care, quality of specialist care, ease of using specialist care, ease of using the health plan as a whole, and value of the health plan. For both managed care and traditional fee-for-service health plans, members reported high rates of satisfaction, with scores of over 80 (out of 100) in all indices except "value of health plan." Overall, scores were extremely similar, although managed care members rated the quality of specialist care lower, with a score of 81 versus 91 for fee-for-service members. Interestingly, while less satisfied with the quality of specialist care, managed care enrollees were more satisfied with the speed of referrals to specialists. Despite their concerns about specialty care services, managed care enrollees were also more willing to recommend their health plans to friends or relatives (Blendon et al., 1994).

Finally, the third survey, conducted by the Commonwealth Fund between January and March 1994, included 3,000 randomly selected adults from Boston, Los Angeles, and Miami (Davis, Collins, Schoen & Morris, 1995). This study also found that Americans are satisfied with their health plans, with over 80% of both fee-for-service and managed care patients ranking their plans as good or excellent. However, the study found greater differences between fee-for-service care and managed care than did the Harvard/Boston Globe survey. As Table 38-1 shows, fee-for-service enrollees were more likely to rate their health plans as excellent overall (38%) than were managed care enrollees (29%). Managed care enrollees were also less likely to rate aspects of access and quality of service as excellent. However, unlike the Harvard/Boston Globe study, which found that fee-for-service enrollees were more satisfied with their plans' focus on prevention than were managed care enrollees (rankings of 67 and 57 out of 100, respectively), the Commonwealth study found that managed care plans were likely to be scored as excellent in their coverage of preventive care.

Table 38-1 Enrollees' satisfaction with their health plans

	Excellent	Good	Fair	Poor
Plan overall[a]				
Fee-for-service	38%	47%	12%	2%
Managed care	29	49	17	4
Quality of services[b]				
Fee-for-service	50	40	5	1
Managed care	37	44	12	3
Choice of physicians[a]				
Fee-for-service	60	32	4	1
Managed care	32	41	18	7
Access to specialty care[a]				
Fee-for-service	45	34	6	2
Managed care	26	38	16	7
Availability of emergency care[a]				
Fee-for-service	50	34	4	1
Managed care	36	39	9	3
Waiting time for appointment[a]				
Fee-for-service	43	39	9	2
Managed care	27	41	19	9
Premium paid for plan[b]				
Fee-for-service	30	35	22	8
Managed care	27	35	22	8
Out-of-pocket costs[a]				
Fee-for-service	27	40	23	7
Managed care	35	37	18	7
Paperwork[a]				
Fee-for-service	36	35	14	5
Managed care	44	27	11	4
Coverage of preventive care[a]				
Fee-for-service	33	38	16	8
Managed care	38	40	13	5

Source: Commonwealth Fund Managed Care Survey, 1994 (Louis Harris and Associates, Inc.)

Notes: Percentages weighted to give each city equal weight. Respondents were also asked to rate plans by sevice location, hours, ease of changing doctors, ease of filling prescriptions, availability of advice by phone, office waiting times, and range of services. On these other dimensions, fee-for-service plans were significantly more likely to receive excellent ratings and less likely to receive fair/poor ratings.

[a] Distribution difference significant ($p < .01$).

[b] Not significant ($p > .05$).

Two major literature reviews also provide insight into the quality of care provided under managed care plans. The first review analyzes the literature on managed care plan performance since 1980 (Miller and Luft, 1994). This review only includes studies on enrollees with either private insurance or Medicare, not Medicaid. The second study, conducted by the Kaiser Commission (Rowland, Rosenbaum, Simon, & Chait, 1995), focuses only on Medicaid and managed care. These reviews draw similar conclusions about the quality of health care delivered under the managed care model.

The Miller and Luft (1994) literature analysis found that managed care organizations and fee-for-service plans provided basically comparable quality of care, with some studies indicating a higher level of care under managed care. The only negative findings on managed care came from a study of enrollees with mental health problems. Managed care enrollees also gave high ratings to most aspects of their health care. However, managed care enrollees were likely to rate their health plans less highly than members with traditional coverage. This finding highlights the image problem that managed care organizations face in promoting their services. Yet managed care enrollees rated most aspects of their health care highly.

The Kaiser Commission also found the quality of care in fee-for-service and managed care models to be roughly equivalent. However, their review found variations in the quality of care in different states' managed care programs. For example, the Kaiser Commission cites a 1990 GAO review of managed care in Chicago, which found inadequate structures in place within managed care organizations to ensure quality of care. On the other hand, the GAO's review of Oregon's program found that equal quality of care was provided. Several studies reviewed by the Commission examined birth outcomes. These studies demonstrate that in important outcomes such as birth weight, complication rates, and cesarean rates, managed care organizations demonstrated equivalent, if not slightly better, outcomes than fee-for-service programs. Finally, the Commission's review demonstrated that managed care can improve overall and after-hours availability of health services, increasing the likelihood that patients can access appropriate and timely health care services (Rowland, Rosenbaum, Simon, & Chait, 1995).

Taken together, the many studies that have been conducted both by clinical reviews of the quality of health care and through patient satisfaction surveys support the notion that the quality of care in managed care has been equal to that of fee-for-service care. At the same time, studies have shown that the cost of care has been contained or reduced. In the past year, for the first time in years, employers' health care costs remained stable. Reviews of the many Medicaid managed care demonstration projects have also demonstrated a cost savings between 5% and 15%. As a model for health care reform, managed care has demonstrated its usefulness in containing costs while maintaining quality services.

While the literature does indicate that managed care has shown promise for reforming the health care delivery system, it has not done so without controversy. In the past few years, the media have focused on the fear that managed care organizations are more concerned with profits than quality of care. In numerous articles, citing individual cases in which patients have been denied appropriate or timely care, newspapers and other media have argued that managed care organizations are reducing costs not by providing more preventive care, but simply by denying access.

Perhaps nowhere has this argument been made more forcefully than in New York City. While the transition to a managed care system has largely been made in many West Coast states, New York is just now in the midst of a rapid transformation. In 1995, all major newspapers and media in New York featured series on the "dangers" of managed care. For example, in September 1995 the *New York Post* ran a full-week series titled "HMOs: What You Don't Know Could Kill You." Several stories each day highlighted the difficulties of individuals with serious health problems in accessing necessary health care through their managed care organizations. A January 1996 story in the *New York Times* chronicled the difficulties of an HIV-positive managed care patient who became increasingly ill as physicians inexperienced in treating AIDS failed to diagnose and treat his ailments (Rosenthal, 1996).

Several of New York's elected officials have joined the forces in criticizing managed care organizations. One official, the city's public advocate, published a report, "What Ails HMOs," outlining what he found to be serious problems in the overall management, service delivery, and marketing of managed care organizations. The report calls for managed care organizations to provide the public with accurate measures reflecting the quality of care they deliver to their members (Green, von Nostitz, Piel, & Petroff, 1996).

The transition to managed care in Medicaid has been no less difficult. Many states, implementing large-scale Medicaid managed care programs, have experienced significant difficulties and setbacks. For example, Florida's Medicaid managed care program has suffered from allegations of fraud coupled with a weak oversight ability. Early in the state's managed care program, some Medicaid-only managed care organizations reported expenditures between 50% and 70% on administrative costs—more than three times the industry-wide average (Schulte & Bergal, 1994). In their efforts to recruit managed care organizations to serve Medicaid recipients, Florida routinely waived insurance requirements that commercial managed care organizations were required to meet, such as a review of administrative costs. Additionally, several Medicaid-only managed care organizations were sold shortly after beginning operations, at large profit to the owners. With limited funds devoted to patient care, allegations of denial of care were rampant.

In summary, while evaluations of managed care have indicated that it is a successful model for containing costs without adversely affecting quality of care, the shift to managed care has been marked by a sense of mistrust and fear. The challenge facing the managed care industry today is to demonstrate that high quality health care can be delivered in a more cost-effective manner.

COMPETITION: AN IMPETUS FOR REFORM

One of the important and much discussed elements of managed care is the concept of "competition" in the health care market. In fact, some experts prefer the term "managed competition" to managed care. Introducing competition to the historically protected health care market was seen as a means to stimulate innovation in the reform of health care. However, in the 1970s and 1980s, the focus of this competition was on cost containment. Managed care organizations found that, despite many public concerns and perceptions of lower quality, they could compete successfully on a cost basis.

As managed care begins to dominate the health care market, demands are being made for better and more complete information on all aspects of performance, not just cost. This increased demand for information should not be a surprise to anyone with even an elementary understanding of competitive markets. In the health care market, consumers (both purchasers and users of services) need information on the performance of health plans in such areas as quality of care, access, utilization, *and* cost in order to make appropriate choices among the health services products available. Overall, as consumers become more savvy and the market matures, the focus is shifting away from price competition and toward competition on quality and outcomes of health care services. In the past 5 years, efforts to respond to this demand have increased significantly.

MEASURING THE QUALITY OF MANAGED CARE

There are a number of methods for assessing quality of care, including external review and accrediting processes, patient satisfaction surveys, and technical reviews of clinical appropriateness of services, timeliness of care, and outcomes. All of these methods are applicable and appropriate for evaluating the quality of care delivered in a managed care model. In 1979, the National Committee for Quality Assurance (NCQA), the first national organization dedicated to developing quality standards specifically for managed care organizations, was founded. In addition to their leadership and participation in the development of standardized performance measures for managed care organizations, the NCQA offers a fairly stringent and respected accreditation process.

Managed care organizations can also seek federal accreditation. The accreditation process is under the authority of the Health Care Financing Administration (HCFA). To be a "federally qualified" health plan, an HMO must participate in an extensive application and site review process that examines the organization's ability to offer health care services and maintain an effective quality assurance program.

While the accreditation process offers purchasers and consumers of managed care services some independent assessment that a managed care organization has appropriate procedures in place to ensure quality, the process does have significant limitations. Most important, the findings of the accrediting agency are not made available to the public. Second, accreditation is necessarily focused more on review of procedures and process than it is on actual health outcomes. Several efforts to supplement the accreditation process and to provide purchasers and consumers of services with more useful information have been in development during the early 1990s.

Perhaps the most widely used and discussed of these efforts is the Health Plan and Employer Data and Information Set (HEDIS). HEDIS was originally developed as a collaborative effort among large corporate purchasers of managed care services, the NCQA, and managed care organizations. Its goal was to develop a set of standardized measures that would provide employers with a reasonable means of assessing the performance of managed care organizations. In 1993, HEDIS 2.0, the first of a continuing series of revisions of HEDIS, was released. HEDIS consists of a set of standardized measures of performance in five areas: membership and utilization, access and satisfaction, quality of care, health plan management, and finance. The HEDIS measures have been widely adopted in the private sector.

Since the release of the HEDIS measures, efforts have been under way to adapt them for use in evaluating the performance of managed care organizations serving the Medicaid population. In early 1994, a working group made up of the NCQA, the HCFA, Medicaid beneficiary advocates, state Medicaid agencies, managed care plans, and others began the process of adapting HEDIS 2.0/2.5 for Medicaid (NCQA, 1996). The results are expected to be widely adopted by state Medicaid managed care programs and have been incorporated by New York City in its recently restructured Medicaid managed care program. The Medicaid HEDIS measures are designed explicitly to serve as elements of a "report card" on health plan performance in order to assist consumers in choosing a quality health plan. It is also designed with the goal of fostering continuous quality improvement.

What kinds of measures are included in HEDIS? HEDIS outlines measures of performance for utilization, quality, access, and patient satisfaction, which should all be factored together in assessing the overall quality of care delivered by a health plan. Specific measures include the following:

- The frequency of selected procedures, such as tonsillectomy
- Utilization of inpatient and ambulatory care
- Immunization rates
- Rates of low birth weight babies
- Initial prenatal care visits
- Mammography rates
- Asthma inpatient admission rates
- Availability of primary care providers
- Waiting times for appointments
- Member satisfaction

The HEDIS measures have provided a solid first step toward providing comparable managed care performance data. However, many leaders in the field of quality review have faulted the data set for too little focus on health care outcome measures. For consumers, outcome measures are more important than process measures. The typical patient is likely to be less interested in the rate of immunizations or mammograms provided than in how these services have improved the health of patients. Outcome measures are increasingly the focus of national efforts to evaluate quality of care.

In preparation for the issuance of HEDIS 3.0, which is expected to be released in fall 1996, the NCQA has convened the Committee on Performance Measurement, which will make recommendations for revisions for HEDIS 3.0. HEDIS 3.0 is expected to include a greater focus on outcomes measurement, member satisfaction, and patient-reported information and should incorporate data on Medicare and Medicaid recipients with that of the commercial population (Edlin, 1995).

Another organization, the Foundation for Accountability, has recently been formed with the goal of increasing the focus on outcomes of health care, patient satisfaction, and overall health status. The foundation's members, who include 3M, Ameritech, GTE Corporation, American Express, Pepsico, the HCFA, and the Federal Employees Health Benefits Plan, represent 80 million users of health care.

The HEDIS data set and other similar efforts to evaluate the performance of managed care organizations have laid the groundwork for the development of "report cards," which should be disseminated widely to fill the current information void for health consumers. Over the next several years, we predict that this distribution of information, together with the large-scale public-private initiatives to improve the measurement of quality of care, will drive managed care organizations to improve their services or be forced out of the market.

NURSING'S CONTRIBUTION TO IMPROVING QUALITY

Nurses are at the center of the managed care revolution in health care delivery. Indeed, they are more critical now than they were under traditional fee-for-service settings. With the influence of managed care, never before has nursing leadership been more crucial to the future of the health care delivery system. Nurses are the key professionals at the nerve centers of managed health care, and in those roles they have extraordinary influence to bring patient advocacy and quality of care priorities to the center of the health care delivery systems. Nurses have particular influence in the two particular roles described below.

Prevention and primary care

Nurses have a long history of competence and dedication in this area of health care. Nurses have long been advocates of elevating the priority of primary care in the U.S. health care system, from visiting nurses at the turn of the century who provided all health needs for new immigrants to today's nurse practitioners and nurse midwives practicing in all parts of the country (including traditionally underserved areas). Moreover, nurses in every setting have differed from the medical model in their approach to health care, preferring to treat the patient throughout the life cycle, instead of intervening only in an instance of illness or disease.

Because the most critical element of managed care is the primary care gatekeeper encounter, nurse practitioners, clinical nurse specialists, and other advanced nurse providers can have a critical role in the delivery system of the future. All of the many studies on the subject have demonstrated that nurses provide a quality of care that is equal to, and in some cases superior to, the care provided by primary care physicians.

Nurses will have to assert leadership both individually

and as a profession in order to assume these crucial roles in today's fast-growing arena of managed care. Some managed care organizations, such as Humana, do not use advanced nurse providers at all, while others use fewer than they could. Meanwhile, policy makers and providers continually call for increased incentives to attract physicians into primary care roles and fund medical education for family practitioners. Nursing is often excluded from discussions that center on improving the primary care infrastructure. As managed care increasingly dominates health care delivery, it will be essential for nurses to assert publicly the value of their services.

In the process, nurses must optimize the value of their services to meet the changing demands of the managed care environment. Primary among these is the need to increase productivity. The capitated payment structure means that each primary care provider under managed care must meet productivity guidelines. The nursing model of care emphasizes spending time with patients and listening to them, skills at which most nurses excel. However, if nursing care is to be competitive and earn its rightful place in the managed health care system of the future, nurses must learn to provide a high level of quality while balancing more severe time constraints than ever before. If nursing practice does not accommodate these new demands, the marketplace will not long accommodate them.

Assessment and utilization review

Another role requiring nursing leadership is the continued development and operation of internal and external regulatory organizations that govern the managed care industry. Within managed care organizations nurses frequently function as case managers, reviewing utilization of services. This is clearly one of the cutting edge jobs in the managed care industry, literally inventing the notion of external review of physicians' decisions. In addition, regulatory agencies and policy-making bodies that oversee managed care require nursing expertise to evaluate managed care companies, develop plans for integrating managed care into existing health programs, and provide the perspective of a health professional known to be a patient advocate. Thus nurses are invaluable authorities in the evolving new health care delivery system.

Ultimately, nurses are at the eye of the storm as the health care system undergoes rapid transformation. Nurses have an option in this new environment. They can quietly go about their business, hoping managed care organizations recognize their talents and include them prominently in the many areas in which nurses have expertise and experience. Or nurses can assert leadership, provide information, and take hold of their rightful place in the delivery system of the future. By taking the latter approach, nurses will secure and expand the role of the profession in the future. More importantly, however, nursing leadership will help to create a delivery system that emphasizes quality of care as much as it does cost-effectiveness. Nurses should not abdicate this responsibility or miss this opportunity to fulfill nursing's mission.

As the nation's health care delivery system converts to managed care, the forces of competition and the increasing demand for consumer information on performance will drive managed care organizations to improve quality continually or be forced out of the market. The nursing profession has a unique but brief opportunity to assume a central role in this transformation.

REFERENCES

Blendon, R., Mebane, F., Brody, M., Benson, J., Taylor, H., Leitman, R., Knox, R. (1994). Managed care: Public and employer perspectives. In R. Blendon & M.M. Brodie (Eds.), *Transforming the system: Building a new structure for a new century.* Washington, DC: Faulkner and Gray, Inc.

Bloch, R. (1995, November 29). Comments at "Cross Training for Medicaid Managed Care" conference sponsored by New York State Departments of Health and Social Services at the Mariott in New York.

Davis, K., Collins, K.S., Schoen, C., & Morris, C. (1995). Choice matters for consumers. *Health Affairs, 14.*

Edlin, M. (1995). How good is HEDIS? *Managed Healthcare, 5,* 30-32.

Green, M., von Nostitz, G., Piel, S., & Petroff, D. (1996). What ails HMOs—a consumer diagnosis and Rx. New York: Office of the Public Advocate for the City of New York.

Miller, R., & Luft, H. (1994). Managed care plan performance since 1980: A literature analysis. *Journal of the American Medical Association, 271,* 1512-1518.

National Committee for Quality Assurance. (1995, July). Medicaid HEDIS. Washington DC: Author.

National Committee for Quality Assurance (NCQA). (1996, February). Medicaid HEDIS. Washington, DC: Author.

Rosenthal, E. (1996, January 15). Managed Care Has Trouble Treating AIDS, Patients Say. *New York Times,* p. A1.

Rowland, D., Rosenbaum, S., Simon, L., & Chait, E. (1995, March). *Medicaid and managed care: Lessons from the literature.* The Kaiser Commission on the Future of Medicaid.

Schulte, F., & Bergal, J. (1994, December 12). Healthy profits: Owners of Medicaid HMOs are making a lot of money—courtesy of taxpayers. *The Sun-Sentinel.*

Shouldice, R. (1991). *Introduction to managed care.* Information Resources Press.

Winslow, R. (1994, June 23). Performance of HMOs is rated higher than fee-for-service plans in study. *The Wall Street Journal.*

Standards and guidelines: Do they make any difference?

SUSAN L. DEAN-BAAR

What is the purpose of having standards and guidelines for nursing practice? Is there any benefit to having a framework for standards and guidelines that has been developed collaboratively among professional nursing organizations? What is the impact of such a framework on current nursing practice? Do standards and guidelines have any relationship to quality? These are just some of the questions that have been raised since the development of a unifying framework for standards and guidelines for nursing practice. Standards can be categorized into three groups related to the source from which they originate: professional nursing association standards, institution-specific agencies, and regulatory agencies (Smith & Popovich, 1993). The framework discussed in this chapter was developed by the American Nurses Association (ANA) in conjunction with more than 30 specialty nursing organizations (ANA, 1991a). For additional information, Schroeder (1991) provides a comprehensive review of other approaches to standards in nursing.

HISTORY OF PROFESSIONAL NURSING STANDARDS

A component of the ANA's core mission is its responsibility for defining nursing, establishing the scope of nursing practice, and setting the standards of nursing practice. In 1952, the ANA established functions, standards, and qualification committees that serve as the roots of today's practice standards.

In 1973, the ANA Congress for Nursing Practice published the generic *Standards of Nursing Practice,* which was based on the nursing process and provided a systematic approach to nursing practice in any setting and in any specialty area. Over the next 15 years there were numerous standards documents published both by the ANA and other specialty nursing organizations. Definitions of standards developed by professional nursing organizations ranged from setting a baseline for practice or minimum expectations to establishing a goal for practice or level of excellence. In addition to the various definitions there were also multiple approaches to the structure and format of standards. Many used a structure, process, and outcome format that reflected the ANA model for quality assurance (ANA, 1975).

An analysis of standards published by the ANA between 1973 and 1989 found that standards related to areas other than the nursing process were being included (McGuffin & Mariani, 1990). These additional areas were theory, organizations, continuity of care, collaboration, professional development and continuing education, quality assurance and peer review, research, community systems, and ethics. There was considerable repetition among these standards and apparent confusion between the concepts of professional development and continuing education and quality assurance and peer review. McGuffin and Mariani (1990) also found that at least four specialty areas had published criteria for selected nursing diagnoses in those areas. The authors recommended that those aspects of practice that consistently appear in or affect practice be shared among areas of nursing to avoid duplication and that agreement be reached on the broad category headings. In addition, they concluded that clarification and consistency were needed in several areas, including how the categories of professional practice and professional performance standards are defined and whether standards indicate a minimum or maximum level of practice.

The diversity of definitions and frameworks for standards during this time resulted in a fragmented approach and confusion over the purpose of standards for nursing practice. In 1988, the ANA began a process of reevaluating the nature and purpose of standards of nursing practice as a result of the concerns that had been raised during this evolution. These concerns included the inability to use standards to evaluate the effectiveness of care, the lack of consistency in the process used to develop professional standards, the proliferation of standards of nursing practice, and the wide range in the intent, format, and scope of standards. The divergent and numerous approaches used in standards limited their usefulness to nurses, other health care providers, payers, policy makers, and consumers for use in a variety of activities such as clinical decision making and quality activities. As a result of other activities within the health care arena, including some of the work being done by the Agency for Health Care Policy and Research (AHCPR), the work on evaluating the nature and purpose of standards was expanded to include the purpose and format of guidelines for practice (ANA, 1991a).

The development of the framework for nursing practice standards and guidelines that resulted from this evaluation began with a critical analysis of the environment internal and external to nursing. This included discussion representing the perspectives of nurses in a variety of practice roles and settings with input from numerous specialty groups, state nurses associations, and ANA structural units. This process and the framework that resulted were substantially different from previous standards work done by the ANA.

MODEL FOR PROFESSIONAL NURSING STANDARDS AND GUIDELINES

The model for standards and guidelines for practice has the potential to serve as a unifying framework to evaluate the quality of nursing in a variety of practice settings. The combined model for standards of nursing practice and practice guidelines is designed to provide direction for nursing practice, a means to evaluate practice, and a way in which the profession can describe its accountability to the public. Each of these is important to building a foundation that ensures quality.

Standards

Within the model, standards and guidelines differ primarily in their scope and intent. The purpose of standards is to provide broad direction for the overall practice of nursing, including the provision of care and professional role activities. *Standards* are authoritative statements that describe a level of care or performance common to the profession of nursing by which the quality of nursing practice can be judged (ANA, 1991a). They reflect the values of the profession and further explicate the definition of professional practice. Standards of clinical nursing practice are divided into two categories: care and professional performance (Table 39-1). The intent of standards of care is to describe an acceptable level of client or patient care; the intent of standards of professional performance is to describe an acceptable level of behavior in the professional nurse's role. Standards of care describe a competent level of care as demonstrated by the nursing process involving assessment, diagnosis, outcome identification, planning, implementation, and evaluation. Standards of professional performance describe a competent level of behavior in the professional role including activities related to quality of care, performance appraisal, education, collegiality, ethics, collaboration, research, and resource utilization (ANA, 1991b).

These definitions of standards clearly delineate their role in setting a competent level of care or performance. This is a significant change from previous standards that were designed to describe excellence and were not intended to define minimum levels of nursing care or legal parameters for measuring the quality of care. Each of the standards of nursing practice includes criteria that will allow them to be measured. These criteria are relevant, measurable indicators of the standard. The framework was developed with the belief that standards are anticipated to remain relatively stable over time but that the criteria may change due to advancements in knowledge and technology.

The framework was intended to be a model for devel-

Table 39-1 Standards of clinical nursing practice

Standards of care	Standards of professional performance
Assessment	Quality of care
Diagnosis	Performance appraisal
Outcome identification	Education
Planning	Collegiality
Implementation	Ethics
Evaluation	Collaboration
	Research
	Resource utilization

Note. From *Standards of Clinical Nursing Practice*, by the American Nurses Association, 1991, Washington, DC: Author. Copyright American Nurses Association.

oping standards of clinical practice for specialty areas. Differentiation among specialty areas could be accomplished by developing criteria that reflected the common level of performance for nurses practicing in a given specialty for each of the standards. These standards of practice would be congruent with the intent, format, and scope of the general standards of clinical nursing practice. Thus the standards would not change, but the criteria will change to reflect the specialty area, in essence creating standards of practice for that particular area. This approach is being used as specialty areas of practice revise their own standards. Community health, gerontology, home health, otorhinolaryngology, psychiatric-mental health, public health, rehabilitation, and respiratory nursing are among those specialties that have adopted the model for the development of standards of practice. Most of these groups have worked with the ANA in the revision of their standards. Only a few specialty groups have used the model in independently developing standards of practice for their specialty. It is still too early to assess whether the collaborative development of the model with over 30 specialty groups will result in all of those groups actually adopting the model when it comes to development of standards in each area. If specialty areas of practice develop standards using different definitions, intents, or formats the strength of the model's application in providing a framework by which to evaluate the quality of nursing across settings and areas will be weakened.

One area into which the model has expanded is advanced practice. The first advanced practice standards using this framework have been published for the acute care nurse practitioner (ANA & American Association of Critical Care Nurses, 1995). Standards for all advanced practice nurses have been developed (ANA, 1996). These could be adapted for specialty areas of practice in much the same way as can be done for the standards of clinical nursing practice.

This model for standards does not incorporate the structure, process, and outcome formats frequently used in the past. However, the deletion of this format does not negate the importance of structure, process, and outcome attributes in evaluating quality of care (Donabedian, 1988). Structure attributes are those related to the setting in which the care occurs. What had previously been labeled as "structure criteria" are more appropriate as separate standards related to the administrative domain. Process reflects the actions taken in giving and receiving care, and in this framework are reflected within both standards and guidelines. Outcomes reflect the effects of care and are patient- or client-focused. Outcomes are more appropriately included as part of guidelines for practice.

Guidelines

In contrast, *guidelines* describe a process of patient or client care management that has the potential to improve the quality of clinical and consumer decision making. The goal of guidelines is to describe a recommended course of action to address a specific nursing diagnosis, clinical condition, or the needs of a particular patient or client population. They guide practice by providing links among diagnoses, treatments, and outcomes and by describing available alternatives.

This approach to guidelines is similar to that in previous work done within nursing that was frequently labeled "standards." This is reflected most commonly in the standardized care plan approach to planning and providing nursing care. Both approaches attempted to describe a course of action to address a specific need or diagnosis, and also have the potential to reduce variation in clinical practice.

However, there are some significant differences in the approaches. One of the major differences is in the change in terminology from "standards" to "guidelines." Standards in health care are commonly interpreted from a legal perspective as written documents that are intended to be applied rigidly and to be followed in virtually all cases. Exceptions to following a standard would be rare and difficult to justify. In addition, standards are considered the foundation for safe health provider practices and not following them would indicate unsafe and incompetent practice (W. Carson, personal communication, 1992). Guidelines are recommendations for patient management and may include a range of interventions or strategies, and as such, would not meet the characteristics just described. Another difference is the intent of guidelines to describe alternatives and to assist nurses in decision making. One of the difficulties frequently encountered in practice is the inability to use standardized care plans because of the individual characteristics of the patient or client situation. Standardized plans of care do not account for the complexity and comorbidity frequently present in individuals. The intent of guidelines is to identify those circumstances in which it is known that the guideline would not be appropriate or would need modification in either interventions or expected outcomes.

Guidelines convert science-based knowledge into clinical action in a form that is accessible to practitioners. They reflect knowledge generated through research and professional consensus by practitioners regarding preferred interventions for a particular problem or select group of patients or clients. Guidelines have the potential for decreasing variability in practice by providing nurses and other providers with a synthesis of published information that can decrease the amount of professional uncertainty that occurs in making diagnosis and treatment decisions.

The development of guidelines is occurring in many arenas. The AHCPR has devoted considerable resources to developing multidisciplinary guidelines (AHCPR, 1993). All of the guidelines developed by the AHCPR have included at least one nurse as a member of the panel developing the guideline. Several guidelines released by the AHCPR have focused on clinical conditions in which nursing makes a significant contribution to the care and outcomes of the affected individuals (e.g., acute pain management, cancer pain management, prediction and prevention of pressure ulcers, treatment of pressure ulcers, and incontinence).

To assist nursing specialty groups and other nursing groups, the ANA published a manual describing a process that could be used in the development of clinical practice guidelines (Marek, 1995). As nursing groups become involved in the development of guidelines the following issues should be considered in choosing a topic for development: nursing's contribution to the care of the client; variation in nursing interventions and outcomes; the impact of the clinical condition on the client's physical, psychological, and social functioning; costs of caring for the client with the clinical condition and variations in those costs; the high incidence or prevalence of the clinical condition; and the extent of the research base. Once these questions have been answered the scope of the guideline must be identified and the client or patient population, care settings, assessment criteria, interventions, and outcomes, and the intended audience for the guideline must be defined.

In the development of practice guidelines, certain characteristics should be taken into consideration to maximize their usefulness. First, they should be reasonable in view of the state of the art. Interventions and outcomes described within a practice guideline should be possible and should not be developed in a way that renders them unreasonable to implement or achieve. They should be comprehensible by nurses, other health care providers, and consumers. They should be consistent in format across specialties. They must be measurable, and they must be validated by research or professional consensus. The process for reviewing and updating guidelines will need to be dynamic so that guidelines can reflect changes in knowledge and technological capabilities.

From the early stages in the discussion of how professional nursing organizations should be involved in guideline development the course has not been as clear and consistent as it has been with the development of standards. The working paper of the original task force (ANA, 1991a) describes an approach to guidelines that underwent almost immediate revision. This included a revised definition that is used in this chapter and the deletion of references to different types of guidelines within nursing (ANA, 1992). It became increasingly clear that the development of guidelines that would meet the attributes proposed by the work of the ANA Committee on Nursing Practice Standards and Guidelines in conjunction with representatives of specialty nursing organizations through the Nursing Organization Liaison Forum would take considerable organizational resources and would probably require collaboration between several nursing organizations.

In contrast to the expectations at the time the model for professional nursing standards and guidelines was developed, no professional nursing organization has yet developed guidelines that meet the definition and characteristics described. Organizational representatives who participated in the development of the model were very encouraging in their assessment that collaborative development of practice guidelines was a realistic goal. Perhaps part of the reason that guideline development by professional nursing organizations has not occurred is the realization by all groups involved that it is a very complex, expensive process if it is to be done well. The U.S. Government Accounting Office (1991) reported in a review of 35 medical specialty societies that guideline development generally took from 1 to 3 years, and costs ranged from $5,000 and $130,000 per guideline and did not reflect the volunteer time required of members.

It has also become clear that most health care practices have no basis in published scientific research. This may be true of 80% to 90% of common practices (James, 1995). The use of published scientific research is a cornerstone of well-developed guidelines. This may be another reason why the development of guidelines by professional nursing organizations is not occurring.

The new model developed collaboratively with the ANA and more than 30 specialty nursing organizations makes clear distinctions between standards and guidelines for practice. These distinctions in intent and definition are important in determining the appropriate use of standards and guidelines. However, they are both equally important in evaluating nursing practice and the quality of care provided. Standards of clinical nursing practice provide a framework to evaluate the individual professional nurse's overall performance. Guidelines provide a means to evaluate the quality of nursing care provided to a specific patient or population. Components of the standards of care should be embedded within guidelines. Within a guideline should be information about assessment, diagnosis, outcome identification, planning, implementation, and evaluation of that specific diagnosis or clinical condition.

USE OF STANDARDS AND GUIDELINES IN PRACTICE

Standards of nursing practice and practice guidelines can serve as the basis for many activities within nursing (Dean-Baar, 1993; Taylor, 1994). Nationally published guidelines and standards can be used in the development of agency-specific documents. Guidelines can serve as the basis for the development of agency-specific policies and procedures and are being used to develop clinical pathways (Brandt, 1994; Duncan & Otto, 1995). Guidelines also can be used to promote patient or client participation in health care decision making by clarifying health care choices (including choice of practitioner) and their consequences for the patient or client.

The standards of clinical nursing practice are being used to develop job descriptions and performance appraisal systems that support quality professional practice. In those agencies with clinical or career ladders, the standards can serve as the framework for the initial step of the ladder with additional stages reflecting increased expectations for practice.

The components of standards embedded in guidelines can be used in conjunction with the Nursing Minimum Data Set (Werley & Lang, 1988) to develop database systems that can provide valuable information on the quality of nursing care. They could also serve as the basis for including relevant nursing information in large database systems such as the Health Care Finance Administration. The inclusion of elements in databases that reflect nursing's contributions to patient or client care can assist in positioning nursing to be included more clearly in discussions of cost and payment for providing health care services.

In addition, the standards of clinical nursing practice and content of guidelines for practice can be incorporated into certification activities. Particularly, those guidelines developed by national agencies or organizations have been the focus of educational offerings aimed at disseminating the information to practitioners so that quality of care can be improved.

Perhaps the most important area in which standards and guidelines are used is quality improvement. Standards and guidelines can be used to develop institution-, agency-, or unit-based quality programs that demonstrate that the organization is delivering safe, effective, and appropriate care. Written, meaningful standards and guidelines are essential to developing quality improvement programs. They can serve as the basis for quality improvement systems by identifying important aspects of performance or care within either the standards or a specific guideline. These can be used to identify indicators of quality nursing care that are then monitored. The AHCPR has described how to translate clinical practice guidelines into evaluation tools and how to use those tools to evaluate the quality of care provided (AHCPR, 1995a, 1995b). The data collected can be used to improve quality of care.

In evaluating nursing's performance in relation to professional standards, organizations can use the standards of practice and the criteria for each to develop their own indicators and make decisions about how and what data should be collected to determine the degree to which the standard is being met. Because of the framework's ability to include general and specialty areas of practice, an institution or agency could use the same approach as the framework in developing its program. This approach provides for many possibilities, including the capability to evaluate practice not only within an agency but also across agencies.

If nursing uses the standards of clinical practice and practice guidelines to develop quality improvement programs, the potential of being able to demonstrate clearly the contribution of nursing in providing quality care within that setting would be considerable. As health care becomes increasingly competitive, information on quality becomes even more valuable.

SUMMARY

Standards of clinical nursing practice and guidelines are essential to professional nursing. They are one mechanism that we use to describe and define the scope of professional nursing practice. Standards and guidelines can make a difference but not if the profession continues to be inconsistent in their development, definition, and use. As the standards of clinical nursing practice are implemented and work continues on the development and implementation of practice guidelines, we must develop ways to translate this work into ways that assist in articulating the contributions of professional nursing practice to the health and well-being of patients and clients.

It is still too early to tell what will be the benefits to having a framework for standards and guidelines that was developed collaboratively among professional nursing organizations. It becomes clearer every day, however, that the potential to speak with one voice about the role of standards and guidelines in describing our practice and our contributions to the outcomes of patients and clients is essential. Common definitions of "standard" and "guideline" can only help to articulate clearly the critical role that nursing plays in the planning and delivering of quality, appropriate, and effective health care.

REFERENCES

Agency for Health Care Policy and Research. (1993). *Clinical practice guideline development.* (AHCPR Publication No. 93-0023). Rockville, MD: Author.

Agency for Health Care Policy and Research. (1995a). *Using clinical practice guidelines to evaluate quality of care: Issue* (Vol. 1) (AHCPR Publication No. 95-0045). Rockville, MD: Author.

Agency for Health Care Policy and Research. (1995b). *Using clinical practice guidelines to evaluate quality of care: Methodology* (Vol. 2) (AHCPR Publication No. 95-0046). Rockville, MD: Author.

American Nurses Association, (1975). *A plan for implementation of standards of nursing practice.* Washington, DC: Author.

American Nurses Association. (1991a). Task force on nursing practice standards and guidelines; Working paper. *Journal of Nursing Care Quality, 5*(3), 1-17.

American Nurses Association. (1991b). *Standards of clinical nursing practice.* Washington, DC: Author.

American Nurses Association. (1992). *Second working paper of the ANA Committee on Nursing Practice Standards and Guidelines.* Washington, DC: Author.

American Nurses Association & American Association of Critical Care Nurses. (1995). *Standards of clinical practice and scope of practice for the acute care nurse practitioner.* Washington, DC: Author.

American Nurses Association. (1996). *Scopes and standards of advanced practice registered nursing.* Washington, DC: Author.

Brandt, M. (1994). Clinical practice guidelines and critical paths-road maps to quality, cost-effective care: Part II. *Journal of AHIMA, 65*(2), 54-57.

Dean-Baar, S. (1993). Application of the new ANA framework for nursing practice standards and guidelines. *Journal of Nursing Care Quality, 8*(1), 33-42.

Donabedian, A. (1988). The quality of care: How can it be assessed? *Journal of the American Medical Association, 260*(12), 1743-1748.

Duncan, S.K., & Otto, S.E. (1995). Implementing guidelines for acute pain management. *Nursing Management, 26*(5), 40-47.

James, B.C. (1995). Implementing practice guidelines through clinical quality improvement. In N.O. Graham (Ed.), *Quality in health care: Theory, application, and evolution.* (pp. 157-187). Gaithersburg, MD: Aspen.

Marek, K. (1995). *Manual to develop guidelines.* Washington, DC: American Nurses Association.

McGuffin, B., & Mariani, M. (1990). Clinical nursing standards: Toward a synthesis. *Journal of Nursing Quality Assurance, 4*(3), 35-45.

Schroeder, P. (1991). *Approaches to nursing standards.* Gaithersburg, MD: Aspen.

Smith, T.C., & Popovich, J.M. (1993). Health care standards: The interstitial matter of quality programs. *Journal of Nursing Care Quality, 8*(1), 1-11.

Taylor, J.W. (1994). *Implementation of nursing practice standards and guidelines.* Washington, DC: American Nurses Association.

U. S. Government Accounting Office. (1991). *Practice guidelines: The experience of medical specialty societies* (Publication PEMD-91-11). Washington, DC: Author.

Werley, H., & Lang, N. (Eds.) (1988). *Identification of the Nursing Minimum Data Set.* New York: Springer.

The use of clinical pathways: Do they improve quality?

SUSAN PARK KYZER

The concept of clinical pathways has been evolving over the past decade. Very appropriate to the title of this viewpoint chapter, the idea for clinical pathways was born out of a concern for quality of care (Zander, 1991b). Although the concept has been used successfully for cost containment, clinical pathways would not have achieved the robust health they enjoy today had they not also held the key to maintaining quality. Economic necessity has forced everyone involved in health care to become cost-conscious. However, the heart of the health care must not be moved from its focus on quality of care for the patient and family.

In 1983 one of the most dramatic changes in modern health care occurred with the enactment of the diagnosis-related group (DRG) legislation. Faced with the first external control of care delivery, the Nursing Department of the New England Medical Center determined to ". . . address the demand to incorporate patient-centered, quality nursing care within the context of DRG's, length of stay and cost-effectiveness" (Zander, 1985). The clinical systems that evolved from that determination—case management plans, critical pathways, and then fully developed clinical pathway systems—require that three questions be answered. These questions aim for the root of providing quality health care: (1) What work is required to get patients within certain case types to desired outcomes? (2) What is the best way to produce these outcomes? (3) Who is accountable for the results? (Zander and McGill, 1994). These basic questions are as relevant today as they were in 1983.

DEFINITIONS

A *clinical pathway* is a multidisciplinary plan for patient care that sequences interventions and clinical outcomes on a timeline (Zander, 1991a). Clinical pathways are developed for homogeneous patient populations and are uniquely different from traditional care plans in the following ways:

- Clinical pathways are multidisciplinary, and therefore truly represent patient care plans rather than nursing care plans.
- A multidisciplinary team is formed to author the clinical pathway; therefore, care is planned in an interrelated, more comprehensive fashion and reflects the care as experienced by the patient rather than by each discipline's separate focus.
- The interventions are planned on a timeline, thereby providing shift-to-shift and day-to-day continuity and coordination of the activities needed to move the patient toward desired outcomes.
- Anticipated clinical outcomes statements at key points on the timeline assist clinicians in evaluating the clinical progress of patients (even if "This is my first day back" or "I was pulled and don't usually work with this kind of patient"), thereby focusing the caregiving team on patient outcomes of care rather than on task completion only.
- Clinical pathways are written for the environment in which the work is done by a team of expert clinicians who will be using them, thereby creating a plan of care that uniquely reflects the resources and working patterns that exist in that delivery setting.

Quality of care has been defined by a working group of the Institute of Medicine as ". . . the degree to which health services for individuals and populations increase the likelihood of desired health outcomes and are consistent with current professional knowledge" (Mitchell, 1993). Traditionally, quality has been measured by negatives such as morbidity and mortality, unexpected returns to surgery, nosocomial infections, iatrogenic complications, and readmission rates. This level of measurement ". . . in essence, quantifies what went wrong in patient care" (Nash, 1993). However, the absence of "something going wrong," while important, does not necessarily equate to quality care. The focus is now shifting to more positive quality measures such as ". . . survival, clinical condition-specific endpoints, health status (physiological, psychological and emotional health), functional status, general well-being and satisfaction with care" (Mitchell, 1993). Increased consistency, continuity, and coordination of care as well as interdisciplinary collaboration are factors underlying improved quality for patients and families. Based on the previous definitions of a clinical pathway and quality of care the view expressed here is that quality of care can be improved by the development and use of clinical pathways.

IMPROVING QUALITY OF CARE

Quality of care can be improved at each step in the process of developing and implementing a clinical pathway for a specific population of patients—during the initial process of clinical pathway development, as the clinical pathway content is written, as clinicians use the pathway to guide patient care, and as data generated from use of the pathway are reviewed and evaluated and changes made to further improve care. There are many specific examples of improved quality that have occurred in various settings in relation to each of these steps.

Quality of care is often improved during the initial process of clinical pathway development. One of the first steps in writing a clinical pathway is bringing together a team of expert clinicians who are involved in caring for a specific patient population (i.e., case-type). This in itself is an exciting event because it is often the first time all of the people involved in caring for these patients are able to sit down together to talk about all of the aspects of that care. This team meeting provides a structure and a time for examining system issues and problems from a patient outcome focus. Caregivers get to know one another and understand each others' disciplines better, think of ways to smooth out communications and coordination of care, and begin to form cooperative and collaborative relationships, thereby enabling them to work toward the same outcomes.

On an orthopedic unit, for example, nurses routinely required patients with total hip replacements to sit up for lunch after their morning physical therapy. During the clinical pathway development meeting it came to light that frequently the afternoon physical therapy session accomplished little as a result of patient fatigue. After some discussion, the unit nursing staff changed their routine and began allowing patients to rest after the morning session. Patients were then able to take better advantage of their afternoon physical therapy sessions. Instead of nursing and physical therapy attempting to obtain a certain level of patient activity individually, they became aware of each others' routines and developed a plan that would best assist the patients in reaching their desired clinical outcomes.

Quality of care can be improved as the content of the clinical pathway is written. These improvements may include better sequencing and timing of interventions, care that is based on current professional knowledge, care that is planned from a patient focus, and better coordination and continuity of care from setting to setting. Following are examples of these improvements.

In planning care for patients with elective total hip replacement the clinical outcome desired was early ambulation in order to prevent deep vein thrombosis, pneumonia, and urinary tract infection. In discussing how soon patients could be expected to ambulate, one problem identified by the physical therapist was the difficulty in teaching patients with postoperative pain to use a walker. It was decided that a physical therapist would see these patients for walker training prior to surgery when this new skill could be mastered without the added distraction of postoperative pain. The altered sequence of events involving a physical therapy consult prior to rather than after surgery resulted in earlier ambulation for this group of patients.

In another group of patients, digoxin levels were drawn routinely at 6 a.m., medication administered at 9 a.m., and reports from morning blood draws posted at 10 a.m., resulting in a day's delay in adjusting medication dosages. When unit staff and laboratory personnel realized that their respective routines were not really focused on the patients, adjustments in timing were made so that results were posted and dosages adjusted prior to the administration of morning medications.

During a team meeting to develop a clinical pathway for cesarean section, a discussion took place regarding the appropriate prophylactic intravenous antibiotic to use. The physicians at the meeting agreed that research would support the use of any one of several first-generation antibiotics, and were quite surprised when the pharmacist reported that many of their colleagues were routinely using third-generation antibiotics for this purpose, contrary to published recommendations. Using the clinical pathway process, the hospital was able to standardize a more appropriate treatment choice among the physicians.

In another example, after establishing a preadmission testing program for elective hip replacement patients, the clinical pathway team examined the provision of care from the patient's perspective. They realized that patients (who usually were experiencing pain on walking already) were being required to go to seven different departments, some of them quite distant from one another, to complete the preadmission program. Further changes were made so that patients could remain in one location to complete all testing. This decreased the average time a patient spent at the preadmission visit from several hours to about 1 hour. Patient and family satisfaction increased dramatically.

The Hospital Association of New York State has developed a model that ". . . extends beyond the acute-care hospital stay in both directions. They (the pathways) begin with pre-admission and continue through post-discharge" (Causey, 1992). The entire episode is included, resulting in well-coordinated continuity of care.

These examples illustrate simple changes that are not difficult to make once the problems have been identified but obviously improve quality of care. The process of getting clinicians together to discuss the kind of continual quality care they would like to deliver produces these kinds of changes. Interdisciplinary collaboration is increased as clinicians get to know one another, begin to appreciate each other's viewpoints, and work together with patient outcomes as the primary focus. Not only is formal collaboration increased (e.g., in team meetings and interdisciplinary rounds) but informal collaboration is also increased, on the phone, at the bedside, and in day-to-day activities. According to Lord, "For pathways to become truly meaningful, you need to define and design the process for the continuum of care—beginning with the patient's entry into the health care system, not just the component that's delivered in the hospital" (Lumsdon & Hagland, 1993). More and more hospitals, physician offices, outpatient settings, and home care agencies are joining together to do just that—plan care from a patient's perspective so that desired outcomes can be identified, achieved, and measured for the entire episode of care across the continuum.

Quality of care is improved as clinicians use the pathway to provide continuity of plan. Creative staffing patterns, more part-time workers, flexible staffing, float pool and agency staff use, and increased use of contract staff for therapies all contribute to the loss of continuity of caregiver; and therefore it is extremely important to maximize continuity of care planning. A clinical pathway provides continuity of plan from shift to shift and from day to day even as caregivers change (Flynn & Kilgallen, 1993). Having a tool that displays the patient's progress visually and states key outcomes to evaluate greatly assists caregivers. When a patient has not met the intermediate outcomes for a particular time interval, caregivers are alerted to look for corrective actions that can help the patient continue to make progress. As a result, care is more proactive and problems are recognized earlier. Details of care that might sometimes be missed or forgotten appear on the clinical pathway to serve as a "cuing mechanism" for staff. Care is complex, and varies from patient to patient; if the essential components of care are not blueprinted they may be forgotten or not done on time. As a result, patient outcomes may be jeopardized (Campbell, 1992).

For example, a dietitian might say, "The drug-food interactions are done before I arrive!" Tasks like this no longer "fall through the cracks" as accountabilities are clarified and the clinical pathway structures the total care. Another problem with regard to the timing of administration of intravenous prophylactic antibiotics prior to surgery was eliminated by listing the time frame and the person (position) responsible for administration of the medication on the pathway. This clarified who was accountable for this procedure and provided the means to track success in meeting the specified time frame.

Another example is that of a patient who is on "post-op day 3" of a total hip clinical pathway. The anticipated intermediate outcome is "Ambulates with assistance 10 feet," but the patient is unable to accomplish this outcome. Prior to having the clinical pathway, staff would not have been particularly focused on evaluating ambulation at this point, but because this has been identified as a key outcome the nurse and physical therapist will discuss the situation and try to determine the reason. Is the patient's inability to walk a result of excessive pain? Is the problem nausea or weakness? What about the hematocrit? Depending on the situation and the answers to these and other questions the caregivers will decide whether there are any corrective actions that can be taken or whether there is a need to involve other members of the health care team. Noting the patient's lack of progression and early intervention promote accomplishing the desired outcomes.

Quality of care is improved as clinicians review data generated by aggregating variance from the clinical pathway over a period of time. The clinical pathway represents the pattern of care and the desired patient outcomes. By measuring how care actually progresses against what is planned, both process and outcome are evaluated. Looking at achievement of outcomes for groups of patients over a period of time can reveal where the plan is working and where improvements can be made.

For example, a clinical pathway for bowel resection has as a postoperative outcome of "Bowel sounds present." A quarterly aggregation and analysis of data from this pathway showed that a number of patients did not achieve the stated outcome during the appropriate time interval and experienced ileus. Further investigation revealed that preoperative bowel preparations were being started too late in the day and therefore were not finished completely. An adjustment of routines and attention to starting and completing the bowel preparations appropriately resulted in a decreased incidence of ileus during the next quarter for bowel resection patients. In another example,

> When statistical analysis found that patients with dysphagia were prone to develop pneumonia, changes were instituted: 'Now the nurse assesses the patient's gag reflex and swallowing on admission. If dysphagia is suspected, the patient is made NPO, and the physician and other team members are notified.' . . . The new protocol for dysphagia has reduced complications and length of stay. (Luquire, 1994)

When data are generated in a systematic, ongoing fashion, evaluated, and changes made based on that data, improvement efforts are more likely to be directed at real rather than spurious issues. A clinical pathway and its associated measurement data provide a logical, methodical approach to quality improvement that is specific to patient populations and is supported by clinicians who really understand the problems.

RESULTS OF CLINICAL PATHWAYS WITH REGARD TO TRADITIONAL QUALITY MEASURES

Traditional quality measures of mortality, morbidity, readmission rates, complication rates, and patient satisfaction, while not the whole story, certainly cannot be overlooked. Here are some examples of the results of established clinical pathway systems.

- In a study done at the Toronto Hospital in Ontario, elderly patients with a fractured hip who managed with a clinical pathway (CareMap) had a statistically significantly better outcome at 6 months and fewer postoperative complications, and a greater number of the patients returned home within 14 days of admission (Ogilvie-Harris, Botsford, & Hawker, 1993).
- Patients having coronary artery bypass graft surgery without cardiac catherization at Scripps Memorial Hospital in La Jolla, California, spend less time on average in the intensive care unit and are extubated sooner—improvements that have in turn reduced the incidence of nosocomial pneumonia (Andersson, 1993).
- At Barnes Hospital in St. Louis, Missouri, using the Thoracotomy CarePath®, pulmonary complications such as atelectasis, pneumonia, and respiratory failure were reduced by 50% (Weilitz & Potter, 1993).
- With regard to the chemotherapy CarePath® at Barnes Hospital, ". . . improved communication between the hospital's outpatient cancer center, the pharmacy, and the nursing divisions resulted in chemotherapy drugs arriving on the nursing unit near the time of the patient's admission rather than several hours later. As a result, the hospital achieved greater efficiency in delivering patient care and improved physician and patient satisfaction" (Weilitz & Potter, 1993).
- The conclusion from a study done by Vanderbilt University Medical Center in Nashville, Tennessee and St. Thomas Hospital on the use of clinical pathways with cerebral revascularization patients states, "The dual approach of case management (clinical pathways) and selective use of the ICU promotes quality patient care, conserves financial resources without adversely affecting morbidity or mortality rates, enhances physician/nurse collaboration, and improves patient satisfaction" (Hoyle et al., 1994).
- At Scripps Memorial Hospital, monitoring of mortality, morbidity, and readmission rates has shown no deterioration in quality outcomes using CareTrac® (Trubo, 1993).
- Using clinical pathways at St. Luke's Episcopal Hospital in Houston, Texas, the readmission rate for neuroscience patients dropped from 5% to 1% (Luquire, 1994).

These are but a few of the published outcomes of the use of clinical pathways. Although much has been written about the use of clinical pathways to reduce length of stay and provide some measure of cost containment, this chapter has focused solely on quality improvement. It is quite evident that the development and use of clinical pathways can be a major quality strategy and that pathways are possibly the most powerful tool health care providers have to maintain and improve quality of care.

REFERENCES

Andersson, D. (1993). Scripps health: Quality planning for clinical processes of care. *The Quality Letter, 5*(8), 2-4.

Campbell, A., & Lakier, N. (1992). Process intervention—applying TQM to clinical care. *Healthcare Forum Journal, 35*(4), 81-83.

Causey, W. (1992). Clinical pathways seen as opportunity to integrate traditional QA with CQI. *Quality Improvement/Total Quality Management, 2*(4), 49-64.

Flynn, A., & Kilgallen, M. (1993). Case management: A multidisciplinary approach to the evaluation of cost and quality standards. *Journal of Nursing Care Quality, 8*(1), 4.

Hoyle, R., Jenkins, M., Edwards, W., Edwards, W., Martin, R., & Mulherin, J. (1994). Case management in cerebral revascularization. *Journal of Vascular Surgery, 20*(3), 396-401.

Lumsdon, K., & Hagland, M. (1993). Mapping care. *Hospitals & Health Networks, 67*(20), 34-40.

Luquire, R. (1994). Focusing on outcomes. *RN, 57*(5), 57-60.

Mitchell, P. (1993). Perspectives on outcome-oriented care systems. *Nursing Administration Quarterly, 17*(3), 4.

Nash, D. (1993). The state of the outcomes/guidelines movement. *Decisions in Imaging Economics*, 11-17.

Ogilvie-Harris, D., Botsford, D., & Hawker, R. (1993). Elderly patients with hip fractures: Improved outcome with the use of CareMaps with high-quality medical and nursing protocols. *Journal of Orthopaedic Trauma, 7*(5), 428-437.

Trubo, R. (1993). If this is cookbook medicine, you may like it. *Medical Economics, 70*(5), 69-82.

Weilitz, P., & Potter, P. (1993). A managed care system: Financial and clinical evaluation. *Journal of Nursing Administration, 23*(11), 51-57.

Zander, K. (1985). Defining nursing . . . roots and wings. *Definition, 1*, 2.

Zander, K. (1991a). CareMaps: The core of cost/quality care. *The New Definition, 6*(3),

Zander, K. (1991b). Critical pathways. In M. Mellum & M. Sinoris (Eds.), *Total quality management* (pp. 305-314). Chicago: American Hospital Association Publishing, Inc.

Zander, K., & McGill, R. (1994). Critical and anticipated recovery paths: Only the beginning. *Nursing Management, 25*(8), 34.

Total quality management, redesign, reengineering: What's the difference?

PAMELA KLAUER TRIOLO, SUSAN O. HENDRICKS, DAWN A. DUNCAN

In response to dynamic changes in the environment and increasing disenchantment with the high cost of health care, health care organizations are redesigning, restructuring, and reengineering themselves, launching quality improvement teams, and sponsoring cost-reduction projects. Terms are often used interchangeably today, and there is general confusion about whether reengineering is the same as redesign or total quality management (TQM) and where these initiatives fit within organizational performance improvement. This chapter presents information from the fields and gurus of TQM, redesign, and reengineering and provides a framework for understanding the similarities and differences among the three. The chapter begins with TQM because our experience leads us to believe that TQM is the "umbrella" for fostering a culture committed to constant, customer-focused performance improvement.

TOTAL QUALITY MANAGEMENT

In his recent book *Leading Change,* O'Toole (1995) observes that although we are willing and quick to accept and use scientific and technologic knowledge, the same cannot be said of social knowledge (O'Toole, 1995). He explores the reasons for this and observes the difficulty we find in accepting ideas that will challenge us to change our own behavior. Although this is a simplistic summary of O'Toole's thinking, it provides a basis for understanding both the great usefulness and the difficulties of pursuing what is most often referred to as TQM.

Total quality management integrates the knowledge and practices of many disciplines, including (but by no means limited to) the following: the marketer's focus on customers, the psychologist's study and facilitation of group dynamics, the statistician's understanding of variation, the sociologist's awareness of group behavior and interaction, the scientist's research methodology, the educator's approach to learning, the management theorist's observations and advice about commitment and accomplishment, the strategic planner's awareness of the market and priority setting, and the engineer's analytical methods. The beauty of this collection is that one need not be an expert in all disciplines in order to take advantage of their knowledge and practice. Over the years, TQM has developed approaches and tools that allow people to come together to improve their own work and to bring to bear upon it the collective wisdom of many specialists. Berwick has described it as enabling us to become "scientists of the work" (Berwick, 1992, p. 1).

Although TQM provides both philosophy and tools for action, it involves us in situations that are unfamiliar and potentially uncomfortable. For example, some of us, particularly those in the highly technologic and scientific world of health care, are more comfortable with individualistic analysis in the company of others in our own disciplines. The team approach, which involves shared data development and analysis as well as creative collaboration with people of diverse backgrounds and perspectives, requires an openness to personal challenge and growth. The rewards, however, are not only the improvement of processes and outcomes but also what Deming came to call "joy in work" (Berwick, Blanton, & Roessner, 1990, p. 148).

History

In most industries there is a long history of quality control. Typically, this has involved inspecting the outcomes of the work, noticing errors and faulty products, and then investigating. This process of inspection has often become one of assigning blame and suggests a theory of "bad apples" (Berwick, 1989). In health care it is known as *quality assurance*. The aims of quality assurance have always been honorable but the practice has often resulted in fear of blame without providing the knowledge and means for improvement. Furthermore, the practice has been reactive rather than proactive, focused backward rather than forward, attending to fixing presumably broken parts rather than providing the means to improve overall systems.

Many of the early thinkers in the shift to a philosophy and practice for improvement (as opposed to inspection) were engineers such as Shewhart, Deming, Juran, and Crosby. Deming found an audience willing to adopt his ideas in Japan during that country's efforts to recover from the economic devastation of World War II. His "Fourteen Points," nicely described in Walton's *The Deming Management Method,* summarize his approach (Walton, 1986). His system of profound knowledge, described in *The New Economics,* provides guidance in the skills needed for the work of improvement: appreciation for a system, knowledge about variation and psychology, and a theory of knowledge (Deming, 1993).

American companies noticed and attempted to apply the improvement philosophy some years later. Most notably, American automobile makers took notice when Japanese cars surpassed American cars in both quality and sales. The first major work to bring this philosophy and practice to health care is described in *Curing Health Care: New Strategies for Quality Improvement* (Berwick et al., 1990). This report on the National Demonstration Project on Quality Improvement in Health Care tells the why, what, and how of the improvement philosophy; it is not merely a project report. Another overall resource focused on health care is *The Health Care Manager's Guide to Continuous Quality Improvement,* by Leebov and Ersoz (1991).

Terms

A word about vocabulary is in order. Deming, upon arriving to speak at a conference, saw a poster labeling the conference a TQM event. He said, as the story goes, that he would not have come if he'd known it was a TQM conference. We cannot blame the jargon on him; he avoided it. We will not try to defend or attack jargon here; it can be both useful and a confusing barrier. Phrases such as TQM, total quality leadership, total quality control, continuous quality improvement (CQI), and many others have been used to refer to what this chapter calls TQM. Although jargon can provide a shorthand to communication, we have found that the *Q* phrases can mean different things to different people. In some organizations it seems to mean little more than a suggestion plan or a training class.

The biggest leap for us in health care is to understand that the shift from quality assurance to quality improvement is not merely a change in name; it is a profound and comprehensive change in principles and practice. Neither is it the layering of a few more ideas or tools onto standard practices; in many ways quality assurance and quality improvement are mutually exclusive. TQM requires us to think differently and therefore to act differently from what may be our habit.

A particular caveat regarding the *Q* phrases is about the phrase "continuous quality improvement." In many health care organizations CQI is used as though it were synonymous with TQM. That's fine if we all share an understanding of what we mean by our terms, but often we don't. The idea that everything can be improved, that we should always be seeking ways to make improvements, and that there are some approaches to help us do it, is, of course, an essential part of TQM; but it is not the total, and its success depends on other managerial and organizational characteristics.

Principles and requirements

The basic principles of TQM are summarized in Table 44-1. As previously discussed, then, CQI is one of the principles underlying TQM. The implications include an acknowledgment that perfection is never reached, that an attempt to improve is not a condemnation of the past, and that circumstances are continually changing and requiring change.

A second focus of TQM is service to customers. There is a sacredness to the relationship between patients and caregivers; the word "customer" is not intended to de-

Table 41-1 Principles and necessary conditions for total quality management

Principles	Development of a culture
• Continuous quality improvement • Knowledge of customer requirements • Processes of customer-supplier relationships • Belief in people • Statistical thinking with facts • Costs of poor quality	• Employee involvement • Empowerment • An environment free of fear • Teamwork • Data collection and analysis skills • Group interaction skills • Structure and management to enable the improvement • Tools to facilitate the improvement

value that. Rather, the intention is to broaden each person's concept of relationships with others in doing work. Just as nurses develop relationships with patients in order to understand their needs and to assess progress and outcomes, others develop a relationship with a secretary in order to supply to him or her what is needed to accomplish the work in which both parties have a share. The work, whether it is nursing care or manuscript preparation, requires a complex interaction in which information, needs, expectations, and assessments occur. If we wish to improve, we must work together—customer and supplier—to negotiate requirements.

If the secretary is our customer—in requiring a legible manuscript from which to work, for example, or in needing to know a due date for the work—then we are the secretary's customers for the prepared manuscript. We interchange roles constantly, and the larger and more complex the organization, the more numerous and complex the customer-supplier relationships.

The third principle of TQM is that work is accomplished through processes, and processes make up systems. To improve the outcomes we must examine and improve the processes. Only in this way can we prevent the adverse events that trigger after-the-fact investigations.

There are numerous hand-offs between customers and suppliers in any process, numerous opportunities for error and inefficiency, and complexities too great for any one person to grasp and understand alone. Therefore, a requirement for this philosophy and practice that we are calling TQM is that the people who are in the process, although they may not even be aware of one another (e.g., the billing clerk for the hospital and the intake clerk in admitting) are the people who must become scientists of their processes and act to make them better. This is usually expressed as employee involvement and empowerment. It also mandates teamwork, and all of the complex sets of skills required for people to work together most effectively. In addition to providing the environment to support involvement, empowerment, and skill development, the organization must also provide the structure and action that can bring those two clerks mentioned above, along with others, to the table to study and improve the process that brings us our hospital bills.

A structure is also essential to enable collaboration among employees. The organization must maintain management approaches that will not hinder learning and innovation. People who fear blame do not make good collaborators or scientists; cannot be depended on to bring openmindedness, creativity, and vulnerability to the table; and cannot be depended on not to "game" whatever systems they are in. Driving out fear is one of Deming's Fourteen Points: Where there is fear, the improvement potential of the organization is crippled.

The fourth principle, then, is a belief in people. With rare exceptions, people are doing their best; they are not saboteurs. Most of us maintain our self-esteem not by doing poor work but by doing work of which we are proud. Even though all of that is true, sometimes things do go wrong because something in a system isn't working as well as it must. Or perhaps there is an unavoidable and singular event, an outlier. Rather than look for where to place blame, discover whether the outcome was merely a matter of normal variation or whether there is truly a process that is inadequate to the needs of its customers. Perhaps there is a knowledge deficit among the admitting clerks that contributes to time-consuming rework in the billing office. Should we blame the admitting clerks for not knowing something? Will that cause them to know it? Will it contribute to their commitment to serving the billing clerks? How can we even discover the deficit without the cooperation and commitment of the admitting clerks themselves? As we study this process we will develop ideas not only to correct the current deficit, but also to prevent recurrence, perhaps by improving the orientation training of admitting clerks or by providing improved job aids.

In order to conduct the analysis and discover what is happening in the system rather than lay blame, people need the skills for collecting and analyzing data. Free of fear or blame, and with the proper skills, people are in a position to develop new shared knowledge of the system, and can work together with facts rather than react to singular events, emotions, guesswork, or arbitrary decisions derived from individuals. This commitment to understanding the facts is the fifth principle in TQM and requires developing an understanding of variation and the knowledge of the statistician as well as system analysis—a skill of the engineer.

Most of us fall easily into thinking that the solution to our problems is to spend more money—on staff, a better information system, or more supplies. These solutions are appropriate in many circumstances, but much more often they are not. Our elaborate work processes are very expensive; our new, improved, streamlined work processes are less expensive. Clearly, our billing clerk friends spend expensive time reworking and repairing the faulty process that provided incorrect and incomplete patient registration information; we expect great time savings and shortened turnaround time in their offices after the admitting clerks begin to key in the patient information differently.

Another principle of TQM is that poor quality is more expensive than total quality.

All of the skills required for TQM must be developed throughout the organization. The way to learn these skills is by doing. Courses in each of the disciplines mentioned at the beginning of this chapter would help but would still only be like reading about riding a bike. What is needed is the bike itself with a coach running alongside, helping to steady it and providing the right information at the right moment. This is the way the learning can and must occur to develop TQM.

Tools for total quality management

Just as there are survey tools for gathering information and statistical tests for analyzing data, there is also an array of tools for enhancing work throughout the TQM process. Virtually all of these tools are accessible to any team. Two of the most practically focused publications are *The Team Handbook* by Scholtes (1988) and *The Memory Jogger II* by Brassard and Ritter (1994). These publications are aids to what Plsek describes as phases of divergent and convergent thinking that are parts of the creative and empirical process of problem solving (Plsek, 1993). Plsek presents problem-solving models used in the improvement process. Models and tools are aids to both the group-process aspects and the task-specific aspects of the improvement and problem-solving process.

Simple as most of the TQM tools are, they present a challenge and provide help on a sophisticated level. For example, brainstorming is something with which most people are familiar, and there are numerous ways to conduct a brainstorming session. It is quite challenging to beginners with different habits and experiences to follow the "rules." The discipline of withholding comments, criticisms, and off-line conversation—all of which would divert the group from the creative task at hand—does not come naturally to everyone. Furthermore, for a group accustomed to deferring to the opinion of a nominal leader, it is unsettling when all opinions are laid out (literally, on pieces of paper) as equals on the table. The "voice of authority" does not stick on the paper, nor does the shyness of another participant.

In hoshin planning a group uses numerous tools in a specific sequence to identify a "hoshin" for their organization. From the Japanese, literally meaning "shiny pointing object," the hoshin is the one focused priority for improvement for the entire organization. One hospital made bed availability their hoshin for a year and achieved results beyond their own expectations. The breakthrough achieved through hoshin planning requires a leadership commitment from which many organization shy away due either to lack of readiness or a fear of letting go. Critics of TQM who describe it as only being able to achieve incremental improvement fail to recognize the power of hoshin planning to achieve leaps in organizational performance through alignment and focus.

Because TQM offers an integration of principles from a variety of fields of knowledge, and guidelines and tools for both task accomplishment and the processes for achievement, it is a framework within which other approaches can be integrated. Lutheran General Hospital in Chicago, for example, worked to instill the quality improvement methodology before initiating reengineering efforts (Ummel et al., 1995). Among the most interesting and exciting ideas evolving in many organizations today are those presented by Senge (1990) in *The Fifth Discipline*. These ideas are congruent with those of TQM and similarly offer breadth and depth. In the chapter, "Thinking Strategically about Building Learning Organizations," in *The Fifth Discipline Fieldbook,* Senge describes a model for the learning organization framework that includes what he calls the domains of enduring change and action (Senge, Kleiner, Roberts, Ross, & Smith, 1994). Building a learning organization, one that is constantly improving in its service to customers—patients and families, students, the community, and all the players in the systems—is not a project with a finish line.

REDESIGN

Every aspect of health care, from concept (disease prevention vs. illness treatment) to delivery systems and outcomes, is being examined, changed, and manipulated. Reengineering and redesign appear often in current health care literature as examples of how various institutions are responding. A specific definition of redesign, as opposed to a specific definition of reengineering, however, is somewhat illusory.

Greenberg (1994) defines *redesign* as "a label or buzzword used to describe a variety of concepts, including variations of reengineering and patient-focused care; it is occasionally used to describe changes made in care-delivery systems, as well as physical plant redesign" (p. 28A). Dienemann and Gessner (1992) suggest that systems redesign is an alternative to job design. Instead of just changing who does what work, systems redesign takes a top-down approach to redesigning the organization from the unit to the larger system. These authors also suggest that organizations use TQM as the systems theory–based approach for their redesign process.

Hammer and Champy (1994) provide abundant information on reengineering, including definitions of what it is and what it is not. They suggest that redesign is one of four phases or reengineering: Redesign occurs after mobilization and diagnosis but before formulating a strategy for transition. They also suggest that process redesign is a step in the total reengineering process, not the end (Hammer & Champy, 1994).

The basic principles of redesign are stated implicitly in most of the literature and are stated explicitly by Minnen et al. (1993). It is dynamic, multidisciplinary, and collaborative. Many state that it must be top-down because the radical changes that are the desired outcomes of such a process cannot be developed by either the clinical staff or grassroots workers. These workers must be involved, however, to elicit critical information and to generate understanding to decrease resistance to implementation.

Many authors of redesign/reengineering literature suggest that the tools and philosophies of CQI provide structure and an organized approach for the process of redesign (Dienemann & Gessner, 1992; Greenberg, 1994; Smith, Adams, Bersante, & Kalma, 1994). Plsek (1993) lists several project models for CQI. He notes that most of the models focus on problem/project selection/definition, analysis, solution generation and selection, and implementation and monitoring. Plsek (1993) has developed a model that describes the process of redesign as transposing the second and third steps, similar to the process of Hammer and Champy. He suggests that redesign is done first and then subjected to systematic analysis, leading to problem prevention and monitoring.

The expected or desired outcomes of redesign (vs. reengineering) are as illusory as its definition. Hammer and Champy (1994) and Dienemann and Gessner (1992) agree that the focus switches from the manager to the professional, from satisfying the boss to satisfying the customer. The redesigned system should create a structure that allows for scanning the environment, working with a multidisciplinary team for highest potential benefit, and flexible adaptation to the ever-changing demands of work. The strength of such an approach is the emphasis placed on productivity and interdependence.

In summary, no absolutes regarding redesign can be found in the literature. Perhaps redesign is a piece of the reengineering process (e.g., redesigning the functions of a few core processes or of one division vs. the entire organization). Perhaps redesign is one phase of reengineering. Redesign may be the appropriate terminology for health care organizations that think they are undergoing reengineering. The discussion and confusion about redesign continue.

REENGINEERING

Reengineering, first introduced in the mid-1980s, is defined by the gurus of reengineering, Hammer and Champy, as "the fundamental rethinking and radical redesign of business processes to achieve dramatic improvements in critical, contemporary measures of performance, such as cost, quality, service, and speed" (Hammer & Champy, 1994, p. 32). Reengineering is not about improving existing processes; it is about starting all over and inventing the future.

As used by Hammer and Champy (1994), the term *business system* encompasses an entire business structure, including the relationships between business processes, job definitions/organizational structure management and measurement systems, and values and beliefs. When these relationships are supported by sound business processes, the resultant synergy enables significant, sustainable performance improvement (Kralovec, 1992).

Reengineering in health care is aimed at producing revolutionary changes to the systems associated with the delivery of patient care. Reengineering is synonymous with reinvention and asks the question, If I were to start this service or system all over again, what would it look like? Reinvention is about creating what is not (Goss, Pascale, & Athos, 1993). The process of reengineering is highly creative, innovative, and breaks with traditional thinking.

Industrial reengineering efforts typically follow similar implementation strategies. Hammer has identified four discrete phases to the implementation process: mobilization, diagnosis, redesign, and transition. As adapted to health care, Kravolec (1992) describes the principle phases of reengineering as business process reengineering plan; process analysis and redesign; and implementation and transition.

An underlying premise of reengineering is that business processes should be designed around related and interdependent tasks that together produce outcomes that fulfill defined customer needs. These customer-focused processes transcend traditional departmental boundaries. Processes and systems within organizations rarely operate in isolation; rather, they are integrated and interrelated. Because reengineering is a global strategy, it impacts multiple aspects of the operation. It does not consider processes in isolation, but focuses on reinventing these pro-

CORE FACETS OF REENGINEERING

- Reinvention
- Quantum change
- Future-focused
- Customer-focused
- Multiple-process–oriented
- Driven top-down
- Organization-wide focus and impact
- Alignment
- Voyage

cesses and systems in an integrated fashion (Flarey & Blancett, 1995). Therefore, a core feature of reengineering is its global, cross-functional approach.

Reengineering drives significant, radical change. It seeks quantum leaps in performance and outcomes. Reengineering efforts generally target a 20% to 50% change in processes, with resultant transformations in cost, quality, and targeted indicators of customer satisfaction (Wachel, 1994).

True reengineering begins with the future and works back to the present (Stewart, 1993). Future-oriented creative thinking and analysis are essential goals that require having a vision of what could be and then developing special goals and objectives for achieving that vision. This concept of rethinking is vital to the success of any reengineering efforts.

Reengineering must be driven by the top leadership (Champy, 1995). By the nature of its radical change, reengineering requires substantial commitments of time, human, and financial resources. It is not a quick-fix for old problems; it is the creation of a new organization. Reengineering efforts impact all aspects of the organization, and commitment must be present and sustained in order for the efforts to be successful.

Reengineering actions are long-term and have been described as a voyage that will last years, possibly lifetimes. For leadership, there are key issues surrounding reengineering, including purpose, culture, process and performance, and people (Champy, 1995). The essence of reengineering is a future-focused, radical, sweeping reinvention of the company culture and processes (see box).

CONCLUSION

One of the barriers to changing our antiquated health care delivery systems is that we do not all speak the same language or mean the same thing with the same terminology. Table 41-2 is our interpretation of the differences and similarities among TQM, reengineering, and redesign.

We believe that any organization that fully commits to TQM by developing the culture, valuing people, driving out fear, focusing on the processes rather than blaming

Table 41-2

Total quality management	Reengineering	Redesign
Culture development		
Customer-focused	Customer-focused	Customer-focused
Driven by top leadership	Driven by top leadership	
Process-oriented	Multiple-process–oriented	Process-focused
Data-driven	Data-driven	Data-driven
Employee involvement	Employee involvement	Employee involvement
Organization-wide focus	Organization-wide focus	
Environment free of fear		
Teamwork	Teamwork	Teamwork
Analysis of environment/market	Analysis of market/environment	
Statistical process control tools		
Slow → rapid	Rapid	Slow → rapid
Incremental to quantum change	Quantum	Step in process
Priorities drive improvement, deployment ensures alignment	Alignment of processes	Episodic
Belief in people		
Group interaction skills		
Management and planning tools		
Scientific problem solving process		
Journey without end	Journey without end	A trip

people, supporting continuous learning, and using the full scope of disciplines that are the foundation of TQM will be highly successful in achieving breakthroughs not only in performance but also in developing an environment in which people take pride in their work. Many of the techniques of reengineering can be integrated to produce quantum change with a futuristic focus. TQM, as a philosophy and approach, is the most universally translatable strategy to virtually any environment from the hospital to the academe. TQM is not the quickest way to success because it requires a tremendous commitment, a willingness to change behavior from the top down, and years to produce substantial results. But TQM, as a way of life, can provide superior satisfaction not only to customers but also to the staff who deliver the service.

REFERENCES

Berwick, D.M. (1989). Sounding board: Continuous improvement as an ideal in health care. *The New England Journal of Medicine, 320*(1), 53-56.

Berwick, D.M. (1992). The clinical process and the quality process. *Quality Management in Healthcare, 1*(2), 1-8.

Berwick, D.M., Blanton, G.A., Roessner, J. (1990). *Curing health care: New strategies for quality improvement* (p. 148). San Francisco: Jossey-Bass.

Brassard, M., & Ritter, D. (1994). *The memory jogger II*. Methuen, MA: Goal/QPC.

Champy, J. (1995). *Reengineering management: The mandate for new leadership* (pp. 6-8). New York: Harper Business.

Deming, W.E. (1993). *The new economics*. Cambridge, MA: MIT Center for Advanced Engineering Study.

Dienemann, J., & Gessner, T. (1992). Restructuring nursing care delivery systems. *Nursing Economic$, 10*(4), 253-258.

Flarey, D.L., & Blancett, S.S. (1995). *Reengineering: The road best traveled in reengineering nursing and health care* (p. 17). Gaithersburg, MD: Aspen.

Goss, T., Pascale, R., & Athos, A. (1993). The reinvention roller coaster: Risking the present for a powerful future. *Harvard Business Review, 71*, 97-108.

Greenberg, L. (1994). Work redesign: An overview. *Journal of Emergency Nursing, 10*(3), 28A-32A.

Hammer, M., & Champy, J. (1994). *Reengineering the corporation: A manifest for business revolution*. New York: Harper Business.

Kralovec, O.J. (1992). Applying industrial reengineering techniques to health care. *The Journal of the Healthcare Information and Management Systems Society, 7*(2), 3-10.

Leebov, W., & Ersoz, C. (1991). *The health care manager's guide to continuous quality improvement*. Chicago: American Hospital Association Publishing, Inc.

Minnen, T.G., Berger, E., Ames, A., Dubree, M., Baker, W.L., & Spinella, J. (1993). Sustaining work redesign innovations through shared governance. *Journal of Nursing Administration, 23*(7/8), 35-40.

O'Toole, J. (1995). *Leading change: Overcoming the ideology of comfort and the tyranny of custom*. San Francisco: Jossey-Bass.

Plsek, P.E. (1993). Tutorial: Quality improvement project models. *Quality Management in Health Care, 1*(2), 69-81.

Plsek, P.D. (1993). Tutorial: Quality improvement project models. *Quality Management in Health Care, 1*(2), 1193.

Scholtes, P.R. (1988). *The team handbook: How to use teams to improve quality*. Madison, WI: Joiner, Assoc., Inc.

Senge, P. (1990). *The fifth discipline*. New York: Doubleday.

Senge, P., Kleiner, A., Roberts, C., Ross, R., Smith, B., (1994). *The fifth discipline field book* (pp. 15-48). New York: Doubleday.

Smith, P., Adams, D., Bersante, S., & Kalma, S. (1994). Planning for patient care redesign: Success through continuous quality improvement. *Journal of Nursing Care Quality, 8*(2), 73-80.

Stewart, T.A. (1993). Reengineering: The hot new management tool. *Fortune, 128*(4), 41-48.

Ummel, S.L., Schaffner, J.W., Smith, B.D., & Ludwig-Beymer, P. (1995). Advancing the continuum of care: The Lutheran General Health System experience. In S.S. Blancet & D.L.O. Flarey (Eds.), *Reengineering nursing and health care: The handbook for organizational transformation* (pp. 261-281). Gaithersburg, MD: Aspen.

Wachel, W. (1994). Reengineering: Beyond incremental change. *Healthcare Executive, 9*, 18-21.

Walton, M. (1986). *The Deming management method*. New York: Perigee.

How can the quality of nursing practice be measured?

KAREN S. MARTIN, DIANN L. MARTIN

The question of how to measure the quality of nursing practice is not new. Nurses in practice, education, and research have asked this question repeatedly, especially since 1961 when Freeman wrote, "There is no problem in public health practice today as important, as haunting, and as frustrating as that of measuring the effectiveness of services afforded the public" (Freeman, 1961, p. 605). Freeman also noted the potential for error when measurement approaches are selected that are too general or specific. A decade later, the dilemma of "quantifying the unquantifiable" was described by Lewis in her 1976 *Nursing Outlook* editorial. Hegyvary (1992, p. 23) concurred, stating, "Yet the assessment of outcomes is one of the greatest challenges in health care research. Their definitions are elusive, difficult to validate, and based on varying perspectives and world views."

As we approach the 21st century, the question of how to measure quality has not been answered. However, exciting progress and promising research have been described. Some chapters in this book clearly identify the increasing demands of regulatory and reimbursement groups and the potential for linking payment to client outcomes, cost-effectiveness, and cost benefits. These authors are among the nursing leaders who recognize that, as a profession, nurses must develop not only skills but also research-based, valid, and reliable instruments to identify, describe, count, and measure the cost and quality of their practice. Furthermore, we are recognizing that we must attempt to measure quality in a manner that is sensitive to both the interdisciplinary nature of our practice and to our clients, who are the reason we practice.

MEASUREMENT BARRIERS

Various barriers contribute to the difficulties experienced by practitioners and nursing administrators as they attempt to measure the effectiveness of nursing practice. One of these barriers involves definitions (Mark, 1995). Freeman defined the effectiveness of nursing services as "the relationship between goals and achievement; it is a measure of the degree to which the service accomplishes the job it sets out to do" (Freeman, 1961, p. 605). When considering health care in general, quality is the degree to which services increase the likelihood of desired health outcomes and are consistent with current professional knowledge (Lohr, 1990).

More recent definitions change the focus of quality as determined by the professional to an emphasis on the client as a consumer or customer of nursing services. Quality in this context has been defined broadly as consistent conformance to customer expectations (Scholtes, 1988). This definition focuses not only on the technical competence and expertise of clinical practice, but also highlights the growing public demand for outcomes that address wants and needs as perceived by clients and their families. For example, customers may expect functional improvements but also want prompt, courteous, and empathetic service. As the health care delivery system becomes increasingly competitive from a business sense, nurses have accepted the challenge of the customer-focused view of quality measurement. Although the definitions of measurement and quality are becoming easier to understand, nurses, especially those in the practice setting, may still have difficulty operationalizing them.

Conceptual issues are closely related to definitions and represent another obstacle in measuring nursing practice. Donabedian (1976) constructed a cubical structure to describe the complex nature of quality. Central to the structure are the client's physiological, psychological, and social functions. The structure also depicts the client and the health care provider on a continuum ranging from the individual client and practitioner to the global community and institution. The literature suggests a shift in emphasis from structure and process to outcomes, that is, a shift from assessing nurses' activities to direct assessment of results or client outcomes (American Nurses Association [ANA], 1988; Lang, 1995; National Center for Nursing Research [NCNR], 1992; Remington, 1990). Again, the practicing nurse faces an overwhelming task of translating a global theoretical perspective into a pragmatic plan of action.

Issues related to methods and cost are the third barrier to measuring practice. The number of methods being developed for nursing by both nurses and nonnurses is increasing dramatically (American Nurses Association [ANA], 1995; Joint Commission on Accreditation of Healthcare Organizations, 1994; Martin & Scheet, 1992a; Shaughnessy, Crisler, Schlenker, & Arnold, 1995; Shaughnessy et al., 1994; Wilson, 1993). Some nursing educators and researchers indicate that measurement of the nurse-client relationship should approach the precision of the chemist in the laboratory or the postal quality inspector calculating the time between pickup and delivery of a package. The methods and procedures these nurses offer are often very complex and consume extensive professional and support staff resources. Designs selected for most measurement research involve a small number of outcome variables that have a narrow focus or limited applicability within acute care and community-focused settings. In contrast, other nursing leaders focus on the art and caring of practice and suggest that actual measurement can only be global or is impossible. They emphasize the unique, human aspect of the nurse-client relationship. The results of global outcome research studies offer practitioners conflicting implications that would be difficult to implement.

Both narrow and global approaches to outcome measurement have led to diverse research and have produced equally diverse models that may not be relevant or cost-beneficial for practice settings (Donabedian, 1988; Marek & Lang, 1993; Shamian, 1993). Thus, selecting the right outcome measures is a critical step in the process. Before beginning outcome measurement, however, staff must also select, use, and document interventions in a systematic manner. "Measurable variables include behavioral changes that occur following participation in educational programs or an intervention, as well as general responses (how a person reacts or feels) to different problem areas (Mateo, 1991, p. 154). Other necessary steps in implementing an outcome measurement program include gaining staff support and maintaining that program. Each of these steps consumes valuable time and financial resources for providers regardless of the service setting. With the current fiscal constraints, neither administrators nor clinicians have the luxury of extra time. Both demand proof of cost-effectiveness and cost benefits before implementing outcome measurement and continuous quality improvement approaches.

The complex definitional, conceptual, methodological, and cost issues offer dilemmas to the practicing nurse and agency or institution as they ask how to measure the effectiveness of practice in their setting. The decision to ignore the entire issue and wait until the "experts" develop a solution is tempting but dangerous. If the profession does not address client outcomes and quality improvement issues energetically, nonnurses are likely to impose their own regulations. In addition, some providers are beginning to use outcome measurement and continuous quality improvement methods with enough precision and consistency that they can demonstrate definite improvements for their clients and cost savings for their service settings. Because nursing is a complex phenomenon and a practice discipline, practitioners not only can contribute extensively to the developing art and science of measurement but also have a vested interest in ensuring that developments are congruent with the realities of practice and the practice setting.

ADAPTING MEASUREMENT TO PRACTICE

Simultaneously, nurses and their agencies or institutions should make a firm commitment to the following recommendations:

1. They should appreciate nursing's history and commitment to quality issues. Other health care professions such as medicine are also struggling with quality issues; in comparison, nursing has made excellent progress (Lang, 1995; NCNR, 1992).
2. They should contribute to agency-institutional models that are practical and valuable. All staff need to be involved in the development and use of quality indicators.
3. They should acknowledge that the existing models are commendable but that extensive work remains.
4. They should become informed about current efforts to increase the science for measuring nursing practice.
5. They should collaborate with educators and researchers to advance scientific rigor. Again, all responsibilities should not be assigned to "experts" outside the organization or to one or two persons within the organization.

Many home care and public health agencies, hospitals, and nursing homes use appropriate approaches or models for measuring the quality of nursing practice. These models are multifaceted and involve formative or ongoing evaluation. Some are comprehensive, and many combine quantitative and qualitative measurement techniques. Such an eclectic approach for all health care professionals is endorsed strongly in the conclusions of the Institute of Medicine study and by other experts (Lohr, 1990; NCNR, 1992; Shaughnessy et al., 1994).

An important goal for service-setting providers is to incorporate the developing sciences of measurement and research into their models. Another goal is to use the approaches consistently, because practice settings often report inconsistent application. Measuring the quality of practice must combine aspects of Donabedian's structure, process, and outcome concepts. These approaches should reflect the following inherent assumptions, realities, and constraints of the practice setting: (1) clients, health care providers, and third-party payers desire consistent, high-quality service delivery; (2) multifaceted, formative approaches strengthen the evaluation of clinical practice because no adequate, single method exists; (3) discrepancies exist between ideal services and available resources; and (4) providers and clients make occasional errors.

MODELS FOR PRACTICE

Interest in outcome measurement models that are useful in practice settings continues to increase (Joint Commission on Accreditation of Healthcare Organizations, 1994; Marek & Lang, 1993; National League for Nursing, 1994). Traditional indicators include mortality, morbidity, and length of hospital stay. Functional status, mental status, stress level, satisfaction with care, burden of care, and cost of care have been described as significant emerging measures (Naylor, Munro, & Brooten, 1991; NCNR, 1992). Recent changes in the health care delivery system suggest reevaluation of outcome indicators and continuous quality improvement techniques for two critical reasons, both of which clearly involve financial incentives.

First, free-standing health care providers are becoming obsolete. Mergers, sales, and contractual agreements are producing huge, integrated provider groups, often referred to as *seamless health care systems*. Many of these systems include the full range of services and providers such as acute, long-term, home health, and physician services. There is a dramatic shift from the acute care setting as the primary site of care to diverse community-focused programs provided by home care and public health agencies, clinics, ambulatory care and nursing centers, and schools. Suddenly, the client is not perceived as a medical diagnosis who receives care during a 3-day hospital stay or infrequent office visits and who can be discharged from a point of care and forgotten. Instead, the client has become a desired customer, a whole person who purchases a variety of preventive and therapeutic services across a continuum of time or even the life span. Furthermore, providers are recognizing the impact of the family and significant others on the client's long-term health care outcomes and the financial impact of those outcomes on the providers within the health care system. A wonderful shift in providers' thinking is occurring: The customer is becoming the focus of service and providers are acknowledging that quality begins with the customer.

Second, the process and results of outcome measurement and continuous quality improvement used to be of little interest to persons outside the institution or agency. Now, outcome data are the basis for critical decisions that affect the growth and even survival of the health care institution. Many providers are using scorecards, report cards, or other quantitative data for making operations more efficient and economical, for publicity, to compete for new business, to meet the regulations of existing contracts with managed care companies and other third-party payers, and to fulfill accreditation requirements. Health care providers have talked about the merits of following leaders such as Donabedian, Deming, Crosby, and Juran. They have talked about collecting accurate individual client data that could be aggregated and analyzed for groups of clients, programs, or entire agencies. However, the advent of integrated health care systems, competition for clients, and managed care contracts has provided the needed incentive to transform words into action. That incentive may be so great that some providers accept methods for generating data that are questionable at best (General Accounting Office, 1994). Quality issues are now serious business in service settings.

The new challenge is to identify outcome measurement and continuous quality improvement models that are capable of providing valid and reliable data that are both clinically significant and financially relevant. In order for traditional and emerging measures to be useful to practitioners, outcomes measures must address comprehensive practice, documentation, and information management issues. For measures to be satisfactory to managed care contractors and other third-party payers, cost needs to be part of the equation. Some outcome data should reflect structure and process variables. Examples include data about the type of health care providers who deliver services, the location at which the services are provided, the choice and timing of interventions, and the cost of equipment, supplies, and overhead. Other outcome data should reflect factors specific to the client. Examples include the client's health history and the number and type of medical diagnoses, as well as the number and type of the client's environmental, psychosocial, physiological, and health-related behavior problems.

IMPLEMENTATION IN THE PRACTICE SETTING

The remainder of this chapter offers an introduction to implementation of outcome measurement, which is the most difficult step in the process. The details necessary for actual application of the following practice, documentation, and information management model are described elsewhere (Martin & Scheet, 1992a; Reif & Martin, in press). This description reflects current realities and constraints and does not represent the ultimate solution for measuring the quality of nursing practice in all settings.

The Omaha System provides the model for the outcome measurement process. This system consists of three research-based, standardized schemes; the Problem Rating Scale for Outcomes is the portion designed to address outcome measurement. The Omaha System is one of the nursing vocabularies recognized by the ANA (Martin & Scheet, 1995). An increasingly diverse number of health care providers are using the Omaha System as the foundation of interdisciplinary professional practice, documentation, and information management (Martin, in press; Martin & Scheet, 1992a, 1992b; Martin, Scheet, & Stegman, 1993). Providers using the Omaha System include staff nurses, nurse practitioners, and other health care professionals employed in home care and public health agencies, nursing centers, clinics, schools, parish nursing programs, as well as case managers in a variety of hospital settings.

The Omaha System was developed and refined during four research projects conducted between 1975 and 1993 by the Visiting Nurse Association (VNA) of Omaha at seven diverse sites throughout the country. The purpose of the research was to identify ways to increase the effectiveness and efficiency of professional practice. The Problem Classification Scheme offers the nurse or other health care provider a holistic, standardized method for client assessment and nursing diagnosis/problem identification. For example, the Problem Classification Scheme can become the basis of the admission form. The Intervention Scheme provides a vocabulary and codes for documenting plans and interventions in the client record. It can also become the basis of evaluation instruments used when managers observe clinicians providing services. The Problem Rating Scale for Outcomes is used to document client progress in the record. This scale can also be used during case conferences such as those conducted by interdisciplinary hospice staff as they discuss the hospice caseload and changes in clients. The Problem Rating Scale for Outcomes was constructed as a relatively simple, criterion-referenced instrument under the guidance of Donabedian. It consists of three 5-point, Likert-type subscales that address the client's problem-specific knowledge, behavior, and status and assist the nurse with the complex task of measuring client progress.

PRACTICE AND DOCUMENTATION

The process of providing orientation for new employees is an important cornerstone in the effort to ensure and measure the quality of nursing practice. The new clinician needs information about assignments and client caseload, client-nurse relationships, procedures, equipment, productivity, agency and community resources, and fees and reimbursement. The employer must provide essential information that matches the new clinician's needs and that enables the clinician to function effectively and efficiently. Employers select various approaches to communicate policies and expectations including competency-based and preceptor programs. When preceptors are used, the goal is to assign each newly employed clinician to one preceptor who has extensive experience and demonstrated expertise. Preceptors can evaluate the clinical, documentation, and communication skills of new staff in comparison with agency standards of competence for a period of several months.

For those agencies that use the Omaha System, it is introduced as part of the agency's client record and quality improvement orientation. Many agencies use a combination of methods including lecture and discussion, handouts or the *Pocket Guide* (Martin & Scheet, 1992b), sample records, and practice. The opportunity to practice is a critical part of orientation and can be accomplished with a videotape, role play, or description of a simulated nurse-client encounter. Working both together and independently, new staff use the Omaha System to select nursing diagnoses/client problems, nursing interventions, and client outcome ratings from the simulated encounter. When new clinicians are able to discuss their decisions with peers and their instructor, they learn more quickly.

The speed with which new clinicians acquire competence applying the Omaha System varies considerably. For many, the idea of documenting outcome measures is a new and sometimes uncomfortable experience.

INFORMATION MANAGEMENT

Managing clinical information in a practice setting presents an enormous challenge to individual nurses and to community health agencies. The Omaha System was implemented at the VNA of Chicago as a tool to assist nurses and other clinicians as they collect data and report on the services they provide. At the time of implementation, the VNA used five different documentation systems across its diverse programs, which served more than 6,600 clients annually and included hospice, home health, home infusion, private duty, and durable medical equipment. VNA nurses were spending up to 30% of their time documenting the delivery of care on a manual client record that lacked a conceptual or theoretical framework to guide practice. No objective mechanism was in place to track client outcomes, and client records were often cited as an area of concern during federal survey and certification and accreditation visits. Other than manual audits conducted quarterly on a sample of records, no systematic methods were used to track or report on the quality of clinical interventions provided by VNA staff.

Managed care organizations and third-party payers are increasingly interested in tracking patient outcomes and in examining the relationship between the cost of care and client improvement. Recognizing that interest prompted the VNA staff to investigate the Omaha System as a mechanism for clinical information management. The Omaha System was selected because systematic research has been conducted and reliability and validity were established in numerous clinical practice settings. It was practical and useful by all disciplines that provide care including nursing, social service, physical therapy, and occupational therapy. The Problem Classification Scheme, Intervention Scheme, and Problem Rating Scale for Outcomes use standard definitions and employ a coding system that can be computerized in the VNA documentation system. Prior to implementation of the Omaha System, several clinical management staff conducted a review of the literature specific to vocabulary and systems, and made a site visit to the VNA of Omaha to determine how the Omaha System could be applied in a large agency.

Implementing the Omaha System required that the assessment database, progress notes, care plans, and discharge summaries be adapted and coded to reflect the numerical taxonomy of the Omaha System. Staff were offered a 7-hour orientation to the Omaha System that consisted of lecture, discussion, and a workshop. A case study was used as an example for simulating the documentation of services. In addition, the VNA information/data processing staff entered the physician orders, interventions, and outcomes into the agency's computer. Having an automated record allows the VNA to track and profile client information.

The automation of the Omaha System allows the VNA to track client outcomes and improvement in knowledge, behavior, and health status. It also allows managers and staff to track the array of client problems that occur for any given medical diagnosis and to tie together utilization information such as the number of visits by discipline to specific client problems. At admission, problems are identified for each client, and the problem-specific knowledge, behavior, and status ratings are recorded. The coded information for the problems, the outcome ratings, and the interventions are entered into the agency computer. At discharge, knowledge, behavior, and status are rated again and compared with the admission ratings. After discharge, the information system provides reports that detail the improvement or deterioration in outcome ratings for each client. When cost information is added, the VNA can track cost per case by diagnostic category and report on what problems were identified in these cases. Over time, the database that has been collected will enable the VNA of Chicago to identify the cost of care for specific problems and to determine which specific interventions are most effective in achieving favorable outcomes.

Figure 42-1 displays a sample of the integrated clinical, statistical, and financial information that is now available at the VNA. At the end of the month, managers receive detailed reports that list the number of clients discharged for each diagnostic category by the International Classification of Diseases-9th Revision-Clinical Modification code. The report includes details about the services and supplies that were used by clients in each diagnostic category and itemizes the cost of services from the agency pricing matrix. For each category, reports are also subdivided by payer source (e.g., Medicare, Medicaid, or private insurance). Figure 42-1 provides a sample of 21 individuals with hypertension who were discharged from Medicare services during a 5-month period. The specific client problems identified for the sample are based on terms and codes from the Omaha Problem Classification Scheme. In this sample, the most frequently oc-

Management Information Using the Omaha System[1]

Diagnostic Category: 401.9 Hypertension

Number of Patients Served: 21

Primary Omaha System Problems Identified:

29. Circulation (16 patients)
42. Prescribed Medication Regime (5 patients)
27. Neuro-musculo-skeletal (5 patients)

Service Use by Discipline:

Nursing	323 Visits
LPN	85 Visits
HHA	202 Visits
PT	293 Visits
OT	110 Visits
MSW	70 Visits

Average Visits/Patient: 51.6

Average Length of Stay in VNA Service: 92 days

Outcome at Discharge by Omaha Problem Rating (Percentage of Patients Improved):

29. Circulation
    Knowledge Improved 75%
    Behavior Improved 81%
    Status Improved 75%
42. Prescribed Medication Regime
    Knowledge Improved 80%
    Behavior Improved 80%
    Status Improved 80%
27. Neuro-Muscular-Skeletal
    Knowledge Improved 50%
    Behavior Improved 25%
    Status Improved 50%

Average Cost Per Case: $3,726.44

[1]Depicts a (5) month period of data generated by VNA of Chicago Medicare clients with a diagnosis of hypertension and their associated Omaha Problems and Problem Ratings

Fig. 42-1. Management information using the Omaha System.

curring problems were Circulation, Prescribed Medication Regime, and Neuromusculoskeletal. VNA staff documented problem-specific outcome ratings for the client's knowledge, behavior, and status at admission and discharge using the 5-point, Likert-type Problem Rating Scale for Outcomes. Based on the discharge ratings, the computer report displays the number of clients who improved, deteriorated, or remained unchanged for each problem. The percentage of clients showing improvement is also listed. In addition to clinical and statistical information, the database allows the manager to track the cost per case by diagnosis and by payer. For the hypertensive sample that was discharged from the VNA during this 5-month period, the average cost per case was $3,726.44. The level of information provided by integrating the Omaha System with the other statistical and financial data is useful in reporting the impact of clinical interventions to managed care organization and other provider groups.

Use of the Omaha System at the VNA of Chicago has improved the level of job satisfaction in the clinical staff. They now speak a common language as they document client status and outcome achievement. Productivity has improved with the introduction of a conceptually based record-keeping system. Compliance with regulatory and accreditation standards has increased since the client record and information system have been modified. Most significantly, the Omaha System has provided a means of reviewing the quality of patient care and has introduced a reliable and valid method of tracking the benefits and costs of VNA service.

SUMMARY

It is critical that administrators and clinicians employed by community-focused agencies, nursing homes, and acute care facilities become concerned about measuring the quality of nursing practice. There is no single correct approach for all settings. This chapter describes a practice, documentation, and information management model that has been adopted by various service providers, including the VNA of Chicago. The model is congruent with the resources, regulations, and contracts of the practice setting. It provides a way to integrate clinical data with other statistical and financial data that are part of a total management information system. When considered as a unit, the model contains aspects of traditional and emerging indicators such as process indicators and client knowledge-behavior-status outcome measures.

The profession is making remarkable progress toward its goal of measuring the quality of nursing practice. Considerable time and commitment will be required, however, before nurses consistently use scientifically rigorous, practical, client-focused models. It is possible that all nurses may never use such ideal models. That possibility, however, should not diminish our collective effort. "The task ahead is arduous; the benefits are far reaching" (Vahldieck, Reeves, & Schmelzer, 1989, p. 107).

REFERENCES

American Nurses Association. (1976). Some basic ideas in evaluating the quality of health care. In A, Donabedian (Ed.), *Issues in evaluation research* (pp. 3-28). Kansas City, MO: Author.

American Nurses Association. (1988). *Classification systems for describing nursing practice.* Kansas City, MO: Author.

American Nurses Association. (1995). *Nursing report card for acute care.* (Publication No. NP-101). Washington, DC: Author.

Donabedian, A. (1988, September). The quality of care: How can it be assessed? *Journal of American Medical Association, 260,* 1743-1748.

Freeman, R.B. (1961). Measuring the effectiveness of public health nursing service. *Nursing Outlook, 9,* 605-607.

General Accounting Office. (1994, September). *Health care reform "Report cards" are useful but significant issues need to be addressed.* (GAO/HEHS-94-219). Gaithersburg, MD: Author.

Hegyvary, S.T. (1992). Outcomes research: Integrating nursing practice into the world view. In *Patient outcomes research: Examining the effectiveness of nursing practice.* (NIH Publication No. 93-3411). Bethesda, MD: National Institutes of Health, National Center for Nursing Research.

Joint Commission on Accreditation of Healthcare Organizations. (1994). *1995 Accreditation Manual for Home Care* (Vol. I). Oakbrook Terrace, IL: Author.

Lang, N.M. (Ed.). (1995). *Nursing data systems: The emerging framework.* Washington, DC: American Nurses Association.

Lewis, E.P. (1976, March). Quantifying the unquantifiable. *Nursing Outlook, 24,* 147.

Lohr, K.N. (Ed.). (1990). *Medicare: A strategy for quality assurance* (Vol. I). Washington, DC: National Academy Press.

Marek, K.D., & Lang, N.M. (1993). Nursing sensitive outcomes. In *Papers from the Nursing Minimum Data Set Conference* (pp. 100-120). Edmonton, Alberta, Canada: Canadian Nurses Association.

Mark, B.A. (1995, Spring). The black box of patient outcomes research. *Image: The Journal for Nursing Scholarship, 27,* 42.

Martin, K.S. (In press). The Omaha System: A data base for ambulatory and home care. In M.E. Mills, C.A. Romano, & B.R. Heller (Eds.), *Information management in nursing and healthcare.* Springhouse, PA: Springhouse.

Martin, K.S., & Scheet, N.J. (1992a). *The Omaha System: Applications for community health nursing.* Philadelphia: Saunders.

Martin, K.S., & Scheet, N.J. (1992b). *The Omaha System: A pocket guide for community health nursing.* Philadelphia: Saunders.

Martin, K.S., & Scheet, N.J. (1995). The Omaha System: Nursing diagnoses, interventions, and client outcomes. In N.M. Lang, (Ed.), *Nursing data systems: The emerging framework* (pp. 105-113). Washington, DC: American Nurses Association.

Martin, K.S., Scheet, N.J., & Stegman, M.R. (1993). Home health clients: Characteristics, outcomes of care, and nursing interventions. *American Journal of Public Health, 83,* 1730-1734.

Mateo, M. (1991). Psychosocial measurement. In M. Mateo & K. Kirchhoff, *Conducting and using nursing research in the clinical setting* (pp. 154-166). Baltimore: Williams & Wilkins.

National Center for Nursing Research. (1992). *Patient outcomes research: Examining the effectiveness of nursing practice.* (NIH Publication No. 93-3411). Bethesda, MD: National Institutes of Health.

National League for Nursing. (1994). *Summary of findings: In search of excellence in home care.* New York: Author.

Naylor, M.D., Munro, B.H., & Brooten, D.A. (1991). Measuring the effectiveness of nursing practice. *Clinical Nurse Specialist, 5,* 210-215.

Reif, L.J., & Martin, K.S. (In press). *Nurses and consumers: Partners in assuring quality in the home.* Washington, DC: American Nurses Association.

Remington, M.A. (1990). Measuring the quality of nursing care among critical care nurses. In C. Waltz & O. Strickland (Eds.), *Measurement of nursing outcomes:* Vol. 3. *Measuring clinical skills and professional development in education and practice* (pp. 69-84). New York: Springer.

Scholtes, P.R. (1988). *The team handbook.* Madison, WI: Joiner Associates.

Shamian, J. (1993). Response to K.D. Marek's and N.M. Lang's paper on nursing sensitive outcomes. In *Papers from the Nursing Minimum Data Set Conference* (pp. 121-126). Edmonton, Alberta, Canada: Canadian Nurses Association.

Shaughnessy, P.W., Crisler, K.S., Schlenker, R.E., & Arnold, A.G. (1995). Outcome-based quality improvement in home care. *Caring, 14,* 44-49.

Shaughnessy, P.W., Schlenker, R.E., Crisler, K.S., Powell, M.C., Hittle, D.F., Kramer, A.M., Spencer, M.J., Beale, S.K., Bostrom, S.G., Beaudry, J.M., DeVore, P.A., Chandramouli, V., Grant, W.V., Arnold, A.G., Bauman, M.K., & Jenkins, J. (1994). *Measuring outcomes of home health care: Vol. I: Final report: Development of outcome-based quality measures for home health services.* Denver, CO: Center for Health Policy Research and Center for Health Sciences Research, University of Colorado Health Sciences Center.

Vahldieck, R., Reeves, S., & Schmelzer, M. (1989). A framework for planning public health nursing service to families. *Public Health Nursing, 6,* 102-107.

Wilson, A.A. (1993). Bridging issues of cost and quality through patient outcome measurement. *Caring, 12,* 40-44.

Validating clinical competence: Old and new approaches

CAROLYN J. YOCOM*

Concern about and recognition of a nurse's level of clinical competence have been ongoing issues throughout the history of nursing in the United States. Initially, in the late 1800s, hospital schools of nursing established registries to assist the public in identifying individuals who had completed a specific nursing education program. However, because educational standards varied greatly, the public continued to experience great difficulty distinguishing between safe and unsafe practitioners (Waddle, 1979). Subsequently, the efforts of early nursing leaders, including Isabel Hampton Robb, Sophia Palmer, and Lavinia Dock, were instrumental to the introduction and passage of legislation establishing state boards of nursing (Goodnow, 1929; Shannon, 1975). The first of these boards were established in 1903 in New York, New Jersey, North Carolina, and Virginia (Goodnow, 1929; National Council of State Boards of Nursing, 1994; Shannon, 1975). A primary function of the boards was and continues to be to protect the public from unsafe practitioners through the establishment of standards for nursing education programs and maintenance of a registry of nurses who meet specified criteria, including graduation from a state-approved school of nursing and passage of a state-recognized examination (Goodnow, 1929; Shannon, 1975; Waddle, 1979).

A nurse's ability to provide competent care to clients continues to be of great importance in today's health care environment. The professional nurse is held accountable for the delivery of safe and effective care to his or her clients in a wide variety of health care settings. Given the increasing acuity levels of clients' health problems within a complex and highly technical health care system, it is crucial to the maintenance of the public's health, safety, and welfare that appropriate mechanisms are available to assess or measure the clinical competence of licensed professional nurses as well as candidates for licensure.

The purposes of this paper are to describe the approaches currently used to determine a nurse's level of clinical competence and to describe new and emerging approaches that may enhance our ability to assess this trait accurately.

The measurement approaches described here are applicable to the assessment of clinical competence of candidates for nurse licensure as well as of those already licensed to practice. They are also applicable to all levels of practice, from the entry-level professional nurse who is, at the least, minimally competent, to the experienced nurse who is licensed and/or certified as an advanced practitioner. Therefore, intertwined throughout this discussion are references to the assessment of individuals both to determine whether they are minimally competent to provide safe and effective nursing care, which is the focus of boards of nursing, and to determine whether they possess characteristics that are indicative of having reached a higher level of expertise, as exemplified by the certification process.

DEFINITION OF CLINICAL COMPETENCE

As with the measurement of any abstract concept, an identification of its attributes is critical. A *competency* can be described as a single, observable or definable skill that can be further classified as consisting of knowledge, skills, aptitudes, attitudes, and intellectual strategies such as problem solving and the ability to deal with ambiguity (Callahan, 1988). Furthermore, a definition of professional competence, introduced by Kane (1992) and based

*The opinions expressed herein are those of the author and are not those of the National Council of State Boards of Nursing.

on the work of LaDuca, Engle, and Risley, (1978), Benner (1984), and McGaghie (1991) is also relevant. Kane (1992) defines an individual's level of competence in an area of practice as ". . . the degree to which the individual can use the knowledge, skills, and judgment associated with the profession to perform effectively in the domain of possible encounters defining the scope of professional practice" (p. 166).

The key phrase in this definition is, "use the knowledge, skills and judgment associated with the profession to perform effectively." An individual can possess specific knowledge and/or be able to demonstrate the ability to perform certain psychomotor, communication, or other skills pertinent to a specific domain. However, for an individual's practice to typify that of a clinically competent practitioner, the exercise of appropriate levels of clinical judgment and decision-making skills that incorporate the use and application of knowledge and skills to meet a client's specific needs must be demonstrated.

It is also important to recognize that demonstration of competence within a profession is not, and should not be, a one-time-only endeavor. Rather, it should be an ongoing process. In 1985, the National Council of State Boards of Nursing's (NCSBN) position paper on continued competence stated, "Continued competence is the ability to continue to demonstrate competence throughout one's career. In nursing, it encompasses the ongoing ability to render direct nursing care or the ongoing ability to make sound judgements upon which nursing care is based" (NCSBN, 1985).

MEASUREMENT CONCEPTS

A naive approach used to judge whether an individual or object possesses a specific attribute is to fall back on the old adage, "I know one (it) when I see it." This approach is commonly used when shopping for artwork or antiques (is it a "good" piece?). It could also be applied to informal evaluations of members of the nursing profession (is he or she a competent nurse?). In either case, arriving at a conclusion is based on a personal, internal set of criteria generated and used as a basis for comparing the characteristics of the object or person to be evaluated.

In situations exemplified by these examples, the reasonableness of the criteria and the generalizability of the evaluation outcomes can be open to question because of the degree of abstractness of the concept being measured, the individual preferences of the evaluator, and the consistency in which the criteria are applied. It is therefore obvious that a more formal, standardized approach is required to obtain consistent, valid judgements about the presence of a trait such as clinical competence.

Within nursing, the development of standardized measurement tools to assess the knowledge, skills, and abilities of professional nurses are exemplified by both licensure and certification examinations. In both cases, empirically grounded indicators (e.g., an examinee's responses to a series of test questions) are compared with predetermined criteria indicative of the desired trait (e.g., clinical competence). The psychometric soundness of the measurement device (e.g., paper and pencil or performance examinations) must be supported by evidence of two desirable qualities: reliability and validity.

Reliability concerns the extent to which a measuring procedure yields the same results on repeated trials (i.e., that there is consistency across repeated measurements) (Carmines & Zeller, 1979). In evaluating the suitability of an examination, its validity is of primary concern. "*Validity* refers to the appropriateness, meaningfulness, and usefulness of the specific inferences made from test scores. Test validation is the process of accumulating evidence to support such inferences" (American Education Research Association, American Psychological Association, and National Council on Measurement in Education, 1985, p. 9).

As Kane (1992) points out, "[t]he validity of an assessment of professional competence depends on the evidence supporting inferences from an examinee's score to conclusions about the examinee's expected performance over the domain of encounters defining the area of practice." Three primary inferences are inherent in this process: determining the quality of the examinee's performance (evaluation); drawing conclusion about general behavior from the observed behavior (generalization); and drawing conclusions about performance in the "real world" from results on the type of assessment performed (extrapolation) (Kane, 1992).

CURRENT MEASUREMENT APPROACHES

Methods used to assess the degree of clinical competence possessed by a professional nurse can be grouped within two different types of approaches: performance testing and objective testing.

Performance testing

Examples of performance testing include the use of skill inventories (checklists), peer evaluations, and chart/record audits. Following a brief description of each approach, their advantages and disadvantages are discussed.

Skill inventories are commonly used in basic nursing education programs and in specialty courses/programs (e.g., nurse midwifery) to determine whether the examinee can demonstrate acceptable levels of performance while interacting with real clients. However, they are not used in professional licensure and certification tests in the United States because of the amount of personnel and fiscal resources necessary to perform performance evaluations on large numbers of examinees.

Peer evaluations of practicing nurses are used in some states to validate the continued competence of advanced practitioners. This involves observation of the targeted nurse by a recognized "expert" colleague during the course of regular work assignments and the use of rating forms or checklists. This approach also requires extensive personnel and fiscal resources if it is to be used in a large-scale testing or evaluation program.

A chart/record audit entails a systematic review of client charts for the purpose of documenting a nurse's accuracy and the thoroughness of client assessments and management. It is also used on a limited basis to validate the continued competence of advanced practitioners. A common concern raised in relation to the use of this approach involves claims that a client's written record includes neither complete documentation of the processes used by the practitioner nor all of the nursing activities in which nurses are engaged.

Evaluation of the performance of a specific skill (checklist/inventory) or a sample of activities commonly used in client interactions (peer evaluations) has a major advantage over objective testing formats because they involve the use of real versus contrived or simulated situations. The examinee's ability to provide competent care can be observed and evaluated directly. To a lesser extent, the same also can be said for chart/record audits.

As mentioned earlier, these approaches currently have limited use in large-scale testing situations because of the need for an extensive number of trained raters and the availability of sufficient fiscal resources to carry out the evaluations in a timely manner. In addition, several other disadvantages of these approaches contribute to their non-use (Kane, 1992; Swanson, 1990). Because of the use of real clients and a lack of examiner control over the client health problems being manifested and the testing environment, standardization of the testing situation across examinees is difficult at best. In addition, the probability of measurement errors is high and contributes to an unacceptable level of reliability in reported scores. This is related to a lack of specificity in evaluation criteria, which is necessary because of the potential for wide variations in client conditions, the use of multiple raters, and consequently the potential for interrater reliability problems.

Objective testing

An objective test usually consists of multiple-choice questions (MCQ), but may also contain true-false or matching-type questions. Standardized MCQ examinations are used commonly in high-volume licensure and certification testing because of their relative ease of construction and administration, the use of objective scoring mechanisms, and, through the use of optical mark scanners or computer-based administration, short turnaround times for score reporting. The test items on these examinations are developed by content experts who have received instruction in item construction and are recognized by peers as expert item writers. Items are developed according to the following specifications: specific knowledge, skill, or ability to be measured; degree of difficulty; and level of competency (e.g., entry-level, expert). Content validation of newly constructed items can be strengthened via documentation of the correct response in reference materials commonly available to prospective examinees, review by a second panel of experts, and pretesting of the item.

The *Standards for Educational and Psychological Testing* (American Education Research Association et al., 1985) identifies specific standards for the compilation of a valid examination from available test items. Included is Standard 11.1, which states that the content domain to be covered must be defined clearly and explained in terms of the importance of the content for competent performance in an occupation.

Adherence to the *Standards* during the process of examination development results in a valid and reliable evaluation of clinical competence to the extent that one believes that an objective-type test question (e.g., MCQ, true-false) can test the knowledge, skills, and abilities inherent in the domain of nursing practice. A carefully constructed MCQ-based examination can evaluate knowledge and the ability to analyze and synthesize selected clinical and theoretical facts, or, for example, knowledge of the procedural steps involved in the performance of psychomotor skills. However, it is difficult to make a strong argument that such an examination can measure competence effectively in the areas of clinical decision making and clinical judgement (Schleutermann, Albano, Miller, Farrand, & Holzemer, 1979). This is partly due to the level of artificiality imposed by a written test and partly due to the "cuing" effect of item response options.

(When was the last time you interacted with a client and found four options for dealing with the client's problem painted on the wall behind them?)

Alternatives to the use of an MCQ examination for the purpose of evaluating clinical decision making and judgement have been explored in both nursing and medicine during the past two decades. These alternative approaches are grouped generally under the rubric of "performance-based assessment." These approaches place an emphasis on "testing complex, 'higher-order' knowledge and skills in the real-world context in which they are actually used, generally with open-ended tasks that require substantial examinee time to complete" (Swanson, Norman, & Linn, 1995, p. 6). According to Moss (1992), many experts in the field of testing maintain that performance assessment is likely to produce more valid interpretations of certain complex domains than do MCQ assessments alone. Performance assessment taps into an individual's ability to apply knowledge of principles, theories, and facts to decision-making activities in situations representative of those encountered in real life, thus increasing the validity of assessment results.

One such alternative, the use of paper-and-pencil–based simulations as an examination technique, was pioneered by McGuire, Solomon, and Bashook (1976) at the University of Illinois at Chicago. This approach, referred to as a patient management problem (PMP), is characterized by the use of a latent image, branched simulation of a clinical situation in which the examinee is presented with a brief client situation. Patient management skills are demonstrated by making judgments about what types of data to obtain and what nursing actions to undertake. Options for data collection and patient management actions are included in long lists of possibilities. Upon selection of the desired option, pertinent client information is revealed by showing the latent, printed material associated with each option. Progression through the PMP is dependent on examinee choices.

Within nursing, Holzemer et al. developed and evaluated a series of PMPs designed to evaluate the performance of graduate students in a nurse practitioner program (Farrand, Holzemer, & Schleutermann, 1982; Holzemer, Schleutermann, Farrand, & Miller, 1981; Noricini, Swanson, Grosso, & Webster, 1985). Subsequently, these investigators and others (e.g., Noricini, et al., 1985) reported continuing concerns regarding the validity of using PMPs for measuring competence in clinical decision making and judgment. Among these were the artificiality imposed by the written format and the linear pathway imposed on the examinee. Another disadvantage of the PMP was the cuing effect imposed by the use of long lists of response options (Yocom, 1985). Therefore, some of the same problems identified with the use of MCQ examinations were not eliminated by PMPs.

A second alternative involves a simulation technique, called Performanced Based Development System, that uses videotaped sequences, usually 1 to 3 minutes in length, to depict either an overt or subtle clinical problem with known nursing and/or medical interventions (Del Bueno, 1983, 1990). Each video sequence contains visual and aural information that is based on signs, symptoms, cues, and clues deemed relevant for problem recognition. Following viewing, the nurse completes a separate answer sheet by recording the patient's priority health risk or problem, the nursing actions or interventions that would be used to correct or reduce the risk, and the rationale for the actions or interventions chosen. Written responses are then compared with a set of criterion answers and a performance rating (acceptable, unacceptable, or partially acceptable) is determined.

This approach permits the nurse to assimilate and process information without the aid of cues as to what data are important (i.e., lists of available data) or their interpretation. It also provides insight into the reasoning underlying the selection of a specific course of action. The disadvantages of this approach to competence assessment include the necessity to review and grade handwritten narrative statements by examiners, thus making it unsuitable for use in large-scale testing programs, and the inability of the examinee to interact with the "patient" in a dynamic manner.

A third alternative, currently being explored by the medical testing community, involves the use of standardized patients. Individuals are taught to portray patients in a standardized, consistent fashion depicting a variety of clinical problems. Examinees interact directly with the "patients," engaging in history taking, physical examination performance, ordering and interpreting diagnostic tests, and counseling behaviors (van der Vleuten & Swanson, 1990; Vu & Barrows, 1994). While other performance evaluation methods are being explored (Blackwell et al., 1991), examinees generally write short answers to open-ended questions about physical findings, diagnosis, and treatment plan following each interaction with a series of standardized patients. Examinee performance is evaluated by examining checklists or rating forms completed by the "patient" or physician raters. This approach, while still being evaluated for use in large-scale competence testing programs, may be a valuable adjunct in small-scale certification programs or institution-based evaluation programs following resolution of issues impacting on the validity and reliability of scoring mechanisms.

USE OF PERFORMANCE ASSESSMENTS IN FUTURE MEASUREMENT APPROACHES

The advent of major advances in computer technology, including interactive audiovisual enhancements, has been instrumental in facilitating exploration of an alternative approach to the evaluation of clinical competence. The use of computer and interactive audiovisual technology opens new horizons in attempts to overcome the disadvantages associated with the use of paper-and-pencil based MCQ examinations, PMPs, and other written response formats for the evaluation of clinical competence in nursing.

In 1988, the NCSBN was the recipient of a major grant from the W.K. Kellogg Foundation for a 3-year study to explore the feasibility of developing computerized clinical simulation testing (CST™) for evaluating the clinical decision-making skills and competencies of entry-level nurses (Bersky, 1991, 1994; Bersky & Brady, 1994; Bersky & Yocom, 1991, 1994; Yocom & Bersky, 1992). The project, conducted in collaboration with the National Board of Medical Examiners (NBME), was designed to adapt technology and software developed by the NBME for the delivery of computer-based clinical simulations for initial nurse licensure; to initiate the development of 20 computerized simulations in nursing; and to examine the validity and reliability of computerized clinical simulation tests as a basis for making nursing licensure decisions.

Computerized clinical simulation testing permits examinees to realistically simulate the problem-solving and decision-making skills used in the management of client needs. In CST, each case begins with a brief description of a client situation, presented on an introductory screen, along with the client's location, the day of care, and the time. The examinee is then free to collect client data through assessment activities and review of client records and to specify nursing interventions through free keyboard entry. At any point in the case, the examinee may advance the clock in simulated time in order to evaluate the client at a later point in time or to specify further interventions. Originally, the client assessment function consisted of a list of 22 options from which any or all could be selected. This approach has been converted to a free keyboard entry format in order to eliminate cuing. No intervention questions or answer options are presented to the examinee.

The simulations are dynamic in that the client's condition changes over time and in response to nursing actions. This permits examinees to evaluate the effectiveness of nursing actions and to provide follow-up care. In response to a request for assessment data (e.g., vital signs), these are reported in a manner and time frame consistent with current practice. The specification of a nursing intervention (e.g., administer Demerol) results in the provision of a printed message reporting that the medication has been given. To evaluate the client's response to the medication, the examinee must first move the simulated "clock" ahead to the desired time and then assess the client's comfort level.

As an examinee proceeds through the case, a permanent record of his or her actions is made. This is then compared with the case's scoring key by a computer program. The case scoring keys, developed by a committee of expert nurses, specify performance criteria with items defined as benefits (is an appropriate action), neutrals (no positive or negative client impact), or as inappropriates, risks, and flags (cause harm to the client). A unique feature of the CST scoring system enables the application of procedures that can award credit for different but equally valid nursing actions. It can also award different amounts of credit depending on the timing, sequencing, and level of correctness of nursing actions.

During the course of the project, 27 nursing simulation cases were developed. Of these, 25 were programmed and had scoring keys developed. In addition, audiovisual augmentation was developed for two cases. A 2,500+ term default nursing intervention database was developed to enable CST to function as a unique uncued examination because it is programmed to recognize a full range of nursing activities specified by examinees through free keyboard entry. A comparable assessment database is currently being developed to support this change in format.

The results of a pilot study using diploma, associate degree, and baccalaureate degree graduates who were candidates for registered nurse (RN) licensure provide preliminary evidence that a valid and reliable CST examination can be constructed to evaluate clinical decision-making competency in nursing. Statistical evidence supported the hypothesis that CST is measuring something different than that measured by multiple-choice questions. While there was no clear documentation of construct validity, examinee comments strongly suggest that they were able to demonstrate use of clinical decision-making skills.

The use of audiovisual augmentation had no statistically significant effect on overall examinee performance in two cases. However, there were differences in how examinees performed on different items within these cases, depending on whether or not the cases were augmented with audiovisual material (Bersky, 1994).

The findings of this initial study provide a basis for continued research on CST. The current phase of the CST Project (1993-1999) includes revision of the simulation authoring system, use of a "windows" software environment, redesign of the CST user-interface screens, additional case development including audiovisual enhancement of selected cases, a test of the simulation software in selected schools of nursing, and a large-scale field study to further examine CST's psychometric characteristics. Results of the field study and other supporting evidence will be used by the National Council's membership to decide whether CST will become a component of NCLEX-RN™.

Additional issues will also be addressed in this next phase of development. Plans include an investigation of the feasibility of expanding the use of CST beyond the originally conceived view that it could be used as an adjunct to the computerized adaptive testing (CAT) methodology used to administer the current MCQ-based NCLEX™. Current thinking is that CST could potentially be used to test licensed nurses returning to practice after a period of inactivity in addition to testing practicing (licensed) nurses to determine their continued ability to apply nursing knowledge to the complex health care needs of clients.

The use of CST as a diagnostic assessment tool also has great potential value. One such application would involve its use in those jurisdictions in which nursing boards mandate that licensees meet specific continuing education requirements. A second application would involve the use of CST to evaluate licensees who have had disciplinary action taken against their licenses. In both of these applications, reeducation could be targeted to identified areas of weakness.

SUMMARY

The ability of a nurse to provide competent care to clients is of primary concern to the profession and to members of the regulatory profession. Several approaches currently used to evaluate clinical competence have been described. These include the use of skill inventories, peer evaluations, chart audits, and standardized, objective tests. With respect to their validity, each approach has contrasting strengths and weaknesses in terms of the reliability of the data provided and the ability to arrive at valid judgments about the quality of an examinee's performance and to draw conclusions about general behavior based on observed behavior and about projected performance in the "real" world based on results on the type of assessment performed. Advances in computer technology have opened up a new avenue of exploration in our attempt to identify a testing methodology that can surmount the disadvantages of using currently available performance and objective testing formats. Preliminary results of research exploring the feasibility of using CST are promising. If strong evidence can be gathered supporting the validity and reliability of CST, it is possible that CST could be used alone or as an adjunct to other testing methodologies to evaluate the clinical decision-making and judgment components of clinical competence.

REFERENCES

American Education Research Association, American Psychological Association, and National Council on Measurement in Education. (1985). *Standards for educational and psychological testing.* Washington, DC: American Psychological Association.

Benner, P. (1984). *From novice to expert: Excellence and power in clinical nursing practice.* Menlo Park, CA: Addison-Wesley.

Bersky, A. (1991). The measurement characteristics of computerized clinical simulation tests (CST). In M. Garbin (Ed.), *Assessing educational outcomes* (pp. 107-112). New York: National League for Nursing.

Bersky, A. (1994). Effect of audiovisual enhancement on problem-solving and decision-making activities during a computerized clinical simulation test (CST) of nursing competence. *Evaluation and the Health Professions, 17*(4), 446-464.

Bersky, A., & Brady, D. (1994). A new generation in competence assessment in nursing: Computerized clinical simulation testing (CST). *Issues, 14*(1), 1, 4-5, 8.

Bersky, A., & Yocom, C. (1991). *Computerized clinical simulation testing project: Year three report.* Chicago: National Council of State Boards of Nursing.

Bersky, A., & Yocom, C. (1994). Computerized clinical simulation testing: Its use for competence assessment in nursing. *Nursing and Health Care, 15*(3), 120-127.

Blackwell, T., Ainsworth, M., Dorsey, N., Callaway, M., Rogers, & Collins, J. (1991). A comparison of short-answer and extended-matching question scores in an objective structured clinical exam. *Academic Medicine, 66*(9) (Suppl), S40-S42.

Callahan, L. (1988). Competence models: From theory to practical application. *Journal of the American Association of Nurse Anesthetists, 56,* 387-389.

Carmines, E., & Zeller, R. (1979). *Reliability and validity assessment.* Beverly Hills, CA: Sage Publications.

del Bueno, D.J. (1983). Doing the right thing: Nurses ability to make clinical decisions. *Nurse Educator, 8,* 7-11.

del Bueno, D.J. (1990). Experience, education and nurses ability to make clinical judgments. *Nursing and Health Care, 11,* 290-294.

Farrand, L., Holzemer, W., & Schleutermann, J. (1982). A study of construct validity: Simulations as a measure of nurse practitioners' problem solving skills. *Nursing Research, 31,* 37-42.

Goodnow, M. (1929). *Outlines of nursing history.* Philadelphia: Saunders.

Holzemer, W., Schleutermann, J., Farrand, L., & Miller, A. (1981). A validation study: Simulations as a measure of nurse practitioner's problem-solving skills. *Nursing Research, 30,* 139-144.

Kane, M. (1992). The assessment of professional competence. *Evaluation & the Health Professions, 15,* 163-182.

LaDuca, A., Engel, J.D., & Risley, M.E. (1978). Progress toward development of a general model for competence definition in health professions. *Journal of Allied Health, 7,* 149-155.

MaGaghie, W.C. (1991). Professional competence evaluation. *Educational Researcher, 20*(1), 3-9.

McGuire, C., Solomon, L., & Bashook, P. (1976). *Construction and use of written simulations.* New York: The Psychological Corporation.

Moss, P. (1992). Shifting conceptions of validity in educational measurement: Implications for performance assessment. *Review of Educational Research, 62*(3), 229-258.

National Council of State Boards of Nursing. (1985). *Position paper on continued competence.* Chicago: Author.

National Council of State Boards of Nursing. (1994). *Profiles of member boards (1994).* Chicago: Author.

Noricini, J., Swanson, D., Grosso, L., & Webster, G. (1985). Reliability, validity and efficiency of multiple choice question and patient management problem item formats in assessment of clinical competence. *Medical Education, 19,* 238-247.

Schleutermann, J., Albano, E., Miller, A., Farrand, L., & Holzemer, W. (1979). *Mr. Ellis, a 48 year old man complaining of chest pain and difficulty breathing.* Chicago: University of Illinois at Chicago, Health Sciences Center.

Shannon, M.L. (1975). Nurses in American history: Our first four licensure laws. *American Journal of Nursing, 79,* 1327-1329.

Swanson, D. (1990). Issues in assessment of practice skills in medicine. *Professions Education Research, 12,* 3-6.

Swanson, D., Norman, G., & Linn, R. (1995). Performance-based assessment: Lessons from the health professions. *Educational Researcher, 24*(5), 5-11, 35.

van der Vleuten, C.P.M., & Swanson, D.B. (1990). Assessment of clinical skills with standardized patients: State of the art. *Teaching and Learning in Medicine, 2*(2), 58-76.

Vu, N.V., & Barrows, H.S. (1994). Use of standardized patients: Recent developments and measurement findings. *Educational Researcher, 23*(3), 23-30.

Waddle, F. (1979). Licensure achievements and limitations. In *The study of credentialing in nursing: A new approach: Volume II. Staff working papers* (pp. 126-164). Kansas City, MO: American Nurses Association.

Yocom, C. (1985). *Influence of initial nursing educational preparation of patient assessment.* Unpublished doctoral dissertation, University of Illinois at Chicago.

Yocom, C., & Bersky, A. (1992). The relationship of critical thinking ability and NCLEX-RN performance on computerized clinical simulation tests. Paper presented at the Tenth Anniversary Conference, Council for the Society for Research in Nursing Education, San Francisco, CA, February 12-14, 1992.

Ensuring quality in a managed care system

DULCELINA ALBANO STAHL

Rapid changes in the managed care arena continue to generate debate on the merits of managed care. Some health care providers blame managed care for the closure of many hospitals in the United States. Many health care executives attribute the reengineering and restructuring of their health care organizations to the effects of managed care capitation. The job security of registered nurses (RNs) is in jeopardy as hospitals cut salary and benefit costs by replacing RNs with patient care assistants and nurse extenders in response to decreased reimbursement under managed care and reduced payment from government-funded health care programs such as Medicaid and Medicare. Amid this scenario, it is significant to note that the public at large has not rallied against managed care. Even the American Nurses Association's demonstration at the Capitol in Washington, D.C. in the early spring of 1995 failed to elicit public support for their contention that quality of care is being jeopardized by the replacement of RNs with nonprofessional workers. What is really going on in managed care? Are the concerns for quality of care valid? What do consumers, providers of services, employers, the government, and payers contend about quality in a managed care system? To answer these questions, it is necessary to examine and critically analyze current trends in the managed care arena.

GOAL OF MANAGED CARE

Managed care is the provision of comprehensive quality services in a cost-effective and efficient manner. Its goal is to ensure access to quality health care services at the lowest possible cost. Thus, in a managed care system, the managed care organization (MCO), as the payer of the services delivered, is looking for value. This primary value is the price of the service. The lower the price, the higher will be the value for the MCO. To ensure a competitive advantage, the MCO also wants to see quality clinical outcomes from the providers of health care services.

TYPES OF MANAGED CARE ORGANIZATIONS

There are different types of MCOs. An understanding of how these different types basically function is beneficial in order to ascertain how they impact the quality of a managed care delivery system. The six key MCOs in the health care industry are the health maintenance organization (HMO), preferred provider organization (PPO), point-of-service (POS) plan, medical service organization (MSO), organized system of care (OSC), and integrated delivery system (IDS). The HMO also has different models, namely the group model, individual practice association (IPA), network health plan, and staff model.

In a group model HMO, the HMO contracts directly with a medical group consisting of physicians who are paid a certain amount of money per HMO member per month regardless of whether the members utilize any services. The physician group is then responsible for providing health care services to the HMO members. This is referred to as *capitation.* There is a financial incentive under this arrangement to control overutilization of services, and there may be instances of underutilization because the lower the utilization, the more monies would be saved for the physician group at the end of the contract year. Consequently, there have been issues raised regarding the long waiting time for HMO members to schedule an appointment with the HMO participating physician or to access services as needed. In fact, the physician, who acts as the gatekeeper of services, must authorize what services the patient can have; otherwise, the provider may not be reimbursed by the HMO. There have been documented cases in which serious injury occurred when the HMO failed to authorize the provision of services needed by a patient.

In a staff model HMO, the physicians are employed by the HMO and are expected to provide services to members. In a similar vein, the HMO-employed physicians are given financial incentives. With control of service utilization, there are more cost savings for the HMO, and part of these cost savings are then shared with the physicians.

In a network model, the HMO contracts with different medical groups as part of the HMO network. HMO members must use these participating physicians for their health care. If a member seeks health care outside the network, the HMO would not necessarily pay for the services. In this case, it is possible that a member may have to switch from his or her own physician of several years to another physician who is a member of the network. When this occurs, there may be a negative impact on the continuity of care because patients need to "start all over again" in establishing patient-physician relationships based on trust and confidence in the physicians' knowledge and sensitivity to their individual needs.

The IPA model entails a contract between the HMO and the individual physician who may be in solo practice but is part of the physician association. In this regard, the IPA functions very much like the group model in terms of control of utilization of services.

In a PPO arrangement, the MCO contracts with a provider who is willing to provide discounts for services delivered to a PPO member (usually about 20% off charges). This discount is passed on to the PPO member in the form of decreased premiums paid for the PPO benefits.

The MCO that allows patients the freedom of choice to seek health care for certain specialty services such as cardiology is the POS plan. The patient who is a member of the MCO can go to another physician who may not be part of the HMO network, but he or she will pay for out-of-pocket expenses as stipulated in the benefit plan. In this regard, access to services is not problematic as long as the patient is willing to pay the difference between what the MCO pays and the copayment required by the plan.

The MSO operates like a foundation. In an OSC, the providers are linked together in an organized system of care with the community and state agencies. The latest trend is the IDS, in which there is vertical and horizontal integration of services so that there is a continuum of care from acute, subacute, skilled nursing, ambulatory, home health care, and assisted living. These MCOs also subscribe to control of utilization of services and cost containment.

How do these different types of MCOs impact the quality of care in a managed care system? The HMO appears to have the most impact on the quality of care delivered to members in three areas: access to health care services, utilization of services, and financial incentives. If a participating provider or physician is concerned about overutilization, then an HMO member may experience delayed access to or even denial of health care services. To prevent financial loss, utilization of services may be controlled. Thus, if a patient needs more therapy than what the HMO is willing to pay for, the patient may not receive the additional therapy. This scenario obviously may create negative consequences for the patient's long-term quality of life. Providers who are given financial incentives may wind up limiting services even though these services may be necessary. These issues are difficult to address because HMOs have established parameters on what they consider "medically necessary" services through an analysis of utilization data of certain disease conditions. This medical necessity criterion is arrived at in consultation with the physician medical director of the HMO.

The major problem posed by a PPO arrangement lies in the denial of payment for services sought by the patient in a hospital, clinic, physician office, or other health care site that is not a participating provider of the MCO. Thus, a patient may not necessarily seek the services of a specialist of a nonparticipating provider, even though he or she may have wanted to do so, because of the financial constraint imposed by the MCO.

While there is freedom of choice under the POS plan, again the financial constraint of paying out-of-pocket expenses may deter the patient from accessing the best possible care. Finally, in an IDS, the patient may also be denied access to care at his or her preferred provider site because the provider is not a member of the IDS.

THE MANAGED CARE SCENARIO

A recent report by the Group Health Association of America (GHAA) revealed that there were approximately 50.5 million HMO members in the United States in 1994, an increase of 5.3 million from 1993 (Managed Care Information Center). It is predicted that by the end of 1995, this number could increase to 56 million. According to the Lewin-VHI study, "States as Payers: Managed Care for Medicaid Populations," about one quarter of all Medicaid recipients, or 7.6 million individuals, were under managed care programs in 1994, more than double the figure of 1993 (Capitol Publications, Inc., 1995). The Health Care Financing Administration (HCFA) had Medicare risk contracts with 154 HMOs as of January 1995 compared with 109 in 1994. Early 1995 HCFA data showed 2.3 million Medicare beneficiaries under a risk-contract HMO, of whom 582,000 were in health care prepayment plans that provide Part B services (noninpatient), 175,000 were in cost-contract HMOs, and about 17,000 were in other managed care demonstration projects (*Managed Care Stats & Facts,* 1995). This represents a 27% increase between 1994 and 1995 compared with a 19% increase between 1993 and 1994. Today, there are more than 3.1 million beneficiaries, or about 9% of all Medicare eligibles, who are enrolled in Medicare managed care contracts (Capitol Publications, Inc., 1995a). On July 9, 1995, President Clinton signed into law the Medicare SELECT bill, which allows Medicare supplemental insurance, or Medigap, in 50 states for another 3 years (Capitol Publications, Inc., 1995b). Employers are increasingly utilizing managed care to curb their health care costs. In 1994, a survey of 2,097 firms with 10 or more workers indicated a 1.1% decrease in their total health benefit costs. There has been a dramatic increase in managed care enrollment of covered workers from 52% in 1993 to 64% in 1994 (Atlantic Information Services, Inc., 1995a). Clearly, these managed care trends indicate that the public at large and the federal and state governments have accepted managed care as a cost-effective delivery system.

In terms of capitation, current data reveal tremendous cost savings for insurers and payers. This is primarily due to the financial incentives built into a capitation arrangement. If utilization of services is high, the provider is likely to incur financial loss because the capitated amount paid by the HMO may be inadequate to cover the provider's costs. Conversely, if there is low utilization of services, the provider would keep the per-member-per-month monies from the HMO. Prior to capitation and managed care, providers were able to bill for services provided in various settings, even though there was duplication of laboratory work, radiography, and the like. Today, HMOs do not pay for any duplication of ancillary tests or procedures. In effect, managed care has forced providers to be more efficient and to control costs.

Undoubtedly, MCOs have successfully decreased the costs of health care. However, today's more informed consumers continue to question the value they are getting from the health care premiums they pay. As HMOs compete to grow their businesses by enrolling more members, they also want quality outcomes from providers of services. The question remains, How can quality outcomes be ensured in a managed care system?

ENSURING QUALITY IN A MANAGED CARE SYSTEM

A definition of quality of care must be understood before any mechanism can be undertaken to ensure quality. For the HMOs, quality of care has been defined in terms of the parameters set by the National Committee on Quality Assurance (NCQA) in Washington, D.C. under the much-publicized Health Plan Employer Data and Information Set (HEDIS) standards. These standards of performance include member satisfaction, quality, access, preventive care, health promotion, and wellness. The HEDIS report provides purchasers and consumers with a tool for assessing the value of managed care plans. For example, under preventive health care, an MCO would be evaluated in terms of the percentage of children under 2 years of age who are immunized, the percentage of women receiving mammograms, and other such parameters. The recently published HEDIS "report cards" of 21 MCOs represented 10 million members and provided information on how well the HMOs met the NCQA standards of performance (Atlantic Information Services, Inc., 1995b). In 1995, Health Partners, a Minneapolis HMO, took bold initiative to provide their members with on-line access to the plan's data on their quality reports and provider directories via computer modem or diskette. In effect, members could then make an informed decision in choosing a provider that not only meets their needs but also provides quality services (Atlantic Information Services, Inc., 1995a).

The NCQA accredits the HMOs, particularly the Medicare-risk HMOs. The HCFA requires that an HMO pass the NCQA standards of performance in order to obtain Medicare-risk contracts with providers. Once an HMO fails to achieve NCQA accreditation, it may not continue to contract with providers until a plan of correction is submitted to the HCFA and this plan is implemented. Thus, it appears that there is already a mechanism in place and endorsed by the federal government to ensure that HMOs adhere to standards of performance that promote quality of care. Nevertheless, corporate and federal government health plan purchasers representing 80 million members recently formed a national Foundation for Accountability to design uniform outcomes-based standards for health plan performance because they believe that the HEDIS measures don't adequately measure the HMO's actual performance in the treatment of a particular case. They contend that the percentage of mammograms done does not provide data on how well the HMO examined the stage of cancer detection, the quality of life after treatment, or the effectiveness of a given procedure such as a lumpectomy versus a mastectomy (Atlantic Information Services, Inc., 1995c). The results of the foundation's efforts will need to be scrutinized in the future. Meanwhile, although the HEDIS report provides some standards of performance that relate to ensuring quality of care, a more critical examination of the day-to-day realities of inpatient acute, subacute, and outpatient (ambulatory) care suggests that the HEDIS standards are inadequate to ensure quality of care from both the providers' and health care professionals' perspectives.

For example, a 17-year-old Hispanic HMO patient was admitted for obstetrical delivery at a local community hospital. This patient has a history of substance abuse and no support systems available at home. As required by the HMO, she was discharged within 24 hours after delivery. Although social service and nursing staff attempted to address the patient's substance abuse problem, the early discharge precluded any intervention that would have made a difference in the quality of life of this teenage mother. Moreover, the patient was ill-prepared to assume the role of motherhood. Again, due to time constraints, the nursing staff could not provide adequate patient teaching.

This case raises both serious issues of quality of care for the patient and her newborn and ethical dilemmas. With no support system at home and inadequate preparation for assuming the role of motherhood, this early discharge cannot be considered quality care. The professional nurses were torn between their moral obligation to provide adequate patient teaching and necessary psychosocial intervention for the patient and the financial constraint posed by the HMO requirement of discharge within 24 hours. This problem is so rampant throughout the country that at least one state, New Jersey, recently passed legislation to require that managed care organizations such as HMOs allow longer hospital stays for mothers and their newborns. These early discharge practices have been labelled "drive-through deliveries," and have prompted Senators Bill Bradley (D-NJ) and Nancy Kassebaum (R-KN) to introduce similar legislation in the U.S. Senate. This bill would eliminate 24-hour hospital discharges, requiring 48-hour and 96-hour minimum stays for vaginal and cesarean deliveries, respectively (*Managed Care Law Outlook,* 1995).

Extant literature reveals that the results of patient satisfaction surveys among HMO members are conflicting. The Commonwealth Fund study, for instance, indicates that HMO members in Boston, Los Angeles, and Miami are less satisfied overall with their health plans than are fee-for-service recipients when focused on care issues rather than cost issues (*Managed Care Stats & Facts,* 1995). The GHAA was critical of this result as not being representative of the national population. Their criticisms notwithstanding, there have been instances encountered by nurse administrators when an expensive procedure such as a magnetic resonance image was not the diagnostic procedure of choice because the HMO would not reimburse the hospital. If quality of care is the goal of a managed care system, then the necessary procedure should be done even though it is expensive.

The latest trend in the health care delivery market is the advent of subacute care. It is in this area that ensuring quality presents major challenges to the providers and the health care industry at large.

What is subacute care? The American Health Care Association, as the leading representative of the long-term care industry, defines *subacute care* as a "comprehensive inpatient program designed for the individual who has had an acute event as a result of an illness, injury, or exacerbation of a disease process; has a determined course of treatment; and does not require intensive diagnostic and/ or invasive procedures" (American Health Care Association, 1994, p. 3). The Joint Commission on Accreditation of Healthcare Organization's (JCAHO) definition of subacute care is

> comprehensive inpatient care designed for someone who has had an acute illness, injury, or exacerbation of a disease process. It is goal-oriented treatment rendered immediately after or instead of acute hospitalization to treat one or more specific, active complex medical conditions or to administer one or more technically complex treatments, in the context of a person's underlying long-term conditions and overall situation. (JCAHO, 1995, p. 3)

Subacute care can be delivered in free-standing skilled nursing facilities, hospital-based subacute care units, or free-standing subacute care facilities (e.g., subacute rehabilitation). The subacute care program presents tremendous cost savings to MCOs because it costs at least 20% to 50% less than inpatient acute care (Stahl, 1994). Thus, many free-standing skilled nursing facilities have jumped on the bandwagon and developed subacute care programs. Many hospitals that are struggling with their occupancy have also adopted the subacute care program as an opportunity for survival. Indeed, the subacute care market is believed to have increased from a $900 million business in 1994 to $2.7 billion in 1997 (Marion Merrell Dow, Inc., 1993).

While many free-standing skilled nursing facilities truly took the time and initiative to ensure that the physical environment of the facility was remodelled to ensure safety and functionality in terms of the different levels of acuity of the patients under their care, there are those that consider themselves subacute care providers simply because they happen to be able to provide nursing care to the subacute care patients without regard to the required safety and environmental features for subacute care. Others have properly hired critical care nurses or nurses with medical-surgical acute care experience rather than utilizing their long-term care nurses who do not necessarily have the expertise to deal with the latest equipment needed by a subacute patient, such as ventilators. Nevertheless, there are some whose staffing levels may not be commensurate with the required nursing care hours for the level of acuity of these patients.

Because subacute care programs are being utilized increasingly by MCOs as a result of the tremendous cost savings, assurance for quality of care in a subacute care program is very important. One mechanism is accreditation by the JCAHO. In 1994, the JCAHO established its accreditation standards for subacute care programs. This accreditation would provide some degree of assurance that subacute care providers are meeting quality standards of care. Another mechanism is for the nursing profession to make a commitment to implement change in the nursing education curriculum to include a course on subacute care standards of nursing practice and attempt to refine the definitions that have been advanced by the American Health Care Association and JCAHO. Moreover, nurse researchers should focus their efforts on clinical outcomes in subacute care settings. Nurse administrators should also begin to address how management of a subacute care program can be enhanced by adapting previous knowledge of inpatient acute nursing service administration within the context of interdisciplinary team management.

Another avenue that would ensure quality of care in a managed care system is the implementation of the principles of case management. In this regard, the RN case manager functions as the coordinator of the services needed by the patient in order to ensure timely access to services and appropriate utilization. The case manager should also serve as patient advocate, educator, and facilitator. When the MCO limits services due to financial constraints, the case manager can present clinical data to support the medical necessity of such services so that approval by the MCO can be obtained. As an educator, he or she not only should provide patient education in terms of achieving desirable clinical outcomes based on critical pathways, but also should educate the members of the health care team regarding variables that impact the quality of care provided as a result of his or her nursing assessment and diagnosis.

Critical pathways are also significant in ensuring quality of care in a managed care system. Because critical pathways are timed sequences of interventions by the interdisciplinary team (e.g., physician, RN, physical therapist, occupational therapist, speech therapist, activity/recreational therapist, nutritionist, pharmacist, business office staff, clergy) that are designed to achieve measurable clinical and financial outcomes, RNs must take on the leadership role within their own organization in paving the way for the development of critical pathways. To date, there are still many health care providers, including subacute care providers, who are just beginning to develop critical pathways. Through critical pathways, the desired clinical outcomes could be better achieved because each member of the health team would have a set of principles that provide parameters for carrying out their respective discipline's objectives in achieving quality of care.

Another strategy for ensuring quality in a managed care system is for all providers of health care services to work in collaboration rather than in competition with each other. This could be achieved through the establishment of IDSs, community health integration networks, and information system networks. The information system networks are very important because they enable providers to access both clinical and financial data for a patient, at any point of entry in the health care system, thereby preventing duplication of tests and procedures as well as promoting quality clinical assessment.

The challenge of health care organizations and health care professionals in the future is to continue to perform continuous quality improvement activities designed not only to ensure quality care but also to improve processes and systems that ultimately impact positively on the managed care system. Processes and systems constitute the infrastructure of a system of care that has quality care delivered in the most cost-effective and cost-efficient manner at the core of its mission. In the final analysis, the assurance of quality care in a managed care system can only be truly achieved when the MCOs, the public at large, federal, state, and local governments, academia, employer groups, and the health professions collaborate in demanding quality as the norm rather than just a benchmark.

REFERENCES

American Health Care Association. (1994). *Subacute care medical and rehabilitation definition and guide to business development.* Washington, DC: Author.

Atlantic Information Services, Inc. (1995a, February 27). *Managed Care Week.* (p. 3). Washington, DC.

Atlantic Information Services, Inc. (1995b, February 27). *Managed Care Week.* (p. 2). Washington, DC.

Atlantic Information Services, Inc. (1995c, July 10). *Managed Care Week.* (pp. 1-2). Washington, DC.

Capitol Publications, Inc. (1995, February 10). *Managed Care Outlook Special Report.* (p. 3).

Capitol Publications, Inc. (1995a, July). *Managed Care Outlook.* (p. 6). Alexandria, VA.

Capitol Publications, Inc. (1995b, June 16). *Managed Care Outlook.* (p. 3). Alexandria, VA.

Joint Commission on Accreditation of Healthcare Organizations. (1995). *1995 Survey protocol for subacute programs.* Oakbrook Terrace, IL: Author.

Managed Care Information Center. The Executive Report on Integrated Care and Capitation. *1*(3), 9. Wall, N.J.

Managed Care Law Outlook. (1995, July). (p. 3).

Managed Care Stats & Facts. (1995, June 19). (p. 3).

Marion Merrell Dow, Inc. (1993). *Managed Care Digest Long Term Care Edition.*

Stahl, D. (1994). Subacute care: The future of health care. *Nursing Management 10,* 34-36.

Self-care nursing as a contribution to quality improvement in health: A Latin American experience

ILTA LANGE, SONIA JAIMOVICH

As they progress, the developing countries of the world are confronted with many of the problems of the industrialized world; as they become urbanized, they begin to share morbidity patterns (Levin, 1983) in addition to dealing with other ongoing problems. As a result of the decrease in fertility and mortality rates, demographic trends show that the adult population is increasing at a higher rate than the total population; thus, the relative importance of the adult population's health problems is also increasing, bringing serious consequences for the family, community, and society. Data from 1990 to 1995 reveal that in several Latin American countries such as Argentina, Chile, Uruguay, Costa Rica, Cuba, and Puerto Rico, life expectancy borders 74 years, while in other countries such as Bolivia, Guatemala, Honduras, and Nicaragua life expectancy is still 65 years or less (OPS/OMS, 1994). Infectious diseases, especially diarrhea, are still the primary cause of infant mortality in many developing countries: In 45% of the world's population infant mortality is still higher than 50 per 1000 live births (Rey, 1989). The main causes of death in the Latin American adult population, just as in the industrialized world, are cardiovascular diseases, cancer, and accidents, and more than half of all health care resources are allocated to treat health problems of this age group (although the implementation of preventive and curative policies are still rudimentary [Feachem, 1993]).

We can conclude then that the biggest health care concerns in Latin America are still related to the maternal-child population; however, as life expectancy increases, the problems related to the adult and elderly populations are becoming more important, especially in countries that are in demographic and epidemiological transition (Giaconi, 1995; Ministerio de Salud de Chile, 1993). In fact, the main challenge of health care in the 21st century will be the prevention and management of chronic diseases for which lifestyle changes and healthy self-care practices are essential (Valdivieso, 1992). Studies (Minesterio de Salud de Chile, 1993) show that health care services have a much lesser impact in reducing morbidity and mortality due to cancer, heart disease, accidents, cirrhosis, diabetes, and cerebrovascular disease than do healthy daily living practices and a healthy environment. There is an urgent need to design and implement health care delivery models that increase self-care capacities in the individuals, families, and communities they serve.

HEALTH CARE IN LATIN AMERICA

In most Latin American countries the funds allocated to health care are insufficient and the health systems do not provide adequate access and continuity of care to the populations they serve. The implementation of a primary health care strategy has been a goal in the Latin-American region since the 1979 World Health Organization conference in Alma Ata in the Soviet Union. Nevertheless, active participation of individuals, families, and communities in health-related decisions is still very limited. When people feel they cannot solve their health problems on their own, they seek professional help. These individuals then become dependent on the "health care providers," who treat their "patients" as though they have little knowledge and give them only minor opportunities to participate in the decisions that affect their own health and well-being. In this traditional health care model, health professionals are considered by society and by themselves as the exclusive owners of the truth regarding health issues. Patients are treated as though they are incapable of making adequate health-related decisions, and so the "experts" decide what is best. The patients' psychological, social, and spiritual needs as well as their self-care practices are usually ignored, and family participation is limited as a result of administrative regulations of the health services (Fig. 45-1).

Great efforts have been made in Latin America to operationalize the philosophical principles of the primary health care strategy—universality, equity, and social participation—in order to humanize quality health care (Aguayo, Chodowiecki, Lange, Ruiz, & Urrutia, 1994). *Universality* is understood as the right of every person to public or private health care according to his or her preferences and economic resources (Giaconi, 1995). *Equity* is the timely access to health care and its technologies, that is, to "give more to whom needs more." *Social participation* is the incorporation of community groups, organizations, or institutions in the identification of health problems and in the decision-making process (Aguayo et al., 1994; Minesterio de Salud de Chile, 1993).

In order to improve access to health care in the most cost-effective manner, the health system is organized in primary, secondary, and tertiary levels of care. The *primary level* of care is the entrance to the health care system; its services are located closest to where the people are, and its responsibility is to offer basic health services to the population through the implementation of health programs that strengthen basic sanitation, foster maternal/child health, improve nutrition, prevent infectious diseases, treat minor illnesses, and manage chronic diseases. This level of care deals with problems of great sociocultural complexity, most of which are related directly to unhealthy lifestyles such as teenage pregnancy, drug addictions, alcoholism, and prostitution, among others, that do not require high technology but rather a wide range of intersectoral commitment and coordination. Although this level of care is supposed to offer coverage to the highest proportion of the population, health services are still failing to reach those who need them most (Maglacas, 1988). The *secondary level* of care offers specialized curative care and diagnostic and therapeutic procedures such as chemotherapy and minor surgery, which require more sophisticated technology, but are required by a smaller proportion of the population. The *tertiary level* of care offers high-cost and high-technological specialist care; only a very small proportion of the population requires this level of care (Aguayo et al., 1994). The three levels of care should be articulated through a reference and counter-reference system to ensure continuity of care, but this goal has not yet been achieved sufficiently in most Latin American countries.

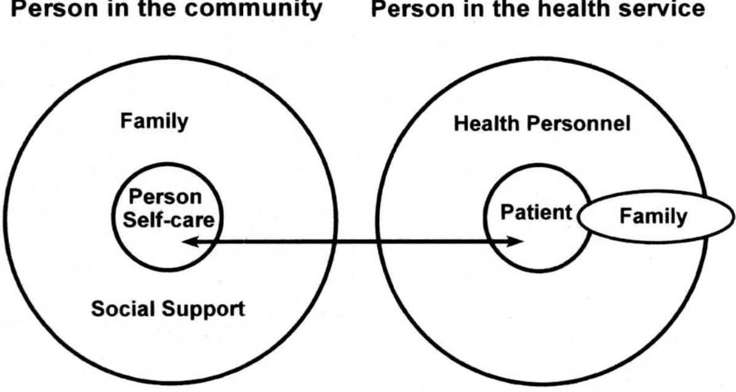

Fig. 45-1. Traditional health care model.

Primary health care is a strategy based on philosophical principles that can be applied in all three levels of care. Its purpose is to ensure universal, participatory, humanized, quality health care to the entire population. The following methodological tools contribute to attaining this goal: health education, self-care, client's participation, reference and counter-reference systems, interdisciplinary work, an intersectoral approach, application of appropriate technologies, risk approach, and strategic planning. Fig. 45-2 shows the primary health care strategy, its philosophical principles, its organizational and programmatic dimensions, and its methodological tools (Aguayo et al., 1994).

Self-care

Self-care is one of the methodological tools used to implement the primary health care strategy. Together with health education and client participation, self-care can be a key factor in improving access, continuity, and opportunity of care.

Self-care can be defined as all voluntary actions or activities in which individuals, families, and communities engage to promote and maintain their health and prevent and cure diseases. Woods (1989) defines self-care as an attempt to promote optimal health, prevent illness, detect symptoms at an early date, and manage chronic illness. Self-care also includes processes of self-monitoring and assessment, symptom perception and labeling, evaluation of severity, and evaluation and selection of treatment alternatives such as self-help, lay-helping resources, or formal health services.

Self-care nursing

Self-care nursing is a particular approach of nursing practice in which special emphasis is given to the clients' ca-

METHODOLOGICAL TOOLS:
· Health education
· Self-care
· Clients' participation
· Appropriate technology
· Reference/counter reference system
· Risk approach
· Interdisciplinary work
· Intersectoral approach
· Strategic planning
EQUITY
QUALITY
HEALTH CARE
UNIVERSALITY
SOCIAL PARTICIPATION
PROGRAMS:
· Health promotion
· Recuperation
· Rehabilitation
ORGANIZATION:
· First level of care
· Second level of care
· Third level of care

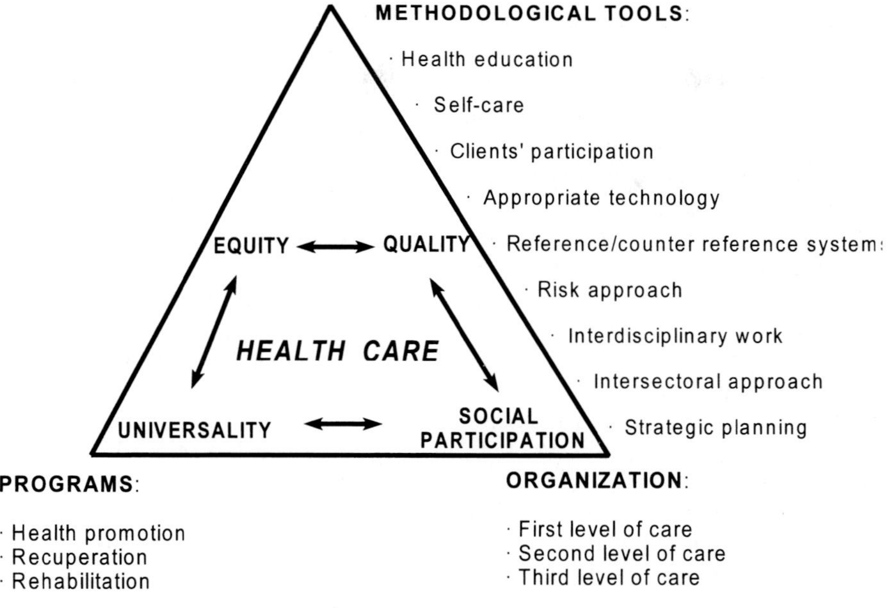

Fig. 45-2. Primary health strategy.

pacities to attain and maintain their own health. Self-care nursing incorporates strategies, methodologies, and activities into nursing care geared toward helping individuals, families, and communities to learn how to care for themselves and when to seek professional help (Hill & Smith, 1985).

Self-care nursing is considered a philosophy of care as well as a specific professional intervention. "It is a perspective that permeates all aspects of care, guiding nurses to consider all the ways clients can care for themselves in illness and in health" (Steiger & Lipson, 1985, p. 16). One of the consequences of this health care approach is that the clients learn to make better health-related decisions and to use health services more efficiently, thus reducing health costs.

Nurses have always been concerned about teaching self-care practices to their patients. Nightingale believed that every woman is a nurse because at some point in her life each woman has been in charge of the health care of someone else (e.g., a child, an elderly parent) (Shortell, 1976).

Orem is undoubtedly the person most commonly associated with the incorporation of the self-care concept into nursing practice. Her basic premise is that people have the potential to take care of themselves in health as well as in illness and that their self-care capacities can be strengthened through education and guidance. The core of Orem's philosophy is the belief that people have an innate ability to care for themselves. According to this philosophy the concept of self-care becomes the focal point of the nurse's thinking and behavior. Self-care contributes in specific ways to human structural integrity, human functioning, and human development (Orem, 1991). Orem defines self-care as ". . . practice of activities a person initiates and performs on his own behalf in order to maintain life, health and well-being" (Orem, 1990, p. 35). *Self-care agency* is the individual's own ability to perform self-care. This includes decisions about self-care as well as the actions required to accomplish them (Woods, 1989). Nursing, therefore, is required when a deficit exists between an individual's self-care needs and his or her self-care abilities. Nursing interventions vary according to the identified deficits of clients. The methods used to help clients include acting or doing for another, offering physical or psychological support, guiding and teaching, and providing a physical as well as a psychological environment that promotes personal development.

The nursing plan is implemented by the nurse who will assess and evaluate the client's progress. As needs and abilities change, the plan is modified. The client should progress until self-care deficits no longer exist and nursing actions are no longer needed (David, Christensen, Hohon,

Ord, & Wells, 1978; Morse & Werner, 1988). Five components can be identified in the self-care process.

1. *Health promotion:* These activities are geared toward maximizing well-being (e.g., exercising regularly).
2. *Health maintenance:* These activities are geared toward maintaining health status (e.g., getting enough sleep).
3. *Prevention of health problems:* Disease prevention activities seek to eliminate risk factors of specific health problems (e.g., eating a low cholesterol diet to reduce heart disease risk).
4. *Detection of health problems:* Disease detection activities seek to increase the consciousness of the individual with regard to signs and symptoms; these include certain self-examination techniques (e.g., breast self-examination to detect breast lumps).
5. *Disease management:* These activities include learning to follow the instructions of the health team and early detection of complications or side effects of treatments.

WHAT SHIFTS ARE NEEDED IN LATIN AMERICA TO IMPROVE THE QUALITY OF HEALTH CARE?

Quality in health care can be defined from two perspectives. From an institutional perspective it is defined as the provision of high-level professional services that are accessible to the population and that, through the use of existing resources, attain compliance and satisfaction in the clients (Palmer, 1990). From the client's perspective, health care is of high quality if it responds or exceeds his or her expectations.

The tangible component within this concept (Moller, 1992) is the quality of a product (e.g., a precise diagnosis or a revealing radiograph). Very often, however, the client evaluates the quality of health care mainly by the personal attributes of the health team that provides the service (e.g., their attitudes, ethical behavior, compromise, loyalty, and respect for the client).

According to the literature, different dimensions are included in the concept of quality health care. We will define eight of these dimensions and comment on how each of them can be strengthened by a self-care nursing model. These dimensions are scientific and technical expertise, accessibility, satisfaction or acceptability of health care services, effectiveness, efficiency, continuity of care, timeliness of care, and job satisfaction of health care providers.

Scientific and technical expertise

This dimension considers the competency of professional and nonprofessional health personnel in applying advances in knowledge and technology within the existing resource base to produce health and satisfaction in the patient population. Expertise is measured not only in the strict technical sense but also in the quality of interpersonal relationships between the client and health care providers.

The self-care nursing model emphasizes a strong horizontal relationship between the nursing staff and clients: Every question that a client or family member asks is considered an opportunity to improve quality, because questions can result in information regarding organizational or administrative deficiencies.

Accessibility

Accessibility is the facility by which health care services are obtained by the population. Accessibility measures consider geographical, organizational, economic, cultural, and emotional barriers. Is health care available for whomever needs it and when it is needed? With a self-care nursing approach cultural and emotional barriers can be reduced, thus increasing access to health care.

Continuity of care

One dimension of quality is defined as the degree to which needed care is provided in an uninterrupted and coordinated manner (Shortell, 1976). In this definition, it becomes evident that quality of care depends on the health team as well as on the clients themselves. In order to have uninterrupted care, self-care is essential.

Satisfaction or acceptability of health care services

This component measures the degree by which health care services satisfy the expectations of the clients (individuals, families, or communities). These expectations may not necessarily match those of the health professionals; for example, scientific and technical expertise, which is highly valued by the health team, is not always acceptable to and does not necessarily produce high satisfaction in the clients.

Acceptability is affected by the following: (a) the effect of health care actions on the specific health problem of the client, family, or community; (b) organizational factors such as physical environment, waiting time, schedules, visiting hours, and continuity of care by the same professional; and (c) the interpersonal relationship established between the client and the health team. Studies show that a good interpersonal relationship between the health team and clients is associated with higher client satisfaction. In Chile, for example, clients usually leave the physician's office unsatisfied if they do not get a prescription for medication. If a positive relationship is established, the gap between the clients' and the health professionals' perceptions and expectations can be minimized.

Within the concept of acceptability, compliance—the degree to which the patient or client accepts and does what the health care team has recommended—is also present. Self-care education tends to improve compliance by increasing the levels of knowledge, motivation, and skill in clients and their families to make health-related decisions.

Effectiveness

Effectiveness measures the degree to which a certain health care activity, which is practiced in a specific health care setting, produces an improvement in the health status of the patient, family, or community.

Efficiency

Efficiency measures the degree to which the highest level of quality can be obtained with the existing resources. Efficient services are those that offer individuals, families, and the community the best rather than the most health care. A self-care nursing model helps to avoid excessive treatments or indications that the client cannot or will not pursue because of economic problems or cultural, social, or psychological barriers. A self-care nursing model can augment efficiency because it considers the clients and their families as health resources. For example, mothers can be taught to stimulate the psychomotor development of their infants, which traditionally is an activity done by nurses during the well baby clinic (Campos et al., 1992). In this model, instead of using time stimulating the infant herself, the nurse shifts her role to teaching, counseling, and reinforcing in the parents how to stimulate normal development in their infants, thereby augmenting the efficiency of the system.

Timeliness of care

The Joint Commission on Accreditation of Healthcare Organizations (1990) has incorporated the dimension of timeliness of care into the definition of quality care. Timeliness of care is defined as the degree to which care is provided when it is needed. Self-care nursing contributes to improved timeliness of care by teaching clients and their families about signs and symptoms that require prompt professional intervention.

Job satisfaction

Some authors (Batalden, Goldfield, & Buchanan, 1989) consider job satisfaction of the health care team as another measure of quality health care because job satisfaction influences the quality of interpersonal relationships between professionals and clients and consequently influences the client's satisfaction with the care obtained.

A self-care model promotes the participation of both clients and employees. The participatory process helps to clarify information and goals and increases the motivation and commitment with the institutional mission.

Data from Santiago, Chile show that approximately half of the health events in the community are solved by the individuals themselves without the support of community health services (Medina, 1984). Approximately 14% of the population suffers from chronic diseases that require professional assistance; nevertheless, the reduced resources within the health institutions, high medical costs, and other problems that affect access to health services limit the population from attaining timely professional health care. These data are not too different from studies done in industrialized countries, where it has been found that only 25% to 50% of those who are sick have contact with professional health care providers (De Friese, Sehnert, & Barry, 1982). For this reason, self-care health practices of individuals and families must be recognized as the first level of care and as part of the primary health care system (Medina, 1984; Williamson & Danaher, 1978). If we believe that self-care practices are the base of the health care pyramid, then we can affirm that to improve health and life expectancy it is not only necessary to modify the organization and structure of health services but it is also essential to increase the motivation, knowledge, and skills of individuals, families, and communities to take better care of themselves and to obtain professional help when needed. Health services must share responsibilities as an integrated system that offers health care and self-care education to the population in the search for improvement of their health (Fig. 45-3).

In Latin America, the primary reasons to incorporate self-care into the health care system are as follows:

- Life expectancy has increased, as has the incidence of chronic diseases in the adult population (Valdivieso, 1992). To manage the health problems that arise in an

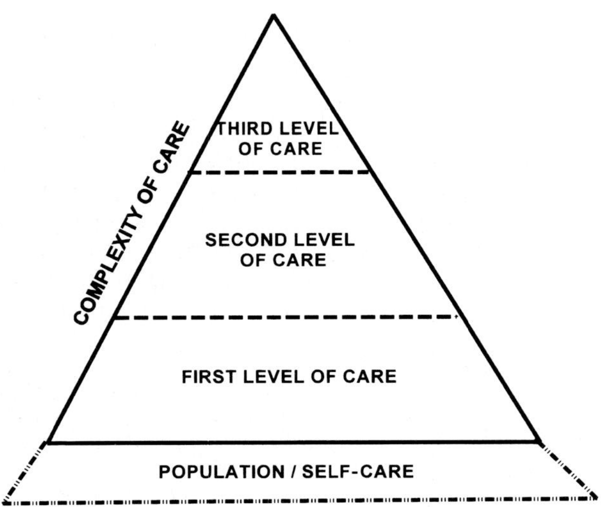

Fig. 45-3. Levels of health care.

older population, compliance to treatment and healthy self-care behaviors are essential.

• The dissatisfaction of the population to highly specialized medical care by a health care team that does not consider the patient to be a human being with psychological, social, and spiritual needs has increased the population's interest in participating in their own health care decisions.

• The recognition that the majority of health problems are solved in the community without the participation of the health care institutions confirms that there is a need to help the population improve their knowledge, attitudes, and self-care skills and to learn when and how to use the available health services more effectively.

• The awareness of the existing relationship between unhealthy lifestyles and morbidity and mortality patterns, with the main causes of death being cardiovascular diseases, cancer, accidents, and liver cirrhosis, all of which are related to health risk behaviors that can be reduced by healthy self-care practices.

Concern has arisen lately among health professionals, the public, and administrators in developing countries about how to improve quality in health care. Professionals are concerned with improving their scientific and technical expertise and correcting certain deficiencies in the health system. The public is worried about the lack of accessibility to health care services and is not satisfied with the interpersonal relationship that is now established with health care personnel. The administrators are concerned about how health care resources are allocated and distributed, how the health system can be made more accessible and equitable for the population, and how health care costs can be reduced (Saturno, Imperatori, & Corbella, 1990).

In institutions in which self-care is considered a permanent component of health care delivery, all activities performed by the health team, mainly by nursing personnel, are geared toward obtaining and maintaining the clients' autonomy, respecting their needs and preferences, and strengthening their self-care practices to make adequate health-related decisions. In this health delivery model, the clients and their families are considered part of the health care team and every interaction between nursing personnel and clients is used to strengthen their self-care capacities and to increase their health promotion and disease prevention behaviors (Fig. 45-4). Clients are taught and encouraged to define their own health status, identify health problems when they arise, and take more control over their own health, either through self-care actions or seeking professional help.

The nursing team considers the clients' self-care practices as well as their lifestyles, beliefs, myths, and values, all of which will undoubtedly affect the way they participate in health care decisions, comply with medical treatment, or change their behaviors. Such a model was developed by the Nursing Service of the Outpatient Clinic of the Catholic University Hospital in Santiago, Chile in partnership with the School of Nursing and with the financial support of Kellogg Foundation (1983 to 1989). This experience has shown that this working philosophy improves the morale of nursing personnel and decreases turnover rates. In this institution, healthy self-care practices are now promoted not only among the clients but

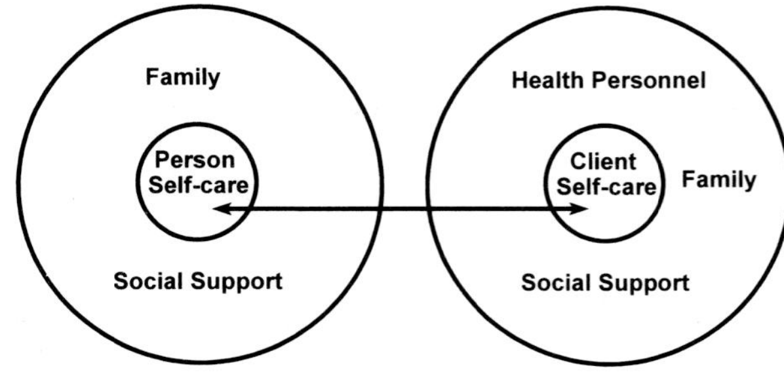

Fig. 45-4. Health care delivery model with emphasis on self-care.

also among the health care workers of the institution who are models for the community they serve. These practices are fostered during working hours by providing time for regular exercise during lunch breaks, and by organizing stress management activities and self-care continuing education programs (Lange & Campos, 1989). The nursing personnel feels proud of this model, has clarity of mission, and strives to improve the eight dimensions of quality in health care. In this system everyone has two jobs: their own and that of helping to improve the patients' job of taking care of themselves (Berwick, Godfrey, & Roessner, 1991).

The Chilean Ministry of Health has stated that to improve the level of health of a population that is in a demographic and epidemiological transition, a shift is needed in the formation of human resources and in the health services from a curative, illness-centered approach to a biopsychosocial, person-centered model that considers the concepts of universality, equity, efficiency, decentralization, and comprehensiveness (Giaconi, 1995). This Ministry has been explicit about its conviction that health care is a shared responsibility between every person, family, and community, the health system, and other governmental and social sectors that can directly or indirectly influence health. Health education should emphasize behavioral changes in children and promote healthy lifestyles. Within the health services themselves, efforts should be made to improve the interpersonal relationship between the health team and the clients and to increase efficiency, equity, continuity of care, and the problem-solving capacity in the three levels of care (Feachem et al., 1993; Minesterio de Salud de Chile, 1993).

CONCLUSIONS

Self-care nursing improves the quality of health care as it works toward a holistic approach of health care and emphasizes human values. In this model, clients move from a passive role toward a more participatory one, increasing compliance with the recommendations of the health team and empowering them to demand their rights, to recognize their responsibilities, and to identify their needs and priorities with regard to their personal and community health.

The self-care nursing model fosters the continuity and timeliness of care by promoting self-responsibility and self-efficacy of clients, families, and communities. It tends to the democratization of professional knowledge. Because the model is centered around the clients' opinions and practices, it increases their satisfaction with and acceptability of health services.

Research is needed in Latin America to measure and improve quality of care. The relationship between health professionals and clients must be explored as a quality measurement, and more clarification is needed on the role of each party in improving health. In addition, much work must still be done to educate both clients and health workers about a more participatory style of health care delivery.

REFERENCES

Aguayo, E., Chodowiecki, C., Lange, I., Ruiz, J., & Urrutia, M. (1994). *Curso atención primaria de salud: Módulo de estudio autodirigido.* Santiago, Chile: Escuela de Enfermería, Pontificia Universidad Católica de Chile.

Batalden, P., Goldfield, N., & Buchanan, E. (1989). Industrial models of quality improvement. In D.B. Nash (Ed.), *Providing quality care: The challenge to physicians.* Philadelphia: American College of Physicians.

Berwick, D., Godfrey, A., & Roessner, J. (1991). *Curing health care.* San Francisco-Oxford: Jossey Bass.

Campos, C., Jaimovich, S., Campos, M.S., Marzolo, L., Cantwel, M., & Herrera, L.M. (1992). Participación de los padres en la evaluación del desarrollo psicomotor de sus hijos menores de dos años. *Educación para el autocuidado de salud, 9*(4), 30-35.

David, J.A., Christensen, D., Hohon, S., Ord, L., & Wells, S. (1978). Implementing Orem's conceptual framework. *The Journal of Nursing Administration, 8*(11), 8-11.

De Friese, G., Sehnert, K., & Barry, P. (1982). Medical selfcare instruction for laypersons: A new agenda for health. *Möbius, 2*(1), 45-51.

Feachem, R., Kjellstrom, T., Murray, C., Over, M., & Phillips, M. (Ed.). (1993). *La salud del adulto en el mundo en desarrollo: Un resumen.* Banco Mundial.

Giaconi, G. (Ed.). (1995). *La salud en el siglo XXI: Cambios necesarios.* Santiago, Chile: Centro de Estudios Públicos.

Hill, L., & Smith, N. (1985). *Selfcare nursing: Promotion of health.* Norwalk, CT: Appleton Century Crofts.

Joint Commission on Accreditation of Healthcare Organizations. (1990). *Quality assurance in ambulatory care* (2nd ed.). Chicago: Author.

Lange, I., & Campos, C. (1989). Atención de salud con énfasis en autocuidado. *Educación para el autocuidado de salud, 6*(4), 10-15.

Levin, L. (1983, February). Self-help: One way to health. *World Health,* 24-29.

Maglacas, A. (1988). Health for all: Nursing's role. *Nursing Outlook, 36*(2), 66-71.

Medina, E. (1984). Importancia de la educación para el autocuidado del paciente. *Educación para el autocuidado de salud, 1*(12), 11-15.

Ministerio de Salud de Chile. (1993). *De consultorio a centro de salud: Marco conceptual.* Santiago, Chile: Author.

Moller, C. (1992). *Calidad personal: La base de todas las demás calidades.* Santiago, Chile: Time Manager International H/S.

Morse, W., & Werner, J. (1988). Individualization of patient care using Orem's theory. *Cancer Nursing, 1*(3) 195-202.

OPS/OMS. (1994). *Las condiciones de salud de las Americas.* Plubicacion Cientifica 549. Washington DC, 49-51.

Orem, D. (1980). *Nursing: Concepts in practice*. McGraw-Hill.

Orem, D. (1991). *Nursing: Concepts in practice*. (4th ed.). St. Louis: Mosby.

Palmer, R.H. (1990). *Evaluación de la asistencia ambulatoria: Principios y prácticas*. Madrid: Ministerio de Sanidad y Consumo.

Rey, C.J. (1989). *Método epidemiológico y salud de la communidad*. Madrid: McGraw-Hill.

Saturno, P., Imperatori, E., & Corbella A. (1990). *Evaluación de la calidad asistencial en atención primaria*. Madrid: Ministerio de Sanidad y Consumo.

Shortell, S.M. (1976). Continuity of medical care: Conceptualization and measurement. *Medical Care*, 14, 377-391.

Steiger, N., & Lipson, J. (1985). *Self-care nursing: Theory and practice*. Bowle, MD: Brady Communications Company.

Valdivieso, V. (1992). Medicina Interna en Chile. *Revista Médica de Chile, 120*(5), 503.

Williamson, J.D., & Danaher, K. (1978). *Selfcare in health*. London: Croom Helm.

Woods, N. (1989). Conceptualization of self-care: Towards health-oriented models. *Advanced Nursing Science, 12*(1), 1-13.

Section Six

GOVERNANCE

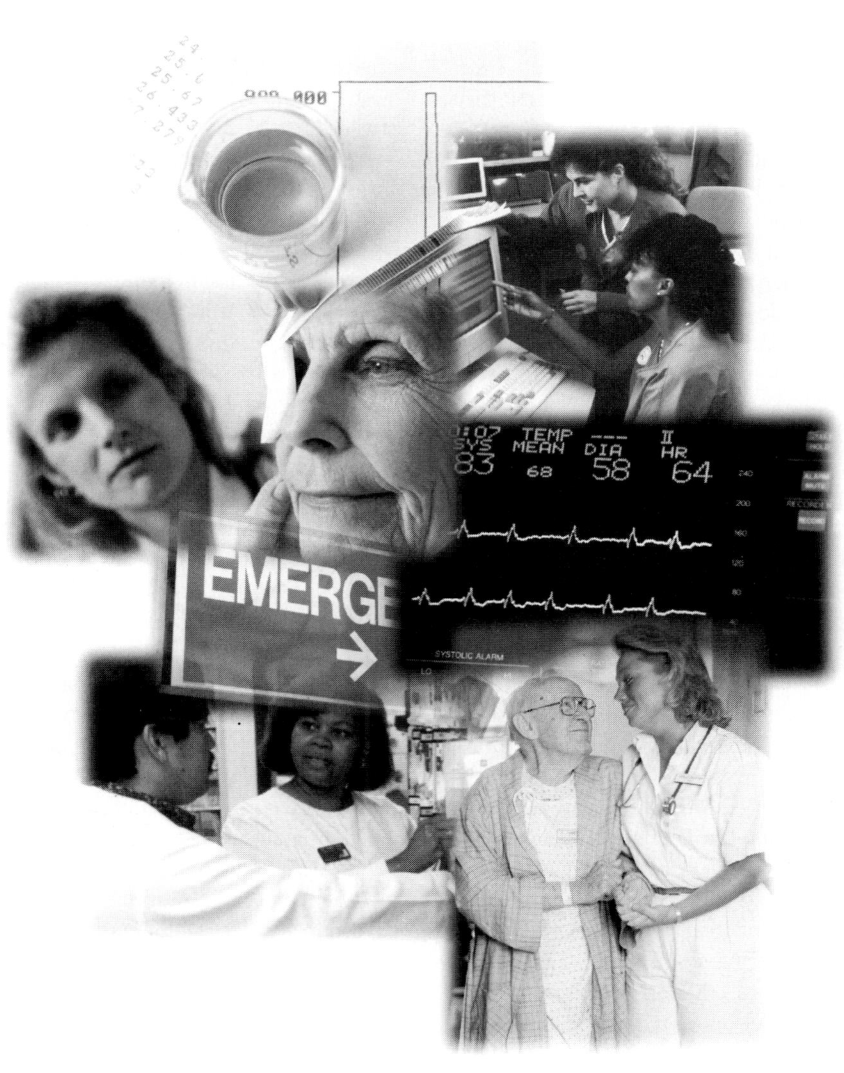

OVERVIEW

Challenges to nursing leadership in a changing practice world

JOANNE COMI McCLOSKEY, HELEN KENNEDY GRACE

The structures in which nursing has been practiced through the years have sometimes been a constraint to the ability of the profession to govern its own practice. In the changing terrain of health care in the 1990s the entire field is shifting, offering unusual challenges for nursing to take a more prominent role in governance issues. The pressures for cost control push nursing leaders to be experts not only in the domain of quality of patient care but also in the economics undergirding the field. Use of less costly personnel to provide patient care has emerged through the years as one way of addressing cost problems. Increasingly, the dichotomy between nursing education and nursing practice is narrowing. As nursing educational programs become increasingly involved in the provision of services, the lines between funding for educational programs and funding for services become blurred. As nursing moves toward more independence, governance models for nursing centers and community-based practices are beginning to emerge. These changes are occurring not only within the United States, but as the international practice terrain changes, nurses are playing increasingly important roles in the governance of the discipline. This section provides an interesting cross-section of issues and points of view related to governance issues in nursing.

In the opening debate paper Zimmermann examines an age-old concern—the use of unlicensed assistive personnel (UAP) to assist in the delivery of nursing care. Arguments for the use of UAP include the potential for reducing the cost of care and for using the skills of nurses more appropriately for performance of nursing tasks by delegating nonnursing work to UAP. But does the use of unlicensed assistive personnel really reduce costs? Or is this another chapter in the ongoing struggle for control of nurses? Legal accountability and the erosion of quality in nursing practice are raised as additional concerns. Recognizing that UAP will continue to be part of the caregiving team, the issue becomes that of delineating the boundaries for use of UAP. Zimmermann summarizes the debate by posing long-standing questions: What does the verb "nursing" mean? Is nursing merely a list of acts that can be prioritized, delegated to anyone, and supervised? Or is it an embodied art and skill that incorporates the whole of patient care, knowledge, assessment, prioritization, and discernment that is bigger than the sum of its parts? She challenges the nursing profession to address this issue.

Kerfoot addresses the issue of the business forces that are shaping the health care field and challenges nurses to be active participants in the transformation so that positive outcomes are achieved. The increased focus on the business side of health care, the shifting focus on health versus illness, the shift from decision making based on individual needs to a broader population-based perspective, and new models for health care are identified as the current trends. These changes in the health care industry provide unusual opportunities for nurses but require a shift in perspective from a "goal-driven model based on idealistic goals set in the abstract to a resource-driven model in which the nurse first takes into account the resources available and then determines what goals one can reasonably develop for a group of patients given these financial parameters."

In today's changing health care terrain, nurses are moving beyond traditional leadership roles to broader governance roles. Malone addresses the challenges faced by nurses who move into and hold nonnursing leadership positions. One of the major obstacles is that of the ambivalence of nursing related to power. Becoming a leader in shaping health care requires the use of power. Characteristics of successful leaders include vision and risk taking along with the ability to manage boundaries, empower others, and mentor followers. Pointing out the numbers of nurses who have advanced into key leadership positions in nonnursing roles, Malone speaks to the challenges of being an effective leader and the ambivalence of nurses in supporting these leaders.

New structures linking nurses in academic settings with those in community-based practices have provided opportunities for nurses to play key leadership roles in shaping practice. The next three chapters address these issues. Meservey addresses a new model for health care, the community-based academic health center. Addressing the challenge of educating providers and researchers in the settings in which care is delivered requires new models in which students learn "in close proximity to where people live, work, play, and pray, providing a new environment for discovery, learning, and care." Making this shift requires a changed orientation from a health care system organized around providers to one that is organized around people and communities. Describing the Boston Center for Community Health, Education, Research, and Service (CCHERS), Meservey identifies a set of leadership challenges in implementing this new model.

While nursing centers have evolved over the past 20 years, Lundeen points out that the roots for this practice model are in community-health nursing. In this comprehensive overview of the current state of development of the nursing center, Lundeen highlights the key role that nursing centers are playing in the provision of health services to the most vulnerable populations. Not surprisingly, one of the major constraints identified is the lack of reimbursement for services. The challenge to nursing leadership is to find effective ways to overcome a series of constraints that limit the demonstrated capacity of nurses to play a key role in a multidisciplinary, collaborative community-based health care delivery system.

Drawing on experiences in developing professional-community partnerships, Farley focuses her presentation on the power of the people to be contributors in the health care system. The Rural Elderly Enhancement Program, established in rural Alabama, has demonstrated the power of the community in joining together to address their priorities. Nurses working with communities can be catalysts in mobilizing this power.

Shifting from community to hospital settings, the next two articles address governance issues within hospitals. Maas, Specht, and Ramler address the broader involvement of nurses in general governance issues related to professional practice in hospitals. Involvement in broad governance issues is essential to the professional practice of nursing. These are a wide variety of models in place—in more than 1,000 hospitals across the United States. It is important that the involvement of nursing be real rather than token.

The collaboration of nursing staff and nursing management in decision making related to their work is critical. Too often management makes unilateral decisions that do not engage nursing staff to participate in problem solving. For nurses to participate in shared governance they must learn skills in negotiation, consensus building, and conflict management. One form of shared governance involves the scheduling of work hours for nurses. Wulff addresses the issues of flex-time and self-scheduling. Through the years, the nature of nursing in institutional settings, which requires an around-the-clock schedule, has been advanced as the reason that management schedules the work hours for nurses. Establishment of the parameters by nursing management, however, and allowing staff nurses to schedule their own work hours within that context are proposed as an approach that can be effective in involving nursing staff in decision making. Wulff poses a challenge to nursing leaders "to provide vision and, through flexible management, to provide a culture that promotes positive patient care outcomes and meets individualized needs of professional nurses."

The final article in this section turns to international nursing governance issues. Ohlson and Styles provide an overview of the two major international voices for nursing. The International Council of Nurses, representing professional nursing organizations around the world, and the World Health Organization, representing the ministries of health of member nations, have a powerful role in establishing standards to ensure quality of nursing practice around the world.

The voice of nursing is being heard more frequently in the broader health care arena. As patient care moves increasingly to the community, nurses are taking a leading role in developing and implementing new practice models. As nursing becomes more professionalized, nurses become much more active participants in governance within hospital settings. In our changing health care environment, the health care needs of people require that nurses be full participants not only in the provision of health care services but also in the decision-making arenas that impact the health of people around the world.

The increasing use of unlicensed assistive personnel: The erosion or elevation of nursing?

POLLY GERBER ZIMMERMANN

The term *unlicensed assistive personnel* (UAP) comprises at least 65 different job titles. This position was created to assist with patient needs under the supervision of the registered nurse (RN). The position statements of professional nursing organizations have allowed a place for such an assistive role in both direct nursing and indirect non-nursing patient care tasks, provided the RN determines, delegates, and oversees the process (American Association of Critical Care Nurses, 1990; American Nurses Association [ANA], 1992; Emergency Nurses Association [ENA], 1993; Tri-Council for Nursing, 1995).

Currently, 97% of hospitals employ UAP (Merker, Cerda, & Blank, 1991). While UAP have existed for decades, they now function increasingly in direct patient care and critical environments. Does this change represent the erosion of nursing and quality health care by delegating nursing's unique essence? Or does it elevate nurses to a respected leadership role by allowing the recognition and use of their advanced capabilities?

The outcome of the debate for and against the increasing use of UAP promises to radically influence the shape of nursing for the future. Debate points focus on why and how UAP are being used, their effect on nursing positions, their effect on patient care, and how the nursing profession should respond to the increasing use of UAP.

BACKGROUND

The nursing shortage in World War II created team nursing—a sharp demarcation of routine tasks under a skill mix ratio of 70% auxiliary workers and 30% RNs. In the 1970s and 1980s, however, primary care by RNs with undivided responsibility dominated, a change that was attributed both to the administration's interest in nurses' abilities for increased productivity and to the professionalization of nursing (Brannon, 1990).

Meanwhile, health care costs were burgeoning out of control, using 14% of the gross national product in 1992. It was predicted that, at the current rate of growth, health care costs would require 25% of the gross national product by 1997 (Curran, 1994). Clearly some type of reform was needed.

RATIONALE FOR INCREASING USE OF UNLICENSED ASSISTIVE PERSONNEL

One response to the need for reform was the introduction of the business concept of "reengineering," a fundamental "rethinking of processes" for health care. In one survey of health care chief executive officers, work reengineering was the most frequently identified tactic (67%) used to save money, and nearly two thirds of those surveyed were satisfied with the results (ANA, 1995e).

In health care's application, this redesign often includes combining several jobs into one and decentralizing operations, because overspecialization and excessive departmentalization is blamed for eroding the efficiency and effectiveness of hospitals (Townsend, 1995). One aspect usually includes hiring less skilled, cheaper auxiliary workers as a way to cut labor expenses, a cost that typically uses 53% or more of the budget (Burda, 1993). The current skill mix is now 69% RN nationwide (Huntington, 1995).

Rationale For Increasing Use: Work design's goal is *better* patient-focused care at *less* cost. Hospitals are under growing pressure to control costs, due, among other things, to significant Medicare and Medicaid payment shortfalls, increasing price competition, governmental health care reform, and the growing use of managed care and capitation (e.g., a fixed fee per member) (Buerhaus, 1995; Smith & Panting, 1995).

The realities are that the average wages of RNs rose 124% from the early 1980s to 1992 (Mills & Tilbury, 1995); the average wage for an RN is 144% higher than that of UAP (Anders, 1995); and our society emphasizes and rewards economic rather than quality incentives in health care.

While start-up costs are still a factor, success stories are already emerging. One study has shown that the use of a team approach increases nurses' productivity (Manuel & Alster, 1994), and California's Stanford University Hospital estimates a savings of $25 million since 1989 by changing the skill mix from 80% to 90% RNs to 69% RNs.

Rationale Against Increasing Use: Concentrating on labor expenses mistakenly misses other larger health care cost drivers such as the costs of physician residency training programs (Japsen, 1994); malpractice (Curran, 1994); administration (averaging 24.8% of total costs) (U.S. Government Accounting Office, 1992; Woodhandler, Himmelstein, & Lewortin, 1993); rapid technology advancement (U.S. Government Accounting Office, 1992); critical care misuse (Bonvissuto, 1994; Smith & Panting, 1995); drugs (Kapinos, 1994); and increasing capital expenditures (U.S. Government Accounting Office, 1992).

Other global alternatives to save costs must be explored. These familiar business strategies include controlling waste globally, facility consolidation, vertical integration, building market share, growth in new markets, standardizing products, negotiating clout with suppliers, or just-in-time (JIT) inventory (Castro, 1994; Smith & Panting, 1995). One Chicago hospital saved over $120,000 per year on intravenous supplies just by entering into a multihospital buying contract with a new supplier.

Nursing labor is only 24% of the hospital budget (Huntington, 1995). But even within the labor costs, considering the hourly wages of RNs in isolation ignores other RN staffing alternatives, such as on-call RNs for fluctuating needs (Zimmermann, 1993); floating cross-trained RNs in-house; "stat" nurses to cover episodic, short-term, hospital-wide critical care needs (Zimmermann, 1995); differentiating between technical and supervisory use of RNs; and payment of RNs according to their education and experience, similar to the levels suggested by Benner (Benner, 1982; Manuel & Alster, 1994; Rowitz, 1995b). A stat nurse system saved one Phoenix hospital $120,000 per year (Taylor, 1991). Using trained triage RNs to redirect nonemergency patients saved the University of California-Davis Medical Center $3,700,000 over 5 years (ANA, 1995g).

Hospitals using UAP often do not realize their projected savings because the hiring and benefits costs (which typically run about 30%) are the same (Rubach, 1995), and there are new training and supervision expenses as well (Burda, 1994a). Overtime use often rises to compensate because RNs cover more patients for nursing functions (Manuel & Alster, 1994).

In addition, productivity varies between the two types of workers. One study found that UAP typically have 27% downtime while RNs have only 8% (Fagin, 1982); another study found 40% downtime for UAP compared with 12% for RNs (Curry, 1992). Overall, only 15% of surveyed CEOs said they saved 11% or more by cutting labor and 25% saved less than 3% (ANA, 1995e).

The arguments for limiting the use of UAP are also compelling. The University of Illinois' elimination of 100 RN full-time-equivalent positions resulted in an eventual loss of $300,000, rather than the projected savings of $6 million, owing to skyrocketing overtime and registry costs (Illinois Nurses Association, 1994). In comparison, The University of Washington Medical Center kept their all-RN staff and only modified processes. They won the magnet status from the American Nurses Credentialing Center while saving $10 million per year (ANA, 1995f; Zimmermann, Wills, Soules, & Fiore, in press).

Another point to consider is that hospital financial desperation is being exaggerated. While some institutions do struggle as the market consolidates, hospitals overall have had a 6.9% increase in total revenues (Burda, 1995). An article by Burda (1994a) reveals that the American Hospital Association's (AHA's) own figures show that only 24% of hospitals had a negative total profit margin because, among other things, outpatient visits (and related income) increased.

Some suggest that hospitals' desire for control is a hidden agenda because they feel more vulnerable to a strike threat when harder-to-replace RNs make up a larger percentage of the workforce (Brannon, 1990). Others suggest that this is a feminist issue, "depowering" the 96% female profession now that the nursing shortage is over (S. Gordon, personal communication, December 4, 1994).

EFFECT ON NURSING JOB POSITIONS

UAP *assist* nurses. Although the number of nurses may decrease, with UAP the number of total caregivers can increase (Elias, 1995).

Data support that nurses want UAP. RN job satisfaction is correlated negatively to performing nonnursing tasks

(Hayes, 1994), and there is no evidence that increased use of UAP heightens RN stress levels (Rowitz, 1995a).

Increasing use of UAP is not affecting RN job positions because there is less need for inpatient hospital nurses. In fact, from 1984 to 1990, an average of two hospitals closed each week in the United States (Smith & Panting, 1995). Hospital overcapacity resulted from increasing managed care enrollments, outpatient procedures, and use of home health care, as well as deferred elective procedures (Castro, 1994; Church, 1993; Ferguson, 1993). One study predicts that the need for inpatient hospital beds could decrease by 34% by 1999 (AHA, 1995). The Pew Health Professions Commission predicts losses of RN hospital jobs to number 200,000 to 300,000 jobs (Lumsdon, 1995).

In response, nursing is transitioning back to its community origins (Brannon, 1990). It has been predicted that by the year 2000, only 35% to 40% of nurses will be working in hospitals (Smith & Panting, 1995). According to the National Association for Home Care, the demand for home care services is estimated to be growing by about 12% each year (Lampman, 1995).

Resistance from nurses actually represents job insecurity, "turf" battles (Rowitz, 1995a), and fear of the unknown (Turner, 1995). It is interesting that the same nurses who protest against physicians blocking expanded advanced nurse practitioner roles want to block UAP from expanding their role.

UAP are *replacing* RNs. Forty-four percent of survey nurses report increased use of UAP performing hospital duties that had formerly been done by RNs (ANA, 1994). In 1994, 27% of surveyed hospitals indicated plans to target RNs for position eliminations, compared with only 19% targeting RNs in 1993 (Burda, 1994b).

Regardless of what may occur in the future, 66% of RNs are currently working in hospitals, giving complex care to those patients who are beyond the scope of community services (Smith & Panting, 1995; Sullivan, 1995). At a time when patients are older and sicker, there is a greater need for professional-level critical thinking and skills in direct care.

In the past, it was recognized that team nursing demoralized the profession and increased nursing turnover (Kapinos, 1994). Data show that nurse job satisfaction decreased when reverting from primary nursing to the newly termed "patient-centered" (team) nursing (Bethel & Ridder, 1994).

Although acknowledging concerns about their future employment, for many nurses this has become a moral and ethical issue (ANA, 1995b). Being a patient advocate now means demanding adequate staffing ratios and job distinctions. Delegating direct patient care to untrained personnel who practice on the nurse's license is radically different from trained, licensed nurses being prohibited from performing some functions on their own credentials.

EFFECT ON PATIENT CARE QUALITY AND SAFETY

UAP Promote Quality Care. Up to 70% of nurses' time is now spent performing nonnursing tasks (Boston & Vestal, 1994; Manuel & Alster, 1994; Mills & Tilbury, 1995). Fifty percent of patients in one major public opinion survey complained that nurses do not spend enough time at the bedside (Begany, 1994). The benefit of using UAP is that they free the RN to actually "nurse" by performing the small details (e.g., getting an extra pillow for a patient) (Bethel & Ridder, 1994). Patients like UAP, and nurses need to respect them as an integral part of the health care team.

The heart of successful UAP implementation is proper delegation (Zimmermann, 1996b). Even in critical care settings, the use of UAP has been successful if UAP delegation is made according to the needs of the nurse directing the patient care rather than assigning generic responsibility by tasks or patients (Raffensberger, 1992). Because many of today's nurses were educated and practiced only under primary care, training for RNs in delegation is probably needed.

The research being quoted is flawed, however; it is outdated and lacks commonality in terms and outcome indicators. Too much "evidence" is isolated anecdotes and opinions that are misleading and melodramatic. The Institute of Medicine's Committee on the Adequacy of Nurse Staffing identified a need for data collection, analysis, and research (Buerhaus, 1995). One consulting firm claims that their own research of 117 hospitals found that reconfiguring jobs improved mortality rates and had no effect on patient morbidity (Elias, 1995).

UAP Diminish Quality Care. Presently, there are no universal standards regarding UAP hiring, training, or job descriptions—all of which contribute to the wide variation in actual UAP performance. The Health Care Financing Administration confirmed that inadequate staffing and poor training of technicians were a major problem at one hospital where five serious patient care incidents occurred (Rosen, 1995).

Some institutions have excellent, extensive programs, while others do not. One survey of acute care hospitals found that 70% do not even require nursing assistant certification or a high school diploma. This survey also found that 59% of acute care hospitals had fewer than 20 hours of classroom orientation, and 41% provided fewer than 40 hours of on-the-job training (Barter & Furmidge, 1994).

There is no argument over the value of UAP in continuing to perform supportive, repetitive, or nonnursing tasks such as stocking, housekeeping, clerical, dietary, and transportation needs. It is quite helpful to have UAP hold a patient during a procedure or obtain a urine specimen.

The issue focuses on UAP qualifications for increasingly assuming skilled nursing functions and working within specialized environments such as a critical care. The staffing ratios and roles that may work in a rehabilitation unit are usually not appropriate in a busy emergency department with unstable critical care patients.

Some confusion remains about the legal accountability in delegating. The nurse retains responsibility for the completion, quality, and outcome of the UAP's performance of a delegated task and legal liability for proper delegation, potential problems, and interventions. Unlike an assignment to a licensed peer, this responsibility remains even when the UAP is deemed qualified (trained and verified competent) (Barter & Furmidge, 1994; Burbach, 1994; ENA, 1994; Hansten & Washburn, 1992). Many RNs feel exhausted by the hypervigilance that is required for proper delegation.

The nursing process cannot be delegated. Yet a convenience sample study found 85% of the RNs witnessed UAP triaging, assessing, discharging, and giving extensive counseling to patients (Zimmermann, 1996a).

Team nursing's ingrained difficulty is the frequent blurring or informal violations of the assigned distinct task delineations and responsibilities as a result of the ever-changing nature of patient needs and interactions. On-the-spot decisions, requiring a depth of knowledge and trained critical thinking, are made at the bedside during "routine" care (Brannon, 1990). Many RNs feel frustration at being responsible for care they don't even witness or at being required to delegate what they are not comfortable delegating but what their employer insists they must.

Up-to-date evidence may be sparse but data available so far points in a clear direction: The number of RNs on staff and skill mix ratio do have an effect on quality and safety:

- Thirteen studies have found that patient morbidity and mortality are adversely affected by changing the number of RNs on staff and the RN component in the skill mix (Aiken & Lake, 1992; Prescott, 1993).
- Hospitals that recognize and institute the provision of excellent care by nurses have lower mortality rates among elderly patients (Aiken, Smith, & Lake, 1994).
- A reduction of RNs and their replacement with UAP have resulted in a reported increase in accidents, including patient falls, medication errors, and lapses in infection control. Eighty percent of the responding nurses who reported staff cuts were convinced that the quality of care had suffered (ANA, 1994).
- A convenience sample study of the effects of restructuring in Massachusetts found a reported 43% increase in unsafe staffing, a 40% increase in incident reports, a 36% increase in injuries to RNs, a 31% increase in patient complaints, and 15 attributable patient deaths (Kong, 1994; Shindul-Rothschild, 1994).
- A 1996 AJN patient care survey by Dr. J. Shindul-Rothschild found that nine out of 10 nurses polled indicate serious concerns that the safety and quality of care is being diminished through RN cutbacks and increase use of UAP; two out of five nurses polled report an increase in patient complications, medication errors, nosocomial infections, skin breakdowns, and injuries to patients.
- The Joint Commission on Accreditation of Health Organizations is receiving four to five complaint calls per day about staffing and safety compared with five to six calls per month a year ago (ANA, 1995d; Anders, 1995).

The health care consumer cannot always judge true quality accurately. The number of patient contacts is not as important as less obvious deficiencies such as lapses in infection control.

Primary care evolved for reasons that are all the more prevalent in today's environment of patient acuity and expected nursing assessments. Complexity of communication, conflict, fragmented care, and patient dehumanization often increase when more caregivers from different backgrounds are involved. Lawsuits are anticipated to rise as a result of errors due to restructuring, staff downsizing, and increased use of UAP (Varro, 1995).

RESPONSES

Responses For Increasing Use: The American Organization of Nurse Executives, a subsidiary of the AHA, emphasizes the need for nursing to adjust to health care's rapid changes. Health care delivery is based on community needs that are unique, and focusing on RN ratios stifles innovation.

It is time to stop "needlessly alarming" the public about quality of health care in hospitals. The credibility of our entire industry and profession is damaged in the public arena by press releases that state that profit is more important than quality.

The reality is that the issue is not *if* these labor changes are inevitable, but *how* they will be made. As the largest group of health care providers, nurses should be at the forefront in these exciting times, providing direction for new models of care, rather than resisting and seeking the status quo. It is time to lose the "codependent," "victim" posture (ANA, 1995c; Cowley, 1995; Mills & Tilbury, 1995; Turner, 1995). The current militant handling of this issue is causing unnecessary division between nursing administration and staff. Nurses degrade their professionalism by assuming a "blue collar," "union mentality."

We need to change the culture of nursing and the nursing role. The answers lie in embracing change, education, and communication (Turner, 1995).

Responses Against Increasing Use: The ANA is concerned about non-RN encroachment and has launched a campaign to educate the public about the link between RN staffing levels and quality care. They have published a brochure, *Every Patient Deserves a Nurse,* for lay people and an overview booklet, *Registered Professional Nurses & Unlicensed Assistive Personnel,* for nurses (for ordering information call 1-800-274-4ANA).

The public *should* be alarmed about these changes because change is not automatically good for forward growth. Are these the changes nurses and society want? Minimizing the differences between staff qualifications is a disturbing trend. Some hospitals are removing the RN distinction from employee identification badges, classifying everyone from environmental service employees to RNs as "health care workers" (Curtin, 1995; Kauffold, 1996).

Public service announcements state that it is nurses who make quality health care available, accessible, affordable, and accountable and that the industry is choosing profit over quality and safety. Patients are encouraged to ask if an RN ("real nurse") will check on them and to report incidents resulting from unsafe staffing. This current practice of proceeding with staff ratio changes and then looking retrospectively at the damage needs to be halted.

Many nurses feel alienated and abandoned by nursing administration that does not deal with their difficult day-to-day realities (ANA, 1995b). Professional collective bargaining has been the only means by which some nurses have been able to hold professional standards while having job protection under the labor law statues (ANA, 1995a). Currently, there are no national laws protecting whistle-blowing (Zimmermann, 1996c).

SUMMARY

Proponents of both sides make strong points that are emotionally fortified by their own experience. Both sides agree on the need to have research on staffing issues and to take leadership in the development and training of the UAP role.

What a point-by-point debate cannot deal with concretely is the element of value judgments. What is "nursing" as a verb? Is it a list of acts that can be prioritized, delegated to anyone, and supervised? Or is it an embodied art and skill that incorporates the whole of patient care knowledge, assessment, prioritization, and discernment that is bigger than the sum of its parts?

Often, nurses in the past have not done a good job of identifying these answers for themselves, let alone for the public. "Unfortunately, many nurses themselves do not appreciate the complexity of their practice. The quality of care does depend on the quality and reliability of the nurse" (R. Benner, personal communication, July 25, 1995).

True nursing goes beyond a skillful performance of isolated tasks under physicians' orders. It is an intuitive, deep perception of the entire patient with an anticipation and meeting of all his or her needs. Anyone can physically count a pulse. An "expert" nurse assesses circulatory, perfusion, hydration, skin integrity, overall physical state, and emotional status in that act as well.

There is a sense for many nurses "against" the use of UAP that while nursing staffing patterns and fads come and go, this trend is more devious. This time the very essence and needs of nursing are at stake. On the other hand, many nurses "for" the use of UAP feel that nurses artificially holding on to the RN-only, "Cadillac care" standards are not accepting of the new financial realities and will end up leaving the profession out in the cold.

This issue is too important to ignore and too broad to deal with alone. Nurses need to join their voices with the support of professional organizations. Yet memberships in these organizations remain paltry. Only 14% of nurses belong to the ANA, compared with 40.8% of physicians who belong to the American Medical Association. Memberships are also low in speciality nursing organizations. Within the emergency care speciality, 32% to 34% of emergency department nurses belong to the ENA, while 71% of full-time emergency department physicians belong to the American College of Emergency Physicians.

All nurses need to join in the debate because this phenomenon has the potential to change the shape of the nursing profession radically. This is still a fluid trend and subject to influence (Gordon & Buresh, 1995). Look what vocal, concerned nurses accomplished in affecting some states' "drive-through" deliveries (i.e., postpartum discharges of less than 24 hours) (ANA, 1995h). The caring essence nurses extend one-on-one to patients must now be extended to the nursing profession itself.

REFERENCES

Aiken, L., & Lake, E. (1992, December). *Summary of empirical literature on the relationship between nursing skill mix or RN-to-patient ratio and hospital mortality.* Philadelphia: University of Pennsylvania, Center for Health Services and Policy Research, School of Nursing.

Aiken, L., Smith, H., & Lake, E. (1994). Lower Medicare mortality among a set of hospitals known for good nursing care. *Medical Care, 32,* 771-787.

American Association of Critical Care Nurses (AACN). (1990). *Delegation of nursing and nonnursing activities in critical care.* Aliso Viejo, CA: Author.

American Hospital Association. (1995, August 5). Currents. *Hospital & Health Networks, 69,*(15), 12-13.

American Nurses Association (ANA). (1992). *Registered nurse utilization of unlicensed assistive personnel.* (Position statement). Washington, DC: Author.

American Nurses Association. (1994). *Layoffs survey.* McLean, VA: Decision Data Collection, Inc.

American Nurses Association. (1995a). In landmark pact, Illinois RNs win staffing guarantees. *American Journal of Nursing, 95*(3), 67, 70.

American Nurses Association. (1995b). Cuts in RN staffing keep escalating; ANA sees patient safety at stake. *American Journal of Nursing, 95*(3), 68, 72.

American Nurses Association. (1995c). Hospitals demand proof that cuts are hurting care. *American Journal of Nursing, 95*(3), 69-70.

American Nurses Association. (1995d). Denouncing cuts, RN groups go public with safety issue. *American Journal of Nursing, 95*(4), 67, 71.

American Nurses Association. (1995e). How hospitals are saving work redesign tops cost-cutting efforts. *American Journal of Nursing, 95*(6), 70.

American Nurses Association. (1995f). Magnet hospital advertises its pride in nurses. *American Journal of Nursing, 95*(6), 70, 74.

American Nurses Association. (1995g). Findings and forecasts. *American Journal of Nursing, 95*(6), 71.

American Nurses Association. (1995h). RNs join backlash against 'drive-through' deliveries. *American Journal of Nursing, 95*(8), 63, 66.

Anders, G. (1995, February 10). Hospitals' Rx for high costs: Fewer nurses, more aides. *The Wall Street Journal,* pp. B1, B4.

Barter, M., & Furmidge, M. (1994). Unlicensed assistive personnel: Issues relating to delegation and supervision. *Journal of Nursing Administration, 24*(4), 36-40.

Begany, T. (1994, October). Your image is brighter than ever. *RN,* 28-36.

Benner, P. From novice to expert. (1982). *American Journal of Nursing, 82*(3), 402-407.

Bethel, S., & Ridder, J. (1994). Evaluating nursing practice: Satisfaction at what cost? *Nursing Management, 25*(9), 41-43, 46-48.

Bonvissuto, C. (1994). Avoiding unnecessary critical care costs. *Healthcare Financial Management, 48*(11), 47-52.

Boston, C., & Vestal, K. (1994, April 5). Work transformation. *Hospital and Health Networks,* pp. 50-55.

Brannon, R. (1990). The reorganization of the nursing labor process: From team to primary nursing. *International Journal of Health Services, 20*(3), 511-524.

Buerhaus, P. (1995). Economics and reform: Forces affecting nurse staffing. *Nursing Policy Forum, 1*(2), 9-14.

Burbach, V. (1994). Delegation in nursing. *Issue, 15*(3), 7-8.

Burda, D. (1993, December 20-27). Cutting down. *Modern Healthcare, 23*(51), 49-58.

Burda, D. (1994a, August 8). A profit by any other name would still give hospitals fits. *Modern Healthcare, 24*(32), 115-134.

Burda, D. (1994b, December 12). Layoffs rise as pace of cost-cutting accelerates. *Modern Healthcare, 23*(51), 33.

Burda, D. (1995, January 2). Hospital profits level off—AHA. *Modern Healthcare, 27*(1), 2.

Castro, J. (1994, March 21). Wanted: Slightly used hospitals. *Time,* 58-59.

Church, G. (1993, November 22). Jobs in an age of insecurity. *Time,* 37.

Cowley, G. (1995, February 13). Intensive care on a budget. *Newsweek,* 86.

Curran, C. (1994). Work redesign: The key to true health care reform. In J.C. McCloskey & H.K. Grace (Eds.), *Current issues in nursing* (4th ed., pp. 460). St. Louis: Mosby.

Curry, J. (1992). Bridge over troubled waters: ED nurses share strategies regarding use of prehospital care providers in the emergency department. *Journal of Emergency Nursing, 18*(6), 30A–35A.

Curtin, L. (1995). Comrade healthcare worker . . . ? *Nursing Management, 26*(4), 7, 8.

Elias, M. (1995, January 1). Caregiving is shifting from RNs to aides. *USA Today,* pp. 1D, 2D.

Emergency Nurses Association (ENA). (1993). *The use of non-RN caregivers in emergency care* (pp. 91-96). (Position statements). Park Ridge, IL: Author.

Emergency Nurses Association. (1994, October). Delegation: What every emergency nurse needs to know! *ENA Management Update, 1*(4).

Fagin, C. (1982). The economic value of nursing research. *American Journal of Nursing, 82,* 1845-1849.

Ferguson, T. (1993, August 9). Hospital charts take a turn for the worse. *The Wall Street Journal,* p. A13.

Foer, S. & Baumann, A. (1996, July/August). RNs voice critical concerns about patient care. *AJN* survey details increasing pressures on nurses. *The American Nurse,* 19.

Gordon, S., & Buresh, B. (1995). Keep the story alive. *American Journal of Nursing, 95*(5), 20-22.

Hansten, R., & Washburn, M. (1992). How to plan what to delegate. *American Journal of Nursing, 92*(4), 71-72.

Hayes, P. (1994). Non-nursing functions: Time for them to go. *Nursing Economic$, 12*(3), 120-125.

Huber, D.G., Blegen, M., & McCloskey, J.C. (1994). Use of nursing assistants: Staff nurse opinions. *Nursing Management, 25*(5), 64-8.

Huntington, J.A. (1995). Restructuring: Safety, quality and cost. Staff nurses' view. *Nursing Policy Forum, 1*(2), 16, 19, 38.

Illinois Nurses Association. (1994, November-December). UIH RNs step up campaign against RN replacement. *Chart,* 12.

Japsen, B. (1994). Teaching hospitals face hard lessons. *Modern Healthcare, 24*(6), 36-40.

Kapinos, T. (1994, July 13). When aides replace RNs at the bedside. *The Chicago Tribune, NursingNews,* p. 3.

Kauffold, M.P. (1996, March 20). RNs protest job rewrites. *The Chicago Tribune, NursingNews,* p. 2.

Kong, D. (1994, October 31). Nurses save patients feeling the pain of staffing cutbacks. *Boston Globe,* p. 37.

Lampman, K. (1995). Getting back to nursing. *AJN Career Guide for 1995,* pp. 30-31.

Lumsdon, K. (1995, December 5). Faded glory. *Hospital and Health Networks, 69,* 30-35.

Manuel, P., & Alster, K. (1994). Unlicensed personnel no cure for an ailing health care system. *Nursing & Health Care, 15*(1), 18-21.

Merker, L.R., Cerda, F., & Blank, M. (1991). *1990 utilization of nurse extenders.* Chicago: American Hospital Association.

Mills, M.E., & Tilbury, M.S. (1995). Restructuring: Safety, quality and cost. Nursing administration's perspective. *Nursing Policy Forum, 1*(2), 17-19.

Prescott, P. (1993). Nursing: An important component of hospital survival under a reformed healthcare system. *Nursing Economic$, 11*(4), 192-199.

Raffensberger, D. (1992, December). Nursing attendants in the ICU? You bet! *RN,* 17-20.

Rosen, M. (1995, April 8). Staff cuts alarm hospital experts. *St. Petersberg Times,* pp. B1, B7.

Rowitz, M. (1995a, June 14). Unlicensed workers in the eye of a storm. *The Chicago Tribune, NursingNews,* p. 3.

Rowitz, M. (1995b, June 28). Differentiated nursing practice. *The Chicago Tribune, NursingNews,* p. 3.

Rubach, L. (1995). Downsizing: How quality is affected as companies shrink. *Quality Progress, 28*(4), 8-14.

Shindul-Rothschild, J. (1994, October). *Impact of restructuring and redesign on the quality of patient care.* Written report to the Institute of Medicine (IOM) Committee on the Adequacy of Nurse Staffing in Hospitals and Nursing Homes, Washington, DC.

Smith, R.N., & Panting, K. (1995, May). The changing and challenging ICU. *Nursing Dynamics, 4*(1), 10-15.

Sullivan, B. (1995, February 2). Nurses on front lines as hospitals restructure. *The Chicago Tribune,* pp. 1, 4.

Taylor, M. (1991). SWAT Team: Aggressive approach to the '90s. *Nursing Economic$, 9*(6), 431-433.

Townsend, M.B. (1995, May). The impact of reengineering on inpatient nursing. *Nursing Dynamics, 4*(1), 16-20.

Tri-Council for Nursing. (1995). *Statement on assistive personnel to the registered nurse.* Chicago: American Organization of Nurse Executives (AONE).

Turner, S.O. (1995, August 20). Perspectives: Reality check. *Hospital and Health Networks, 69*(16), 20-22.

U.S. Government Accounting Office. (1992). Hospital costs: Adoption of new technologies drive costs growth. Washington, DC: U.S. Government Accounting Office.

Varro, B. (1995, May 17). We will see more lawsuits. *The Chicago Tribune, NursingNews,* pp. 1.

Varro, B. (1996, July 24). The "V" words. ANA pushes vision, visibility, value, voice; Clinton stumps for victory. *The Chicago Tribune, Nursing News,* p. 1.

Woodhandler, S., Himmelstein, D., & Lewortin, J. (1993). Administrative costs in U.S. hospital. *New England Journal of Medicine, 329*(6), 400-403.

Zimmermann, P.G. (1993). How we do it: "On call" staffing. *Journal of Emergency Nursing, 19*(6), 529-531.

Zimmermann, P.G. (1995). How we do it: Use of "STAT" nurses in the ED. *Journal of Emergency Nursing, 21,* 335-337.

Zimmermann, P.G. (1996a). *Nursing's perceptions of the effects of unlicensed assistive personnel in hospital emergency departments.* Unpublished master's thesis, North Park College, Chicago.

Zimmermann, P.G. (1996b). Delegating to assistive personnel. *Journal of Emergency Nursing, 22,* 206-212.

Zimmermann, P.G. (1996c). Use of unlicensed assistive personnel: Anecdotes and antidotes. *Journal of Emergency Nursing, 22,* 42-48.

Zimmermann, P.G., Wills, T., Soules, D.M., & Fiore, T. (in press) Avoiding RN layoffs: Three hospitals show how it is done. *Journal of Emergency Nursing.*

Leadership in transition

KARLENE KERFOOT

The work of leaders in health care today is much different than that of work only a few years ago. Our health care system is undergoing a dramatic restructuring that amounts to nothing short of a major revolution. The health care field is experiencing the greatest reorganization of any industry since the Industrial Revolution. We are quickly moving from an industry built around disease and small, independent organizations into an industry focused on health and comprised of large corporate organizations. Mergers and acquisitions are restructuring health care into large regional and national networks and organizations. The era of stand-alone hospitals and solo physicians' practices is gone. Instead, consolidations are taking place rapidly and small "mom and pop" operating units of any kind are quickly being eliminated and merged into large organizations.

People in the workforce today have much different expectations and values than they had in years past. Diversity has brought many changes to the workplace. Gender, ethnicity, and the diversity of skill sets in the workforce challenge even the most capable leader's ability to mold divergent mental models into a shared vision for the mission of the organization. Consequently, the work of leadership in nursing and health care is undergoing a great transformation. An entirely new system of health care requires a different kind of leader. These are some of the most exciting times to be a part of the world of health care and also the most challenging. We are witnessing a major transformation in which we have the opportunity to participate. More than just participating, however, we can help build and mold the new era of health care with leaders committed to making the transformation a positive one. This chapter surveys only a few of the major trends in health care and provides suggestions for the kind of leadership that is needed in this new era.

TRENDS

Health care is a business

Health care is rapidly transitioning from what has been primarily a not-for-profit, service-based industry into one that is driven by the corporatization of health care. The entry of for-profit organizations in the world of hospitals, nursing homes, and other health-related organizations has transferred the discipline of business from the for-profit to the not-for-profit sector. Both types of organizations must now compete against each other on the same playing field for enrolled lives, patients, and health care dollars. Sophisticated financial analysis is now a survival skill for everyone in health care. Corporate restructuring, competing to gain market share, measuring success via sophisticated financial ratios, marketing techniques, and acquisition strategies are now a part of everyone's repertoire whether they work in a for-profit or a not-for-profit organization. Consequently, knowledge of business concepts is essential for leaders to function in this new era. Also important are the ability and skills to work in a large, complicated corporate structure as opposed to the small, independent organizations of the past.

Focusing on health as opposed to illness

The health care system that has evolved in the United States has been heavily geared toward the process of performing procedures rather than maintaining health. There has been little money available in the system for the maintenance of health and the prevention of illness. Instead, financial reimbursement has only been available when a disease was present and specific treatments were possible. The "more is better" philosophy therefore evolved because financial gains were only realized when more procedures, more tests, and more interventions were done. Programs to prevent disease, such as patient teaching, and to provide surveillance and early detection, such as mammography, were not traditionally reimbursed.

Also in evidence is the move toward developing healthier communities rather than focusing on the treatment of disease and performance of procedures. Not-for-profit hospitals are under much greater scrutiny to justify their tax-exempt status. Many organizations are thoughtfully rethinking how they can articulate their "community benefit" by demonstrating an ability to improve the health status of the community. For-profit hospitals, in their quest to be "good citizens," are also committing to provide benefit to the community and are involved in the drive to develop healthy communities. Nurses are well positioned to work effectively in this area because of the profession's emphasis on health promotion and illness prevention in the curriculum of nursing schools.

The leaders of the future will be in the business of maintaining health rather than running hospital "repair shops." Some leaders will be able to make this transformation to the new kind of business and others will not. The transformation is similar to laundering oneself out of the mainframe business in the world of computers to personal computers; some leaders made the transformation while others could not.

Population-based versus individual-based care

We all grew up in a world of nursing focused on individual patients and learned that we must do everything we possibly could for each patient we encountered. We learned to be advocates for individual patients and knew less about advocating for large groups of patients or for society as a whole. The emerging public health model that is competing with the traditional medical model is now demanding that the allocation of health care dollars consider the greater good for the entire population, not just for one individual patient. Consequently, there are many ongoing ethical discussions about providing highly technical, expensive care to individual patients who have no hope for the restoration of health while other groups of people lack immunizations and prenatal and other preventive services because the scarce health care dollars have been diverted to people with poorer outcomes. Oregon has taken the lead in these tough issues and has blazed the trail between the difficult choices of denying access to transplants for indigent patients in favor of using those dollars for health promotion activities such as immunizations. We are definitely witnessing a trend toward making decisions about health care based on aggregate data of the population and focusing on the health status of the population versus the expensive treatment of complicated terminal diseases for a few individual patients who likely will not survive. Consequently, knowledge of the public health model is essential for leaders in this transformation, and grounding in epidemiology and public health principals will be necessary.

Changing reimbursement strategies

With the onset of changes in reimbursement patterns (e.g., capitation), the financial incentives are there to spend the dollars on health maintenance and illness prevention rather than only on the treatment of disease. Under capitation, the insurance company shares dollars from each enrollee's monthly premium with a physician's organization and a hospital. The amount of money does not vary if a person becomes ill, is hospitalized, or incurs any kind of health problems. Therefore, it is cost-effective to prevent hospitalization and illness from happening because a healthy group of enrollees will provide the best financial returns. The success measures in the future will, in many cases, be the opposite of what they are in the current system. For example, filling intensive care units at one time meant profit under the fee-for-service reimbursement system. Under capitation, however, this leads to a financial loss. Consequently, leaders must be able to work in a totally different system of care and transform everyone's thinking to new models quickly.

New organizational models

With rightsizing, downsizing, corporate restructuring, and reengineering, health care institutions look very different than they did a few years ago. New, innovative models have created fewer departments, flatter organizations, and the concept of cross-divisional project teams as a vehicle by which much of the work is done. These new organizational models place much less emphasis on managing vertically in isolated, stand-alone departments such as pharmacy, nursing, or respiratory therapy. Instead, vertical management has given way to the concept of horizontal management (Denton, 1991), in which cross-divisional teams that focus on the patient/family/client and the flow of care versus individual departments are now common. Organizational charts are no longer represented by the common top-down, pyramidal-type organization. Instead, organizational charts are designed to look like pepperoni pizzas, shamrocks, star bursts, and other models that show that companies have grown flatter, have decentralized, utilize teams to get the work done, and have fewer reporting layers (Byrne, 1993). Autocratic, bureaucratic organizations are quickly falling by the wayside, being replaced by innovative, agile, team-based designs that provide for much more flexibility and agility to meet the demands of a rapidly shifting industry. Sophisticated knowledge of teams will be a requirement for the future.

LEADERSHIP FOR THE NEW ERA OF HEALTH CARE

Obviously, with these kinds of trends in the health care industry, the traditional role of nursing and nursing leadership is undergoing dramatic change. The competencies required to manage in this new era of health care are much different than they were a few years ago when the nurse executive was responsible only for the department of nursing services. Consequently, many nursing leaders have had to retrofit their skills to meet these new challenges or fall by the wayside. Leadership in nursing is in transition. There will be survivors and there will be those who do not survive. There are great opportunities out there for those who can adapt quickly. There are several essential competencies for this new era.

NURSING AS A BUSINESS

Marketing, financial analysis and management, and other concepts from the business world must be a part of every leader's repertoire in order to thrive in this new era. Each month brings more and more information about how new concepts of business are being integrated into the practices in this health care industry. The leaders who will survive will be those who can make the transition to integrating the financial management with the care processes. It is no longer good enough just to have quality outcomes. The same quality outcomes must be achieved at a lower cost. Therefore, each leader is challenged to be able to understand the financial bottom line, and to work backwards from that bottom line to design new care systems. Barnum and Kerfoot (1995) describe this transition in thinking and leadership styles as moving from a goal-driven model based on idealistic goals set in the abstract to a resource-driven model in which the nurse first takes into account the resources available and then determines what goals can reasonably be developed for a group of patients given these financial parameters. Resource-driven care means that the leader knows how to calculate the cost per case, knows what the revenue will be per enrolled life, and can work backwards from that to calculate the cost at which the care must be delivered. Nurses can no longer work in isolated departments. Instead, they must see health care across a continuum of services within an integrated delivery system because this is where almost all of the health care of the future will be delivered. Nurse leaders must now transition from seeing themselves as the leaders in a setting such as a hospital or nursing home to considering themselves members, participants, or executives in an integrated delivery system that includes alliances, ownership, partnerships, and other models of a large group of organizations that provide health care throughout the continuum, which ranges from increasing the health status of the community to hospice care.

The leader of the future will be part of an integrated delivery system that operates as a vertically organized corporation. The extent of this organization can be local, regional, or eventually statewide. Having a voice among thousands, rather than among few, is a different experience for a leader and requires different skills. The ability to work in large corporations will be a skill in high demand.

DETERMINING THE GREATEST GOOD FOR THE GREATEST NUMBERS

Leaders are challenged to provide evidence of effectiveness that shows the greater good for the most number of patients or people. Competencies in outcomes management, outcomes measurement, and disease management will be essential. Nurses are usually quite well schooled in the areas of disease prevention and health promotion. When working in an acute care setting, however, these principles can sometimes be forgotten and must be updated because of the tremendous emphasis on illness. Concepts of epidemiology and determining risk are also important competencies for this new era. The ability to demonstrate value continually to the greatest number will be essential.

MANAGING HEALTH, NOT ILLNESS

The shift from treating illness to maintaining health will demand that the leader of the future is well schooled in wellness, disease management (Gonzalez, 1995), and demand management sophisticated patient teaching (Vickery & Lynch, 1995) and can clinically convert hospitals and illness systems into systems of health maintenance. Excellence in clinical knowledge will be very important in the future. Nurses are well positioned to take leadership roles in this new era because clinical knowledge will be required to obtain the necessary outcomes. Helping people transition from the world of ill care to the world of health care is the work of leaders in this new era.

INTEGRATION

Mintzberg (1994) has written that the research on leadership has overlooked the most important part of the integration/synthesis role of the leader. He notes that the list of individual behaviors, such as leading and controlling, overlook the integration of many roles and behaviors that must take place to be effective. Mintzberg builds a model of leadership on a core of the agenda of the job, the frame of the job, and the person in the job who is surrounded by the roles of managing information, managing people, and managing action. Mintzberg posits that the components cannot be examined as singular linear functions and separated behaviorally. The job cannot be actualized as independent parts. He concludes that the role of managing must be well rounded. Perhaps this is the most important message that one can take into the new world of health care—that of integrating and synthesizing a variety of complicated roles defined by a diversity of situations into a synergized, interactive style of leadership. The new world is more complicated and leaders will have to address more complicated situations of greater diversity at one time. Leading many concentric interacting circles at one time as opposed to the linear "five things list" of the organized model of leadership will be the norm.

NEW ORGANIZATIONAL MODELS REQUIRE NEW SKILLS

Autocratic leadership styles are giving way to the transformational styles of leading, coaching, and teaching that are necessary in the new organizational models. Leading a team effectively, creating learning, and encouraging innovation and entrepreneurship are all new kinds of leadership activities. Senge, in *The Fifth Discipline* (1990), states that organizations must become learning organizations with the following essential disciplines: systems thinking, personal mastery, mental models, building shared vision, and team learning. Senge tells us that leaders must become designers, teachers, and stewards. The successful leader of the future is one who can work outside the walls of the traditional departmental organization and to synergize teams that can direct projects.

SUMMARY

The American Association of Critical Care Nurses (AACN) has described six key transformational competencies and values needed to lead the 21st century health care organization (AACN, 1994). These serve as excellent road maps to the kind of leadership we need in the future.

- **Mastering change:** To help organizations view change as an opportunity for new alternatives and calculated risk-taking
- **Systems thinking:** To understand interrelationships and patterns in solving complex problems
- **Shared vision:** To craft a collective organizational vision of the future
- **Continuous quality improvement:** To engender a never-satisfied attitude that supports an ongoing process to improve clinical and service outcomes
- **Redefining healthcare:** To focus on healing, changing lifestyles, and the holistic interplay of mind, body, and spirit
- **Serving the public and community:** To weld a social mission to organizational goals, objectives, and actions

REFERENCES

American Association of Critical Care Nurses. (1994, April). Call for nominations letter to members from Nancy Molter.

Barnum, B., & Kerfoot, K. (1995). *The nurse as executive* (4th ed.). Gaithersburg, MD: Aspen.

Byrne, J. (1993, December 20). Congratulations: You're moving to a new pepperoni. *Business Week,* 3351, 80-81.

Denton, D. (1991). *Horizontal management: Beyond total customer satisfaction.* New York: Lexington.

Gonzalez, E. (1995). Designing a disease management program. *Formulary, 30*(6), 326-340.

Mintzberg, H. (1994). Rounding out the manager's job. *Sloan Management Review, 36*(1), 11-26.

Senge, P. (1990). *The fifth discipline: The art and practice of the learning organization.* New York: Doubleday.

Vickery, D., & Lynch, W. (1995). Demand management: Enabling patients to use medical care appropriately. *Journal of Occupational & Environmental Medicine, 37*(5), 551-557.

Nurses in nonnursing leadership positions

BEVERLY L. MALONE

Nurses have a very special role in today's society. In addition to providing holistic care, nursing is the test case for women's issues in the 1990s. The interconnectedness of nursing and feminism places the nursing profession in the nonnursing leadership position for women's issues worldwide (Roberts & Group, 1995). As a profession, nursing is familiar with taking on nonnursing leadership positions; likewise, as individuals, nurses, are growing accustomed to assuming nonnursing leadership positions in pursuing the development of their full potential.

With the complex interaction as women in a male-dominated society and as nurses in the traditional health care world—dominated by male hospital administrators and physicians (Moss, 1995)—nurses confront the issues of women who are pursuing careers of purpose. Not being a part of the dominant society places nurses in double jeopardy as a result of the compound factors of being both female and nurses. The consequences of society's myopic view of women and nursing can influence nurses and the nursing profession to choose powerless behavior reflective of an oppressed group rather than proactive behavior dedicated to change and growth.

Stereotypes of nurses flourish with images of the physician's handmaiden and a motherly, spontaneously altruistic, caregiver needing constant direction and supervision. Adding to the complexity are nurses who buy into these traditional stereotypes by their words and actions.

Interestingly, the real nursing leaders have never accepted these stereotypes, but by their words and actions have negated them, thereby expanding the nurse's role into new territory. This chapter considers the acquisition of new territory or old space redesigned. While, entitled, "Nurses in Nonnursing Leadership Positions," this chapter is about power.

To examine this expansionary strategy fully, the traditional roots of nursing are explored along with issues of leadership and power and nursing's ambivalent relationship with power. Finally, advantages and disadvantages of nurses in nonnursing leadership positions are presented.

THE TRADITIONAL NURSING LEADERSHIP POSITION

The nurse executive, vice president for nursing, or director of nursing is the chief nurse in a hospital. The individual in this position is ultimately responsible for all of the nursing care—24 hours a day—that is provided in and more frequently out of the hospital. The educational preparation for these individuals usually includes a master's degree in nursing administration or business administration (Chitty, 1993). While supervising the largest group of health care personnel in the institution, nurse executives are frequently limited in their power base. These limitations may include exclusion from the board of trustees, where major policy decision-making occurs, and less stature and clout than the chief of the medical staff.

While nurse executives are identified as leaders in health care settings, their origins are similar to all nurses, and all women, with the common bond of Victorian roots (Moss, 1995). From these Victorian roots grew branches of stereotypes that disqualified women from engaging in business with men outside the home. Some of these stereotypes were biologically based because women were perceived as not being intelligent enough to manage commerce or the professions (Altick, 1973). As Nightingale demonstrated in the reengineering of the military health care system of Britain, nurses can be brilliant, strategic administrators and leaders (Shames, 1993). However, the Victorian society transformed Nightingale from a gutsy, unrelenting visionary into a stereotypical ministering angel who reinforced the assumptions about women and their abilities.

These stereotypes are the underpinnings for the glass

ceiling that serves as an unseen boundary to the career aspirations of nurses and women. Nurses in nonnursing leadership positions are frequently the first crack in the glass ceiling. Due to the invisibility of the glass ceiling and its lack of smell, taste, or other indications of its existence, nurses are usually surprised and confused when they bump or crash into the reality of the barrier.

The rumor of its existence has been shared throughout nursing folklore. However, the accomplished nurse leader who has surmounted obstacles ranging from irate and irrational physicians to the lack of adequate resources to provide optimum care is quite comfortable in tackling and overcoming barriers. Therein lies the surprise. The glass ceiling is an unusual barrier that has unique properties that attack the internal core self-esteem. The inability of nurses to break this barrier is typified by the following unstated areas:

- *Diagnosis:* Nurse leader dysfunction, with an origin based on being female, and early nurse-related social development
- *Symptoms:* Inability to run an organization or to make the hard decisions; lacking in depth in critical thinking and fortitude in risk taking and not fluent in the organizational culture's language
- *Treatment and prognosis:* Terminal unless the individual can reject the "nurse" descriptor and convert to the generic term of administrator/leader, which has a more acceptable, male-based origin.

All is not lost. This diagnosis is laced with sexism, which affirmative action guidelines began reproving and addressing in the 1960s and 1970s as a result of the Civil Rights and Women's Movements. These symptoms have not been documented in nurse leaders, and the mastery of leadership competencies is not gender-related. The prognosis is clearly not terminal and there exist other options than the rejection of one's nursing identity. In fact, the following action plan can allow one to crack the glass ceiling without capitulating one's nursing identity (adapted from Moss, 1995):

1. **Overcome hidden agendas.** Acknowledge the existence of an informal structure with unwritten expectations and stereotypes related to women, nurses, and others who are culturally different. Establish power networks of support both internal and external to the organization. Seek out mentoring relationships.
2. **Understand the existing power structure.** Learn the history of the corporate structure. Study the pathways and gatekeepers to organizational ascendancy. Develop your mentoring relationships.
3. **Learn the corporate language.** Moss (1995) suggests that corporate language stems from the military, sports, and sexual allusions. Developing a comfort level and familiarity with the language and its hidden meaning is a critical skill that does not necessarily require imitating men in the use of the language. While comprehending the language, a nurse leader can be selective but fluent in communicating the issues to colleagues.
4. **Memorize the play book.** For example, know the consequences of winning too frequently without sharing the perceived rewards with others. Underground societies have emerged to control the success of nurses and nursing departments who, in the eyes of the beholder, receive the lion's share of resources in the organization. One such organization rumored to exist is SPNGE, the *S*ociety to *P*revent *N*ursing from *G*etting *E*verything. Develop a strategic plan to write new sections to the play book.
5. **Establish business and financial credibility.** Seek out validation of your business and financial skills from the head of the finance department. If these skills are absent develop or polish them through continuing education or additional graduate study. In the interim, hire someone with the expertise required to affirm this critical area of knowledge.
6. **Utilize gender-specific communication styles.** This step involves acknowledging the basic differences in the communication of men and women. The premise is that men and women view the world differently: Men see the world as a hierarchial social structure while women view it as a network of connections. As a result, to men, dialogue is meant to achieve and maintain the upper hand; for women, it is a process meant to achieve closeness, confirmation, and support. Once these differences are acknowledged, one can choose the type of dialogue and the outcomes preferred. Heim and Galant (1993), on the other hand, suggest that women should limit rapport building with male colleagues to business topics because the discussion of personal experiences may leave a man feeling vulnerable. In other words, women should hide their differences. However, with today's global perspective and economic environment, diversity is being managed, not denied, through the acknowledgment and valuing of differences (Carnevale & Stone, 1994). Health care institutions and educational institutions have been the slowest learners in this new model of valuing diversity. In a recent study, six of six health care institutions were found to be lagging behind corporate industrial America in proac-

tively managing diversity (Muller, 1994). Instead, these health care institutions were described as pluralistic organizations with compliance-oriented strategies that address routine, modern human resource management practices. As the sociopolitical economic environment continues to demand management of diversity, health care institutions will choose to change or will not survive.

LEADERSHIP AND POWER: NURSING'S AMBIVALENT AFFAIR

While nursing is enamored with leadership, it is hesitant about its relationship with power. Nurses in nonnursing leadership positions must have a clear understanding of the intangible connectedness between leadership and power. Ambivalence is distracting and disempowering. Leadership and power are attached at their core, are inseparable, and are used most effectively with conscious, deliberate purpose. Leadership has been described as both a process and a property (Jago, 1982). The process of leadership is the use of power, the ability to move self and others toward a shared vision that becomes a shared reality. Depree (1989) describes leadership as an art form that empowers people to do what is required of them in the most effective and human way possible. Power is the action word for leadership.

As a property, leadership is a set of qualities attributed to those who are perceived as successfully achieving, with and through others, the outcome of a new shared reality. Nurses in nonnursing leadership positions need to have the following characteristics: vision, boundary management skills, risk taking, empowerment of followers, and mentoring (Bennis & Nanus, 1985, Grohar-Murray & DiCroce, 1992; Malone, 1984). A vision is a relative of a dream; it is not constrained by logic, time, or place. However, it is the sharable vision that is meaningful and achievable. In a study by Dunham and Fisher (1990), a nurse executive described the visioning process this way: "I always use the analogy of the artist who sketches a scene on a piece of canvas. It doesn't have to have all the colors. A tree doesn't have to have all the leaves (p. 3)."

Boundary management is of particular importance to nurses in nonnursing leadership positions. Nurses in these roles frequently exhibit cutting edge behavior. An edge is a boundary that separates entities and immediately alerts a leader to the need to design transactions across the boundary. Depree (1987) described living and dying edges. Nurses who have moved into nonnursing leadership positions are functioning at the living edge of the nursing profession. A nurse leader who was chief executive officer of an academic institution stated that a nurse in a nonnursing leadership position is an oxymoron. Once a nurse enters the position, it automatically becomes a nursing position, claimed new territory for the nursing profession.

Like all leaders, the nurse prior to or in a nonnursing leadership position must define the current reality, which includes the identification of existing boundaries. Once boundaries are located and noted, they are extended through risk taking. These nurse leaders are adept at temporarily overlapping boundaries with other entities while maintaining the integrity of their own boundaries.

The use and empowerment of followers is at the heart of nursing's reluctance to embrace the concept of power as an irretractable part of leadership. The idea of using and manipulating followers to achieve an outcome is not philosophically palatable to most nurses. Using followers implies a traditional hierarchial system of leadership that is based more on the male model than on a woman's way of knowing (Belenky, Clinchy, & Tarule, 1986). Yet in the process of leadership, the leader and followers are all used in service to the vision.

Perhaps what nurses uniquely bring to nonnursing leadership positions is the ability to achieve the outcomes of a new reality in a humanistic, caring manner. This requires not only the use of followers, but also the empowerment of these followers. Depree (1987) used the term "roving leadership" to describe a participatory process that emphasizes situational leadership by empowered followers through the support and approval of the hierarchial leader. In support of this line of thought, Senge (1990) described leaders as designers, stewards, and teachers responsible for building organizations in which people continually expand their capabilities to understand complexity, clarify vision, and improve shared mental models. Nurses in leadership nonnursing positions come well prepared for this type of leadership behavior.

The final characteristic ascribed to a leader is mentoring. Mentoring is an intense career building, mutually beneficial relationship between two individuals of unequal power in an organization (Levinson, 1978). Nurses in nonnursing leadership positions require a mentor. They need a guide, coach, advocate and sponsor in formal and informal settings who is committed to maximizing their success. At the same time, in order to continue the expansion of nurses in nonnursing leadership positions, the nurse leader must be mentoring other potential nurse leaders, preparing them for a successful encounter with the invisible glass ceiling of career opportunity.

ADVANTAGES AND DISADVANTAGES

The advantages of nurses in nonnursing leadership positions are multifaceted. There are rewards for both the individual nurse leader and for the nursing profession and humankind in general. These rewards include the affirmation of one's ability to lead, increased compensation potential, and increased political, policy, and decision-making power. These rewards result in an empowered and expanded image of the nurse.

Advantages: Affirmation, compensation, and power

Affirmation For the individual nursing leader, the affirmation of one's ability to lead represents a step toward self-actualization, the ultimate building block in Maslow's (1954) hierarchy of needs. For nurses, who belong to a predominantly female profession, to be able to maximize their career potential within and beyond the traditional boundaries of nursing, thereby successfully breaking through the glass ceiling, is revolutionary. The individual nurse is affirmed. The profession, with all of its self-doubts about its professional status, is reaffirmed. Women, biologically different than men but capable of serving as leaders and partners in visionary organizational growth, are also affirmed.

Compensation In concert with nursing's ambivalence to embrace power is the parallel reluctance to publicly value financial gain. Within every stratum of nursing (staff nurse, nurse manager, nurse director, school of nursing educator, and nurse executive), there is the issue of salary compression. Salary compression results in limited pay increases during a typical nursing career. Nurses tend to "top out" early in their careers, with more experienced nurses making little more than their less experienced counterparts. Chitty (1993) points out that salary progression in other professions is much greater than in nursing. For example, attorneys can expect a 226% salary progression during a typical career span, while nurses average a 69% progression. Moving nurses beyond the typical nursing career provides a greater opportunity for salary progression for all nurses as the "typical" nursing career is redefined with new and expanded boundaries.

The opportunity for greater financial compensation serves as an individual, professional, and public reward. The fact that 96% of the 2.2 million nurses in the United States are women translates into every step forward for nursing is a step forward for women throughout the nation and world.

Power: Policy shaping and decision making Nurses in nonnursing leadership positions are based in legislative bodies, major health care entities, academic settings, foundations, entrepreneurial small businesses, and industrial corporate institutions. For example, Eddie Bernice Johnson, Democratic State Representative from Texas, is the first nurse in Congress. Sheila Burke, as the Chief of Staff for Senator Bob Dole, the Senate Majority Leader, wields tremendous influence on the shaping of public policy. Irma Goertzen, President and Chief Executive Officer of Magee Women's Hospital in Pittsburgh, has the option to shape a system that empowers as well as delivers care to women. Gloria R. Smith, past Director of the Michigan Department of Public Health and presently Program Director and Vice President-Program within the Kellogg Foundation, works from a national and international frame to empower communities by structuring partnerships in primary health care, healing, and learning between providers and consumers. Rhetaugh Dumas, past Deputy Director of the National Institute of Mental Health and now as Vice Provost of Health Affairs at the University of Michigan, has provided leadership in the expansion of nursing's image to include the successful management of complex health-related organizations that extend beyond nursing. For a more comprehensive listing of nurses in nonnursing leadership positions, see Table 48.1.

These nurse leaders affect the availability of resources and opportunities for other nurses and the general public. Nurses at the bedside benefit from deliberations occurring in the halls of Congress, hospital board rooms, and other decision-making forums that include nurses in nonnursing leadership positions. These nurses can advocate not only for other nurses, but most importantly for the individual consumer's quality of life.

Bringing a nursing perspective of healing and collaboration to a traditionally nonnursing leadership position has far-reaching consequences for the health of this nation. Whether the health of the nation is defined in physical, psychological, spiritual or economic terms, nurse leaders add value to organizations critical to its well-being.

Disadvantages: tokenism, competition, and passing

Tokenism The burden of tokenism is intense. As a token, the female nurse is brought in as an artificial, transitional intervention intended to give management a

Table 48-1 Examples of Nurses in Nonnursing Leadership Positions

Name	Position
Andersen, Marcia	President Personalized Nursing Corporation Ann Arbor, Michigan
Biester, Doris	Senior Vice President Childrens Hospital Patient Care Services Denver, Colorado
Burke, Sheila	US Senate, Chief of Staff Office of the Majority Leader Washington, DC
Camphina-Bacote, Josephina	President Camphina-Bacote Associates Cincinnati, Ohio
Canton, Denise	Lawyer Public Health Service Department of Health and Human Services Washington, DC
Charter, Shirley	Commissioner of Social Security Social Security Administration Washington, DC
Daniel, Elnora	Provost and Executive Assistant to the President Hampton University Hampton, Virginia
Dow, Karen H.	Director of Education Geffern Cancer Center Vero Beach, Florida
Dumas, Rhetaugh	Vice Provost for Health Affairs, University of Michigan Ann Arbor, Michigan
Fishman, Dorothy	Manager, Business Development and Health Care Interconnection Services Group Southern New England Telephone Meridian, Connecticut
Fleming, Juanita	Executive Assistant to the President University of Kentucky Lexington, Kentucky
Floyd, Gloria Jo Wade	President Floyd & Associates Texas
Gaskin, Frances	President Cosmetics for the Black Women Albany, New York
Goertzen, Irma	President and Chief Executive Officer Magee Women's Hospital Pittsburgh, Pennsylvania
Grace, Helen	Senior Consultant W.K. Kellogg Foundation Battle Creek, Michigan
Haber, Judith	Family Therapist, Private Practice Stanford, Connecticut
Hanley, Catherine	Hospital Administrator Tuba City Indian Health Center Ada, Oklahoma
Hansen, Barbara	Director University of Maryland-Baltimore Graduate Studies and Research Baltimore, Maryland
Hanson, Catherine	Director Georgia Southern University Center Rural Health and Research Statesboro, Georgia
Koerner, JoEllen	Vice President, Patient Services Sioux Valley Hospital Sioux Falls, South Dakota
Lamb, Gerri	Clinical Director, Community Services Tucson, Arizona
Leavitt, Judith	Director, Generations United Ithaca, New York
Ledray, Linda E.	Director, Sexual Assault Resource Service Minneapolis, Minnesota
McClure, Margaret	Executive Director NYU Medical Center New York, New York
Nash, Mary G.	Vice President for Patient Care Services University of Alabama Birmingham, Alabama
Pierce, Patricia	President and Chief Executive Officer Health Care Focus, Inc. Tampa, Florida
Quinn, Joan	President Connecticut Community Care Bristol, Connecticut
Richards, Hilda	Chancellor, Indiana University-Northwest Indiana
Saltzer, Eleanor	President, Cancer Counseling Services Orange, California
Simpson, Roy	Executive Director, Nursing Affairs HBO & Company Atlanta, Georgia
Smith, Gloria R.	Vice President for Programs for Health Care W.K. Kellogg Foundation Battle Creek, Michigan
Sorrells-Jones, Jean	Patient Care Services Officer University of Virginia Health Sciences Center Charlottesville, Virginia

Table 48-1 Continued

Name	Position
Sparks, Susan	Research Education Specialist National Library of Medicine Division of Extramural Programs Bethesda, Maryland
Stetler, Cheryl B.	Project Director, Patient Centered Redesigner Hartford Hospital Hartford, Connecticut
Trofino, Joan	President Trofino Associates Holmdel, New Jersey
Tucker-Allen, Sallie	President Tucker Publishing Company Lisle, Illinois
Vestal, Katherine	Managing Partner Health Care Counsulting Hay Management Consultants Coppell, Texas
Walker, Duane	Vice President, Patient Services Queens Medical Center Honolulu, Hawaii
Weaver, Diana	Senior Vice President for Patient Services Yale New Haven Hospital New Haven, Connecticut
Wellons, Retha V.	President Wellons and Associates San Francisco, California
Wheeler, Robinetta	Co-President Wheeler and Associates Fremont, California
White, Suzanne	Vice President CV SVS/Clinical Affairs St. Joseph's Health System Atlanta, Georgia
Whitman, Gayle	Director Cleveland Clinic Foundation Cleveland, Ohio

chance to correct an imbalance (Thomas, 1991). The nurse in the nonnursing leadership position may be identified as only one of few and thereby becomes representative of what women and nurses can do or becomes a stand-in for all women and nurses. While one may receive significant visibility in organizations in which success is dependent on becoming known, the more likely scenario is one of loneliness or exclusion. Kanter (1977, p. 207) describes it as "a stranger who intrudes upon an alien culture." Dumas (1985) describes the dilemmas of black female leaders in a way that is reminiscent of nurses in nonnursing leadership positions:

> There is a general resistance to having black women perform competently in formal, high status positions. . . . The black woman in leadership is expected to comfort the weary and oppressed, intercede on behalf of those who feel abused, champion the cause for equality and justice—often as a lone crusader. She is expected to compensate for the deficits of other members of her group, speaking up for those who are unable or unwilling to speak for themselves. . . . Expected to be mother confessor, she counsels and advises her superiors and peers as well as her subordinates, often on matters unrelated to the tasks at hand. (p. 326)

Bayes and Newton (1985) state that a woman given primary authority for an organization faces a basic incongruity between role requirements of the leadership position and the sex-linked role conception of a woman. This incongruity is magnified when a nurse occupies a nonnursing leadership position.

Competition Nurses in nonnursing leadership positions are automatically in competition with other males, females, or nurses. The success of having cracked the glass ceiling is frequently envied rather than applauded and supported. Men assume that there is one less position available for them. Women have been socialized to compete with other women for favored positions with powerful men. It may appear difficult for women to join in supporting or protecting another woman who has achieved success (Bayes & Newton, 1985).

Competition is not necessarily negative. In corporate America, competition is the spice of organizational work life that leads to the prize. However, competition can be painful when the prize is gained only at the expense of other players. Nurses usually do not identify themselves as competitive. Therefore, they tend to be unaware of their own competitive urges and unprepared to compete in a healthy yet protective manner. Competition, especially from other female nurses, may be perceived as a malicious assault rather than a natural process of organizational life.

Passing "Passing" is usually discussed in relationship to passing over the color line. In the days of slavery, children born to racially mixed parents, depending on the lightness of their skin color, had the opportunity to slip from the bonds of slavery into the mainstream of white America. This process was described as passing. For nurses in nonnursing leadership positions, the same opportunity is presented. By simply dropping the credential of Registered Nurse and all references to a nursing background, women and men are afforded the opportunity to wipe the presence of nursing from their career portfolio. This denial of one's educational and professional preparation eliminates another voice from being heard and identified as part of the nursing tradition. It nullifies the advantages that were discussed earlier and reinforces stereotypes of low status and mobility that surround the nursing profession. It is an individual decision with system-wide repercussions.

SUMMARY

Nurses in nonnursing leadership positions are of great value to the individual nurse, to the profession, and to society. These leaders clearly operate at the edge of the profession, balancing on the precipice of change and power. They have the opportunity to expand the dimensions of the profession, to be the holistic voice in redesigning the health care system, the welfare system, or other policy shaping processes.

We in the nursing profession are aware of the potential isolation and loneliness for those who function at the edge of any activity. We must nurture our nurses in nonnursing leadership positions. Nursing and its organizations must find ways to continue to include our colleagues without demanding the sacrifice of their nonnursing positions; without requesting an exception from the role requirements of the position; and with an understanding that those who perform at the edge of the profession are just as essential to the wholeness of the profession as those who function at its core.

In nursing's role as an exemplar for women's issues worldwide, nurses must step forward to embrace this nonnursing leadership position. It is for the good of humankind that nursing must choose to lead.

REFERENCES

Altick, R. (1973). *The weaker sex in Victorian people and ideas.* New York: Norton.

Bayes, M., & Newton, P. (1985). Women in authority: A sociopsychological analysis. In A. Colman, & M. Geller (Eds.), *Group relations reader 2.* Washington, DC: AK Rice Institute.

Belenky, M.F., Clinchy, B.M., & Tarule, J.M. (1986). *Women ways of knowing.* New York: Basic Books.

Bennis, W., & Nanus, B. (1985). *Leaders: The strategies for taking charge.* New York: Harper & Row.

Carnevale, A., & Stone, S. (1994, October). Diversity beyond the golden rule. *Training and Development.*

Chitty, K.K. (1993). *Professional nursing: Concepts and challenges.* Philadelphia: Saunders.

Depree, M. (1989). *Leadership is an art.* New York: Doubleday Currency.

Dumas, R. (1985). Dilemmas of black females in leadership. In A. Colman & M. Geller (Eds.), *Group relations reader 2.* Washington, DC: AK Rice Institute.

Dunham, J., & Fisher, E. (1990). Nurse executive profile of excellent nursing leadership. *Nursing Administration Quarterly 15,* 1-8.

Grohar-Murray, M.E., & DiCroce, H.R. (1992). *Leadership and management in nursing.* Norwalk, CT: Appleton and Lange.

Heim, P., & Galant, S.K. (1993). *Hardball for Women: Winning at the Game of Business.* New York: NAL/Dutton.

Jago, A. (1982). Leadership: Perspective training and research. *Management Science,* 28. 315-336.

Kanter, R. (1977). *Men and women of the corporation.* New York: Basic Books.

Levinson, D.J. (1978). *Seasons of a man's life.* New York: Knopf.

Malone, B. (1984). Strategies and approaches to policymaking: A nursing perspective. *Occupational Health Nursing, 32*(1), 24-27.

Maslow, A. (1954). *Motivation and personality.* New York: Harpers & Row.

Moss, M.T. (1995). Developing glass breaking skills. *Nursing Administration Quarterly, 19*(2), 41-47: Aspen Publishers.

Muller, H. (Winter, 1994). Managing diversity in health services organizations. *Hospital & Health Services Administration.* 415-433.

Roberts, J., & Group, T.M. (1995). *Feminism and nursing. An historical perspective on power, status and political activism in the nursing profession.* CT: Praeger Publishers.

Senge, P. (1990). *The fifth discipline.* New York: Doubleday.

Shames, K.H. (1993). *The Nightingale conspiracy.* NJ: Enlightenment Press.

Thomas, Jr., R. (1991). *Beyond race and gender.* New York: American Management Association.

Community-based academic health centers: The CCHERS model

PATRICIA MAGUIRE MESERVEY

How do we ensure that today's students will contribute to and thrive as practitioners in tomorrow's radically different and ever-changing new health care environment? (Clare & Richardson, 1991, p. vii)

In the confusion of vertical integration, health care networks, and corporate linkages, we find our health care system becoming a seamless organization in which a person's care crosses traditional boundaries. Years ago a person might have been admitted into the hospital for a "diagnostic work-up," remain in the hospital for treatment, and prolong the hospital stay with an extended recovery. Today, we see same-day admissions for the most complicated of treatments, rapid discharges, and recovery occurring at home or in an extended care facility.

Added to the complexity, all of the standard health indicators in the United States point to an inefficient health care delivery system with inadequate outcomes. A few examples are our infant mortality rate, which ranks 29th in the world, life expectancy, which ranks 7th, and the majority of premature deaths in the country being linked to behavior (e.g., substance abuse, smoking, AIDS, cardiovascular disease). All of this occurs despite the fact that the United States spends more money per person on health care than any other country in the world. We do not have a health care system in the United States; we have a medical intervention system that is not providing the comprehensive health care our communities need. *Health* encompasses a broader definition than the absence of illness. It encompasses the availability of resources for the family, for the environment in which they live, for the knowledge they possess to prevent disease, and for the belief system guiding their choices. All of these factors contribute to the health status of our society; all are aspects of health that doctors, nurses, and social workers must know.

How then do we educate a workforce to attend to this broad definition of health? How do we teach the diagnosis and treatment of physical, mental, and social illness when the consumers are the population and not patients in a hospital bed? How do we validate our approaches to care, ensuring quality in both cost and care?

Health professions education and health services research must respond to the changing environment of health care by educating providers and researchers in the settings in which they will deliver care. No longer can medical, nursing, and social work education remain exclusively in the hospital institution. Students of all health professions must learn their practice in the arena in which care will be rendered. Research must address the integration and application of knowledge in the broader community. Community-based academic health centers capture the functions of education, research, and service in close proximity to where people live, work, play, and pray, providing a new environment for discovery, learning, and care.

COMMUNITY-BASED ACADEMIC HEALTH CENTERS

Training of professionals should occur increasingly in community-based centers that emphasize prevention, maintenance of a state of health and management of chronic diseases, as well as the patient's broader health needs. (Shugars, O'Neil, & Bader, 1991, p. 21)

Noting these changes emerging in the health care disciplines, the W.K. Kellogg Foundation developed the

Community Partnership with Health Professions Education Initiative. The intent of this initiative was to reduce the gap between the culture of the community and the culture of academe and hospitals through partnerships (Richards, 1995). These partnerships would yield an organizational structure that would be academic, community-based, and have a primary care focus (see the box). This community-based academic health center may take many forms (e.g., a nursing center, school-based health center, homeless shelter, or community health center). It shares common characteristics with the traditional academic health center through its role in education, research, and service. Yet it is the emphasis on the community and the implementation of education, research, and service in this setting that differentiates the community-based academic health center from its traditional counterpart (see Fig. 49-1).

Shifting education and research to the community requires significant change in our academic and health care systems. First is a change in the orientation of health care from a system developed for providers and organizations to one centered on people (i.e., communities). Communities must be engaged as full partners in health care and health profession education, providing greater assurances that the outcomes will address community needs.

A second change is developing the academic nature of the health center in the community environment. Historically, many community health centers drew away from teaching programs because they resented the sense of being regarded as "teaching material" rather than as human beings (Zuvekas & Rosenbaum, 1995). More recently, health centers have recognized that for new practitioners to choose a community-based practice they must be exposed to and socialized into the practice arena. Further, students must view their community experiences as challenging and fulfilling, requiring community-based education to receive the same time and quality emphasis in curricula that institutionally based care receives. Universities and community-based health care centers must develop experiences together, in partnership, and focused on the essential knowledge and skills needed for the practice environment.

Health services should emphasize prevention and early intervention through a multidisciplinary approach. One example of the need for prevention and early intervention is captured in the study conducted by the Commonwealth of Massachusetts Rate Setting Commission in 1994. This study revealed that from 1989 through 1990 1 in every 10 hospital stays was preventable—a cost to the Commonwealth of over $473 million (Massachusetts Rate Setting Commission, 1994). Each of the illnesses and conditions was sensitive to ambulatory care (i.e., conditions that are treatable in an outpatient setting). Had care been available, hospitalization could have been avoided.

CHARACTERISTICS OF COMMUNITY-BASED ACADEMIC HEALTH CENTERS

- Are community driven
- Are a partnership between communities and academic health systems
- Undertake equal responsibility for service, teaching, and research
- Undertake a major responsibility for teaching and learning
- Provide comprehensive health services that are multidisciplinary, preventive, and focused on early intervention
- Undertake research that is community-responsive and meets the highest standards of scholarship

Note. From Meservey, P.M., & Richards, R.W. Creating new organizational structures. In *Building Partnerships: Educating Health Professions for the Communities they Serve,* by R.W. Richards (Ed.), 1995, San Francisco: Jossey-Bass. Copyright 1995 by Jossey-Bass. Reprinted with permission.

Community-based academic health centers should focus their practices in the areas of prevention and early intervention through a multidisciplinary model. It is important to bring health professionals together with the community to provide care. Much has been written about the advantages of teaming and coordinated care, yet most organizations promote a "turn" care system instead. *Turn care* is care delivered through patient panels that are shared by multiple providers, with some consultation across the disciplines. Multidisciplinary care blends the knowledge and skills that medicine, nursing, social work, and other health professions have to offer to improve health outcomes through a team approach, which reflects a true collaboration and coordination of care.

Community-based research is a shift from the traditional notion of research. As health service research has transformed our delivery system, community responsive research will bring the talents of the scientist to the pragmatic needs of the community. Boyer (1991) describes it as the "scholarship of application." Taking knowledge believed to be true, applying it to practice in the community, and determining its effectiveness makes the scholarship of use to society.

Finally, there are large groups of people who are not receiving the health care services they need. Within the

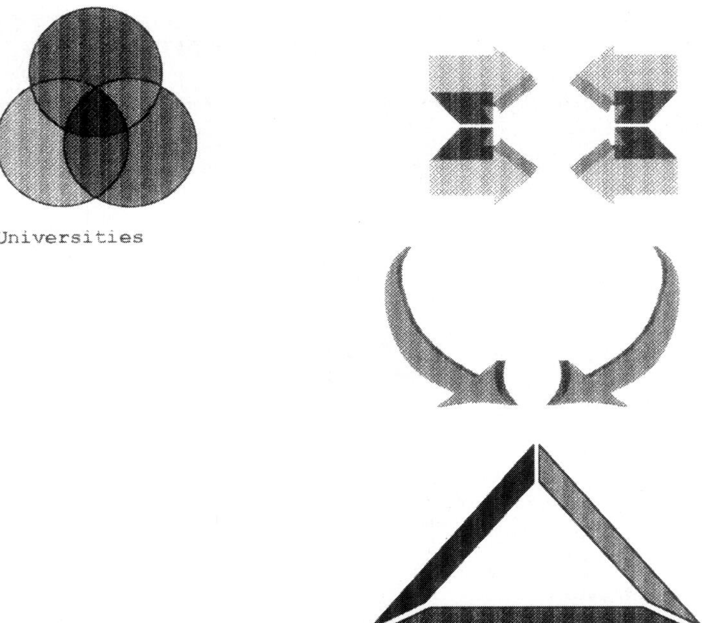

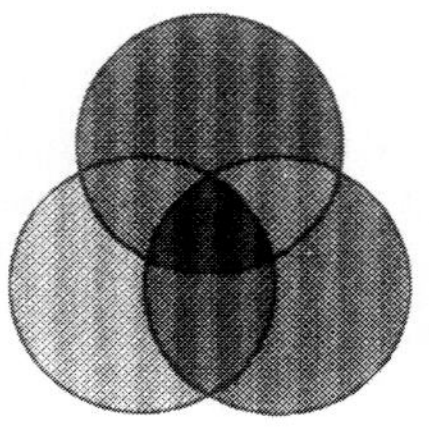

Fig. 49-1. Community-based academic health centers.

overall frame of the community-based academic health center is a focus on communities that are underserved and whose needs place them in high-risk health categories. This increases the services available in the community and socializes students to work in settings in which the clinical needs are high through a service-learning approach. The assumption is that students will gain an appreciation for the strengths and challenges of both the communities and the providers who have chosen to serve them, increasing the likelihood of their choosing careers in underserved areas (Zurvekas & Rosenbaum, 1995).

CCHERS—A W.K. KELLOGG COMMUNITY PARTNERSHIPS PROGRAM

Boston's Center for Community Health, Education, Research, and Service (CCHERS-pronounced "cheers") is a community-based academic health center, one of the seven programs partially funded through the W.K. Kellogg Community Partnerships Initiative. The membership of CCHERS includes 2 universities, 12 health centers and their communities, and the city's hospital and public health department (see Fig. 49-2). The primary purposes of this partnership are to create academic health centers in the community for primary care and to redirect health professional education into the primary care sector. These goals must be fulfilled with the full participation and involvement of the residents of these communities.

CCHERS is a nonprofit organization governed by a board of directors (see Fig. 49-3). The membership of the board includes representation from all constituents: universities, health centers, communities, hospital and public health departments. The board sets the policy direction, allocates resources, and oversees the implementation of the various programs of the organization. Reporting to the board is an executive director who is responsible for the daily work of the programs. Each organization (health center, university, and health department) has a coordinator on site to facilitate the work of the program offerings and to ensure that the goals are met.

CCHERS is a community-based academic health system with 12 participating health centers. Each health center has advanced its mission to include an active role in education and research to complement the strong service base that was their original mission. The communities served by the health center have active roles in the education and research of CCHERS, with many community-based organizations outside the health center joining the

Membership of the Center for Community Health Education, Research, and Service Boston, MA.

Community Health Centers and Communities	Universities / Government
Bowdoin Street Health Center Codman Square Health Center Dimock Community Health Center Dorchester House Multi-Service Center East Boston Neighborhood Health Center Harbor Health Services, Inc. *Geiger-Gibson Community Health Center* *Mary Ellen McCormick Health Center* *Neponset Health Center* Little House Health Center Mattapan Community Health Center South Boston Community Health Center Whittier Street Neighborhood Health Center	**Universities** Boston University Northeastern University **Government** Boston's Department of Health and Hospitals

Fig. 49-2. CCHERS organization. (Courtesy Center for Community Health Education, Research, and Service)

efforts in educating students and participating in research endeavors.

Education

The lead educational activity of CCHERS has been participating in the curricula transformations and implementation for the undergraduate nursing program and the medical school. Inherent in the philosophy of the CCHERS partnership is the belief that the health services of the community are owned by the community, that the power of the community to direct its health and welfare is the right and responsibility of the community. Curriculum is owned by the university faculty, with the faculty maintaining the responsibility for providing a sound educational experience for students. These two worlds converge because the curriculum must be designed to prepare graduates to meet the needs of the community's health.

The partnership enables the faculty and community to share information, expectations, and limitations across traditional boundaries in order to create a responsive educational experience for students that benefits the community in both the short and long term. Residents of the neighborhoods are direct partners in the education of the students, in the development of service projects to meet community needs, and in the identification of research problems that the community wants and that need attention.

To accomplish the goal of community benefits in depth, clinical assignments are organized so that students return to the same community and neighborhood health center over the course of their educational program. In this manner a genuine partnership can be developed between the students and the families and clients they serve. Further, it is expected that the students will develop partnerships with each other and with community staff that is reflective of a genuine collaborative model (Meservey & Zungolo, 1995).

Extending beyond the nursing and medical programs, the community representatives of the CCHERS partnership sought opportunities for the children of the neighborhoods to have greater access to the university programs. It is their intent to "grow their own" and have the students in the health professions programs be the children of the community. In response to this need the CCHERS partnership has joined with the Boston School Department and Boston and Dorchester High Schools to establish a Health Careers Academy. The Academy is a full high school curriculum enriched with career exploration, mentoring, youth development, family supports, and academic enrichment. Students in the Academy work with the medical and nursing students in the communities to learn about the opportunities of higher education and health professions careers. It is expected that the Academy will serve as a pipeline for inner-city children to pursue health careers.

Research

To achieve all the dimensions of an academic health center traditionally found in hospitals, the partnership must address other aspects of the shared relationship in addi-

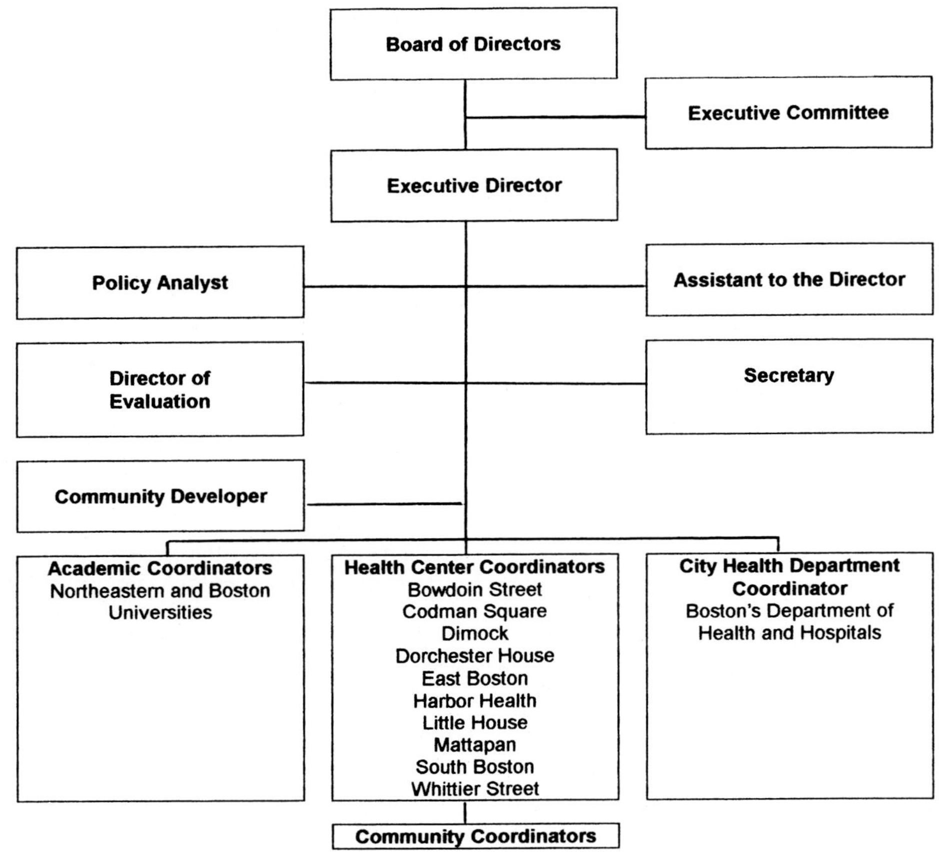

Fig. 49-3. CCHERS organizational chart. (Courtesy Center for Community Health Education, Research, and Service)

tion to the learning experiences. The research-rich environment of the traditional settings must be captured to enable the communities to attract top-notch clinicians for their centers and to communicate a value in the advancement of knowledge. Essential to these perceptions is the recognition of the void in knowledge about the efficacy of many of current health practices, the effectiveness of interventions, the cost-benefit ratio of preventive therapies and diagnostic screenings, and the whole range of investigations necessary to explore the effectiveness of the health service delivery mechanisms. The role of the community residents in the approval and acceptance of research activities is pivotal to the success of the project as well as to the integrity of any research undertaking (Meservey & Zungolo, 1995).

CHALLENGES OF A COMMUNITY-BASED ACADEMIC HEALTH CENTER

The community-based academic health center creates linkages that produce new organizations or—at the very least—new, stronger relationships. There is a blurring of traditional boundaries that is a source of confusion, fear, and risk. There are differences in primary orientation between the health centers and universities. Universities have a primary mission to educate students, while community health centers, nursing centers, and school-based health centers have as their primary mission to provide health services. The transition to the new organizational model demands a shifting of focus from the organization of origin to the partnership organization that has as its primary concern the blending of community and educational needs. Issues that will surface can be captured in the concept of a "boundaryless" organization. The four principal boundaries to be considered are authority, task, politics, and identity (Hirschhorn & Gilmore, 1992).

Developing strong communication, evolving trust, and creating positive organizational self-esteem are essential to the success of the new organization (Kawamoto, 1994). The traditional lines of authority are changed. The particular person or organization responsible for aspects of the work varies depending on the piece of work and how the work has changed with the new linkages of the organization. This, as with the next arena of the task boundaries, creates tensions in the organization.

The task boundary is that of the work to be done. This may be the most directly threatening aspect of the new organization because an individual's or organization's past responsibilities are shifted in the new environment. The normal expectation that university faculty will do the teaching is changed. Community providers, community members, and a variety of other people participate in the new educational model. Similarly, delivery of care changes. The faculty and students are new additions to the community setting, and there are shifts of responsibility, authority, and control.

The new organization blurs our past definitions and creates a sense of confusion for the members of the original organizations. A new identity is needed. Emphasis on the common goals of the group and efforts to create a new model of both education and service are examples of strategies to foster the identity of "us." Multiple fields of expertise are needed. Neither of the original organizations alone could achieve the same level of success in the new model as could the combined talents of both health centers and universities. Excellence in each part of the organization is essential for the blended system to succeed, and the recognition of the need for collective excellence becomes the team's motivation.

The merging of organizations is very difficult work and will certainly give rise to the question: "What is in it for us?" The common vision or shared goals are an essential element of the political boundary. Guiding the groups to an understanding of how mutual gains will be achieved and how, absent the new consortium, such gains could not be realized, is the basis for success in this area (Meservey, 1995).

PATHWAYS TO SUCCESS

Vision, leadership, and power are the keys elements for success in the new health care organization. With these elements, the new model of education will find a new locus of operation that will interconnect the needs of communities with the learning needs, knowledge, and skills of students. Learning can occur as service is provided, yielding a gain-gain outcome for the organization.

Vision is the ability to move toward a collective goal. It requires an understanding that the principal orientation of each participating organization and individual will be shifting to a new arena. We do not know at this time what the future holds for health care. With change occurring at a very rapid pace, the system is in chaos. In this environment, creating and holding a vision is challenging. The cornerstone of the community-based academic health center is understanding that however the system evolves there will be communities and the need to educate new health professionals, and that these two needs can be mutually supportive.

Leadership plays a pivotal role in the success of these new organizations (Meservey & Richards, 1995). Leadership must evolve from each part of the new organization, including service, education, and community. Having a cadre of leaders who can understand the needs and demands of the multiple aspects of the organization and provide the "bridge" for the organization is important. Leaders can create a climate of openness in the organization to transcend the cultures of community and academe.

Finally, power. Control over resources is essential. The current educational system is supported by a long tradition of funding pathways. This system must change to support community-based education, multiprofessional education, and primary care. To become a permanent part of the educational system, to be an essential care provider, the mainstream support must be redirected to provide the funds necessary for all aspects of education.

CONCLUSION

Outcomes sought with the new community-based academic health centers are an assurance of responsiveness and quality of services for the community. There must be a process of community assessment and mechanisms for community evaluation of programs. Because education is a cornerstone of such programs, ensuring quality education is also essential. The new community-based academic health centers facilitate the delineation of new roles for health professionals, establish mechanisms for policy changes in health care systems, and determine outcomes measures for successful programming.

REFERENCES

Boyer, E.L. (1991). *Scholarship reconsidered: Priorities of the professorate.* Princeton, NJ: The Carnegie Foundation.

Clare, D.R., & Richardson, W.C. (1991). Preface. In D.A. Shugars, E.H. O'Neil, & J.D. Bader (Eds.), *Healthy America: Practitioners for 2005* (p. vii). Durham, NC: The Pew Health Professions Commission.

Hirschhorn, L., & Gilmore, T. (1992, May-June). The new boundaries of the boundaryless company. *Harvard Business Review.* pp. 106-115.

Kawamoto, K. (1994). Nursing leadership: To thrive in a world of change. *Nursing Administration Quarterly, 18*(3), 1-6.

Massachusetts Rate Setting Commission. (1994). *Preventable hospitalization in Massachusetts.* Boston: Commonwealth of Massachusetts.

Meservey, P.M. (1995). Fostering collaboration in a boundaryless health professions education organization. *Nursing & Health Care: Perspectives on Community, 16*(4), 234-236.

Meservey, P.M., & Richards, R.W. (1995). Creating new organizational structures. In R.W. Richards (Ed.), *Building partnerships: Educating health professionals for the communities they serve.* San Francisco: Jossey-Bass Publishers.

Meservey, P.M., & Zungolo, E. (1995). Out of the tower and onto the streets: One college of nursing's partnership with communities. In P.S. Matteson (Ed.), *Nursing in the neighborhoods: The Northeastern University model.* Philadelphia: Springer Publishing Company.

Richards, R.W. (1995). From problems to solutions: A bridge between cultures. In R.W. Richards (Ed.), *Building partnerships: Educating health professionals for the communities they serve.* San Francisco: Jossey-Bass Publishers.

Shugars, D.A., O'Neil, E.H., & Bader, J.D. (Eds.). (1991). *Healthy America: Practitioners for 2005* (p. vii). Durham, NC: The Pew Health Professions Commission.

Zurvekas, A., & Rosenbaum, S. (1995). *Teaching community health centers: A guide.* Washington, DC: National Association of Community Health Centers.

Nursing centers: Where are they and what are they doing?

SALLY PECK LUNDEEN

Nursing centers have been discussed in the professional nursing literature for nearly 2 decades (Branstetter & Holman, 1989; Fehring, Schulte, & Riesch, 1986; Hauf, 1977; Henry, 1978; Jones, 1976; Lang, 1983; Lundeen, 1986; Riesch, Felder, & Stauder, 1980). In fact, the nursing centers of today share common roots with the birth of community health nursing under the leadership of Wald and others over a century ago (Glass, 1989). The nurse practitioner movement and the expansion of other advanced practice nursing (APN) roles have been important factors in recent nursing center development. There are indications that the number of nursing centers across the country has increased during the last decade, but the definition and purpose of these innovative health care delivery models continues to evolve. The development of a definition of what nursing centers are and what they do is definitely still a work in progress.

AN EVOLVING DEFINITION OF NURSING CENTERS

The progressive development of a definition of nursing centers has been undertaken by several professional groups during the past 15 years. A Delphi technique was used during the first Biennial National Conference on Nurse Managed Centers (Fehring et al., 1984) to develop one of the earliest published nursing center definitions. The American Nurses Association (ANA) Task Force on Nurse-Managed Centers, which convened in 1986, reaffirmed the key elements of the 1984 definition and modified it to read:

> Nursing centers—sometimes referred to as nursing organizations, nurse-managed centers, nursing clinics and community nursing centers—are organizations that give the client direct access to professional nursing services. Using nursing models of health, professional nurses in these centers diagnose and treat human responses to actual and potential health problems, and promote health and optimal functioning among target populations and communities. The services provided in these centers are holistic and client centered, and are reimbursable at a reasonable fee level. Accountability and responsibility for client care and professional practice remain with the professional nurse. Overall accountability and responsibility remain with the nurse executive.
>
> Nursing centers are not limited to any particular organizational configuration. Nursing centers may be freestanding or may be affiliated with universities or other service institutions, such as home health agencies or hospitals. The primary characteristic of the organization is responsiveness to the health needs of the population. (ANA, 1987, p. 1)

The National League for Nursing (NLN) Council on Nursing Centers adopted a more simplified working definition of a nursing center as a criteria for membership in 1990: "A nursing center is defined as an organization whose primary mission is to provide nursing services, may provide other services, and is owned, operated or controlled by nurses" (NLN, 1994b). This same NLN Council is currently distributing a national survey using a snowball sampling technique in order to establish a national database on nursing centers. The following criteria are being used for inclusion in this database:

- It provides direct access to nursing services for clients.
- Nurses are the major service providers with access to other health services.
- Nurses control the budget.
- A nurse is chief executive officer or operations officer (NLN, 1995b).

These definitions of nursing centers share several common themes that are important to the continued conceptual work of nurses who develop and study nursing centers. Common elements in these definitions underscore the need for nursing centers to do the following:

- Provide consumers direct access to nursing services (no referrals from other health care professionals are necessary)
- Provide nurse clinicians a high level of professional autonomy
- Place professional nurses in administrative control
- Develop mechanisms for nurses to receive direct payment for nursing services
- Use nursing models of health as the core element of the conceptual service delivery framework

Two other criteria frequently included in these definitions suggest that most nursing centers do the following:

- Provide opportunities for the education of nursing students
- Promote the conduct of nursing research

It is important that these key features be used as a frame of reference when describing the work of nursing centers today. These characteristics have been identified inductively by nurses who develop and practice in these centers. They serve as important criteria that can be used to differentiate nursing centers from other practice settings in which nurses may also play a prominent role. Conversely, there is great variation in the settings that qualify as nursing centers under these criteria; the nature of the clientele, the staffing patterns, the administrative and organizational structure, even the missions and goals of nursing centers vary widely. To paraphrase Stein, a nursing center is *not* a nursing center is *not* a nursing center. In fact, it has been said that there are as many models of nursing centers in the country today as there are centers themselves. This is undoubtedly an exaggeration; however, it is becoming increasingly important to sort out just what nursing centers are and what they are doing in order to determine their impact on the health care arena.

Unfortunately, much of the current change in the nature of health care delivery is occurring at a rapid pace that has been precipitated most directly by economics. Scores of programmatic changes in health care delivery that are being proposed and implemented across the country are based on short-term cost factors without concern for long-term improvements in the health status of whole communities. In many cases, "new delivery models of community-based care" are simply the same old institutional models transported to community locations. Frequently, these rapidly developing community networks are implemented without a clear understanding of either the nature of community systems or the needs and desires of various community constituencies. There is clearly a need for substantive research on issues related to the delivery of more effective and efficient methods to organize and deliver primary health care to the residents of many different types of communities. There is also a need to know more about the values and lifestyles of the constituents of health care services if services are to be developed that more appropriately meet their needs. This suggests that much more research is needed to promote a better understanding of the diverse nature of health care consumers as well as the health care interventions and models of delivery best suited to met these diverse needs. Nursing centers are well positioned to contribute new knowledge to providers and policymakers in these areas.

As the paradigms on which health care delivery has been predicated shift, there is a great need for field research in community-based practice settings. Nursing centers provide a rich source of data for researchers and public policymakers who wish to determine the impact of community-based, primary health care models on the health outcomes of specific populations (Frenn et al., 1996; Lundeen, 1993; Lundeen, 1994). The literature does not yet reflect clearly the articulated conceptual models of practice and health care delivery on which many nursing centers are built. Ultimately, nursing centers will need to be defined in large measure on the nursing models of care on which they are based and the degree of professional autonomy afforded nursing in the organization and delivery of services. Further conceptual work needs to be done in this area and specific nursing center models need to be explicated. This process is important not only to achieve conceptual clarity within professional nursing but also to maximize the impact nursing centers might have on health care policy in the rapidly changing health care arena.

Efforts to capitalize on the potential impact of nursing centers in the public policy arena have been hampered somewhat by a lack of clarity within the profession about the nursing center concept. There is a lack of specificity when trying to define and identify nursing centers across the country. Practice settings that perceive themselves as "nursing centers" continue to be called by many different names, including nurse-managed centers, nursing clinics, community nursing centers, and community nursing organizations. Other practice settings that qualify as nursing centers according to the current criteria have identified themselves more specifically with either a particular practice model (parish nurses) or with a particular practice site or targeted population (school-based clinics). The acknowledgment of a strong identification with the nursing center movement on the part of various nursing practice models, particularly those without academic affiliation, would undoubtedly increase the collective impact that these nurse practice settings might have on public policy.

Legislative efforts to define and recognize nursing centers as a key organizational element in health care reform have always received the persistent and extensive support of a few key legislators led by Senator Daniel Inouye (D-Hawaii) and his staff. In the early 1980s, many nursing center supporters (with the assistance of the ANA and others) lobbied for federal legislation that would support reimbursement for nurses providing services through nursing centers to Medicaid populations, including women and children, elders, and postdischarge psychiatric patients who need long-term care, including a large percentage of the nation's homeless. Several years later, after many major disappointments, federal legislation finally was crafted and passed to implement the national demonstration project funding of community nursing organizations (CNOs), which would be capitated to provide comprehensive, community-based health care services to Medicare recipients. After extensive delays in the development of the rules and regulations necessary to implement this legislation, the Health Care Financing Administration implemented a competitive application process (completed in 1992) and a 5-year project was begun. The applicants for this project included an interesting array of visiting nurse organizations, hospital-based nurse case management units, neighborhood nursing organizations, and primary care clinics. Four CNOs, including the Visiting Nurses Association of New York, St. Mary's Carondelet Hospital in Tucson, the Block Nurse Program in Minneapolis, and the Carle Clinic in Urbana, Illinois, were selected for this project. The results of this experiment in capitated managed care delivery to Medicare recipients through nursing center models are anticipated before the turn of the century.

AVAILABLE SURVEY DATA ON NURSING CENTERS

Determining the answer to where nursing centers are and what they do has always posed a challenge to researchers because there is no comprehensive national database on nursing centers. The actual identification of these centers, therefore, continues to pose problems and make any attempts to survey them difficult. Currently, the NLN Council for Nursing Centers is developing a database for nursing centers that will be as inclusive as possible of these centers and will be modified as appropriate to include additional sites as they are developed. This should improve the ability to collect and analyze data on where nursing centers are and what they are doing. Despite the acknowledged limitations imposed by the inability to identify the total population of nursing centers, a number of national surveys have been conducted over the years. Early efforts include surveys by Barger (1986), Higgs, (1988), and Roehring (1989). More recent studies, including those of the American Academy of Colleges of Nursing (AACN, 1993) and others (Rosenkoetter, 1994; Barger & Bridges, 1990) have focused predominantly on academic centers. The NLN Council on Nursing Centers has supported several surveys that have attempted to broaden the base to include nonacademic centers as well. Several of the more recent surveys are reported here (NLN, 1994a; NLN, 1995b).

NLN/Met Life survey

In 1992, the NLN, with the support of the Met Life Insurance Company, conducted a survey that was reported by Barger and Rosenfeld in 1993. They identified 170 nursing centers from professional organizations, funding sources, government mailing lists, and snowball sampling. Fifty-seven percent of these centers responded to the survey, resulting in 80 usable surveys. Their study documents that nursing centers are relatively new organizations to health care delivery, with many (53%) established within the 5 years prior to the survey. The median annual budget for these centers for 1990 was $222,500. Sixty-three percent of the respondents were affiliated with schools of nursing.

This survey found that the number of nurses working in these settings ranged from 1 to 115, with a mean of 8 and a median of 3 nurses per center. The nurses who work in nursing centers are highly educated, with 44% in this study prepared at the master's or doctoral level and 31% prepared with baccalaureate degrees. It is also noteworthy that two thirds of those eligible are certified in some area of advanced practice.

The racial composition of the clients reported indicates that a disproportionate number of minorities are served by community nursing centers. Over 50% of all clients served were persons of color while less than 25% of the total U.S. population held minority status during the study period. It is also interesting to note that nursing centers serve a high percentage of individuals with lower incomes as compared with the population as a whole. Nearly 63% of all clients earned incomes of $15,000 or less in 1990, while the median income in the United States was $29,943.

There were several differences noted among centers that were more established (i.e., in operation more than

5 years) and newer nursing centers (i.e., those in existence 5 years or less). Newer centers were more likely to provide a majority of services to the most vulnerable populations such as the frail elderly, homeless, or HIV-infected population, while older centers served predominantly the health needs of women and families. Payment for services also varied according to the length of time the center had been in operation. Nearly 30% of all services provided by newer centers are "uncompensated," while 57% of all service provided in older centers was paid for out of pocket or covered by insurance. The average of uncompensated care for all centers was very high (20%). Clearly, nursing centers are providing care to the most vulnerable populations, which are typically underserved in other health care delivery organizations. However, if adequate reimbursement through either public or private insurance sources cannot be obtained, these findings highlight the vulnerability of the nursing centers themselves.

AACN survey

A recent AACN survey (AACN, 1993a) reported data on 60 nursing centers operated by schools of nursing. These academic nursing centers were summarized as follows:

> The average nursing center had been in operation for slightly more than 5 years with a range from just over 1 month with one center that had been in operation for 16 years. Most responding centers (59%) were located off the nursing school's campus, in urban areas (75%), with nearly 40% operating in inner city locations. Eight centers (13%) were located in rural sites. While many centers were based at nursing schools (21%), others cover a wide range of locations, such as senior or neighborhood centers (16%), storefronts (16%), public housing projects (12%), churches (8%), schools (7%), and mobile van or home visits (3%). Most centers (70%) operated on a year-round basis with more than a third (37%) open between 21-40 hours per week. Eighteen clinics (30%) offered evening or weekend hours.
>
> The vast majority of centers in the AACN survey (91%) were staffed by nurse practitioners, clinical nurse specialists, and certified nurse-midwives with faculty appointments to the nursing school. Staff also included undergraduate and graduate students, registered nurses, physicians, laboratory technicians, and support and administrative personnel. . . . Forty-one centers (66%) reported that special populations comprise more than 15% of clients, such as the frail elderly, low birth weight and preterm infants, substance abusers, persons with developmental abilities, HIV positive individuals, homeless populations, victims of abuse and persons with mental illness. (AACN, 1993a)

This survey also found that financial constraints were reported by 76% of respondents as the greatest barrier to center operations. Because most reimbursement policies are tied to Medicare provisions, most nursing centers are not recognized as providers and therefore are denied reimbursement for services. The results of this report stimulated AACN President Janet A. Rodgers to conclude that the "limited or lack of reimbursement for nursing centers is a lingering issue hampering the access of many other Americans to quality, affordable health care" (AACN, 1993b).

NLN Council on Nursing Centers member survey

A survey conducted in 1994 by the NLN Council on Nursing Centers indicated that of the 52 member centers responding 61.5% were academic centers, 25% had an affiliation with another health care institution, and 19.2% were freestanding. The mean number of staff working in these centers was 4.8 full time equivalents, and centers were open an average of 36.6 hours a week. Services provided by these centers were broad and included health education (96%), health assessment (92%), health promotion (92%), information and referral (71%), primary care (63%), care coordination (53%), mental health counseling (23%), and home health care (22%). A database is currently being established by the NLN Council on Nursing Centers to track descriptive data on nursing centers across the country on an annual basis. This database will include both academic and nonacademic centers. It is critical to continue to describe and define these centers empirically if they are to serve as models for restructuring the health care delivery system.

FACTORS AFFECTING WHAT NURSING CENTERS ARE DOING

There are a number of factors that currently affect nursing centers significantly. The changes in the practice climate in health care delivery in general obviously has had an effect on all health care delivery settings including nursing centers. The sharp reduction in resources has been experienced in both service and academic settings during the past several years. The need for outcome data presents significant challenges to nursing centers and must serve to refocus research efforts in these settings. Challenges to nursing centers in the areas of practice and research must be explored further.

THE PRACTICE CLIMATE

Key factors related to the practice climate include issues related to the nature of the philosophies underpinning nursing center practice, the health care delivery models being developed by the centers, and the nature of compensation in nursing centers. As a result of the high percentage of APNs in nursing centers (Barger & Rosenfeld, 1993), many of these issues are also strongly related to the roles and functions that are being carved out by APNs—particularly clinical nurse specialists, nurse practitioners, and certified nurse midwives—in the practice arena.

There are some indications that positive changes are occurring in some regions with regard to collaborative practice models. Federal funding has supported interdisciplinary models of health care delivery through the special project grants of the division of nursing, rural and urban health center initiatives, area health education centers, and many local and national initiatives that are supported by private funders such as the W.K. Kellogg and Robert Wood Johnson Foundations. There has been some interest by public policymakers and health care organizations in the need to increase the number of educational programs for the preparation of APNs, particularly those with a focus on primary care. Prescriptive authority and direct reimbursement of nurse practitioners for selected services has also become a part of most state laws across the nation. These factors certainly support and encourage the maintenance and expansion of nursing centers and provide signs of the potential for substantive change in this area.

However, although most nursing centers are built on collaborative, interdisciplinary models of practice, the predominant practice climate in most parts of this nation is neither truly interdisciplinary nor collaborative. Most communities are in the throes of a widely competitive climate in the delivery of health care services that has adversely affected both consumers and providers. Health care systems have generally been unsupportive of truly expanded practice roles for APNs in many parts of the country. Hospital privileges, including delivery privileges for certified nurse midwives, have been slow in coming in most regions. These and other essential elements for independent nursing practice, including direct compensation, are not routinely a part of the community practice environment where nursing centers are located. This has caused the failure of more than a few nursing centers that were largely dependent on "soft monies" from grants and limited-term contracts for funding. In fact, many centers continue to seek models for organizational survival in which a major goal continues to be fiscal viability (Lundeen, 1989; Walker, 1994). Although nurses continue to persist in their struggle to develop and maintain viable nursing center models throughout the country, there is substantial evidence to suggest that developing nursing centers in most communities necessitates that nurses allocate considerable time and energy (which might be better spent in practice, education, or research) battling antiquated policies that support only an illness-dominated medical model of health care delivery and compensation simply in order to survive. Nursing center survey data indicate that the majority of centers responding had been in operation for 5 years or less. Current policies have had a negative effect on the ability of nursing centers to develop and implement effective models of practice and health care delivery over sustained periods of time in many communities in the past. The implications of these continued policies on fledgling centers seems obvious.

In this practice climate, some nursing centers have found that survival depends on the ability to develop practice models and define roles for APNs that are focused predominantly on providing care that closely resembles that provided by physicians. This "substitutive model of nursing center practice" is particularly attractive and well supported in communities in which an adequate number of physicians is not available in the workforce. For instance, public funding is available through legislative action to support rural health centers that are staffed by APNs even though nursing centers staffed by APNs in urban areas are not covered by similar legislation. Presumably this is because there is considered to be adequate physician availability in urban areas despite the fact that maldistribution of physician providers in most urban areas has been established for some time. In other words, nursing centers are less likely to be supported by current funding policies in areas in which they are perceived to provide greater competition to physicians. In areas where there is a "physicians shortage," on the other hand, APNs will be compensated by public monies for the provision of traditional medical services.

There are currently very different opinions on the most appropriate mix of providers necessary for a rational, efficient, and effective restructured health care delivery workforce in this country. The implementation of models of care that are based on truly collegial relationships between nurses, physicians, and other health care providers in order to ensure a full range of services to clients has proved to be another real challenge for many nursing centers. Collaborative demonstration sites, which are actually testing models of health care delivery that rely on an interdisciplinary framework that includes APNs, physicians, allied health workers, social workers, and other human service providers, although under development, are rare. Therefore, even when nursing centers are tolerated or encouraged, the practice models supported by health care policies are based typically on relatively traditional medical models of care. These policies frequently do not recognize or provide compensation for more innovative, collaborative, complementary primary health care models such as nursing centers.

The practice climate simply does not support these newer paradigms of health care delivery in many communities, yet until there are more nursing centers and other alternative practice settings that do provide alternative models of health care delivery and collect the data necessary to evaluate these new models, major changes in the practice climate are not likely to occur. Long-term follow-up of providers to determine satisfaction, retention, and evaluation of the impact of such models on community health indicators is also impossible without long-term center viability. The "catch 22" is that sustaining these new models, which are actually based on nursing models of care with interdisciplinary staffing, long enough to evaluate them requires exceptional skill, energy, and perseverance devoted to maintaining an extramural funding base that will support nursing center operations over time. This is perhaps the greatest challenge facing nursing centers today.

Effects of the current compensation policies on nursing centers

Although there is considerable research to support the position that primary care provided by nurses is cost-effective and that the clients' outcomes in selected populations are at least equal to (and in many cases greater than) those produced through physician interventions (Safriet, 1992 U.S. Congress, Office of Technology Assessment, 1986), the struggle to secure third-party reimbursement for APNs has been hard fought. This has been a major concern for many nursing center advocates for more than a decade. Pursuant to the Omnibus Reconciliation Act of 1989, reimbursement from Medicaid for the services of family and pediatric nurse practitioners was finally mandated to be part of each state's health care policies. Although a few states have avoided this mandate successfully for years by delaying the development and implementation of state rules and regulations, others have implemented liberal interpretations of this policy. Some have even set the reimbursement rate for nurses at 100% of the physicians' rate for selected services and have defined eligible nurses as all master's-prepared nurses who are certified as APNs, including nurse practitioners, certified nurse midwives, and clinical nurse specialists. These changes in reimbursement policies so long sought by those involved in the nursing center movement and others have not had an overwhelmingly positive effect on many nursing centers, however.

In most states, there is little or no recognition in the currently approved third-party reimbursement mechanisms of differences in nursing and medical practice. That is, the policies that determine which services are reimbursed (whether provided by physicians or APNs) are based solely on an illness-focused, medical model of care. Only a subset of those services deemed reimbursable for physicians in the traditional medical model are reimbursable to nurses in nursing centers or other practice settings. In fact, those services that have been approved as reimbursable for nurses are based on selections from the Current Procedural Terminology (CPT) codes developed to reimburse medical practitioners. This has had the net effect of encouraging many nursing centers concerned with fiscal stability to adopt a practice model that emphasizes the provision of these medical model services so that they can develop stable funding streams. In fact, it might be argued that the emphasis on the need to develop and maintain nursing centers as viable businesses threatens to supercede the original nursing center concept that emphasized that centers base practice on "nursing models of care" (ANA, 1987).

Nursing centers that emphasize primary prevention programs, especially those with a population-focused orientation, are also ineligible for compensation for many of the services that are provided in a health-oriented practice model. Services that are complementary to medical interventions and consistent with the World Health Organization (WHO) definition of primary health care (WHO/UNICEF, 1978) include community assessment, community education, health teaching and counseling, care coordination activities, and long-term surveillance of health- and safety-related phenomena. Although it can be argued that the long-term outcomes of communities are most improved through community-wide prevention activities of the nature long provided by community-based nurses, these interventions rarely receive compensation except through project-related extramural funds.

A recent study of over 14,000 nursing interventions coded in an inner-city nursing center (Lundeen, 1995b) indicates that less than 12% of all interventions provided by nurses were coded as treatments or procedures (i.e., those traditionally reimbursable for physicians through CPT coding). The remainder of the interventions provided by nurses in this community nursing center were health teaching, guidance, and counseling (49%), case management (21%), and surveillance (18%). These *nursing* interventions, arguably those that contributed most to healthier outcomes in the client population, were not considered reimbursable services for Medicaid clients. Thus, less than 12% of the interventions provided through this nursing center can be reimbursed through traditional payment mechanisms. Policies supporting only those elements of practice in nursing centers that are essentially based on more traditional medical practice may be having the effect of diluting the nursing models of care developed as a part of the original nursing centers. This has incredible implications for the fiscal viability of nursing centers that are based on nursing models of practice and warrants considerable further investigation.

Reimbursement policies as discussed to this point are probably not the critical issues related to compensation for nursing center services for the future, however. Increasingly in many states, particularly in urban areas, the penetration of managed care practice settings has increased dramatically. Managed care plans are in effect in most states for Medicaid populations, and there is every indication that Medicare recipients will also be members of capitated systems. Unfortunately, there seems to be more emphasis in most managed care environments on productivity related to episodic, acute care indicators (volume of clients seen per provider) and other short-term, cost-saving indicators than on the health maintenance philosophy of keeping people well that characterized early managed care systems. Again, these policies have influenced many nursing centers to focus almost exclusively on *substitutive* models of nursing practice rather than the *complementary* elements of nursing practice that were originally characterized by nursing center practice. The energy expended by professional nursing organizations and individual nurses in the state-by-state battles fought to ensure that APNs have "prescriptive authority," while extremely important, serves to highlight the emphasis by many on the substitutive elements of APN roles. A shift in the emphasis of advanced nursing practice, which embraces these medical skills of APNs and nursing centers to the exclusion of their nursing skills, will result in the loss of the unique contributions that *nursing* interventions can offer center users.

The administrative aspects of the current practice climate can prove devastating even to those nursing centers that are organized with a traditional episodic primary care approach. In many communities, centers must develop contracts for a specific set of services with as many as half a dozen managed care networks in order to operate independently. The subsequent administrative burdens of documenting discrete client descriptors and service delivery elements for each health maintenance organization in order to secure compensation nearly preclude this as a possibility for some community nursing centers. Nursing centers need to develop more sophisticated systems for clinical documentation of services and update their billing procedures if they are to be prepared to compete in the current competitive managed care environment.

There are some positive changes in the practice climate. Some states have developed programs for specific populations (e.g., pregnant women on Medicaid) that have embraced primary prevention strategies and case management as cost-effective intervention strategies that can be reimbursed as a part of the state's Medicaid program. These policy decisions provide nursing centers with excellent opportunities to bid for provider contracts and demonstrate the effectiveness of nursing centers as mainstream providers of care. Once again, however, nursing centers must be prepared to compete with other providers in order to secure contracts for these services. In many instances in which these programs are considered demonstration or pilot projects, it will also be important for nursing centers to collect adequate program evaluation data in order to demonstrate the effectiveness of nursing center delivery models.

In summary, direct reimbursement to APNs has been supported by the federal government and policymakers in many states for specific services. This has facilitated an improved practice climate for nursing centers that are delivering a significant proportion of reimbursable services. However, there are continuing challenges related to compensation for nursing services that affect the practice climate for nursing centers. These problems include focuses on the current limitations on the definitions of reimbursable services and the domination in many areas of large managed care networks that are frequently unwilling to contract with nursing centers for the provision of specific primary care services. The trend toward managed care networks probably holds the key to the future of nursing centers in this country. In order to be recognized as important provider organizations in managed care networks, nursing centers must provide outcome data on issues related to access, quality, and costs that demonstrate their value as effective and efficient health care providers. In fact, it may be argued that there will be a relatively narrow window of opportunity for nursing centers to prove their worth as partners in the health care delivery arena as these managed care networks emerge and stabilize in the next wave of health care delivery restructuring. This will require an increasing emphasis on nursing center research and program evaluation in the immediate future.

ISSUES RELATED TO NURSING CENTER SCHOLARSHIP AND RESEARCH

In her review of research conducted in nursing centers, Riesch (1992) identifies a great need for additional nursing center studies that focus on the outcomes of care. She argues that the documentation of a positive nursing impact on client outcomes through additional nursing research is necessary to define the position of nursing centers as providers of effective and efficient health care. To date, descriptive studies that focus on the nature of the nursing centers themselves have dominated the professional literature. These studies must now be balanced with studies on the health and health-related issues and concerns of various undersampled populations; the nature of nursing practice in these innovative, autonomous settings; the outcomes of nursing interventions with a wide variety of populations; and the impact of nursing models of practice on a restructured health care delivery environment. The high level of trust coupled with the high percentage of APNs prepared at the master's or doctoral level in most nursing centers provides the opportunity for research and practice missions to be integrated in these community-based settings. Nursing centers have a unique opportunity to contribute much to our knowledge about the issues and concerns *as well as the strengths* of many populations not frequently included in health research studies. The perspectives of participants should always be considered in the development and implementation of such research activities. The close relationship between nursing center staff and their clients forms the basis for the conduct of much needed studies on vulnerable populations.

Clinicians, administrators, and researchers have sometimes concluded that practice and research roles are incompatible, separate entities. In fact, in some settings, administrators and clinical staff may view research as an intrusion on the rights of patients or as an interference with clinical care (Oberst, 1985). This separation of research and practice agendas in many practice settings can impede the process of conducting important, clinically relevant studies. Perhaps the single most important element that nursing centers can contribute to the implementation and completion of meaningful research studies is the potential for merging these agendas by including the same trusted nurse clinicians who provide safe and effective nursing care to clients in the research process. A practice-oriented research agenda can be woven through the continuum of programs and services at nursing centers. Research should not be developed in isolation from either the clinical providers or consumers. Blending the research and practice roles in nursing center settings enables nurses to build on the nurse/client relationship of trust established over time and can enable the investigation of even the most sensitive issues, such as high-risk behavior, sexual and domestic violence, and loss of loved ones.

In many cases, particularly in academic nursing centers, the roles of nurse researcher and nurse clinician naturally overlap. The expertise of the clinical team is, therefore, better appreciated by the research team and the expertise of the researchers can be acknowledged and respected by the clinical team. Overlapping roles ensure that the insights from clinical work guide the formulation of research questions and the research process, and the findings of research studies can be integrated quickly into practice to be further tested or clinically modified.

Nursing centers are settings in which the outcomes of nursing interventions can be tested on a wide variety of populations. Based on available survey data, nurses practicing in nursing centers have access to a large number of clients who are underrepresented in the service populations of many other health care settings and in most research samples. Because so few health care settings exist where the model of care delivery can be developed, implemented, and controlled by professionals nurses, it is, in fact, the responsibility of nursing centers to evaluate client outcomes related to nursing models of care. Issues of quality, access, and cost are more amenable to nursing research in many nursing centers as a result of the ability of nursing to control both the practice and the data—a situation that is infrequent in most other health care environments.

Nursing centers provide the opportunity for teams of nurse clinicians and researchers to systematically document and analyze the nature of nursing practice in community-based settings. Very limited primary care research has been conducted that evaluates the effects of nursing models of health care delivery. In this area, perhaps more than any other, research activities must be integrated as part of the practice model. Researchers need to be prepared to adopt nontraditional and creative strategies in designing and conducting studies on the nature of nursing practice that are compatible with practice realities. They must translate the research language with ease and clarity so that it can be understood and applied by those in the practice arena. This integration of the research and practice elements can serve to greatly increase the chances of successful research activities in nursing centers (Zachariah & Lundeen, in press).

A core group in the nursing center movement has been involved actively in efforts to develop and implement computerized clinical documentation systems based on nursing taxonomies (Lundeen, 1995a). These efforts include a working group within the NLN Council on Nursing Centers that has been developing a common set of data elements appropriate for implementation across all nursing center settings (NLN, 1995a). This group is also investigating the development and modification of computerized nursing information systems that include established nursing taxonomies. These systems will be able to integrate administrative, clinical, and research applications in order to support the integrated research and practice agendas. Nursing centers are also well represented in the work being done by the International Council of Nurses on the establishment of an international nursing classification system for primary health care. Both the work on nursing classification schemes and the development of information systems are examples of the cutting edge conceptual work and applications of information technology that nursing centers are contributing to primary health care settings.

SUMMARY

What are nursing centers doing? In addition to providing excellent sites for the education of nursing and other health professional students, it appears that nursing centers are doing quite a bit. Survey data indicate that nursing centers provide primary care and nursing services to predominantly vulnerable populations who are underserved by other health care organizations. Nursing centers provide health care services in nontraditional, accessible settings. In addition, many are developing new paradigms for the delivery of health care based on nursing practice models. Several of these models are the focal point of demonstration projects to determine the effect of these centers on the outcomes of client care. Nursing centers are in the forefront of the development and testing of new techniques to document community-based nursing practice. Innovative programs of integrated research are being developed at many nursing centers. These centers are implementing computerized data systems that will support extensive programs of longitudinal clinical and health services research. Nurses who work in nursing centers are visible in the public policy arena providing leadership in implementing change in health care delivery. Nursing centers continue to provide a vision of the future of health care in this country.

Despite their accomplishments, these centers continue to struggle with a number of issues. Despite legislative changes in reimbursement for nurses, many are underfunded and resource-poor to the point that viability is a continuing problem. "Patchwork funding" (Lundeen, 1989) seems to be the mechanism that many centers, particularly those with the strongest nursing practice models, continue to utilize in order to survive. Adequate outcome research has not yet been conducted or disseminated to demonstrate appropriately the impact of nursing center services on the access, quality, and cost indicators that are so important in health services research today.

Nursing centers have different philosophies of practice and models of health care delivery. They may be affiliated with schools of nursing or with other health care organizations, including hospitals, group practices, and community health centers. Nursing centers may be nursing practice sites that are subunits of or totally dependent on another service organization, independent nurse organizations, or nursing organizations that are interdependent with other organizations such as schools, churches, work sites, homeless shelters, community centers, or social service agencies. The philosophy and models of practice in nursing centers vary and staffing patterns are not always similar. In addition, the defining characteristics of the nursing centers established to date are neither site- nor population-specific; nor are they dependent on any one specific and clearly articulated conceptual model. Although the key elements presented earlier have provided an important beginning to the definition and description of nursing centers, it is my opinion that there are many different types of nursing centers. This is a strength in a change-oriented health care environment, but there is a need to clarify within nursing and in interdisciplinary circles what nursing centers look like in their various forms. A sample of some questions that must continue to be addressed by leaders in the field include the following:

- What populations should be served by nursing centers? Should centers target only vulnerable populations or is there a need for these centers in all communities?

• What is the nature of the client problems addressed by providers in nursing centers? Does this constellation of problems vary significantly from center to center? Does it vary significantly in comparison with other practice settings?

• What is the nature of nursing practice in nursing centers? Does it vary significantly by the population served? Does the nature of practice vary significantly from center to center? Does nursing practice in nursing centers vary from practice in other primary are settings?

• What are the outcomes of nursing centers on access, quality, and cost of health care delivery?

• What impact do nursing centers have on health professionals' education?

• What impact do nursing centers have on the health status of the communities in which they are located?

• What is the potential of nursing centers to contribute to the reform of health care delivery in this country?

Ultimately, the success of nursing centers will be determined by the nursing models of care they develop and the degree of professional autonomy they afford nurses in the organization, delivery, and evaluation of services. These centers must be evaluated on the impact they have on the clients whom they serve (access and quality) and the systems with which they link (cost). It is important that further conceptual work be done and specific nursing center models explicated. This process is critical not only for conceptual clarity within the nursing community but also in order to maximize the impact that nursing centers might have on health care policy in our rapidly changing health care delivery environment.

REFERENCES

American Association of Colleges of Nursing. (1993a). *1992-93 Special Report on Institutional Resources and Budgets in Baccalaureate and Graduate Programs in Nursing.* Washington, DC: Author.

American Association of Colleges of Nursing. (1993b). *News release, September 22, 1993.* Washington, DC: Author.

American Nurses Association. (1987). *The nursing center: Concept and design.* Kansas City, MO: Author.

Barger, S.E. (1986). Academic nursing centers: a demographic profile. *Journal of Professional Nursing, 2,* 246-251.

Barger, S.E., & Bridges, W. (1990). An assessment of academic nursing centers. *Nurse Educator, 15*(2), 31-36.

Barger, S.E., & Rosenfeld, P. (1993). Models in community health care. *Nursing & Health Care, 14*(8), 426-431.

Branstetter, E., & Holman, E. (1989). A nursing model of health care: a 10-year trend analysis. In A. Arvonio (Ed.), *Nursing centers: Meeting the demand for quality health care* (NLN Publication No. [1993] 21-2311). New York: National League for Nursing.

Fehring, R.J., Schulte, J., & Riesch, S.K. (1986). Toward a definition of nurse-managed centers. *Journal of Community Health Nursing, 3*(2), 59.

Frenn, M., Lundeen, S.P., Martin, K., Riesch, S.K., & Wilson, S.A. (1996). Symposium on nursing centers: Past, present, and future. *Journal of Nursing Education, 35*(2), 54-62.

Glass, L.K. (1989). The historic origins of nursing centers. In A. Arvonio (Ed.), *Nursing centers: Meeting the demand for quality health care* (NLN Publication No. 21-2311). New York: National League for Nursing.

Hauf, B. (1977). An evaluation study of a nursing center for community nursing student experiences. *Journal of Nursing Education, 16*(8), 7-11.

Henry, O.M. (1978, October 15). *Demonstration centers for nursing practice, education, and research.* Paper presented at the annual meeting of the American Public Health Association, Los Angeles, CA.

Higgs, Z. (1988). The academic nurse-managed center movement: A survey report. *Journal of Professional Nursing, 4*(6), 422-429.

Jones, A. (1976). Nursing center for family services: Overview of a nursing center for family services in Freeport. *Nurse Practitioner, 1*(6), 26-31.

Lang, N. (1983). Nursing centers: Will they survive? *American Journal of Nursing, 83*(9), 1290-1294.

Lundeen, S.P. (1986). An interdisciplinary nurse managed center: The Erie Family Health Center. In M.D. Mezey & D.O. McGivern (Eds.), *Nurse, nurse practitioners: The evolution of primary care* (pp. 278-288). Boston: Little, Brown.

Lundeen, S.P. (1989). Strategies for community nursing center survival. In A. Arvonio (Ed.), *Nursing centers: Meeting the demand for quality health care* (NLN Publication No. 21-2311). New York: National League for Nursing.

Lundeen, S.P. (1993). Comprehensive, collaborative, coordinated, community-based care: A community nursing center model. *Journal of Family and Community Health, 12*(2), 59-67.

Lundeen, S.P. (1994). Community nursing centers: Implications for health policy reform. In J. McCloskey & H.K. Grace (Eds.) *Current issues in nursing* (4th ed.). St. Louis: Mosby.

Lundeen, S.P. (1995a). Information systems for community nursing center: Issues of clinical documentation. In B. Murphy (Ed.), *Nursing centers: The time is now.* New York: National League for Nursing.

Lundeen, S.P. (1995b, May 17). *Redesigning primary health care: A community nursing center model for the integration of public health, social services and primary care.* Paper presented at the Community-based Primary Care Conference sponsored by East Tennessee State University, Asheville, NC.

National League for Nursing. (1994a). *Initial results for 1994 Council on Nursing Centers Annual Survey of Members.* Unpublished report.

National League for Nursing. (1994b). *Council for Nursing Center Membership Directory.* New York: Author.

National League for Nursing. (1995a). *Report on the Council on Nursing Centers Nursing Information System Task Force.* Unpublished report.

National League for Nursing. (1995b). *Nursing Centers Database Survey.* New York: Author.

Oberst, M.T. (1985). Integrating research and clinical practice roles. *Topics in Clinical Nursing, 7*(2), 45-53.

Riesch, S.K., Felder, E., & Stauder, C. (1980). Nursing centers can promote health for individuals, families and communities. *Nursing Administration Quarterly, 4*(3), 3-4.

Riesch, S.K. (1992). Nursing centers. In J.J. Fitzpatrick, A. Jacox, & R.L. Taunton (Eds.), *Annual review of nursing research, Vol. 10, Part II: Research on nursing care delivery* (pp. 145-161). New York: Springer Publishing Company.

Rosenkoetter, M.M., Zakutney, M.A., Reynolds, B.J., & Faller, H.S.

(1994). *A Survey of Academic Nursing Centers.* Wilmington, NC: The University of North Carolina at Wilmington School of Nursing.

Roehring, M.J. (1989). Nursing centers: State of the art-survey results. In A. Arvonio (Ed.), *Nursing centers: Meeting the demand for quality health care.* NLN Publication No. 21-2311. New York: National League for Nursing.

Safriet, B.J. (1992). Health care dollars and regulatory sense: The role of advanced practice nursing. *Yale Journal of Regulation,* 417-488.

U.S. Congress, Office of Technology Assessment. (1986). *Nurse practitioners, physicians, assistants and certified nurse midwives: A policy analysis.* Washington, DC: U.S. Government Printing Office.

Walker, P.H. (1994). Dollars and sense in health reform: Interdisciplinary practice and community nursing centers. *Nursing Administration Quarterly, 1*(1), 1-11.

World Health Organization/UNICEF. (1978). *Primary health care.* Geneva: Author.

Zachariah, R., & Lundeen, S.P. (In press). Research and practice in community nursing centers. *Image.*

Developing professional-community partnerships

SHARON FARLEY

Community-based primary health care is like motherhood and apple pie: Everyone praises it. Yet there are various interpretations of how community-based programs should be implemented. In addition, despite public rhetoric, some health professionals may be ambivalent toward the concepts of community partnerships and citizen empowerment that must accompany successful community-based primary health care.

Some public and private agencies physically place community health centers, mental health centers, nursing care centers, and the like in the community but keep them responsible to the system instead of to the citizens they serve. McKnight (1985) believes that outreach programs are a way for systems to expand themselves and diminish communities. In these programs, health and social service providers view people as clients instead of citizens; the clients are people who are defined by their needs and are dependent on the programs to fix their problems (Dewar, 1990).

Sometimes these systems promise partnerships with the community to identify needs and design programs to fill the gaps in services. However, these powerful outside groups and bureaucracies are not willing to share power with their citizen partners or to give up the supervisory role. These "partnerships" perpetuate the paternalistic health and social service delivery system and, consequently, the community-based programs often are not successful.

Many social and health reformers are advocating that citizens become genuinely involved in making decisions about programs and policies that affect their health and quality of life (Braithwaite & Lythcott, 1989; McKnight, 1985; Williams, 1991). This community empowerment is a process of increasing control by groups over consequences that are important to their members (Fuchs, 1983). Research by McKnight (1985) indicates that it is impossible to produce health among the powerless but that it is possible to allow health by transferring tools, authority, budgets, and income to those with the malady of powerlessness.

The health status of those with the least power—minorities and the poor—remains unconscionably low. The *Report of the Secretary's Task Force on Black and Minority Health* (U.S. Department of Health and Human Services, 1986) noted that minorities experienced approximately 60,000 "excess deaths" annually. Signs of the health costs of powerlessness among the poor and disenfranchised are interpersonal violence, dangerous housing, drug overdose, alcoholism, and teenage pregnancy, among others. Powerlessness and poverty of the spirit and of resources are the antecedent risk factors of preventable disease (Braithwaite & Lythcott, 1989).

Nurses and other health professionals need new actions and allies to solve the health problems of the year 2000 and beyond. Communities have an abundant capacity for caring about their citizens. When people are enabled to work with professionals in real partnerships in which decision making is shared, changes that improve health and quality of life will occur. Nurses, traditionally committed to involving individuals in decision making, can play a key role in empowering citizens for participation in community-based health care programs.

BUILDING COMMUNITY-BASED PARTNERSHIPS

The Rural Elderly Enhancement Program (REEP) in Alabama, which is partially funded by the W.K. Kellogg Foundation, is a nurse-initiated project administered by Auburn University at Montgomery School of Nursing. It is developed on a model of community participation and empowerment. REEP's initial goal was to maintain the health and independence of the elderly, but in response to citizens' demands, it was expanded to include a family focus with a strong commitment to youth. The majority of the population in the two targeted Alabama counties is black, poor, and medically underserved. The project views health according to the World Health Organization's definition:

- Access to adequate food, shelter, and clothing
- Access to medical care when needed
- An opportunity to participate
- A safe healthful environment

Therefore, nurses work with other health and human service professionals, local and state government units, agencies, volunteer coalitions, and schools to do the following:

- Stimulate rural development involving community volunteer coalitions, leadership training, infrastructure improvement, job training, and public education
- Foster health care systems that include family-centered, community-based service and collaboration among multiple sectors
- Conduct family assessments and respond to needs with linkage to services, education, and appropriate volunteer coalitions
- Establish school-based community health and resource centers

The REEP staff help communities organize volunteer coalitions and foster links between these coalitions and health and human service organizations. Although the needs are great and the resources are few, volunteers are giving many hours of free services to assist their neighbors and friends. The tradition of "neighbor helping neighbor," long recognized as a hallmark of rural life, forms the value base for these volunteer coalitions. These citizens, many impoverished themselves, recognize their interconnectedness and responsibility for the well-being of each other and believe in their capacity to act to solve their communities' problems. Volunteers provide friendly visiting, homemaking, personal care, and respite for the elderly and their families. They also raise funds to assist the elderly in buying medications, obtaining transportation, and getting public water to their homes. These volunteers are graduates of the home health aide/nursing home assistant training classes taught by nurses in the project. They also assist the project nurses with case findings and referrals as well as helping families gain access to the health care system. Sixty percent of the graduates are employed by home health agencies and nursing homes.

In 10 small communities, volunteers are assisting school-age children with mathematics, reading, and science in after-school and summer programs. They also offer recreational activities for families and implement programs in the arts and humanities. In four of the communities, the parents receive adult basic education and job training and are taught parenting skills. Retired school teachers and other older residents use story telling to connect children to their history, culture, and values.

In collaboration with a community health agency, the school of nursing established school-based community health and resource centers at a middle school and an elementary school. Community advisory boards at both schools approve policies and plan and evaluate activities of the centers. A nurse practitioner coordinates the centers and works with volunteers and other health and human service agencies to provide comprehensive family-focused services.

Links between volunteer coalitions and professionals are provided through interagency councils that have representatives from health, social service, and education agencies. The councils serve four purposes: (1) to plan and implement cooperative programs with the volunteer coalitions that assist the communities; (2) to assist with volunteer training; (3) to play an advisory role to the coalitions and provide linkages between community initiatives and available services and resources; and (4) to communicate with each other and decrease duplication of services. Project staff provide leadership and educational activities for council members that enable them to implement a community empowerment model and to assume an advisory instead of a supervisory role for community-based programs.

The following story illustrates how citizens working in partnership with professionals can make a difference in community-based programs:

> A volunteer called one of the project staff members because she was concerned about a 14-year-old boy and his 78-year-old grandmother who lived together in an isolated area. The boy was the main caregiver for his grandmother, who had many chronic illnesses. The volunteer believed the boy to be depressed, anxious, and angry about his lack of freedom to pursue his interests because of his responsibilities for the grandmother.
>
> The project nurse visited the home and did an assessment. She obtained an order for home health services and contacted a volunteer who provided respite care and housekeeping. A male volunteer spent time with the teenager and involved him in a

recreation and tutoring program also staffed with volunteers. The grandmother's health improved so she could take care of her activities of daily living. The teenager's grades improved from *Ds* to *Bs* and *Cs*, and he remained active in basketball and soccer.

FACTORS CRITICAL TO SUCCESS

Cooperative goals, trusting relationships, and commitment are the foundation for coalition building and partnerships. Increasingly, collaboration becomes a necessity as individuals and groups seek to develop individual competencies, solve problems, and respond to a rapidly changing world. Some factors are critical to building successful coalitions and partnerships for community-based primary health care programs.

Competent communities

Citizens in communities often feel helpless and unable to address problems or improve their quality of life. People who live in poverty are especially disenfranchised and have no voice or any organization to represent them. When the REEP project began people made statements such as "We don't have any drinking water and we aren't likely to get any" and "These young boys take our money each month and we are afraid to say anything." A critical part of the coalition building process is to develop empowered and competent communities. Iscoe (1974) defines a competent community as "one that utilizes, develops, or obtains resources so that members of the community may make reasoned decisions about issues confronting them" (p. 608). The community is able to gain mastery over its life and mobilize to solve problems.

Effective partnerships develop when communities and professionals possess relatively equal power to influence decision making. However, professionals usually possess the most power because they control information, resources, knowledge, and money and they do not want to share. The dominant belief is that service planning and delivery are the role of professionals. McKnight (1989) states that, "It isn't until the capacities of people are recognized, honored, respected and lifted up that outside resources make much difference" (p. 5). Egan and Cowan (1979) suggest that, "The challenge of the professional is to develop the humility, willingness and methodology to give away the philosophy, knowledge and skills pioneered in the past" (p. 128).

Focus on issues that matter most

The place to begin is with what matters most, that is, what matters most to the people in the community. Of course, this must be tempered with rational thought and the probability of success. To build community competence, it is important that first projects be achievable. Persons in a constant battle with poverty look for immediate visible goals. Given that consideration, the choice of types of coalitions and the projects they undertake should be left to the discretion of the group. The guidance and advice of the project staff can prevent the selection of first projects that will be difficult to complete or that will not allow the group to experience an early success.

It is essential to remember that communities have many problems and that it is very likely that they will always have problems. The goal is not to eliminate all problems; rather, it is to focus the community's energies toward those problems that they are willing to work together to solve. These problems then become issues, which should be grouped in related categories around which volunteer coalitions can be developed. The development of successful coalitions and the selection of successful projects will depend on the following factors: the selection and grouping of issues into possible projects for the different volunteer coalitions and concentration on developing only two or three coalitions at first.

The first community meeting of REEP was a joint meeting of community leaders from both counties. Before this meeting, the project staff had listed opportunities for volunteer involvement related to each project goal and grouped these opportunities into fields of interest such as transportation, housing rehabilitation, water, health education, fund-raising, nutrition, recreation, chore services for the elderly, and clerical support for the project staff. The project staff envisioned that each field of interest would be the basis for a possible volunteer coalition, and they developed job descriptions for each possible coalition. The project staff also had definite opinions about those coalitions they felt were most needed and were surprised when their opinions were not shared by all present at the meeting. The additional surprise came when these two counties, very similar in demographic profiles, also had differing opinions concerning the coalitions they wanted to form. From the outset, the project staff learned a valuable lesson: Never assume that you know what the community needs and is willing to work together to achieve; always ask them what their needs are and what they want to work to achieve.

Respect for individual and community values

The underlying goal of a successful coalition is to improve the quality of life, and the underlying value is to maintain the dignity of every individual. Health professionals who respect the dignity of people emphasize the concept of possible change created by local leaders and volunteers versus the fantasy of "saviors." The issues, solutions, and programs flow from the people. Alinsky (1971) said, "Denial of the opportunity for participation is the denial of human dignity and democracy" (p. 122).

The community's sense of dignity and confidence in directing its own efforts is an essential element in developing community-based programs. The community existed long before the community organizer came into it, and it will exist long after the community organizer is gone. Time in rural communities is measured not in days or weeks but in decades and centuries; time in rural communities is a smooth, ever-flowing big river. From this perspective, community-based programs become mere ripples in the stream—they come and they go.

Many rural communities, having seen community-based programs come and go, have little faith in the longevity of such projects, and this is an obstacle to overcome. Because the underlying purpose in developing volunteer coalitions is to create both an organized approach to the community's problems and a leadership group that will survive or evolve into another group when the project's goals are completed, the issue of time and making lasting changes is a major concern. REEP chose to address this concern by selecting staff community development coordinators who were natives of the counties. These coordinators gave the project credibility with the local population. Their commitment to their communities, their sterling characters, and their willingness to listen and learn enhanced the possibility of lasting changes.

Continuous leadership development

Leadership development for citizens is one of the most important activities for building community competence. Leadership development for local community leaders often consists of an organized program of meetings, seminars, and workshops that last 1 or 2 days, 1 week, or several weeks. Leadership development is seldom viewed as a continuous need. When one-shot leadership training is the mode of instruction, several problems occur. If the leadership program is not relevant to the leader's current situation, the knowledge and skills gained in the training will suffer from a lack of application and will often be forgotten. Leadership development, for both community leaders and coalition members, should be ongoing, and the topics of the development programs should meet the participants' current needs.

Oftentimes, one training session on a particular topic will not be sufficient. For the REEP project, planning workshops were held in both counties, and project staff *assumed* that all coalition members understood both the elements of the planning process and the methods used in developing strategic and long-range plans. During the training, all coalition members received instruction in how to construct charts which included goals, interventions, projected dates of completion, and persons responsible for the interventions. The coalition's use of these planning charts in subsequent meetings convinced the project staff that they understood the planning process. Only 9 months later did they realize that the coalition members may have understood how to use some planning tools but had not completely internalized what they knew about the planning process. Following a second planning workshop, one participant said,

> I attended the first workshop you did on this, but I didn't realize that we were going to have to keep doing this. I was used to our getting together to help someone when their house burned. I didn't realize that we were going to have to continuously develop plans to reach all the people who are in need.

The cyclical nature of planning as it related to their coalition and their county was slowly becoming an accepted fact of life, but it was not the result of one-shot leadership training and development.

Experimental learning is the most effective type of learning. It is only in repetition that one gains confidence and belief in newly gained skills. Learning reinforced with positive experiences is also most successful. All leadership training should focus only on the skills the coalition members need to develop at that time, and it should allow for the successful practice of newly gained skills. Allowing the coalition members to determine the projects they want to undertake, helping them to set realistic goals, and giving them the training they need to accomplish these goals is essential to the long-term success of any volunteer community development project.

Leadership development should also be open to everyone; it is not a blessing given to few. All members of coalitions should participate in the leadership development events, which should be scheduled with their attendance in mind. Essential topics for all leaders and members of volunteer coalitions include group management skills, including conflict resolution, methods of encouraging participation, and group dynamics; organizational skills, including planning, delegation, fund raising, and budgeting; problem resolution skills, including problem identification and analysis, setting goals, and group decision making; and evaluation skills, including assessment of results and revision of approaches. In addition, all leadership programs should include a reiteration of basic values: the improvement of the quality of life and the maintenance of the dignity of every individual.

Natural leaders have emerged in most of the REEP coalitions, but leadership in some is sporadic. Lack of strong local leaders is a problem facing many communities, and the causes of this problem are often similar. Many communities have lost their strong leaders of the past, and the opportunities for leadership development have not been readily available to the young. Many communities have "risen to the bait" only to be disappointed, and they are reluctant to rise again. Much time and patience are required to develop the leadership strength needed by communities, and this can be a problem that at times seems unresponsive to outside intervention. Yet leadership training is the key—leadership training that provides opportunities for practice and success with newly learned skills, that does not push the coalitions into efforts they are unready or unwilling to undertake, and that continually reaffirms the possibility of actual change is essential. At the same time, organizers should be aware that communities have not reached the state they are in overnight and that state will not be changed overnight.

Remember to celebrate

A fringe benefit of working with REEP is the experience of participating in community celebrations. People in rural communities constantly incorporate parties and social events into their activities. Every REEP coalition meeting begins with social chatter and food and ends with more food. McKnight (1987) believes, "You will know that you are in a community if you often hear laughter and singing. You will know you are in an institution, corporation, or bureaucracy if you hear the silence of long halls and reasoned meetings" (p. 54).

Social events and celebrations are effective tools for building trust between health professionals and citizens and for recruiting volunteers and motivating community participation. REEP staff sponsor two or three community parties each year to thank volunteers, to celebrate progress, and to laugh and play together. One of the most successful events was a Christmas parade and party organized by a helping hand coalition for the elderly they served. Ten 80- and 90-year-olds, some in wheelchairs, rode on floats blowing kisses and throwing candy to the children.

BARRIERS TO SUCCESS

When REEP was implemented in the counties, many health and social service providers were skeptical about its chances for success. One health provider's comments illustrate this attitude: "These people don't care, and they really don't want any change. They won't volunteer. We are giving them plenty of services and welfare. You are really spinning your wheels." So, the first barrier encountered was professionals who did not trust the capacity of community people to work as equal partners. McKnight (1987) says that they see communities as collections of "parochial, inexpert, uninformed, and biased people" (p. 54).

Another barrier is the resistance of hierarchical social service institutions to share power and decision making with citizens. They do not want to lose control and supervisory power over community-based programs. A social service professional was willing to support "using" REEP volunteers to support the agency's programs, but was not willing to "include" volunteers in planning and establishing priorities for those programs. A competent and empowered community is bound to cause trouble for service institutions. The citizens begin to make "outrageous" demands such as health and service agencies being open in the evenings and on weekends, parent-teacher association meetings in the evening, safe water and sewage, and decent housing. Iscoe believes that "powerlessness means safety for some" (p. 609).

In addition, health and service agencies do not tolerate the uncertainty that is inherent in community-based programs. This is understandable because agencies' funding often is tied to successful programs. However, in the process of helping communities becoming competent, these will be failures because of the lack of leadership and experience among the citizens. When programs are not successful, instead of evaluating efforts and trying new strategies, the professionals often want to abandon the effort.

The interagency councils are assisting to break down barriers. Members participate in the leadership training with the coalition members as well as participating as advisers and partners in the coalition's programs. They experience the capacity of the volunteers to make a difference when citizens become empowered. When they embrace the concepts of partnerships and empowerment, they spread the word to their colleagues in the agencies. Many agencies are now eager to participate as partners in REEP's community-based programs.

PHILOSOPHICAL ADMONITIONS

Health professionals should enter communities with the goal of mobilizing the capacities of people to respond to issues. However, communities are not managed, orderly environments; disenfranchised people are sometimes the least organized; and their voices are sometimes the most angry or despondent (Dewar, 1990). Some philosophical admonitions are offered as a foundation for developing community-based primary health care programs that empower citizens.

Community development is a process, not an event

Evolutionary change is not an event that happens on one day like Christmas. All evolutionary change takes time but more often results in a stable organization. Revolutionary change will create an organization that exists only a short time for a purpose that, when achieved, leads to the dissolving of the organization.

Avoid developing a "Messiah complex"

Community empowerment is a process that enables but does not impose. For community members to recognize and meet the needs of their community may require the intervention of persons or institutions outside the community. This intervention may be teaching the methodology of problem resolution, but the specific solutions to specific problems must be decided by the citizens. Professionals do not simply provide communities with set "answers."

Iscoe (1974) writes that "achieving the goal of independence does not guarantee similarity of actions and attitudes between initiators and those who presumably have benefitted" (p. 613). As communities become competent, citizens become independent and may start their own programs without the professional partners. When coalitions started holding meetings on their own, the REEP staff's first reaction was that the volunteers were ungrateful for the help they had received. However, the staff quickly realized that like mothers whose children leave the nest, they were feeling abandoned but happy that the volunteers could act independently.

Maintain a policy of inclusion

Respecting the dignity of the individual and community means opening the door to all "stakeholders" who want to participate. There must be a policy of inclusion, not exclusion. During leadership training, words must be chosen carefully and key ideas repeated constantly:

- "Working together we can do wonderful things."
- "Involve others, do not use others."
- "Who else should we involve in this?"
- "Develop resources, develop people, build communities."
- "When you help to build a cathedral, you may not see it completed in your lifetime."

Go beyond promises

Universities as well as government and private agencies have started many community-based programs to improve citizens' health and quality of life. Some have been very successful, whereas many have failed. At an organization meeting for REEP an elderly woman said

> Other universities have promised to help us. They have used statistics from our county to get funding for themselves. We've been studied and written up. People have created charts and figures and told us that we'll hear from them later. We've never heard from them again. All we want is water, better houses, and jobs. We don't need any more studies. Don't promise if you can't help us.

Nurses can assist communities to organize successful programs that improve health and quality of life. To go beyond promises and to build programs that flourish, nurses must form partnerships with citizens and share power and decision making. George (1983) writes, "Successful organizers are those willing to enjoy the reflected glow of others' successes, those who find satisfaction, not in their own production, but in the production of others. We can starve ourselves and others with promises or we can feast together" (p. 86).

REFERENCES

Alinsky, S.D. (1971). *Rules for radicals.* New York: Vintage.

Braithwaite, R., & Lythcott, N. (1989). Community empowerment as a strategy for health promotion for black and other minority populations. *Journal of the American Medical Association, 261*(2), 282.

Dewar, T. (1990). 'Systems' talk turns off citizens. *Metro Monitor, 21*(7), 3.

Egan, G., & Cowan, M. (1979). *People in systems: A model for development in the human service professions and education.* Monterey, CA: Brooks Cole.

Fuchs, V.R. (1983). *Who shall live.* New York: Basic.

George, I.R. (1983). *Beyond promises: A guide for rural program development* (p. 42). Montgomery, AL: Alabama Office of Voluntary Citizen Participation, State of Alabama Commission on Aging.

Iscoe, I. (1974, August). Community psychology and the competent community. *American Psychologist,* 607.

McKnight, J.L. (1985). Health and empowerment. *Canadian Journal of Public Health, 73,* 37.

McKnight, J.L. (1987, Winter). Regenerating community. *Social Policy,* 54.

McKnight, J.L. (1989, Spring). Do no harm: Policy options that meet human needs. *Social Policy,* 5.

U.S. Department of Health and Human Services. (1986). *Report of the secretary's task force on black and minority health.* Washington, DC: Author.

Williams, D.M. (1991). Policy at the grassroots: Community-based participation in health care policy. *Journal of Professional Nursing, 7*(5), 271.

Shared governance models in nursing: What is shared, who governs, and who benefits?

MERIDEAN L. MAAS, JANET P. SPECHT, CHERYL L. RAMLER

Governance or self-regulation has long been recognized as a privilege given to professions that earn the public trust by demonstrating accountability for their specialized practices (Crocker, Kirkpatrick, & Lentenbrink, 1992). To ensure that professionals do not misuse autonomy for their own interests, rather than those of their clients, society requires professionals to demonstrate accountability for their actions (Maas & Jacox, 1977). Nursing has developed many self-regulating mechanisms (e.g., codes of ethics, standards, credentialing and accreditation criteria, and guidelines for peer review) that demonstrate the ability to govern its members in the public interest (McCloskey et al., 1994); however, the privilege of governance has been slow in coming. Professional nursing governance in practice settings, where physicians and administrators who benefit from the subordinate employee status of nurses have dominated, has been especially constrained.

Although there have been isolated examples of the implementation of professional nursing practice models over several decades (Horvath, 1990; Jacoby & Terpste, 1990; Johnson, 1987; Maas & Jacox, 1977; McDonagh, Rhodes, Sharkey, & Goodroe, 1989; Rose & DiPasquale, 1990), recognition of the need for nursing governance in hospitals became most focused during the nursing shortage in the 1980s. The value of nursing to the delivery of health care in hospitals has also become more visible as a result of relentless technological and medical advances and their associated costs. After a period of widespread use of registered nurses (RNs) to provide a variety of services in order to downsize other departments and workers, hospitals began to reconsider the best use of nursing knowledge and skills. The folly of using nurses to perform functions for which they are highly overqualified became clearer as the undersupply of nurses compared with demand reached critical proportions. While the demand for nurses grew, increasing numbers of nurses demonstrated dissatisfaction with their jobs and careers by moving to part-time work, leaving nursing for other careers, or moving to other practice settings after a brief period of employment in one hospital (Prescott, 1987). A decreasing number of persons entered the nursing field owing to low pay, limited career advancement opportunities, and a greater number of other career options for women (American Nurses Association [ANA], 1992).

Finally, demands for more accountability for the outcomes of care have accompanied the pressures to control costs. As a result, nurse and hospital administrators are recognizing that the staff nurse, at the point of contact with the patient, is in the critical position to ensure the delivery of quality care (Spitzer-Lehmann, 1989).

These and other factors have encouraged nurse executives in hospitals to move to models of nursing practice that increase nurse autonomy for clinical decision making and participation in decision making throughout the organization. Shared governance models have been a popular strategy in the 1980s and early 1990s to increase nurse job satisfaction and retention and to achieve cost-effective quality outcomes (Sticker, 1992). Empowering nurses within the hospital decision-making system, particularly with regard to increasing nurses' authority and control over nursing practice, has been the stated aim of shared governance models. There are a number of issues, however, that are apparent as increasing numbers of hospitals initiate changes to implement shared governance. These issues include the lack of clearly defined criteria for shared governance, mixed motives for the implementation of nursing shared governance, disagreement about how shared governance can and should be implemented, and concerns about the effects of shared governance on different roles within nursing and hospital systems.

WHAT IS SHARED GOVERNANCE?

Clarification of the concept of shared governance and the structures and processes that must be in place for implementation in employing organizations is needed if the nursing profession is to honor its contract with society as described in the ANA's *Social Policy Statement* (ANA, 1980). The concept of shared governance comes from the recognition of the need to accommodate two systems of authority when professionals are employed in organizations. In organizations, authority is ordinarily vested in positions arranged in a hierarchy, with positions higher in the hierarchy assigned a greater scope of authority than lower positions. Although professionals employed by organizations occupy positions with corresponding organizational authority, they also have authority as a function of membership in their profession (Minzberg, 1979). For a profession, this authority is based on specialized knowledge. Society gives professionals autonomy to get important jobs done effectively by experts who are also competent judges of the needed expertise. When professionals are employed by organizations, there is always the danger that the societal needs that are entrusted to the profession will become subordinated to the organization's needs. This is the critical reason why governance shared by the organization and its employed professionals has evolved.

Nurse-shared governance in organizations is synonymous with professional nursing practice in organizations that employ nurses (Mass & Specht, 1990). In nursing, shared governance means that nurse employees and the organization are partners in meeting the goals of the organization and the mandates of the nursing profession (Porter-O'Grady, 1991a; 1991b). However, descriptions of the requisite structures and processes for claimed shared governance models are often incomplete or unclear. Professional nurse shared governance does not exist unless the authority and accountability of professional nurses is codified in the organization and decision-making structures and processes already in place that enable nurses to define and regulate nursing practices and share decisions with administrators regarding the management of resources.

As illustrated in Figure 52-1, specialized knowledge and commitment to a service ideal are the foundation for professional nurse autonomy and accountability (Maas & Specht, 1990). *Professional nursing autonomy* means that professional nurses have the authority to define and decide what services they will provide and what constitutes safe and effective practice. *Professional nurse accountability* means responsibility and answerability to authority for the services rendered. The profession must take action to ensure that the practice of its members is safe and effective. Thus organizational structures of decision making, coordination, and control, which are set forth in a constitution and bylaws, are needed (1) to enable nurse peer definition of the scope of nursing practice, standards of practice, nursing delivery systems, qualifications for the selection of staff, and knowledge and resources required; and (2) to enable peer evaluation of the practice, promotion, and retention of individual nurses, evaluation of the department (collective) practice, peer consultation, dissemination of knowledge, and development of knowledge through research. Contrary to some definitions that describe shared governance as a structure for staff nurse autonomy (Pinkerton, 1988), the structure must enable professional autonomy and accountability of all professional nurses, as individuals and as a collective, if governance is to be shared by the organization and employed professional nurses (Maas, Jacox & Specht, 1975). All RNs, regardless of their position in the organization (e.g., staff nurse, clinical nurse specialist, nurse researcher, nurse educator, nurse manager, nurse administrator), must have professional autonomy and accountability as individuals and as a collective of peers (Maas & Jacox, 1977).

More than 1,000 hospitals in the United States have implemented shared governance during the past decade (Porter-O'Grady, 1994). However, there is much variation in the organizational models implemented under the label of shared governance. A number of different terms, such as participation in decision making, participative management, self-governance, empowerment, and professional practice, are used at times to be synonyms with shared governance and at other times to indicate different organizational models with varying degrees of nurse participation in decision making. There appears to be consensus that shared governance means some amount or type of shared decision making by staff and nursing management. There is less clarity and agreement regarding what specific decisions are made or shared by nurses and management, what staff are included in the shared governance, and whether nurses as individuals or as a collective have authority and accountability for certain decisions. Thus, models of practice implemented under the label of

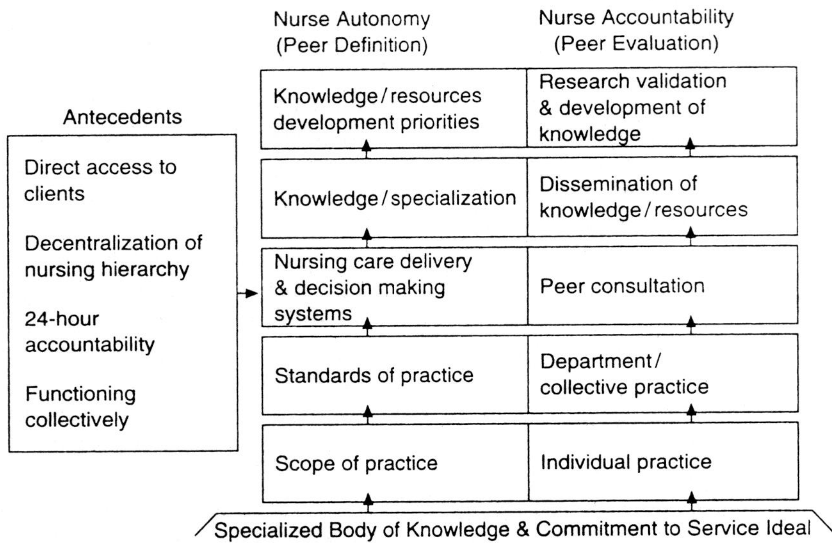

Fig. 52-1. Iowa Veterans Home model of professional nursing practice. (From Maas, M.L. [1989]. Professional practice for the extended care environment: learning from one model and its implication. Journal of Professional Nursing 5(22), 66-76.) © W.B. Saunders Company. Used with permission.

shared governance range from those with minimal, ad hoc, or informal participation by some or all nursing staff in a very limited number of decisions with little or no expectation for nursing staff accountability, to models in which the profession and the organization truly share authority and accountability for the profession's mandates and the organization's mission.

Because all nursing staff do not have the specialized knowledge and socialization to the service ideal that professional nurses do, it should be obvious that democracy in the workplace is not nursing shared governance. Nursing staff who assist RNs in the delivery of care are clearly not qualified to govern the profession, although they can participate in decision making.

There has been increased discussion recently of whole-systems shared governance (Evan, Aubry, Hawkins, Curley, & Porter-O'Grady, 1995; Porter-O'Grady, 1994). Whole-systems governance models are more similar to democracy in the workplace than to professional nurse governance. The basis for sharing in these models is doing the work rather than being a member of the profession. While whole-systems governance schemes increase participation in decision making for all workers, they do not address control of professional practice by the profession. Whole-systems shared governance reinforces the need for nurse shared governance and does not supplant it.

The confusion between the concept of participation in decision making and professional governance has contributed to the view advanced by Porter-O'Grady (1994) that whole-systems governance is a progression beyond nurse shared governance. However, this is not the case. The goals of whole-systems shared governance and professional nurse shared governance are distinctly different. Integration, equity, and communication among the disciplines within the organization are fundamental objectives of whole-systems governance, while nurse shared governance is a partnership between the professional nurses and the organization to meet the mandates of the profession for autonomy and accountability of nurses and the goals of the organization. These two approaches to governance come from different theoretical bases. From an organizational behavior perspective, whole-systems shared governance does not address the development of the profession as does nurse shared governance, which is derived from the sociology of professions literature. The two systems are not mutually exclusive and both can contribute positively to patient outcomes and effective organizations.

It is less obvious and more controversial to assert that all RNs are qualified to assume autonomy and accountability. All RNs share the profession's mandates; however, there is great variation in their knowledge, education, and experience. Implementation of shared governance requires that RNs who are expected to assume professional autonomy and accountability are prepared to do so. This means that the first shared decisions of the organization and nursing leadership must be the definition of criteria for admitting RNs to professional decision-making privileges and agreement on the programming and resources needed to assist RNs who desire to meet the criteria.

The controversy over what decisions professional nurses and organization management should make mostly focuses on a debate about whether nurses who are not managers can decide matters of resource distribution. This is simply a concern about loss of control on the part of managers and reflects a lack of commitment to professional nursing governance. The importance of this issue is underscored by the results of a survey of 1,100 RNs from 10 hospitals that was conducted from June 1993 to April 1994 (Hess, 1995). The study revealed that out of six aspects of governance, including control over professional practice, the nurses rated as most important the influence over organization resources that support practice.

Professional shared governance requires that all nurses in the organization develop a consensus about goals and priorities and the expectations that available resources will be allocated accordingly. All nurses are kept aware of the available resources and share the planning of their allocation and the responsibility to develop alternatives when there is shortfall. Specific areas of authority and responsibility for different roles (e.g., managers, educators, and clinicians) are defined, and control for decisions is placed with those who carry them out (Jenkins, 1991). Disagreements about decisions are resolved through negotiation. Although the development of the consensus, structures, and expectations for shared governance is not easy, resistance to doing it because of concern about who will make what decisions is most often a lack of commitment to professional nursing practice and an unwillingness to relinquish nursing control.

Professional nurse participation in decision making, empowerment of nurse professionals, participative management, and work redesign each are coincident and necessary for professional nurse shared governance, but none are synonymous with it. The goals of work redesign are often to enhance the authority of nurses and rectify organizational problems that contribute to suboptimal use and turnover of professional nurses (Strasen, 1989). Thus, the goal of work redesign efforts may be directed toward implementation of shared governance models. However, the goals of many work redesign efforts are also to increase the participation of nurses in decision making without providing the structures whereby they have professional authority and accountability for all decisions affecting nursing practice. Some work redesign efforts actually obscure nursing's identity as a professional discipline with obligations of accountability to clients for services rendered. The current emphasis on interdisciplinary efforts and team building, while laudable, often is interpreted as shared authority and accountability without recognizing the necessity of retaining mechanisms for demonstrating the accountability of disciplines other than medicine. A recent study of the implementation of nurse shared governance in one hospital described the concurrent implementation of patient-focused care, which resulted in the removal of the term "nursing" from all nurse shared governance documents (Ramler, 1995).

Many nurse executives have become vice presidents for patient care services (or some similar title), promoting the change in language from "nursing" to "patient care services," and in many instances eliminating departments of nursing (Specht, 1995). While most nurses applaud the need for a nurse executive to administer all patient services, few seem to analyze the implications critically if the nursing discipline is not a visible and accountable entity. In these circumstances, it is perhaps most critical to have professional nursing shared governance operational, but least likely to be implemented.

It is nurses who must be astute about the distinctions among these concepts, so that they are not misled into believing that they are sharing governance with management as professionals, when in fact they are not equal partners in meeting the mandates of the profession or the goals of the organization. If the structures enabling professional autonomy and accountability outlined in Fig. 52-1 are not implemented, nursing shared governance is not operational. Fig. 52-2 provides one example of decision making, coordination, and control structures defined in a constitution and bylaws that enable nursing shared governance in an organization (Maas & Specht, 1990).

Clarity about shared governance for nurses is essential if it is to be more than one more "bandwagon" that is jumped on without being anchored to a clear theoretical base and commitment to enabling professional nursing practice. Some argue that nursing's knowledge base is insufficient to support control of practice as professionals and that the majority of nurses do not want professional authority and accountability. Others complain that shared governance is little more than a philosophy, a fad, or a nursing self-aggrandizement and that there is no empirical evidence that benefits accrue when nurses have more professional autonomy. A few even assert that shared governance even sounds like a religion when the converted

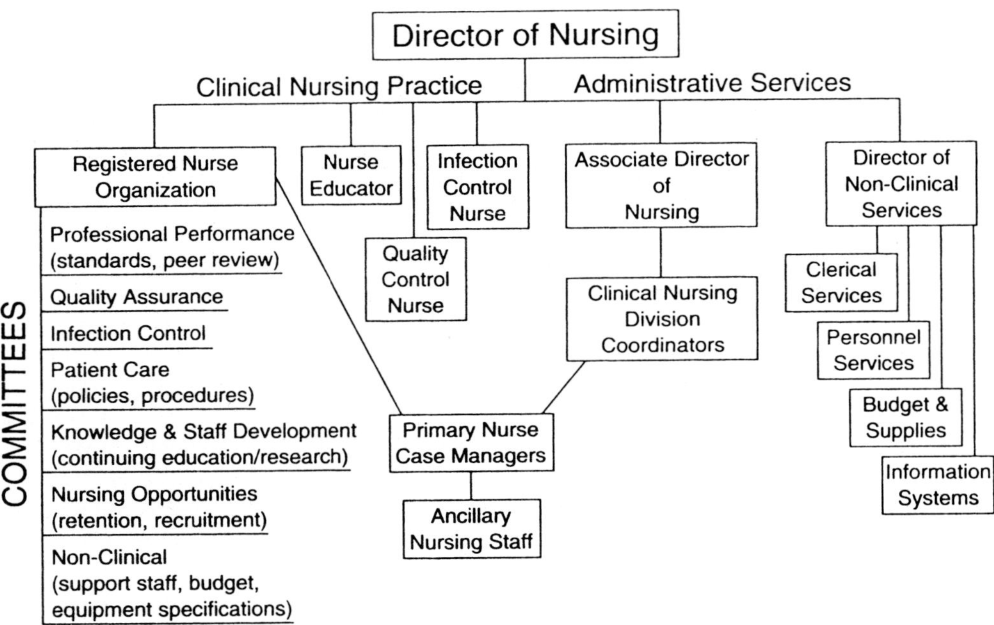

Fig. 52-2. Iowa Veterans Home department of nursing. (From Maas, M.L. [1989]. Professional practice for the extended care environment: learning from one model and its implication. Journal of Professional Nursing 5(22), 66-76.) © W.B. Saunders Company. Used with permission.

argue its merits. Admittedly, the recent description of change to shared governance as "transformation" may sound a bit like "being born again," connoting a spiritual experience rather than a functional model of social organization that has been derived from sound theory and validated empirically (Porter-O'Grady, 1992).

The claim by some (Schwartz, 1990) that nurses are unwilling to exercise self-discipline and act in the public's interest is unfounded. As a profession, nursing has demonstrated over and over that it is worthy of the public's trust and that it is able to govern its members in accord with that trust (Peplau, 1985). Nurse administrators who observe that staff nurses appear to be unwilling to assume professional authority and accountability are too often noting the behaviors of nurses who have been used and abused to benefit others. These nurses have typically experienced capricious changes, a lack of power and control over a heavy workload, and a lack of socialization in the knowledge and skills needed for organizational and interdisciplinary politics. There is evidence that professional nurses welcome shared governance if it is implemented with their participation, with ample opportunity to gain the needed knowledge and skills for consensus decision making, and with the appropriate organizational structures for professional authority and control of practice in place (Maas, 1989). Further, there is evidence that nursing's knowledge base is sufficient to support control of practice and that nurses participate more actively in the development and dissemination of knowledge in a professional model of practice (Maas, 1989; McDonagh et al., 1989). The recent increased focus on outcomes effectiveness is an opportunity for nursing to demonstrate its accountability for client outcomes. It is unfortunate that structures and processes for the assessment of outcomes effectiveness are often not linked to the structures and processes for professional nurse shared governance.

MOTIVES FOR SHARED GOVERNANCE: IS IT AN OPIATE?

While it is assumed that the motives for implementing all shared governance models are to enhance the delivery of care in hospitals, these motives are mixed with regard to the commitment to enabling the work of the professional nurse. Because shared governance is currently a popular concept among nurses, many hospitals boast shared governance as a desirable feature of their organization with minimal structures of shared governance actually in place. In some cases, the motive seems to be to increase nurses' perceptions of empowerment for practice without actually divesting power from the organization hierarchy to nurses as professionals (Porter-O'Grady, 1991a; 1991b). Clearly, organization and nurse managers have been reluctant to relinquish power and control over decisions that influence nursing and the organization. Recently, because of nurse dissatisfaction with the practice environment, collective bargaining and collective action has become more of a threat to nurse and hospital administrators (Kerfoot, 1992). Thus administrators' decisions to implement shared governance may be based on a selection of the better of two less than desirable choices: shared governance rather than collective bargaining. When collective bargaining or some other collective threat is perceived, wise nurse administrators seek models that integrate the "threat" with structures of shared governance (Crocker et al., 1992).

Too often, nurses have had their hopes raised that they are gaining authority and control over the circumstances of their work and their ability to effect patient care priorities, only to have those hopes dashed by the whims of those who hold the real power in the organization. Implementation of shared governance may simply be a strategy to gain what management wants without actual gains in decision-making authority for nurses. Nurses may not initially recognize that what is portrayed as shared governance does not provide them with authority and control over their practice or enable nursing and the organization to meet the professional mandate and organizational goals as partners. However, they soon recognize their lack of power and become frustrated and disillusioned. This is when nurses are apt to leave employment or withdraw to the safety of the traditional hierarchy, where they seek minimal accountability and investment of time, energy, and risk in their jobs. These circumstances underscore the importance of what shared governance entails in terms of nurses' authority and accountability for decision making as well as how shared governance is best implemented in organizations.

IMPLEMENTATION OF SHARED GOVERNANCE: IS THERE A BEST WAY?

It has been noted that shared governance models are not the same in all settings and that this variation is appropriate because of cultural and system operational differences (Porter-O'Grady, 1987; Wilson, 1989). However, there is debate about whether implementation is best orchestrated from the top down or from the bottom up and whether shared governance can be operational as separate unit-based as opposed to department-wide models. Certainly, there is agreement that the nursing and hospital administrations must be supportive of the changes in any case (Jenkins, 1988; Maas, 1989; Porter-O'Grady, 1991a; 1991b). There is less agreement, however, about how to involve the whole staff in the change process and about which is better—unit-by-unit implementation or simultaneous, phased-in implementation of change to shared governance throughout an entire nursing department (Carmanica & Rosenbecker, 1991; Fagan, 1991; Porter-O'Grady, 1991a; Porter-O'Grady, 1991b). Although unique issues must be addressed with each approach, either is appropriate, depending on the situation and assuming that principles of participative change and socialization are not violated.

Leadership from nursing administration and from clinical nurses who have a vision regarding nurse shared governance is essential. These persons must begin to define the objectives and expectations of nurses and create the organizational circumstances whereby all nurses can participate to conceptualize and implement shared governance. Planned change, rather than directed change, is necessary (Hersey & Blanchard, 1986). Paradoxically, bureaucratic methods are used at the outset to reinforce expectations about professional practice, participation, and change. However, participation of all nurses to gain an understanding of shared governance and new organizational goals, develop new meanings about the nurse's role and work, and acquire new skills and behaviors needed to enact shared governance soon shifts the predominant decision-making methods to collaboration, negotiation, and consensus. Whether implementation of shared governance is top down throughout the whole organization or bottom up, unit by unit, nursing administrators and managers become consultants, teachers, coaches, and facilitators.

In either approach, nurses must learn the skills of confrontation, negotiation, collaboration, and consensus decision making (Maas, 1989). They must also understand the requirements of professional practice and what it means to be accountable as a professional (Wilson, 1989). Through consensus decision making combined with the expectation of accountability, nurses must develop shared beliefs and values about standards of practice and the structures and processes that will best ensure their enactment (Maas, 1989). Consensus decision making promotes collegiality and the responsible use of collective action by all nurses, regardless of position.

If the unit-based approach to the implementation of

shared governance is chosen, one advantage is that more nurses involved in the change will likely be committed to it from the outset. Implementation is more focused and involves fewer nurses. Following success on one or more units, other units are apt to become interested, choose to implement shared governance, and profit from the experience of the pioneering units. However, nursing administration and the nurses on the pioneering units will need to be cognizant of the effects of shared governance in one or a few units on the rest of the nursing department and organization. Different patterns and modes of communication and decision making will necessarily exist between the nurses on the units with shared governance and nurses on other units, nurse administrators and managers, persons in other departments, and members of other disciplines. Finally, the scope of shared governance implemented on single units will be constrained at the outset because collective authority and accountability cannot include all nurses in the organization. With unit-based shared governance, the collective, central power and influence of nursing are diluted. Nursing administration will need to retain the prerogative for any decisions that affect the nursing department or organization as a whole until all units implement shared governance and the partnership for decision between all nursing professionals and the organization is defined. For this reason, unit-based implementation may be more appealing to some nurse administrators who wish to dilute the collective power of nurses. Because of the limited scope of unit-based shared governance, progress to a full partnership of shared governance between nursing and the organization may be very slow and may never evolve. Shared governance is not fully implemented until there are structures for all professional nurses to make collective department-wide decisions and negotiate these decisions with administration (Foster, 1992).

With the department-wide approach, the issues focus on how to involve large numbers of nurses in the change process so that they learn the skills of consensus decision making, participate in decision making, develop shared meanings, and actualize the behaviors of professional autonomy and accountability. If shared governance is implemented throughout an entire system, individual nurses should be deprived of the choice not to participate and not to be accountable professionals. This can present difficult problems because nurses will have different amounts of understanding and commitment to professional practice. Nursing administration must expect all nurses, regardless of position, to plan and implement the changes needed for nurses to share governance with the organization. In this regard, nursing administrators must depend on middle- and first-line managers to support the change to shared governance and to alter their roles to become facilitators, teachers, and consultants for each other and for staff nurses. If middle managers are not committed to shared governance and resist the needed changes, many problems will ensue. The effects of shared governance on middle- and first-line managers, as well as on nursing and organization line and staff roles, staff nurse roles and the roles of members of other disciplines must be anticipated with plans carefully made to prepare position occupants for the needed changes and skills (Wilson, 1989).

ROLE AND SYSTEM EFFECTS OF SHARED GOVERNANCE

Little empirical data have been reported about the effects of shared governance models on the roles of staff nurses, managers, and administrators, or on the structures and processes of organizational systems (Wilson, 1989). Discussions focus on the effects of shared governance on the role of the nurse manager and on the authority and accountability of the staff nurse (Ludemann & Brown, 1989; Maas & Jacox, 1977; Porter-O'Grady, 1991a; 1991b).

There is agreement that management styles must change along with organizational structures to enable professional nurse shared governance (Maas & Jacox, 1977; Porter-O'Grady, 1991a; 1991b). As stated earlier, the role of management becomes one of consulting, teaching, collaborating, and creating an environment with the structure and resources needed for the practice of nursing and shared decision making between nurses and the organization (Stickler, 1992). This new role is foreign to many managers. Although managers will retain responsibility for specified functions, they will share accountability with all nurses and act in accord with the consensus among nurses about goals and priorities. Because rules about sharing decisions between management and professional nurses are ambiguous, managers experience stress and anxiety especially in the early stages of implementing shared governance (Wilson, 1989). Managers also experience role stress because of the added time and costs required to enable consensus decision making among nurses (Jenkins, 1988). If not supported by organization and nursing administration, middle- and first-line managers—even though they are committed to shared governance—may not choose to expend the effort or take the risks needed to enable nurses to develop the needed consensus. Nurses need to be able to meet together for consensus decision making, and it is managers who must facilitate their doing so. Administrators who are serious about implementing shared governance will prepare managers for the new role and support them throughout the lengthy change process, and they will also relinquish control of the decisions for which professional nurses are accountable.

For staff nurses, the critical role changes with shared governance are increased accountability and risk. Problems can no longer be blamed on others because all nurses share decisions and accountability for their outcomes. As noted earlier, new understandings and skills are needed. Perhaps most stressful to nurses is the accountability for knowledge to support the decision making authority of professionals. However, role conflict and ambiguity are also stressors. An important example of role conflict with management is when resources are not considered appropriate for quality care (Porter-O'Grady, 1991a; 1991b). Rather than being avoided or ignored as sources of dissatisfaction, shared governance provides the structures and processes for conflict resolution and role clarification through confrontation, negotiation, and consensus decision making.

Staff nurses should be salaried rather than paid an hourly wage, with salaries commensurate with the added accountability and investment required of a participant in shared governance (Johnson, 1987). Further, salaried staff nurses should have more flexible hours and greater control over their time, with accountability shared among nurses for patient care coverage. Staff nurses often fear being salaried because they believe administration may take advantage of them and make inordinate demands on their time. Likewise, administrators often resist paying staff nurses set salaries because they fear they will lose control and will not be able to hold nurses accountable for an equitable exchange of investment and productivity for salary. Shared governance, with staff nurses salaried, provides the means for the most benefits to accrue to all parties—nurses, the organization, and patients—if nurses are also afforded the rights and privileges ordinarily enjoyed by salaried professionals and are held accountable for cost-effective practice.

CONCLUSION

Because almost all practicing nurses are employed, nurse shared governance in employing organizations is imperative if the profession is to fulfill its social contract (ANA, 1980). Implementation of shared governance models that enable professional nursing practice is jeopardized, however, when there is lack of clarity about what shared governance is and when shared governance is confused with other organizational innovations that are similar but not exactly the same. Likewise, it is important that the motives of those who implement nurse shared governance be consistent with the commitment to professional nursing authority and control over nursing practice so that the profession can meet its commitments to clients in all practice settings. As Hess (1995) notes, nurses and administrators need to agree on the meaning of shared governance and resolve their different views as to what aspects of authority and accountability are most important for nurses. Shared governance requires that nurses are accountable to define and control nursing practice. Nurses must also be accountable to understand what shared governance is, expect that the necessary structures and processes are present if implementation of shared governance is claimed, be discerning about the motives for implementation, and take the risks and develop the knowledge to support the privilege of professional practice. If the aim of all nurses in an organization is to implement structures that enable the profession to define and control practice, the approach to unit-based versus department-wide implementation does not matter as long as mechanisms for collective nursing authority and accountability are developed for the nursing department as a whole. Nurses committed to professional nursing practice will also be committed to the role adaptations and corresponding stresses that accompany implementation of shared governance, recognizing the benefits of supportive collegial relationships and consensus decision making among nurses in all roles.

Finally, nurses must also be accountable for demonstrating the benefits of shared governance to patients, other nurses, and the employing organizations. There is some research linking shared governance to improved job satisfaction and social integration of nurses (Hinshaw, Smeltzer, & Atwood, 1987; Maas & Jacox, 1977; McCloskey, 1990), improved patient outcomes (Maas, 1989; Maas & Jacox, 1977), and decreased cost to the organization (Jenkins, 1988). In a search of dissertation abstracts, 43 dissertations or theses were completed on the subject from 1993 through September 1995. Although this indicates increased efforts to study shared governance, more systematic evaluation of shared governance and publication of the results are needed. As with all organizational innovations, strategies and tools must be developed so that nurse administrators and clinicians can conveniently initiate the collection of data to systematically evaluate the outcomes of shared governance (McCloskey et al., 1994). Foremost among the needed strategies is a standardized definition of the operations that must be observed for nurse shared governance to be implemented (Hess,

1995). Accountability for systematic evaluation of shared governance, as well as other innovations, would prevent the adoption of every "new idea" presented as a panacea for nursing and provide the data to refine the innovations and their implementation.

REFERENCES

American Nurses Association. (1980). *Nursing: A social policy statement.* Kansas City, MO: Author.

American Nurses Association. (1992). Standards of nursing practice. Code for nurses with interpretive statement. The nursing shortage in the 1990's: Realities and remedies. In *Best sellers.* Kansas City, MO: American Nurses Publishing.

Carmanica, L., & Rosenbecker, S. (1991). A pilot unit approach to shared governance. *Nursing Management, 22*(1), 46-48.

Crocker, D.G., Kirkpatrick, R.M., & Lentenbrink, L. (1992). Shared governance and collective bargaining: Integration, not confrontation. In T. Porter-O'Porter (Ed.), *Implementing shared governance: Creating a professional organization.* St. Louis: Mosby.

Evan, K., Aubry, K., Hawkins, M., Curley, T.A., & Porter O'Grady, T. (1995). Whole systems shared governance: A model for the integrated health system. *Journal of Nursing Administration, 25*(5), 18-27.

Fagan, M.J. (1991). Can unit-based shared governance thrive on its own? *Nursing Management, 22*(7), 104L-104P.

Foster, B.E. (1992). Models of shared governance: Design and implementation. In T. Porter-O'Grady (Ed.), *Implementing shared governance: Creating a professional organization.* St. Louis: Mosby.

Hersey, P., & Blanchard, K. (1986). *Management of organizational behavior: Utilizing human resources.* Englewood Cliffs, N.J.: Prentice-Hall.

Hess, R.G. (1995). Shared governance: Nursing's 20th-century Tower of Babel. *Journal of Nursing Administration, 25*(5), 14-17.

Hinshaw, A.S., Smeltzer, C.H., & Atwood, J. (1987). Innovative retention strategies for nursing staff. *Journal of Nursing Administration, 17*(6), 8-16.

Horvath, K.J. (1990). Professional nursing practice model. In G.G. Mayer, M.J. Madden, & E. Lawrenz (Eds.), *Patient care delivery models.* Rockville, MD: Aspen.

Jacoby, J., & Terpste, M. (1990). Collaborative governance: Model for professional autonomy. *Nursing Management, 21*(2), 42-44.

Jenkins, J.E. (1988). A nursing governance and practice model: What are the costs? *Nursing Economic$, 6*(6), 302-311.

Jenkins, J.E. (1991). Professional governance: The missing link. *Nursing Management, 22*(8), 26-30.

Johnson, L.M. (1987). Self-governance: Treatment for an unhealthy nursing culture. *Health Progress, 5,* 41-43.

Kerfoot, K. (1992, March). *Unit-based shared governance: The federation model.* Paper presented at Shared governance: Sailing towards success, San Diego, CA.

Lawrenz, E., & Mayer, G.G. (1990). In G.G. Mayer, M.J. Madden, & E. Lawrenz (Eds.), *Patient care delivery models.* Rockville, MD: Aspen.

Ludemann, R.S., & Brown, C. (1989). Staff perceptions of shared governance. *Nursing Administration Quarterly, 13*(4), 49-56.

Maas, M. (1989). Professional practice for the extended care environment: Learning from one model and its implementation. *Journal of Professional Nursing, 5*(2), 66-76.

Maas, M., & Jacox, A. (1977). *Guidelines for nurse autonomy/patient welfare.* New York: Appleton-Century-Crofts.

Maas, M., Jacox, A., & Specht, J. (1975). Nurse autonomy: Not rhetoric but for real. *American Journal of Nursing, 20,* 2201-2208.

Maas, M.L., & Specht, J.P. (1990). Nursing professionalization and self-governance: A model for long term care. In G.G. Mayer, M.J. Madden, & E. Lawrenz (Eds.), *Patient care delivery models.* Rockville, MD: Aspen.

McCloskey, J.C. (1990). Two requirements for job contentment: Autonomy and social integration. *Image: The Journal of Nursing Scholarship, 22*(3), 140-143.

McCloskey, J., Maas, M., Gardner Huber, D., Kasparek, A., Specht, J., Ramler, C., Watson, C., Blegen, M., Delaney, C., Ellerbe, S., Etscheidt, C., Gongaware, C., Johnson, M., Kelly, K., Mehmert, P., & Clougherty, J. (1994). Nursing management innovations: A need for systematic evaluation. *Nursing Economic$, 12*(1), 35-45.

McDonagh, K.J., Rhodes, B., Sharkey, K., & Goodroe, J.H. (1989). Shared governance at St. Joseph's hospital of Atlanta: A mature professional practice model. *Nursing Administration Quarterly, 13*(4), 17-28.

Minzberg, H. (1979). *The structure of organization.* Englewood Cliffs, NJ: Prentice-Hall.

Peplau, H. (1985, February). Is nursing self-regulatory power being eroded? *American Journal of Nursing, 85*(2), 141-143.

Pinkerton, S.E. (1988). An overview of shared governance. In S.E. Pinkerton & P. Schroeder (Eds.), *Commitment to excellence: Developing a professional nursing staff.* Rockville, MD: Aspen.

Porter O'Grady, T. (1987). Shared governance and new organizational models. *Nursing Economic$, 5*(6), 281-286.

Porter O'Grady, T. (1991a). Shared governance for nursing. Part I: Creating the new organization. *AORN Journal, 53*(2), 694-703.

Porter O'Grady, T. (1991b). Shared governance for nursing. Part II: Putting the organization into action. *AORN Journal, 53*(3), 694-703.

Porter O'Grady, T. (1992). Shared governance: Looking toward the future. In T. Porter-O'Grady (Ed.), *Implementing shared governance: Creating a professional organization.* St. Louis: Mosby.

Porter O'Grady, T. (1994). Whole systems shared governance: Creating the seamless organization. *Nursing Economic$, 12*(4), 187-195.

Prescott, P.A. (1987). Another round of nurse shortage. *Image: The Journal of Nursing Scholarship, 19*(4), 204-209.

Ramler, C.L. (1995). *Evaluation of the implementation of a professional nurse shared governance model.* Unpublished doctoral dissertation, University of Iowa, College of Nursing, Iowa City.

Rose, M., & DiPasquale, B. (1990). The Johns Hopkins professional practice model. In G.G. Mayer, M.J. Madden, & E. Lawrenz (Eds.), *Patient care delivery models.* Rockville, MD: Aspen.

Schwartz, R.H. (1990). Nurse decision-making influence: A discrepancy between the nursing and hospital literatures. *Journal of Nursing Administration, 20*(6), 35-39.

Specht, J. (1995). *Shared governance: Development and features.* Unpublished doctoral dissertation, University of Iowa, College of Nursing, Iowa City.

Spitzer-Lehmann, R. (1989). Middle management consolidation. *Nursing Management, 20*(4), 59-62.

Stickler, J.F. (1992). A conceptual basis for shared governance. In T. Porter-O'Grady (Ed.), *Implementing shared governance: Creating a professional organization.* St. Louis: Mosby.

Strasen, L. (1989). Redesigning patient care to empower nurses and increase productivity. *Nursing Economic$, 7*(1), 32-35.

Wilson, C.K. (1989). Shared governance: The challenge of change in the early phase of implementation. *Nursing Administration Quarterly, 13*(4), 29-33.

Flex-time and self-scheduling: Transitional leadership tools

KAREN S. WULFF

Nurses today are being challenged not only by the cost-containment environment of health care and the resulting rapid continuous change but also by increased expectations of consumers for involvement in their care and for quality outcomes. Faced with these challenges, nurse leaders need for every staff nurse to be a responsible decision maker. Additionally, staff nurses want to be treated as professionals and to be given a more active role in the decision-making process. Studies have shown that implementation of self-scheduling can result in increased professional accountability by staff nurses (Bischof, 1992; Tully, 1992; Zimmerman, 1995). Self-scheduling represents a complex form of worker participation in decision making. Flex-time requires increased organizational and management flexibility.

BACKGROUND

The profession of nursing is in another major transition. Patient care is being shifted to outpatient and home settings with a need for professional nurses to coordinate their patients' care. Continued advances in technology are in some cases making the transition to outpatient care possible and in other cases demanding increased nursing care and vigilance in monitoring patients' responses to the high-technology drugs and therapies in order to prevent complications. Nurses are needed less often for tasks and more often for their knowledge, critical thinking, and decisions related to high-technology care and to coordinating patient care and enabling that care to be done in alternative settings.

Organizational research by Lawrence and Lorsch (1967) documents that to cope with the uncertainty of an unstable and changing environment, successful organizations need to be both highly differentiated and highly integrated. Rather than rely on managerial hierarchy, organizations must decentralize decision making and use liaison roles to facilitate cross-departmental task forces and teams. With the current uncertainty and rapid changes in the health care environment, nursing leaders need to decentralize decision making and foster staff nurses' involvement in cross-departmental teams. To meet the quality demands of patients and their families, nurses must be empowered to make decisions and coordinate interdisciplinary treatment plans for their patients. Both self-scheduling and flex-time are congruent with staff empowerment and foster both professionalism and mutual respect and trust between staff and managers (Hawkins & Sutton, 1991; Ringl & Dotson, 1989). Additionally, the negotiation skills required of staff nurses to successfully implement self-scheduling can also contribute to their success on interdisciplinary teams.

Charles Handy (1990) describes the current changing environment as being different not only because of the pace of change but also because the change is discontinuous and not part of a pattern. Change no longer is a single event that can be planned for and managed. The current changing environment calls for transitional leaders who coach, facilitate, and empower their staff (Noer 1993). Brookfield (1991) reports that in settings in which democratic participation and worker control are the norm, prime conditions for critical thinking exist. Empowerment will dramatically increase the sense of responsibility and ownership at every level of an organization, especially where services are delivered and customers are served (Block, 1987; Byham, 1989). The transitional leader's primary responsibility is to facilitate meaning and provide overall direction (Noer, 1993) as staff assume increased responsibility for decisions.

Self-scheduling results in the transition of the manager

role from controller to facilitator and increases the professionalism of nursing staff. Follow-up studies have shown that self-scheduling leads to professional growth, enhanced collaboration among staff, and increased participation in decision making (Bischof, 1992; Griesmer, 1993; Hensinger, Harkins, & Bruce, 1993; Tully, 1992). Professional nurses routinely handle life-threatening situations and decisions and are capable of self-scheduling and of assuming more responsibility for operational decisions. Past management approaches dealing with scheduling often left nurses feeling undervalued and mistrustful of management. Both flex-time and self-scheduling can contribute to a participatory environment with increased staff accountability and a sense of empowerment and enhanced mutual respect and trust between staff and management (Hawkins & Sutton, 1991; Ringl & Dotson, 1989; Tully, 1992). Flex-time and self-scheduling can contribute to a professional relationship that helps move the organization from a reactive to a proactive position in health care (McCoy, 1992).

Regarding the staff's desire for a more participatory work environment, Jamieson and O'Mara (1991) describe a workforce that is more diverse in six perspectives: age, gender, culture, education, disabilities and values. They go on to prescribe flexible management to meet the needs of this more diverse workforce. Flexible management requires a shift in focus from the worker being expected to conform to the organization's norms to the employer being expected to make adjustments to meet the individualized needs of a more varied workforce (Geber, 1993). Management practices are based on accepting individual differences, valuing people, and providing choices. Policies are minimal and expectations are focused on outcomes rather than on constraints and rules about how to do things (Jamieson & O'Mara, 1991).

Higher levels of education, along with more leisure time and greater affluence of American workers, have shifted workers' values, priorities, and expectations of work to greater autonomy, respect from superiors, open communication, and opportunities to participate in decision making (Yankelovitch, 1982). Based on Maslow's theory of motivation, the lower needs of food, shelter, and security are met, and workers now desire conditions that provide for increased esteem (recognition from superiors and others they respect) and self-actualization (challenge, learning, and achievement).

During the past decade, three separate national studies have been commissioned to focus on recruitment and retention issues of the nursing profession. As documented in these studies, the values and expectations of nurses for their work were similar to those described for the general workforce. As partial solutions to the issues of recruitment and retention, all three studies recommended that nurses be given more involvement in decision making and be provided a work environment that is conducive to professional growth and autonomy (American Academy of Nursing, 1983; Department of Health and Human Services, 1988; National Commission on Nursing, 1983).

The realization that nurses "love their work, but hate their jobs" (Wyatt Company, 1989) has led health care administrators to adopt more flexible management practices and to restructure to provide nurses more involvement in the organizations in which they work. Flex-time and self-scheduling are two management practices that have been adopted in an attempt to increase the job satisfaction of registered nurses and to reduce nurse turnover. These practices also enhance staff's sense of empowerment and professionalism and increase their participation in decision making. With the increased uncertainty in today's health care environment, flex-time and self-scheduling can be used by nurse leaders to decentralize decision making and to prepare nurses to be more effective on interdisciplinary teams.

FLEX-TIME

Flex-time is a system of scheduling work that allows each employee to select a starting and quitting time that best meets his or her personal needs and preference while still meeting work responsibilities. In some work situations, employees may have the discretion to report to work at varying times each day within some established parameters. This generally is only possible within management and leadership roles or in instances in which the work done by the individual is independent and does not interface directly with other work. Work that requires continuous coverage, is interdependent to work performed by other employees, or interfaces with other work within or outside the company generally requires a predictable schedule and is incongruent with daily employee discretion regarding work hours.

While nurses in administrative, management, consultation, academic, and research roles have some discretion in selecting daily work hours, most staff nurses—because of the nature of their work, which requires continuous coverage—do not have this discretion. Staff nurses work either as members of a group practice in a hospital setting, where continuous nursing coverage is required, or within an outpatient setting, where nursing care is administered by appointment. Because of the continuous coverage required within staff nursing, flex-time is accomplished by providing variable prescheduled shift start times, shift lengths, and percentages of work.

Because of the numbers of patients requiring care and the fact that patients' care requirements are not evenly spread over the hours in a shift or a day, the number of nurses needed differs from time to time. This provides an opportunity for both the organization and individual nurses to implement and benefit from variable prescheduled start times and shift lengths. Nurses in many hospital settings can now find work schedules that vary from the traditional shift start times of 7:00 a.m., 3:00 p.m., and 11:00 p.m. Variations from the traditional shifts may be start times of 1:00 a.m., 3:00 a.m., 5:00 a.m., 6:00 a.m., 9:00 a.m., 11:00 a.m., 1:00 p.m., 5:00 p.m., 7:00 p.m., 9:00 p.m., 10:00 p.m., and 12:00 a.m. These variable start times are usually associated with either shorter or longer shift lengths than the traditional 8 hours. Some nursing units offer shorter 4-, 5-, or 6-hour shifts to meet peaks in workload that occur in the middle of the traditional shifts or to match the gap between two 10-hour shifts that other nurses on the unit are working. These shorter shifts with variable start times allow nurses to match their work schedules with their children's school schedules, with their spouse's availability for care of children or other family members, or with other social, job, or school commitments.

Many nursing units are offering longer work shifts to accommodate nurses' desires to consolidate their work time into fewer days and to provide longer stretches away from work while maintaining full-time work status. These longer shifts include 9-, 10-, and 12-hour shifts, a mix of 12- and 8-hour shifts, or 16-hour shifts. The 9- and 10-hour shifts usually start an hour or two before the traditional shifts or extend an hour or two beyond them. Sixteen-hour shifts are usually just two consecutive traditional shifts. Although 12-hour shifts could start at any time of the day, provided the nurses were paired and assumed each other's patient care assignments, they are usually restricted to just a few start times within any unit to minimize confusion and disruption of the unit group process. Extensive use of 12-hour shifts is most easily done in critical care settings, where the number of nurses required for patient care remains about the same during the 24-hour period. At times when this is not the case, the number of 12-hour shifts that can be accommodated is usually restricted by the number of staff required to cover the evening and night shifts. Popular start times for 12-hour shifts include 7:00 a.m. and 7:00 p.m., 9:00 a.m. and 9:00 p.m., 11:00 a.m. and 11:00 p.m., and 1:00 a.m. and 1:00 p.m. The two shifts must be equally attractive and tolerable for staff in order for the combination to work.

Factors contributing to the use of variable percentages of work or job sharing among nurses include the continuous coverage required by staff nurses to meet patient care needs, the repeated shortage of nurses, and the predominance of women in nursing. Without the flexibility of working part time, the lifestyle demands of managing a household, raising children, or attending graduate school would force many nurses to quit work. Given the ongoing demand for and the short supply of nurses, organizations adapted to these lifestyle needs by offering nurses part-time work, job sharing opportunities, and flexible schedules. This benefit lessens the impact of the nursing shortage for organizations, retains nurses in the profession, and offers nurses options to increase and decrease the amount that they work at different times in their careers as their lifestyles demand change.

Benefits

Flex-time in the forms of variable prescheduled shift start times, shift lengths, and percentages of work required offer benefits to both the organization and individual nurses. For the organization, being able both to increase the number of nurses at peak workload times and to decrease the number at low workload times results in more efficient and cost-effective patient care. For example, with some predictability of when a surgical patient will be admitted postoperatively to the unit, surgical units can schedule nurses to begin their shifts at those peak times rather than increasing staff for the whole shift in anticipation of the surgical patient admissions.

Flex-time has been shown to increase productivity and job satisfaction and to improve employee morale and motivation (Christensen, 1990; Sullivan, 1994-95). Flex-time is most successful when implemented in a culture that fosters independence and self-motivation, which in turn contributes to increased nurse satisfaction and retention and enhanced professionalism. Increased nurse satisfaction and retention help organizations meet the increased demands for nurses in the face of repeated nursing shortages. Moreover, decreased turnover resulting from flex-time reduces orientation costs and contributes to more cost-effective patient care.

For nurses, prescheduled variable shift start times, variable shift lengths, and the ability to share jobs or work part time offer more choices for balancing work responsibilities and personal lifestyle priorities. For example, the ability to work part-time while children are young, to match children's school hours, or to work evening or night shift or only weekends so spouses are available to relieve them of child or elder care are all advantages of the flex-time variations offered in nursing. Flex-time contributes positively to nurses' perceptions of increased control, increased involvement in decision making, and an enhanced feeling of being valued as an individual. Negativism and burnout are less likely to result with flex-time benefits because of a decreased sense of being trapped without choices for balancing lifestyle.

When attempting to recruit individuals into the profession, nurses have not marketed flex-time options effectively as one of the unique, positive features of nursing. Given the priorities of the workforce for balancing work and lifestyle, these abilities to work variable schedules to match changes in lifestyle needs throughout a career should be publicized.

Difficulties

Flex-time can also present difficulties for both individual nurses and for the organization. Because successful implementation requires a balance between meeting nursing care needs of patients as well as nurses' work scheduling preferences, not all nurses will always be able to work the flex-time option they desire. Thus, it is important that nurses agree with the expectations for required coverage to meet patient care needs and that they feel scheduling decisions are made fairly. Ease of transfer to other nursing units within the organization where the preferred scheduling options are available also should be facilitated.

Introducing a new role for involvement in work unit decisions and for negotiation of scheduling options with peers will result in staff difficulties unless needed education and skill development are provided. Any change in scheduling patterns can initially be disruptive and require time for staff adjustment. Thus flexible schedules should be initiated as a trial for both the unit and the individual.

Without careful planning and evaluation, flex-time schedules can result in disruptions to the unit routines and nursing practice as well as decreased continuity of care for patients. The number of different shifts tried on a single unit should be limited initially to determine the effects on nursing unit routines and to make appropriate adjustments to prevent any negative impacts on nursing practice, patient care, and individual staff. Patient assignments, communications between nursing staff, and physician rounds are examples of unit routines that might need adjustments with flex-time schedules. For example, if primary nursing was accomplished by the full-time staff because of its frequency of being at work when 12-hour shifts are initiated, adjustments may be needed to ensure nurse accountability for coordination and continuity of patient care and for patient outcomes via multiple nurses rather than a consistent nurse.

One of the consequences of job sharing and increased use of part-time staff is a net increase in the number of staff members a manager supervises. This may necessitate an adjustment in management communication methods. It also increases the numbers of staff requiring feedback, orientation and education, and performance evaluations. Depending on organizational benefits policies, the increased number of staff may result in increased benefits being paid. Hopefully, these increased benefit costs are offset by the decreased orientation expenses of reduced turnover and the increased productivity gains associated with flex-time. Follow-up studies have reported that successful implementation requires a change in attitude and management methods (Christensen, 1990; Mullins, 1994).

SELF-SCHEDULING

Self-scheduling is the process by which nurses and other staff on a nursing unit collectively decide and implement the monthly work schedule (Ringl & Dotson, 1989). Self-scheduling requires staff involvement to develop rules and guidelines for staffing and scheduling that seem fair and equitable to each staff member. Staff also set parameters for minimum numbers and mix of staff required to deliver care to the average number and acuity of patients on each shift for each day of the week. These parameters must also meet budget requirements. The guidelines include procedures for scheduling, requirements for weekend and shift rotations, and rules for handling requests, vacations, and holidays. They also may define consequences for staff members who do not follow the guidelines set for self-scheduling.

Successful implementation of self-scheduling requires staff commitment to the concept and participation in its development on the individual nursing unit. Adequate time must be allowed initially for staff to learn needed concepts about scheduling, to increase interpersonal and negotiation skills, and to participate adequately in every aspect of self-scheduling. The actual scheduling process usually involves staff initially sharing their ideal schedules and then making changes and negotiating with each other until a schedule is produced that optimizes staff desires while still meeting the staffing parameters required by patient care (Griesmer, 1993; Ringl & Dotson, 1989). Evaluation of the success of this process is based on each staff member feeling that the scheduling process and outcome were fair and that the patient care staffing needs are met.

Self-scheduling represents a complex form of nurse involvement in unit-level decision making. The goals for self-scheduling include increased nurse recognition, increased perceived autonomy and involvement in decision making, and an increased sense of control over the work environment by nurses. As with flex-time, self-scheduling is a management practice aimed at increasing nurse satisfaction, improving recruitment into the profession, and decreasing nurse turnover. Self-scheduling can also contribute to increased professionalism and staff involvement in decision making.

Benefits

Self-scheduling offers benefits to both individual nurses and the organizations for which they work. Several follow-up studies of the effects of self-scheduling report a positive impact on recruitment and retention of nurses, increased awareness of nursing staff for the unit's needs for nursing care, a new team spirit among staff, and a more cooperative attitude between staff nurses and nursing administration (Hausfield et al., 1994; Hawkins & Sutton, 1991; Hensinger et al., 1993).

Self-scheduling offers the staff nurse increased individualization and creativity in scheduling, an increased sense of control and involvement in unit decisions, and an overall sense of increased autonomy. The individual nurse also benefits from the required change in style of the unit manager because of the self-scheduling process from a negative controlling style of supervisor to a facilitating style of coach. This style change promotes a professional, participatory environment of mutual respect.

The organization benefits from increased nurse satisfaction and retention as a result of the self-scheduling process. Another benefit is increased staff awareness of the difficulties of balancing individual staff scheduling desires with the nursing care requirements of patients. This increased awareness results in increased nurse acceptance of accountability for not only meeting the scheduling needs required for patient care but also for other professional contributions toward the success of the nursing unit and the specialty patient program. Self-scheduling refocuses the nurse manager from schedule development to individualized mentoring of staff toward increased professionalism and accountability.

Difficulties

Self-scheduling is not an easy concept to implement. Success depends on the nurse manager's strong support, patience, and perseverance with implementation. Success also requires staff acceptance of the concept and participation in every aspect of the change to self-scheduling. As stated earlier, adequate time must be allowed for discussion and negotiation at every stage of the process to facilitate staff taking ownership for the schedule. Management must be flexible and allow staff to learn and to be creative with the schedule. The time spent initially in getting ready to implement self-scheduling will be saved later with a smoother implementation.

Self-scheduling is easier to implement with a stable staff in whom team efforts, trust, and participation are already established norms than with a staff who is experiencing turnover and not yet functioning as a team. Because extensive staff participation, discussion, and negotiation are required to implement self-scheduling successfully, implementation is more easily accomplished with small staffs than with large staffs. If extensive shift rotation is not required for coverage, large staffs might be more successful in implementing self-scheduling among the staff on each shift rather than among the entire staff. Because of the complex communication and interpersonal skills required to implement self-scheduling, this should not be the first participatory concept attempted in any work area. Self-scheduling is more likely to be successful in an already established high-involvement, professional environment in which participatory leadership, open communication, trust, and peer support are norms.

CONCLUSION

Flex-time and self-scheduling are being implemented within organizations employing nurses in response to ongoing recruitment and retention issues that contribute to a nursing shortage. Additionally, with the need to decentralize decision making to meet the demands of an uncertain health care environment and the heightened expectations and involvement of patients, both flex-time and self-scheduling can serve as tools to enhance professionalism and staff participation in decision making. Flex-time and self-scheduling are two management practices that increase nurse involvement in unit-level decisions, promote autonomy, and enhance flexibility and nurse control of the work environment. Implementation of these concepts has proven to increase nurse satisfaction and reduce nurse turnover.

Health care is experiencing a rapid succession of changes spurred by concern for escalating health care costs and compromised health care access. Nurse practice models are changing and patient care is being planned and administered as a continuum of care rather than as a hospital episode. These rapid changes and others yet to be defined will result not only in altered nursing practice models but also in further changes in nurse work patterns and in nurse-employer relationships. The key to effective leadership to meet the future needs of nurses is flexibility. Nurse leaders need to encourage flexible management with a primary focus on the needs of patients and staff nurses and with anticipation of potential ongoing changes in the health care environment.

While flex-time and self-scheduling are congruent with increased nurse involvement in decision making and with an environment conducive to professional practice and autonomy, these are only two management practices. The challenge of nurse leaders is to provide vision and, through flexible management, to provide a culture that promotes positive patient care outcomes and meets the individual needs of professional nurses.

REFERENCES

American Academy of Nursing. (1983). *Magnet hospitals: Attraction and retention of professional nurses* (Report of Task Force on Nursing Practice in Hospitals). Kansas City, MO: American Nurses Association.

Bischof, J. (1992). Self-scheduling in critical care. *Critical Care Nurse, 12*(1), 50-55.

Block, P. (1987). *The empowered manager.* San Francisco: Jossey-Bass.

Brookfield, S.D. (1991). *Developing critical thinkers.* San Francisco: Jossey-Bass.

Byham, W.C. (1989). *Zapp! The lightning of empowerment.* Pittsburgh: Development Dimensions International Press.

Christensen, K. (1990). Here we go into the "high-flex" era. *Across the Board, 27*(7-8), 22-23.

Department of Health and Human Services. (1988). *Secretary's Commission on Nursing: Final report* (Vol. 1). Washington, DC: Author.

Geber, B. (1993). The bendable, flexible, open-minded manager. *Training, 30*(2), 46-53.

Griesmer, H. (1993). Self-scheduling turned us into a winning team. *RN, 56*(12), 21-23.

Handy, C. (1990). *The age of unreason.* Boston: Harvard Business School Press.

Hausfeld, J., Gibbons, K., Holtmeier, A., Knight, M., Schulte, C., Stadtmiller, T., & Yeary, K. (1994). Self-scheduling: Improving care and staff satisfaction. *Nursing Management, 25*(10), 74-80.

Hawkins, T., & Sutton, K. (1991). Self-scheduling in a CVICU. *Nursing Management, 22*(11), 64A–64H.

Hensinger, B., Harkins, D., & Bruce, T. (1993). Self-scheduling: Two success stories. *American Journal of Nursing, 93*(3), 66-74.

Jamieson, D., & O'Mara, J. (1991). *Managing workforce 2000: Gaining the diversity advantage.* San Francisco: Jossey-Bass.

Lawrence, P., & Lorsch, J. (1967). *Organization and environment: Managing differentiation and integration.* Cambridge: Harvard Graduate School of Business, Administrative Division of Research.

McCoy, A.K. (1992). Developing self-scheduling in critical care. *Dimensions of Critical Care Nursing, 11*(3), 152-156.

Mullins, R. (1994). Flex time—and frustrations with it—continue to grow. *Business Journal, 11*(30), 8A.

National Commission on Nursing. (1983). *Summary report and recommendations* (Trust Catalog No. 654200). Chicago: Hospital Research and Education Trust.

Noer, D.M. (1993). *Healing the wounds: Overcoming the trauma of layoffs and revitalizing downsized organizations.* San Francisco: Jossey-Bass.

Ringl, K.K., & Dotson, L. (1989). Self-scheduling for professional nurses. *Nursing Management, 20*(2), 42-44.

Sullivan, S.A. (1994-95). Flexibility as a management tool. *Employment Relations Today, 21*(4), 393-405.

Tully, K.C. (1992). Self-scheduling: A strategy for recruitment and retention. *Focus on Critical Care, 19*(1), 69-73.

Wyatt Company. (1989). *I love my work. I hate my job: The nursing crisis in America. A report.* Atlanta: Wyatt Asset Services.

Yankelovitch, D. (1982). The work ethic is underemployed. *Psychology Today, 16*(5), 5-8.

Zimmermann, P.G. (1995). Self-scheduling in the emergency department. *Journal of Emergency Nursing, 21*(1), 58-61.

International nursing: The role of the International Council of Nurses and the World Health Organization

VIRGINIA M. OHLSON, MARGRETTA MADDEN STYLES

Does nursing have the power to change the health care system? There are two major organizations—one governmental and one nongovernmental—whereby nursing's influence can be mobilized at the international level.

The International Council of Nurses (ICN) and the World Health Organization (WHO) play significant roles in nursing and health care worldwide and promote the global goal of health for all by the year 2000. In view of questions frequently raised by nursing students and practicing nurses, however, it seems that some nurses know relatively little about either of these international organizations. Common remarks include "I would like to attend an ICN Congress. How can I become a member of the ICN?" and "I am interested in working with the WHO some day. How do I apply for membership?"

The inquirer is usually surprised to learn that direct membership in either of these organizations is not open to them as individuals. Members of the ICN are national nurses associations (NNAs); when an individual nurse holds membership in a NNA belonging to the ICN, that individual is qualified to participate in many of its activities and programs. Similarly, members of the WHO are affiliated by country. Although certain WHO activities are at the government level, opportunities exist for individual health professionals to participate in working assignments in various parts of the world and to utilize many of the programs and resources of the organization.

This chapter provides a brief description of the ICN and the WHO and their respective roles in international health and nursing. Selected examples from the current agendas of these organizations are used as case studies of the healthy interaction between the professional and governmental sectors in bringing about needed change. We draw from a wealth of experience in international nursing through the ICN, the WHO, and other agencies.

It is not difficult to discuss the role of ICN in international health from a nursing perspective because the ICN is a federation of NNAs managed and primarily financed by nurses. The WHO, in contrast, includes many health disciplines; nevertheless, nursing has always had an active role in the WHO, and its influence has been felt in numerous ways worldwide.

INTERNATIONAL COUNCIL OF NURSES

The ICN was founded in 1899 (Bridges, 1965) as an independent, nongovernmental federation of NNAs. It is the oldest international professional organization in the health care field and the only body that represents the nursing profession worldwide.

Organizations and administration

The NNAs of 112 countries comprised the 1996 membership of the ICN. In addition, the ICN is in contact with nursing bodies or groups of nurses in many countries that are not as yet in affiliation with the organization. Only one NNA per country can belong to ICN. For example, the American Nurses Association is the sole U.S. member of the ICN. However, as nursing and the conditions under which nurses practice continue to change, consideration was given to possible adjustments in the organizational structure of the ICN that might more appropriately accommodate its growing relationship with other organizations. In 1991 the first international nursing specialty organization qualified as a resource group to the ICN, an official designation recently approved by the organization.

The governing body of the ICN is its Council of National Representatives (CNR), which is composed of two delegates from each of the member associations. Each member association has one vote in the conduct of ICN business, regardless of membership size. The largest NNA currently belonging to the ICN is the Japanese Nursing Association followed by the United Kingdom's Royal College of Nursing and the American Nurses Association.

The CNR meets once every 2 years. In the interim, program decisions are made by an elected board of directors that meets annually or as frequently as necessary. Membership on the board includes a president, three vice presidents, seven area representatives, and four members at large. Area representatives are elected from the seven ICN areas—Africa, Europe, North America, South and Central America, Southeast Asia, the Eastern Mediterranean, and the Western Pacific.

The ICN has only one standing committee, the Professional Services Committee (ICN, 1973), which is a very active group that considers problems and trends in nursing education and practice and makes recommendations to the board for further exploration by the CNR. Ad hoc committees or task forces are appointed as needed to deal with matters pertinent to the concerns of the ICN.

Headquartered in Geneva, Switzerland, the ICN employs an international corps of five nurse consultants and other professional and support staff. Oulton of Canada is the current Executive Director, succeeding Holleran of the United States, who held the post from March 1981 to March 1996.

Purpose and objectives

The purpose of the ICN is the same today as it was when it was founded: "to provide a medium through which the interests, needs, and concerns of member national nurses associations can be addressed to the advantage of the public and nurses" (Bridges, 1965; Quinn, 1981). The ICN's program is based on four objectives (Quinn, 1981):

1. To promote the development of strong nursing associations
2. To assist NNAs in improving the standards of nursing and the competence of nurses
3. To assist NNAs in improving the status of nurses
4. To serve as the authoritative voice for nurses and nursing internationally

Objective one: the national associations. Promotion of the development of strong NNAs is a prime objective of the ICN. All ICN programs and activities are planned by the member associations, their elected representatives (the CNR), and the highly qualified staff at headquarters. Collectively, the member associations and their representatives set goals for nursing education practice and research and authorize the staff to use resources to assist member associations, singly and collectively, in ways that will enhance or strengthen their development.

Staff consultation is provided on request to member associations by telephone, correspondence, or in person, as well as through assistance with the implementation of projects pertinent to ICN goals. Manuals, guidelines, and other resource materials are made available to member associations. All aspects of the ICN's programs and activities are directly or indirectly related to the attainment of the organization's prime objective—the development of strong NNAs.

Objective two: education and practice. Since 1978, a main program emphasis of the ICN has reflected the organization's commitment to primary health care and the global goal of health for all by the year 2000, which was adopted by 134 nations at the WHO/United Nations International Children's Emergency Fund (UNICEF) conference in 1978 at Alma Ata in the then Soviet republic of Kazakstan (WHO, 1978). In collaboration with its member associations, the ICN has endeavored to influence and prepare nurses and nursing services to participate more effectively in a primary health care system. Recognizing that nursing has the potential to influence decision making for health at all levels of government and in the society at large, the ICN committed staff and resources to the sponsoring of numerous workshops in primary health care in all seven ICN regions. Workshops were directed to the NNAs' potential for leadership in their countries, with the purpose of strengthening nursing's role in achieving the goal of health for all. Great emphasis is placed in ICN workshops on the continuing education needs of nurses working in rural primary health care settings. A good example of how nurses can be mobilized to participate in country health programs was the ICN-WHO 2-year project to establish appropriate continuing education for nurses in eight African countries and to increase their involvement in AIDS prevention and care. Following train-the-trainer workshops, NNA representatives trained their colleagues to reach communities and coordinate activities with national action plans and with the WHO's General Program on AIDS.

Throughout its existence, the ICN has maintained an interest in the regulation of nursing education and practice worldwide. High priority has been given to encouraging and assisting NNAs in their efforts to establish and update nursing standards. Periodically, the ICN has conducted studies and seminars related to nursing regulations and standards and has published many reports on these efforts (ICN, 1960; 1969; 1970; 1971; 1975; 1987; Styles, 1986).

In recognition of the need for an official statement of position regarding regulatory mechanisms affecting standards for nursing education and practice, an ICN study was conducted by Styles in 1983 and 1984. Overall findings of the study revealed that the structure of the profession is ill-defined and diverse; educational requirements and legal definitions of nursing are generally inadequate for the complexity and expansion of the nursing role as it is emerging in response to health care needs; and the goals and standards of the profession worldwide are less apparent than they were 50 years ago. Although they may be well crystallized in some countries, the conclusion is inescapable that the welfare of the public, the profession, and the practitioner will be better served if greater relevance, rationality, consistency, and clarity are brought to bear on the regulatory system (Styles, 1986).

In response to these findings, in 1987 the CNR adopted an official statement of position on regulation of nursing, guided by 12 principles of professional regulation and associated policy objectives for nursing (ICN, 1960). An opportunity to test and implement these guidelines has been provided through a series of workshops held in all of the ICN's regions from 1986 to 1992, with funding from a variety of governmental and philanthropic organizations. During this extensive decade-long Regulation for Nursing project, the ICN cultivated an international network of experts in nursing regulation. The valuable lessons and practical aids that came from the experts and participants at the numerous workshops have been clearly outlined in the ICN (1992) publication *Nursing Regulation Guidebook: From Principle to Power,* and are being shared by nurses in both developing and developed nations. As a result of these efforts, nursing laws, regulations, and standards have been enacted or revised in many countries, providing greater uniformity and authority for nursing to reach its potential impact on health care.

The ICN has also been at the forefront in developing ethical standards. Its *Code for Nurses—Ethical Concepts Applied to Nursing* (ICN, 1970), which was adopted in May 1973 and reaffirmed by the CNR in 1989, is used as a worldwide resource and as a model for national codes. The ICN's recently updated guide to ethical decision making—*Ethics in Nursing Practice* by nurse ethicist Fry (1993)—is helping nurses solve the difficult ethical dilemmas in today's complex and changing health care environment.

Objective three: social and economic welfare of nurses. The ICN gives high priority to assisting NNAs in matters relating to the socioeconomic welfare of nurses. Great stress is placed on the importance of providing assistance and resources to those associations that are able to initiate and implement socioeconomic welfare programs in their countries through collective bargaining and other approaches, as appropriate.

The ICN's socioeconomic welfare program has four major objectives: (1) to identify information and data about socioeconomic welfare; (2) to provide information, educational programs, and consultation on socioeconomic welfare to NNAs; (3) to work and communicate with other international organizations with regard to the social and economic welfare of nurses—particularly the International Labor Organization (ILO) and WHO; and (4) to examine and determine how the present socioeconomic situation affects the health services and the lives and working conditions of nurses (ICN, 1987). Pertinent information about socioeconomic welfare is shared with member associations through a regularly published newsletter, the *Socio-Economic News.* Launched in 1988, the ICN's Negotiation in Leadership program has been preparing nurses to respond effectively to the crises in their countries by making them knowledgeable in negotiation, interviewing, recruitment, and retention techniques. To better assist NNAs in their response to planned or ongoing changes in reward strategy, the ICN and the United Kingdom's Royal College of Nursing organized an international workgroup in June 1995 to study the trends in remuneration of nurses and strategies being used by NNAs in addressing this complex issue. The association's dedication to the socioeconomic status of nurses has had a tremendous influence on the improvement of working conditions of nurses worldwide.

Objective four: a unified voice for nursing. The ICN, composed of 112 member associations, has the unique potential, opportunity, and responsibility to serve as the authoritative voice for nursing and nurses internationally. The extent to which it honors and accepts this responsibility has been demonstrated and documented on many occasions and in various ways. Frequently at the WHO's annual Executive Board meeting and World Health Assembly (WHA), which convenes in Geneva, Switzerland. The ICN has presented statements on issues relevant to health care and nursing. Examples include the ICN's statements on infant feeding nursing in primary health care, the role of nursing in the WHO, the state of the health of women in today's world, and the lack of protective equipment in some countries for health workers caring for patients with infectious diseases such as AIDS. Although the ICN is a nursing organization and the WHO is an interdisciplinary health organization, the high degree of camaraderie and collaboration that exists between the two and their nursing staffs has contributed immeasurably to a unified voice for nursing in the international arena.

The ICN has maintained an active publishing program, issuing books, manuals, monographs, reports, and guidelines relative to nursing education, practice, and research. Its official organ is the *International Nursing Review,* a bimonthly journal published in Switzerland. Another publication, *ICN News,* provides up-to-date information on ICN activities, programs, meetings, and members.

The ICN has published (in English, French, and Spanish) numerous statements reflecting the organization's stance on issues related to nursing, health care, and societal matters of concern to the profession. Periodic listings of these position statements in the *International Nursing Review* reflect the ICN's broad range of concerns.

It is important to recognize the extent to which the ICN's staff must interact with other international organizations and agencies—such as WHO, UNICEF, ILO, and other governmental and nongovernmental philanthropic agencies—to achieve these objectives. For example, the ICN assisted the ILO in research on nursing salaries that resulted in two publications: *Nurses' Pay: A Vital Factor in Health Care* (ILO, 1994a) and *The Remuneration of Nursing Personnel, An International Perspective* (ILO, 1994b). The ICN also worked with the International Federation of Red Cross and Red Crescent Societies to create a teaching module on the Geneva Conventions and ethical dilemmas for nurses.

Recognition also should be given to the ICN's work with the International Committee for the Red Cross, the International Commission of Health Professionals for Health and Human Rights, Amnesty International, and other organizations, in efforts to trace nurses who have disappeared or have been imprisoned because of their work.

ICN's strategic plan

As it approaches its 100th anniversary in 1999, the ICN is rethinking its priorities and has mapped out a strategy so that nurses can play an even greater role in health care. The ICN's Strategic Plan 1994-99 has set the framework for initiation of new ICN programs both to address issues crucial to international nursing and to strengthen the capabilities of NNAs. The Strategic Plan emphasizes the need for nurses to respond and adapt to the changing environments worldwide, and comprises two goals: (1) to influence matters of health, social policy, and professional and socioeconomic standards worldwide; and (2) to empower NNAs to act on behalf of nurses, nursing, and the public well-being.

Since 1991, the ICN has been involved actively in developing an International Classification for Nursing Practice, which will make nursing practice more understandable to the lay public, other health professionals, and policy makers; more visible in health care settings and lexicons; and capable of being valued and documented in reimbursement systems. The intent is to describe what nurses do relative to certain human needs to produce certain outcomes and to explain what nurses do in response to particular human situations which enable individuals, families, and communities to achieve and maintain good health.

To keep nurses abreast of new methods, new knowledge, and new needs in health care, the ICN is emphasizing the importance of nursing research. In 1990, the ICN set up a task force on international nursing research to develop strategies to promote and facilitate nursing research and to improve access to relevant education that prepares nurses to conduct research. In 1994, the ICN held an international invitational conference in Japan that focused on strategies for transfer of relevant research findings in HIV/AIDS into nursing practice. In 1996, the theme of International Nurses Day, which is celebrated annually on May 12, was "better health through nursing research." International Nurses Day activities, which take many forms such as health fairs, parades, seminars, and media features, lend themselves to continuing education for nurses while at the same time educating the public about the multiple responsibilities and concerns of nurses. To help nurses plan and carry out activities, the ICN prepares a kit with up-to-date information, planning guidelines, fact sheets, suggestions for activities, and a poster.

A new promising ICN initiative has established the International Council of Nurses Foundation, which aims to raise the necessary funding base for educational programs to prepare nurses to assume new leadership roles. Information and advice for individuals and NNAs interested in assisting with this endeavor are available from ICN headquarters in Geneva, Switzerland.

THE WORLD HEALTH ORGANIZATION

The WHO was established in 1948 as a specialized agency of the United Nations in Geneva, Switzerland, where it is still headquartered. It came into existence as the world was attempting to recover from World War II and as millions were falling victim to poverty and disease.

It was in these troubled times that the constitution of the WHO was formulated. The preamble of that historic document gives evidence of the concern for social justice on which the organization was founded. For almost 50 years the WHO has firmly stood on its commitment to the belief that the enjoyment of the highest attainable standard of health is the fundamental right of every individual without distinction of race, religion, political belief, economic, or social condition.

Organization and administration

The WHO is an intergovernmental agency. In 1948, there were 56 member countries; by 1995, membership had increased to over 180 countries. The highest policy-making body of WHO is the World Health Assembly (WHA), which is responsible for the execution of WHO policies in collaboration with its employed staff, referred to as the WHO secretariat. The highest officer in the WHO is the director general, elected for 5-year terms by the WHA on nomination by the executive board. Currently, this position is held by Nakajima of Japan. Numerous administrative and technical personnel with diversified knowledge and skills are employed at WHO headquarters in Geneva.

The WHO's program is decentralized into six regional offices: the African regional office, located in Brazzaville, Congo; the Pan American Health Organization, which serves as the regional office for the Americas, in Washington, D.C.; the Eastern Mediterranean regional office, in Alexandria, Egypt; the European regional office, in Copenhagen, Denmark; the Southeast Asian regional office, in New Delhi, India; and the Western Pacific regional office, in Manila, Philippines. The WHO's activities are financed by annual mandatory contributions from its member countries and by voluntary contributions from government and private agencies.

Functions of WHO

The WHO constitution specifies 22 functions, summarized as follows:

- Coordinating international health work undertaken by national and international groups, both governmental and voluntary, or by scientific and professional groups
- Assisting governments in strengthening health services through technical assistance, through direct aid as requested, or by providing counseling or personnel support in the development of programs
- Fostering action in specific fields of particular need such as maternal and child health and welfare, mental health, disease eradication, nutrition, and improvement of water supplies
- Developing or promoting international agreements and standards including policies and regulations; standards of teaching and training in health, medical, and related fields; and standardization of the international nomenclature of disease and of diagnostic procedures and standards
- Conducting, encouraging, and supporting studies and research in the field of health, including studies of administration and social techniques for health care (Freeman, 1965; WHO, 1948)

Although the constitution of the WHO was written almost 50 years ago, its 22 statements of function have not changed. However, the programs necessary for their implementation have been modified considerably as a result of its increased understanding of the world's health problems. Similarly, the administrative structure of the WHO and the size and nature of the secretariat have also changed as new policies have been formulated by the WHA and new priorities established.

Health for all by the year 2000

Fulop and Roemer (1982) describe the ways in which the WHO's policies and programs have been influenced over time by the variety of social forces operating within the organization and its member countries. Certainly, the changing nature of WHO membership has influenced program directions. In 1948, 57% of WHO member states were developed countries and 43% were developing countries. By 1978, many new countries had become sovereign states and joined WHO, considerably changing the nature of its membership. Interestingly, it was not until 1977 that growing concern over the health conditions in many countries resulted in establishing the year 2000 as the target date for reaching WHO's long-standing objective of the highest possible level of health for all people (Fulop & Roemer, 1982).

In the following year, an international conference on primary health care was convened by WHO and UNICEF in Alma Ata, bringing together representatives of 134 governments and 67 United Nations' organizations and other specialty agencies and nongovernmental organizations. It was at this conference that the renowned Declaration of Alma Ata was formulated, recognizing primary health care (PHC) as the key to attaining health for all by 2000. The conference declared that the health status of hundreds of millions of people was unacceptable and could only be rectified by a new, equitable approach to health and health care that would close the gap between the world's haves and have-nots. In 1979, the 32nd WHA endorsed the Declaration of Alma Ata (WHO, 1978). In 1981, the WHA established the Global Strategy for Health for All by the year 2000 (WHO, 1981), and countries were encouraged to formulate their own national policies, strategies, and plans of action for attaining this goal. Since that time, the pursuit of health for all and the PHC approach have continued to be a central focus for WHO policies and program strategies. However, it has increasingly been recognized that the social, economic, and political changes throughout the world, as well as the differing priorities of the various countries, have had implications for the attainment of this important goal.

Nursing in WHO

Where does nursing fit into this complex intergovernmental, interdisciplinary health organization? What is nursing's role in the WHO in this decade, and what will it be by the fast-approaching year 2000? Some understanding of the structure of nursing within the WHO may assist in answering these questions.

Structure for nursing in WHO. The highest administrative post for nursing in the headquarters of WHO is the position designated as chief scientist for nursing. Hirschfeld from Israel has held this position since 1989. As the chief administrator for nursing in WHO, the nursing chief reports to the director general through the assistant director general, as do other administrative position chiefs. Simultaneously, the nursing chief also holds a position in the Division of Development of Human Resources for Health and in this role reports to the director of that division as well.

The chief scientist for nursing is the primary voice for nursing in the organization and in this capacity must interpret the potential, contributions, and needs of nursing within an interdisciplinary context. In carrying out the responsibilities of the office, the chief scientist for nursing maintains contact with numerous international agencies and organizations concerned directly or indirectly with nursing as well as with nursing personnel in the six WHO regional offices. The administrator reviews program plans and projects of the regions, provides technical assistance as feasible, and participates in conferences and workshops at the request of the regional offices. Possibly the greatest responsibility of the nursing administrator in this interdisciplinary organization is that of communicating, interpreting, stimulating, and planning nursing's contributions to various WHO programs.

Each WHO regional office has its own nursing and other health-related personnel whose responsibilities and programs of work are designed and implemented within the regional areas. The relationship between the WHO headquarters and the regional offices is advisory rather than administrative, because the WHO operates on a decentralized basis that permits autonomy within broad policy guidelines. As a result, nursing may be organized quite differently in each region. The WHO's primary commitment at all levels is to its member countries and to the strengthening of those countries' institutions. Although problems in nursing in various countries are to some extent quite similar, they differ significantly in degree in various areas of the world. WHO nurses in these regions deal with a wide range of programs and problems related to nursing practice, education, training, organization, administration, and research. Duties have encompassed such activities as the analyses of nursing needs in a country or area, the design of projects to meet a particular need, the recruitment or assistance with recruitment of personnel for various projects of the organization or a member country, and evaluation of project outcomes.

Nature of nursing in WHO. Nursing has had an important role in the WHO since the organization's founding. The nursing programs have been carried out through long- and short-term projects in many parts of the world with goals and objectives that have varied according to place and time; through workshops, conferences, and committees that have enabled the development and dissemination of reports, recommendations, and guidelines; and through a wide variety of administrative functions and activities.

Projects have been developed for implementation at the local, regional, and interregional levels. Although some projects have related specifically to nursing, many have been interdisciplinary. In the early years of the WHO, nurses were involved in projects as members of specialized teams concerned with treatment and control of diseases such as malaria, venereal diseases, and tuberculosis, as well as with maternal and child health programs. In later years, a higher priority was placed also on programs of nursing and midwifery education. Although consideration is still given to such projects, a prime emphasis in recent years has been on projects that are particularly relevant to the achievement of the goal of health for all by the year 2000 through PHC.

The WHO maintains a system of expert panels, representative of the various disciplines, that function as advisory bodies to the organization. The expert panel in nursing includes representatives of various disciplines that function as advisory bodies to the organization. The expert panel in nursing includes representatives of various specialty areas in nursing and of the geographic regions. The panel does not meet as a group, but from time to time representatives from the panel meet to deliberate and make recommendations on a matter of concern to nursing and the WHO. A few examples of their action are reflected in the reports of the expert committees of 1984 and 1994—*The Education and Training of Nurse Teachers and Managers with Special Regard to Primary Health Care* (WHO, 1984), and *Nursing beyond the Year 2000* (WHO, 1994). Each time an expert committee on nursing is convened, a report summarizing its deliberations and recommendations is published and made available to governments, professional organizations, educational institutions, and other interested agencies and individuals.

Throughout the years, a wide variety of guide reports and materials relevant to nursing, education, administration, and research have been prepared and disseminated by WHO headquarters and the regional offices. Numerous statements have been developed and published as summaries and recommendations of conferences or workshops convened to deliberate on specific aspects of nursing. These publications frequently represent the work of an individual or group commissioned by the WHO to conduct a specific study. Many are available through the WHO headquarters and regional offices; and in some of the regional areas, bibliographies of studies are available.

As a discipline within the WHO, nursing supports and affirms the programs of the organization and the attainment of its goals. Health care planning and implementation uses the team approach, and within this context nursing must carve out its directions, its functions, and its role.

WHO collaborating centers for nursing development

For many years, the WHO has designated a number of health professional colleges or departments in universities and other health-related agencies and institutions as WHO collaborating centers. This designation has been given in recognition of the institution's or agency's potential to participate in the furtherance of WHO goals and objectives. The first nursing centers to be so designated were in Europe. Two of these centers were named in 1980: the Collaborating Center for Nursing Research and Education, located at the Danish Institute for Health and Nursing Research in Copenhagen, Denmark, and the Collaborating Center for Nursing associated with Hospices Civils de Leon, in Lyon, France. By 1996, 31 such centers had been designated as WHO nursing centers in various parts of the world, including Africa, Australia, Bahrain, Botswana, Brazil, Canada, Colombia, Denmark, Finland, France, Hungary, Italy, India, Japan, Kazakhstan, Korea, Philippines, Scotland, Solvenia, Thailand, the United Kingdom, and the United States. The eight WHO Collaborating Centers for Nursing Development in the United States are as follows: the College of Nursing of the University of Illinois at Chicago (1986); The School of Nursing of the University of Pennsylvania, Philadelphia (1988); the School of Nursing of the University of Texas Medical Branch, Galveston (1988); the School of Nursing of the University of California at San Francisco (1991); the School of Nursing of George Mason University, Fairfax, Virginia (1991); the Frances Payne Boulton School of Nursing of Case Western Reserve University, Cleveland, Ohio (1993); the School of Nursing of the University of Alabama, at Birmingham (1994); and the School of Nursing of Columbia University, New York City, New York (1996).

In April 1988, the historic first general annual meeting of the Global Network of the WHO Collaborating Centers for Nursing Development was convened in Maribor, Yugoslavia (now Slovenia). Representatives of the designated and potential collaborating centers were in attendance. Subsequent meetings have been held in Copenhagen, Denmark (1989), Galveston, Texas, (1990), Geneva, Switzerland (1991), Fermey Voltaire, France (1992), Botswana, Africa (1994), and Manama, Bahrain. The work of the Network is facilitated by the WHO, although the Network itself is not a component of the WHO. When the Network was first established, the College of Nursing of the University of Illinois at Chicago was voted as the first secretariat of the Network and continued to function in this role until 1994, when, by election, the College of Nursing of Yonsei University in Korea assumed this responsibility. From its inception, the Network has served as a conduit for information sharing and the exchange of materials and expertise between members and their individual centers. Two publications, *Women's Health and Development: A Global Challenge* (Elmurry, Norr, & Parker, 1993) and *Primary Health Care: Nurses Lead the Way: A Global Perspective* (Kim, 1993) describe the work of the individual centers that have been initiated since their designation as a WHO Collaborating Center and their membership in the Global Network. Network members, representing all areas of the world, have set down common goals of high priority and strategic plans of collaborative action toward the accomplishment of these goals. Achievement of these goals will strengthen the capacity of each center, as well as that of the Network, to move forward with the particular primary health care mission for which they were established (Duxbury, 1988).

INTERACTING ICN AND WHO AGENDAS

Throughout their history, the ICN and WHO have pursued mutual goals and engaged in collaborative projects. Only a few contemporary examples, among many, are mentioned here.

In 1985, recognizing that regulatory reform was essential to maximize nursing's role in primary health care, the ICN and WHO undertook parallel and cooperative initiatives in nursing regulations. The ICN commissioned the study outlined previously (Styles, 1986), and the WHO convened an expert group on nursing regulation to which the ICN consultant was appointed. Complementary sets of guidelines ensued. The regional workshops on nursing regulation conducted by the ICN from 1986 to 1992 included teams of representatives from the two sectors—the NNAs and the ministries of health. Only through such cooperation could the profession demonstrate its accountability for standards of nursing practice and could governments evidence their commitment to nursing's contribution toward health for all.

In 1989, the 42nd WHA adopted a very significant resolution on Strengthening Nursing and Midwifery in Support of the Strategy of Health for All (WHO, 1992). The resolution called on the WHO and member nations to engage in strategic planning of their nurse workforce; to develop sound policy, management, and supervision at all levels; and to improve standards of nursing education along the lines of PHC. The resolution further mandated a progress report in 1992. The ICN mobilized its NNAs to bring this resolution to the attention of their governments, to press for action on the specific recommendations, and to pursue every avenue to achieve more representation on the member delegations to the 1992 WHA. Nurses showed up en force in close to 20 delegations at the 45th WHA in 1992 and were very active and effective throughout the discussions. With respect to the report on strengthening nursing, they were successful in getting facts on the table regarding nursing's involvement in health care policy and planning throughout the WHO and its member nations. As a consequence, a Global Advisory Group, reporting to the highest level of the WHO secretariat, was established (WHO, 1992). The Global Advisory Group meets annually to develop mechanisms for assessing national nursing and midwifery service needs; to assist countries in the development of national action plans for nursing and midwifery services including research and resource planning; and to monitor progress on the utilization of nurses and midwives in strengthening the WHO goal for all people. Based on Global Advisory Group reports and findings, the WHO director general was requested to report on progress of the 1992 Resolution WHA45.5 to the WHA in 1996.

In 1993 a WHO Study Group on Nursing Beyond the Year 2000 was convened in Geneva, Switzerland. This Study Group was challenged to provide advice and direction regarding a forward move in meeting the global health care service needs and demands beyond the year 2000—and to provide a clear perspective on the perceived role of nursing and midwifery in the 21st century. The work of this Study Group was closely aligned to the work of the Global Advisory Group (WHO, 1994). Recommendations of the Study Group set down three strategic aims relating to a greater collaboration of health care personnel at all levels; a clearer focus on the health needs of specific countries and their vulnerable population groups; and the reorganization of nursing and midwifery education and practice to meet the challenges of the 22nd century (WHO, 1994). Affara of the ICN staff was a participant in this meeting.

As a follow-up to the WHO Study Group on Nursing Beyond the Year 2000, an Expert Committee on Nursing Practice was convened—also in 1993—to focus on PHC delivered by nurses in countries with different levels of socioeconomic and epidemiological development. The ICN President Styles attended as an observer and participated in the discussions.

At the 1996 WHA in Geneva, the WHO director general reported on the progress of the 1992 resolution (WHA45.5) outlining the continuing problems confronted by nursing and midwifery in the countries of the world, as had been identified by the WHO Global Advising Group (GAG). In reference to the report Styles, who was representing the ICN at this meeting, expressed serious concern about the decreased number of nurse/midwife positions in the WHO which had dropped from 46 posts in 1991 to 28 in 1996. The WHA formulated a continuing resolution on Strengthening Nursing and Midwifery (WHA49.1) urging the member states of WHO: to regularly involve nurses and midwives in health care reform and national policy development; to increase fellowship opportunities for nurses and midwives in nursing and health-related fields; and to support nursing/midwifery educational programs and practice in PHC. Included in the resolution was a request to the WHO director general: to provide for the continued work of the GAG; to support the education of nurses and midwives in research methodology to enable them to participate more effectively in health research programs; to keep the Health Assembly advised about the progress of this resolution and to report on it at the 54th WHA in 2001.

SUMMARY

This chapter has described the role of the ICN and WHO in relation to nursing internationally. Much more could be said of the many ways in which the nurse leaders of these two organizations have worked in collaboration with one another and with other international organizations, with diverse groups and individuals through their office headquarters in Geneva, and with the many regions and countries of the world. Nurses in the ICN and WHO are few in number, yet their accomplishments on behalf of nurses, nursing, and the health care of all people have been far-reaching and impressive.

Does nursing have the power to change the health care system and bring the world closer to the goal of health care for all? Certainly the WHO and ICN have influenced directions and patterns for nursing and health care delivery all over the world. *Nursing has led the way!* However, the eternal question is still before us: Can health for all ever become a reality in today's world? The year 2000 is not far away. After 2000 what will our nursing agenda be—globally, in our own countries, and in our workplaces?

REFERENCES

Bridges, D. (1965). *A history of the International Council of Nurses, 1899-1964.* Philadelphia: Lippincott.

Duxbury, M. (1988). *The Global Network of World Health Organization Collaboring Centers for Nursing Development.* Unpublished manuscript.

Elmurry, B.J., Norr, K.F., & Parker, R.S. (1993). *Women's health and development: A global challenge.* Boston: Jones and Bartlett.

Freeman, R. (1965). *Nursing in the World Health Organization.* Geneva: World Health Organization.

Fry, S. (1993). *Ethics in nursing practice.* Geneva: International Council of Nurses.

Fulop, T., & Roemer, M. (1982). *International development of health manpower policy.* Geneva: World Health Organization.

International Council of Nurses. (1960). *Nursing legislation report on survey of nursing legislation.* London: Author.

International Council of Nurses. (1969). *Principles of legislation for nursing education and practice: A guide to assist national nursing associations.* New York: S. Karger.

International Council of Nurses. (1970). Code for nurses: Ethical concepts applied to nursing. Geneva: Author.

International Council of Nurses. (1970, 1971). *Report on an international seminar on nursing legislation, Warsaw.* Geneva: Author.

International Council of Nurses. (1973). *Report of the Professional Services Committee.* Geneva: Author.

International Council of Nurses. (1975). ICN adopts definition of nursing. *International Nursing Review, 22*(6), 184.

International Council of Nurses. (1975). *Nursing legislation in Latin America the last half of the 20th century.* Geneva: Author.

International Council of Nurses. (1987). *Report of the Social Economic Welfare Committee, Council of Nurse Representatives.* Geneva: Author.

International Council of Nurses. (1987). Nursing's priorities set at New Zealand. *International Nursing Review, 34*(6), 276.

International Council of Nurses. (1992). *Nursing regulation guidebook: From principle to power.* Geneva: Author.

International Labor Organization. (1994a). *Nurses pay: A vital factor in health care.* Geneva: Author.

International Labor Organization. (1994b). *The remuneration of nursing personnel: An international perspective.* Geneva: Author.

Kim, M.J. (1993). *Primary health care: Nurses lead the way: A global perspective.* Washington, DC: American College of Nursing.

Quinn, S. (1981). *What about me? Caring for the carers.* Geneva: International Council of Nurses.

Styles, M. (1986). *Report on the regulation of nursing: A report on the present, a position for the future.* Geneva: International Council of Nurses.

World Health Organization. (1948). *Constitution of the World Health Organization.* Geneva: Author.

World Health Organization. (1978). *Alma Ata, 1978: Primary health care.* Geneva: Author.

World Health Organization. (1981). *Global strategies for health for all by year 2000.* Geneva: Author.

World Health Organization. (1984). *Education and training of teachers and managers with special regard to primary health care.* Technical report #708. Geneva: Author.

World Health Organization. (1992). *Strengthening nursing and midwifery in support of strategies for health for all.* Geneva: Author.

World Health Organization. (1994). *Nursing beyond the year 2000: Report of a WHO Study Group.* Technical Report #842. Geneva: Author.

Section Seven

HEALTH CARE SYSTEMS

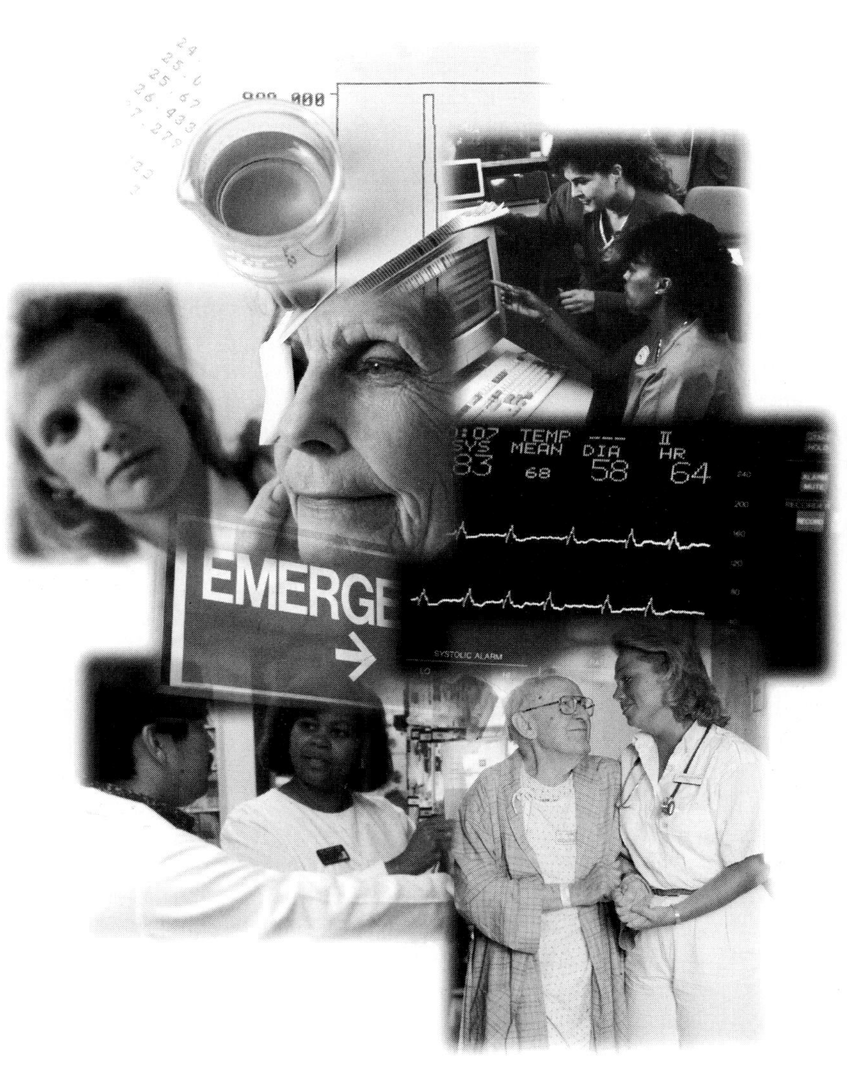

System reform—opportunity or threat?

JOANNE COMI McCLOSKEY, HELEN KENNEDY GRACE

The health care systems of the United States and many other countries are undergoing rapid change. Cost containment efforts and the move toward managed care have raised questions about everything from the setting where care is delivered to the provider of care to the payer and even to the status of the patient. The evolving situation is creating a good deal of disturbing turmoil. Jobs are being threatened and the security of the past is gone. During times of great change, however, there is also opportunity as people look for new solutions. What will nursing's attitude and behavior be during these next years of system change?

In the debate chapter for this section Grace clearly outlines the old medical care system from which we are slowly moving away and the new comprehensive community-based health care system into which we are evolving. She demonstrates the wisdom of this evolution by presenting the arguments for both systems. She first gives the reasons for keeping our current medical care system of illness treatment, then outlines the reasons for refocusing toward health promotion and disease prevention. Arguments for keeping what we have include the following: (1) we know how to treat illness and we do it well; (2) the education of our practitioners requires the challenges of complex medical problems; (3) our hospitals are designed efficiently to use the expertise of highly trained professionals; (4) the economic welfare of communities rests on the viability of hospitals; and (5) there are few proven alternatives. Arguments for refocusing our efforts toward health promotion and disease prevention include the following: (1) more than half of all diseases are a product of unhealthy lifestyles; (2) educating the young will result in healthier adults; (3) community-based monitoring programs can detect problems at an early stage when intervention is most likely to have an effect; and (4) the closing of some hospitals and the change in financing of health care would save money. Grace discusses the need for a more integrated health care system whereby there is less fragmentation of services. She finishes her chapter with an example of three communities in Michigan that are beginning the process of restructuring their health care systems. The importance of educating communities about health care is central to the revisioning of new systems and the identification of barriers that constrain them. Grace believes that "quality affordable health care for all is an attainable goal" if community members are brought into partnerships with providers. This is a hard-hitting and interesting chapter that is a must-read for everyone.

The first three viewpoint chapters in the section describe approaches to a comprehensive health care system. Lawrence describes the beginning efforts of one Michigan community to develop health status through citizen participation. (This is one of the communities that Grace includes in her example.) A 48-member advisory committee representing consumers, providers, and payers oversees a larger grassroots effort to determine the health needs of the community. Problems in the existing delivery system were identified as uneven access to services, fragmentation of care, rising costs, inadequate performance measurement, and inadequate primary and preventive care. A profile of the health status of the citizens of the community has helped to identify community health needs. Lawrence describes the difficulties as well as the benefits of this grassroots effort. She also includes some aspects of her own decision-making process as she moved from a career in hospital nursing to a commitment to community-based care. Lawrence believes that all nurses must take a community development approach in order for health care to work.

Next, Walker describes how a comprehensive health care system is being built through the development of coalitions. Walker states that the development of coalitions, alliances, mergers, and partnerships is a global phenomenon that is occurring in response to cost containment and a need to be more competitive. Various groups are trying to "shape the structures" for managed care through the development of coalitions. Because no one structure has yet emerged as dominant, Walker believes that this is an opportunity for nurses to become active players in shaping the managed care organizational structures of the future. This chapter serves as a crash course on organizational structures and coalition building. Walker gives several examples of newly formed health care coalitions, including the community nursing center in the School of Nursing at the University of Rochester, which joined with Strong Memorial Hospital and established coalition relationships with several other local groups to provide school-based care for adolescents in the state under a grant by the New York State Department of Health. An important point made by Walker is that partners in coalitions share risk. Managed care coalitions offer opportunities for providers who can blend business knowledge with clinical practice. New roles, according to Walker, include disease specialist, case manager, nurse informaticist, and outcomes manager. Walker challenges nurses to seize the opportunity created by this time of great change. She says that the prerequisites to our doing this are to "stretch beyond our clinical focus" to acquire more business knowledge and skills and to embrace the financial side of health care.

A comprehensive statewide health care system is described next by Capuzzi, who begins her chapter with an overview of the major types of health care reform being proposed by various states. These include multiple cost-containment strategies, insurance and financing reform, and changes in service delivery. Advantages and disadvantages to states initiating reform are listed. This information sets the stage for a review of state reform in Oregon, which enacted the Oregon Health Plan in 1989. Capuzzi reviews the additional legislation in the ensuing years and the revisions to the initial plan. Oregon is a "laboratory to test the process of ranking health services." According to Capuzzi, the experiment is continuing with "seeming success," but health care reform in Oregon has had some setbacks. She reviews the setbacks and then discusses both the positive and negative impacts on nurses. As health care reform efforts gear up in other states, nurses will want to pay close attention to the case study of Oregon. Capuzzi urges nurses to become involved in state reform efforts to ensure control of their practice and good outcomes for consumers.

The next chapter by Salmon makes the case that all nurses must take more responsibility for shaping the political forces that direct health care in the United States. Salmon wants her chapter to challenge each reader to examine his or her own participation in health policymaking. It does. She begins by describing how the current health care system is a product of politics. The movement to a health care system that is market-driven makes the politics less clear but perhaps more important. New questions related to quality and control of health care and roles and licensure of health professionals are emerging. While nursing has achieved a good deal of political sophistication in the past decade, Salmon says this is not enough. She calls for nursing to expand beyond our own boundaries and to make alliances with physicians and organized medicine and with consumers and communities. "The alliance of organized nursing with organized consumer groups is the political equivalent to the individual nurse serving as the patient's advocate." Salmon ends her chapter by reviewing the specific steps of public policymaking and places where nurses could take a more active role. While the chapter relates to the political process in the United States, the message and ideas are relevant to nursing and the nursing profession worldwide.

Next, Fagin and Binder describe nursing's opportunities and challenges in the new managed care delivery settings. They begin their chapter with some facts about managed care. While costs have decreased, they say, it is unclear whether managed care arrangements enhance quality. They point out that the focus on cost containment has risks for quality and, indeed, safety. While advising caution, they believe that managed care is a promising solution to many of the nation's health problems. They also point out that the philosophies of nursing and managed care are the same—holistic primary care. Yet despite a sharing of beliefs, nurses, especially hospital-employed nurses, are being marginalized by managed care. Fagin and Binder are disturbed by several current trends to discount nursing, including downsizing of nursing staff, replacement of nurses with unlicensed assistants, and elimination of nursing credentials in staff identification. They explore reasons that may account for others ignoring nursing and devaluing nursing contributions. They also point to some successes and some enhanced opportunities, and they outline some possible goals around which coalitions can emerge. In addition, they address challenges to nursing leadership including partnership with consumers and a more active, assertive voice for nursing participation in the new and emerging systems.

Market forces are challenging academic health centers in the United States to rethink and reshape their missions and structures. Curran does a nice job of laying out the challenges that face the 126 academic health centers that are attached to universities. Due to current forces that are enhancing competition in health care, each element of the academic health center's mission, research, education, and practice is threatened. In order to change, academic health centers must understand the growth and requirements of managed care. Curran overviews the four stages of managed care as identified by the University Hospital Consortium. She discusses integrated networks and whether it is best that an academic health center join one. While there are still many unknowns, one thing is clear: Health care is moving toward managing health rather than illness. Academic health centers must be more concerned with the health of the public and the community as well as that of individuals, and university-based physicians must unite with each other and with hospital governance and operations. Curran suggests that some academic health centers will separate from universities and others may close. In this challenging situation, Curran believes that nursing has many opportunities if we respond appropriately. She then discusses implications for nursing in education, research, and practice. She ends her chapter with eight critical success factors that she believes will determine the future of academic health centers.

In the international chapter in this section, Kerr provides an overview of the Canadian health care system. Provisions of the Canadian plan include universality of coverage to all people, comprehensiveness of medically necessary services, accessibility of health services to all segments of the population, portability of coverage from one province to another, and public administration of the program at the provincial level. Kerr traces the development of health care in Canada from the 1800s and overviews the tax-supported system that has evolved over the last 40 years. Approximately 75% of health expenditures are paid for by Medicare. Introduction of the system has produced stability in health care costs in relation to the gross national product, in contrast to the situation in the United States, where health care costs have escalated at a far more rapid pace. Physician fees, however, have been difficult to control, and new methods are being explored. Optimal size of medical school enrollments is another issue with recent small decreases in class sizes. Noting that the Canadian system has been built primarily around medical service, Kerr points out that nursing has been most affected in relation to hospital services, where nursing is viewed as one of the high costs. Nurses are vulnerable within the system. There is a growing emphasis, however, on maintaining patients in community-based settings, stressing prevention and health promotion. As this change in emphasis develops, opportunities for nurses should open up. Although they are different, the U.S. and Canadian health care systems share many similarities.

While the need for health care reform is obvious, the shape of the reform is not yet clear. There is a definite movement from hospital-based and illness treatment care to community-based and health promotion care. Building coalitions among providers and with consumers is a part of this shift in emphasis. The changes are threatening to many, and politics plays a big part of the success or failure of new efforts. While the future shape of the health care system is unknown, it is clear that nurses must take an active role in being part of the solution.

From a medical care system for a few to a comprehensive health care system for all

HELEN KENNEDY GRACE

This is the story of a village on top of a mountain. The children of the village loved to play near the ledge at the top of the mountain, but they sometimes fell off the ledge to the bottom and suffered broken legs and other injuries. Eventually a hospital was built at the bottom of the mountain to treat the injured children. The doctors set up their offices and emergency care centers, and the parents would struggle to the bottom of the mountain to visit their injured children. One day at a meeting called for another purpose, the villagers began to reflect on the problem of the injured children. One young mother asked, "Why haven't we put a fence around the top of the mountain ledge so the children won't fall off?" After considerable discussion of how this might impair the panoramic view for the villagers, they agreed that an attractive fence could be built and that they could prevent the injuries. They did so, and eventually the hospital at the bottom of the mountain was closed and a comprehensive health care clinic opened in the village because the villagers, having solved the problems of childrens' injuries, then thought of numerous other ways that they might work together to keep their community healthy. They mounted a campaign to clean up the environment, paying special attention to toxic waste from the nearby chemical factory and testing of the water to be sure that it was pure. Every expectant mother had access to quality prenatal care that recognized the culture and values of the community, and there was a comprehensive immunization program so that all infants and children were protected from childhood illnesses. Every villager had access to a program of periodic monitoring of their health status; and whenever an illness was detected, the villagers were referred to the appropriate practitioner with expertise needed to address the problem. A small, efficient short-term-care hospital was part of the clinic, and a well-developed system of referral to the regional tertiary care center was in place. Use of information technology provided links between available knowledge and information to all within the network, and a system of transportation was in place to ensure that people in need of advanced medical treatment could access these services. The elderly were cared for in their homes through a comprehensive eldercare program. When they were unable to remain in their homes for some reason, they entered a nursing home that was located in the center of the village. The nursing home had a wide range of volunteer programs that brought the community—its young people and others—into partnerships to provide humane, caring services for the elders and served as a vital community communication link in transmitting the wisdom of the elders to future generations.

Is this utopia possible? Is it desirable? If so, how do we move from our current system of "hospitals at the bottom of mountains" (i.e., fixing problems only after they have developed) to one with a primary emphasis on keeping people healthy (i.e., preventing people from "falling off of the mountain")? This paper poses two sides of this argument. Should the emphasis be on maintaining and enhancing our current medical care system, or should the focus be shifted to health promotion and disease prevention? The closing argument suggests that we have both the capacity and the resources to merge our current medical care system into a comprehensive health care system and proposes steps that will move us down this road.

SUSTAIN AND IMPROVE OUR CURRENT MEDICAL CARE SYSTEM

The United States has the best medical care system in the world. We have the best-educated doctors and nurses and the most sophisticated hospitals in the world. Don't tinker with what isn't broken. We don't know how to prevent illness but we do know how to treat it. We just need to find a way to finance the existing system. Those who have the means should have the right to "the best."

Our current medical care system is a reflection of values in American society. No one should be denied access to the "best" care if they have the ability to pay or if insurance coverage is provided by their employers. These values are reflected in the way our society invests its resources. Over the years we have made substantial societal investments in scientific and medical research that has resulted in the most advanced knowledge related to the etiology and treatment of diseases. When organs are severely diseased and irreparable, we have the capacity for transplantation of hearts, livers, lungs, kidneys, or a combination of body parts. The ability to overcome the body's tendency to reject transplants has been addressed by a wide array of immunosuppressive agents. A great variety of drug treatments are available for the most complex of diseases. If a body part is "broken," our medical care system has a high level of capability for "fixing" it, either surgically or medically. We can keep people with a plethora of problems alive for prolonged periods of time. For example, cancer sufferers now have a much longer life span and a better quality of that life as a result of advances in the treatment agents given as well as those used to compensate for the numerous side effects of the treatment. Superpowerful antibiotics have given us the capability to overcome ever-increasing numbers of infectious diseases.

The training of medical doctors and nurses in the United States is the most sophisticated and arduous in the world. Extreme competition to get into medical schools in particular ensures that we are capturing the brightest minds in the country. These individuals need to be challenged continuously, both in their medical training and as they move into practice settings. The major challenges lay in finding ways to deal with the most complicated medical care problems. The medical school curricula, based on ever more complex decision-making trees, challenges the ability of the students to diagnose problems and devise treatment plans. Given the extensive investment of resources in medical education by the public, which supports most medical education through their tax dollars, and the extensive investment of time, energy, and money to support 4 years of postbaccalaureate study followed by residency programs, it would be a misuse of these dollars if specialty training were not the end product. This extensive an education to treat the commonplace colds, flus, broken arms, and aches and pains that plague most patients would be a misuse of these valued resources. The commonplace problems of people offer an insufficient challenge to the brilliantly honed minds of medical practitioners that is the end product of their rigorous education.

While in nursing there has never been the clamor to gain entrance to the field as there has been in medicine, many of the same arguments might hold. The "excitement" of an intensive care unit with its many sophisticated pieces of equipment, the challenge of interpreting the laboratory reports and correlating them to the clinical status of the patient, and the hovering over monitors to detect changes in the physiological status of the patient are all intellectually challenging. Investment in highly specialized advanced practitioner training dictates that this training be used in the intensive care environment of a hospital setting.

Hospitals are the centerpiece of our medical care system. They are the specially designed workplaces that use the expertise of our highly trained health professionals most efficiently. Further, they constitute a significant economic development resource in any community. With 6% of people employed in health-related fields, and the majority of these employed by hospitals, the economic welfare of communities frequently rests on the viability of hospitals and health-related institutions. Society has made a tremendous investment in the building of highly sophisticated hospitals with advanced technology equipment. It would be a tremendous waste of resources to see these facilities disintegrate or disappear; it is a wise investment to see that they are used to benefit all.

Perhaps one of the strongest arguments for maintaining and improving our current medical care system is that there are few proven alternatives. While some argue that it would be a better use of resources to invest in prevention, our highly trained health professionals and our highly developed technology are not designed to deal with health promotion and disease prevention. Most aspects of health promotion and disease prevention are contingent on the capacity of individuals to change their health-related behaviors, and it is in this area that highly educated medical practitioners are the most helpless. In addition, unless individuals are motivated to change their behavior there is little that can be done. Our hospital facilities and our highly trained health professionals can be better utilized for the diagnosis and treatment of disease than in a misuse of this capacity in the area of health promotion and disease prevention.

REFOCUS OUR EFFORTS TOWARD HEALTH PROMOTION AND DISEASE PREVENTION

Despite our sophisticated technology and highly trained health care professionals, the efforts to diagnose and treat disease are far more costly than if the focus was on prevention of disease. Approximately 52% of all diseases are a product of unhealthy lifestyles and behavioral choices that result in ill health. Resources would be better used to focus on prevention of disease than on the very costly approaches to treatment.

We should divert the large amounts of money going to

research for the treatment of diseases and for development of technology and redirect these funds to focus on health promotion and disease prevention. For example, huge amounts of research and treatment dollars are spent on leukemia. The effects of the treatment approaches are limited at best, yet the cost of treating one leukemia patient can reach astronomical figures. Resources could be used much more effectively to reduce the toxic waste in our environment, control the use of chemicals that lead to bone marrow damage, and prevent disease rather than invest in treatments of unproved worth. We should spend some of the money that is currently being spent on medical care and research to clean up the environment.

Instead of our current focus on treatment, the emphasis should be shifted to education. We should focus on instilling within young people healthy lifestyles that will contribute to long and productive lives, and we should ensure that all citizens receive appropriate preventive health care. Every school curriculum in the country should contain content on the effects of the abuse of alcohol and drugs (including tobacco) and the impact of lack of exercise and poor nutrition on the health of the individual. A program designed to promote physical fitness in young people should be built into all educational programs. Fitness levels of school children should be tested periodically, and test scores should be reported much as academic achievement is now reported. Fitness trails, recreational facilities, and support groups that encourage healthy lifestyles should be part of each community.

Systematic programs of health monitoring should be set up in each community, with the expectation that different population groups would have periodic health screening to detect problems at the earliest possible stages and at the level at which intervention is most likely to have a profound effect. Prenatal care for expectant mothers, monitoring of both physical and psychological growth and development in children, adolescent health monitoring, periodic health examinations for adults, health and fitness assessment for seniors, and monitoring programs for chronic illnesses of the elderly would be components of this comprehensive preventive system.

The numbers of highly specialized health care providers should be decreased and the numbers of primary care practitioners increased. Additionally, practitioners from the education and behavioral science fields should be integrated into the health professions teams. Educational programs for health professionals should be refocused on early diagnosis and prevention and away from the heavy emphasis on physical sciences to a more balanced study of the behavioral sciences with a heavy emphasis on methodologies of teaching for adult learners.

The payment incentives within the system should provide rewards for keeping people well rather than paying for treatment of illnesses. This could best be achieved through funding on a capitated basis for communities. Because most public funds flow into communities through county governments, counties might well be the base for a capitated system. In instances in which a county is comprised of a large metropolitan area, the capitated system might be drawn along smaller geographic boundaries. The particular funding base for a community would need to be calculated based on the demographics of the particular area and would take into consideration the age spread of the population, the level of income and the racial and ethnic composition of the community, and the association of these demographics with known health risks. If the health care dollars flowing into the community were based on the numbers of people living in that community, the incentives would be to maintain the health of the people rather than to pay for treatment of costly illnesses. A capitated system that pays for building health promotion into the fabric of the community and one in which the health care "providers" are salaried rather than paid on a fee-for-service basis would be one way in which the incentive systems could be changed.

The majority of hospital beds in this country should be closed. Community hospitals in both urban and rural settings could become the hub for organizing the comprehensive system of health promotion and disease prevention activities across the community. A capitated system would dramatically decrease the numbers of people involved in the processing of paperwork related to financing the system (now estimated to be about 25% of health care dollars). These community hospitals would have facilities for short-term stays for "normal" conditions such as delivery of babies, handling of accidents and fractures, and simple surgery. The numbers of people displaced from paper-processing jobs could be absorbed into new, more productive roles within the community such as health promoters. A few highly specialized hospitals would remain to treat the limited number of acute care problems that develop despite all efforts at maintaining health in the community.

DEVELOP INTEGRATED COMPREHENSIVE HEALTH CARE SYSTEMS

This debate is posed most frequently as an either/or argument—that one must make a choice between a quality medical care system versus a system focused on the maintenance of health. The argument is generally made on the basis of available resources and is grounded on a premise that lack of resources constrains the system. The arguments develop based on what would appear to be a faulty premise, that is, that lack of resources are the problem. If one views the problem as one of lack of resources, the response is that of exerting efforts to get more resources out of the existing system. However, if one looks at the situation as one in which the problem is *use* of *existing* resources, the focus changes to looking at ways to achieve greater efficiency.

The United States spends more on medical care than any other country in the world. Yet our health indices do not reflect that this investment is paying off with the improved health of the people. Rarely is the question addressed from the perspective of how the resources flow and the use of these resources in the most cost-effective ways. Money for health and human services flows into communities through a wide array of funding tracks, each carrying with them their own rules and regulations, and a plethora of individuals is employed as gatekeepers to ensure "compliance." This results in inefficient use of the resources that are available in that funding "packages" are difficult to put together to meet the needs of individuals and families and that a disproportionate amount of the resources are used to pay for the paper-processing to maintain all of the separate funding streams. In a typical community there would of course be federally funded programs such as Medicare and Medicaid, but within these general programs there would be a variety of funding streams for a variety of programs. For example, prenatal care would have several components, often provided by multiple agencies. The Women, Infants, and Children programs are administered typically through health departments. A mother receiving prenatal care from a community health center may need to go to the public health department to receive funds from the Women, Infants, and Children program. If an expectant mother has other human service problems, such as being abused or abusing substances, she would then typically be referred to another agency that offers these programs. Most frequently the funding for these programs would be through a department of social services or mental health department. The department of child and family services might also be a possibility. However, all of these agencies carry with them their own unique rules and regulations and a set of functionaries to maintain the multiple "systems." This results in fragmentation of services, difficulty for patients in obtaining the help that they need (frequently a case manager is added to help the patient navigate through the morass), inefficient use of the human resources, (the providers) within the system, and a plethora of paperwork that would be unnecessary if the system was put together as a system. In addition to publicly funded programs, a multitude of insurers provide several insurance plans to individuals and workers within the community. A typical community hospital may deal with up to 50 insurers, all with different reporting requirements and different forms to fill out. Hospitals have added to their financial and administrative staffs to process claims and to respond to the challenges. It is estimated that at least 25% of the resources within the system currently goes to administration. In private discussions with chief executive officers in community-based health service organizations such as visiting nurse associations it is estimated that up to one third of their resources are spent on administrative overhead to manage the multiple funding streams on which their survival is dependent. Noting how very limited resources are used for health care in other countries and the misuse of our comparatively abundant resources within the United States, it is hard to accept the premise that the problem is one of lack of resources.

Some might argue that use of human resources in the medical care system is integral to the economic well-being of communities, and therefore one should not tinker with the system. In a number of both rural and urban communities, the health care sector is one of the major employers in the community. Closing a rural hospital is viewed as a major threat to the economy of the community, and this concern takes precedence over concerns for the impact of hospital closure on the health of the community. The health care industry is a major economic force within this country, and maintenance of the nonsystem may be crucial to our economic well-being. Seldom is this issue addressed in a straightforward manner, however. If we wish to have resources directed toward health as an industry and maintenance of the economy it would be far better to address this issue directly rather than couching the arguments in terms of concern for the well-being of individuals who use the health care system. My personal argument would be that there are more productive ways of using the human resources that are now engaged in "paper processing," and that if we wish to develop integrated, comprehensive health care systems, some of the human resources need to be diverted to more productive lines of work that would have a more direct pay-off in terms of improved health of people.

In recent years, the W.K. Kellogg Foundation has provided funding to three communities in Michigan to begin the process of reconceptualizing and restructuring their health care to achieve a comprehensive integrated system.

In one of these communities, the total amount of funding coming into a county with 135,982 residents was $402,401,000, which translates to $3,000 per individual. A basic assumption underlying the Comprehensive Community Health Models of Michigan (CCHMs) program is that these resources, if they were put together in a different way, would be adequate to fund a comprehensive integrated health care system that would be accessible to all. During the transition, there may be a limited period of increased costs, but over time the benefits to be achieved from linking comprehensive health care to the current medical and human services, pooling the resources within the community to fund an integrated health care system, and placing the emphasis on maintaining the health of the community will result in a much more cost-effective system.

In the process of working with these three communities many lessons are being learned, the first and foremost of which is the importance of educating communities about health and medical care so that they can begin to exercise their decision-making power in a rational manner. A primary factor that inhibits significant change within the health-related fields is the degree to which the system has been a mystery to the general public. By engaging in an extensive community "visioning" process the communities have begun to shift their views of health care away from the medical system as it is commonly defined toward a comprehensive health care system. For example, one of the results of this reconceptualization is that each of the three communities has placed a high value on the health of children and has concluded that an essential component of a comprehensive system is school nurses. In each community they have found ways of funding school nurses who are responsible for health monitoring and other health-related functions in the school. After defining a set of guiding values and identifying essential characteristics of a comprehensive health system, a process of electronic town meetings has been useful in building group consensus, identifying areas that are conflicting, and focusing discussions to resolve differences. As a wide range of community participants have become engaged in the visioning process, the tertiary medical care system is no longer the central focus, sometimes to the consternation of hospital administrators and physician specialists who view themselves as the center of the universe.

Each of these communities has engaged in a process of surveying the health of their residents, identifying preventable health problems within their community, prioritizing areas of concern, and addressing ways in which problem areas might be addressed. As communities begin to understand that a comprehensive, integrated health care system includes comprehensive health promotion programs for target groups throughout the community (i.e., pregnant women, children, adolescents, working adults, women, impoverished groups, and elders), weaving health promotion into the fabric of the community becomes a major facet of the system. Health monitoring of key groups such as pregnant women, children, and adults and elderly then becomes another key component. As the focus shifts to health promotion and maintenance, the locus of services moves out of traditional health settings into community-based institutions such as schools, churches, Y centers, senior citizen centers, and worksites. The importance of primary health care providers also rises to the surface as communities build their vision of a comprehensive health care system.

As all sectors begin to come together around a common vision for health care in their community, a natural realignment of working relationships begins to occur. For example, the local public health department, which in most communities has become quite isolated from other sectors, becomes the source of data on the health of the community and has a key role to play in monitoring progress. As the health of all members of the community becomes the business of the community as a whole, no longer does the health department become relegated to being the providers of "last resort." Social service agencies and health providers find new ways of working together. Engaging members of the community in the dialogue and dealing with "real life" situations that people face in getting health care for themselves and their family members adds a new dimension to the discussion.

As these discussions progress, new voices emerge. In the community discussions in Michigan, a wide array of "alternative health care providers" have emerged, adding yet another dimension to the discussions. For example, a young woman described her problem with migraine headaches. She could tell when a migraine was coming on, and if she went for massage therapy, the migraine could be averted. Her health insurance would not pay for massage therapy, however. If she went to her doctor, she couldn't get an appointment until the headache had developed, and she would need to take time off from work and take medication. Yet this much more costly (both physical and financial) course of action was reimbursable. This situation precipitated an interesting debate in the visioning process as to what should be reimbursable in an "ideal" health system. A prominent oncologist agreed that "only scientifically validated treatments" should be reimbursable. This was countered by a question of how many of his treatments were scientifically proven to be beneficial.

As the community becomes engaged in a new type of dialogue, and the health of the community becomes "community business," the barriers that constrain the system inevitably become much more evident. Community governing boards have been constituted in the three communities involved in the CCHMs process. These boards become engaged in ways that they may begin to have an impact on changing public policy, particularly that relevant to the funding for health and human services. An underlying premise of the CCHMs effort is that if communities could "pool" the dollars that are currently coming into communities through the funding stream, and that if this funding could be redirected to fund health promotion and preventive services as well as treatment for diseases, then there are sufficient resources to ensure an adequate level of health care for all. Using state-of-the-art information technology and an understanding of how a comprehensive, integrated system works, the fragmented pieces that are currently out there could function in a much different way. In the end, then, each part of the system would be a "winner." Appropriate use of the expert skills of specialists, scaled-down hospitals, an organized system for monitoring health, a comprehensive health promotion program integrated into community-based organizations such as schools, churches, senior citizen centers, and a system in which community members and health workers work as a team to improve the health of the community would benefit all members of the community.

All can be winners. To achieve this goal, however, requires putting aside the traditional boundaries that have served to divide the "turf." Community members must be brought into the partnerships, and all parties must give up some additional areas of control. For example, physicians alone can no longer be the gatekeepers for the system. The health system of the future must be one in which the worth of all individuals—be they providers or patients—is valued and the human resources that collectively might work together are used to their full potential. Quality, affordable health care for all is an attainable goal.

Toward a comprehensive health care system: Using a grassroots consumer effort

MARLENE LAWRENCE

The American health care system didn't get into its present condition as the result of one bad idea, and it will not get out of its current state on the strength of one good idea. The health care system has reached a crisis point as a result of a complicated mixture of social and economic forces. To move beyond it will require many good ideas and institutions that not only stand on their own but that also interact with other good ideas and institutions.

All players in the health care system—consumers, purchasers, and providers—have historically acted in their own best interests. This myopic philosophy has led us to our current dilemma, in which health care reform, for good or bad, is inevitable. All three participants of the health care system have legitimate fears from abrupt and massive change (T. McLaughlin, personal communication, August, 1995).

BACKGROUND

Upon earning my associate degree in nursing in 1968 I worked as a staff nurse in a hospital setting. Over the next 10 years I held a variety of positions in nursing and hospital administration. In 1978 I enrolled in the University of Michigan where I obtained my bachelor's of science degree in nursing. During the completion of a clinical rotation in community health, for the first time in my career I was entering clients' homes. This rotation, my faculty, and contact with consumers outside of the hospital refocused my view of the health care system.

I returned to the hospital as Director of Education and after 1 year advanced to Vice President of Nursing Services, and ultimately to Assistant to the President, where my duties included physician recruitment, management of ambulatory care clinics, and physician practice management. Although I remained in an acute care setting, I no longer viewed the hospital and acute care as the center of the health system. I recognized that community and community interests needed to be central for the health system to be effective.

In 1982, when our community was faced with a high infant mortality rate, it became apparent this community issue could only be solved by engaging broad community segments. In the midst of this crisis, we sought help from the W.K. Kellogg Foundation, and with support and mentoring from Dr. Helen K. Grace we were able to establish the Family Health Center. This Center provides an interdisciplinary model of care that includes physicians, family nurse practitioners, pediatric nurse practitioners, nurse midwives, nutritionists, and social workers. It now has an annual caseload of 40,000 visits per year. This was a milestone in our community because it began to decentralize the way we viewed and provided care.

In 1992, I traveled to the People's Republic of China with Dr. Hanmin Liu, President of the United States/China Educational Institute, and Mr. Robert DeVries, Program Director/Director of International Study Grants at the Kellogg Foundation, and a delegation of representatives from education and health from our country. As I

The author wishes to acknowledge the assistance of Greig Grey, Author/writer, Ann Arbor, Michigan studied the culture and developed personal relationships with the people we met I was again faced with the narrow view of our health care system and its lack of focus on prevention and primary care. These experiences prompted me to inventory my priorities and to focus my career to be more inclusive of community.

COMPREHENSIVE COMMUNITY HEALTH MODELS OF MICHIGAN

In 1991, the W.K. Kellogg Foundation concluded that, although they were receiving innovative grant requests related to health issues, none of the requests addressed all of the elements necessary to improve health status and influence public policy. The Foundation identified what they believed to be six critical components that must be addressed concurrently at the local level to improve health status and bring about systemic change: (1) community decision making (governance); (2) community-wide coverage; (3) a comprehensive integrated health delivery system organized around primary prevention and primary care; (4) an integrated administrative structure; (5) a community-based health information system; and (6) community health assessment.

The Foundation believed that the only way for health reform to occur was at the local level because health care is a local product—delivered, consumed, and paid for locally. They established an initiative known as Comprehensive Community Health Models of Michigan (CCHMs) to provide a vehicle for communities to initiate health reform at the local level. Through this initiative, the Foundation is partnering with three geographic communities in Michigan: Calhoun, Muskegon, and St. Clair counties. The focus of the project is to nurture community decision making and improve local preventive and primary care services ("An In-Depth Look at CCHMs," 1995).

The CCHMs approach is to assemble a community-wide forum representing the spectrum of people with a stake in the community's health (civic and business leaders, providers, payers, employers, unions, and consumers) to assess local health problems and needs and develop a vision and plan for addressing them. The CCHMs project objectives are to develop community-wide efforts to improve community health and to use participation in community-wide structures to create collaborative approaches and solutions for strengthening illness prevention and primary care delivery. The depth of the citizen involvement goes to the heart of the process. Consumers in all three counties are at the table with providers and payers.

In order to attract all parties to the table, the Kellogg Foundation sought a neutral body without a specific stake in the health care system to host and facilitate the process. In Calhoun County, Battle Creek Community Foundation, a private, nonprofit philanthropic organization, expressed interest in the project. The Calhoun County Health Improvement Program (CCHIP) began in July of 1993 and operates as a special project of the Battle Creek Community Foundation.

COUNTY PROFILE

Calhoun County has a population of 135,982 and encompasses 712 square miles. It is located in the southwest quadrant of Michigan's lower peninsula, 90 miles due west of Detroit. Following a period of rapid development and prosperity in the early 1900s, economic growth in the area leveled off following the Great Depression. In the late 1970s and 1980s, the region experienced a modest recovery, but the booming expansion of industry that characterized its earlier growth has not developed. Farms occupy half the land in the county, with three fourths of the farmland under cultivation. Eighty-three percent of businesses in Calhoun County have fewer than 20 employees. The unemployment rate currently hovers around 5%.

Eighty-seven percent of Calhoun County's population is white; 10% are black; 2% are Hispanic; 1% are Asian/Pacific Islanders; and .07% are American Indian. One federally recognized American Indian tribe, the Nottawaseppi Huron Band of Potawatomi, is located in Calhoun County. Thirteen percent of Calhoun County's citizens are 65 years of age or older (U.S. Bureau of the Census, 1990 Census of Population).

I was offered the opportunity to direct the CCHIP. After over 20 years' experience in hospitals, I accepted the challenge to move into a community setting. We established a 48-member advisory committee that represented consumers, hospitals, physicians, other providers, payers, human service organizations, and diverse racial and geographic communities to initiate a broad-based review of health in the county. We also set up five working subcommittees and three task groups, which brought the total number of citizens directly involved to 250. To reach beyond the formal representation of those directly participating, CCHIP participants conducted an initial survey of 1,000 additional citizens across the county to assess their perceptions of the health needs of the community. To date we have interviewed over 7,000 citizens, with their input and participation driving a new model of care.

We also developed an overview of the problems in the current delivery system: uneven access to health services, fragmentation of care, rising costs, inadequate information for measuring performance of the system, and shortfalls in the availability of primary care and prevention.

One of the significant things we did was to profile the health status of the citizens of Calhoun County. As a result of this profile and the citizen interviews it was decided that Calhoun County would have an integrated delivery system that makes primary care and prevention a priority. Based on the health status and needs of our community, we would build on existing health and human services resources to modify delivery and reimbursement systems to support a primary care focus. Linkages with health professionals and health organizations would be in place to expand the local availability of primary care providers as the system moves to prevention and primary care. Services would be organized from the consumer perspective and built on existing strengths (Calhoun County Health Improvement Program, 1996).

Early in the project we realized that providing health services to those who are less vocal, underserved, and more vulnerable cannot be achieved from a centralized point. Besides outreach, CCHIP realized that our effectiveness depends on providing a forum for all points of view to be articulated and not allowing any single interest to dominate the process or decision-making. We have tried particularly to bring together people and organizations that had operated independently or competed, rather than collaborated, in the past. Galvanizing relationships between competitors remains a challenge.

Strategies have been developed to address the six areas identified by the Kellogg Foundation. In addition, project staff are engaged in a process of intensive community outreach to validate and further define the community's health needs. The focus of this outreach is to achieve a high level of community participation and awareness and to develop realistic mechanisms to address those needs.

One of the major problems we identified was the reimbursement system. As we began to address this problem, we discovered that it gave us an opportunity to educate consumers in understanding their benefits. The proposed system will allow a consumer of health services to know exactly what services are covered and how much payment will be required out of pocket before the services are delivered. This system will also help lower administrative costs by reducing the "claims paper trail," and will free additional dollars. According to estimates by a CCHMs consultant, a 4% reduction in duplicate coverage, achieved through up-front coordination of benefits, coupled with a 2% decrease in duplicate payment, will result in over $10 million in savings for Calhoun County (Calhoun County Health Improvement Program, 1995).

We have determined what minimal health benefits should be guaranteed to all Calhoun County members and defined a minimal and core set of benefits marketable in our current system. A matrix of current benefit levels of consumers in the county was developed. Through information from public agencies, a survey conducted by the area employers association, local benefit brokers, and primary research conducted by staff, this matrix compared both public and private plans according to the services covered. The minimal benefit recommended was developed to protect individuals from the high cost of health services through catastrophic coverage, while also providing coverage for primary and preventive services, including preventive dentistry for children. At $45 per month, or $105 per month for a family, the plan is affordable to many who are currently uninsured or underinsured. This minimal plan is not intended to be a standard for the community.

Financing alternatives for the minimal and core benefits have been explored. As noted above, administrative waste accounts for over $10 million alone. In addition, it is estimated that another $7 million is wasted through cost shifting in the private sector. For example, employers offer "opt-out" programs to employees who can be covered under their spouses' plans. The incentive normally consists of a flat dollar amount if coverage is sought elsewhere, and it shifts the burden (and cost) from one employer to another. We have focused on strategies for utilizing these savings.

To maintain community control and involvement, the power within the community decision-making structure is balanced among three groups—consumers, payers, and providers—all equally represented on a 15-member Governing Board. This board reports to a community group of 650 citizens from across Calhoun County.

Conflicting viewpoints must be welcomed for the stimulation of new ideas, possible problems, and shortcomings. We listen, and listen again, to the negative viewpoints, seeking out any merits they may contain, not simply dismissing them. Indeed, we are traveling into uncharted territory, and having no "history to ignore," we can ill afford to dismiss any ideas, suggestions, or criticism.

Our ultimate success will hinge on continued community involvement and input. One of our toughest challenges at CCHIP is getting people to the table who have conventionally had no voice in their health concerns and remain distrustful of our attempts to get them involved.

One of CCHIP's assets is its position as a neutral facilitator, organizer, and convener, with no economic stake in our mission and only the improvement of our community's health as our focus. This effort is obviously important to Calhoun County. However, it is also important on a national level. There is a need for models that offer reference and direction to local initiatives that too often seek answers through a narrow program focus rather than through a broadly defined systems approach. The greatest proof of the need for the CCHMs initiative is the fragmentation of clinical services and information and financing and delivery systems that are the legacy of past top-down federal and state initiatives.

In Calhoun County we are committed to having institutions that are responsive to the community. We have relied on the work of Kretzmann and McKnight (1993) in formulating a new approach to consumers: an asset-based rather than a need-based focus. Their work at the Center for Urban Affairs and Policy Research at Northwestern University has had a marked effect on the development of the Health Improvement Program. McKnight has offered guidance on the difficult transition of a provider-driven focus on a community's needs, deficiencies, and problems to discovering a community's capacities and assets. When needs are the focus, community residents come to believe that their well-being depends on being a client, with special needs that can only be met by people and organizations outside the community. Stated simply, the community focus on its own assets leads to the development of policies and activities that are based on the capacities, skills, and assets of people and their neighborhoods. The research has been done in lower-income urban areas. In Calhoun County, we have attempted to identify neighborhood associations that can provide information, guidance, and direction for the Health Improvement Program. Breaking from a traditional deficit perspective, the models operate from an asset-based belief system that places priorities on experiences such as training and mentoring that can expand self-sufficiency, enhance problem-solving skills, and promote leadership. We are beginning the implementation of a community-focused health plan in our county, including the following:

- Establishment of a purchasing cooperative
- Addressing seven high-risk behaviors through the establishment of existing and new coalitions
- Helping people regain the confidence to be in charge of their own health
- Continuing to bring consumers, providers, and payers together to achieve a balanced perspective

CONCLUSION

Community nursing must not be confined to those nurses who work in traditional community health agencies (e.g., public health departments). For health reform to occur, nursing must subscribe to a community development approach. I am fortunate to have been able to join a project where I can utilize my nursing degree in a field that is breaking new ground, centered and focused around community health. There is no magic formula for success other than the privilege of working with highly qualified and motivated staff and community volunteers. My initial plunge into community health was the mechanism that has allowed me to pursue a career that has been more fulfilling than I could have imagined. I challenge each of you to examine your individual communities and question the status quo. Don't be afraid to ask questions and don't be afraid to make a difference.

REFERENCES

An In-Depth Look at CCHMs [Pamphlet]. (1995).

Background on Comprehensive Community Health Models of Michigan [Pamphlet]. (1995).

Calhoun County Health Improvement Program to the W.K. Kellogg Foundation. (1995, April/June). *Quarterly Report.*

Calhoun County Health Improvement Program for the W.K. Kellogg Foundation Comprehensive Community Health Models of Michigan Project. (1996). *Grant Proposal.*

McKnight, J.L., & Kretzmann, J.P. (1993). *Building communities from the inside out: A path toward finding and mobilizing a community's assets.* Evanston, IL: Northwestern University.

U.S. Bureau of the Census, 1990 Census of Population.

Toward a comprehensive health care system: Business and provider coalitions

PATRICIA HINTON WALKER

The United States spends nearly 14% of its gross national product on health care, which is significantly more than any other country. Over $3,000 per capita was spent on health care in 1992 (which is at least $1,000 higher than any other country), and costs continue to rise uncontrollably (Schroeder, 1994). However, U.S. clinical outcomes compared with other countries are not significantly better. In some cases (e.g., infant mortality), the outcomes are clearly worse. Although rising costs and documented overuse of the medical care delivery system caused great concern and political debate in 1994, there was no consensus about what approach to adopt (from a legislative perspective) to solve the health care problem.

Although health care reform was not legislated, changes driven by market forces are occurring in the health care delivery system at an unprecedented rate. As business and state governments strive to find ways to control health care costs, managed care is emerging as the most prevalent choice for change. The term *managed care* is used to describe many different types of health care delivery system approaches. It may be described as a health maintenance organization (HMO), such as Kaiser Permanente; an integrated delivery system (IDS), which includes some of the attempts to link hospitals, home health agencies, and group primary care practices; or some form of preferred provider organization (PPO). Regardless of the particular model or approach, there are at least four common goals of any type of managed care organization: (1) to control costs, usually by controlling utilization of services; (2) to use sound business approaches to ensure efficiency, which is resulting in significant reductions in the health care labor force and work redesign; (3) to ensure quality through the measurement of outcomes (clinical indicators, customer satisfaction, and cost); and (4) to do all of the above by trying to form coalitions, alliances, or partnerships that will "manage care" across the wellness-illness continuum for a specified dollar amount (usually negotiated up front in a managed care contract).

These changes have significant implications for the nursing profession in practice, education, research, and administration. This chapter is designed to help nurses better understand the business side of these new approaches to health care delivery and to provoke serious thought about the implications for nurses both individually and collectively. Lastly, this chapter provides incentives to look at this time of change as a time of great opportunity for nurses and the nursing profession. This change is highlighting the importance of many of the values held and advocated by nurses throughout history: coordinated care across the continuum, attention to prevention and health promotion, attention to the role of the family and community, empowering the voice of the patient (or client/consumer/customer) in his or her own care, and developing interdisciplinary practices that truly focus on patient-centered care versus the needs and interests of the provider and institution. Nurses have the values and much of the knowledge and skills needed in this time of change; however, we must stretch beyond our clinical focus and expertise to embrace the relationship of business to practice, research, and administration. Nurses must be involved in the negotiations for *care, costs,* and *outcomes,* and must actively prepare individually and collectively to understand and articulate the *value* of patient/client-centered care as the *ratio of cost to quality* (measured in outcomes) (see Fig. 57-1).

CONTEXT FOR COALITIONS

When health care costs rose significantly in the 1980s, one of the ways that businesses and employers tried to control these costs was through the development of coali-

$$Value = \frac{Quality\ of\ Care}{Cost}$$

Fig. 57-1. Formula for value of health care.

tions (Rooney, 1992). Usually these coalitions were developed on a community-wide basis in an attempt to contain costs on a widespread basis and to control cost-shifting from employer to employer. Although this approach met with marginal success, the use and development of many forms of coalitions to address many of the health care problems of today has continued. We are now seeing many forms of coalitions spring up, including alliances and affiliations (coalitions) of providers, hospitals, and other health care delivery agencies; networks developed to address fragmented care of specific populations; quality improvement and outcomes research consortiums; and finally, community, business, and government partnerships (coalitions) designed to enhance population-based, community-sensitive care for underserved groups. What is a coalition? How does a coalition differ from an alliance, a partnership, a merger, or a network? What do we need to know about coalitions? Finally, how will coalitions affect nursing and interdisciplinary practice, administration, and research?

The literature contains many references to coalitions but uses different terms to label them. A thesaurus lists alliance, network, partnership, affiliation, and consortium in connection with the term *coalition*. Merriam-Webster (1995) specifically defines a *coalition* as "a temporary alliance of distinct parties, persons, or states for joint action" (p. 30). *Partnership* refers to a legal relationship usually involving a close cooperation between parties with specified and joint rights and responsibilities; an *alliance* is an association that furthers the common interests of its members; and a *consortium* is an agreement, combination, or group formed to undertake an enterprise beyond the resources of any one member. In this chapter, these terms are used somewhat interchangeably, depending on the particular reference.

Is a coalition an organization? Can we study coalitions and learn how to work within them and manage them in the same way we study traditional organizational structures? Can we better understand how to work in this newest evolution of organizational change in response to rapid changes in the delivery of health care? The answers are yes, yes, and yes! Tichy (1983) indicates that we must understand organizational models in order to understand how organizations change. He describes a *model* as a set of assumptions or beliefs that guide managerial action, assist in diagnosing organizational problems, and focus the people who work in the organization. Three models, classical/mechanistic, human resource organic, and political, were described by Tichy (1983). These models will sound familiar to most people who have lived and worked in organizations. The classical/mechanistic model focuses on structure, span of control, and specialized task functions. This is like a typical bureaucratic organization with detailed job descriptions and a rigid chain of command by which decisions are made along vertical lines with minimal flexibility. The human resources organic model is more concerned about the human side where there are more democratic decisions made, with lots of interaction both vertically and laterally in the organization. The supervisor is more of a motivator and facilitator who communicates through expectations rather than strict orders and tasks. There are clearly strengths and weaknesses within each of these two approaches. Third is the political model, which can be viewed as a political arena in which multiple coalitions vie for control of the organization through ongoing processes of bargaining and negotiation. This model is best studied from the perspective of understanding internal coalitions (usually full-time employees) and external coalitions (partners, alliance members, or networked groups) that make up the larger organization (Mintzberg, 1977). We need to better understand the type of organization in which change strategies are based on making political adjustments, understanding where the greatest power and influence are held, and mastering the skills of negotiation, bargaining, and coalition building (Tichy, 1983).

The political model is developing rapidly in the health care field in order to respond to competition for health care dollars, because it is the most flexible, adaptive, and responsive. However, two weaknesses must be noted in this evolving model; sometimes the technical production with attention to detail and cultural problems between different organizations in a coalition are difficult to resolve (Tichy, 1983). Consequently, attention to the structure, processes, and outcomes of quality care (production) and the merging of different organizational cultures and values may create problems in these new health care delivery structures.

PURPOSES AND REASONS FOR COALITION DEVELOPMENT

Why is the political model or the development of coalitions dominating the health care delivery organizational structures at this time? Why do we even need to understand this new phenomenon in health care? Again, we look to the business literature for answers because if we understand the nature of the organizational change in which we are all participating (either by choice, chance, or requirement), nursing can position itself as a profession and ourselves as professionals. The evolution of alliances, coalitions, mergers, and partnerships is a global phenomenon. Many companies in a variety of industries are choosing alliances, coalitions, and partnerships as vehicles for change in a tight market economy, and this phenomenon is occurring worldwide. Competition is the name of the game. In a timely book, *Competing for the Future,* Hamel and Prahalad (1994) write that, "Competition for the future is competition to create and dominate emerging opportunities—to stake out new competitive space" (p. 22). Further, the authors say that organizations must not only compete within the boundaries of existing industries (e.g., hospitals, home health, insurance industries), but they must also shape the structure of industries that will be able to compete and dominate the market in the future. This means that "competition will take place within and between coalitions of companies, and not only between individual businesses" (Hamel and Prahalad, 1994, p. 23).

Why is it so important to understand these business trends? It is clear that those nurses and other clinical professionals who are willing to "unlearn" old ways and to assist the organization in its efforts to remain competitive will be valued and will survive in a changing workforce. Because competition is so high in health care and many other industries today, no one organizational structure has evolved to be the solution. As nurses, if we understand that many companies are trying to "shape the structures" for managed care through development of different kinds of alliances and coalitions, then we can position ourselves within these evolving structures to have more influence on quality of care and customer satisfaction—two of nursing's strengths. This also helps us understand why some coalitions develop into IDSs, physician/hospital organizations (PHOs), independent provider associations (IPAs), or a variety of consortiums or network structures. Because most managed care organizations are in the early stages of development, no particular structure has yet emerged as the best way to compete and do business. Consequently, regardless of the type of structure, it is important for nurses to decide to be active players in shaping the organization and contributing meaningfully to new ways of doing things.

One key to assisting our health care organizations in developing successful coalitions for change is to understand the reasons for coalition development and the process of building coalitions. Coalitions develop for several reasons, most obvious of which is the fact that no one organization has all the required resources, skills, knowledge, and expertise to produce the product. In health care, the product must provide cost-effective quality care across the continuum. A second reason that coalitions are formed is for political advantage. In some cases, a coalition is a good way to co-opt potential future competitors or, through partnering, to prevent resources from getting in the hands of a competitor. A political coalition may also provide access to new markets. A third reason for coalition development is to share risks and costs. "Alliances allow participation in highly volatile industries, where knowledge spreads rapidly, at substantially lower investment and risk than would be the case for a single organization" (Kaluzny, Zuckerman, & Ricketts, 1995, p. 3).

Because there is a combination of needs to acquire resources, skills, and knowledge as well as political reasons, many business coalitions may seem to be linkages without logic. Coalition building follows no distinct pattern. The company with the most relevant competencies and resources to the product is usually the center of the coalition and has the most influence and power. Therefore, it is not unusual to see physicians and hospitals enjoy relatively strong positions in this changing health care market because of their importance to the provision and management of medical care. However, with the shift in emphasis from medical to health care, the value of nursing's relevance to outcomes care holds potential for increased power and influence as these managed care organizations mature. Nursing's knowledge, skills, and competencies in health promotion and prevention, care across the continuum as cost-effective providers, and attention to customer satisfaction will hold increasing value in the ratio of cost to quality regardless of the type of coalition.

TYPES AND FORMATION OF COALITIONS IN HEALTH CARE

According to Kaluzny et al. (1995), there are two general types of alliances or coalitions in health care: lateral and integrative. Similar types of organizations come together to achieve economies of scale by pooling resources, sharing information and human resources, group purchasing, and increasing collective power. When this occurs, it is called a *lateral* alliance or coalition. Examples include hospitals merging or networking together based on type of service, geographic distribution, or religious preferences. Rural hospital networks or consortiums and community hospital partnerships are two specific examples. Conversely, the *integrative* alliance or coalition is more related to market, strategic positioning, and competitive advantage. Kanter (1989) uses the term "stakeholder alliance" to describe linkages among buyers, suppliers, and customers. This type of alliance usually calls its members stakeholders. In these coalitions, both vertical and horizontal integration is evident. Such integration includes the clinical, administrative, financial, and delivery components of the organization. An example of this type of coalition in health care is the emergence of corporate partnerships linking providers (physicians), suppliers (medical supply companies or pharmacies), provider organizations (hospitals), and consumers (insurance companies or industry purchasers of health care). In the literature this may be described as an HMO, a PHO, or an IDS.

Other coalitions that are emerging or affecting health care have been reported in the literature. Many of these are not necessarily known as "business coalitions" but clearly impact health care delivery. With the shift from hospital to community-based care, there will be increasing numbers of coalitions that will bring together the business side of the health care industry, such as volunteer-run community coalitions and in some cases state and local governmental groups that assume responsibility for changing access, cost, quality, and health care policy. Russell (1992) describes the role of a nurse in mobilizing a racial-ethnic minority community to impact public policy. In this case study, a black community, through the development of a coalition, was able to change state-level child care policies by linking mothers to a child care advocacy group, a welfare watch coalition, and a welfare reform advisory committee to the state welfare department. McCray (1986) describes another example of a political coalition comprised of members from nursing speciality organizations to ensure passage of nursing specific legislation.

Rosenstein and Stier (1991) state that "health care purchasers have now begun to a take more active role in scrutinizing the actual process and outcome of health care delivery, demanding to know the indications and justifications for health care actions and interventions" (p. 175). Rooney (1992) describes the development and evolution of business coalitions among employers that are concerned about both rising costs and quality of care. Approximately 140 employers from nine states formed the Midwest Business Group on Health. This coalition developed educational programs and quality measures and conducted research designed to assist purchasers of health care.

Two examples of coalitions have linked providers, local communities, and state government to address consumer, provider, and political issues related to population-based care. First, fragmentation of care for specific populations such as technology-dependent children and their families stimulated the development of a community coalition in New York to coordinate services for this at-risk population (Lobosco, Eron, Bobo, Kril, & Chalanick, 1991). This coalition is an interagency, professional, and community collaboration at the state, regional, and local levels for the purposes of improving coordination of services for children and families. Coalitions were established through local agencies (i.e., a hospital, a pediatric pulmonary center, and a health systems agency) in which providers, parents, and community-based agencies worked together to achieve common goals. Secondly, another report of a community-wide coalition formed to promote farm health and safety was reported by Lexau, Kingsbury, Lenz, Nelson, and Voehl (1993). The Occupational Health Nurses in Agricultural Communities Project was developed by a professional organization, the state department of health, and local public health agencies to design intervention strategies using education, engineering, and enforcement in an attempt to reduce farm accidents and influence the health of agricultural families and workers. These two examples exemplify the trend toward population-based care and the potential roles for nurses in the development of and participation in coalitions to improve care.

COALITION CASE STUDY: A COMMUNITY NURSING CENTER AND SCHOOL-BASED HEALTH

The Community Nursing Center (CNC) in the School of Nursing at the University of Rochester was created to facilitate faculty practice in the community. Over a 5-year period (from 1990 to 1995), a number of community partnerships were developed for urban and rural community-based care. Advanced practice nurses provided a variety of services through community settings such as rural community hospitals, a rural hospital consortium, group homes for troubled teens, primary care offices, county health departments, and a rural county jail. With a growing reputation for development of true community-based care and commitment to community partnerships, an opportunity was presented to compete for a school-based health center grant sponsored by the New York State Department of Health.

A major ingredient for proposals and subsequent funding was the development of alliances with physician providers for referral and consultation for advanced practice nurses; with other provider organizations (such as a hospital) for 24-hour care; with the county health department that provided some school health services; with the high school where the school-based center would be housed (including students, parents, teachers, and administrators); and with the city school system. Because New York State was using these grants to stimulate development of capitated care arrangements for school-age and adolescent populations, the participation of insurance companies in these coalitions was a clear expectation. The development of coalitions in this case study reflect the purpose, reasons, and type of organizational structure previously described in this chapter.

One reason already mentioned for the development of coalitions is the need to share risk. In this coalition for school-based care, financial risk is shared primarily between the school of nursing CNC and Strong Memorial Hospital. Rosenstein (1994b) explains that financial risk to providers is not new and discusses the importance of controlling utilization along with strict monitoring of resources and costs as ways of managing risk. It is clear that the hospital agreed to share the risk and participate in this coalition, primarily to penetrate the market, develop positive community-based care partnerships, and participate in future Medicaid managed-care contracts for adolescent care initiated by the State of New York. The CNC was interested in developing a coalition with the physicians because their knowledge and competency were needed. The coalition with the hospital provided access to 24-hour care, emergency room access, and inpatient care for enrollees. Additionally, using administrative and financial services of the hospital such as billing, purchase of supplies, pharmaceuticals, and laboratory and radiography services was the most financially feasible and cost-effective approach.

Coalition relationships with the Monroe County Health Department, the Rochester City School System, East High School, and the Adolescent Medicine Department in the University of Rochester School of Medicine were developed for the purposes of coordinating activities among provider and consumer groups. Memoranda of agreement were generated and signed by each of these coalition players that identified roles and responsibilities, payment where appropriate, and an ongoing liaison structure established for quality assurance and problem-solving. These memoranda clarified relationships among all these important players in the consumer and provider community.

Key stakeholders and players from each of the coalition groups were identified early in the process, and ongoing meetings were held to involve the players in the development, implementation, and evaluation of the school health center. Additionally, expectations, authority, financial risk sharing, and roles and responsibilities of the different groups in the coalition were clarified through a combination of letters of agreement, memoranda of understanding, and contracts. An advisory committee structure was designed to facilitate involvement of the consumers in the community (students, parents, faculty, and administrators), contracted physicians, stakeholders from the health department, the school system, and the school of nursing. The advisory group is very active in policy development and review, marketing, quality assurance, and problem solving, especially related to student and parent issues. Nurses provide the leadership at the clinic site, nurture the relationships in this alliance for care of adolescents, negotiate financial arrangements and contracts, and assume full responsibility for the care of this underserved, at-risk population. The CNC is at the center of this coalition, with the strongest power and influence because this population needs the skills, knowledge, and competencies of nurses such as nurse practitioners and psychiatric–mental health clinical nurse specialists. The community expressed a need for a preventive model of care with a psychiatric–mental health component, and the CNC had practitioners with expertise in adolescent care available for this population, along with the business knowledge and expertise to put this coalition together.

IMPLICATIONS FOR NURSES AND THE NURSING PROFESSION

Rosenstein (1994a) reports that "newer industry initiatives have begun to focus on the value for the health care dollar where large health care coalitions have begun to selectively contract with those providers who deliver more effective care" (p. 53). Is nursing ready for this challenge? Nurses have a unique opportunity to position themselves for places of influence in the development of new coalitions. New roles are emerging that offer nurses opportunities to move from the traditional care provided in hospitals into entrepreneurial roles.

One new role in managed care coalitions is a disease management specialist. These specialists are often nurses who have the knowledge and expertise to manage populations of chronically ill adults and children with illnesses such as asthma, diabetes, and cardiac problems. These roles are emerging in the more mature managed care markets to do the following: (1) coordinate care across the continuum, (2) educate providers and consumers regarding prevention and health promotion, (3) facilitate interdisciplinary practice, and (4) develop outcome indicators and link processes of care to outcomes that make a difference in the cost:quality ratio. A similar role that may not be disease-specific is that of case manager or care manager. This role is often filled by baccalaureate-prepared nurses and involves development and implementation of care maps or clinical pathways. Other roles developing on the business side of these new organizations involve the management of groups of practitioners. In some settings, advanced practice nurses are already managing primary care practices with physicians in a collaborative way. Some of the managed care organizations are hiring nurses who have advanced knowledge and skills in business (master's in business administration [MBA] or master's in health administration degree) to manage some of the provider networks or coalitions associated with the managed care organization. There is a unique niche in the future for blending business and clinical practice. This is evidenced by increasing numbers of physicians now getting MBA or law degrees in order to continue to control clinical decision making instead of just defaulting to the business expert in the organization.

Other new roles that are emerging are related to the data and research needed to measure cost and quality outcomes of care. Some disease management teams in mature managed care organizations have an expert in data and information analysis on the team as an equal player with the clinician. New roles for nurse informaticists are clear, particularly those interested in tracking and analyzing relevant data specifically related to the processes and outcomes of care. There are new roles for nurse researchers, particularly those interested in practice-based research, and cost and quality outcomes research. More comparative studies demonstrating the cost-effectiveness of nurse-managed models of care such as birthing centers and nursing centers with sound methodological approaches are needed. Stone and Hinton Walker (1995) used decision analysis to demonstrate the cost-effectiveness of free-standing birthing centers versus traditional hospital care.

Whether nurses are employed in one of the new nurse-managed care structures, in hospitals, home health agencies, physicians' offices, public health departments, or are self-employed, each person must strengthen his or her knowledge of reimbursement, costs, and quality and negotiate carefully in the managed care arena. It is important for nurses in community-based organizations, like the nursing center described in this chapter, to position themselves for participation in managed care contracts. There are also faculty practices at the Frances Payne Bolton School of Nursing of Case Western Reserve University in Ohio, and in nursing centers in Arizona, Tennessee, Texas, and Wisconsin that are planning for managed care contracts. However, beyond coalitions for practice, there is a need for education and research coalitions. Practice-based research networks, specifically linking processes of care to nurse-sensitive outcomes (cost, quality care, and customer satisfaction) must be developed. The nursing profession must also develop new coalitions to facilitate both informal and formal education for managed care in innovative ways, such as coalitions between academic institutions and managed care organizations. The Frances Payne Bolton School of Nursing of Case Western Reserve University has taken a leadership role in developing coalition relationships with managed care organizations for research and education. At this time, joint research projects have been submitted for national funding, and a Managed Care Institute is in the planning stage with organizations such as the Henry Ford Health System and Group Health Association of America.

> Many of tomorrow's most intriguing opportunities—interactive television, on-board navigational systems for cars and trucks, cell therapy, remote at-home medical diagnostics, satellite personal communication devises, a national video register of homes for sale, an alternative to internal combustion engine—will require the integration of skills and capabilities residing in a wide variety of companies. (Hamel and Prahalad, 1994, p. 276)

Business coalitions will dominate all markets, including health care. Managed care and the new competitive arena in health care offers intriguing opportunities for nursing within the traditional health care industries (e.g., hospitals, home health, long-term care) as well as in insurance companies, industries struggling with the management of their own health costs (occupational medicine), and within a variety of new managed care organizational structures. Currently, many organizations are downsizing to manage costs, but mature managed care organizations are more concerned about what drives costs, particularly outside of the acute care setting. Nurses know how to address many of the problems driving cost of care through holistic approaches to care, integration of the family, and addressing community-based care issues.

Are nurses ready for the challenge? Will nurses seize this opportunity to provide population-based care? Nurses must accept and use this new way of delivering health care and prepare. The time is now! Choose to take the following steps. Be more knowledgeable about business processes and priorities. Embrace and actively learn about the financial side of health care. Measure both cost and quality outcomes of the health care value coin. Strengthen your interpersonal and facilitating skills for interdisciplinary care. Develop negotiation and bargaining skills for contracts and coalition. Courageously develop both internal and external coalitions in order to be a full member/player in the future of health care in the United States.

REFERENCES

Hamel, G., & Prahalad, C.K. (1994). *Competing for the future: Breakthrough strategies for seizing control of your industry and creating the markets of tomorrow* (p. 23). Boston, MA: Harvard Business Press.

Kaluzny, A.D., Zuckerman, H.S., & Ricketts III, T.C. (with Walton, G.B.) (Eds.). (1995). Strategic alliances: A worldwide phenomenon comes to health care. *Partners for the dance: Forming strategic alliances in health care* (pp. 1-15, pp. 199-218). Ann Arbor, MI: Health Administration Press.

Kanter, R.M. (1989, August). Becoming PALs: Pooling, allying, and linking across companies. *Academy of Management Executives,* 3, 183-193.

Lexau, C., Kingsbury, L., Lenz, B., Nelson, C., & Voehl, S. (1993). Building coalitions: A community wide approach for promoting farming health and safety. *American Association of Mental Health Nurses, 41,* 440-463.

Lobosco, A., Eron, N., Bobo, T., Kril, L., & Chalanick, K. (1991). Local coalitions for coordinating services to children dependent on technology and their families. *Childrens Health Care, 20,* 75-86.

McCray, N. (1986). Networks and coalitions: Tools for strength. *Oncology Nursing Forum, 13,* 103-104.

Merriam-Webster Collegiate Dictionary. (1995). (10th ed., pp. 30, 219, 247, 848). Springfield, MA: Merriam Webster.

Mintzberg, H. (1977). Policy as a field of management theory. *Academy of Management Review, 2,* 88-103.

Rooney, E. (1992). Business coalitions on health care: An evolution from cost containment to quality improvement. *American Association of Occupational Health Nurses, 40,* 342-351.

Russell, K. (1992). Strengthening black and minority community coalitions for health policy action. *Journal of National Black Nurses 6,* 42-47.

Rosenstein, A.H. (1994a). Cost-effective health care: Tools for improvement. *Health Care Management Review 19,* 53-61.

Rosenstein, A.H. (1994b). Financial risk, accountability and outcome management: Using data to manage and measure clinical performance. *Hospital & Health Services Administration, 9,* 116-121.

Rosenstein, A.H., & Stier, M. (1991). Health resources management and physician control in a San Francisco, California hospital. *The Western Journal of Medicine 154,* 175-181.

Schroeder, S.A. (1994). The President's message: Cost containment. *The Robert Wood Johnson Foundation Annual Report: Cost containment* (pp. 6-23). Princeton, NJ: Robert Wood Johnson Foundation.

Stone, P.W., & Hinton Walker, P. (1995). Cost-effective analysis: Birth center vs. hospital care. *Nursing Economic$ 13,* 299-308.

Tichy, N.M. (1983). *Managing strategic change: Technical, political and cultural dynamics.* New York, Chichester, Brisband Toronto, Singapore: John Wiley and Sons.

Toward a comprehensive health care system: Example of a statewide system

CECELIA CAPUZZI

STATE HEALTH CARE REFORM

Historically, states have led the movement in health care (Rogal & Helms, 1993). Several bellweather states began health care reform in the mid-1980s (e.g., Massachusetts, Oregon), and in 1992, the National Governor's Association made health care reform a priority (Curley, Omata, & Luehrs, 1992).

There are several reasons why states have initiated their own health care reforms. One compelling factor was the rising costs of health care in conjunction with state budget limitations (Blankenau, 1994; Coopers & Lybrand Health Decisions Resource Group, 1994; Curley et al., 1992). In addition, in most states there were rising numbers of uninsured individuals (Coopers & Lybrand Health Decisions Resource Group, 1994; Curley et al., 1992) and significant problems with small businesses providing health insurance (Rogal & Helms, 1993). Moreover, some states were experiencing an increase in the number of immigrants (Coopers & Lybrand Health Decisions Resource Group, 1994).

When federal changes in health care did not materialize quickly in 1993, many states believed that there was no option but to advance their own health reforms (Blankenau, 1994). In addition, many states did not want health care reforms passed down from the national level; they wanted to craft their own systems (Friedman, 1994). Lastly, some states are currently initiating reforms and seeking waivers from the federal government to lock into place their base budgets in the anticipation of increasing federal budget problems in the future (Blankenau, 1994).

Types of reforms

There are a variety of health care reforms being proposed by individual states (Barrand & Schroeder, 1994). While most states agree on the need for universal coverage, proposals for meeting this goal are varied and controversial (Rogal & Helms, 1993). Some states are enacting limited changes, while others are attempting to be comprehensive (Curley et al., 1992; Palmer, 1994). Additionally, most states initiating reform are building on existing public and private systems (Curley et al., 1992). Those states that are reforming the current system are creating market incentives to encourage providers, insurers, and consumers to be cost-conscious. They are also increasing regulations to ensure fairness in the insurance and health care markets and to increase the efficiency of Medicaid (Curley et al., 1992).

Health care reform also includes altering the composition of the health provider workforce because this too affects health care costs, access, and quality (Weissert, Knott, & Stieber, 1994). The box lists the major types of health care reform being proposed by various states.

Advantages and disadvantages of state reform

There are both advantages and disadvantages to states initiating health care reform. One advantage is that these states can act as laboratories to test different types of changes before reforms are enacted on a wider scale. In addition, these state "experiments" show how the major players—employers, providers, insurers, and consumers—react to the varying initiatives (Barrand & Schroeder, 1994; Rogal & Helms, 1993). Secondly, states can adapt health care reforms to meet their specific needs and conform to their historical, social, demographic, and infrastructural variations (Barrand & Schroeder, 1994; Friedman, 1994). Further, states can adopt reforms more quickly than the federal government and can get better

TYPES OF HEALTH CARE REFORM

- **Coverage** (universal)
- **Benefits**
  - Basic
  - Prevention
- **Cost-containment**
  - Limiting administrative costs
  - Utilization control
  - Technology assessment
  - Certificate of need
  - Practice guidelines
  - Tort reform
  - Global budgeting
  - Expenditure targets
  - Managed competition
  - Consumer education
- **Insurance reform**
  - Rate restrictions
  - Prohibiting the use of medical underwriting criteria such as preexisting conditions
  - Establishing small group market plans
  - Improving portability
  - Establishing state reinsurance pools and high-risk pools
  - Community rating
- **Financing**
  - Employer mandates
  - Individual mandates
  - Expanding Medicaid
  - Subsidizing insurance premiums for low-income individuals
  - Single-payer and multipayer systems
  - Cost-sharing
- **Service delivery**
  - Encouraging primary care providers through regulation, reimbursement, targeted programs, and education
  - Organizing systems of care (e.g., managed care)
- **Data enhancement**
  - Developing shared data sets
- **Quality**
  - Consumer score cards
  - Requiring quality assurance

(Compiled from Coopers & Lybrand Health Decisions Resource Group, 1994; Curley et al., 1993; Rogal & Helms, 1993; Weissert, et al., 1994.)

consensus for implementation because the designs are of their own making (Friedman, 1994).

There also are some major disadvantages to having states initiate health care reforms. The biggest disadvantage is that individual state initiatives continue the patchwork system of health care (Friedman, 1994). Specifically, individual state initiatives that change health insurance laws create problems for businesses that operate in several states (Barrand & Schroeder, 1994). Also, some states will not develop reforms, and adjoining states that do are at a disadvantage (Friedman, 1994). Another disadvantage is that most states lack the financial resources to enact major changes (Barrand & Schroeder, 1994; Friedman, 1994; Rogal & Helms, 1993) and lack the data systems necessary for making rational reforms (Barrand & Schroeder, 1994). Thirdly, some federal laws such as the Employee Retirement Income Security Act (ERISA), which focuses on employer insurance, inhibit state reforms (Barrand & Schroeder, 1994). Fourth, some believe health care reform at the state level will be as difficult to implement as reform at the federal level because it is a political issue at both levels (Barrand & Schroeder, 1994). Moreover, it is difficult to maintain a commitment to specific health reform strategies over time because of high turnover in many state legislatures, especially now that some states have enacted term limits (Friedman, 1994). Lastly, some critics believe state reforms will delay federal actions and will be difficult to operate once federal reform occurs (Barrand & Schroeder, 1994).

HEALTH CARE REFORM IN OREGON
The Oregon Health Plan

With enactment of The Oregon Health Plan in 1989, Oregon began health care reform that changed the financing for health care, the delivery system, and the health policy process. The goal was to ensure universal access for all citizens to a basic set of health services (Kitzhaber, 1990).

The impetus for this health care reform was the increasing numbers of people who were uninsured and the rising costs of health care (Kitzhaber, 1991). In addition, policymakers were dissatisfied with the then current process for making health care resource decisions. There was the realization that legislators and administrators were implicitly rationing health care each time a health care allocation decision was made. The Oregon Health Plan changed the decision-making process so that explicit policy outcomes would be derived with input from a broader array of individuals.

The current Oregon Health Plan is a compilation of several bills enacted over a 6-year period. Three keystone bills were enacted during the 1989 legislature (Oregon Department of Human Resources, 1993). Senate Bill 27 expanded the numbers of people covered by Medicaid by increasing eligibility to 100% of the federal poverty level.

SUMMARY OF SENATE BILL 27

1. Provide medical assistance to those in need whose family income is below the federal poverty level.
2. Establish a Health Services Commission that will develop a list of health services ranked by priority (with certain exemptions).
3. Submit a report on the list of health services ranked by priority, from the most important to the least important, representing the comparative benefits of each service to the entire population to be served, to the Joint Legislative Committee on Health Care and to the governor in the following session.
4. Conduct public hearings prior to making the report.
5. Solicit testimony and information from advocates for seniors; handicapped persons; mental health services consumers; low-income Oregonians; and providers of health care including but not limited to physicians licensed to practice medicine, dentists, oral surgeons, chiropractors, naturopaths, hospitals, clinics, pharmacists, nurses, and allied health professionals.
6. Solicit public involvement in a community meeting process.
7. Obtain an actuarial report to determine the rates necessary to cover the costs of services.
8. Services are offered under prepaid managed care contracts when feasible.

A summary of Senate Bill 27 is outlined in the box. Senate Bill 935 required all businesses, including small businesses, to offer health insurance to their employees and dependents or to contribute to a state insurance pool by 1994 (this date has subsequently been extended); and Senate Bill 534 mandated the state to establish a high-risk insurance pool. The intent of Senate Bills 534 and 935 was to provide the same benefits derived from the prioritized list of health services that governs Medicaid (Senate Bill 27).

In order to implement Senate Bill 27, Oregon needed a waiver from the federal government. After submitting a proposal and then modifying it, a 5-year waiver was granted by the Health Care Financing Administration, and the expanded Medicaid program began February 1994.

In the ensuing 6 years, additional legislation has been enacted to increase the comprehensiveness of the health reform. Table 58-1 summarizes this legislation.

Besides this legislation, several other health reform events occurred in Oregon during this time. In 1993, the Office of Health Policy (a state agency) received a 2-year Robert Wood Johnson grant to conduct a series of activities to further health care reform (Office of Health Policy, 1992). In addition, the governor reactivated the Oregon Health Council (OHC), a 16-member board comprised of health providers, purchasers, and consumers, and charged the group to "present a State Health Plan for Oregon that will assure universal access to quality health care at a reasonable cost to all Oregonians by the year 1996" (OHC 1995 p. 7). Furthermore, the Health Service Commission began a project to develop and utilize practice

Table 58-1 Legislation comprising the Oregon health plan

Year	Bill No.	Description
1989	Senate Bill 27	Expanded Medicaid
	Senate Bill 935	Developed employer mandate and small business insurance pool
	Senate Bill 534	Developed high-risk insurance pool
1991	Senate Bill 44	Added mental health services and the elderly and disabled populations to the Medicaid expansion
	House Bill 1076	Initiated select health insurance reforms for small businesses
	House Bill 1077	Created the Health Resources Commission to develop alternatives to the certificate of need process. (In 1993, the legislature redefined the mission of the Health Resources Commission to medical technology assessment.)
1993	Senate Bill 5530	Created the position of Administrator of the Oregon Health Plan and initiated activities to further develop a comprehensive health care system; also delayed implementation of the employer mandate until 1998
1995	House Bill 1079	Consolidated the health reform activities under the Administrator of the Oregon Health Plan
	Senate Bill 152	Enacted additional insurance reform including the establishment of standardized benefit plans
	Senate Bill 1155	Repealed the employer insurance mandate (was vetoed by the governor)

(Compiled from Gates, 1994; Mapps, 1995; Oregon Department of Human Resources, 1993.)

guidelines in conjunction with prioritizing health services for the basic benefit package. Although cost containment and increasing the quality of care were underlying goals of the Oregon Health Plan, these later activities brought these issues of cost and quality to the forefront.

CURRENT OUTCOMES: ONE STEP FORWARD, ONE STEP BACK

Outcomes for Oregonians

The case of Oregon's health care reform is a true study of incrementalism. Although the 1989 legislation appeared radical, it was just one step in initiating comprehensive health reform. Subsequent legislation has added other needed components. As with incrementalism, parts of the original plan have been modified in response to new information.

On the positive side, with the Medicaid waiver, Oregon became a "laboratory" to test the process of ranking health services. This experiment is continuing with refinements in the process and with seeming success. Despite dire predictions of rationing care, more Oregonians now have access to health care. As of August 1994, more than 81,000 new people were enrolled in the plan (Oregon Health Plan Monitor, 1994). In addition, these individuals now have access to preventive services.

On the down side, health care reform in Oregon has also had setbacks. In 1989, the legislation appeared to take a big step forward in providing universal health coverage for all Oregonians. Today, the step is less gigantic. As predicted with any state initiative, the impetus for health care reform has waned, particularly on the issue of an employer mandate. Many of the major players in the legislature in 1989 have since left, and the current members are less enamored with the original plan. Fortunately, the originator of the legislation is currently the state's governor.

Federal regulations (e.g., ERISA) have also delayed implementation of the employer mandate legislation. At this time, Oregon is awaiting a federal waiver. If the waiver is not received by January 1996, the state mandate is automatically repealed; and it does not appear that the federal government with its Republican majority will be inclined to grant this request (Mapps, 1995).

Additionally, a property tax limitation measure passed in 1991 decreased state revenues for the past 4 years. This legislation, along with the "no new taxes" environment, has seriously affected further health care reform that requires additional revenues.

The Oregon health care "experiment" also has demonstrated how the major players would respond. When it became clear that those with health insurance might have reduced benefits if all health insurance plans in Oregon used the same guidelines specified by Senate Bill 27, there was major backtracking. The first group to retreat was the state legislators, who voted down legislation affecting their health care benefits. When the lobbying became fierce, these legislators also backed off from requiring those insured through the small business insurance pool to receive benefits identical to those of the Medicaid population.

Outcomes for nurses

The Oregon Health Plan has had both a positive and negative impact on nurses. On the positive side, Senate Bill 27 changed the policy decision-making process to an explicit process and mandated the involvement of nurses. (Other articles describe nurses' involvement [Capuzzi, 1993, 1994]). Subsequently, nurses also have been involved with the Office of Health Policy, the Oregon Health Plan Administrator's Office, and the OHC.

On the down side, health care reform has created new problems for nurses. A major component of Senate Bill 27 was that of providing care through managed care organizations (MCOs). Again, the response of the major players became clear. Initially, there was a flurry of activity to form MCOs, with the major providers (e.g., hospital systems) seeking the best alliances to secure the largest market share. Additionally, other smaller clinics and individual providers needed to align themselves with MCOs or they would be blocked from being reimbursed for care provided to this population.

The move to managed care had a major impact on nurses in Oregon. Advanced practice nurses, unless associated with an MCO, could no longer get reimbursed for services provided to the Medicaid population. Additionally, many advanced practice nurses found that despite being part of an MCO, they were not receiving referrals from primary care providers, particularly if these providers had negative economic incentives to refer.

Nurses working in hospitals were also impacted by this trend. Hospital administrators attempting to lower costs are hiring more nonnurse personnel and are decreasing patient:nursing staffing ratios. Hospital administrators also attempted to eliminate the board of nursing's control over nursing practice in the 1995 legislative session so as to have more freedom in using nonlicensed patient care personnel. The hospital association lobbyists were formidable and nearly won this battle despite solid nursing opposition.

CONCLUSION

There are many components to comprehensive health care reform. Some reform efforts are explicitly directed toward nurses and other providers (e.g., ratio of primary care providers to specialists); while other reforms have indirect effects (e.g., limiting access of nurse to clients). State health care reform efforts provide nurses with more direct opportunities for shaping a new system. Health care reform will occur at the state level whether nurses are involved or not. It is imperative for nurses to become involved so that they can control their practice as well as shape a desirable system for consumers.

REFERENCES

Barrand, N.L., & Schroeder, S.A. (1994). Lessons from the states. *Inquiry, 31,* 10-13.

Blankenau, R. (1994). Forging ahead with no national reform, states look to tackle Medicaid issues. *Hospitals & Health Networks, 68*(22), 40, 43.

Capuzzi, C. (1993). Rationing health care: The Oregon story. In D.J. Mason, S.W. Talbott, & J.K. Leavitt (Eds.), *Policy and Politics for Nurses* (pp. 208-220). Philadelphia: Saunders.

Capuzzi, C. (1994). The Oregon model of decision making and its implications for nursing practice. In J. McCloskey & H.K. Grace (Eds.), *Current Issues in Nursing* (4th ed., pp. 711-717). St. Louis: Mosby.

Coopers & Lybrand Health Decisions Resource Group. (1994). Health-care reform: Innovations at the state level. *Nursing Management, 25,* 30-42.

Curley, T., Omata, R., & Luehrs, J. (1992). *State progress in health care reform, 1992.* Washington, DC: National Governors Association.

Friedman, E. (1994). Getting a head start: The states and health care reform. *Journal of the American Medical Association, 271,* 875-878.

Gates, V. (1994, February 2). *Oregon health plan status report.* Salem, OR: Office of the Health Plan Administrator.

Kitzhaber, J. (1990). *The Oregon Basic Health Services Act.* Salem, OR: Oregon Senate.

Kitzhaber, J. (1991, August). *Presentation at the 1991 Conference on Health Care: The Oregon solution.* Portland, OR.

Mapps, J. (1995, June 7). Kitzhaber struggles to save health insurance requirement, *Oregonian,* pp. B1, B4.

Office of Health Policy. (1992, March 2). *Planning for universal access: The Oregon health plan.* Portland, OR: Department of Human Resources.

Oregon Department of Human Resources. (1993, August 23). *The Oregon health plan.* Salem, OR: Oregon Department of Human Resources.

Oregon Health Council. (1995, February). *Recommendations for a fair and affordable health system: Report to Governor John A. Kitzhaber.* Portland, OR: Office of Health Policy.

Oregon Health Plan Monitor. (1994, July/August). More than 81,000 enroll in 6 months. *Oregon Health Plan Monitor, 1*(2), p. 1.

Palmer, P.N. (1994). Attention shifts to state health care reform efforts. *AORN Journal, 60,* 989.

Rogal, D.L., & Helms, W.D. (1993). State models: An overview. Tracking states' efforts to reform their health systems, *Health Affairs, 12,* 27-30.

Weissert, C.S., Knott, J.H., & Stieber, B.E. (1994). Education and the health professions: Explaining policy choices among the states. *Journal of Health Politics, Policy and Law, 19,* 361-392.

Nursing practice in a political era*

MARLA E. SALMON

The point of view to be explored in this chapter is fairly simple and reflects a chain of logic that is fundamental to understanding nursing and health services in the United States. First, politics and public policy play major roles in shaping the current and emerging state of health care in the United States. Second, any shift toward a more health-oriented system will be driven largely by political and market forces. Third, professional nurses, whose primary orientation is toward promoting and protecting health, have a major stake in shifting the system toward one in which health is a primary goal.

These three statements should lead to a simple conclusion: If the system of health care in the United States is to become one in which nursing plays a major professional role, then nurses will need to assume responsibility for directing the political forces that are driving this system. In other words, professional nursing practice cannot exist in a politicized health care system without nurses practicing politics.

This chapter explores these three statements and the conclusion drawn from them regarding the necessity of nursing's political action. This chapter should challenge all nurses to examine their own engagement in the practice of health policy.

THE HEALTH CARE SYSTEM AS A PRODUCT OF POLITICS

In examining the history of the health care system of the United States one does not see a neat evolution of an organized mechanism for responding to the health care needs of the people. In the tradition of individualism and entrepreneurialism that characterizes the development of this country, the development of health care in the United States has been anything but systematic. Whether this disorder is explained through the lenses of a Norman Rockwell–like image of the fatherly physician guiding health care on a person-by-person basis or through a picture of a system shaped by professional dominance, shifting political agendas, and individual and corporate greed, it is clear that the delivery of health care in this country does not reflect a well-thought-out approach to meeting peoples' health care needs.

The rather chaotic nature of health care in the United States, however, is the very reason why politics and public policy are so important to its future. Throughout this century, government has been asked again and again by society to fix the system in a number of ways—including protecting people from unsafe medical practice, ensuring access to care, setting limits on how industry behaves, financing research to move health care forward, and constructing health care facilities, among others.

The involvement of government in health care, which actually began in 1798 with compulsory hospital insurance for merchant seamen (Mullan, 1989), initially focused on the development of public health interventions. Efforts to develop a social insurance-based system of health care in the early part of this century did not succeed (Starr, 1982). As a result, a pattern of fragmentation of financing and health care delivery was set into motion that has continued through today. The role of government inevitably has been sporadic, ranging from active intervention to invisibility. This is not to say that there have not been forces driving what we see today. On the contrary, our health care "nonsystem" is the direct result of such factors as professional self-interest, corporate interest, and political action—none of which have been mutually exclusive. Political action has been the vehicle for both professional and corporate self-interest. In addition, it has been the single most important voice for the consumer—the mechanism for the people to have a voice.

*The views expressed here are solely those of the author and not necessarily those of the Department of Health and Human Services.

To understand how these forces have worked, one need only consider what has transpired with national health care reform since 1993. National health care reform was a major plank in the Clinton presidential campaign. With nearly 40 million Americans lacking health care insurance, millions of others uninsured, and growing concern about the runaway costs of health care, national health care reform was seen as a critical problem for the United States. Americans seemed to want the federal government to "fix" the problems of health care. As a result, the Clinton Administration launched its Task Force on Health Care Reform and developed a proposal for comprehensive national health care reform that was formalized in the President's proposed Health Security Act.

The national debate on health care reform during that period was also heavily influenced by professional and corporate interest. Organized nursing, for example, was a very vocal advocate for national reform and had set its interests in motion with the development of Nursing's Agenda for Health Care Reform in 1991 (American Nurses Association, 1991). Other professional groups were less supportive of overall health care reform. Corporations, particularly those with a stake in the current system (e.g., insurers and pharmaceutical manufacturers), weighed heavily in the final outcomes of the national health care reform effort.

One major lesson that was learned from the defeat of national health care reform was that health care had become unquestionably politicized. Through the political process, the nature of the health care system made a major shift to a highly market-driven system in which the role of government became less, rather than more, directive.

MOVEMENT TO A HEALTH-ORIENTED SYSTEM

The overall goals of national health care reform were aimed at increasing access, reducing cost, and ensuring quality of services. These are not equally addressed by the emerging market-driven system. The goal of reducing cost combined with the related interest in enhancing corporate gain and profit are the most heavily reflected in today's medical marketplace. There are some who believe that the competitive forces of the market will eventually result in the improvement of quality of care. There is also a belief that reduction in the overall cost of health care will allow public resources to be stretched further to enhance access. Others are not nearly as sanguine. What is clear, however, is that the reduction of cost and increase in profit in the health care system has moved provider organizations to take a closer look at earlier and less expensive health care interventions.

The critical question, of course, relates to whether the current wildfire corporatization of health care will actually result in enhancement of health. Unlike the national health care reform proposal of the Clinton Administration, the system that we see evolving does not yet have clear mechanisms in place relating to quality of care and access. The traditional relationship between patient and provider, which was shaped by professional and legal checks and balances, has been overshadowed by a less well-understood relationship between payers and health care organizations. In the past, health professionals have been major determinants of the quality and nature of health care. Licensure, state practice acts, education, and professionalization have been viewed as mechanisms for ensuring quality and expressing the public's endorsement of health professionals' roles.

With the movement away from provider-patient control of health care delivery, there is uncertainty on the part of patients and providers regarding the control of health care. As a result, emerging concerns are becoming expressed politically. One indicator of this type of political activity is the passage of state legislation dictating the minimum length of hospitals stays for new mothers and babies. Other political efforts seem to be aimed at putting into place some legislative checks and balances at state levels relating to accountability for quality and access.

There are also major political efforts underway relating to the roles and licensure of health professionals. The health care system that is emerging, again primarily market driven, is seeking to achieve as much flexibility and as many efficiencies as possible relating to health workers. As a result, the traditional health professions, including medicine and nursing, are potential targets for major change. Questions are emerging about the needs for state licensure and its role in the new health care system; interest in "institutional" licensure appears to be increasing. A fundamental question that is surfacing in health care is who is responsible for the quality of health care and what mechanisms need to be in place to ensure the quality of care. An underlying question, of course, is if health care providers do not have control over the delivery of care, how can they actually ensure its quality?

If this discussion creates some discomfort in the nurse reader, it should. While nursing as a profession has made major gains in the last century in its ability to function as a profession (Keeling & Ramos, 1995), its impact on the delivery of services may be in serious jeopardy. To be sure, there will always be nurses. The more important question is whether or not they will play the roles for which they are prepared. The simple relationship between nurse, patients, and families is no longer simple. The major players in the health care system—care organization, payer, politics, and public policy—are increasingly determining whether or not a nurse even comes into contact with the patient and his or her family. If nursing has as its fundamental purpose the enhancement and preservation of the health of people, it can no longer do so only through the interactions of those people it "sees." Nursing must move its practice to a broader social level and involve itself with the forces that are, in fact, shaping that system.

NURSING AS A POLITICAL PROFESSION

The notion that politics and health are intrinsically linked is not new. In fact, Nightingale herself clearly made the connection between the political decisions of Parliament in England and the conditions in which soldiers found themselves in the Crimea. American nursing has also known of this link and has involved itself in shaping the political forces that impact health. Health policy in the early part of this century was influenced by the voices of such remarkable nurses as Sanger, Wald, and Dock, who understood clearly that the plight of those whom they hoped to serve was influenced heavily by the presence or absence of sound public policy (Hall-Long, 1995). They were consummate political activists who were clear that their advocacy was on behalf of the people whom they served. Their common goal was to enhance the health of these people through constructive public policy.

The realization of the importance of political activism in nursing has not been restricted to the notables of the beginning of this century. These last nine decades in nursing have seen a dramatic increase in the numbers of professional organizations and the rise in organized political activism in nursing. Nursing has recognized the importance of political activism to its own survival and to the health of the people it serves. Nursing's prominence in the national health care reform debates is a strong indicator of nursing's political successes (Clinton, 1993; "Health Care Reform," 1993; Sprayberry, 1993).

Given nursing's political sophistication, one might question why it is now necessary to call for political action on the part of nurses. The imperative rests in the recognition that this emerging health care system is unlike any we have seen before; the roles of nurses and other health professionals in the system are increasingly less clear; and the impact of this system on the health of people has yet to be demonstrated. In short, the stakes are very high for both the health of people and the future of nursing.

So what should nursing do? First, it is essential that nursing accept political responsibility for the current and future health care system. This is not to say that nurses alone are responsible for what has or will transpire. Rather, if nursing is to play a crucial role in the health of people in the future, it must assume responsibility for the system on a larger societal level. It is not enough to be responsible for only those people we touch in the everyday delivery of care. Because the marketplace and politics are key venues for making an impact, nursing must "weigh in" politically. Because so much of the political action in health care will occur at state and national levels, these should be the primary foci for major nursing political activity.

Secondly, nursing must examine critically what it has done in the area of political action and where it wishes to go. The tradition of nursing political action has been one in which nursing has focused largely on unifying its own political forces within the profession and on issues relating to the profession itself or to specific proposed legislative agendas. It is important to analyze these dimensions of political activity carefully.

There are a number of examples of the unification of nursing's political clout. Perhaps the most prominent is the formation of the Tri-Council for Nursing in 1981, composed initially of the American Nurses Association, the National League for Nursing, and the American Association of Colleges of Nursing and, later, the American Organization of Nurse Executives. This alliance and others have been instrumental in galvanizing the various interests across organized nursing into consolidated political action. Certainly each of the professional organizations representing nursing or subsets of nursing is a form of organizing nursing's political clout.

While nursing has become quite sophisticated about alliances across nursing and consolidating its own political power, the political challenges facing the profession call for expanding effectively beyond nursing's own boundaries. Although nursing has at times developed alliances with other groups in both state and national political arenas, this has not been the hallmark of its ongoing political activism. This must change. As the impact of the marketplace increasingly overshadows the roles that health professionals and patients play in the determination of care, two types of natural alliances seem to be emerging.

The first natural alliance is probably the least comfortable for organized nursing and its potential counterpart, organized medicine. Although there are clearly longstanding chasms in the political landscape between the two groups, there is a rapidly expanding common ground that needs to be cultivated by both. Nursing, medicine, and other health professional groups are experiencing major threats to both their professional autonomy and the quality of care for which they have traditionally been responsible. If the emerging health care system is to achieve a reasonable set of checks and balances in which cost is part of a larger equation that includes quality and access, it will be because of social and political activism. It makes great sense that nursing and medicine should lead in these efforts, given their longstanding shared social mandate of caring for the health of people.

The second natural alliance is with consumers and communities. As our health care system emerges, major changes are taking place in the ways in which care is delivered and its impact on communities. For example, the community hospital or clinic may be a very important institution to the community in which it is located. Unfortunately, these very resources may cease to exist in the face of new ways of delivering service. So also is the case with the individual physician or other provider. Systems of service also means systems of providers. The fabric of communities will increasingly be affected by the changes in the overall system.

For the individual consumer, the emerging health care system also indicates major change. As individual concerns become more public, individual activism will also become better organized. The history of health policy nationally is one in which consumers have organized and weighed in on the debates. One only need examine the debates around the restructuring of Medicare and the grave and growing concerns about the financing of health care for older Americans to see this type of consumer activism.

As the concerns and involvement of consumers become better organized, nursing has an opportunity to amplify and focus its own political power. Nursing has claimed that one of its key roles is that of patient's advocate. The alliance of organized nursing with organized consumer groups is the political equivalent to the individual nurse serving as the patient's advocate.

Let's look again now at what nursing should be concerned with politically. The themes of the Clinton health care reform agenda are still compelling and valid—high-quality, affordable health care for all people. Nursing's political agenda should continue to focus on these key goals and it should do so in partnership with others who share those commitments.

NURSING'S ACTIVISM IN HEALTH POLICY: GOING BEYOND A NARROW VIEW OF POLITICAL ACTIVISM

Any discussion of the impact of nursing on a societal level must go beyond the rather restrictive view of political activism. Nurses need to see themselves as politically responsible—well beyond the basic function of voting. Nursing must also see itself as politically responsible beyond influencing the legislative process through lobbying and grassroots efforts. These are certainly essential and a part of all that has been discussed here. Nursing, however, must view itself as engaged in all of the processes that result in public policy relating to health. This is a far broader agenda and requires consideration of ground that is probably not very familiar to nurses.

Perhaps the easiest way to describe where nurses should "weigh in" is to describe the dimensions of public policy that affect health care today. The first is the identification of problems that need policy solutions. Surely there is no better time than now to begin to identify what is not working well about the emerging system of health care. What is important to note here is that initially identifying problems in a politically relevant way is frequently best done through use of media and anecdotal evidence. This is not to say that one should not attempt to document problems carefully. Rather it is to suggest that the political system is highly media-sensitive and tends to be more responsive to those issues that receive the attention of the media. Now is the time for nurses to tell their stories and the stories of those they serve. One cannot expect policymakers to become concerned about problems that are not brought to their attention. This is an area in which nurses should become better equipped. For better or worse, Americans look to media such as talk-radio, exposé reporting, and afternoon talk shows to inform their opinions. Nurses need to become "fluent" in the ways in which people get and give information.

Once problems are identified, the transition to developing viable policy agendas can be difficult. Policy agenda setting in the area of health care benefits tremendously from having people in public office and public service who understand the problems related to health care delivery and are knowledgeable about and committed to health issues. Nurses need to participate actively in the development of health agendas, not just in influencing legislation. Because these agendas generally precede the development of legislation and involve policymakers, nurses should become involved in agenda setting through service in political office and other roles directly related to this process at all levels. For example, the U.S. Congress has been heavily influenced in health-related policy matters by the Physician Payment Review Commission, a national advisory body composed of health care experts, and other national advisory groups. Membership in such groups is very important to nursing. As well, serving in Congress or state legislatures is a role that nurses should play, and congressional and legislative staff positions are also roles in which nurses can make major contributions. The message here, of course, is that nurses should seek public policy careers in both elected and career types of service.

Once a policy agenda is developed, it may then move to the stage of developing program proposals and supportive legislation. In the area of health, this means that nurses should be playing active roles in developing the actual strategies for addressing the problems and implementing an agenda. Again, active, ongoing roles in Congress and state legislatures are very important for nursing involvement. As proposals and actual legislation move forward, it is also important that nurses be prepared to serve as experts in informing the process by providing testimony and input to legislators. (However, if this is all that nurses do, it is simply not enough.)

It is important to note here that not all policy is enacted through legislation. Most presidents and governors come into office with their own policy platforms and seek to accomplish these through both the executive and legislative branches of government. Their choices of political appointees for key positions can have a major impact on the nature of governmental action. Nurses should seek political appointment and understand the type of political activism that is required to become positioned for these types of appointments.

For policy that is enacted through legislation, though, the stage following enactment is one in which nursing should also play a key role. The actual implementation of legislation moves the law into the "machinery" of government and relies on the bureaucracy to do what is intended legislatively. There is usually latitude in the interpretation and implementation of legislation; most laws are not microscopic in their language. The old adage about "the devil is in the details" is very true when it comes to actually making laws work. Implementation of health legislation can benefit greatly from the advice and involvement of nurses. Most nurses probably do not consider moving into careers in government. However, the important knowledge and skills that nurses can bring to moving legislation into actual implementation should not be overlooked. Nurses interested in policy should consider both the executive and legislative branches of government as career options.

Finally, laws that have been enacted generally have some requirements or expectations for assessment of impact. Frequently, assessments of this type are undertaken as studies or projects by contractors outside of the government itself. This is an area in which nurses can also play roles. Schools of nursing, for example, might begin to look at evaluation research contracts as an area in which their nurse researchers might be involved. Nurse researchers themselves should consider conducting health services research that can shed light on the impact of policy on the delivery and effectiveness of health services. Nurses should actively seek opportunities to become involved in all dimensions of the assessment of government program effectiveness.

SUMMARY

The ability of nurses to practice nursing and have a positive impact on health is no longer primarily determined by the capabilities of the individual nurse and the health status of individual patients and families. Nursing, as with all that is health care today, is being shaped by the societal forces found in the marketplace and the public policy arena. If nursing is to be all that it claims—the patient's advocate and a profession with a commitment to achieving, protecting, and preserving health—then it must strive to direct those forces that are shaping the system of health care delivery in this country. In other words, the practice of nursing at all levels should include the practice of public policy.

REFERENCES

American Nurses Association. (1991). *Nursing's agenda for health care reform.* Kansas City, MO: Author.

Clinton, H.R. (1993). Nurses in the front lines. *Nursing & Health Care, 14*(6), 286-288.

Hall-Long, B.A. (1995). Nursing's past, present, and future political experiences. *Nursing & Health Care: Perspectives on Community, 16*(1), 24-28.

Health care reform: A politically high-risk venture, Washington focus. (1993, May). *Nursing & Health Care, 14*(5), 236-237.

Keeling, A.W., & Ramos, M.C. (1995). The role of nursing history in preparing nursing for the future: Nursing policy forum. *Nursing & Health Care: Perspectives on Community, 16*(1), 30-34.

Mullan, F. (1989). Plagues and politics (p. 14). New York: Basic Books, Inc.

Sprayberry, L.D. (1993). Nursing's dual role in health care policy. *Nursing & Health Care, 14*(5), 250-254.

Starr, P. (1982). *The social transformation of American medicine* (p. 241). New York: Basic Books, Inc.

Dangerous liaisons: Nursing, consumers, and the managed care marketplace

CLAIRE M. FAGIN, LEAH F. BINDER

The Clinton Administration's ambitious attempt to restructure the nation's health care delivery system failed in Congress in 1994. Yet the progress of reorganization of health care delivery continues unabated and appears to be accelerating at state and national levels, notwithstanding the federal government's inability to reach a consensus and take a leading role on how it should occur. The central characteristic of this reorganization is the growth of private sector managed care networks. The growth of managed care brings opportunity and threat for both the nursing profession and the public.

Traditional roles have changed in the new managed delivery settings. Physicians are no longer unquestioned authorities; administrators are involved in clinical decision making; and consumers are expected to be active proponents—not passive recipients—of quality care. As advocates, leaders, and educators, nurses will be valuable allies for consumers making the transition to managed care environments. This chapter examines the managed care phenomenon and its implications for nurses and consumers of care. We argue that consumers need to develop partnerships with nurses, and that nurses should be taking an active leadership role in helping to evaluate the current organizational "reforms" in order to ensure quality and safety of care.

MANAGED CARE

Managed care networks come in numerous forms, including preferred provider organizations (PPOs), health maintenance organizations, coordinated care arrangements, and other so-called integrated systems. All managed care organizations (MCOs) share some fundamental characteristics. They limit the range of providers available to members, and they monitor and sometimes restrict the health services that enrolled members are permitted to utilize. Unlike traditional fee-for-service plans that reimburse providers for each patient visit, managed care arrangements often pay providers a set (capitated) monthly rate for each patient assigned to them, regardless of how often the patient visits, if at all. Thus, in managed care providers have a financial incentive to provide the smallest quantity of services necessary to preserve their patients' health. Many managed care arrangements require members to affiliate with a case manager or primary care provider, who may serve as a gatekeeper by referring patients to specialists and for other services as needed. As a result of the financial incentives and policies to coordinate care and monitor utilization of services, most managed care networks are able to offer cost savings to members (Congressional Budget Office, 1994).

Increasing numbers of Americans are enrolling in MCOs. As of 1994, 47 million Americans were enrolled in HMOs, and another 50 million were members of PPOs (Health Insurance Association of America, 1995). Even traditional fee-for-service arrangements have begun to implement a process borrowed from managed care called "utilization review," in which insurance companies and not providers have the final say on the services enrollees utilize. Almost all employees covered by employer-based private insurance are now subject to some form of utilization review (Congressional Budget Office, 1994).

Since the early 1990s, managed care arrangements have grown very rapidly in the private sector and have become increasingly the mode of choice in the public sector. In 1994 for example, 8 million Medicaid participants were enrolled in MCOs, up from 1 million a decade earlier (Health Care Financing Administration, Office of Managed Care, 1994). Nearly half of the states have applied for Medicaid waivers to enable them to require portions of their Medicaid participants to join MCOs (Alan Guttmacher Institute, 1995).

The jury is still out on whether managed care arrangements enhance the overall quality of care. The literature is contradictory on managed care's impact on the number of provider visits per patient (i.e., Hurley, Freund, & Paul, 1993), but there is strong evidence that managed care enrollees are far less likely than people in other kinds of plans to visit specialists (Rowland, Rosenbaum, Simon, & Chait, 1995). There is a decline in emergency room use and some evidence of decline in overall hospitalization rates (Rowland et al., 1995). To date, studies have not found evidence that managed care improves utilization of preventive services. Among Medicaid participants, managed care has not improved the number of prenatal visits, immunizations, or well-child visits (Rowland et al., 1995). These findings are particularly disappointing for this most vulnerable population.

There have been incidences of abuse and fraud in MCOs, particularly in those serving Medicaid participants. A series of investigative pieces in a Florida newspaper gained national attention when they unveiled a host of abuses in several HMOs that enrolled Medicaid participants. Problems cited included neglectful providers allowing illnesses to go undetected and untreated; administrative costs exceeding 50%, and in some cases 60%, of revenues; fraudulent marketing techniques; and in one case the employment of a convicted felon as chief executive officer (Schulte & Bergal, 1994). Questions about MCOs with publicly funded enrollees prompted the Health Care Financing Administration to adopt new regulations to curb abuses ("GAO Questions HCFA," 1995). More recently, reports from New York State and New York City indicate that ". . . sweeping efforts to turn over health care for Medicaid recipients to private managed care companies had been moving too quickly with too little government oversight" (Fisher & Fein, 1995, p. B1).

Today's managed care industry is dominated by the private sector. The combination of fiscal responsibility to shareholders and government payers, with the focus on *cost containment* (rather than *cost-effectiveness*) and control over patient utilization of care, has some risk potential. Recognition of the deficits in evaluation of managed care practice suggests that regulation and oversight may be important to ensure that quality of care is not sacrificed to profit considerations. Discussions and actions with regard to such regulation are under way in several states (e.g., New Jersey, Maryland).

Despite the foregoing cautionary notes, we believe that MCOs ultimately offer the most promising solution to the nation's health care problems. As the population ages, accelerating health care costs necessitate better coordination of care for Americans. Fee-for-service arrangements, in which providers are reimbursed for every service provided, offer patients wide choices, and for those workers who have generous health benefit plans it is natural that these arrangements are the package of choice. However, there is little evidence in the aggregate that these expensive benefit packages are any more effective than managed care at ensuring quality of care.

THE NURSING MODEL OF CARE

The philosophy undergirding managed care is, in many respects, consonant with the nursing model of care. Like nursing, managed care philosophy emphasizes the whole patient, coordination of care, and prevention and primary care. Most managed care arrangements monitor, and some disclose data on, quality and cost-effectiveness of providers and services; and most emphasize collaboration between health professionals (Appleby, 1995).

The convergence of the managed care philosophy with the professional belief system of nursing might suggest that nursing's moment has arrived. We believe that this is indeed the case. However, vast changes in hospitals caused by reductions both in patient stay and in hospital usage are having severe effects on nurses. Because more than two thirds of nurses work in hospitals, radical reductions in the numbers of hospital beds have had a direct impact on nursing staff. In addition, hospitals are attempting to lower costs in ways that may prove noxious to both nurses and patients by layoffs of nurses regardless of patient need, reduction of nurse:patient ratios in many delivery settings, and reclassification of nursing responsibilities into more ambiguous categories of patient services (Manthey, 1995). In short, despite the centrality of nursing philosophy to the emerging managed care delivery systems, nurses themselves appear increasingly marginalized.

The facts that hospitals have become increasingly reliant on MCOs to supply patients, and that the financial incentives under managed care to minimize the amount of care provided result in efforts to reduce per-patient costs, not militate against excellent-quality nursing care. Rather, these circumstances present opportunities for nurses to develop and articulate to hospital management and to the public strong patient care systems that are cost-effective and not harmful to the patient. Nurse specialist transitional care, for example, helps counter the fragmentation of care that many consumers experience as they navigate among different providers, treatments, and settings. Nurse-managed, hospital-based programs that provide transitional care for patients diagnosed with cancer, perinatal care for new mothers and their infants, care for the frail elderly, and care for patients with AIDS and for many other populations have been shown to be extremely effective.

Study after study reinforces the value of nurses in enhancing quality and cost-effectiveness. Aiken et al. (1994) found a significant correlation between the organization of nursing and mortality rates at the hospitals they studied. A much earlier study by Draper (1987) found that strong collaboration between registered nurses and physicians resulted in 58% more patients surviving than expected. Research has demonstrated lower mortality rates in hospitals with higher nurse:patient ratios (Hartz, Krakauer, & Kuhn, 1989) and a correlation between levels of nursing and quality of patient care (Carter, Mills, & Homan, 1987; Krakauer, Bailey, & Skellan, 1992).

The newest model of the advanced practice nurse (APN) is one consumer-oriented, cost-effective solution for hospitals. In this model, the role of hospital-based tertiary nurse practitioner (TNP) blends the nurse practitioner role with that of the clinical nurse specialist (Keane & Richmond, 1993).

The development of the APN role was stimulated by two parallel forces: (1) nursing's recognition that care should be offered by the most cost-effective providers familiar with therapeutic options in the most appropriate setting and (2) the decrease in the size of medical specialty residency programs resulting from an excess of physician specialists in the United States. The TNP programs are designed to provide care to hospitalized patients with complex, specialized needs. These nurses have in-depth knowledge of the specialty, are technologically expert, and utilize the generalist approach reflecting nursing's holistic view of the individual (Keane & Richmond, 1993).

An excellent example of the implementation of the TNP role is at the Columbia-Presbyterian Medical Center in Manhattan. On selected units of the hospital, TNPs do initial assessments, write admission orders, work with attending physicians to review plans of care, and work with the nursing staff to interpret clinical information and explain the rationale for treatment plans. Silver, a pioneer in the nurse practitioner movement, predicted and recommended the development of a hospital-based nurse practitioner role in a 1988 article. Silver and McAtee (1988) believed that these nurses would perform many functions and provide many services given by first-year residents in teaching hospitals.

However, despite the proven effective contributions of nurses in these roles and others and the obvious compatibility of nursing's professional identity with the goals and priorities of managed care, nurses appear increasingly marginalized within MCOs, and, even more serious, are often excluded from the process of planning change in the organization of hospital patient care. Because nursing care is the essential ingredient of patients' hospitalization, the lack of involvement of nurses in planning patient-oriented change is incomprehensible.

A survey by the American Nurses Association found that nearly 70% of nurse respondents claimed that there were cutbacks in the number of registered nurses employed in their institutions, with no other staff or service area cut back as often. Nearly half cited the employment of unlicensed assistive personnel, some with training as minimal as 4 to 6 weeks, and a few (2.3%) claimed that patients have died as a result of nursing absence ("Survey Finds Loss of RNs," 1995). Recent publicized deaths and morbidities in hospitals in Boston, Florida, and Michigan (among others) seem to be related to major changes in hospital organization, including downsizing of the nursing staff and change of responsibilities.

The troubling absence of nurses is compounded by the increasing removal of word "nurse" in the title of the administrator of nursing; titles increasingly refer to "patient care services" instead. Describing these new administrators of patient care services, Beyers of the American Organization of Nurse Executives explains that the title change is not merely semantic but a reorientation of the mission of nursing leaders: "Whereas they previously had to focus on making the nursing service work, they now have to focus on making patient care services work" (Beyers, 1995, p. 22). Yet exactly what is the difference between the goal of good nursing and the goal of good patient care? Why is it necessary to erase the professional identity and heritage of nursing when nursing is arguably more compatible with the mission and goals of managed care than any other element of the delivery system?

The message that nursing is incidental and not integral to the goal of good patient care services appears to have been heard. The recent trends in hospitals—downsizing nursing staff without downsizing the patient population, replacing nurses with unlicensed personnel, eliminating mention of nursing credentials in the identification of staff, increasing reports of resignations or removals of directors of nursing, and eliminating positions for clinical nurse specialists—are clear signs of intent to minimize the role of professional nursing in our nation's hospitals.

Hospitals are not the only delivery settings discounting nursing resources. Although primary care and case management are central to the managed care model, and physician shortages are cited frequently, nurses' ability to provide cost-effective primary care is also being compromised (i.e., Clark, 1995). For example, in many states implementing Medicaid managed care, waivers override federal directives requiring direct reimbursement for certain advanced nurse providers to require physician-only case management (Keepnews, 1995).

Even as the role and experience of nurses are marginalized, the responsibilities traditionally attributed to them are being extolled as central to the delivery of care. Health policy expert Shortell from the Kellogg School of Management at Northwestern University put it this way:

> We need to take responsibility for more of the whole process of patient care. That is what total quality management is all about. We need more cross-training, more multi-disciplinary teams, better information systems, and new ways to treat the 'entire' patient. (Shortell, 1995, p. 28)

This quote could have come from any nursing textbook or nursing research journal from 10 or 20 years ago. Yet as the delivery system moves to embrace this model, it frequently reinvents the wheel instead of turning to the providers with the proven experience to implement it—nurses.

What accounts for the paradox that nurses are devalued while the emerging model of health care delivery replicates the nursing model of care? At least one explanation lies in the classic conundrum of the nursing profession: Nurses control their own education but not their practice. Thus nursing has never been able to adequately reinforce a wholly independent professional identity in the practice setting. A brief list of characteristics of independent professions usually includes the power to control the terms, conditions, and content of work (Friedson, 1994). The power to control one's work has been the principal differentiation between the way medicine and nursing have progressed and organized their systems.

Two additional explanations seem as cogent. First, nurses' writings are generally not read by anyone but nurses. Thus the teaching that nurses do with regard to their models of care reaches nurses but not the professional or lay public. Second, when nurses bring up the fact that the newer organizations or ideas were discussed and taught by nurses years ago, their comments are often dismissed by words or nonverbal behavior. After all, what powerful group wishes to hear a group without power say that it has invented what they are taking credit for?

Without full and independent control over the practice of nursing, nurses are a group without direct power, and nursing can appear to be a wholly dependent component of the practice setting. Managed care reformers may then identify nurses as hospital representatives, part and parcel of the delivery setting, instead of independently credentialed professionals with a set of coherent values and goals. The tendency to see nursing as part of the old ways may be compounded by the fact many of the changemakers are not providers themselves, but business executives and policymakers with little experience in direct patient care and unfamiliar with the role of nurses and the needs of patients.

COLLABORATIONS THAT WORK

Not all MCOs overlook nursing expertise and resources. We are witnessing increasing interest in nurse practitioners in MCOs and other innovative community-based practice settings. There have also been signs that MCOs are employing more nurses as direct primary care providers and case managers. There are two kinds of case manager roles in which advanced nurse providers can be found. One type utilizes APNs to deliver and manage the care of various populations such as the chronically mentally ill, medically fragile patients, patients with AIDS, and clients with preventive or maintenance needs. These APNs coordinate the care of these clients and manage their entry into other parts of the health care system. Others use the term "case manager" to indicate gatekeeper roles without direct care responsibilities. These gatekeeper roles call on the nurse to make decisions about the kind of care, the length of the treatment, and the appropriateness of care.

Furthermore, the potential for nursing leadership in collaboration with MCOs has never been as dramatic. There are at least 300 nurse-managed health centers such as community clinics nationwide, many of which are affiliated with schools of nursing and other institutions (Barger & Rosenfeld, 1993; Hothaus, 1993). A family health center in South Carolina managed by a nurse practitioner was developed as a community alternative to inappropriate use of the emergency room. In a 6-month period the nurse practitioners had seen almost 5000 clients. In Arizona, one nurse-managed center is projecting cost savings of $500,000 in its first year, based on fewer inpatient days and emergency room visits for 18,500 enrollees. The program utilizes APNs to provide both direct care and integrated case management to patients with multisystem, chronic diseases requiring extensive health care interventions; the program tends to focus on patients with limited socioeconomic, familial, and cultural resources (Barger & Rosenfeld, 1993).

Among the many nurse-managed centers of the University of Pennsylvania School of Nursing, the West Philadelphia Community Health Corner is an interesting model. Started by a faculty member and students from the University of Pennsylvania Division of Pediatric Nursing, with strong cooperation from neighborhood groups, the Corner addresses the specific health needs of the community in its neighborhood setting. It offers services to children and adolescents as well as adults, including immunization services, physicals, screening, walk-in pregnancy testing, birth control advice, sexually transmitted disease testing, driver's license, and sport physicals. The nurses are reimbursed directly for their services through federal and state programs.

Other current nurse-managed centers at the University of Pennsylvania include a day care hospital and a recreation center–based family health care service. Additional centers are being developed at this and other university schools of nursing in the United States.

School and community center clinics, expanded home health visits, and work site health programs have mushroomed in recent years and utilize nurse practitioners almost exclusively. The settings may differ with regard to the type of services and the background of the nurse provider. Stress prevention and maintenance of health provide opportunities for innovation on the part of nurse leaders, many of whom involve the community in planning and monitoring services. The notion of marketing prevention and risk reduction in vulnerable populations is an implicit or explicit part of many nursing centers.

THE NEXT STEP: NURSING AND CONSUMERS

It is interesting to note how rapidly the health care scene has changed in recent years. In our earlier article (Fagin & Binder, 1994) we noted that ". . . the health care system frequently offers incentives for high-technology, high-skill operations, procedures and interventions without addressing some of the preventive mechanisms that would eliminate demand for such services" (p. 450). The incentives today are vastly different, although they still do not offer sufficient opportunities for preventive services. In addition, consumers have become more concerned about what is available to them and more active in seeking appropriate interventions. Unfortunately, that does not mean that the public's power and control over the health care system has increased. In fact, it would appear that there will be more rather than less power, at least in the short term.

So where does that leave the potential of the nurse-consumer partnership? ". . . The challenge of public health calls for consumer participation as full partners in the health care system, actively responsible for their own ongoing health maintenance and vigilant in demanding quality and cost effectiveness" (Fagin & Binder, 1994, p. 453). That is where nursing must come in.

Given the current pace of change, the need for consumer participation is crucial. No system that is changing as fast as health care delivery can be all good, completely safe, or even of the highest quality. How is the consumer to have any idea of what to look for or how to evaluate what they are getting without a regular source of information and support? Consumers are ready to act and in the managed care arena will be less intimidated because the "deity" power of the physician will not be transferred to the more mundane businesslike atmosphere of the organized care system. The systems themselves view patients and the public as customers, and it will be in their best interest to respond to customer wishes and concerns.

We stated earlier that nurses in MCOs may be in two different roles of case management—one as a direct provider and the other as gatekeeper. In the gatekeeper position it is crucial that nurses see themselves as patient advocates who can translate complex information into concrete options and formulas for customer decision making.

> The consumer makes the decision, but nurses are in the position of (1) spearheading consumer usage of valuable information, which if implemented on a widespread basis would likely lead to innovations in the delivery setting aimed at enhancing efficiency, quality, and cost-effectiveness and (2) discouraging on a mass scale the habits of patient subordination that are ingrained . . . and perpetuated in part by the current health system structure. (Fagin & Binder, 1994, p. 457)

Nurses have had a very hard time being whistle blowers in the current environment, despite their concern with what they see and experience. It is hard to be a whistle blower when your family relies on you for support and you and all of your colleagues are employees of the change makers. However, in coalition with other nurses, other health care providers, and consumers—in neighborhoods where the nurse works or lives—building coalitions around health care and its quality is quite another matter.

In our previous paper we outlined several possible goals around which such a coalition might rally. We have reexamined the goals and revised them somewhat. Some useful ideas for discussion of goals for coalitions are:

- Release information about quality of care in local hospitals, nursing homes, community health care agencies, and private practice providers. Personal stories will be helpful.
- Promote healthy lifestyles in the local community such as smoking cessation, fitness, diet, and disease prevention. The key here is to suggest alternative behaviors to targeted populations.
- Look into the potential of nursing centers for the community. Invite speakers from successful centers and determine whether this community is an appropriate setting for a community nursing center and who can help it get started.
- With the help of community members, start an informal file of the needs of the community in terms of demographics and the most likely health problems. Once you have this basic data, try to address the major needs by getting volunteers from local health professional schools to give some time to working with your group.

If we are trying to increase power in any sphere we need knowledge, in this case knowledge of the system, its constraints, and options; the varieties of insurance benefits we can obtain; cost-effective providers; and information about the most common health problems affecting us in our age group and about appropriate self-care. All changes currently under way call for the development of personal accountability for one's health and medical choices.

Two principles that are essential for the consumer to have a rational choice in the health care market are:

1. Consumers should have a variety of choices of health care plans to match a variety of preferences and needs. These choices should include preventive and counseling services, alternatives to hospitalization such as home care, nonphysician providers, ambulatory surgicenters where appropriate, ambulatory diagnostic centers, birthing centers, and hospice centers.
2. We cannot make intelligent choices in a competitive health care system without information. Information must be widely available through an array of media.

NURSING LEADERSHIP

The nursing profession is experiencing chaos in the current downsizing. We believe that major adjustments are needed in relation to the size of the nursing student population and where the students are being educated. It has become clear in recent years that in a greatly reduced nursing marketplace nurses with only an associate degree will not have the opportunities that had previously been present in the health field during times of expansion and nursing shortages. The current chaos should not get in the way of nursing's recognition of the potential of a managed care system for patients and for the nursing profession if quality is monitored and assured. Nursing's proven expertise and cost-effectiveness suggests that the future can be bright for nursing's involvement in new delivery systems. Yet there is opposite potential as well. If nurses are too preoccupied with the current problems, they may be unable to collaborate aggressively to help develop the best future models. Unless nurses assert the authority and knowledge base of the profession it is possible that the changing system will soar forward without them.

While we have argued that the nursing model of care coincides with the philosophy of MCOs, the two philosophies differ in one crucial respect. Nursing has no profit motive, while most MCOs—whether simply to survive or for the accumulation of wealth—are guided in large part by the demands of the dollar. Certainly nurses have enjoyed the more recent fair earnings and deserve to be paid equitable salaries. Because their primary focus is on patient care, however, nurses may occasionally diverge from their managed care colleagues when they seek to esteem the quality of patient care over and above the cost of that care. Often enough, quality and cost-effectiveness go hand in hand, such as in gatekeeping functions that help patients avoid unnecessary and dangerous procedures. When they do not, it is critical that nurses remain patient advocates.

Unless nurses assert the value of nursing as a voice for cost-effective, quality care, and a profession with ideals compatible to managed care, the contributions of nurses and the profession will be at risk, and the safety and well-being of patients will be compromised. There are immediate, sometimes severe, consequences to patients when nursing leadership is devalued, when per-patient nursing staff levels are lowered, when inadequately trained workers are placed at the bedside, and when nursing's experience and knowledge are excluded from provider collaborations, planning, and coordinated care.

Nurse educators have an obligation to prepare nursing students for the world of managed care, including both clinical aspects and issues of financing and administration. Concurrently, nurse educators need to understand the techniques of community organization and leadership and the importance of building partnerships and coalitions with the public. These concomitant and sometimes conflictual learnings are crucial if nurses wish to effect quality care. Providers without an understanding of the business of managed care are at a distinct disadvantage in the new cost-dominated delivery systems; providers without an understanding of the role of the active consumer will be equally disadvantaged. Nurse researchers should reflect how their research can be applied to managed care and develop proposals to investigate and uncover best practices. Despite its prevalence, managed care is in many respects in its infancy, when new research and data can offer pioneering new directions with the potential to shape health care reform. It is interesting, for example, that managed care has been largely unable to improve certain kinds of preventive care such as prenatal visits. Can nurse researchers learn how to improve the record? We think so.

No group of professionals better understands the philosophy of managed care and how to implement it than nurses. Gardner's views (1964) on the tasks of leadership describe what leaders must do and offer a blueprint for nurses to consider in their daily work:

1. Envision goals.
2. Affirm values.
3. Motivate.
4. Manage.
   —Plan and set priorities.
   —Organize and build institutions.
   —Keep the system functioning.
   —Set agendas and make decisions.
   —Exercise political judgement.
5. Achieve workable unity.
6. Explain.
7. Serve as a symbol.
8. Represent the group.
9. Renew.

Nurses must take leadership roles to preserve the vision, goals, values, and symbols of good health care that brought them into the health care system. Nurses should not step aside quietly to give others an exclusive forum to educate the public and set direction on issues like preventive care and coordination of care, all of which are the lifeblood of nursing experience and knowledge. By upholding the autonomy and professionalism of the nursing role—recognizing that autonomy is not lost in partnership with consumers—and asserting that health care quality is the raison d'etre for professionalism, nurses have the opportunity as never before to help set the direction for and implement positive health care reform.

REFERENCES

Aiken, L., Smith, H., & Lake, E. (1994). Lower Medicare mortality among a set of hospitals known for good nursing care. *Medical Care, 32*(8), 771-787.

Alan Guttmacher Institute. (1995). Special analysis: How family planning services fare under state bids to restructure Medicaid. *State Reproductive Health Monitor, 6*(2), 3.

Appleby, C. (1995, June 20). The measure of medical services. *Hospitals & Health Networks,* 26.

Barger, S., & Rosenfeld, P. (1993). Models in community health care: Findings from a national study of community nursing centers. *Nursing & Health Care 14*(8), 426-431.

Beyers, M. (1995). The consequences of change. *Nursing Management, 26*(5), 22.

Carter, J.H., Mills, A.C., Homan, S.M., et al. (1987, December). *Correlating the quality of care with nursing resources and patient parameters: A longitudinal study.* NLN Publications (20-2191), 331-345.

Clark, C.S. (1995, January). Defining primary care. *Healthcare Financial Management,* 19.

Congressional Budget Office. (1994). *Effects of managed care: An update.* Washington, DC: Author.

Draper, E.A. (1987). Effects of nurse/physician collaboration and nursing standards on ICU patient outcomes. *Current Concepts In Nursing, 1*(4), 2-8.

Fagin, C.M., & Binder, L.F. (1994). Nursing and consumerism: How can we get decision making closer to the consumer? In J. McCloskey & H. Grace (Eds.), *Current Issues in Nursing* (pp. 450-459). St. Louis: Mosby.

Fisher, I., & Fein, E.B. (1995, August 28). Forced marriage of Medicaid and Managed care hits snags. *The New York Times,* p. B1.

Friedson, E. (1994). Professional reborn. Chicago: University of Chicago Press.

Gardner, J.W. (1964). *Self renewal.* New York: Perennial Library.

Hartz, A.J., Krakauer, H., & Kuhn, E.M. (1989). Hospital characteristics and mortality rates. *New England Journal of Medicine, 321,* 1720-1725.

GAO Questions HCFA vigilance against quality violations by Medicare risk contract HMOs. (1995). *Managed Medicare & Medicaid News, 24*(31), 1.

Health Insurance Association of America. (1995). *Source book of health insurance data 1994.* Washington, DC: Author.

Health Care Financing Administration, Office of Managed Care. (1994). *Medicaid managed care enrollment report: Summary statistics as of June 30, 1994.* Washington, DC: U.S. Department of Health and Human Services.

Holthaus, R. (1993). Nurse-managed health care: An ongoing tradition. *Nurse Practitioner Forum, 4*(3), 128-132.

Hurley, R., Freund, D., & Paul, J. (1993). *Managed care in Medicaid: Lessons for policy and program design.* Ann Arbor, MI: Health Administration Press.

Krakauer, H., Bailey, R.C., Skellan, K.J., et al. (1992, August). Evaluation of the HCFA model for the analysis of mortality following hospitalization. *Health Services Research, 27*(3), 317-335.

Keane, A., & Richmond, T. (1993, Winter). Tertiary nurse practitioners. *Image, 25*(4), 281-284.

Keepnews, D. (1995, April/May). State Medicaid waivers: Issues for nurses. *American Nurse,* 16.

Manthey, M. (1995, March/April). Marie Manthey interviews Norma Lang. *Creative Nursing,* 7.

Rowland, D., Rosenbaum, S., Simon, L., & Chait, E. (1995). *Medicaid and managed care: Lessons from the literature.* Washington, DC: The Henry J. Kaiser Family Foundation.

Schulte, F., & Bergal, J. (1994, December 11-15). Florida's Medicaid HMO's: Profits from pain. *Sun Sentinel.*

Shortell, S.M. (1995). The future of integrated systems. *Health Care Financial Management, 24,* 28.

Silver, H.K., & McAtee, P. (1988, December). Should nurses substitute for House staff? *American Journal of Nursing, 88*(12): 1671-1673.

Survey finds loss of RNs jeopardizes patient safety. (1995, January/February). *American Nurse,* p. 1.

The future of academic health centers in a cost-driven market

CONNIE CURRAN

There are 126 academic health centers (AHCs) in the United States, each comprising a hospital and at least one health professional school. These institutions function as the primary resources for research in biomedical and health services, for education in the health professions, and for the provision of many aspects of patient care in the United States (Association of Academic Health Centers, 1992).

Over the past 40 years, AHCs have been extremely successful in adapting to health care–related changes in public policy. Most of these changes, prompted by government and the health care industry, have allowed time for extensive planning and consideration. Today, the market is dictating a change in policy. Competition from alternative providers is pressuring AHCs to lower costs and improve the quality of care, and to do so with greater speed and versatility. AHCs have been slow to respond, however, and the future for many of them is threatened. Each element of the AHC tripartite mission—research, education, and patient care—is vulnerable:

- *Research:* A new emphasis is being placed on multidisciplinary and clinical outcomes research. As hospital systems form, health maintenance organizations (HMOs) grow, and physicians join large group practices, there are fewer referrals to teaching hospitals, which threatens the AHC research mission (Allison & Dalton, 1982). In addition, new requirements challenge the traditional model and suggest a need for new forms of organization.
- *Education:* The financing that has traditionally available for education through payments by the Health Care Financing Administration (HCFA) and through implicit subsidies in commercial insurance is evaporating in the path of capitated payments for clinical services and a drive to control government spending. In addition, the national shortage of primary care providers is pressuring AHCs to shift the priorities of their programs from training subspecialists to training primary care physicians. Further, as increasing amounts of care are provided outside hospital walls, AHCs must devise programs with a substantial proportion of their training in outpatient settings.
- *Patient care:* AHCs increasingly compete with integrated delivery systems that are highly effective in price-sensitive marketplaces. At the same time, reimbursements are being cut and AHCs are compelled to provide increasing levels of uncompensated care.

These trends threaten the base of clinical income to faculty and hospitals that provide support for education and research endeavors. Facing these challenges requires AHCs to create a closer alignment between their faculty practice plan and university hospitals so they can share a capitated revenue stream. The goals of broad-based, integrated systems are consistent with AHC missions to serve the needs of buyers, consumers, referring physicians, students, and residents. In developing systems AHCs can realize (1) an "economic dividend" to the school and departments for funding education and research; (2) new educational opportunities within the clinical delivery structure to train primary care physicians, other providers, and specialists in hospital and ambulatory settings; and (3) broad access to patients for population-based clinical research.

Of course, not all AHCs will benefit from these partnerships and some may seek other opportunities. Some may be better served by focusing on creating excellence within a particular specialty. These centers of excellence often can offer reductions in costs of as much as 35% to 40% compared with procedures done elsewhere (Wise,

1993). Others may choose to downsize and refocus on specific elements of their mission; some will change governance and organizational structures to have more control over their destinies; and some may choose to merge or close. Massachusetts General Hospital surprised Boston's medical community by agreeing to merge with longtime rival Brigham and Women's Hospital, creating the nation's largest hospital.

As centers of excellence in teaching and research, AHCs are one of our country's national treasures and the envy of the world. AHCs are positioned to be leaders in preparing practitioners for the next century and to shape the values and direction of the entire health care system—if they are willing to reconceptualize their systems for research, education, and patient care. New approaches to the funding of teaching and research may emerge from this reconceptualization. For instance, smaller, more specialized medical schools may result (i.e., the University of Minnesota at Duluth School of Medicine, established in 1972 as a 2-year school devoted to producing rural primary care practitioners) (Friedman, 1993), and some AHC functions may be absorbed by other, better organized entities.

The implications are clear: AHCs will have to change their ways. The traditional tripartite mission still applies, but in a new, competitive environment. Consumers and payers are confronted with a diversity of choices and are demanding providers with lower costs, increased access and availability, and verifiable quality. AHCs must rise to the challenge.

MARKET NEEDS AND EVOLUTION

Consumer needs

In determining a course of action for the 21st century, AHCs must begin by taking an in-depth, studied look at the needs and desires of the market (i.e., the buyers of care). The first of these health care consumers is the American public.

Despite the inability of the Clinton Administration and Congress to agree on a plan for universal health coverage, the American public increasingly seems to endorse the idea. A recent poll conducted by the *New York Times* showed that 8 of 10 Americans are now as concerned about health care as they are about crime (Dowd, 1994). A majority also felt willing to pay higher taxes to achieve this goal. Still, at both the public and governmental levels, there is disagreement about what portion of this care is to be paid by employers, employees, and the government.

In the spring of 1994, the W.K. Kellogg Foundation funded a bipartisan national opinion survey of the nation's health care consumers. The poll found that American consumers overwhelmingly believe that the country should make use of more family health care providers—family doctors, nurses, and other basic health care providers—rather than medical specialists, and a solid majority also believe the current health care system fails to meet the needs of most Americans. A majority said they were very satisfied with the care they received from health care professionals other than doctors, particularly nurses, nurse practitioners, and physician assistants. Based on their experience, consumers prefer a system that places more emphasis on basic health care and teams of providers like doctors and nurses. The consumer's view is very much in line with both the direction of proposed health care reform and the commitment that AHCs must make to fulfill their mission. It suggests that if a restructuring of priorities and goals in health care takes place as proposed, the public faith in medicine is sure to be restored.

Payer needs

The other consumers to consider are the payers—federal and state governments as well as employers—who represent the majority of buying power. In today's market, these entities seek providers with lower costs, increased access, and verifiable quality. Interviews with payers and insights gained from successful AHC-payer relationships indicate the need for AHCs to (1) build an attractive network with strong primary care capabilities and skills to effectively manage patient populations; (2) incorporate managed care-oriented education and research into the AHC mission; and (3) significantly improve the unit cost structure to support competitive pricing and maintain and secure managed care contracts.

Payers, especially sophisticated ones, are quickly becoming skillful at negotiating significant discounts. The unfortunate reality for an AHC is that it is not an issue of "if" but rather "when" these actions will be carried out. In the new health care environment, payers will be confronted with a choice in providers, all of whom will have implemented these actions.

The evolution of managed care

The managed care market is evolving as a result of payer demands. In many markets, the evolution is occurring so quickly that many hospitals, especially AHCs, are finding themselves unprepared to act. In order to effect action, AHCs must fully understand the characteristics and evolution of this market.

The development of managed care across the country

is highly influenced by the characteristics of local markets, in particular the penetration of managed care and the mechanisms through which managed care payers contract for provider services; the extent of group practice development among physicians; the financial security and administrative support offered to primary care physicians by hospitals, payers, and proprietary companies that a developing network must match or enhance; and the number of family practitioners in the market as they tend to be more willing to consider new models and participate in larger organizations.

On the surface, local market conditions appear to be highly individualized. Research conducted in approximately 50 markets across the country by the University Hospital Consortium and APM Management Consultants, however, show a pattern of evolution through four stages.

Stage 1: Unstructured. Stage 1 can be characterized as fragmented health care delivery. Managed care is in its introductory phase and primarily involves preferred provider organization (PPO) products that offer large panels of hospitals and physicians at discounted rates (generally in the 5% to 10% range). When offered at all, managed care plans are generally a benefit option with little or no economic or social pressure by employers to encourage employees to select them.

Stage 2: Loose framework. The market becomes more competitive as HMOs and PPOs become increasingly accepted among employers and employees and grow larger and more powerful. Hospitals become nervous during the annual negotiations process because they cannot afford to lose the larger contracts. Discounting for hospitals typically ranges in the 15% to 25% range. Utilization management efforts by payers lead to reduced hospital occupancy and create financial pressures for hospitals. At the end of Stage 2, enrollment in HMOs reaches a plateau of 35% to 45% of the population. Managed care plans recognize that they are now competing with each other rather than with indemnity insurance, suggesting a greater ability to shrink networks and shift risk to providers.

Stage 3: Consolidation. Stage 3 often causes concern for providers because HMOs become powerful enough to move large blocks of patients. The strongest HMOs continue to contract with individual providers, but they also limit panels to the most cost-effective providers and shift utilization risk through capitated payment arrangements or payments for inpatient care. In this stage, it becomes clear who will take leadership in creating new networks. This can lead to significant hospital merger activity. Depending on local circumstances, AHCs need to determine whether to sponsor a developing network, team up with other hospitals to develop a network, evolve in such a way as to become central to any local network development, remain independent, or close.

Stage 4: Managed competition. In Stage 4, most providers contract in a more integrated fashion as part of a provider network. The norm is for networks to accept and manage fully capitated contracts. In order to encourage the development of such systems, employer coalitions often contract as a block. Networks that include insurance functions can contract directly with these employer coalitions. During this stage, AHCs face the possibility of losing input into the mission of the developing network. Their influence in determining the portion of reserves used to invest in network-based services for the community may be lost.

The evolutionary stage of an AHC's local market helps define whether it is best for an AHC to join an integrated network, create one of its own, or simply form an alliance with other community hospitals. Variations in the functioning of local health care markets means that AHCs in different areas will be held accountable for their performance through different mechanisms. Two paradigms are likely. In localities that have little experience with competition and little prospect of its development (i.e., rural states), the equivalent of government-operated single-payer systems may take hold. In these situations AHCs will find themselves dealing with public agencies in matters vital to their well-being. In highly competitive localities, private health care systems will hold AHCs accountable in at least some critical areas, most notably cost of care. AHCs may themselves form such systems, but in those cases the pressures to restrain costs will only be internalized.

Some argue that managed care will not develop to the extent that many envision. By virtue of its ability to reduce costs, however, managed care is sure to continue to expand. A 1991 study by A. Foster Higgins & Co., an employee benefit consulting firm, showed that HMOs significantly reduce corporate health care costs ("Health Plan Savings," 1992). In the study, employers saved an average of $527 per employee. As further proof, by 1992, when managed care had made significant inroads, corporate health care costs rose only 10%, the smallest increase in 5 years (although still triple the inflation rate) (Winslow, 1993). Growing numbers of Medicaid patients are joining managed care organizations. In 1993, 12% of the total Medicaid population (3.6 million people) were in managed care, and one study found that the per-member-per-month costs were 5%-15% less than in fee-for-service plans (Anders, 1993). The number of Medicare patients in managed care is also on the rise. This is especially significant because it is projected that those over 65 years of age, who account for only 11.1% of the population, consume 35% of all health care services (Wise, 1993). The most significant implication of this evolution is that it further shifts the focus onto issues already of concern to AHCs—issues of quality, cost and access.

THE MARKET'S DIRECTION

Moving toward a population perspective

Academic health centers and the industry at large are moving toward health care practices that emphasize managing health rather than managing illness. Although there are cost savings inherent in this paradigm, more importantly the goal is to improve the overall health status of our population by reducing illness, disability, and premature death. While some AHCs have already begun embracing this paradigm, it will be necessary for academic organizations as a whole to do so for a significant shift to occur.

In 1993, the Health of the Public program was initiated by a group of 17 AHCs concerned with the unfocused mission that is characteristic of AHCs. The goal of this program was to present academic medicine with a mission less preoccupied with high-technology medical care and biomedical research and more concerned with meeting the basic health care needs of the public. One of the most important outcomes of the group's research was the understanding that this new perspective required the reorientation of AHC mission statements. A Health of the Public Mission Statement has as its goals that AHCs be concerned with the health of the public and adopt a broad construct of health that emphasizes individuals' social and personal resources as well as physical capacity. Institutions dedicated to this goal need to establish a thorough integration of population and clinical perspectives into their tripartite mission (Kaufman & Waterman, 1993). The program developed a set of five goals necessary to successfully integrate a population perspective into clinical medicine: (1) maximize the health of a defined population; (2) achieve collaboration among the broad array of professionals needed to meet the health needs of that population; (3) provide appropriate preventive and therapeutic services; (4) conduct population-based research studies and apply the results to shaping and enhancing care; (5) use the social and behavioral sciences and humanities to gain a richer understanding of the individual patient, the roles and responsibilities of providers, and the performance of the health care system.

The integration of these goals will have several defined benefits to both the community and the AHC. From the community's perspective, such a system will graduate physicians who can subsequently improve the health of their communities, not just the health of their individual patients. With closer ties to the community, these physicians are more likely to stay in the community beyond their residency. This is particularly important in rural and underserved areas. The system will also realize higher-quality, more cost-effective care for patients both inside and outside the AHC. From an AHC perspective, adoption of these goals creates new venues for service and education, such as new collaborations or joint ventures in providing care for underserved populations, population laboratories, and more effectively developed policies. This system also generates new sources of funding for AHC research, such as clinical outcomes research and the effectiveness of community and practice-based care. Perhaps the most important benefit of these new initiatives is that a Health of the Public program enhances the public's trust in AHCs, a benefit that is needed in today's competitive market.

A commitment to a population health perspective requires AHCs to redefine education, putting more emphasis on the needs of their population and restructuring their focus on research and patient care quality.

Integrated delivery network development

While the philosophical direction of the market is to a population perspective, it is manifested through the creation of integrated delivery networks (IDNs). Outside of reform, the most significant development of the industry has been the formation of these diversified and integrated systems of health care delivery. It is the market, not government, that is driving this development.

Larger than HMOs, IDNs often include outpatient clinics, freestanding physician offices, nursing homes, hospices, home health agencies, retail pharmacies, drug treatment centers, and medical equipment suppliers in addition to hospitals. By definition, an IDN is a set of providers, operating under contractual or ownership arrangements, organized to render a coordinated continuum of care to an enrolled population in return for capitated revenue. Capitation provides new incentives to reduce duplication, coordinate care across settings, and ensure that enrollees receive care in appropriate and cost-effective settings. IDNs differ from the current system in that they focus on community wellness, require a coordinated continuum of care, and align economic incentives for hospitals and physicians. IDNs shift the focus from providing acute care, treating illness, and caring for individual patients to coordinating care, maintaining wellness, and improving the health of a population. IDNs provide an effective way to fulfill the central goals of health care reform. According to the Association of American Medical Colleges, these goals are (1) giving all Americans the chance for a healthy living; (2) providing universal access to health care; (3) recognizing that once health care excellence is achieved, the necessary resources must be provided so that quality and capacity are maintained; (4) instituting cost-containment measures that do not compromise health care quality; and (5) supporting essential medical and other health professional education as well as biomedical, behavioral, and health services research (Knapp, 1993).

The development of these networks will have a significant impact on the future of AHCs, ultimately forcing many out of the market. In many advanced markets, AHCs are not yet players. Most have neither the primary care patient base necessary to build a network nor staff trained to the needs of an IDN. Because community hospitals are starting to provide the same tertiary care available from AHCs at a lower cost, many IDNs do not feel obligated to AHCs. Further, AHCs are ill prepared to compete alone against these networks. As markets evolve, AHCs will be faced with larger, more numerous and powerful health care systems as competitors in their regions. Because community hospitals serve as referral sources, AHCs must carefully examine the impact of competition with them.

Nor should changes be made for the sake of making change. Changes in the autonomy of an AHC should be made to facilitate a specific strategy. To adapt to a changing environment, AHCs must assess the environment, evaluate organizational strengths and weaknesses, and consider strategies in light of competitive advantages and disadvantages (Zuckerman, D'Aunno, & Vaughan, 1990). Although 45% of community hospitals belong to some kind of multihospital system, relatively few AHCs have followed suit. Instead, many have joined or formed hospital alliances that do not require a change in corporate ownership and allow AHCs to retain legal status as independent, university-owned firms (Japsen, 1994).

The strategy chosen by some AHCs is the creation of an individual managed care entity. A 1992 study by the Association of Academic Health Centers showed that 43% of the nation's 102 AHCs own or operate an HMO, PPO, or independent practice association (IPA) (Japsen, 1994). In order to attract employers, AHCs must be able to share the risk and provide a continuum of care to the members of their plan. AHCs need new methods of relating to a much larger base of providers and of organizing themselves to achieve rapid and consistent institutional decision making. Because of the rapid encroachment by managed care, some believe that a new, smaller teaching hospital is likely to emerge out of those AHCs that do not devise their own managed care system (Japsen, 1994). The most important element of the AHC managed care development process is the involvement of physician staff in negotiations and discussions to prevent physician resistance and failure. For example, doctors at one Los Angeles hospital have joined various groups that could eventually redirect patients to rival hospitals. With a lack of unity among the doctors, insurers and employers are given an opportunity to use one faction against another to negotiate lower rates (Olmos, 1994).

Across the nation, communities are witnessing the rapid consolidation and integration of health care providers. This environment provides AHCs with an opportunity to influence delivery by creating or affiliating with an IDN. To participate in an IDN, AHCs are generally required to share power with community providers and to integrate the traditionally separate faculty practice organization with hospital governance and operations. Most faculty practices do not function as group practices. The faculty group often provides centralized scheduling and billing to autonomous departmental practice groups. In order to function effectively within an IDN, faculty groups must form and be structured similarly to nonacademic group practices (e.g., with centralized revenue capture and resource allocation and institutionally retained earnings).

The two most important steps AHCs can take in this direction are to encourage integration among physicians and between hospitals and physicians. It is easier for AHCs to negotiate with a limited number of larger physician groups than with hundreds of independent physicians. Because a significant number of physicians may not be ready to participate in a network, one solution is to offer a range of physician integration options that build IDN capabilities that are consistent with market requirements and community needs (i.e., IPA, group practices without walls, and management service organizations). A coordinated continuum of care can only be achieved by AHCs if physicians, hospitals, and other providers work together through formal arrangements. Because physicians typically act as the primary contact for patients—by determining what care is delivered, coordinating among disciplines, and determining the utilization of hospital resources—their aligned participation is a prerequisite to successful managed care contracting.

New forms of governance and organization

In determining the right relationship between university hospitals and their sponsors, one author wrote: "The question regarding university hospitals may not be one of how well they are managed, but how they can be made manageable" (Westerman, 1980). The speed with which the creation of systems is occurring represents a real challenge for AHCs. Many find themselves constrained by ownership and governance, unable to rapidly make and implement decisions and limited in their attempts to operate as businesses that maximize opportunities and resources. Most AHC hospitals cannot enter into contracts without bringing in the entire university governance structure. For the same reasons, it is also very difficult for these hospitals to borrow money.

The trend toward greater autonomy stems from a hospital's inability to be market-oriented as long as it is controlled by university boards, whose primary objectives are evaluation and accountability. A study by Kaufman, Shortell, Becker, and Neuhauser in 1979 found that hospitals with boards emphasizing oversight and accountability were the least efficient (Allison & Dalton, 1982).

In particular, IDNs require a different kind of governance. Approximately 55% of university hospitals are directly owned by the universities, which constrains the ability of the hospital to move aggressively into a regional system because the universities are often concerned about the risk of owning a large health care system. The specific needs of the hospital must be understood along with the various models of hospital ownership and governance that are likely to ensure the continued success of both the academic and clinical missions.

A strong case can be made for separation of university hospitals from their sponsors. Over the past 15 years, a steady stream of university hospitals have done so, with at least 13 achieving significant autonomy from their sponsors. University leaders may oppose separation if they think they can remain profitable by maintaining the status quo. In state universities, employees are civil servants or are unionized and may well oppose separation because of potential losses in entitlements. Munson and D'Aunno (1987) found that deans often favored separation as a way to minimize bureaucratic controls, secure capital for new patient care facilities, increase hospital revenues, increase practice plan revenues, and stem the loss of paying patients. They tended to oppose separation out of concern for maintaining the quality of clinical research and residency experience and maximizing state financial support. Separation is not viewed as an end in itself but rather as a vehicle to help improve the AHC, given its resources, problems, and local market conditions. Some medical school deans support separation to preserve the strengths of a good situation, not to make the best of a bad one.

Separation from the university can facilitate joining an IDN. While it maintains its affiliation with the university, the medical school pays for services used at the hospital, focuses on teaching and research, and is supported by tuition and grants flowing through the university. It is separate to the extent that it has control over management policy decisions. The separation is a matter of relative perspective: University hospitals may be separate from some groups (i.e., state agencies) but not others (i.e., university administrators) (Munson & D'Aunno, 1987).

CONFRONTING THE MARKET AND THE MISSION: IMPLICATIONS FOR NURSING

Requirements for success in the new market are centered around three key factors: cost, quality, and access. Nursing has innumerable opportunities to influence these three factors—if it reorients education, research, and practice around these variables. It is essential that rigorous analysis be applied to every aspect of nursing.

Education

The issue of basic educational preparation to practice nursing in this new environment is, once again, a serious factor. Eighteen months of education is not adequate preparation for many of the practice opportunities in IDNs, nor do many of our IDN programs provide the education necessary for the new market. The Health of the Public recommendations should be used to review curricula. Programs should be identified clearly in terms of how and how much they are devoted to cost, quality, and access. Does the curriculum reflect a true population health perspective? Most curricula are still organized around diseased body parts (orthopedics), types of hospital units (medical-surgical), or the profession of nursing (nursing theory). The role of education within health care organizations usually expands during times of rapid change, expanding faculty opportunities in the community as well as in the AHC.

Medicare funding of nursing education is insufficient and misdirected. Approximately 15% ($174 million) of

Medicare funding for health care professional education is directed to hospitals for the training of nurses and paramedical personnel, although there are roughly three times as many practicing nurses as physicians in the United States (Aiken, Gwyther, & Whelan, 1994). This funding supports primarily professional education in nursing, with 66% going to hospitals operating diploma programs and graduating less than 10% of nurse graduates. Graduate education for nurses, including the preparation of advanced practice nurses (APNs), does not generally qualify for reimbursement under existing Medicare policy (Aiken & Gwyther, 1995). Starting to recognize the importance of nurses, the federal government proposed increased funding for their support through The Health Security Act of 1993, which would have provided $200 million in financial support for nurses in graduate study, but the legislation was not implemented (Aiken & Gwyther, 1995).

Research

Many of the research subsidies that have traditionally been encompassed in Medicare and Medicaid pass-throughs and private insurer premiums have come under increased scrutiny and will no doubt be decreased. The allocation of overhead allowances has tightened, further restricting funds. Additionally, competition for research funding will undoubtedly increase.

To compete effectively, researchers will have to change their focus to clinical outcomes. Researchers who create multidisciplinary, multisituational teams will have an advantage in this new environment. Nursing's proximity to patients and the community is very advantageous in designing and successfully executing outcomes research. Faculty must encourage graduate students to move their research focus from nurses and nursing issues to patients and population health.

Nursing practice

Nursing practice is the key to addressing cost, quality, and access. As the largest group of health care professionals, nurses can greatly expand and improve access. Although nurses have been employed primarily in acute care settings, they have also been the largest group of health professionals in long-term care, home care, ambulatory care settings.

In assessing an organization's ability to move from intervention during episodes of illness to assuming responsibility for covered lives, the importance of nursing becomes obvious. Although acute care volume will continue to decline in most markets, acute care cost and quality are essential to success in an IDN. Nursing is also the key to restructuring clinical operations to achieve targets for service, clinical outcomes, and cost. In addition to eliminating waste and duplication, nurses must also develop clinical practice guidelines to restructure clinical practice. These guidelines must move beyond acute care to be enterprise-wide. Typically, APNs will assume the case management roles necessary to manage patients across the continuum.

There will be significantly more positions for APNs in IDNs. APNs provide a simple, high-quality, cost-effective approach to the shortage of primary care providers. Many organizations are creating collaborative practices for APN/MD pairings. Because of the high cost of subspecialist physicians, hospitals will increasingly employ APNs to leverage the subspecialists.

Because patient satisfaction is one of the key variables that managed care organizations monitor, it is essential for nurses to take the lead in developing and refining report cards. It will be increasingly important for nurse managers to create unit-specific report cards that monitor cost, service, and outcome measures for their units and for nurse executives to create incentives and rewards for nurse performance based on these report cards.

Because nurses are essential to providing access to the IDN, as IDNs seek closer partnerships with their communities, nurses can assist in forging these relationships through roles in school nursing, occupational health nursing, and congregational nursing. In addition to school, work, and place of worship, nurses are the primary providers of home health services. Opportunities in all of these nonacute care sites will increase significantly in the near future. To continue to dominate these markets, nurses must continue to strive for better clinical outcomes, increased satisfaction, and lower costs.

The survival of many of the nation's AHCs is uncertain. While the American public values their innovation, research, and high-quality education, it is clear that AHCs must refocus their mission for research, education, and patient service on pressing public health care needs. This refocussing will require the AHC to transform itself from a system that has served well to one that will lead the way for improved health for the nation.

CRITICAL SUCCESS FACTORS

As AHCs prepare themselves to deliver services in a prepaid, inclusive health care market, there are a number of critical success factors that will determine whether they achieve the transformation required:

- AHCs must have a vision of integrated delivery, closely shared among the leadership of the school, the faculty practice, and the hospital, as well as a strong concept of how to achieve it.
- AHCs must be capable of rapid decision making in order to implement external strategies, including partnering with other providers and investing in building a managed care system.
- AHCs must create greater efficiency in internal operations, including contracting, capital investments, faculty recruitment, funds management, and medical center cost management.
- AHCs must achieve excellent utilization of services and have the management systems in place to cross departmental and organizational boundaries.
- AHCs must create an integrated information system that spans all medical center operations and ultimately links with community providers and potentially with buyers.
- AHC leadership must understand the current economic interrelationships and flow of funds between the teaching, research, and patient-care components of the organization, and they must define how it will be managed in the future.
- AHCs must partner with community organizations and create mechanisms to mutually integrate practice methods to field a superior health services system together.
- AHCs must work with their universities and other constituents (including state legislatures) to craft the ownership and governance structures that support these success factors.

REFERENCES

Aiken, L.H., & Gwyther, M.E. (1995). Medicare funding of nurse education: The case for policy change. *Journal of the American Medical Association, 273*(19), 1528-1532.

Aiken, L.H., Gwyther, M.E., & Whelan, E.-M. (1994, July). *Advanced practice nursing education: Strategies for the allocation of the proposed graduate nursing education account.* Philadelphia: University of Pennsylvania Center for Health Services and Policy Research/School of Nursing.

Allison, R.F., & Dalton, J.W. (1982, Spring). Governance of university-owned teaching hospitals. *Inquiry,* 3-17.

Anders, G. (1993, June 11). Health initiatives. *The Wall Street Journal.*

Association of Academic Health Centers. (1992, November). *Critical data about academic health centers survey report.* Washington, DC: The Association Health Centers.

Dowd, M. (1994, July 20). Strong support for health plans. *The New York Times,* p. A1.

Friedman, E. (1993). Whither medical education? *JAMA, 270*(12), 1473-1476.

Health plans savings. (1992, April 8). *The New York Times,* p. D11. Associated Press.

Japsen, B. (1994). Teaching hospitals face hard lessons. *Modern Healthcare 24*(6), 36-40.

Kaufman, A. & Waterman, R. (1993). *Health of the public: A challenge to academic health centers: Strategies for reorienting academic health centers toward community health needs.* Albuquerque, NM: University of New Mexico School of Medicine.

Kaufman, K., Shortell, S., Becker, S., & Neuhauser, D. (1979). The effects of board composition and structure on hospital performance. *Hospital and Health Services Administration, 24,* 37-63.

Knapp, R. (1993). *Academic medicine and health care reform: Goals and principles for healthcare reform.* (p. 3). Washington, DC: Association of American Colleges.

Munson, F.C., & D'Aunno, T.A. (1987). *The university hospital in the academic medical center: Finding the right relationship* (vol. 1.). Washington, DC: Association of Academic Health Centers and Association of American Medical Colleges.

Olmos, D. (1994, August 15). *A dose of reality hits Cedars. The Los Angeles Times,* p. A1.

Westerman, J. (1980). A requiem for the university hospital. *Health Care Management Review,* 5, 17-24.

Winslow, R. (1993, March 2). Corporate health-cost rise is called lowest in 5 years. *The Wall Street Journal,* pp. B2-B3.

Wise, D. The state of health care in America. (1993). *Business and Health Magazine, 13,* 57.

Zuckerman, H.S., D'Aunno, T.A., & Vaughan, T.E. (1990, Spring). *The strategies and autonomy of university hospitals in competitive environments.* Hospital and Health Services Administration.

The Canadian health care system: Overview and issues

JANET C. ROSS KERR

Canadians have come to believe passionately in health insurance coverage as a right of citizenship, and the tax-supported Medicare program remains one of the most highly valued and popular initiatives of the Canadian government. Public opinion polls reflect this support, which is reported to be as high as 85% (Inglehart, 1990). Even though costs have skyrocketed in recent years, Canadians are unsympathetic to the possibility of a return to the private arrangements for health care that were common prior to federal legislation for hospital care almost 40 years ago. Despite the high level of public support for Medicare, several provinces have challenged the provisions of the Canada Health Act by allowing private clinics to charge "facility fees" while allowing physicians to be reimbursed for their services through publicly funded Medicare, a federal program that is administered jointly by the federal and provincial governments. While the high cost of federal health care expenditures has led to a rethinking and reconsideration of funding arrangements by the federal government, the Liberal government elected in 1992 has maintained that it has a fundamental commitment to the principles of Medicare. It has further denounced the facility fees as a contravention of the Canada Health Act and gave provinces a firm October 15, 1995 deadline to eliminate facility fees or face severe financial penalties. Such penalties were imposed on provinces that did not comply by the deadline. The establishment of the National Forum on Health on October 20, 1994, chaired by the Prime Minister, put in the forefront the issues surrounding "public and private financing of health care." Its purpose was to study the issues and make recommendations for action (National Forum on Health, 1995, p. i).

PHILOSOPHICAL BASIS OF THE CANADIAN SYSTEM OF UNIVERSAL HEALTH CARE

The rationale for the evolution of the federal health legislation program can be found in five basic principles of health care from which the standards for the legislation are derived. The first principle, *universality,* refers to extending coverage to the population as a whole rather than to selected groups. *Comprehensiveness* ensures that all medically necessary services included in the plan are covered. Although extrabilling and user fees were allowed prior to 1984, since that time differential charges may no longer be applied on a private basis for services covered by the plan. *Accessibility* is perhaps the most difficult principle to satisfy, particularly with a sparse population scattered over a vast territory. However, reasonable access to services is seen as essential even in view of the need to constrain costs. *Portability,* or coverage for residents of one province when they require services just after a move or during a visit to another, must be ensured in plans. *Public administration,* nonprofit operation by an organization fiscally responsible to the provincial government, is also required. In the various acts passed by the federal government relative to health insurance since 1957, progressive refinement of the standards applicable to provincial health plans based on the basic principles has been evident.

The incorporation of a system of health care in legislation ensures that certain defining characteristics will emerge from the philosophy and principles on which it is based. Because the system itself is entrenched in law, if change is desired then full legislative review is required. This could be either an advantage of a disadvantage depending on the issue of concern and the nature of any change deemed necessary. Approximately 75% of health care expenditures in Canada fall under Medicare, while about 25% fall outside Medicare in services not reimbursed by the plan. At the outset, the Canadian health care system evolved in a manner not unlike systems in other Western countries. The fact that the provincial plans insure hospital care and physicians' services means that the hospital and the physician are paramount in the system. It is not surprising to find that the number of hospital beds increased at a rate much higher than the rate of population increase until legislation appeared to end the 50/50 federal/provincial cost sharing. Outpatient care, home care, and community health services were areas not eligible for federal cost sharing at the outset. The exclusion of these forms of care from federal financing encouraged the physician-centered, in-hospital care that have been dominant features of the system that evolved over 40 years (Ross Kerr, 1996). The high cost of these methods of providing care has led to a search for more effective and efficient lower-cost alternatives. The consumer movement has also heightened awareness of the need for consumers to be active participants in matters pertaining to their health. The Alma Ata agreement by countries who are members of the World Health Organization—of health for all by the year 2000—has carried with it an implicit challenge to encourage genuine community involvement in planning for health in ways that have been neither recognized nor explored previously in health care delivery systems. The challenge for health care in Canada is to tailor the legislative arrangements for health care to encourage community-based measures facilitating health maintenance, health promotion, and prevention of disease and to balance these with measures to restore health.

> Many believe that it will not be possible to sustain the current system without major modifications. Task forces and commissions in most provinces are looking at ways to shift the heavy focus on physician and institutional care to "community based" alternatives and non-physician providers. (Deber, Hastings, & Thompson, 1991, pp. 73-74)

THE ESTABLISHMENT OF THE CANADIAN HEALTH INSURANCE SYSTEM

In a society in which life is deeply valued, the health of people becomes an issue of fundamental importance. Responsibility for health was granted to the provinces in the British North America Act, which established the Canadian Confederation in 1867. Health was reserved as a federal prerogative for marine and quarantine hospitals and for aboriginal peoples. The Constitution Act of 1982, which superseded the original legislation, confirmed and continued this division of powers. Social democratic traditions along with Canada's growth and development as a colonial empire perhaps contributed more than other factors to the perception of the need to ensure the availability of health care for the entire population. In the aftermath of social upheavals created by the Great Depression and two world wars, many factors converged to create a receptive climate for consideration of public financing of individual health care expenditures. Federal/provincial agreements emerged from public debate and discussion and culminated in the implementation of a system of national health insurance to cover health care costs for all Canadians.

Although the Canadian program of insurance for hospital services at the federal level was not enacted until 1957, the stage was set for the federal legislation in previous supportive developments in the provinces. The province of Saskatchewan was clearly in the forefront of provincial developments, and after World War I passed legislation enabling municipalities to raise taxes to support the employment of physicians (the municipal doctor plans), the establishment of hospitals, and the development of hospitalization plans. The window of opportunity created by the Canadian Medical Association's firm support for publicly financed health insurance in 1934 was lost through government inaction, and the Canadian Medical Association later withdrew its support in favor of private plans initiated by physicians in several provinces. Saskatchewan decided to "go it alone" when it became the first jurisdiction in North America to enact legislation establishing a prepaid plan of hospital insurance in 1947. Although it fell short of the objective of establishing a prepaid hospital insurance plan, the first legislation dealing with health was passed by the federal government in 1948. The National Health Grants Act included funds for hospital construction, professional training, public health, and other provincial services, areas seen as providing the basis for the later establishment of national health insurance.

When the Hospital Insurance and Diagnostic Services Act was passed in 1957, it provided for comprehensive inhospital patient care services with universal coverage for residents of participating provinces. Because health fell within provincial jurisdiction, the government of each province had the right to decide whether or not to develop a plan to insure hospital services conforming to the federal guidelines outlined in the legislation. However, because the plan involved 50/50 cost-sharing with the provinces, any province deciding to opt out of the arrangement would forego any tax dollars that the federal government would otherwise contribute to health care in that province and would effectively subsidize the plans of other provinces. Five provinces initially agreed to participate when the Act came into force in 1958, and by 1961 all provinces were full participants in the program. Excepted from the national hospital insurance program were tuberculosis and mental hospitals and certain other institutions.

In adding prepayment for medical services to the hospitalization plan in 1962, Saskatchewan again became the first jurisdiction to implement such legislation. It did so over the loud protests of Saskatchewan physicians who went on strike for 23 days beginning July 1, 1962, the date the legislation was implemented. In the face of vehement opposition from physicians, the Saskatchewan government was forced to make concessions to the medical profession in the form of allowing opting out of the plan and extrabilling. Implementation of the federal agenda to add medical services to its program of prepaid health insurance was undoubtedly hastened and facilitated by the lessons learned from the Saskatchewan experience. The federal Medical Care Act was thus passed in 1966, and the controversial nature of the legislation may explain the participation of only two provinces at the time the legislation came into force on July 1, 1968, as well as the 5 years it required for all provinces to enter into an arrangement with the federal government for the prepayment of medical services. The plan allowed for coverage of physicians' services both in and out of the hospital but did not prevent the provinces from allowing physicians to opt out of the plan, bill patients directly, or impose surcharges on the established fee for a particular service.

In the early 1970s, the escalation of expenditures and the growing size of the federal deficit caused concern over the open-ended nature of some health expenditures, in particular those for physicians' services. In 1977, the system of federal/provincial cost sharing was amended with the passage of the Fiscal Arrangements and Established Programs Financing Act. This ended the open-ended 50/50 cost sharing and introduced block funding, which involved transfer of some tax points to the provinces and reduced to 25% the federal contribution to health care with additional federal contributions based on increases in the Gross Domestic Product. In the years following the passage of this legislation, concern mounted over the increased use of copayments, termed *user fees,* for institutional services and extrabilling practices among physicians in provinces where this was allowed. The Liberal federal government responded to these perceived erosions of Medicare by disallowing extrabilling and user fees in the Canada Health Act of 1984. Although physicians mounted a strong and vocal campaign to prevent the prohibition of extrabilling, it was to no avail. A measure of the popularity of Medicare in Canada may be seen in the fact that the Progressive Conservative government elected later in 1984 did not make any attempt either to amend the legislation or to develop new proposals, either immediately or in the 8 subsequent years. This government, however, did turn a blind eye to the Canada Health Act in allowing facility fees, charges imposed by private clinics for care by physicians who were also reimbursed by fees for their services through the public Medicare program.

ISSUES IN COST CONTAINMENT

Costs of medical care

Analyses of the Canadian experience with Medicare have concluded that the introduction of a system of universal health insurance has led to relative stability in health care costs in reference to the Gross National Product (Barer, Evans, & Labelle, 1988; Van Loon, 1980). Whereas Canadian health care costs were equivalent to those in the United States prior to the full implementation of Medicare in 1971, "by 1985 the United States was spending over two percentage points of GNP more (and growing) on health care" (Barer et al., p. 44). Despite the Canadian record, it is widely concluded that fine-tuning is required to control escalation of costs in the system. The focus of the most attention is that of physicians fees: "Payments for physician services, which in most countries run a significant second to institutional care in their share of total health costs, tend to be the most difficult and controversial to control" (Barer, p. 1). Because physicians are remunerated primarily on a fee-for-service basis in Canada, "the rate of increase of those fees is a natural target" (p. 1).

Although physicians are reimbursed through fees paid for individual services, they bill the health insurance plan in each province for their fees rather than billing the individual patient. Because the health insurance plan is billed, physicians' fee schedules have been the subject of negotiation between provincial governments and the medical profession in each province since the full implementation of Medicare in 1971. In the interest of containing costs, there is considerable pressure in most provinces to keep the rates of increase in physicians' fee schedules to a reasonable level. Expenditures for physicians' services constitute approximately 16% of health expenditures, a figure that is considerably higher (20%) in the United States

(Barer et al., 1988). Analyses of fee increases have noted that, "since 1971 physicians' fees in all the provinces of Canada have risen no more rapidly than general inflation rates, and in some provinces and/or time periods have lagged well behind" (Barer et al., 1988, p. 4).

The negotiation of fee schedules between governments and physicians has often produced considerable conflict and from time to time is carried out in the public eye with intense media attention. Although strikes are rare, physicians have not hesitated to employ threats of service withdrawal in negotiations in order to support their fee demands. A strike lasting 25 days occurred in Ontario in 1986; however, as in the 1962 Saskatchewan physicians' strike, it "failed in its fundamental political objective—the obstruction of government's resolve to extend its control over health insurance" (Stevenson, Williams, & Vayda, 1988, p. 71). However, the notion of solidarity within physician ranks to maintain "autonomy and dominance in the health care system" (p. 71) has been challenged. It has been suggested that:

> "the degree of organization and commitment" of the medical profession is less than is commonly assumed, and that the political weight of the profession is greater than it need be because governments and other political actors hold exaggerated assumptions about its organization and commitment. (Stevenson et al., 1988, p. 71)

This national survey of Canadian physicians conducted in 1986 and 1987 found that 61% agreed that "Medicare 'has positively influenced the health status of Canadians' by improving access to medical services" (Stevenson et al., 1988, p. 79). It also found that just over "60 percent of physicians are satisfied 'in the practice of medicine' under Medicare and only 24 percent are dissatisfied" (p. 79). Finally, a finding that "60 percent of physicians disapprove and only one-quarter approve of 'the withdrawal of nonemergency services' in support of income demands" (p. 85) lends credence to the premise that solidarity and commitment among physicians to "an unregulated medical marketplace" (p. 84) is not as firm as is commonly believed.

Other concerns in relation to the costs of physicians' services are physicians' billing activity, the supply of physicians, and specialization. Controls on fees produced increased billing activity as physicians sought to respond to fee controls by increasing their activity. However, a number of studies have shown that physicians have not been able to offset the impact of fee controls on their incomes, and "the extent to which they are able to do so depends critically on the fee negotiation context" (Barer et al., p. 44). In addition, because fees are negotiated between physicians and provincial governments on an annual basis, there is an ongoing opportunity for removing "'loopholes' in the fee schedule that provide the opportunities for procedural multiplication" (p. 44). The supply of physicians is another factor that interacts with other variables relative to containment of medical costs. Thus, while

> billing activity per physician has increased more rapidly in Canada [than in the United States], utilization per capita has not, at least since 1975. In that year Canada cut back sharply on physician immigration, with the result that while prior to 1975 physician supply was growing more rapidly in Canada, since then it has grown more slowly. (Barer et al., p. 45)

Access to specialization has been strictly limited in Canada, and as a result half of all Canadian physicians are general practitioners, as compared with 10% in the United States (Terris, 1991). Because specialists perform more procedures and carry out more tests, allowing the ratio of general practitioners to specialists to change will cause increases in costs and may not serve the public good. Indeed, the optimal size of medical school enrollments is an issue of concern in Canada: If the ratio of physicians to population size increases, it is likely that medical services and costs will also increase. An agreement by the provincial ministers of health to curtail medical school enrollments has produced some downsizing of medical school capacity. Because higher education receives significant operating support from provincial and federal governments, pressure placed by government on universities is considered very seriously by the institutions. The recent experience is that political pressure did produce a small decrease in the size of medical school enrollments. Whether or not the decrease was sufficient, however, remains to be seen. In any case, it must be recognized that all of the variables of concern in containing physician costs become more difficult to deal with because of the open-ended nature of expenditures for medical care.

Alternative methods of paying physicians are increasingly being sought in Canada as a means of constraining expenditures for physicians' services. Under consideration in a number of provinces are salaries and capitation, a method of remunerating general practitioners whereby they are paid a fee for providing services to a certain number of people. In a recent report commissioned by the provincial ministers of health, the development of primary care organizations was promoted (Kennedy, 1995). Physicians would be grouped in these large clinics where they would practice in conjunction with a number of other health professionals. In the primary care organizations, physicians would be paid an annual fee for each person registered with the organization; hence, there would be a built-in incentive for promoting health and keeping people well. Other methods such as capping of incomes and other provisions have been used in some provinces as additional regulations imposed on the fee-for-service system, but it would appear that in the face of dramatic health care reform across the country, Canada is moving quickly to find more satisfactory ways of remunerating physicians, and in an era in which governments are determined to eliminate debt and avoid deficit financing, expenditures for medical care have come under close scrutiny. The aging of the population, increasing rates of health care utilization, and mounting costs have given impetus to health care reform and have ensured that the debate over payment for medical services will have a high profile in the public arena once again. As Northcott (1994a) has reflected: "And so the debates continue. Canada's health-care program is currently neither free-enterprise medicine nor socialized medicine. Rather it is something in between" (p. 79). It is defining that "something in between" that has presented challenges to practitioners, policymakers, and the Canadian public alike.

Costs of hospitalization

The problems of escalating expenditures for hospitalization are not of the same magnitude as those for physicians' services as budgets for hospitals are established and strictly followed. There are important issues of cost control here, and provincial governments hold responsibility for establishing and maintaining a health system that will not only serve consumer needs but will also be affordable. Hospitals are provided with a global budget to cover operating costs on an annual basis by provincial governments. Capital expenditures are considered separately, but the process is again one of negotiation with the government. This does not allow for expansion of hospitals or the purchase of expensive equipment without a process of rationalization. Although hospitals have generally operated under the direction of boards of directors, in the matter of annual budget determination and approval the government clearly has the upper hand. This centralized process by which the annual total expenditures of hospitals are established is clearly a political one, and the debate is often highly public. Hospital administrators increasingly have been going public with their case for maintenance of or increases in funding. This can sometimes paint a false picture of the situation, however, because what appears in the media may be simply posturing in a public debate over the advisability of expenditures in one area or another. Thus,

> The difficulty for health policy and funding is that, since the boy always cries wolf (and must do so, given the political system of funding), one does not know if the wolf is really there. The political dramatics should not mislead external observers into believing that the wolf is always at hand. (Evans et al., 1989, p. 574)

Costs for nursing form a significant portion of the costs of hospitalization, although they are hidden within the global budget of the hospital. Despite the intense and prolonged public debate over hospital costs, the nursing workforce forms the element of hospital expenditures that can perhaps be most easily manipulated. The all too familiar scenario of closing beds and laying off employees, principally nurses, in response to government cost-cutting measures is played out frequently in tough economic times. However, in view of changing emphases in the health system, with the focus moving from acute, in-hospital care to community-based care and treatment emphasizing prevention, promotion of health, and consumer initiative, nurses must face the prospect of radical changes in the nature and structure of care that will have a profound impact on the profession. All too often, nurses are not at the table when cost-containment decisions are made, or if they are there, they may find themselves in a vulnerable and compromised position in relation to the hard decisions being made. In contrast to the process of determining remuneration for physicians, for whom the fee schedule is directly negotiated between physician organizations and the government, the situation is very different for nurses. Because nurses are largely employees of hospitals, they answer to their superiors, nursing administrators, and ultimately the chief executive officer of the employing institution. While nursing unions exist in all provinces with a mandate from nursing members in local hospitals to bargain collectively for salary levels for various categories of nursing employees, individual hospital administrators acting on direction from boards have the right to determine the number of nursing positions needed in an institution. Under enlightened administrations, representatives of nursing unions may sit on advisory councils that consider nursing issues and recommend solutions to the chief nursing administrator; however, it is unlikely that this is the case in the majority of hospitals. Therefore, the nursing workforce in hospitals can be made to contract or expand rather quickly by changing the number of positions. Issues relative to the supply of nurses are important because it is essential to prepare an appropriate number of nurses with the educational background necessary to allow them to contribute to the health system in an important and meaningful way.

While they find their positions disappearing in substantial numbers from the acute care system, nurses are finding themselves at the forefront of the increasing emphasis on community-based care. While community health agencies have employed a small part of the nursing workforce, nurses working in the community form a highly educated group and have historically worked relatively autonomously in collaboration with other health professionals. Although initial health legislation only allowed for remuneration in provincial plans for physicians and dental surgeons, the Canada Health Act of 1984 contained a provision to allow for payments to "health practitioners." The Canadian Nurses Association lobbied intensively and successfully for the inclusion of this clause, which no provincial government to date has implemented as a part of its plan. However, the opportunity is there for the development of community health centers that could be reimbursed for the services of a variety of health professionals, including nurses. A small group of nurses is engaged in independent practice in most provinces; however, a nurse in independent practice must bill the client directly for services, because no provincial plan will currently allow this. In an era when there is a movement toward salaries or contracts for all health professionals, it is unlikely that nurses would be paid on a fee-for-service basis by provincial health plans. Nevertheless, in the move to an increased focus on community-based health care services, nurses will undoubtedly be called on to play important and continuing roles.

ALTERNATIVE HEALTH SYSTEM

It must be recognized that there is a thriving alternative health system in Canada with patients seeking the services of the providers of these services in relatively large numbers. While some alternative services fall partly within and partly outside (e.g., chiropractic) the official health system, most fall completely outside the official system. Northcott has observed that about 10% of the population uses alternative health care and that about 5% to 15% visit a chiropractor annually. Other alternative providers include acupuncturists, reflexologists, herbalists, and many others including those practicing certain forms of folk medicine. The hostility between the two systems has been present historically. However, while it has become increasingly recognized that a number of the treatments and practices that have developed within the alternative system are valuable, some providers have crossed the boundaries and have acquired the skills to offer treatments from both systems (Northcott, 1994b). It is likely that this part of the system will continue to grow and at least some part of it may be subsumed within the official system.

FUTURE DIRECTIONS

The tax-supported system of health care that has evolved in Canada over the last 40 years, while not flawless, is nevertheless highly regarded by consumers who react negatively to any suggestion that the system is imperiled. Such suggestions are the order of the day and simply part of business as usual in a not-for-profit system operated in the public sphere where interest groups and institutions alike have the opportunity to argue for funds and programs that they see as being beneficial. It is recognized today that there are limits to the nature and amount of care that can be provided and limits to growth. In order to ensure the continuation of the system, measures must be taken to ensure that universal availability and access to needed services are balanced by the provision of reasonably comprehensive services in a publicly funded, nonprofit, affordable system.

The system must respond to perceptions of a need for change in the nature and context of health care. It has been pointed out that Canada "provides a test case in the limits of medical care *per se,* and the health problems which still confront Canadians cannot, in general, be improved merely by improving access to medical care" (Deber et al., 1991, p. 74). Canada has had a hospital and physician–centered system of health care entrenched in its universal health care legislation for some 40 years. The social determinants of health such as income, education, and the environment are important elements in the health of a nation. Universal health insurance has provided some assistance to vulnerable populations, but other measures to address some of these problems are needed. Health is increasingly seen more broadly than simply the absence of illness, and in the presence of new approaches to the meaning of health, the nature and context of health care must change as well.

The needs of professional groups must be balanced by the needs of society. In the evolving health care system in Canada, there is a need for the health professions to work collaboratively in the best interest of the consumer. The system that has developed in Canada has provided high-quality medical and hospital care and has contributed significantly to improvements in the health of people. However, despite new and impressive technological adjuncts to care, rational judgements must be made concerning the nature and context of health and health care. Social and cultural determinants of health require much study and attention in order to produce improved health outcomes. The political framework within which the issues relative to health care insurance plans are debated and determined will be conditioned by the economic and social realities of effecting fundamental change in the system. Decisions to move to a community-based model emphasizing prevention of disease, promotion of health, and partnerships between professionals and consumers will be difficult ones but will ultimately hold the greatest potential for impacting health positively. Issues surrounding hospital governance, education of health professionals, integration of boards of health agencies on a regional basis, and restructuring the systems for providing care and for remunerating health professionals in a reasonable and rational way must be considered in a collaborative manner to allow the health care system in Canada to meet the challenges that lay ahead in this century and beyond.

REFERENCES

Barer, M.L., Evans, R.G., & Labelle, R.J. (1988). Fee controls as cost control: Tales from the frozen north. *The Milbank Quarterly, 66*(1), 1-64.

Deber, R.B., Hastings, J.E.F., & Thompson, G.G. (1991). Health care in Canada: Current trends and issues. *Journal of Public Health Policy, 12*(1), 72-82.

Evans, R.G., Lomas, J., Barer, M.L., Labelle, R.J., Fooks, C., Stoddart, G.L., Anderson, G.M., Feeny, D., Gafni, A., Torrance, G.W., & Tholl, W.G. (1989). Controlling health expenditures—the Canadian reality. *New England Journal of Medicine, 320*(9), 571-577.

Inglehart, J.K. (1990). Health policy report: Canada's health care system. *New England Journal of Medicine, 315*(12), 778-784.

Kennedy, M. (1995, September 16). Fee for service under attack from all quarters. *Edmonton Journal,* p. G1.

National Forum on Health. (1995). The public and private financing of Canada's health system: A discussion paper. Ottawa: Government of Canada.

Northcott, Herbert A., (1994a). Threats to medicare: The financing, allocation, and utilization of health care in Canada. In B. Singh Bolaria & H.D. Dickinson (Eds.), *Health, illness, and health care in Canada* (2nd ed., pp. 65-82). Toronto: Harcourt Brace.

Northcott, H.A., (1994b). Alternative health care in Canada. In B. Singh Bolaria & H.D. Dickinson (Eds.), *Health, illness, and health care in Canada* (2nd ed., pp. 487-503). Toronto: Harcourt Brace.

Ross Kerr, J. (1996). The organization and financing of health care. In J. Ross Kerr & J. MacPhail (Eds.), *Canadian nursing: Issues and perspectives* (2nd ed., pp. 216-227). Toronto: Mosby.

Stevenson, H.M., Williams, H.P., & Vayda, E. (1988). Medical politics and Canadian Medicare: Professional response to the Canada Health Act. *The Milbank Quarterly, 66*(1), 65-104.

Terris, M. (1991). Global budgeting and the control of hospital costs. *Journal of Public Health Policy, 12*(1), 61-71.

Van Loon, R.J. (1980). From shared cost to block funding and beyond: The politics of health insurance in Canada. In C. Meilicke & J.L. Storch (Eds.), *Perspectives on Canadian Health and society services policy: History and emerging trends* (pp. 342-366). Ann Arbor, MI: Health Administration Press.

Section Eight

HEALTH CARE COSTS

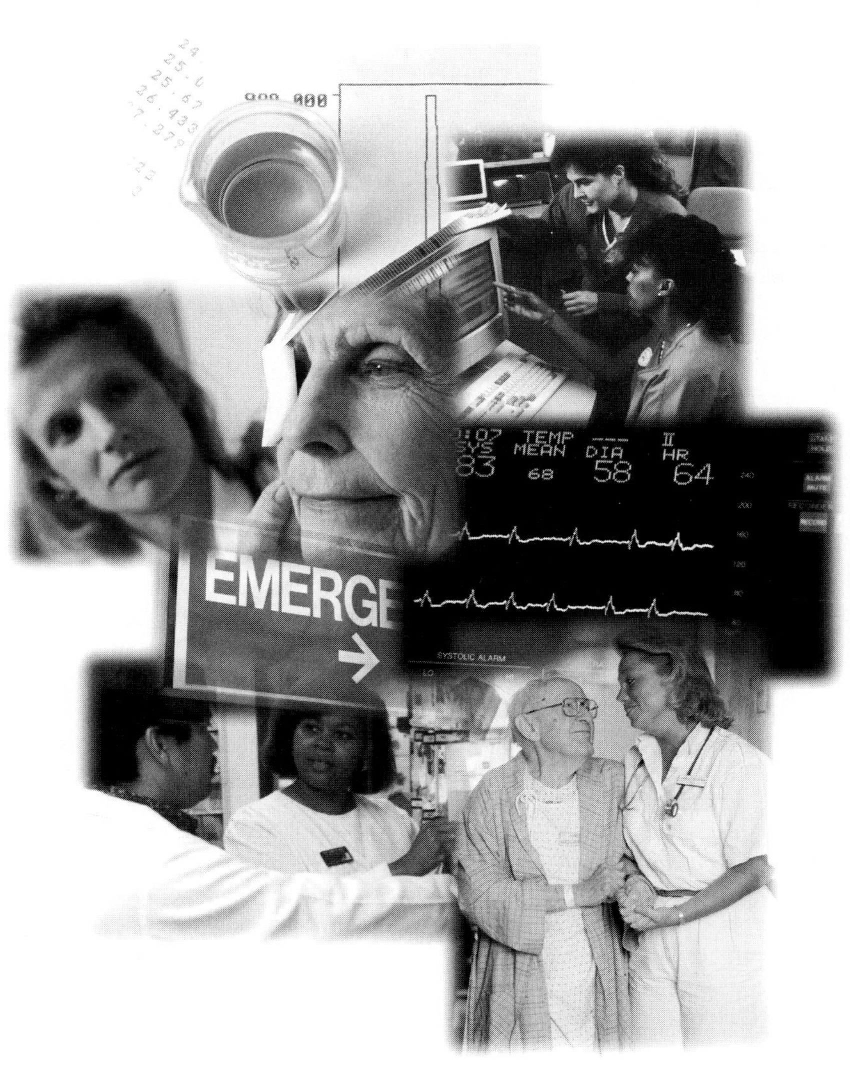

OVERVIEW

A concern for costs

JOANNE COMI McCLOSKEY, HELEN KENNEDY GRACE

It is interesting to note that even though cost containment is the driving force in health care, we always have a difficult time identifying enough people who can write good chapters about health care costs related to nursing. Few nurses have developed programs of research or careers around nursing economics. Until recently, this was neither a subject taught in many schools of nursing nor a source of concern for many nurses. Things have changed. Today's concern for costs is determining a number of decisions that affect nurses and our patients. This section introduces some of the issues surrounding the costs of nursing and health care.

In their debate chapter, Garg, Pinsker, and Grace overview the two major approaches to the control of health care costs: regulation and competition. This very informative chapter contains a clear overview of a number of cost-control initiatives. Total U.S. health expenditures grew from $41.9 billion in 1965 to $425 billion in 1985. The authors review the various regulatory (government intervention) initiatives of the past 30 years: certificates of need, economic stabilization programs, professional standards review organizations, prospective rate setting, and prospective payment systems. Over the past two decades, competitive approaches such as competitive contracting, managed care and health maintenance organizations, preferred provider organizations, cost sharing, medical savings accounts, and managed competition have been used to supplement or supplant regulatory approaches. Each of the regulatory and competitive approaches is described with some information about its advantages and disadvantages. Despite all of the approaches taken, the major problems remain: escalating costs, increasing numbers of individuals without health insurance, and uneven access and quality of care. The solutions to these problems, according to Garg, Pinsker, and Grace, do not lie within government, insurers, providers, or employers but with the consumers of health services. Yet they point out that the consumer is not part of the debate. Garg, Pinsker, and Grace want to end the "outdated model of health care" in which "professionals are the all-knowing" and empower the people. They believe that until the consumer becomes an active partner in the system the problems are insoluble. Their chapter provides an excellent overview of past measures to control costs and raises many important issues that should be carefully digested and debated today.

In the next chapter Buerhaus explains how five interrelated economic pressures are driving the evolution of the health care system. The pressures are: (1) rising health care expenditures, (2) growth of the federal budget deficit, (3) growth of managed care organizations, (4) competition among managed care organizations, and (5) evolution of integrated health delivery systems. Buerhaus says that competition in health care is beginning to lower the rate of health care expenditures. In order to raise their value during this competitive time, nurses must be innovative in contributions that allow the employing organization to lower costs. Buerhaus also sees that changes in the payment system are stimulating a closer alignment between practice and education. All in all, this is a good, clear overview of the economic changes in health care and the impact these changes are having on nursing.

Many believe that shifting care delivery to the home will reduce health care expenses, but there is confusion about the nature of home care. The cost-effectiveness of home care is discussed by Aronow, Gold, Yuhas, Alessi, and Beck. They first classify in-home interventions into three purposes: substitution for institutional-based acute or long-term care, transition from institutional care to the community, and prevention of the onset of disability and the need for institutional care. Each of these purposes—substitution, transition, and prevention—are discussed with regard to goal, population, range of services, benefits, and evidence for cost-effectiveness. The chapter includes an excellent review of the research studies that have evaluated care for each of the three purposes. Building on this background, the authors then describe a 5-year demonstration project in Santa Monica, California. Two hundred fifteen persons 75 years of age or older received a comprehensive geriatric assessment visit plus three additional home visits for 3 years from a geriatric nurse practitioner. The purpose for the care was prevention, and the individuals included in the project had no known terminal diseases or severe functional impairments. Compared with a control group the persons who received the geriatric nurse practitioner visits had fewer nursing home admissions and were more independent in activities of daily living. While the costs of the program offset the lower cost of nursing home days, the effectiveness of care in terms of disability reduction was improved. As the number of elderly persons increases in our society, the initiation of innovative prevention-oriented home care programs is desirable. This chapter helps to clarify the confusion about types of home care services and overviews one possible model for preventive services.

One of the chief costs in health care is the salaries of providers. Havens and Mills address the wage and remuneration practices in nursing. They address the question of whether nurses are paid what they are worth. They present data and examine issues so that readers will debate the question and search for answers. The authors also present many interesting facts including the following: most staff nurses are paid according to an hourly wage; nurses working in the West and Northeast earn more than those employed in the Central states; and differences among specialties amount to less than $2.00 per hour. Nurses, they say, are paid for the time they work rather than for their skills, expertise, or accomplishments. Employers value *when* a registered nurse works (shift) more than his or her knowledge, skills, and job requirements. The authors compare the salary gains of nurses with those of other occupations. Although salaries improved dramatically in the early 1990s, nursing still lags behind in overall gain. Nursing salary increases have slowed, and recent cutbacks in hospitals are likely to result in further losses. The authors also discuss the issues involved in economic equity and call for new methods of evaluating and recognizing job worth.

Although regulations are used to control costs, we must not forget that compliance with regulations also incurs costs. The costs of a specific regulation are addressed by McPherson and Jackson, who examine the costs of safety precautions to protect health care workers from bloodborne pathogens. This is a confusing situation because the guidelines for the U.S. Centers for Disease Control and Prevention (CDC) and the Department of Labor's Occupational Safety and Health Administration (OSHA) address different aspects of infection control and have changed over time. Health care agencies are faced with the dilemma of implementing CDC universal precautions for everyone while also implementing another isolation system. One system expects health care workers to act the same for all patients, while the other expects caution only when caring for patients with known or suspected infections. The costs of complying with the OSHA regulations are estimated at $146 per employee per year, or around $813 million per year. The chief cost is the necessary protective equipment, especially gloves. The annual cost for implementing CDC universal precautions is estimated at about $336 million. Universal precautions use chiefly barrier techniques (gloves, gowns, masks, eyeglasses) based on traditional isolation techniques. While these may minimize nosocomial infections, there is little evidence to support the effectiveness of universal precautions in preventing bloodborne infections in health care workers. These authors say that the best risk reduction strategies to prevent HIV or hepatitis B infection are engineering controls to reduce risks from needles and other sharp equipment as well as work practice modifications in the use of sharp devices. They give an example of using injury data to change products and practices associated with intravenous access devices. The costs of administering a dose of hepatitis B vaccine and the costs of a follow-up program for an employee exposed to hepatitis B are addressed in detail.

The international chapter in this section is authored by Bichel, who describes health care and health care financing in Australia. The historical influence in Australia is British because Australia was established as a penal colony of the United Kingdom. The concept of "mateship," which developed out of the early experiences of convicts, bushrangers, and gold miners, has evolved into a national social conscience to provide for all citizens. Health care in Australia is intimately tied to politics and the party in power. Bichel overviews the health platforms of the Australian Labor Party and the Liberal-National Coalition Party. Australia's Medicare system was formed in 1984 with the principles of universality, access, equity, efficiency, and simplicity. Bichel overviews the benefits and disadvantages of the system from the perspectives of the users, who are generally in favor; the medical profession, which continues to be opposed; and the government, whose members have differing opinions depending on the party in power. Australian diagnosis-related groups were introduced in 1992 to enhance efficiency in hospitals. Future improvements in the health care system are needed in aboriginal health, for the aging, rural services, women's health, and preventive services. It is always helpful to compare health care systems. A reading of Bichel's chapter will give nurses from all countries both information about the Australian situation and insight, through comparison, into the systems in place in their own countries.

Nursing's ability to identify and deal with economic issues has come a long way in the past decade. More and more, nurses and nursing students are gaining knowledge about the costs of health care, but nursing is still not a major player in health care cost-containment efforts. We need to make the concern for costs a nursing concern and voice this concern and appropriate actions whenever the opportunity arises.

Controlling health care costs: Regulation versus competition

MOHAN L. GARG, EVE PINSKER, HELEN KENNEDY GRACE

The issue of controlling health care costs hits at the heart of a major social dilemma that grows out of the American character and the values surrounding the practice of medicine: the rights of the individual versus responsibility for the larger social group. The tensions between balancing individual rights against the common social good become compounded in the area of medical care because the physician becomes the arbiter between the individual and society. While there was a time when the physician could make decisions largely based on what was deemed best for the patient, today's concerns over the rising costs of medical care services and the large numbers of people without access to these services have made it increasingly difficult to practice in this simplistic manner. With the costs of health care rising far more rapidly than those of other parts of the economy, the concern for controlling these costs has become an increasing preoccupation in recent years.

Prior to the 1960s, most medical care costs were covered by insurance that was provided as part of the benefits package paid by employers for their workers. This system worked effectively for those who were employed and provided reimbursement to physicians and hospitals in a satisfactory manner. Over the years, however, an aging population, increased numbers of people who are not part of the workforce, and increasing costs of insurance to employers have resulted in a situation open for governmental intervention. The enactment of Medicare and Medicaid legislation in 1965 signaled the beginning of a new chapter for medical care in this country. The intent behind Medicaid and Medicare was to provide health care to the two most vulnerable groups—the elderly and the indigent who were not covered by employer-provided health care insurance and were unable to pay out of pocket. In effect, the federal government became the insurer for these uninsured populations. Soon after the enactment of these programs it was realized that health care expenditures were rising much faster than the economy, and initiatives were undertaken to address the issue. The agreed payment system based on "reasonable" costs for hospitals and "reasonable prevailing charges for physicians" provided little incentive for patients or providers to control health care costs. Over the past 30 years a variety of legislative approaches have been taken to try to control escalating costs. A systematic display of major initiatives is presented in Figure 63-1. These approaches can be classified either as *competitive,* describing a condition of the workings of the free market in which the unfettered private sector forces of supply and demand determine the most efficient allocation of resources, or *regulatory,* which assumes that market forces function imperfectly and that government intervention is required to control costs.

REGULATORY APPROACHES

The reimbursement system of Medicare and, to some extend, Medicaid, which was based on reasonable charges, created intense inflationary pressure on health care costs. While much of the health care for the elderly had been offered as charity, it was not reimbursable. In addition, there had been no incentives to add new expensive procedures prior to Medicare; that has also changed. Substantial reimbursement was available for increasing hospital revenue for additional procedures requiring new staff and equipment. By creating a surplus of income over revenues, this money went back into further expansion of facilities and staff, ultimately resulting in increased cost. This increased cost, which was not retrievable from public sources, was then passed on to private patients and their insurers, creating inflationary pressures on the entire

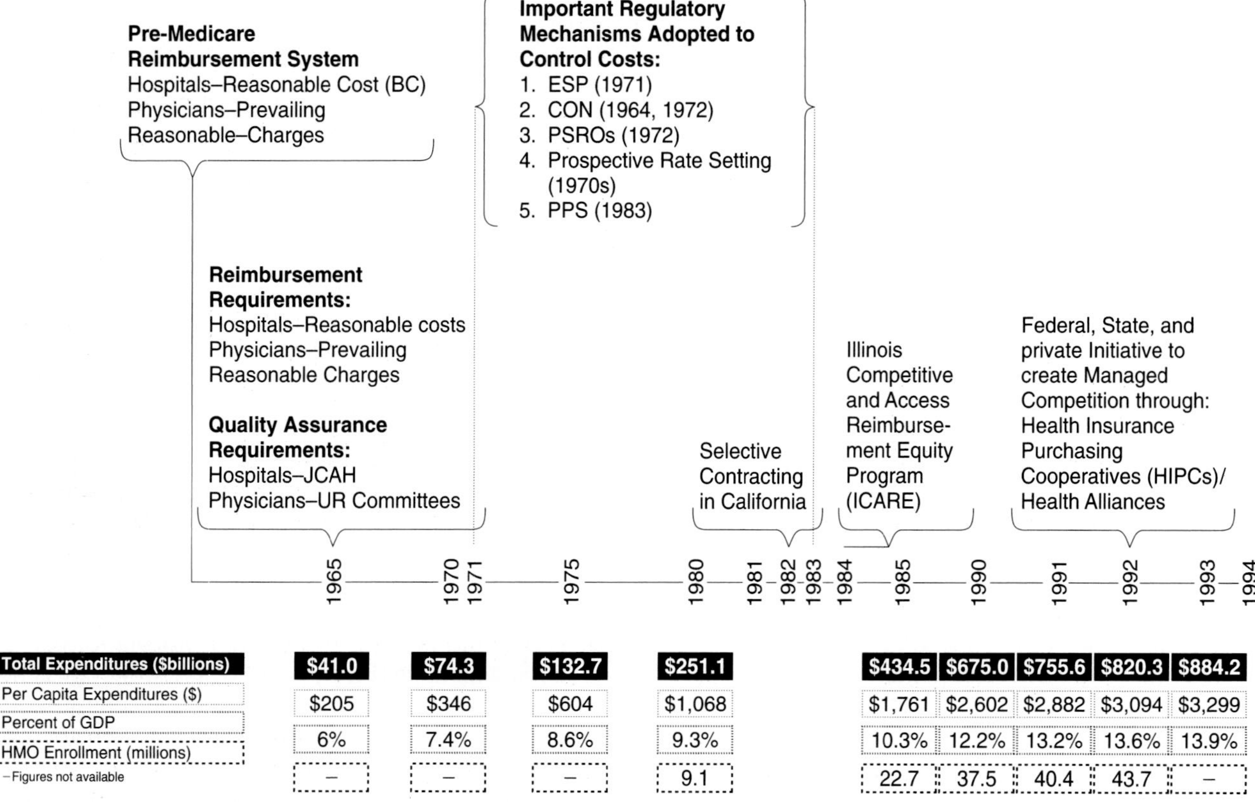

Total Expenditures ($billions)	$41.0	$74.3	$132.7	$251.1	$434.5	$675.0	$755.6	$820.3	$884.2
Per Capita Expenditures ($)	$205	$346	$604	$1,068	$1,761	$2,602	$2,882	$3,094	$3,299
Percent of GDP	6%	7.4%	8.6%	9.3%	10.3%	12.2%	13.2%	13.6%	13.9%
HMO Enrollment (millions)	–	–	–	9.1	22.7	37.5	40.4	43.7	–

Fig. 63-1. An overview of cost-control initiatives in U.S. health care.

system. Total health expenditures grew from $41.9 billion in 1965 to $425 billion in 1985. This increase occurred despite governmental efforts to control costs. From 1971 to 1983 the major efforts to control costs were through regulatory efforts. None has appreciably slowed the growth in total health care costs (Fig. 63-2).

Certificate of need

One type of intervention used the strategy of controlling the structure of medical care (i.e., the settings and instruments available and used for the provision of care), particularly by limiting the development of hospital capacity. Built on a certificate of need (CON) law initiated in New York State in 1964, Congress in 1972 passed amendments to the Social Security Act to give planning agencies more authority. In 1974, Congress passed the National Health Planning and Resources Development Act, which required every state to pass a CON law allowing it to review plans by any institutional provider for capital expenditures over $150,000 or a change in the number of beds and services. The impact of CON programs was minimal. A number of studies indicate that the review boards passed nearly everything that was brought to them (Begley, Schoeman, & Traxler, 1982; Lewin Associates, Inc., 1975; Salkever & Bice, 1976; Sloan & Steinwald, 1980). However, one side effect of the CON program was that hospitals gained sophistication about market conditions, long-range planning, and resource use—expertise easily adapted to a competitive market.

Economic stabilization program

The Economic Stabilization Program, introduced during the Nixon administration, was developed in two phases. Phase I (August 15, 1971 to November 13, 1971) involved a 90-day freeze on all wages and prices, and phase II (November 14, 1971 to April 30, 1974) limited institutional health care providers to a 6% annual limit in price increases in aggregate revenue, subject to cost justification. These controls applied to both hospital and physician fees. The Economic Stabilization Program appears to

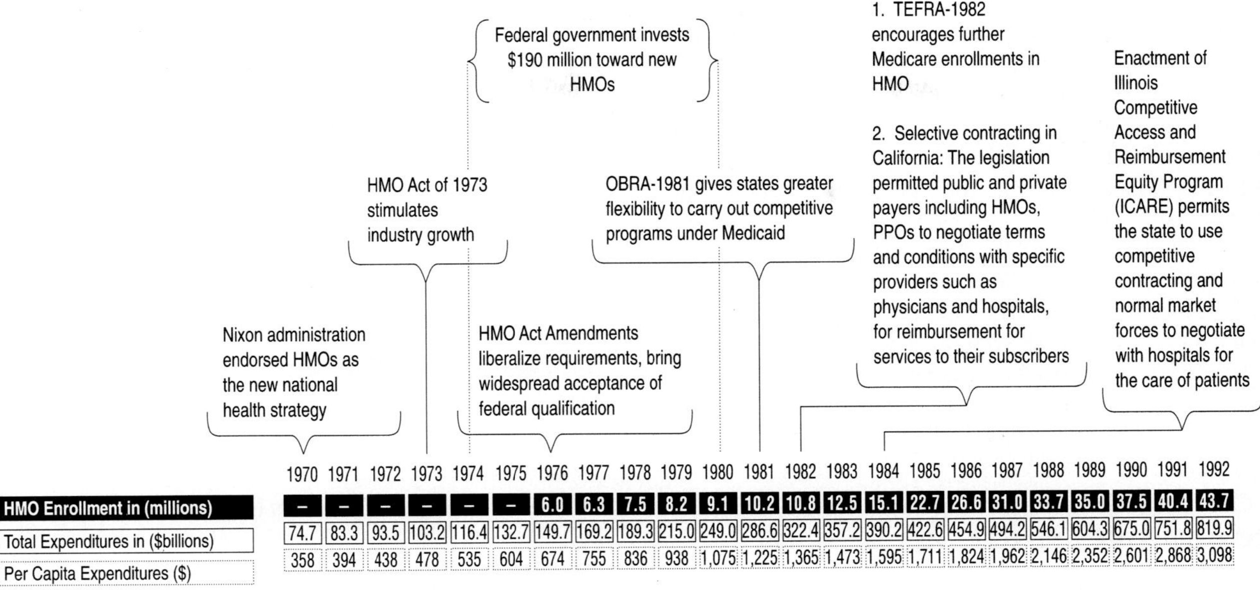

Fig. 63-2. An overview of legislative initiatives and the emergence of managed care and accompanying escalation of cost.

have moderated both the increase in average cost per hospital day (Salkever, 1979) and also the growth of physician fees; but there is some evidence that while fees were frozen, physicians classified visits into more expensive categories, thereby holding the line on price while allowing revenues to increase (Holahan & Scanlon, 1978).

Professional standards review organization

The quality, quantity, and cost of hospital care provided under Medicare was to be monitored primarily through mandatory establishment of utilization review committees in participating hospitals. Through review processes conducted under the supervision of physicians, their function was to control medical services such as admissions, diagnostic investigations, and therapeutic interventions provided by physicians to their hospitalized patients. A 1970 Senate Finance Committee Report judged the utilization reviews to be of a token nature and ineffective as a curb to unnecessary use of institutional care and services. The criticism of the utilization review led the American Medical Association to propose a Medicare peer review system to be controlled by the medical societies. Legislative action led to the establishment of professional standards review organizations with responsibility to review hospital care under their jurisdiction, with particular emphasis on the appropriateness of admission and the length of stay for hospitalization. Evaluations of the program are mixed, with one study concluding that the savings to Medicare and Medicaid exceeded the cost of the program by 10% to 15% (Smits, 1981), while another study concluded that it cost Medicare and Medicaid an estimated $1.80 for every $1 the program spent (Alpern, 1980).

Prospective rate setting

By 1980, most states had some form of hospital rate-setting program, but the programs varied considerably. Most were voluntary, with hospitals choosing whether to participate or comply. Only eight states had programs that involved mandatory review and compliance with rates set by a rate-setting authority. Mandatory rate-setting programs initiated by several states resulted in slowing the rate of growth of expenditures per patient day.

Prospective payment systems

In 1983, Congress established the Medicare Prospective Payment System (PPS), which replaced retrospective cost-based reimbursement for hospital care with the primary objective of controlling escalating hospital costs. Under the PPS, inpatient hospital services for Medicare eligibles were bundled into 468 diagnosis-related groups, with a fixed reimbursement schedule and adjustments for important factors such as case severity, rural/urban and regional labor cost differentials, teaching costs, and disproportionate shares of uncompensated care. During the first 3 years of the PPS, inflation in hospital expense was reduced by about 5% to 7% from the pre-PPS double-digit levels.

Despite these major regulatory programs, health care costs continued to escalate at a higher rate than the general economy. Expenditures for health care in 1985 totaled $420.1 billion as compared with $74.4 billion in 1970. The share of health care expenditures as a percentage of the gross national product increased from 7.3% in 1970 to 10.5% in 1985, with hospital expenditures accounting for 40% of all health care spending.

COMPETITIVE APPROACHES

As health care costs have continued to escalate in the past two decades, attempts to contain costs by restructuring the health care market to make cost-effective competition possible have supplemented, and in some cases supplanted, the regulatory programs described above. For economists, competition in a perfectly competitive or "free" market implies rivalry between sellers of *comparable* goods for customers. Customers will then choose the goods that cost less, knowing that they are not sacrificing quality, and thus the operation of the market encourages suppliers to keep prices down. The model of free market competition fully applies only when all product attributes other than prices are standardized. Obviously, many of the products in health care are not standardized.

A modified form of competition can occur between suppliers of noncomparable products in a particular market, but there is no guarantee that this kind of competition will result in lowered prices. This modified form of (nonprice) competition did occur among health care providers during the regulated era that followed the enactment of Medicare in 1965. During this period, hospitals competed for doctors and patients primarily on the basis of availability of sophisticated diagnostic and therapeutic technology. Patient comforts such as food quality, friendliness of staff, and cleanliness also played a major role in attracting patients to a particular facility. Despite nonstandardized "products" (in this case medical services), prices may have played a role in the competition if patients paid their own bills. However, during this period most patients had insurance so price did not play any role in their choices. Thus, relevant competitive variables included service offerings and amenities but not price. Furthermore, as third-party payers, health insurance companies did not promote price competition because they were not able to exclude providers on the basis of price. Hospitals and physicians were reimbursed on a "reasonable costs" and "reasonable charges" basis, respectively, but there was no competitive mechanism preventing "reasonable costs" from rising over time, and several factors such as collusion within the medical profession did promote increasing costs.

Competitive contracting

This situation began to change in 1982, when the State of California enacted legislation providing a mandate for "selective contracting," that is, reshaping the health-care market by enabling third-party payers to legally exclude providers from their list of participating providers without significant risk of antitrust prosecution. Under this legislation, both private and public payers, including health maintenance organizations (HMOs) and preferred provider organizations, could negotiate terms and conditions with specific providers such as physicians or physician groups and hospitals, who they would reimburse for services to their subscribers. Two hundred fifty hospitals that negotiated agreements with the state to provide services to Medi-Cal eligibles (Medicaid) accepted reductions in their normal payments ranging from 5% to 20%. As a consequence of the selective contracting, California saved an estimated $470 million in fiscal year 1983-84 (Iglehart, 1984). Following the trend set by California, other states began to follow various forms of competitive contracting.

Managed care and health maintenance organizations

The main feature of managed care that distinguishes it from retrospective and fee-for-service payments is that payment under managed care is prospective and capitated. Under such a system, the financial risk no longer resides with the patient or the third-party payer as distinct from the provider; instead the managed care entity becomes a financial riskbearer as well as a patient care provider. This means that the organizational focus of care shifts from individual illness care to concern for the health of a defined population; namely, the membership of the plan or HMO, and that the incentives shift from performing unreviewed, high-intensity patient care to a case management/gatekeeper function in which primary care providers coordinate all care and limit access to costly specialization and hospitalization.

Preferred provider organizations

Changes in state insurance laws have permitted payers in large cities to contract selectively with providers such as hospitals and physicians groups, including those not run by HMOs. Under such schemes a majority of payers have started identifying a subset of hospitals and physicians to be "preferred providers" on the basis of a predetermined rate of reimbursement and steering patients to those hospitals and physicians through financial incentives such as lower copayments and deductibles. The providers signing agreements with payers to deliver services to their enrollees are designated as preferred providers and those organizations as preferred provider organizations. To select these preferred providers, payers generally demand price discounts or strict utilization review procedures from the providers.

Cost-sharing

Cost-sharing through increased coinsurance and larger deductibles is a relatively simple plan for providing disincentives for overuse of the system by insured individuals by requiring them to pay more out of pocket. This approach addresses the concern that third-party payment shields the patient from the costs of his or her care.

Medical savings accounts

If cost-sharing means that individual consumers have to pay more out of their own pockets it becomes a matter of concern how deep those pockets are, cost-sharing as a form of cost containment will not work if consumers cannot pay their bills. The concept of medical savings accounts (MSAs) was developed as a type of cost-sharing program that encourages individuals to save for their own health needs, thus ensuring that the money to pay health bills will be there when they need it. This is how the MSA would work. Currently, on average, nearly $4,500 per year per worker is paid by employers for health insurance. Of this amount, the employer would put $3,000 annually into each employee's MSA, which the employee would use him- or herself to pay the first $3,000 of their medical costs. For the remaining $1,500 the employer would purchase an insurance policy that would take care of medical expenses above $3,000. It is recommended that MSAs (1) would be the personal property of the employee, so that it would be portable if the individual changed jobs; (2) would be allowed to grow tax-free, and (3) the employee would draw from them to pay for medical expenses. Under this arrangement, MSAs will provide consumers with built-in incentives to control health care expenditures because they will benefit directly if they spend less.

Problems of competitive systems

In a competitive environment, it is the firm or organization that maximizes profits that succeeds at the highest level. Health insurance companies wishing to maximize their profits can do so either by operating at a higher level of efficiency and effectiveness than their competitors, or by practicing risk aversion to the highest level possible. Finding ways to avoid insuring the few very sick people can be very rewarding. Insurers practicing risk aversion as their main profit-making approach exclude individuals on the basis of preexisting conditions or by having coverages canceled midtreatment when unexpected illnesses become too large a financial liability to the firm. HMOs are accused of taking only young, healthy members of the workforce, while some firms have had their coverage canceled if one worker or his or her dependent is too great a financial risk.

The costs of health insurance have escalated commensurate with increases in the cost of care. An increasing percentage of the population has no health insurance coverage. Of those earning less than $10,000 per year, 32% are uninsured (Wicks, Curtis, & Haugh, 1994). Many businesses that once provided health insurance can no longer do so. Increasing numbers of individuals are employed on a part-time basis, and thus employers avoid paying costly health insurance benefits.

A considerable proportion of the increased costs are a result of the inefficiencies in the system and the high administrative costs for managing the plans. It is estimated that one third of all fees paid for health insurance are used for costs other than for the direct provision of coverage.

Finally, one of the most commonly voiced concerns of the public is the lack of choice of plan or of provider. The rise of managed care systems, with restrictions on self-referral to specialists by employing a given panel of generalists as gatekeepers increasingly diminishes individual choice, a value ingrained in the American ethos.

MANAGED COMPETITION

In the late 1980s the dynamics and difficulties described above became increasingly problematic, and health care costs continued to escalate despite the innovations in health care financing. A proposal was made by Enthoven on behalf of an ad hoc group called the Jackson Hole Group, espousing a concept called "managed competition." Under managed competition, costs would be controlled by reshaping the health care market through establishing health alliances (sometimes called health insurance purchasing cooperatives), which would represent large groups of consumers, and thus have the clout to negotiate lower costs with providers. Furthermore, these health alliances would offer not just one health care plan, but a variety of plans, providing consumers with adequate information to choose between plans based both on cost and on standardized benefit levels. This would foster price competition—and, more inclusively, what Enthoven (1993) calls "value-for-money competition"—at the level of individuals making choices about plans. Value-for-money competition emphasizes that what cost-conscious health consumers seek isn't simply the least expensive health care services or health care package available, but the ones that give them the most for their money. The ability of the consumer to make informed choices is crucial. If consumers do not have adequate information, available in a form that makes comparing alternatives easy, then competitive market processes cannot work effectively in containing costs and promoting high-quality health care.

Limitations of managed competition

One of the major limitations of managed competition grows out of the fact that it requires competing health plans in order to work: Where this is a population insufficient to support several health plans functioning independently without collusion, this model cannot apply. While information technology could be used to overcome some of the problems of serving isolated communities, transportation technologies are also important when it comes to getting people to tertiary care in a timely fashion or for paying specialists to be flown to remote areas when needed. In all of these plans there would be a mandated minimum benefit package. Those who choose the low-cost benefit package will be those who cannot afford a higher level of coverage or those who feel that they do not need more. This leaves room for a new type of "adverse selection," even within managed competition. A further concern is found in the fact that managed competition relies on managed care to achieve much of its savings. Data on the effectiveness of doing so is far from definitive or complete. While it is clear that HMOs operate at lower costs than traditional fee-for-service plans, it is not yet clear how much of the savings they achieve are due to higher levels of efficiency and how much is due to selection bias (enrolling healthier members) in the markets where they exist. Low-income individuals will still be at a relative disadvantage.

OTHER MODELS

President Clinton made health care reform a major element in his election campaign. In the summer of 1993 he revealed his plan for national health care reform, which he titled the Health Security Act. This Act is based on the model of health insurance purchasing cooperative–driven managed competition, employing regional health alliances (to be established by the states) and large-firm (more than 5,000 employees) corporate alliances as market managers. Among the key features of this proposal were universal coverage for all Americans, portability of coverage from employer to employer, and payment via a mechanism called "employer mandate," by which all employers would be required to provide health insurance for their employees, with subsidies to small businesses to help absorb the costs. As proposed, the Health Security Act was extremely complex, attempting to embrace virtually every aspect of the health care delivery system in the United States. Its complexity and the problems in communicating it to the public, together with the successful lobbying efforts of the insurance industry and others who felt their interests threatened by the bill, led to the failure of the Act or any of the comprehensive reform proposals that came out of Congressional committees to gather enough votes to pass in either house of Congress.

With the federal effort for reform at a standstill, local states and communities are now in the vanguard of innovation. A number of states (e.g. Minnesota, Washington, California, Florida, Tennessee) and local communities (Rochester and Cleveland) are taking a variety of approaches to address the problems. The major problems remain escalating health care costs despite efforts at control through management or competition, increasing numbers of individuals without any health insurance (15% of the population, with most of that group the working poor), and uneven access and quality of care dependent on ability to pay. With capitated health care plans and greater financial monitoring of health care in general, the uninsured find fewer health care providers open to them. Additionally, constant market segmentation by risk-averse health insurers, whether operating in a managed care environment or not, means the number of uninsured and underinsured is likely to increase. This places an increasing burden on the few health care providers willing to provide expensive emergency care to the un- or underinsured; these costs, one way or another, get passed on to the rest of the community.

Are there any answers to these dilemmas? The answers do not lie within the federal government, insurers, physicians (who in the debate are synonymous with providers), or employers, yet these are the only people sitting around the tables. It is noteworthy that the biggest stakeholder of all, the consumer of health care services, is never mentioned as part of the debate. The problems are defined consistently as those having to do with the financing of health care, without any examination of the health care per se. As long as there is such excess capacity within the system—too many specialists, too many hospital beds, overuse of highly trained specialists for work that could more effectively be managed by other practitioners (i.e., nurse practitioners)—and as long as the consumer is left out of the equation, the problems cannot be solved. As a society we are in conflict over health care as an industry serving as a major place of employment for large numbers of people versus health care as a needed service for all people. As long as industry is running the debate, the problems will not be solved. If the public becomes part of the solution, however, rather than being perceived as part of the problem, a whole new dynamic may be brought to bear on the system. As we look to the 21st century as a time of massive shifts from an industrial to an information and increasingly diverse society, in which increasing numbers of people will not be employed or employable in the way to which we have become accustomed, the "third sector" of nongovernmental organizations and community volunteers becomes a potent political force for change. Solving the problems of infant mortality, adolescent pregnancy, and young people who die as a result of violence in their communities will not be achieved through our current health care system no matter how much we invest. The costs of emergency room care for the teenager shot in a gang fight will continue to escalate until we engage communities in a new way to become part of the solution. In a country as wealthy as the United States, to take a posture that we cannot afford to provide access to health care for all is reprehensible. As long as we use an outdated model of health care in which the "professionals" are the all-knowing and controlling seers, we will be unable to solve our problems. If people can be empowered with knowledge, and communities empowered as caring networks of people who will not tolerate the drug dealers and the gangs that would rob them of their children, then we can begin to solve our problems. Our problems are not those of financing the outdated system that currently exists, but to reconstruct a *health care system* that truly emphasizes the maintenance of health for all people. It is only when we have a health system for all that our problems can be solved.

REFERENCES

Alpern, D. (1980, December). Reagan, New directions. *Newsweek,* 1-33.

Begley, C.E., Schoeman C., & Traxler, H. (1982). Factors that may explain interstate differences in certificate of need decisions. *Health Care Financing Review, 3,* 87.

Enthoven, A.C. (1993, Fall). Why managed care has failed to contain costs. *Health Affairs,* 27-43.

Health care: Rochester's community approach yields better access, lower costs. (1993). Washington, DC: General Accounting Office.

Holahan, J., & Scanlon, W. (1978). *Price controls, physician fees and physician incomes.* Washington, DC: The Urban Institute,

Iglehart, J.K. (1984). Cutting costs of healthcare for the poor in California. *New England Journal of Medicine, 311*(11), 745-748.

Lewin Associates, Inc. (1975). *Evaluation of the efficiency and effectiveness of Section 1122 Review Process. National Technical Informational Service,* Washington, U.S. Department of Commerce.

Salkever, D.S. (1979). *Hospital-sector inflation.* Lexington, MA: Lexington Books.

Salkever, D., & Bice, T. (1976). The impact of certificate of need on hospital investment. *Milbank Memorial Fund Quarterly, 54,* 185.

Sloan, F.A., & Steinwald, B. (1980). *Insurance, regulation and hospital costs.* Lexington, MA: Lexington Books, D.C. Heath and Company.

Smits, H.L. (1981). The PSRO in perspective. *New England Journal of Medicine, 305*(3), 253-359.

Wicks, E.K., Curtis, R.E., & Haugh, K. (1994). *Designing health purchasing alliances/cooperatives: Federal policy issues and options.* Washington, DC: Institute for Health Policy Solutions.

How changes in payment systems are affecting nurses

PETER I. BUERHAUS

The inability to enact comprehensive national health care reform in 1994 meant that the evolution of the health care system would be driven by five interrelated economic pressures: (a) efforts to reduce the rate of increase in total national spending on health care; (b) actions to reduce the annual increase and total amount of the federal budget deficit; (c) growth of managed care organizations (MCOs); (d) economic competition among MCOs; and (e) the evolution of integrated health delivery systems competing within a capitated payment environment. Because these pressures are dramatically altering the amount and the way that organizations are paid for producing health care services, they are directly affecting employers' demand for nurses and transforming the economic environment in which nurses work. This chapter briefly discusses each of these pressures and how they are shaping employers' behavior and the practice of nursing.

RISING HEALTH CARE EXPENDITURES

At the heart of much of the pressures changing the health care system is the relentless rise of health care expenditures. Since the introduction of Medicare and Medicaid, the amount of national health care expenditures has increased rapidly. Moreover, the proportion of total expenditures financed by the public sector (federal, state, and local governments) has increased while the proportion of private sector spending has decreased. As shown in Table 64-1, in 1965 public sector payers financed only one quarter of the nation's consumption of personal health care ($10 billion), while private payers and individuals paid the remaining 75% ($31 billion). However, the Congressional Budget Office (CBO, 1995) estimates that 48% ($702 billion) of national health care expenditures will be paid by the public sector in the year 2000, and 52% ($770 billion) will come from private payers. The CBO projects that 5 years later, in 2005, public and private sector financiers will each pay half of all health care expenditures. Table 64-1 also shows that as health care expenditures have increased over the past three decades, the proportion of the nation's gross domestic product (GDP) devoted to health care has risen from 5.9% in 1965 to 14.1% in 1995, a significantly higher percentage than in other industrial nations. In the year 2005, health care spending is estimated to climb to 18% of the GDP (CBO, 1995).

Total health care spending will continue to grow mainly because the forces increasing the demand for health care are expected to continue unabated. The rapid rate of technological advances, population growth, and the aging of the population will mean that more people and more of the elderly will want to take advantage of improvements in early diagnosis, technology, and new treatment methods. Thus, it is important for nurses to appreciate that the main issue with respect to rising health care expenditures is not that total health care spending will increase, but rather how public and private payers can make changes in payment systems that will alter the delivery of health care services so the *rate* of increase in future spending can be constrained.

GROWTH OF FEDERAL BUDGET DEFICITS AND IMPACT ON GOVERNMENT HEALTH CARE SPENDING

Closely related to the rise in health care expenditures, especially the increase in the amount of public sector spending, is the extraordinarily rapid rate of growth in the federal government's budget deficit. Over the past two decades annual budget deficits grew significantly, reach-

Table 64-1 Increasing expenditures on health care

Year	Total spending (in billions$)	Percent of gross domestic product	Total spending government/private (in billions$)	Percent of total spending
1965	42	5.9	10/31	25/75
1985	434	10.8	175/259	40/60
1995	1,008	14.1	455/552	45/55
2000	1,472	16.1	703/770	48/52
2005	2,119	18.0	1,068/1,051	50/50

Note. The sum of government and private sector spending may not equal total spending due to rounding; private includes individual out-of-pocket spending, private insurance, and other sources. Data from "U.S. Congress, Health and Human Resource," by Congressional Budget Office, 1995, February.

Table 64-2 Rising federal budget deficits

Year	Spending on Medicare (in billions$)	Spending on Medicaid (in billions$)	Amount added to the deficit (in billions$)	Debt held by the public (in trillions$)
1995	176	90	176	3,617
1997	217	111	224	4,077
1999	262	136	253	4,589
2001	314	164	297	5,207
2003	379	196	351	5,917
2005	460	234	421	6,757

Note. Data from "U.S. Congress, Health and Human Resources," by Congressional Budget Office, 1995, February.

ing a total of $3.617 trillion in 1995 (CBO, 1995). What's more, fully 16% of the fiscal year federal budget was required simply to pay for interest payments obligated by this amount of debt. As shown in Table 64-2, annual federal deficits are expected to increase steadily, and if there are no actions taken to reduce them, they are expected to reach $6.757 trillion in the year 2005 (CBO, 1995). This rate of increase in the public's debt has elicited a serious effort by elected officials to reduce annual budget deficits. This will require extraordinary changes in spending by federal programs and, over time, a net reduction in the size of the federal government as many programs and entire agencies are eliminated.

Because federal spending on Medicare and Medicaid consumes nearly 20% of each year's federal budget, and because spending by both programs is expected to grow rapidly (see Table 64-2), nurses can anticipate that federal government payments for health care will be a prime target for achieving a significant portion of needed budget savings. Furthermore, because Medicare payments to hospitals are the single largest source of hospital revenue (Prospective Payment Assessment Commission [ProPAC], 1994), these changes will exert a substantial impact on the financial position of hospitals (as well as other providers, namely nursing homes, community health agencies, ambulatory care facilities, home health care programs, and physician offices), who employ the vast majority of the nation's nurses. Thus, nurses can anticipate that reduced federal payments to organizations, born out of the urgent need to reduce the size of annual budget deficits, will place unprecedented cost-containment pressures on health care organizations and providers for years to come.

DEVELOPMENT, GROWTH, AND IMPACT OF MANAGED CARE

Managed care plans and MCOs integrate the financing and delivery of health care services by arranging with selected providers to furnish a comprehensive set of health services to its members (ProPAC, 1993). These services are usually obtained by negotiating discounted fee-for-service payments or agreeing on a capitated amount (a predetermined set payment per subscriber). Although MCOs have evolved considerably over the past two decades, they generally seek to eliminate unnecessary and inappropriate health care services with utilization review programs (e.g., prior authorization for hospital admission, using primary care physicians as "gatekeepers," or requiring second opinions). Most MCOs also attempt to lower costs by limiting an enrollee's choice of provider, offering a closed panel of providers or a select network of providers, and charging enrollees the full costs or a percentage of the costs for using an out-of-plan provider.

Health maintenance organizations (HMOs) contract with large employers (and individual subscribers) to provide basic and supplemental health maintenance and treatment services at a predetermined price for each patient. The price can take the form of a premium or can be capitated. Under capitation, the HMO and the provider contract to furnish a comprehensive set of services for a flat per-member-per-month fee. If the cost of health care exceeds the amount received (the capitated fee) from the payer, the provider loses money; but if the cost is less, the provider will profit from the arrangement.

In addition to HMOs, other forms of MCOs have evolved. Preferred provider organizations (PPOs) were developed in the 1980s among physicians and hospitals who were willing to discount the price of their services. PPOs have become popular because they give subscribers greater freedom of choice of provider. The most recent evolution of managed care is known as point-of-service plans, which combine certain aspects of HMOs and PPOs. To varying degrees, both of the latter forms of MCOs use similar checks and balances to contain costs and utilization inherent in the HMO structure. The population enrolled in these organizations has grown substantially over the past 15 years, with an estimated 100 million people enrolled in some form of MCO in 1993. Of these, it is estimated that in 1993 42 million people were enrolled in roughly 600 HMOs, and 54.4 million were members of approximately 900 PPOs (ProPAC, 1994).

In addition to changing traditional relationships among physicians, hospitals, insurers, and government, the growth of MCOs has had a profound impact on eroding the demand for hospitals. For example, HMO enrollees use considerably fewer and different kinds of services. ProPAC (1994) reports that HMO members both under and over the age of 65 have fewer inpatient hospital discharges (81.4) and inpatient days (379) per 1,000 enrollees than the national average (124.1 and 795, respectively). Additionally, HMO members' average length of stay is about 2 days less than the national average, regardless of age group. Among those over the age of 65, HMO members have a lower rate per 100,000 enrollees for coronary artery bypass surgery, cardiac catheterization, and cholecystecomy compared with the national rate.

In their effort to control health care expenditures, federal and state governments have started new programs to encourage enrollment of Medicare beneficiaries and Medicaid recipients into MCOs. About one quarter (9 million) of Medicare beneficiaries were enrolled in MCOs in 1995, but enrollment is expected to rise substantially in the remaining years of the decade as a result of anticipated legislation to restructure the Medicare program and offer new incentives for beneficiaries to enroll in MCOs. Moreover, with the huge increase in the number of people receiving Medicaid in the early 1990s (Coughlin, Ku, Holahan, Heslam, & Winterbottom, 1994) and subsequent skyrocketing in spending (e.g., between 1988 and 1992, total spending on Medicaid increased from $51 billion to $114 billion), the vast majority of states developed managed care programs and began to rapidly enroll a large number of their citizens receiving Medicaid. Thus, as more Medicare and Medicaid beneficiaries move into MCOs, there will be negative pressure on the demand for hospitals and the amount they are paid for services consumed. Obviously, as fewer patients are admitted and length of stay decrease, fewer nurses will be demanded and employed by hospitals.

Beyond public sector initiatives to bolster enrollment in MCOs, nurses can expect that more American businesses and large employers will shift their employees' choice of health plans toward MCOs. In the early 1990s, large employers finally discovered that they could use their purchasing power to stimulate hospitals and MCOs to start competing and to lower their premium prices. Part of the reason that the business sector awakened is because they and others in health policymaking positions lost faith in government regulations to constrain rising health care costs. The loss of confidence reached a high point with the rejection of the Clinton health plan in 1994. In addition, as Medicare and Medicaid payments to hospitals and doctors were constrained in the late 1980s and early 1990s, providers charged private payers higher prices to make up for government payment shortfalls. Large employers realized that the only way to control cost shifting and promote greater efficiency in the production of health care was to force MCOs to compete based on the price of their premiums.

ECONOMIC COMPETITION AMONG MANAGED CARE ORGANIZATIONS

Businesses and large employers exert their market power when they select the lowest-priced, highest-quality health insurance plans. This action places financial pressure on MCOs to find ways to minimize the costs of providing services for their enrollees. Because MCOs receive a fixed payment per enrollee, they have financial incentives to reduce members' consumption of services, especially high-cost services such as hospital care. As more employers demand lower health insurance premiums for their employees, MCOs face greater pressure to keep costs low so they can offer a competitive premium price. (In contrast, paying providers on a fee-for-service basis leads to too much consumption of services and inflation of costs and medical care prices.) However, if a managed care plan skimps on the quality or quantity of services provided to its members, then it risks alienating enrollees who can either leave the plan or persuade their employers to drop the MCO altogether.

Thus, to be competitive and win contracts with employers, MCOs are taking increasingly vigorous actions to lower their costs and guard against poor quality. MCOs are passing these financial pressures on to hospitals and other organizations by contracting with only the lowest-priced and highest-quality providers. In turn, to win contracts and thereby gain access to members of the MCO, hospitals, home health care agencies, nursing homes, and other providers must lower their prices by becoming more efficient and decreasing their costs. In addition, they must demonstrate high quality and compare favorably on the production of clinical patient outcomes. In this way, the competitive pressures that start with employers demanding lower-priced premiums and improved quality from health care plans offered by MCOs are passed along to hospitals and other health care organizations that need access to the MCO's subscribers.

These changes in payment systems and financial arrangements have already begun to slow the rate of increase in total national spending on health care (Levit et al., 1994). Thus, nurses should realize that competition in health care, even in its formative stages, is beginning to achieve the socially desirable objective of lowering the rate of increase in health care expenditures. In addition, the more health care spending is constrained, the more likely it will be that competitive forces will gain favor.

Competition among MCOs directly affects nurses in both positive and negative ways. Because it reduces the demand for costly hospital-based care, the employment of nurses in these settings is negatively affected. Many organizations have decreased the total number of registered nurses on their nursing staff and have substituted cheaper nursing-related personnel for professional nurses, in addition to restructuring the way that nursing care is organized and provided. At the same time, the search by HMOs and hospitals for ways to lower their costs without harming quality has resulted in an increased demand for nurse practitioners. In addition, nurses can anticipate that organizations will continue to merge and form networks of providers to eliminate excess capacity (too many beds) and costly duplication of facilities and services, and will take other needed actions to achieve lower costs and enhance their chances of surviving in a competitive marketplace.

DEVELOPMENT OF INTEGRATED HEALTH CARE DELIVERY SYSTEMS

The actions of employers to pressure MCOs to constrain their premiums has, in turn, led MCOs, hospitals, and physicians to align themselves through various forms of affiliations into what have become known as integrated health systems (IHSs). Defining an IHS depends on the specific organization and the needs in the geographic area it serves, but some elements are common to these systems.* In general, patients receive a full range of health care services from providers who are affiliated with the system, and there is coordinated case management and information flow among the providers and health professionals. The services provided by IHSs may include wellness programs, preventive care, ambulatory clinics, outpatient diagnostic and laboratory services, emergency care, general and tertiary hospital services, rehabilitation, long-term care, congregate living, psychiatric care, home health care, hospice care, and outpatient pharmaceutical care. Coordination is aimed at reducing duplication of tests and services and making sure that appropriate providers are used instead of more costly ones. In this way the costs of both routine care and expensive specialists and services, such as organ transplants, can be more easily controlled (Feldstein, 1994). By integrating the various providers that comprise the system, it is easier and less expensive to exchange and update patient care information using uniform patient record systems and electronic information systems. Similarly, the ability to develop cost, quality, and outcomes monitoring systems is made easier and cheaper.

Incorporating different providers and achieving effective coordination among them permits the IHS to direct patients to the most appropriate providers and health professionals according to the needs of the patient. The IHS is also better able to monitor costs, quality of care, and patient satisfaction and to obtain and analyze information on the patient's clinical outcomes and the treat-

*In the way that IHSs are discussed here, they are synonymous with community care networks or organized systems of care.

ments provided by specific providers. Additionally, the IHS is able to develop improved projections of the costs of serving different patient populations, more accurately estimate the price of insurance premiums, obtain other economic advantages such as lower liability and malpractice insurance and lower interests rates on loans (Feldstein, 1994). Most importantly, these design features are expected to permit IHSs to be better able to assume the financial risk involved in capitated contracts.

By sharing the same financial incentives, the goals of hospitals and health care professionals that make up the IHS are changed significantly. Because they receive the same capitated rate regardless of the number of admissions, hospitals will no longer profit from increased admissions and expensive new inpatient facilities. Likewise, physicians cannot increase their incomes by performing more procedures because capitation arrangements would motivate them to provide only the care required and promote wellness. Most importantly, because hospitals would become cost centers in an IHS, the goal is to minimize admissions to the IHS's affiliated hospitals.

As small employers and individuals accelerate the formation of coalitions to purchase health care benefits, MCOs and IHSs can be expected to enroll more and more of the patient population, thus substantially impacting the rate of inpatient admissions to hospitals. Yet at the same time that more patient care will be shifted to less expensive ambulatory sites, the inpatient population will be comprised of sicker patients, and hospitals will be seen as largely reserved for critical care.

CHANGING PAYMENT SYSTEMS' EFFECT ON NURSES

Public sector cost-containment efforts, together with the development of economic competition among MCOs and hospitals, the formation of IHSs, and the adoption of capitated payments mean that organizations must carefully select the resources (capital and labor) needed to produce health care services. With respect to employing health professionals, including various types of nursing personnel, employers will face strong economic incentives to spend their dollars only on those who are most valuable to the production of patient care. In the eyes of an employer, the most valuable employees will be those who contribute the most to the organization's ability to survive in an increasingly competitive and rapidly changing financial environment. Cost containment and competitive pressures mandate that organizations become much more efficient, minimize their costs, offer services at competitive prices, and improve the quality of care and production of desired clinical outcomes. The ability to produce health care services in this way will be essential for individual organizations, managed care plans, and IHSs to compete successfully and thrive.

To raise their value and thereby increase their own employment security, nurses will have to continue to innovate and find new ways to lower the costs of producing nursing care. Pressure will not let up on nurses to critically examine their practice and discover new ways to eliminate unnecessary and inappropriate activities, as well as to experiment with new models of organizing and providing nursing care. Nurses must make visible contributions to enable the organization to lower its costs or those organizations will find other health personnel who can produce health care at a lower cost.

Nurses can also increase their value by ensuring that they are integral to the improvement of high-quality health care and clinical outcomes that purchasers desire and are willing to pay for. This means that nurses must constantly ascertain how the interventions and activities of their practice contribute toward raising quality and producing desired outcomes. Nurses must demonstrate a very close link between their actions on behalf of patients and families and the production of high-quality personal health care services. Because the development of a competitive marketplace in health care means that organizations must satisfy consumers' wants and desires at prices they are willing to pay (vs. satisfying their own interests, as was the case in the regulatory years of the 1970s and 1980s), nurses must ensure that they are being responsive to both consumers' and employers' constantly changing needs and preferences. To thrive in the years ahead, nurses must practice the profession of nursing in ways that increase their value.

Finally, changing payment systems mean that nursing education programs must be alert and responsive to the changing needs of the nurse labor market. It is the responsibility of schools of nursing to expand the body of nursing knowledge and ensure that nurses are well prepared to practice in the future. The ability of new graduates to become employed is increasingly determined by their perceived value in helping employers meet their survival needs. Thus, executive leaders of schools of nursing, practice settings, and national organizations need to make changes continually in the curriculum of nurse education, improve the quality of faculty, and develop new partnerships with employers if they are to respond to the needs of employers and ensure the continued advancement of the practice of nursing. If nothing else, the changes in payment systems described in this chapter are stimulating a tighter alignment between the nurse education and nurse labor markets. Much of the future well-being of the nursing profession depends on nurses being more aware of and responsive to each others' needs and the forces driving them.

REFERENCES

Coughlin, T.A., Ku, L., Holahan, J., Heslam, D., & Winterbottom, C. (1994). State responses to the Medicaid spending crisis: 1988 to 1992. *Journal of Health Politics, Policy and Law, 19*(4), 832-864.

Congressional Budget Office. (1995, February). *U.S. Congress, Health and Human Resource.* Washington, DC: Author.

Feldstein, P.J. (1994). *Health policy issues: An economic perspective on health reform.* Ann Arbor, MI: AUPHA Press/Health Administration Press.

Levit, K.R., Cowan, C.A., Lazenby, H.C., McDonnell, P.A., Sensenig, A.L., Stiller, J.M., & Won, D.K. (1994). National health spending trends, 1960-1993. *Health Affairs, 13*(5), 14-32.

Prospective Payment Assessment Commission. (1993). *Medicare and the American health care system: Report to the Congress.* Washington, DC: Author.

Prospective Payment Assessment Commission. (1994). *Medicare and the American health care system: Report to the Congress.* Washington, DC: Author.

An in-home program of disability prevention and health promotion for older persons

HARRIET UDIN ARONOW, MARCIA N. GOLD, KAREN E. YUHAS, CATHY A. ALESSI, JOHN C. BECK

It is often said that we live in an aging world. The elderly population in the United States is expected to double between 1990 and 2025 from 31 million to 59 million. This represents the expansion of the elderly population from about 13% today to over 20% in the next 35 years (U.S. Bureau of the Census, 1989). Furthermore, the oldest of the old, those 85 years of age or older, represent the fastest-growing age group (Rosenwaike, 1985).

As we approach the 21st century, the growth rate in this population is causing concern in the health and social services communities as well as in all levels of government. Evidence suggests that persons of advanced age will place a disability burden on society. Home and community-based care programs are being evaluated as potential cost-effective solutions to the expected increased demand for institutional services.

This chapter describes the results of a 3-year demonstration project that evaluated an in-home preventive health care program for older people. We present the prevention program as an alternative model of home-based health services that shows promise to reduce demand for long-term care services among the rapidly growing oldest population.

THE DEBATE OVER THE COST-EFFECTIVENESS OF HOME CARE FOR THE ELDERLY

Home care services grew rapidly in the decades after the 1960s as the goals of President Lyndon B. Johnson's "Great Society" and the inception of Medicare promoted broad access to comprehensive health care services. Over the past decade, there has been an increased demand for home care to provide a less costly alternative to institutional-based health and long-term care services. We now face the challenge to demonstrate the cost-effectiveness of services delivered in the home setting (Sherry, 1992).

The economic analysis of home care has suffered from the lack of a clear analytic framework to classify the multiple purposes of home care interventions. Ten years ago the home health care industry distinguished between chronic-care, an established industry focused primarily on the long-term care needs of the older population, and technology-based home health services (Moxley & Roeder, 1984). Technology-based services delivered in the home were described as direct substitution for services provided previously in acute care settings (e.g., home dialysis, total parenteral nutrition, cancer chemotherapy). In addition to the effectiveness of the intervention, two widely accepted secondary benefits promoted the growth of home care services: comfort, convenience, and preference for the patient and family and reduced costs for the payer (self or insurance). While no one has challenged the importance of these goals, the home health care industry has been challenged to demonstrate its ability to achieve them.

Several authors describe the difficulty in analyzing the cost-effectiveness of home care because of variations among studies in cost measurement and methods (Green, 1989; Green, Lovely, & Ondrich, 1993; Smith & Wright, 1994; Varricchio, 1994; Williams, 1994). In addition, these studies fail to explicitly articulate the goals of home care interventions in the context of the larger health care system, so that cost trade-offs can be fully accounted for. In 1985, Rogatz directed the home health industry to take a larger focus,

> Home health care should not be analyzed as an isolated modality, but as a component of an integrated health care system

> which operates as a continuum, assuring coordination among hospitals, nursing homes, home care and other health care resources, with the patient transferring from one to another in accordance with his or her needs. (Rogatz, 1985, p. 39)

In this broadened health services framework, home care interventions may have appropriate applications to other valued health goals, such as maintaining and promoting the healthy status and well-being of a community.

The debate on the cost-effectiveness of home care can be clarified by classifying in-home interventions into three underlying programmatic purposes: (1) *substitution* for institutional-based acute or long-term care; (2) *transition* from institutional care and *reintegration* into the community; and (3) *prevention* of the onset of disability and need for long-term care. Each program—substitution, transition, and prevention—can be described with a distinct primary goal, target population, range of services, additional benefits, and evidence of cost-effectiveness.

SUBSTITUTION

Primary goal

The goal of substitutive home care services is to provide comparable quality acute and long-term care services in the home setting as an alternative to acute or long-term care institutions. For home care to be a substitution for acute or long-term care, the target population, services, and outcomes of care should be the same as those of a program of care that would otherwise be offered in the institutional setting. The benefit to the patient and society is derived from the assumption of a higher quality of life (comfort, convenience, and preference) for the patient and family as well as lower costs (associated with institutional overhead and/or shifts to informal unpaid caregivers) for the payer.

Target population

Recipients of substitutive home care services include persons with multiple dependencies requiring personal care services or regular medical monitoring and patients receiving a protracted course of treatment for which a portable technology is available. For these patients, the treatment itself is not life-threatening within 1 day; therefore, the patient does not require frequent monitoring during a 24-hour period.

Range of services

Typical services provided at home include personal care services (e.g., bathing, skin care, daily hygiene), feeding and the delivery of food, social services (e.g., social work, friendly visitor), and skilled nursing services (e.g., physical examination, monitoring vital signs, managing medications, chronic wound care, assessing the patient response to treatments, and teaching the patient and family). A recent distinction for many substitutive home care programs is the presence of a case manager or care coordinator. Typically performed by a nurse or social worker, the role of case manager is to assess the multiple needs of the home care recipient and coordinate the care and services among recipient, his or her family and other informal caregivers, and the network of community resources in the most cost-effective configuration possible.

Additional benefits

In addition to substitution for institutional-based services (and disease-specific recovery goals for acute care programs), the goals of this type of home care are to increase quality of life and satisfaction for recipients and prevent health complications associated with prolonged institutionalization (e.g., physical debilitation, disorientation and social disruption, and increased risk of infections).

Evidence for cost-effectiveness

Although the issues of what needs to be measured in a complete cost analysis have not been addressed fully in the home care literature, there is growing evidence suggesting that certain medical services traditionally provided in the acute care setting are both less expensive to provide in the home and valued by the recipient and his or her family. For example, programs that provide long-term ventilator-dependent care or other respiratory therapy in home versus acute care settings have demonstrated their cost-effectiveness (Dunne, 1994), as have parenteral nutrition (Detsky et al., 1986) and antibiotic therapy (Balinsky & Nesbitt, 1989; Milkovich, 1993). Terminal care has also been demonstrated to be no more expensive at home than in the hospital (Gray, MacAdam, & Boldy, 1987). These promising results should be interpreted with caution. Unmeasured costs of lost opportunities, physical and emotional burdens for informal home caregivers, and less tangible benefits to those same caregivers have not been well measured in studies of the cost-effectiveness of home care (Smith & Wright, 1994; Varricchio, 1994).

Community-based programs providing long-term care in the home have been studied more extensively and have not generally demonstrated cost savings, primarily due to the problems associated with targeting populations truly at risk of institutionalization. Weissert (1985) analyzed the results from a large national study of the delivery of long-term care services in the home as an alternative to nursing home placements (the Channeling Demonstrations). He showed that home-based programs added on services for people who were not at risk of nursing home placement. Only short nursing home stays were diverted, and only a small proportion of these were identified. The high screening costs to find such a small number, paired with the likelihood of delivering diversion services to persons not at risk, made the programs very expensive. Hedrick and Inui (1986) argued that rather than decrease costs, the population targeted for in-home services includes a growing number of older persons who are not at risk for institutionalization, thereby increasing costs but substituting for neither acute or long-term institutional care.

More recently, on the other hand, well-targeted programs of long-term care substitution have demonstrated cost savings. In Minnesota, where eligibility for in-home and community-based programs of long-term care are applied after identifying applicants eligible for institutional long-term care, home-based programs have demonstrated savings (Jamieson, 1990; Lindberg & Monson, 1989). A reanalysis of the National Long-Term Care Channeling Demonstration control group (Greene et al., 1993) suggested that the application of careful screening criteria could increase the cost-effectiveness of long-term care substitution. Forty-one percent of the control group were identified as being at risk for specific long-term care needs that could have been met with substitution by home and community-based services.

TRANSITION AND COMMUNITY REINTEGRATION

Primary goal

The goal of transitional home care programs is to promote the successful reintegration of patients from institutional care into home and community living. When applied to an acute inpatient hospital stay, the use of a home program may also substitute for the last days of the inpatient stay. Advocates of transitional care propose that in-home transitional care programs can be a mutually advantageous situation, where the service is less expensive, more appropriate, and more effective than if it were delivered in the hospital.

Target population

Transitional home care programs have been designed to meet specific treatment needs for patients recovering from life-threatening illnesses and are usually associated with ongoing chronic treatment needs or the onset of specific functional disabilities in the activities of daily living. In addition, according to Kramer, Shaughnessy, and Pettigrew (1985), transitional programs have been posited to benefit the general population of frail older Medicare patients. For this population, the home setting provides an even greater motivation for rehabilitation and shortens the period of dependency and disability after an acute life-threatening condition. Transitional rehabilitative care has been proposed to benefit patients with sudden-onset cognitive disability (e.g., brain injury) who experience difficulty in translating skills learned in an institutional or clinic setting into the home or community setting.

Range of services

Transitional home care focuses on the constellation of rehabilitation services including physical, occupational, and speech therapies with nursing interventions targeted to patient education, health maintenance in the context of disability, and self-management. Services are delivered typically by home health agencies that have developed multidisciplinary rehabilitation programs.

Additional benefits

Enhanced functional status and successful reintegration into the home and community are the expected outcomes of transitional home care. In some cases, transitional care will be a substitute for the end of an acute hospitalization (Drummond, Boucher, Drummond, & Geraci, 1986; Kramer et al., 1985). Additionally, transitional home care programs may prevent long-term institutional placement for many patients.

Evidence for cost-effectiveness

While transitional home care has not been studied extensively, some reports have been published. An early study in Sweden (Jarnlo, Ceder, & Thorngren, 1984) suggested that early at-home rehabilitation of patients with hip fractures was less costly while demonstrating comparable results in restoring functional independence. Two more recent randomized studies found significant cost savings in home-based rehabilitation programs for patients with hip fractures (Hollingworth, Todd, Parker, Roberts, & Williams, 1993) and for the frail elderly (Melin, Hakanssan, & Bygren, 1993). In addition to reduced acute inpatient use, the study by Melin et al. reported other important outcomes, including improved functional status, outdoor mobility, fewer diagnoses, and fewer medications used at 6 months. A third study of stroke rehabilitation compared home physical therapy with day hospital therapy and found better outcomes and less cost for the home-based program (Young & Forster, 1993).

PREVENTION

Primary goal

The purposes of in-home prevention programs are to maximize health, independent functioning, and self-management of health among older persons residing in the community and to prevent or delay the onset of disability and the need for formal or informal caregiver services. Prevention of the onset of illness and disability includes primary prevention (to educate and change health behaviors before the onset of disability risks), secondary prevention (to screen for early signs of risk factors and treat them before they manifest in disability), and tertiary prevention (to rehabilitate and return to independent functioning in the context of existing chronic disease and disability).

Target population

The appropriate population for preventive home care includes persons living independently (or with minimal social and functional supports) in private residences, who by advanced age alone or by the presence of identified chronic illness are at increased risk of acute illness or loss of independence.

Ranges of services

Like transitional care, preventive services are more educational and behavioral. Health risk and health problem identification, recommendations for remediation, and promotion of self-care and self-management are the main interventions. Risk assessment methods vary from in-home comprehensive geriatric assessment (with physical examination) to self-administered questionnaires.

Evidence for cost-effectiveness

Home outreach strategies take place before the target client seeks medical or other attention for a problem, and they permit early preventive interventions. Providing risk assessment in the home setting permits insight into a person's living environment (such as hazards and nutritional support) and provides an excellent social environment for communication. The relatively small number of controlled studies of in-home prevention programs have shown promising results, but most of these programs have been conducted outside of the United States.

Results from the first two controlled experiments with home prevention programs were published in 1984—one from the United Kingdom (Vetter, Jones, & Victor, 1984) and one from Denmark (Hendriksen, Lund, & Stromgard, 1984). Both experiments demonstrated that individuals visited by nurses at regular intervals had lower mortality and made greater use of community services than those who were not visited regularly. The Danish study showed a decrease in hospital days and emergency room visits, whereas the study in the United Kingdom reported improved quality of life.

More recent studies tend to confirm these results, although not all findings are consistent. One U.K. study reported a reduction in long-term care institutionalization (McEwan, Davidson, Forster, Pearson, & Stirling, 1990). Another study reported no service reduction, but improved mood among subjects who received in-home visits and referrals by community health workers or volunteers (Carpenter & Demopoulos, 1990). A 1992 U.K. study of a home-visit case-finding surveillance program (Pathy, Bayer, Harding, & Dibble, 1992) demonstrated reduced mortality and fewer hospital days at 3-year follow-up. In 1992, a Canadian study of an in-home, nurse-administered health promotion program demonstrated an increased 3-year "living at home" rate (Hall et al., 1992). A group from the Netherlands (van Rossum et al., 1993) reported mixed results from a 3-year randomized, controlled trial of visiting nurse home visits (without physical assessment). They concluded that this type of intervention might be effective only for persons in ill health.

Hendriksen (1994) has recently reported continuing positive effects of the original Danish study 7 years after the cessation of the home visits (unpublished results). These effects include less nursing home placement, fewer days of acute care hospital use, and a higher level of functioning among specific subgroups. A recent meta-analysis of comprehensive geriatric assessment programs (Stuck, Sui, Wieland, Adams, & Rubenstein, 1993) suggested that in-home prevention programs increase the likelihood of persons living at home rather than in a nursing home (odds ratio = 1.20, 95% confidence interval = 1.05 to 1.37). The growing experience of European countries with home-based preventive strategies recently led to the convening of a meeting of Western European nations under the Organization for Economic Cooperation and Development (OECD) auspices to discuss implementation of in-home prevention strategies in all OECD countries.

Two studies in United States have reported promising results suggesting the cost-effectiveness of health promotion and prevention programs for older persons. Fries, Bloch, Harrington, Richardson, and Beck (1993) reported changes in health behaviors, reduced health risks, and lowered medical costs in a health promotion program for retirees from the Bank of America in California. Fabacher et al. (1994) reported the results of an intervention that followed subjects for just 1 year. They found that their program of home screening, recommendations, and in-home follow-up was successful in detecting treatable problems, promoting good health behaviors, and maintaining functional status.

In-home prevention programs targeted at special populations at high risk have also been reported with positive results. Kornowski et al. (1995) examined the effects of an intensive home-care surveillance program for elderly patients with severe congestive heart failure. They found a reduction in hospital admissions and length of hospital stay, and suggested that the service could have a large effect on reducing acute care expenditures. Tinetti et al. (1994) evaluated an in-home program to reduce the risk of falling among older community residents who exhibited at least one risk factor associated with falls. In the 1 year of follow-up, the intervention group had significantly fewer falls and reduced risk factors. Finally, a randomized controlled trial of a home-based program versus hospital care for nonelderly persons with severe mental illness found that the home program was significantly less expensive than usual care and had good outcomes over a 20-month study period (Knapp et al., 1994).

THE IN-HOME PREVENTIVE HEALTH CARE PROGRAM FOR OLDER PERSONS

Between 1989 and 1994, the University of California, Los Angeles Multicampus Program in Geriatric Medicine and Gerontology and Senior Health & Peer Counseling, a multipurpose senior center in Santa Monica, California, collaborated on a 5-year demonstration project funded by the W.K. Kellogg Foundation—the In-home Preventive Health Care Program for Older Persons. A program in the Foundation's community-based problem solving strategy, the purpose of our demonstration project was to evaluate the effectiveness of an in-home preventive health care program for older persons living in Santa Monica. The 3-year intervention included comprehensive geriatric assessments performed annually and three additional home visits during each program year.

Target population

Participants for the project were recruited from the voter registration list for Santa Monica, California. Included were community-living persons 75 years of age or older with no known terminal disease or severe functional impairment. We explained that our project would address important questions about maintaining health in older years, and that they would either be participants in the program or be part of a comparison group interviewed periodically so that we could keep track of their health, well-being, and use of services. The total number of participants was 414, with 215 randomly assigned to the intervention group.

Details of the intervention

Participants in the intervention were visited by gerontological nurse practitioners (GNPs) four times a year for 3 years. At the first visit, the GNP established a personal relationship and completed a comprehensive multidimensional health assessment with physical, social, psychological, and environmental components. The GNP then completed a medical history and structured physical examination, medication review, cognitive assessment, vision and hearing testing, gait and balance assessment, and social and nutritional assessment. Participants also received functional status assessment screening for depression. Additional tests included fingerstick hematocrit and glucose, dipstick urinalysis, and mail-in fecal occult blood testing. This comprehensive evaluation was repeated annually for 3 years.

Based on these evaluations the GNPs identified specific problems (e.g., medical, social, emotional, environmental or economic) and, with consultation with project geriatricians, made specific recommendations to the participants. Recommendations consisted of specific actions the older person might take to address health risks or problems identified by the comprehensive assessment. Recommendations were highly variable and tailored to individual needs, but could be classified into three broad categories: referral to a physician (e.g., for a specific symptom, finding, medication review or change), referral or recommendation to use another specific community-based health professional or community service (e.g., podiatrist, counseling or health education class), or recommendation to implement or change a self-care behavior in response to a specific health risk (e.g., exercise, remove throw rugs, take medication per instruction). All participants continued to receive their usual health care from their community physicians. However, their use might be modified by the GNP recommendations.

The GNPs made in-home follow up visits every 3 months to monitor health status and detect new problems, to reinforce adherence to prior recommendations, and to provide general health education and health promotion guidelines (e.g., for immunizations and cancer screening). Throughout the intervention, participants were encouraged to be active in their relationship with the GNP and to take a primary role in the management of their health. GNPs encouraged participants to take the lead in completing recommended actions, and only in situations of extreme complexity or urgency did the GNP initiate a contact with the participant's primary care physician after obtaining the participant's explicit permission.

Ramsdell et al. (Ramsdell, 1991; Ramsdell, Jackson, Renvall, & Swart, 1989) have written of the value of home visit in terms of the amount of available information pertinent to the health of an older person and increased yield of identified problems. We found that the home setting created an atmosphere of shared decision making and allowed the GNP to see how the participants functioned in their own environment. Access to the home also permitted evaluation of the environment for accessibility and for safety hazards such as risks for falls created by poor lighting, electrical and phone cords, clutter, and uneven surfaces. The GNP inspected the home pharmacy for appropriateness and for potential drug interactions. By observing the participant in the home setting, the GNP could make recommendations that were more practical and appropriate for each participant's unique situation.

Other authors have identified problems in providing care in the home environment (Newman, 1985; Rogatz, 1985). Rogatz (1985) listed the disadvantages of home care (difficulty in maintaining a sanitary environment, inability to closely monitor a clinical condition, lack of access to diagnostic services and therapies). We also encountered some difficulties in home assessment such as dim lighting, social interruptions, external environmental noise, discomfort and limitations in the physical examination, as well as the inefficiencies of scheduling appointments and commuting.

Evaluation methods

In addition to an in-home interview completed with all participants at the time of their enrollment, our evaluation team followed both the intervention and comparison groups with an annual interview containing structured questions and established scales measuring health, functional status, quality of life, social networks and supports, and self-reported use of health and community services. We also made interim (every 4 months) telephone calls to obtain more frequent recall of use of services. To gather objective data on the use of health services and long-term care we: (1) accessed Medicare intermediary's claims files and the medical records and patient information systems for subjects who were members of health maintenance organizations to measure use of physicians' services; (2) reviewed the computerized master patient index of the five local hospitals that accounted for over 90% of all self-reported hospitalizations; and (3) verified all self-reported admissions to nursing homes.

Because there were complete data available on all participants regarding survival and use of acute and long-term care services, intervention and control groups could be compared directly. However, because there were missing data in other outcomes (i.e., functional status), multivariate statistical models were used to adjust for any baseline differences between the two groups that might have arisen due to differential drop-out from the annual interview.

Results of the demonstration

The main results of the demonstration of the In-home Preventive Health Care Program for Older Persons appeared in the *New England Journal of Medicine* in November, 1995 (Stuck et al., 1995). Following is a brief summary.

The average age of all participants was 81 years. Approximately 70% were women, and two thirds lived alone. The participants were largely European-American, well educated (over 75% high school graduates), and had fairly low fixed incomes (38% received $11,000 per year or less). Over 90% were completely independent in basic activities of daily living (e.g., eating, walking, bathing) at the beginning of the project.

At the end of 3 years, the intervention group had significantly fewer long-term nursing home admissions and fewer long-term nursing home days (means 3.9 vs. 24.6 days). In addition, after 3 years the intervention group participants were significantly more independent in their activities of daily living. The intervention group was both more independent in their instrumental activities of daily living (e.g., cooking, cleaning, shopping) and less likely to be dependent in the basic activities of daily living (e.g., bathing, grooming, walking).

The intervention group was found to have increased use of physician services and reported increased use of specific community-based services that promote socialization such as senior transportation, self-help, and special community college programs. There were no differences between the two groups in their use of in-home support services such as home health care, personal care services, meals-on-wheels, or case management. There were no differences between the intervention and control groups for use of acute hospital inpatient services or short-term nursing home use.

The cost of the preventive program services and increased physician visits offset the lowered costs associated with fewer long-term nursing home admissions and days. However, the effectiveness of the program to promote independence in daily activities and to delay the onset of disability suggests that program was cost-effective. We estimated that the cost for each year of disability-free life gained was $6,000, or put another way, the cost for each prevented nursing home day was $35.

Characteristics of the preventive intervention

The intervention process was carefully studied to help us understand the nature of the complex preventive intervention (Alessi et al., 1995). Over the 3 years of the program, we documented an average of 19.2 specific health problems for each participant. All participants had at least one medical problem that was identified as active. Almost two thirds had at least one active geriatric syndrome identified (e.g., deconditioning, gait or balance disorder, falls). Over half had a mental health or psychiatric problem identified (e.g., depression, stress, grief or loss), and more than three quarters had at least one social or environmental problem identified (e.g., social isolation, financial difficulty, unsafe home environment). Of the 5,694 recommendations that were recorded for all participants, 51% involved a self-care activity, 29% involved a referral to a physician (typically the participant's primary care physician), and 30% involved referral to a nonphysician professional or community service or program.

We analyzed the identified health problems, GNP recommendations to clients to improve their health, and client adherence to the recommendations. We found that three fourths of the clients had at least one major problem identified that was previously unknown or suboptimally treated. One third of subjects had additional major health problems identified during the second and third years. The number of recommendations made to clients during each of the 3 years of the program did not diminish over time (average of 11.5 per client per year). Adherence to recommendations varied significantly by the type of recommendation, with referrals to see a physician about a problem having the highest rate of follow-through, and self-care activities (especially those that required a sustained behavioral or habit change) having the lowest adherence rate. Participant adherence to mammography, influenza, tetanus, and pneumococcal vaccinations increased during the intervention years. We concluded from these results that repeated annual in-home comprehensive geriatric assessment continued to produce important health information over the entire period of the intervention.

Discussion

The In-home Preventive Health Care Program was successful in reducing long-term nursing home use. This may have been related to better maintenance of independent functioning in daily activities. While we demonstrated no change in overall hospital use, subgroup analyses suggested that the intervention may have promoted increased use among underusers by discovering previously undertreated health problems, while at the same time promoting decreased use among overusers of hospital services.

We concluded that in-home preventive health care, including comprehensive multidimensional health assessment, education, and motivation to act on recommendations to improve or maintain health is a promising strategy for prevention of functional decline.

IMPLICATIONS OF THE DEMONSTRATION

It is important to understand the model underlying the program described here as it relates to the overall picture of home care. The model is preventive. It does not share the case management model (with its premise of dependency sufficient to justify supportive care) that underlies programs that offer home-based long-term care. The method of intervention in this program was assessment, communication, education, and promotion of self-management. The target population is at risk of functional decline; they are not already on a downward spiral of functional disability and health impairments.

Ramsdell (1991) noted the possible benefits of supplemental home-based comprehensive assessment for primary care physicians with large numbers of older patients. With the rapid transition of the primary health care system in this nation from fee-for-service to capitated and at-risk contracts to provide care, more and more physicians are combining their practices into large medical groups. These groups will have the critical mass of older patients to be able to support innovative programs of comprehensive health assessment and home-based preventive interventions.

The future success of preventive home-based programs will depend on targeting enough eligible participants, a clear understanding and implementation of the chosen home care model, and development of low-cost, effective interventions. Compared with substitutive and transitional models of home care, prevention programs will require a different type of intervention and will be appropriately targeted at a population that is quite different from the other programs. The In-home Preventive Health Care Program for Older Persons is a promising home care model developed to address the national problem of growing numbers of older persons living in our communities and increasing demands for long-term care.

REFERENCES

Alessi, C.A., Stuck, A.E., Aronow, H.U., Yuhas, K.E., Bula, C.J., Madison, R., Gold, M., Fanello, R., Rubenstein, L.Z., & Beck, J.C. (1995). *Annual yield and subject adherence with a program of in-home comprehensive geriatric assessment.* Manuscript submitted for publication.

Balinsky, W., & Nesbitt, S. (1989). Cost-effectiveness of outpatient parenteral antibiotics: A review of the literature. *American Journal of Medicine, 87,* 301-305.

Carpenter, G., & Demopoulis, G.R. (1990). Screening the elderly in the community: Controlled trial of dependency surveillance using a questionnaire administered by volunteers. *British Medical Journal, 300,* 1253-1256.

Detsky, A.S., McLaughlin, J.R., Abrams, H.B., Whittaker, J.S., Whitwell, J., L'Abbe, K., & Jeejeebhoy, K.N. (1986). A cost-utility analysis of the home parenteral nutrition program at Toronto General Hospital: 1970-1982. *Journal of Parenteral & Enteral Nutrition, 10,* 49-57.

Drummond, R.C., Boucher, J.D., Drummond, L.J., & Geraci, R.C. (1986). A cost-effective surgical program: Collaboration among an HMO, hospital, and home care agency. *Home Healthcare Nurse, 4,* 37-41.

Dunne, P.J. (1994). Demographics and financial impact of home respiratory care. *Respiratory Care, 39,* 309-317.

Fabacker, D., Josephson, K., Pietruszka, F., Linderborn, K., Morley, J.E., & Rubenstein, L.Z. (1994). An in-home preventive assessment program for independent older adults: A randomized controlled trial. *Journal of the American Geriatrics Society, 42,* 630-638.

Fries, J.F., Bloch, D.A., Harrington, H., Richardson, N., & Beck, R. (1993). Two-year results of a randomized controlled trial of a health promotion program in a retiree population: The Bank of America Study. *American Journal of Medicine, 94,* 455-462.

Gray, D., MacAdam, D., & Boldy, D. (1987). A comparative cost analysis of terminal cancer care in home hospice patients and controls. *Journal of Chronic Diseases, 40,* 801-810.

Green, J.H. (1989). Long term home care research. *Nursing Health and Care, 10,* 138-144.

Greene, V.L., Lovely, M.E., & Ondrich, J.I. (1993). The cost-effectiveness of community services in a frail elderly population. *Gerontologist, 33,* 177-189.

Hall, N., De Beck, P., Johnson, D., Mackinnon, K., Gutman, G., & Glick, N. (1992). Randomized trial of a health promotion program for frail elders. *Canadian Journal of Aging, 11,* 72-91.

Hedrick, S.C., & Inui, T.S. (1986). The effectiveness and cost of home care: An information synthesis. *Health Services Research, 20,* 851-880.

Hendriksen, C. (1994). Personal communication.

Hendriksen, C., Lund, E., & Stromgard, E. (1984). Consequences of assessment and intervention among elderly: A three year randomized controlled trial. *British Medical Journal, 289,* 1522-1524.

Hollingworth, W., Todd, C., Parker, M., Roberts, J.A., Williams, R. (1993). Cost analysis of early discharge after hip fracture. *British Medical Journal, 307,* 903-906.

Jamieson, M.K. (1990). Block nursing: Practicing autonomous professional nursing in the community. *Nursing & Health Care, 11,* 250-253.

Jarnlo, G.B., Ceder, L., & Thorngren, K.G. (1984). Early rehabilitation at home of elderly patients with hip fractures and consumption of resources in primary care. *Scandinavian Journal of Primary Health Care, 2,* 105-112.

Knapp, M., Beecham, J., Koutsogeorgopoulou, V., Hallam, A., Fenyo, A., Marks I.M., Connolly, J., Audini, B. & Muijen, M. (1994). Service use and costs of home-based versus hospital-based care for people with serious mental illness. *British Journal of Psychiatry, 165,* 195-203.

Kornowski, R., Zeeli, D., Averbuch, M., Finkelstein, A., Schwartz, D., Moshkovitz, M., Weinreb, B., Hershkovitz, R., Eyal, D., Miller, M., Levo, Y., & Pines, A. (1995). Intensive home-care surveillance prevents hospitalization and improves morbidity rates among elderly patients with severe congestive heart failure. *American Heart Journal, 129,* 762-766.

Kramer, A.M., Shaughnessy, P.W., & Pettigrew, M.L. (1985). Cost-effectiveness implications based on a comparison of nursing home and home health case mix. *Health Services Research, 20,* 387-405.

Lindberg, G., & Monson, T. (1989). Long-term care initiatives: Success in Hennepin County, Minnesota. *American Journal of Public Health, 79,* 519.

McEwan, R.T., Davidson, N., Forster, D.P., Pearson, P., & Stirling, E. (1990). Screening elderly people in primary care: A randomized controlled trial. *British Journal of General Practice, 40,* 94-97.

Melin, A.L., Hakansson, S., & Bygren, L.O. (1993). The cost-effectiveness of rehabilitation in the home: A study of Swedish elderly. *American Journal of Public Health, 83,* 356-362.

Milkovich, G. (1993). Costs and benefits: Outpatient parenteral antibiotic therapy. *Hospital Practice, 28 (Suppl 1),* 39-43.

Moxley, J.H., & Roeder, P.C. (1984). New opportunities for out-of-hospital health services. *New England Journal of Medicine, 310,* 193-197.

Newman, S.J. (1985). Housing and long-term care: The suitability of the elderly's housing to the provision of in-home services. *Gerontologist, 25,* 35-40.

Pathy, M.S.J., Bayer, A., Harding, K., & Dibble, A. (1992). Randomised trial of case finding and surveillance of elderly people at home. *Lancet, 340,* 890-893.

Ramsdell, J.W. (1991). Geriatric assessment in the home. *Clinics in Geriatric Medicine, 7,* 677-693.

Ramsdell, J.W., Jackson, J.E., Renvall, M., & Swart, J.A. (1989). The yield of a home visit in the assessment of geriatric patients. *Journal of the American Geriatric Society, 37,* 17-24.

Rogatz, P. (1985). Home health care: Some social and economic considerations. *Home Healthcare Nurse, 3,* 38-43.

Rosenwaike, I. (1985). A demographic portrait of the oldest old. *Milbank Memorial Fund Quarterly, 63,* 187-205.

Sherry, D. (1992). Cost effectiveness and home care: Myth or reality? *Home Healthcare Nurse, 10,* 27-29.

Smith, K., & Wright, K. (1994). Informal care and economic appraisal: A discussion of possible methodological approaches. *Health Economics, 3,* 137-148.

Stuck, A.E., Aronow, H.U., Steiner, A., Alessi, C.A., Bula, C.J., Gold, M.N., Yuhas, K.E., Nisenbaum, R., Rubenstein, L.Z., & Beck, J.C. (1995). Effect of annual in-home comprehensive geriatric assessments and other interventions in elderly people living in the community. *The New England Journal of Medicine, 333,* 1184-1189.

Stuck, A.E., Siu, A.L., Wieland, G.D., Adams, J., Rubenstein, L.Z. (1993). Effects of a comprehensive geriatric assessment on survival, residence and function: A meta-analysis of controlled trials. *Lancet, 342,* 1032-1036.

Tinetti, M.E., Baker, D.I., McAvay, G., Claus, E.B., Garrett, P., Gottschalk, M., Koch, M.L., Trainor, K. & Horwitz, R.I. (1994). A multifactorial intervention to reduce the risk of falling among elderly people living in the community. *The New England Journal of Medicine, 331,* 821-827.

U.S. Bureau of the Census. (1989). Projections of the population of the United States by age, sex and race: 1988-2080. *Current Population Reports* (Series P-25, No. 1018).

van Rossum, E., Frederiks, C.M.A., Philipsen, H., Portengen, K., Wiskerke, J., & Knipschild, P. (1993). Effects of preventive home visits to elderly people. *British Medical Journal, 307,* 27-32.

Varricchio, C. (1994). Human and indirect costs of home care. *Nursing Outlook, 42,* 151-157.

Vetter, N.J., Jones, D.A., Victor, C.R. (1984). Effect of health visitors working with elderly patients in general practice: A randomised controlled trial. *British Medical Journal, 288,* 369-372.

Weissert, W.G. (1985). Seven reasons why it is so difficult to make community-based long-term care cost-effective. *Health Services Research, 20,* 423-433.

Williams, B. (1994). Comparison of services among different types of home health agencies. *Medical Care, 32,* 1134-1152.

Young, J., & Forster, A. (1993). Day hospital and home physiotherapy for stroke patients: A comparative cost-effectiveness study. *Journal of the Royal College of Physicians of London, 27,* 252-258.

Are nurses getting paid what they are worth?

DONNA SULLIVAN HAVENS, MARY ETTA MILLS

This chapter provides recent data describing wage and remuneration practices in nursing and presents key issues in determining the worth of nursing work. The question is not whether nurses are paid enough, but whether they are paid what they are worth. From this perspective, we present relevant data and examine issues that can assist readers to participate knowledgeably in the debate and research answers to this question.

COMPENSATION FOR NURSING WORK

Salaries are frequently viewed as a reflection of everything from social values to business and market economics. The value that a society places on a particular job is most often demonstrated by the salary and benefits assigned to that job. Salary is measured through a combination of elements including tangible remuneration (salary and benefits), professional rewards, and personal satisfaction. Traditional registered nurse (RN) compensation has included hourly wage, benefits, overtime, differentials, and holiday pay. More recent additions to this list include bonuses, incentive pay, and pay-for-performance programs (Bell & Bart, 1991; Havens, 1990; Havens & Mills, 1992; Wasylak, 1991; York & Fecteau, 1987; Youngkin, 1985).

Benefits such as time available to meet personal needs (i.e., annual leave, sickness leave, personal, education, and retirement needs); reimbursement for work-related efforts such as education, research, and clinical development; and incentives such as paid transportation, housing, and elder and child care options also have monetary value. While these compensation mechanisms have been available to hospital-employed RNs to some degree, there is evidence to suggest that as health care organizations search for measures to manage costs and contain expenses, benefit/compensation programs such as these may be targeted for cutbacks ("Cost Management Critical," 1995). However, the discussion in this chapter focuses primarily on base wages (excluding benefits) for RNs working in acute care hospitals. According to most recent available data, this includes two thirds of all employed RNs (Joel, 1992). Because data pertaining to this group are collected uniformly across national samples by professional organizations, corporate analysts, and the U.S. government, the chapter focuses on RNs employed in acute care hospitals.

SALARY DETERMINATION

There are several means by which salaries are determined. These include job worth evaluation using a criterion-based rating system developed around knowledge, skills, responsibilities, effort, and working conditions; pay according to productivity; pay according to supply and demand; and same pay for all, in which all employees receive the same wages without regard for the nature of the job or the level of productivity of the employee (Brett, 1983; Youngkin, 1985). Negotiation through collective bargaining and methods that employ a combination of these strategies are also used.

While a variety or combination of methods may be used to determine rate of pay, most staff nurses today are paid according to an hourly wage (Havens, 1990). A 1990 randomized national study with 221 responding acute care hospitals suggested that only 5.9% of staff RNs were salaried, with that number projected to increase to 19.0% by 1995 (Havens, 1990). Replication of this research revealed that in 1994, 9.6% of hospital-employed staff RNs were on salaried status, with that number projected to increase to 13.6% by 1996—falling short of the 1990 projection for 1995 (Havens, 1995). This implies that while there has been some increase in the number of salaried RNs, generally nurses are paid for the time they spend at work, not necessarily for their skills, expertise, or accomplishments.

SALARY LEVELS

Available salary data for RNs generally represent only the two thirds of staff RNs who work in hospitals and usually do not include the other one third working in other settings who have traditionally been paid lower salaries (Joel, 1992). With this caveat in mind, the National Association for Health Care Recruitment Survey reported average staff RN salary data based on a 40-hour workweek excluding differentials. Starting hourly rates were reported from a high range of $15.92 to $24.60 per hour ($33,116 to $51,167 annually) in the western United States to a low range of $12.78 to $20.90 per hour ($26,585 to $43,604 annually) in the South. The Northeast reported a range of $15.45 to $23.10 per hour ($32,145 to $48,048 annually), and the North Central United States reported a range of $13.48 to $20.48 per hour ($28,035 to $42,594 annually). Reported hourly wages did not include premium pay for overtime or for work on weekends, holidays, and late shifts. Also excluded were bonuses such as performance bonuses and profit-sharing payments. Pay increases under cost-of-living allowances and incentive payments were included.

The geographical variability in RN salaries suggests a "territorial market" in terms of salaries and salary gains. According to the Health Care Recruitment Survey, RNs working in the West earned nearly 25% more than RNs employed in the South in 1994. Therefore, when interpreting regional variations, geographical cost-of-living differences must be considered.

Due to the need to limit the growth of health care costs, there is now an increased focus on ways in which health care delivery might be restructured. The results of Havens' 1995 research revealed that 73% of the respondents (n = 183) from a randomized national survey reported implementing changes in staffing that targeted altering the use of RN resources. This restructuring initiative has generally involved using a smaller core of professional staff with redesigned roles supported by a larger cadre of nonprofessional assistive care personnel (Eastaugh, 1990; Kirby & Garfink, 1991). Adjunctively, some institutions have implemented pay-for-performance and incentive-based professional practice programs (Havens & Mills, 1992). These latter arrangements are not included in base wage rates and, as a result, are not reported as part of the salary statistics normally collected by salary surveys such as those conducted by Monitrend II and the Bureau of Labor Statistics.

Because salary advances are economy driven (Brider, 1992), most forecasters now suggest that they will continue to slow. While gains made through contract negotiations that extend several years into the future will continue to increase salaries, there are indications that the trend toward raising nursing salaries may be leveling off. Between 1994 and 1995, medical-surgical nurses experienced a 0.51% decrease in average salary while the average for all staff nurses rose 1.73% ("Executive Summary," 1995).

DIFFERENTIALS

Survey data indicate that hourly earnings also vary according to eight different specialty areas (medical-surgical, intensive care unit, coronary care unit, emergency room, obstetrics-gynecology, pediatrics, operating room, and psychiatry), with staff RNs working in the emergency room earning the highest mean average hourly wage—$18.38 ("National Association," 1994). However, hourly wage differences among the eight specialty areas amounted to less than $2 per hour within the lowest, average, and highest hourly wage categories. In previous studies, the specialty area in which an RN worked did not influence hourly pay as much as did number of years of experience. Interestingly, while there were hourly differences according to different lengths of service within a specialty area, on average, an RN could expect to earn only a maximum of $4 to $5 more over a career than the starting hourly rate (Brider, 1992).

While many nurses have the opportunity to work more lucrative (often undesirable) shifts and overtime hours, this is not an option for all because of age, health status, or other responsibilities. For instance, a nurse working the night shift for 1 year might add $4000 to $5000 to his or her annual salary (Joel, 1992). What this might imply is that those able to enhance their base wages by adding the differentials and bonuses are generally those who do not have additional responsibilities, such as family, outside of the work arena. It has been suggested that those most apt to take advantage of these salary enhancements might be the younger, less experienced nurses. The implication is that younger, less experienced RNs may earn as much or more on an annual basis than their more experienced colleagues (Brider, 1992). This leaves room for interesting speculation as the RN workforce continues to age, with the average age of the employed RN being 41 years (Moses, 1992).

Differentials may also be offered for education or specialty certification. In 1990, only 20% to 27% of hospitals offered salary differentials for RNs with a bachelor's of science in nursing (BSN) or master's degree (Havens, 1990). In 1994, 29% of hospitals reported salary differentials for

Table 66-1 Salary progression in selected occupations (in dollars)

Occupation	1991 Average starting salary	1991 Average maximum salary	1991 Percentage of salary progression	1993 Average starting salary	1993 Average maximum salary	1993 Percentage of salary progression	Percentage rate of gain or loss
Attorney	40,302	125,855	212.3	56,836	135,564	138.5	(34.7)
Accountant	24,809	75,347	203.7	27,248	80,548	193.6	(4.4)
Engineer	32,459	95,058	192.9	35,204	110,084	212.7	(1.0)
Personnel director	45,018	101,922	125.9	55,120	106,236	92.7	(1.2)
General clerk	11,791	23,133	96.0	13,312	25,376	80.6	(5.6)
Registered nurse	27,225	48,924	79.7	29,478	45,549	54.5	(31.8)
Personnel clerk	15,659	27,599	76.3	16,328	27,924	71.0	(6.9)
Secretary	19,844	34,085	71.8	21,372	39,156	83.2	(15.9)
Accounting clerk	14,639	24,787	69.9	15,288	28,340	85.4	(23.2)
Computer programmer	20,103	42,533	62.9	27,144	50,960	87.7	(39.4)

Note. Modified from U.S. Department of Labor, Bureau of Labor Statistics. (1993). *Occupational Compensation Survey: National Summary, 1993.* (Bulletin 2458), Washington, DC: Author; and National Association for Health Care Recruitment Survey (1994), Springhouse Corporation. U.S. Department of Labor, Bureau of Labor Statistics. (1992, January). *Occupational wage survey: Hospitals* (Bulletin 2392), Washington, DC: Author.

RNs with a BSN or master's degree, with that percentage projected to increase to 35% by 1996 (Havens, 1995). The reported increase in base hourly wage for baccalaureate education ranged from $.10 to $1 per hour, with $1 reported most often (Brider, 1992; Havens, 1990). In 1994, the National Association for Health Care Recruitment Survey found an average BSN starting salary of $29,834 and an average associate degree/diploma nurse salary of $29,487. This represents a 1.2% higher salary for BSN graduates. The average maximum BSN salary of $45,526 was only 2% higher than the average maximum associate degree in nursing/diploma salary of $44,649. Of note is the fact that attainment of educational credentials may be built into clinical ladder advancement criteria, and often ladder advancement is associated with higher hourly earnings. Nevertheless, while some institutions report a variety of means to recognize the RN for this educational achievement, the attainment of a BSN degree is at best considered to add $1 per hour to the worth of the work of nursing. In general, educational differentials are less than shift differentials, implying that *when* an RN practices may be more valued by employing institutions than the knowledge, skill, and credentials he or she possesses.

Specialty certification may also be rewarded in a variety of ways, including financial support for preparatory courses and bonuses and awards for passing. Upon certification, bonuses were reported to range from $150 to $1,000 annually (Havens, 1990).

COMPARISON OF NURSING SALARIES WITH THOSE OF OTHER PROFESSIONS

The U.S. Department of Labor Bureau of Labor Statistics surveys wages for selected professional, administrative, technical, and clerical occupations in private hospitals and private industry. A comparison of average starting salaries and average maximum salaries for selected occupations for the years 1991 and 1993 is reported in Table 66-1.

It is interesting to note that over this 2-year period, nursing as a profession showed the second most significant rate of salary loss (−31.6%) when compared with other selected occupations. The percentage of salary progression for nurses, while almost at the midpoint of the rates reported in 1991 (+79.7%), had dropped to the lowest quartile by 1993 with a rate of 71.0%. Further examination reveals that the mean rate of salary progression for the selected occupations equaled 105.7%. Applying this figure to the average starting nursing salary would create an average maximum salary of $60,636, suggesting that nursing salary levels reflect a lag behind the average occupational progression level. Salary compression, therefore, remains a serious issue in nursing corporations. In addition, wide variation in salary levels between certain geographical areas reflects a territorial market ("National Association," 1994). For example, the average maximum RN salary in the north central United States is $42,594 as compared with $51,167 for the western United States—a difference of 20.1%.

Table 66-2 Educational requirements and salaries in selected health care occupations

Occupation	Educational requirements	1991 average salary ($)	2000 average salary ($)
Registered nurse	Associate degree, diploma, baccalaureate, or master's degree	27,000	50,000
Physician assistant	2 years of college and 2 years of physician assistant study (baccalaureate and graduate study available)	35,000–60,000	47,250
Physical therapist	Baccalaureate—master's degree preferred	31,421–66,150	45,000–96,000
Pharmacist	Graduation from a 5-year college of pharmacy	44,000	60,605
Occupational therapist	Baccalaureate or master's degree	29,796	51,000
Speech pathologist	Master's degree	31,421	46,000
Dietitian	Baccalaureate	27,562–71,662	40,000–80,000

Note. Compiled from information in *"The 100 Best Jobs for the 1990s and Beyond,"* by C. Kleiman, 1992, Dearborn, MI: Dearborn Financial Publishing. Adapted with permission.

Other interesting comparisons can be made between the educational requirements and salaries of RNs and other health care professionals as depicted in Table 66-2. Examination of this table suggests that in 1991, RNs had the lowest minimum educational requirements to practice and the lowest average salary.

Combining this with salary data that demonstrate the relatively minor influence of education on current nursing salary levels, there does not appear to be a direct meaningful relationship between the two. Educational level seems to be a greater factor in obtaining promotional positions such as middle manager or clinical specialist for which salary levels have not been reported here.

FACTORS AFFECTING THE WORTH OF NURSING WORK

Worth is defined as "monetary value . . . the value of something measured by its qualities or by the esteem in which it is held" (Webster's, 1988). Calculation of worth here may be dependent on the perspective of the individual or entity making the determination of monetary value or usefulness of nursing. Factors that may influence determination of the value of the services of the nursing profession include the nursing labor market and the concept of economic equity.

The labor market for hospital-employed RNs

In an ideal situation, the value or worth of a good or service (in this case, professional nursing practice) is determined by the demand for that good or service. Before 1988, the shortage of nurses was a key factor in driving salary considerations relative to the recruitment and retention of staff. Since that time, several factors have combined to impact the way in which salaries are viewed. In the late 1980s and early 1990s, RN salaries increased in response to the hospital demand for staff to care for an ever-increasing population requiring acute care (Styles, 1985). However, in the recent past, environmental influences outside of the hospital industry and debate over health care reform have created new pressures for health care organizations. Economic pressures such as price competition, the growth of managed care, capitated payment systems, and projected Medicare/Medicaid shortfalls are providing incentives for hospitals to implement initiatives to manage costs and control expenses (Buerhaus, 1995). In response, many hospitals are adopting strategies to decrease numbers of inpatient beds, anticipating that in this new era more services will be provided on an ambulatory basis. Other organizational strategies include reorganizing, restructuring, or "reinventing" care delivery systems as a means to decrease the numbers of professional staff needed, in some cases relying on nonprofessional, unlicensed personnel to take on some duties formerly performed by RNs. Viewing these events from the perspective of an ideal labor market, one could surmise that in this current economic environment, the demand for hospital-employed RN labor in the traditional sense may be lessened, and that this will be reflected in wages and wage increases. What needs to be kept in mind is that this same economic environment will raise the demand for new and nontraditional RN roles both internal and external to hospitals.

However, the labor market in health care, and in nursing in particular, is not perfect. Potential nursing labor market imperfections affecting the worth of nursing work include an undervaluation of the work of nursing (Dawes, 1989), (2) the existence of a monopsony, and (3) the mobility factor.

The general public does not clearly understand the education needed, the skills required, and the hazards associated with professional nursing practice (Dawes, 1989). Confusion may also exist among the public and employers when not all nurses can clearly describe the nature and value of the services they provide. The existence of multiple educational pathways leading to practice of a single role compounds the confusion both internal and external to the profession. As a result, when performing a wage evaluation of nursing work, it is difficult to build a case for enhanced job worth as a result of the need for a rigorous educational background when those with and without BSN degrees perform the same roles. Strasen (1992, p. 16) noted that "nursing compensation is equitable with other professions that require two years of college education." This multiplicity in educational requirements, with the minimum educational requirement factored into the job worth equation, is not in the best interest of nursing when the worth of the work is analyzed.

A second imperfection in the nursing labor market is the existence of a monopsony. A monopsony exists when there is only one buyer or supplier of goods or services. In today's health care arena, hospitals are the prime employer for over 66.5% of professional nurses (Moses, 1992). This fact carries great importance, especially considering evidence that wages paid to nurses in hospitals often determine noninstitutional nursing wages (Dean & Yetter, 1979). In some geographical areas, there is only one hospital that employs nurses. Even in cases where there are several hospitals in a geographical region, the literature suggests that agreements have been made among institutions to set nursing wages at a particular level (Styles, 1985). When formal agreements are not made, it is not unusual for nursing wages to be set based on the market value of the wages paid by others in a particular region (Brett, 1983; Youngkin, 1985). This has the effect of determining nursing wages according to what is currently paid (whether or not that level is appropriate) rather than assessing critical factors to determine the actual worth of the service.

A third imperfection in the nursing labor market is the fact that the majority of professional nurses are women (96%). Some argue that as women, many nurses are geographically limited in terms of employment. Dawes (1989) points to the fact that many nurses grow up, attend school, and eventually work in the same geographical area. This "immobility factor" may serve to further promote monopsony in the nursing labor market.

Economic equity

According to Brider (1980), women and nurses have been struggling for equitable compensation for many years. This struggle is highlighted by a report from the U.S. Department of Labor Women's Bureau, which notes that when 1992 median weekly earnings of full-time male and female workers were compared, women earned only $.75 for every $1 earned by men (U.S. Department of Labor, 1993). The same source reports that men with an associate's degree working full time earned nearly the same as similarly employed women with a master's degree (U.S. Department of Labor, 1993). Sex-based wage discrimination may occur when less than 30% of either sex is employed in a certain job (Weingard, 1984). In the nursing profession, 96% of all workers are female.

Pay equity is "a broad concept [and] refers to the movement to assure that all disadvantaged groups . . . are compensated on the basis of the inherent value or worth of the work they perform, rather than on the basis of historically depressed pay levels or other discriminatory factors" (Brider, 1980, p. 25). Pay equity is often used to encompass the concepts of comparable worth, sex-based wage discrimination, and equal pay for equal work (Mahrenholz, 1987).

The Equal Employment Act of 1972 focused on "comparable pay for comparable work," and this is the crux of the problem—how and by whom is comparability of work determined? Comparable worth "refers to equal pay for work done by females and males that is of comparable value to the employer. Value to the employer is defined by skill, effort, and responsibility required to do the job" (Mahrenholz, 1987, p. 25).

Nursing salaries have been affected by pay equity issues. Examples include the following (Brett, 1983): Minnesota, 1982—RN work was rated as equivalent to that of vocational instructors, but RNs were paid $537 less per month; California, 1980—electrical foremen were paid $2268 per month for work rated equal to that of nurses, who were paid $839 per month; Washington, 1982—RNs received $1368 per month for work rated higher than that of highway engineers, who were paid $1980 per month (from testimony of American Nurses Association president Eunice Cole to the U.S. House of Representatives Subcommittees on Human Resources, Civil Service, and Compensation and Civil Service, September 21, 1982).

The comparability of nursing wages to those of other professions has also served as the focus for litigation (Cook, 1990; Creighton, 1984; Mahrenholz, 1987). In a landmark comparable worth case (*Lemmon v. City and County of Denver,* 1980) in which the ruling went against nurses, the judge claimed that the comparable worth issue had the potential to "disrupt the entire economic system of the United States" (p. 111). This is symbolic of the environment in which nursing is addressing issues of compensation relative to worth.

CONCLUSIONS

The measure of job worth has often been described in terms of salary. There is evidence that health care organizations have addressed salary levels through an examination of the effect of wage compression within and between professions, use of job evaluation methods, and implementation of programs such as pay for performance.

These factors have been instrumental in changing the dynamics of nursing compensation. The rate of nursing salary growth slowed between 1986 and 1993. For example, in 1986 the average starting salary for RNs was reported at $20,340, with a maximum of $27,744. In 1991, starting salaries averaged $27,225, with an average maximum of $48,924. This represented a 34% increase in average starting salaries and a 76% increase in average maximum salaries over a 5-year period. In 1993, starting salaries averaged $29,478, with an average maximum of $45,549. This reflected an 8% increase over the 1991 starting salary level and a 6.9% decrease in average maximum salary.

Still, there appears to be little relationship between salary and educational level or work experience. Furthermore, a comparison of the average rate of salary progression for selected occupations suggests that, while advances have been made, the rate of nursing salary level change lags behind the progression rate averaged across several occupations.

The real question is how to establish an appropriate means to measure job worth other than "current market rates." Wage levels are currently the best standard measure of comparability. However, they do not account for the variable trends impacting compensation. These might include business-specific demands or downturns, auxiliary roles subsumed by specific careers that impact perceived worth, and changes in professional autonomy. Furthermore, additional means of calculating comprehensive benefit packages inclusive of available bonuses, gain sharing, and other options having a monetary benefit should be developed.

REFERENCES

Bell, E., & Bart, B. (1991). Pay for performance: Motivating the chief nurse executive. *Nursing Economic$, 9*(2), 113.

Brett, J. (1983, June). How much is a nurse's job really worth? *American Journal of Nursing,* 877-881.

Brider, P. (1980, October). The struggle for just compensation. *American Journal of Nursing,* 77-88.

Brider, P. (1992, March). Salary gains slow as more RNs seek full-time benefits. *American Journal of Nursing,* 34-42.

Buerhaus, P. (1995). Economic pressures building in the hospital employed RN labor market. *Nursing Economic$, 13*(3), 137-141.

Cook, A. (1990). Comparable worth: An economic issue. *Nursing Management, 21*(2), 28-30.

Cost management critical. (1995). *Nursing Economic$, 13*(3), 141.

Creighton, H. (1984). Comparable worth cases. *Nursing Management, 15*(11), 20-22.

Dawes, R. (1989). The economics of comparable worth. *Nursing Management, 20*(1), 80B, 80F-80H.

Dean, R., & Yetter, T. (1979). Nurse market policy simulations using an econometric model. In R. Scheffler (Ed.), *Research in health economics* (pp. 255-300). Greenwich, CN: JA1 Press.

Eastaugh, S. (1990). Hospital nursing technical efficiency: Nurse extenders and enhanced productivity. *Hospital and Health Services Administration, 35*(4), 561-573.

Executive summary. (1995). *Hospital salary & benefits report* (25th Ed). Oakland, NJ: Hospital and Health Care Compensation Service.

Havens, D. (1990). Analysis of the nature and extent of implementation and projected implementation of a model proposed to support professional nursing practice in acute care hospitals (Doctoral dissertation, University of Maryland, 1991). *University Microfilms No. 91-100096.*

Havens, D. (1995). [Professional recognition/compensation mechanisms for hospital employed RNs]. Unpublished raw data.

Havens, D., & Mills, M. (1992). Professional recognition and compensation for staff RNs: 1990 and 1995. *Nursing Economic$, 10*(1), 15-20.

Joel, L. (1992). Nursing salaries: Recurring themes and new insights. *Journal of Nursing Administration, 22*(3), 13, 15, 17.

Kirby, K., & Garfink, C. (1991). The university hospital nurse extender model. *Journal of Nursing Administration, 21*(1), 25-30.

Kleiman, C. (1992). *The 100 best jobs for the 1990s & beyond.* Dearborn, MI: Dearborn Financial Publishing.

Lemmon v. City and County of Denver, 620 F.2d 288 (U.S. 10th Cir. Ct., 1980). Cert. denied 499 U.S. 880 (1980).

Mahrenholz, D. (1987). Comparable worth: Litigation and legislation. *Nursing Administration Quarterly, 12*(1), 25-31.

Moses, E. (1992). *The registered nurse population: Findings from the national sample survey of registered nurses, March 1992.* Rockville, MD: Health Resources Services Administration, Bureau of Health Professions.

National Association for Health Care Recruitment Survey. (1994). Springhouse, PA: Springhouse Corporation.

Strasen, L. (1992). Nurses' salaries are adequate! *Journal of Nursing Administration, 22*(3), 12, 14, 16, 18.

Styles, M. (1985). The uphill battle for comparable worth. *Nursing Outlook, 33*(3), 128-132.

U.S. Department of Labor, Bureau of Labor Statistics. (1992, January). *Occupational wage survey: Hospitals* (Bulletin 2392). Washington, DC: Author.

U.S. Department of Labor, Bureau of Labor Statistics. (1993). *Occupational compensation survey: National summary, 1993.* Bulletin 2458 Washington, DC: Author.

U.S. Department of Labor, Women's Bureau. (1993, June). *20 facts on working women* (Publication No. 93-2). Washington, DC: Author.

Wasylak, T. (1991, April). Pay for performance. *Canadian Nurse,* 30-31.

Webster's Ninth New Collegiate Dictionary. (1988). Springfield, MA: Merriam-Webster.

Weingard, M. (1984). Establishing comparable worth through job evaluation. *Nursing Outlook, 32*(2), 113.

York, C., & Fecteau, D. (1987). Innovative models for professional nursing practice. *Nursing Economic$, 5*(4), 162-166.

Youngkin, E. (1985, January-February). Comparable worth: Alternatives to litigation and legislation. *Nursing Economic$, 3,* 38-43.

The costs of safety precautions to reduce risk of exposure to bloodborne pathogens

DIANA C. McPHERSON, MARGUERITE McMILLIAN JACKSON

It has long been recognized that health care workers (HCWs) are at risk for a variety of bloodborne infections, but the epidemic of HIV and AIDS has brought this issue to the forefront.

In late 1986 several labor unions petitioned the Occupational Safety and Health Administration (OSHA) to establish emergency regulations to mandate health care employers to provide a variety of safety measures for HCWs. OSHA did not agree to the emergency regulations, but it did initiate a rule-making process that culminated in the publication of the OSHA bloodborne pathogens standard on December 6, 1991 (U.S. Department of Labor, 1991). The standard marked the completion of more than 4 years of work by OSHA and verbal and written testimony by thousands of health care professionals, labor union representatives, and members of a concerned public. In 1987 when the standard was first proposed, there was a great deal of emphasis on barriers such as gloves, gowns, masks, and protective eyewear as safety measures; however, as the standard evolved, it became apparent that other strategies were much more likely to reduce bloodborne pathogen risks to HCWs (Jackson & Pugliese, 1992).

WHAT ARE SAFETY PRECAUTIONS?

Safety precautions for bloodborne pathogens include a variety of strategies that are intended to reduce or eliminate the risk of exposure of HCWs or patients to potentially infectious biological agents.

Using the traditional industrial hygiene approach, the risk reduction hierarchy of controls is as follows: (1) engineering controls (design out the problem), (2) work practice controls (modify the behavior), and (3) personal protective equipment (barriers).

Engineering controls isolate or remove the bloodborne pathogen hazard from the workplace. Examples include sharps disposal containers, self-sheathing needles, and needle-free intravenous access devices.

Work practice controls are modifications in procedures that reduce the likelihood of exposure by altering the manner in which a task is performed. Examples include using a one-handed recapping technique for used needles; requiring any person (whether nurse, physician, or technician) who uses a sharp device to discard it into a sharps disposal container immediately after use; providing adequate lighting for tasks involving sharps; and lifting all bags of trash and linen so that they are always away from the body in case a sharp has been discarded incorrectly into the bag.

Personal protective equipment is specialized clothing or equipment worn by an employee for protection against a hazard. Examples include gloves, gowns, masks, eye protection, and devices that permit resuscitation without mouth-to-mouth contact.

Universal precautions are an approach to infection prevention and control that was developed by the Centers for Disease Control and Prevention (CDC, 1987, 1988). Universal precautions treat all human blood and certain body fluids as if they are infectious for hepatitis B virus (HBV), HIV, or other bloodborne pathogens. Universal precautions do not apply to feces, nasal secretions, saliva, sputum, sweat, tears, urine, or vomitus (unless they contain visible blood) because these body substances have not been associated epidemiologically with transmission of bloodborne pathogens. The OSHA standard applies only to blood and body fluids to which universal precautions apply. That is, other body substances are not *regulated* under the standard.

There is little evidence to support the effectiveness of

universal precautions in preventing bloodborne infections in HCWs (Gerberding & Henderson, 1987). Universal precautions have their origins in traditional isolation techniques intended to reduce risks of cross-transmission of organisms between and among patients and personnel (CDC, 1970, 1975, 1983). The primary strategy for traditional isolation techniques is the wearing of personal protective equipment, especially gloves, gowns, and masks. In 1987 the CDC responded to increasing concern of HCWs about bloodborne diseases by recommending that the precautions outlined in the 1983 isolation category "blood and body fluid precautions" be used consistently for all patients rather than only for those in whom a bloodborne infection had been diagnosed or was suspected. They titled these new recommendations "universal precautions" or "universal blood and body fluid precautions" (CDC, 1987). Originally these precautions also applied to all blood and body fluids (e.g., feces, urine, saliva) but in 1988 were modified to *exclude* those body substances that had not been associated epidemiologically with transmission of bloodborne pathogens (CDC, 1988). Universal precautions recommend specific precautions to be taken with soiled linen, trash, and used sharps, as well as a comprehensive post-exposure management strategy for persons experiencing mucous membrane, parenteral, or nonintact skin exposures to blood or body fluids. Universal precautions also emphasize the importance of HBV immunization, employee education and training, and monitoring for compliance. Engineering controls and work practice modifications are not strongly emphasized in isolation precautions because the intent is to use a barrier to interrupt transmission of organisms from one person to another.

An important aspect of universal precautions, as defined by the CDC, is that they must be combined with another strategy of precautions intended to reduce risks of infection to patients and HCWs with other types of biological agents. Thus health care agencies are faced with the dilemma of implementing universal precautions for everyone, based on taking specific precautions with certain body fluids of all patients while also implementing another isolation system. The traditional isolation systems commonly in use involve assigning a patient to a category of isolation (category-specific isolation precautions) or using specific barriers based on the diagnosis or suspected diagnosis of a particular disease in the patient (disease-specific isolation precautions). Thus one system expects HCWs to act the same for all patients when handling blood or certain body fluids, while the other system expects HCWs to act with caution only when caring for patients with diagnosed or suspected diagnosed infections caused by other infectious agents. This leads to considerable confusion!

Many health care agencies have elected to consider *all* blood and body substances as potentially infectious because infectious agents other than HIV, HBV, and other bloodborne pathogens may be transmitted by feces, urine, saliva, sputum, vomitus, wound, and other drainage. This broader strategy of generic infection precautions has been named body substance isolation (BSI) (Jackson, 1989; Jackson & Lynch, 1984; Jackson, Lynch, McPherson, Cummings, & Greenawalt, 1987; Lynch, Jackson, Cummings, & Stamm, 1987; McPherson & Jackson, 1987) and is also called body substance precautions, universal body substance precautions, or a variety of other names. When evaluated, BSI has proved to be much easier to teach and implement than a combination of other strategies. In addition, its primary purpose is to reduce risks of cross-transmission of organisms among and between patients, with the secondary benefit of reducing risks to HCWs (Birnbaum, Schulzer, Mathias, Kelly, & Chow, 1990; Jackson & Lynch, 1991; Lee, Marvin, Heimbach, Grube, & Engrav, 1990; Lynch et al., 1990; Troya, Jackson, Lovrich-Kerr, & McPherson, 1991).

COSTS OF SAFETY PRECAUTIONS

There are a variety of ways to calculate costs for safety precautions. Costs are incurred when vaccines are administered, tests are performed, supplies are purchased, and treatment and follow-up for exposures are prescribed. These costs are usually referred to as direct costs. Direct costs attributable to safety programs also include the salaries and benefits for personnel who provide training, monitor for compliance, and provide the services of post-exposure follow-up. In addition, the costs of space to provide the services and equipment needed to maintain the office (e.g., computers and telephones) are also measurable costs.

Indirect costs include the cost of illness incurred primarily due to lack of implementation of risk reduction strategies. These costs also include decreased earnings resulting from lost time from work and lost wages due to premature death or disability from occupational illness or injury.

Cost savings from prevention of avoidable injuries, exposures, infections, and illnesses are difficult to measure. Although it is possible to measure the costs of providing prevention services (e.g., the personnel, space, and equipment for an employee health service and a hospital epidemiology unit), it is not possible to directly assess savings from an infection prevented in either a patient or an employee. McPherson, Jackson, and Rogers (1988) stated it well:

> What is it worth to a worker *not* to get an infection? We can measure the cost of hepatitis B vaccine and the compliance rate. We cannot measure the value of life lost due to hepatitis B because the worker failed to get hepatitis B vaccine. What does it cost to provide other prevention strategies to reduce worker risk? How well do they work? Again, because the outcomes (infections in workers) are so rare, it is nearly impossible to measure a before-and-after change in worker infection rates.

It is also difficult to measure the positive effects of educational programs about safety. Common strategies include pre- and posttest measurement of knowledge of the information presented, but observation of behavior change is rarely done because of the costs of the labor required for such observational evaluations. Nonetheless, when observational studies have been done (Lynch et al., 1990), it has been clearly shown that education and monitoring for compliance can have a positive effect on employee behavior.

OSHA included costs of compliance in their rulemaking process (U.S. Department of Labor, 1991). Annual costs of compliance were estimated in association with the following components of the standard:

$97,523,109	Engineering and work practice controls
$106,710,705	Vaccination and postexposure follow-up
$32,587,446	Exposure control plan
$101,937,270	Housekeeping
$326,877,357	Personal protective equipment
$134,405,018	Training
$17,253,151	Record keeping
$812,703,560	Total

OSHA also estimates that there are 5,576,026 HCWs in the United States to whom the OSHA standard applies. This means that the annual cost per HCW for compliance with the standard is $145.75. Of the affected HCW population, 68% are employed in hospitals, physicians' offices, dentists' offices, and nursing facilities (nursing homes). These settings also represent about half of all affected establishments. Other settings where the standard applies include medical and dental laboratories, residential and hospice facilities, home health agencies, drug rehabilitation centers, hemodialysis centers, government and industry clinics, blood-plasma-tissue centers, and sites performing personnel services for temporary help, funeral services, medical equipment repair services, and linen services. Also affected are public service workers in law enforcement, fire and rescue, correctional facilities, lifesaving, schools, and waste removal.

The cost of providing personal protective equipment is clearly one of the major expenses of implementing the OSHA standard. Several years before implementation of the standard, McPherson et al. (1988) evaluated the cost of supplies associated with implementation of the BSI system at a large teaching hospital. The system was fully in place by May 1987. In this study of changes in supply costs before, during, and after implementation of the BSI system, we found that about 80% of the costs were for nonsterile gloves. Glove use, estimated on a per-patient-per-day basis, increased from 7.8 pairs per patient per day before implementation to 15.7 pairs per patient per day when the system was fully implemented. The use of gloves in the BSI system is primarily intended to reduce risks of cross-transmission of organisms between and among patients, and secondarily to reduce risks to HCWs. The positive effect of appropriate use of gloves in reducing risks of cross-transmission between and among patients as evaluated by Lynch et al. (1990) was evidenced by a measurable decline in the frequency of certain marker organisms during and after implementation of the BSI system at their large teaching hospital.

Several investigators have evaluated the costs of supplies associated with implementation of the CDC's universal precautions (CDC, 1987; 1988). Doebbeling and Wenzel (1990) studied the direct costs of universal precautions in a large teaching hospital by calculating costs per patient admission. Costs increased from $13.70 to $22.89 per admission after implementation of universal precautions. Two thirds of the increase was due to the cost of nonsterile gloves. Extrapolating the data to all U.S. hospitals for fiscal year 1989, they estimated total costs to be at least $336 million. This is very close to the $322 million estimated for hospitals by OSHA (U.S. Department of Labor, 1991).

Stock, Gafni, and Bloch (1990) conducted an economic analysis of universal precautions in a large hospital in Canada. They estimated the incremental cost of implementing universal precautions to be about $315,000 for their hospital for 1 year. Using these data combined with estimates of the low frequency of occupationally acquired HIV infection among HCWs, they estimated that more than $8 million would be spent to prevent one case of HIV seroconversion. These costs are well above the usual amount our society spends on prevention of death from any other disease. Most importantly, Stock et al. (1990)

Table 67-1 Estimated cost per dose for hepatitis B vaccine*

Element of cost	Time involved per dose (min)	Cost per dose ($)
Vaccine	—	37.00
Supplies, forms, immunization record, etc.	—	1.00
Nurse practitioner: salary = $24/hour; benefits (25%) = $6/hour†	10	5.00
Practical nurse: salary = $12/hour; benefits (25%) = $3/hour‡	10	2.50
Clerk: salary = $9/hour; benefits (25%) = $2.25/hour§	12	2.25
Totals	32	47.75

*Estimated costs of administering a single dose of hepatitis B vaccine to a health care worker in an employee health service of a health care facility in a metropolitan area on the West Coast of the United States. This estimate does not include overhead costs such as space, computers for scheduling and data management, refrigerator space for storage of vaccine, and physician backup for the nurse practitioner. These additional overhead costs for administration of hepatitis B vaccine by a private physician's office can add an additional 40% to 60% to the overall cost per dose, making it $75/dose or more.

†Nurse practitioner functions: Medical evaluation, interview for contraindications, record completion (including consent) consistent with requirements of the Occupational Safety and Health Administration. Note: Nurse practitioner may not need to see employee for second and third doses; initial intake may take longer than 10 minutes; employees may call nurse practitioner for questions before or during vaccine series.

‡Practical nurse functions: Preparation and administration of vaccine, completion of immunization record for medical record and for employee, blood drawing for postvaccine screening (if requested by employee or nurse practitioner).

§Clerk functions: Scheduling of initial and subsequent appointments, data entry into employee health database, pulling and refiling medical records, completion of other forms as required by agency, reordering vaccine from supplier.

concluded that the universal precautions implemented in their hospital were neither efficacious nor cost-effective if their purpose was to prevent bloodborne infections in HCWs. However, they noted that the impact of universal precautions on nosocomial infections in patients may be the most appropriate and effective measure of their usefulness. Proponents of the BSI system have made this point consistently since 1987 (Jackson & Lynch, 1991; Jackson et al., 1987; Lynch et al., 1987).

McPherson et al. (1988) and Stock et al. (1990) suggested that rather than placing emphasis on barriers that have little proved efficacy in reducing risks of HIV or HBV infection, prevention strategies should focus on those circumstances in which risk is greatest: puncture injuries. Strategies to reduce these risks primarily include engineering controls to reduce risks from needles and other sharp equipment and work practice modifications in the use of sharp devices.

HEPATITIS B AND HEPATITIS B VACCINATION

Thousands of HCWs have been infected with HBV over the years, and HCWs are a primary target for the HBV vaccine, first licensed in the United States in 1982. A number of studies have quantified the risk of HBV infection from a single needle puncture to be between 6% and 30% (CDC, 1985), yet as recently as 1990, researchers at the CDC estimated that fewer than half of all at-risk HCWs had been immunized against HBV (Alter et al., 1990). The OSHA bloodborne pathogens standard (U.S. Department of Labor, 1991) mandates that employers provide the vaccine at no expense to the employee, beginning in 1992. The costs for this safety measure are variable, ranging from $40 to $75 per dose or more. To be fully protected, each employee should receive the three-dose series; some will need a fourth dose. Table 67-1 presents an estimate of cost per dose for HBV vaccine that can be applied generally to this issue.

HIV AND POSTEXPOSURE MANAGEMENT

The first case of occupational transmission of HIV to an HCW was reported in the United Kingdom in 1984 (Anonymous, 1984). Since that time 14 studies have enrolled about 2,000 HCWs at the time of an HIV exposure and followed them for at least 90 days and up to more than 1 year after the exposure (Beekman, Fahey, Gerberding, & Henderson, 1990). In these studies through 1990, six HCWs were reported to have seroconverted, for a seroconversion rate of 0.32% (or about 1 chance in 300). All of these exposures were percutaneous; none of the subjects in the studies have seroconverted from mucous membrane or nonintact skin exposures. There are also case reports of HIV-infected HCWs identified in prevalence surveys or as incidental findings when blood was

Table 67-2 Estimated costs for postexposure management of HIV exposures (with and without AZT)*

Visit	Postexposure follow-up costs($)	Postexposure follow-up and AZT prophylaxis costs ($)
Initial visit	Visit[†] = 125 Lab[‡] = 50	Visit = 125 Lab[§] = 80 AZT[¶] = 450
Week 2		Visit = 50 Lab = 30
Week 4		Visit = 50 Lab = 30
Week 6	Visit = 50 Lab = 50	Visit = 50 Lab = 80
Week 8		Visit = 50 Lab = 30
Week 12 (3 months)	Visit = 50 Lab = 50	Visit = 50 Lab = 50
Month 6	Visit = 50 Lab = 50	Visit = 50 Lab = 50
Month 12 (1 year)	Visit = 50 Lab = 50	Visit = 50 Lab = 50
Totals Totals	Visits = 325 Lab = 250 $575	Totals Visits = 475 Lab = 400 AZT = 450 $1325

*Estimated costs of a postexposure follow-up program for an employee exposed to blood or body fluids who is known to be immune to hepatitis B virus (HBV), either due to completion of the HBV vaccine series or with evidence of natural HBV disease. This program for postexposure follow-up is consistent with requirements of the Occupational Safety and Health Administration (U.S. Department of Labor, 1991) and the Centers for Disease Control and Prevention (CDC, 1987). These estimates are for an occupational health specialist's office located in a metropolitan area of the West Coast and include overhead, salaries, benefits, computer support, and confidential storage and maintenance of medical records for the exposed employee.

[†]Costs of office visit; primary care provider is nurse practitioner working under physician-approved protocol.

[‡]Cost for an HIV antibody test.

[§]Cost for an HIV antibody test ($50) plus laboratory costs for monitoring AZT use according to CDC (1990) protocol.

[¶]Estimated costs for the drug administered for 4 to 6 weeks, depending on protocol followed.

Note. AZT = azidothymidine.

tested for other reasons (e.g., for blood donation). By April 1990, 27 documented seroconversions had been reported in the medical literature or to the CDC, including the 6 seroconversions in the 14 studies (Beekmann et al., 1990). When the routes of exposure were evaluated, 22 of 27 were found to have resulted from percutaneous exposures (punctures or cuts). Mucous membrane or cutaneous exposures were implicated in the 5 remaining cases. Almost all of the cases (25 of 27) were associated with blood or a body fluid containing visible blood; the other cases were in laboratory workers exposed to concentrated virus. In many of these cases, it is difficult to be certain that the only exposure is an occupational one. In addition, because there are many workers' compensation issues, including financial compensation, that are associated with attribution of an illness or injury to the workplace, case reports must be evaluated with caution.

Postexposure management for HIV exposures is variable, largely because of the controversy about whether or not azidothymidine (AZT), zidovudine, or retrovir should be offered as a prophylaxis. Although it is not yet clear whether AZT administration will prevent HIV infection in HCWs, it is clear that if it is to be of any value, it must be initiated as soon as possible after the exposure event.

Guidelines for administration of AZT have been published by the CDC (1990). Table 67-2 presents estimated costs for postexposure management of exposures to HIV with and without the costs of AZT. Because AZT administration requires laboratory testing at several intervals, as well as purchase of the drug itself, the overall postexposure costs with AZT are considerably higher than those without AZT.

It is also important to realize that even if engineering and work practice controls result in a reduction in the number of needle puncture injuries, it is unlikely that the personnel required to run programs for employee health, hospital epidemiology, and postexposure follow-up can be eliminated from the payroll. The major costs for these programs are personnel costs (salaries and benefits). Accordingly, the principal direct cost savings from reducing the numbers of puncture injuries will be costs of laboratory tests and drugs (e.g., AZT). A benefit of fewer injuries to employee health programs is that if fewer HCWs need to be seen for postexposure management, the time saved can be used by program personnel to provide health promotion and disease prevention services and perform other activities usually relegated to less important time slots than acute and follow-up management of injuries. In other words, if there are fewer injuries to care for, the program manager might be able to get "caught up" on his or her other responsibilities!

USING DATA TO REDUCE INJURY-EXPOSURE RISKS

What kind of a price tag does an agency put on disease prevention when measured against the bottom line? One consideration is regulatory requirements. That is, the agency has no choice but to comply with the OSHA bloodborne pathogens standard (U.S. Department of Labor, 1991). Other federal agencies, such as the Food and Drug Administration and the CDC, can also have considerable influence on decisions made by health care agencies. Requirements for accreditation by the Joint Commission on Accreditation of Healthcare Organizations, as well as state licensing and certification requirements, are also influential factors.

OSHA has given some latitude in choices of engineering controls, work practice controls, and personal protective equipment. Clearly, if the best risk reduction strategies are provided by engineering controls, then emphasis should be placed on selection and evaluation of newly designed products intended to reduce percutaneous injury risks. We and others have used our own data to direct selection of risk reduction products. By analyzing our puncture injury-exposure data for 1989 to 1990, we determined that many of our injuries were associated with intravenous access devices. In 1990 to 1991, we obtained information on the devices available and conducted product trial evaluations that led to the selection of several risk reduction devices. During late 1991 to early 1992, these devices were purchased, training was provided, and supplies were made available throughout the facility. In addition, a major training program in the OSHA bloodborne pathogens standard was initiated in early 1992 that is repeated annually. The effects of these risk reduction strategies were seen in 1992 in a reduction of reported puncture injuries-exposures. These injury-exposure data are collected continuously and will be analyzed carefully to direct our risk reduction interventions in the future. This is an important example of continuous quality improvement to make the health care workplace a safer one for HCWs.

REFERENCES

Alter, M.J., Hadler, S.C., Margolis, H.S., Alexander, W.J., Hu, P.Y., Judson, F.N., Mares, A., Miller, J.K., & Moyer, L.A. (1990). The changing epidemiology of hepatitis B in the United States: Need for alternative vaccination strategies. *Journal of the American Medical Association, 263* (9), 1218-1222.

Anonymous. (1984, December). Needlestick transmission of HTLV-III from a patient infected in Africa. *Lancet, 2* (8416), 1376-1377.

Beekmann, S.E., Fahey, B.J., Gerberding, J.L., & Henderson, D.K. (1990). Risky business: Using necessarily imprecise casualty counts to estimate occupational risks for HIV-1 infection. *Infection Control and Hospital Epidemiology, 11,* 371-379.

Birnbaum, D., Schulzer, M., Mathias, R.G. , Kelley, M., & Chow, A.W. (1990). Adoption of guidelines for universal precautions and body substance isolation in Canadian acute-care hospitals. *Infection Control and Hospital Epidemiology, 11,* 465-472.

Centers for Disease Control. (1970). *Isolation techniques for use in hospitals.* Atlanta: Author.

Centers for Disease Control. (1975). *Isolation techniques for use in hospitals* (2nd ed.). Atlanta: Author.

Centers for Disease Control. (1983). Guideline for isolation precautions in hospitals. *Infection Control, 4,* 245-325.

Centers for Disease Control. (1985). Recommendations for protection against viral hepatitis. *Morbidity and Mortality Weekly Report, 34,* 313-335.

Centers for Disease Control. (1987). Recommendations for prevention of HIV transmission in health-care settings. *Morbidity and Mortality Weekly Report, 36* (Suppl. 2S), 3S-18S.

Centers for Disease Control. (1988). Update: Universal precautions for prevention of transmission of human immunodeficiency virus, hepatitis B virus, and other bloodborne pathogens in health-care settings. *Morbidity and Mortality Weekly Report, 37,* 378-388.

Centers for Disease Control. (1990). Public Health Service statement on management of occupational exposure to human immunodeficiency virus, including considerations regarding zidovudine postexposure use. *Morbidity and Mortality Weekly Report, 39* (Suppl. RR-1), 1-14.

Doebbeling, B.N., & Wenzel, R.P. (1990). The direct costs of universal precautions in a teaching hospital. *Journal of the American Medical Association, 264,* 2083-2087.

Gerberding, J.L., & Henderson, D.K. (1987). Design of rational infection control policies for human immunodeficiency virus infection. *Journal of Infectious Diseases, 156,* 861-864.

Jackson, M.M. (1989). Implementing universal body substance precautions. *Occupational Medicine: State of the Art Reviews, 4* (Special issue), 39-44.

Jackson, M.M., & Lynch, P. (1984). Infection control: Too much or too little? *American Journal of Nursing, 84,* 208-210.

Jackson, M.M., & Lynch, P. (1991). An attempt to make an issue less murky: A comparison of four systems for infection precautions. *Infection Control and Hospital Epidemiology, 12,* 448-450.

Jackson, M.M., Lynch, P., McPherson, D.C., Cummings, M.J., & Greenawalt, N.C. (1987). Why not treat all body substances as infectious? *American Journal of Nursing, 87,* 1137-1139.

Jackson, M.M., & Pugliese, G. (1992). Regulations: The OSHA bloodborne pathogens standard. *Today's O.R. Nurse, 14,* 11-16.

Lee, J.J., Marvin, J.A., Heimbach, D.M., Grube, B.J., & Engrav, L.H. (1990). Infection control in a burn center. *Journal of Burn Care and Rehabilitation, 11,* 575-580.

Lynch, P., Cummings, M.J., Roberts, P.L., Herriott, M.J., Yates, B., & Stamm, W.E. (1990). Implementing and evaluating a system of generic infection precautions: Body substance isolation. *American Journal of Infection Control, 18,* 1-12.

Lynch, P., Jackson, M.M., Cummings, M.J., & Stamm, W.E. (1987). Rethinking the role of isolation practices in the prevention of nosocomial infections. *Annals of Internal Medicine, 107,* 243-246.

McPherson, D.C., & Jackson, M.M. (1987). Isolation precautions for a changing environment . . . a new approach. *Journal of Healthcare Material Management, 5,* 28-32.

McPherson, D.C., Jackson, M.M., & Rogers, J.C. (1988). Evaluating the cost of the body substance isolation system. *Journal of Healthcare Material Management, 6,* 20-28.

Stock, S.R., Gafni, A., & Bloch, R.F. (1990). Universal precautions to prevent HIV transmission to health care workers: An economic analysis. *Canadian Medical Association Journal, 142,* 937-946.

Troya, S.H., Jackson, M.M., Lovrich-Kerr, M., & McPherson, D.C. (1991). A survey of nurses' knowledge, opinions, and reported uses of the body substance isolation system. *American Journal of Infection Control, 19,* 268-276.

U.S. Department of Labor, Occupational Safety and Health Administration. (1991). Occupational exposure to bloodborne pathogens: Final rule, 29 CFR Part 1910:1030. *Federal Register, 56,* 64003-64182.

This chapter was written originally for the 4th edition of this book, published in 1994. It reflects information current through 1993. However, since 1995, two important articles have been published that readers will find pertinent to the topic; unfortunately, publishing deadlines precluded revising the chapter to incorporate them:

Centers for Disease Control and Prevention: Guideline for isolation precautions in hospitals. AJIC Am J Infect Control 1996;24:24-52.

Centers for Disease Control and Prevention: Update: Provisional Public Health Service recommendations for chemoprophylaxis after occupational exposure to HIV. MMWR 1996;45:468-472.

Financing health care costs in Australia

JENNIFER MARIA ANN BICHEL

As the 20th century draws to a close, Australia faces the real possibility of major reform in two areas—sovereignty and health care delivery. One would imagine that the former task would be the more difficult in terms of complexity and consensus; however, this is not the case. The current government appears strongly committed to replacing the hereditary office of the monarchy with a republican head of state by the year 2001, a century after the enactment of The Constitution of the Commonwealth. The Commonwealth Constitution can only be amended by the people, and as such, ultimate sovereignty rests with the public. Because Australia is already regarded by some as a "crowned republic," the only constitutional change required to make the nation completely republican is to remove the monarch (Republic Advisory Committee, 1993). Altering Australia's health care system is another matter entirely, given its history of health care delivery, particularly in relation to health insurance and health care financing. With Australia's present health care system deeply rooted in social justice ideals, it is reasonable to purport that our system and the model practiced in the United States have relatively little in common. The one similarity between the systems of these countries is that health insurance and health care financing have been recurring themes within the political arena for nearly half a century. In fact, these two concepts have been an issue in every Australian federal election since 1969 (Palmer & Short, 1994).

HISTORICAL INFLUENCE

To ease the pressures on the overcrowded jails in the United Kingdom, Australia was established as a penal colony, so it comes as no surprise that we readily accepted many of the British institutions. Australia adopted the British language, legal and parliamentary systems, religious philosophies, education and health systems, and most other forms of British culture. By the late 19th century as the nation began to develop, characteristics unique to Australians began to emerge. One such characteristic that cannot be overemphasized when addressing the underpinnings of the nation's social fabric is the concept of "mateship." This ideology seems to have "developed out of the cumulative experience of convicts, bushrangers and gold diggers, and it evolved into some sort of egalitarian sentiment among outback workers" (Sax, 1984, p. 31). In addition to this concept, the beginning of this century witnessed a humanitarian movement within Australia, and a growing social conscience to provide for those less fortunate. By 1930, Australians expected the government to take responsibility for the social welfare and economic planning of its population, "and to be seen 'doing things for people'" (Sax, 1984, p. 35).

Trying to establish a health care system that pleased both the users of the service and the health professionals who provided the care, but did not place excessive pressure on government expenditure, has proved to be a difficult task. Two attempts to legislate for national health insurance in the early 1900s failed, mostly due to fierce opposition by the medical profession who were advised by their British counterparts to avoid any system remotely linked to nationalized medicine. Following two Royal Commissions in the 1930s addressing national insurance and health, the emotive consequences of reorganizing health care became apparent. By 1950, Australia had two major political parties, the Labor Party and the Liberal-National Coalition Party, and both had significantly different ideologies on health financing. Their fundamental disagreement concerning the cost burden on the users of health services still exists today and has led to a certain amount of instability in relation to the delivery of health care.

The Labor Party was formed as the political arm of the trade union movement, although its original working class support later broadened to include middle class professionals and other white collar workers. The party's basic ideology suggests that societal institutions promote injustices and inequality, and it is the government's responsibility to redress them for the benefit of the people (Australian Labor Party, 1991). Health care, therefore, is viewed as a basic human right, and all persons ought to have access to health care regardless of their capacity to pay. Their constant support for national health insurance and equitable financing arrangements has antagonized the medical profession to the point that any proposed policy changes to health care are automatically viewed with suspicion.

Support for the Liberal-National Coalition Party stems predominantly from the middle class, although sections of the working class have gradually begun to align themselves with the party. The Coalition emphasizes individual strengths, aspirations, and creativity (Liberal Party of Australia, 1982) and focuses more on free enterprise and competition. Health is viewed as an individual responsibility for which the burden of cost should fall on the user. While the Labor Party believes that the government ought to participate actively in the provision of social goods, the Coalition's philosophy is to promote professional autonomy, reduce the role of government, and consequently reduce government expenditure (Duckett, 1992). As a result of these opposing ideologies, Australians experienced a puzzling assortment of financial arrangements for health care until the introduction of Medicare in 1984. Every 3 years, health professionals await the election outcome, wondering whether a new infrastructure will be proposed. The only reason Australians have enjoyed the recent phase of permanence in health care financing is the continuation in office of Labor governments for the past 11 years.

THE MEDICARE PROGRAM

Medicare, Australia's system of national health insurance, came into operation in early 1984, and has remained relatively unchanged in its structure and function. Under the authority of the Health Insurance Act, the Health Insurance Commission administers the Medicare program, the Medical Benefits Scheme, and the Pharmaceutical Benefits Scheme. The five principles underpinning Medicare are universality, access, equity, efficiency, and simplicity (Department of Health, Housing, and Community Services [DHHCS], 1992). All residents of Australia are eligible for benefits and are issued a Medicare card that identifies each person by name and registered Medicare number. The program is self-funded through taxation—originally 1% but currently a 1.5% levy on personal taxable income. However, persons deemed to be economically disadvantaged and those earning low incomes ($AUS12,689 per year in the 1993-94 financial period, equivalent to $US9,235 in June 1994) are exempt from the levy. Medicare provides a safety net for multiple users of the system and is adjusted each year in accordance with the Consumer Price Index. The program consists of two arms—access to free inpatient and outpatient treatment in public hospitals and the provision of benefits for the cost of private medical services. Both outpatient and emergency treatment as well as inpatient treatment and accommodation in a shared ward are provided without charge in any Australian public hospital when the services are provided by a doctor appointed by the hospital. The hospital side of Medicare is funded through block grants to the six states and two territories. Services to veterans, workers' compensation patients, automobile third-party insurance cases, and industrial medical services are funded separately, and thus are excluded from the program's statistical data (Deeble, 1991).

Individuals who do not wish to use the public hospital services can seek the services of a private medical practitioner of their choice and will receive a benefit of 85% of the schedule fees. A schedule of fees has been established by the Health Insurance Commission, but doctors, who still operate on a fee-for-service basis, are not required to adhere to this schedule and as such can charge in excess of the schedule. Doctors are assigned a unique provider number and can either bill the patient or bill the Health Insurance Commission directly. In the former arrangement, the patient is entitled to seek reimbursement from Medicare for 85% of the scheduled fee and is responsible for the remaining 15% and any additional monies resulting from the doctor charging in excess of the schedule. If the doctor chooses the latter arrangement, commonly referred to as "bulk billing," he or she accepts the 85% of the schedule fee as total payment without any financial contribution by the patient. In the 1993-94 period, 68.1% of all medical services were bulk billed (Commonwealth Department of Human Services and Health [CDHSH], 1995). For the purposes of Medicare, a "medical service" can be either a diagnostic procedure (such as pathology and radiology) or a treatment visit ordered by a person assigned a provider number, which, under the current system, encompasses mostly medical practitioners.

Medicare also provides benefits of 75% of the schedule fee for medical services encountered in public or private hospitals as a private patient, but the gap is insurable through membership to a private health insurance fund. Private health insurance is currently available through more than 70 organizations in Australia (Copell, 1994), offering ancillary benefits only, hospital benefits only, or a combination of the two. Hospital insurance essentially competes with Medicare-funded public services by providing benefits for private hospital accommodation, while ancillary insurance provides reimbursement for services not funded under Medicare, such as private dentistry, physiotherapy, chiropractic, and appliances, and for prescribed medicines not covered by the pharmaceutical benefits. All private health insurance must be in accord with the community rating principle—that is, everyone must pay the same premium rate, regardless of age, sex, family size, or medical condition, with the only regulation being that a single person pays half of the family rate. All insurance companies have waiting periods, with up to 2 months for general services, 9 months for obstetric services, and 2 years for any preexisting condition. Under the Health Insurance Act, insurance to cover amounts paid in excess of the schedule fees is forbidden, apart from the gap for hospitalized private patients.

MEDICARE ACCORDING TO THE USERS

To the average Australian, Medicare means guaranteed access and free service at the point of delivery in public hospitals as well as financial assistance for medical services provided by private medical practitioners. Opinion polls conducted 4 years after its introduction indicate that close to 70% of the population favors Medicare (Palmer & Short, 1994). However, these results need to be interpreted in light of how health care was organized in the decade prior to Medicare. Health insurance legislation proposed by the Whitlam Labor government was initially rejected in 1973 and finally accepted in 1975 amid fierce and overt opposition by the Australian Medical Association (AMA). Medicare's predecessor, Medibank, was established in July 1975. However, the government was dismissed in November of the same year, and the Coalition caretaker government returned to office. Concerned with rising health care costs and a rapidly rising federal expenditure, the Fraser government slowly began to dismantle the national health insurance scheme. Prior to its demise, Australians were subjected to no fewer than five major changes to its infrastructure, until it ceased to exist in September 1981 when Australia returned to voluntary health insurance. No version of Medibank was in existence long enough for its intended benefits to be realized. Prior to the 1984 election, national health insurance was again a major part of the Labor Party platform, and once again Australians found their financing arrangements for health care altered.

This decade of instability in terms of health care arrangements has almost certainly had an effect on the level of understanding of health services by most of the population, with studies conducted in 1991 revealing significant confusion throughout society about whether certain health services are covered under Medicare or private health insurance and a poor knowledge about the real costs of private health insurance and private hospital care (Wilcox, 1991). There has been a steady decline in private insurance membership since the introduction of Medicare (38.4% in 1993 compared with 50% in 1982) (Australian Institute of Health and Welfare [AIHW], 1994), with the greatest variation occurring across income groups, indicating that income rather than age or family type is a more important predictor of private health insurance status (Willcox, 1991). Reasons for procuring private health insurance include coverage of ancillary services, individual choice of doctor and hospital, avoidance of excessive costs, and the ability to receive immediate attention for hospital care, while the major reason for not insuring is cost (Willcox, 1991). The highest incidence of private health insurance is found in the 35- to 54-year age group, and the lowest is in the under 25-year age category (Willcox, 1991).

Additional studies carried out in 1991 indicate that most Australian households have relatively few out-of-pocket expenses for health and medical care, and low-income households are more likely to spend nothing at all (McClelland, 1991b). In the 1992-93 period, 12% of those enrolled in Medicare used no services, 50% used fewer than six services, 25% used 13 or more services, and 8% used more than 25 services (CDHSH, 1995). The 75-year and over group uses the greatest number of services by both sexes, and the 10- to 14-year group accounts for the least (CDHSH, 1995). Excluding the 0- to 4-year age group, females account for more services than males in all age categories, with females using twice as many services than males in both the 20- to 24-year and 25- to 34-year age groups (CDHSH, 1995). The value of benefits in the 1993-94 period accounted for nearly $AUS5.4 million ($US3.9 million in June 1994), representing $AUS301.36 ($US219.33 in June 1994) in benefits per capita, consistent with an average of 10.1 services per capita (CDHSH, 1995).

MEDICARE ACCORDING TO THE MEDICAL PROFESSION

The introduction of Medicare did not receive as emotive a response by medical practitioners as did its predecessor (Medibank), but the opposition to it focused once again on the concept of moral hazard. Medical opponents asserted that free care at the point of delivery would result in an increase in the number of hospital admissions, an increase in the rate of use of medical services, overservicing, longer waiting lists in public hospitals, and an overall increase in health care expenditure. In addition to these objections, doctors were convinced that Medicare would threaten their private practice in public hospitals, and the seeds of suspicion regarding removal of the fee-for-service structure were once again planted.

The assumption that hospital admissions would rise was difficult to accept, given that hospitalization is controlled by the provider of the service and not the user and that the economic model of supply and demand does not appear to be totally appropriate to health care. In fact, the rate of usage of hospital beds steadily declined during Medibank's existence, and occupied bed days have continued to decrease following Medicare's inception (Commonwealth Department of Health, 1987; CDHHCS, 1992). Although no evidence exists to support the predicted increase in demand for beds, one must take into account the backdrop of events during that time. In the 7 years following Medicare's introduction, Australia experienced a decline in the ratio of private to public patients in public hospitals, a major nursing shortage, and decreases in the supply of beds as a result of the nursing shortage and hospital rationalization policies (Palmer & Short, 1994). The situation was further compounded in Australia's most populated state, New South Wales, by a demonstration of solidarity among doctors against the Labor government in 1985. Fearful that sections of the Medicare legislation would limit their scope for private practice in public hospitals, procedural specialists (led by the orthopedic surgeons) resigned their public hospital appointments and withdrew all but emergency services. Four years later, a third of the orthopedic surgeons still had not returned to the public system (Sax, 1990).

The introduction of Medicare, however, was associated with a small increase in the average use of health care services per person, but the rate of increase has subsequently slowed (Prager, 1995). In the first 6 years of the Medicare program, medical service use per person increased by 23%, with 25% of the increase originating from a higher proportion of the population using the services and the remaining 75% resulting from more services per user (Deeble, 1991). This period has also witnessed an increase in the number of doctors with private practice billing rights, indicating a 15.4% increase relative to the population (Deeble, 1991). Minimal situations of overservicing via direct billing abuse were evidenced and were mostly limited to the use of pathology and radiology services (Deeble, 1991).

Access to hospital services and the prioritizing of the need for these services are controlled by a waiting list system. However, waiting times have been difficult to assess in Australia due to a lack of comparable data between states. Available data in the first 6 years of Medicare indicate that orthopedic surgery, ophthalmology, ear/nose/throat, urology, and plastic surgery demonstrated the longest waiting times (National Health Strategy [NHS], 1991), whereas in 1993 the categories remain the same except for the deletion of ophthalmologic surgery and the inclusion of vascular surgery (AIHW, 1994). Statistics available in 1994 indicated a national clearance time for elective surgery of 2.3 months, with the majority of people receiving elective surgery within 3 months and only a small percentage waiting in excess of 12 months (CDHSH, 1995). The recent federal budget has allocated funds for the publication of national waiting list data and the development of nationally consistent urgency ratings for the prioritization of procedures according to clinical need.

Lastly, an increase in health expenditures as a result of Medicare did not happen, with health expenditure as a percentage of gross domestic product (GDP) remaining fairly constant in the immediate pre- and post-Medicare periods (AIHW, 1992). Total real health expenditure as a proportion of the GDP was 6.4% in 1970-71; rose to 7.6% following the introduction of Medibank; and remained constant until 1982-83, when it increased 0.2% as a result of the recession (AIH, 1988). Following the introduction of Medicare, health expenditure has increased at a rate roughly consistent with the economy as a whole, and is currently 8.5% of GDP, representing AUS$34.3 billion ($US24.5 billion in June 1995) (AIHW, 1994).

MEDICARE ACCORDING TO THE GOVERNMENT

Greater simplicity of health services has undoubtedly been achieved through the administration of services by a single government authority, and has resulted in reduced overhead due to economies of scale and a useful tracking system to detect fraud and overservicing. The current government, however, is still concerned with the health expenditure pressures and attributes these pressures to doctors, in terms of the fee-for-service payment structure, and hospitals in relation to capped budgets that do not provide incentives to improve service efficiency (Organisation for Economic Cooperation and Development [OECD], 1995). Direct billing was initially seen as a way of controlling fees charged by doctors, but this has not been totally successful in part as a result of doctors' nonadherence to the schedule fees. In the current climate, any attempts to erode the fee-for-service system will only result in industrial action by the medical profession, and as such, the government has focused on the hospital side of the program.

In 1993, Australia had 1,099 hospitals (including public, private, and day hospital facilities), representing 77,669 hospital beds and a ratio of 4.4 beds for every 1,000 people (CDHSH, 1995). Health expenditure is funded from three sources—commonwealth government (44%), state and local governments (24%), and the private sector (32%) (AIHW, 1994). The majority of recurrent health expenditure is directed toward institutional care (51%) and medical services (19%), while administration accounts for 3.4% and research 1.5% (AIHW, 1994). In comparison with other OECD countries, Australia's health expenditure rates favorably; however, in the current economic climate we must question whether this is in fact a sound investment. Public hospitals in particular have come under scrutiny for their lack of linking expenditure to actual service outputs.

Medicare agreements between the commonwealth and the states during 1988 and 1993 allocated funds for casemix-related research and encouraged the adoption of a case payment system. The Australian National Diagnostic-Related Groups (AN-DRG) system was established in 1992, and is an adaption of the U.S. classifications. Currently there are 527 AN-DRGs, which are grouped into 25 major diagnostic categories (CDHSH, 1995); and it is anticipated that this type of hospital reimbursement will focus on output of services and result in increased productive and allocative efficiency within hospitals. An overall framework for the introduction of case payment has not been decided on, and each state is continuing to support its development.

One other major problem that the government must address in relation to Medicare is the significant disparities in health status among some subgroups of the population, and the recent budget has allocated additional monies in an attempt to improve these areas. Despite the fact that Australia is one of the healthiest countries in the world (AIHW, 1994), substantial improvements are needed in the areas of aboriginal health, care of the elderly and rural services, women's health, and preventive services. A longstanding concern for the government has been the fact that aboriginality has been strongly associated with the worst health status in the country (McClelland, 1991a). Aboriginal infant mortality rates are close to three times those for the whole of Australia, and standardized Aboriginal death rates are between two and four times those of the whole of Australian population (NHS, 1992). Major infrastructure changes, from both within and outside of the health system, will be necessary to eliminate the inequities experienced by these population subgroups, particularly in the areas of service coordination and funding allocation.

MEDICARE AND NURSING

Not surprisingly, the largest health profession in Australia is nursing, with the 1991 census indicating that of the 482,609 persons employed in the health industries, 188,640 (39%) were nurses (AIHW, 1994). Prior to 1984, the profession only gained significant political, medical, or media attention through severe nursing shortages, which invariably resulted in public hospital bed closures and a reduction in specialty medical services such as availability of operating rooms. In response to numerous reports from expert committees that investigated the increasing dissatisfaction with the nursing profession, and in particular the inherent problems of hospital-based educational preparation of general nurses, the federal government announced its support for the full transfer of nurse education into the higher education sector. This process commenced in 1985 and was fully completed 8 years later, with all nurses now gaining registration only following successful completion of a 3-year bachelor of nursing university degree. Not all sectors of the health industry, nor indeed the community sector, supported this transfer, and it caused major state and federal budgetary shifts in both the health and education sectors.

Although the majority of nurses are salaried employees, independent practitioner services are currently emerging, and the question of third-party direct reimbursement is again being raised. As yet, nurses have not been successful in obtaining provider numbers from the Health Insurance Commission, although not from lack of trying. Internal factors (i.e., changes to the educational preparation of nurses, the introduction of career structures in all states, and the trend toward competency-based practice) and external factors (i.e., increasing difficulty in recruiting and retaining medical personnel in rural and remote areas, the cost burden of medical services in rural and remote areas, and the current emphasis by government authorities on cost-effectiveness and cost efficiency) have augmented support within the nursing profession for the development of the nurse practitioner role. While key health service stakeholders are more receptive to examining alternative service strategies, resistance is still being displayed by some sectors of the health care industry in relation to extending the role of nurses. Nurses, however, are continuing to pursue this path, and it is hoped that this development will soon be realized. The profession eagerly awaits the recommendations from the Public Health Nurse Practitioner Trial, currently being conducted by the New South Wales State Health Authority.

THE FUTURE OF MEDICARE

The next federal election in Australia is scheduled for 1996, and already the issues of health insurance and health care financing have emerged, with the government and the medical profession engaged in intense political conflict. Lengthy waiting lists for elective surgery, evidence of "queue jumping" by private patients to receive more immediate treatment than public patients, and preliminary findings from the Quality in Australian Health Care Study have captured media attention. National results extrapolated from the study indicate that approximately 1% of all hospital admissions experience a preventable adverse event that leads to some degree of permanent disability, and 0.5% of hospital admissions die (Taskforce on Quality in Australian Health Care, 1995).

The government has also uncovered the practice of "double dipping," whereby states are privatizing public hospital outpatient clinics and placing pressure on doctors to bulk bill these services in an attempt to shift state costs to the commonwealth government. Because the Health Insurance Act does not permit reimbursement for public hospital services on an individual basis under the Medical Benefits Scheme, the commonwealth is moving to prosecute the doctors who have become the pawns in this cost-shifting battle.

Ironically, Australia now finds itself in a situation where the Coalition Party is the least likely of the two parties to make major changes to the system. Prior to the last election, the Coalition Party announced their desire to retain Medicare, albeit with increased private sector involvement, rather than repeating history and dismantling the scheme. Their health policy statement indicated that they planned to increase private health insurance membership through a taxation incentive system and to extend the availability of gap insurance (Liberal Party of Australia, 1991). While this proposal was eagerly supported by contributors to private insurance, who have complained for some time about being doubly charged (private insurance contributions plus the taxation levy), the gap insurance was associated with individual copayments. Australians have been down that road before in the early 1990s, when the Labor government initially proposed the issue of consumer copayments and then rejected it on the basis that its importance was overstated and unlikely to solve any existing problems (Richardson, 1991). Taxation rebates have also been trialed in the past under the Fraser Coalition government, but were quickly abandoned once it was realized that they severely disadvantaged the lower-income earner and created gross inequities between the lower- and higher-income groups. Consistent with Coalition ideology, bulk billing was also earmarked for reform, in that it would only be offered to pensioners and the economically disadvantaged. Their current platform does not appear to have deviated far from the previous health policy, and it is difficult to foresee a reduction in health care expenditure based on their modifications to the existing scheme. The Coalition Party has been criticized in the past for its lack of initiative when proposing health policy, and it seems to be forever searching for alternative schemes that fail to take account of the popularity of Medicare within the community and focus more on encouraging cooperation from the medical profession and higher-income groups.

Although the Labor Party has mooted fairly radical changes to the system, it has been plagued by a lack of consistency in retaining the same minister in the health portfolio. Prior to his resignation in 1994, Senator Richardson laid the groundwork for the introduction of case payment and the Private Health Insurance Bill following concerns that private health insurance membership was falling below 40%. This is an important issue for the Labor government, as the taxation levy can only support the system if 40% of the community holds private coverage, and the population is already voicing its dissent about the recent trend by the government to increase the levy in each annual budget. The Private Health Insurance Bill introduces the concept of the purchaser-provider split and creates insurance companies as a third party in health care. Dr. Carmen Lawrence, the current Federal Health Minister, unsuccessfully attempted to rush the Bill through parliament earlier this year. The medical profession again responded quickly to this move, believing that

Australia will end up with the worst features of both the American and British systems (AMA, 1995). The Victorian branch of the AMA believes that the proposed reform will lead to a further reduction in private health insurance membership and that the private health system will collapse, with the hospitals, insurance funds, and themselves being blamed for the inevitable deterioration in medical standards (Prager, 1995). The AMA is prepared to veto the proposal and will attempt to gain support from the community who, according to Mackay (1995, p. 355), "still accept the medical profession as the dominant authority in health care, and the AMA as its collective voice."

The year 1996 will prove to be very interesting for the average Australian. The groundwork for becoming a republic is likely to commence, and taking into account the popular opinion at present, it is highly probable that this aim will be achieved with minimal bloodshed by both politicians and voters. The same cannot be said for health care reforms. Only time will tell whether the nation moves to a system more like that of the American model. One thing is assured, however: The next federal election is likely to be won or lost by the party that presents the health portfolio in the best light to the taxpayers and the providers of the service—and no doubt casualties will fall during the pre-election period. So what else is new in the land down under?

REFERENCES

Australian Institute of Health. (1988). *Australian health expenditure: 1970-71 to 1984-85.* Canberra: Australian Government Printing Service.

Australian Institute of Health and Welfare. (1992). *Australia's health 1992: The Third Biennial Health Report of the Australian Institute of Health and Welfare.* Canberra: Australian Government Printing Service.

Australian Institute of Health and Welfare. (1994). *Australia's health 1994: The Fourth Biennial Health Report of the Australian Institute of Health and Welfare.* Canberra: Australian Government Printing Service.

Australian Labor Party. (1991). *Platform, resolutions and rules.* Barton: Author.

Australian Medical Association. (1995). *Doctors meat-in-the-sandwich in cost shifting war.* Canberra: Author. [News release]

Commonwealth Department of Health. (1987). *Health statistical supplement 1986-87.* Canberra: Australian Government Printing Service.

Commonwealth Department of Human Services and Health. (1995). *Budget 1995-1996.* Canberra: Australian Government Printing Service.

Commonwealth Department of Human Services and Health. (1995). *Department of Human Services and Health: Statistical overview 1993-94.* Canberra: Australian Government Printing Service.

Commonwealth Department of Health, Housing & Community Services. (1992). *Medicare: So much stronger now—Budget 1992-3.* Canberra: Australian Government Printing Service.

Commonwealth Department of Health, Housing and Community Services. (1992). *Annual Report 91-92: Statistical supplement.* Canberra: Australian Government Printing Service.

Copell, B. (1994). *Australia in facts and figures.* Ringwood, Victoria: Penguin.

Deeble, J. (1991). *Medical services through medicare, background Paper No. 2.* Melbourne: National Health Strategy.

Duckett, S.J. (1992). Financing of health care. In Gardner, H. (Ed.), *Health policy: Development, implementation and evaluation in Australia* (pp. 137-161). Melbourne: Churchill Livingstone.

Liberal Party of Australia. (1991). *Fightback! It's your Australia: The way to rebuild and reward Australia.* Canberra: Liberal and National Parties.

Liberal Party of Australia. (1982, May). *Federal Platform.* Canberra: Author.

Mackay, D. (1995). Politics of reaction. In Gardner, H. (Ed.), *The politics of health: An Australian experience* (2nd ed., pp. 344-370). Melbourne: Churchill Livingstone.

McClelland, A. (1991a). *In fair health? Equity and the health service, background paper No. 3.* Melbourne: National Health Strategy.

McClelland, A. (1991b). *Spending on health: The distribution of direct payments for health and medical services, background paper No. 7.* Melbourne: National Health Strategy.

National Health Strategy. (1991). *Hospital services in Australia: Access and financing, issues paper No. 2.* Melbourne: National Health Strategy.

National Health Strategy. (1992). *Enough to make you sick: How income and environment affect health, research paper No. 1.* Melbourne: National Health Strategy.

Organisation for Economic Cooperation and Development. (1995). *OECD economic surveys 1994-95 Australia.* Paris: Author.

Palmer, G.P., & Short, S.D. (1994). *Health care & public policy: An Australian analysis.* Melbourne: MacMillian Education Australia Pty Ltd.

Prager, S. (1995). *She won't be right, mate: Australian Medical Association Victorian Branch News, May.* Melbourne. [Media release]

Republic Advisory Committee. (1993). *An Australian republic: The options—the report.* Canberra: Australian Government Printing Service.

Richardson, J. (1991). *The effects of consumer copayments in medical care, background paper no. 5.* Melbourne: National Health Strategy.

Sax, S. (1984). *A strife of interests: Politics and policies in Australian health services* (pp. 31-35). Sydney: Allen & Unwin.

Sax, S. (1990). *Health care choices and the public purse.* Sydney: Allen & Unwin.

Taskforce on Quality in Australian Health Care. (1995). *Quality in Australian health care: Preliminary findings.* Canberra: Australian Government Printing Service.

Willcox, S. (1991). *A healthy risk? Use of private insurance, background paper no. 4.* Melbourne: National Health Strategy.

Section Nine

ROLE TRANSITIONS

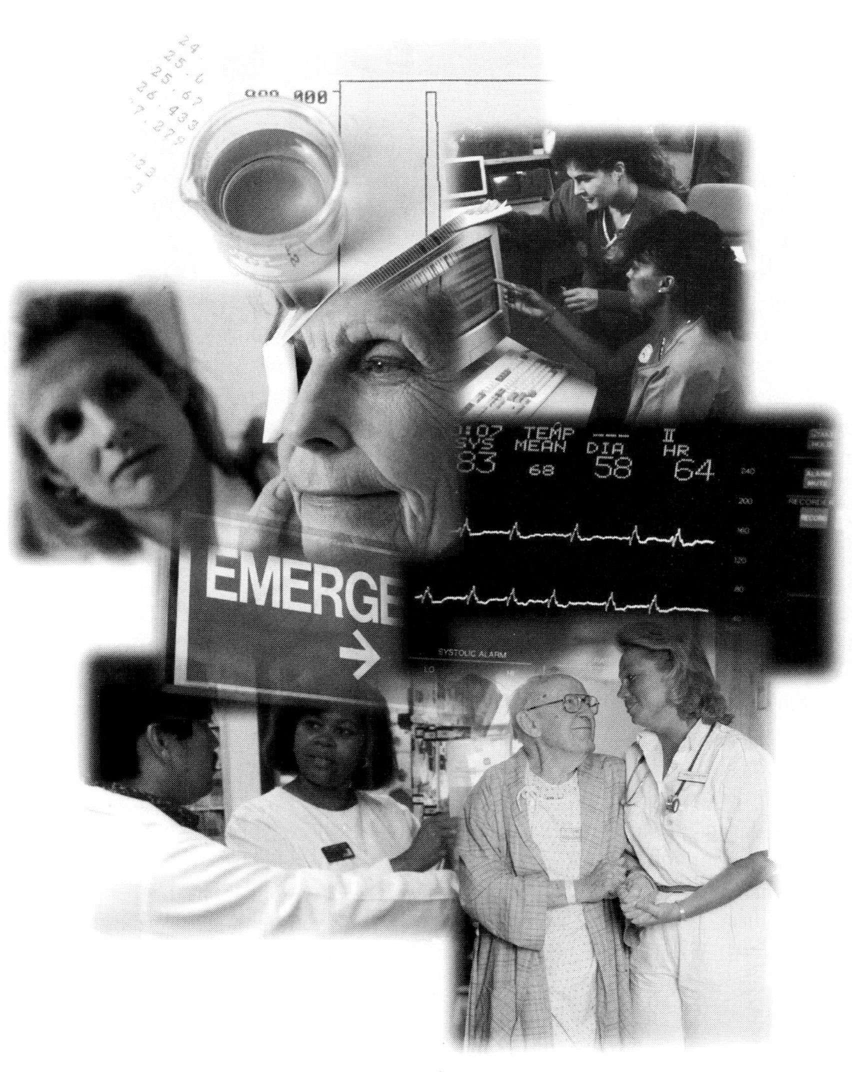

OVERVIEW

Colleagues and conflict

JOANNE COMI McCLOSKEY, HELEN KENNEDY GRACE

The past few years have introduced many new and some unwelcome changes in nursing. Old roles are evolving and new roles are emerging. These roles involve both collaboration and conflict—two topics that are explored in some detail in this section.

The debate chapter for the section is about collaboration between nurses and physicians. Nurse leaders have long desired more collaborative roles and relationships with physicians, but do these exist? Baggs begins her assessment of the situation by noting that the terminology of collaborative practice has different meanings in medicine and nursing. Most of the writing related to collaborative practice has been done by nurses. Loss of power by physicians and gain of power by nurses is a threat to traditional medical practice. Although collaborative practice was advanced through the National Joint Practice Commission some 20 years ago, the guidelines developed then are not implemented to any marked degree in practice settings today. Despite evidence that collaborative practice results in improved patient outcomes, an astoundingly low percentage of physicians (14%) and an even lower percentage of nurses (7%) report using collaborative problem solving in clinical settings. Obstacles to collaborative practice include traditional communication patterns, decision-making prerogatives of physicians, and a reluctance on the part of nurses to accept greater responsibility for decision making. Changes in educational programs to promote collaborative learning and changes within practice settings to facilitate collaborative problem solving are beginning to emerge but, as Baggs concludes, "collaboration is not the usual mode of practice."

The changing roles of nurses reflect the changing roles of women in society. In the first viewpoint chapter, Chinn explains that because most nurses are women and because nursing's role of caring for the sick has been assigned to women worldwide, feminism and nursing are inextricably connected. Chinn structures her chapter around a statement by Nightingale's: "Passion, intellect, moral activity—these three have never been satisfied in women." She discusses these three values both historically and in modern times. She relates passion to feminism as a culture grounded in women's experience and a political stance to right injustices against women; intellect to feminism as a discipline seeking to give voice to women's experience; and moral activity to feminism as an ethic of valuing women and women's experience. Feminism, she says, is not an ideology but a perspective that values diversity. She concludes her chapter with a set of suggested readings and questions to further explore some of the ideas that she has raised. Chinn's chapter is highly recommended for all women and men in nursing who value the contributions of both sexes.

The unique perspective and contribution that nurses bring to patients is labeled by Pike in the next chapter as "nurses' voice." Pike urges nurses to choose colleagueship over silence. She says that nurses' voices have been silenced by both external and internal forces. Among the new external constraints is the restructuring of health care in the United States. These constraints, says Pike, have inflicted wounds on nurses' professional self-esteem. Rather than acting out the appealing victim role and remaining silent and blaming physicians, Pike urges nurses to speak out and to define themselves as colleagues. Taking up this conflict requires, she says, an understanding of the uniqueness of nursing, a breadth of clinical experience, a language to communicate to others the nature of nursing, and an understanding of the constraints imposed on nurses. Using two case studies, she illustrates that nurses' silences have significant implications for patient care as well as for nurses' roles and satisfaction. All nurses should read and act on this thought-provoking and important chapter.

Edwards addresses collaboration between nursing and medicine in the delivery of services to the community. According to Edwards, community-based care requires a shift in power from the hospital and expert professionals to community members. A new collaborative approach to the education of medical and nursing students is necessary in order to embrace the new philosophy. Edwards says that collaboration is about three things: empowerment, relationships, and synergy. She discusses some of the societal, professional, and economic forces that work against collaboration between doctors and nurses. A few successes of effective collaboration are beginning to be documented. In the last part of her chapter, Edwards describes the successful collaborative education model between the Colleges of Nursing and Medicine at East Tennessee State University designed to provide health care to the Blue Ridge Mountain community. A large community need and a grant from the W.K. Kellogg Foundation have enabled community leaders and health professionals to work together to establish a successful multidisciplinary education and practice model. While the setting and driving forces may not be the same as in other parts of the country, the accomplishments of this group are clearly visionary and admirable. In this day of rapid change in health care and the recognized need to refocus our education and services to the community, everyone should read this chapter.

A specific case in which collaboration is needed is between nurse practitioners (NPs) and physician assistants (PAs). Fowkes and Mentink overview the history of PA programs, which began in the 1960s, then discuss the roles of PAs and issues related to their work vis-à-vis NPs and other nurses. In 1994 there were 67 PA programs, with the majority awarding a baccalaureate or a master's degree. PA students typically have previous experience in health care and over half hold a bachelor's degree prior to entry. The PA program of study is similar to the NP program. PAs do not have a separate license and function legally under the supervision of a physician. Fowkes and Mentink point out, however, that they have an "independent role within a dependent practice arrangement." The authors compare PAs and NPs in several areas: functions, educational preparation, and legal, professional, and political differences. Role conflict results from gender issues, competition, and confusion about policies or laws. This is a very informative chapter about a relatively new health care provider that many nurses encounter in their work settings. All nurses who work with PAs will find this chapter helpful.

Turning from practice to education, Copp addresses conflict among faculty. She is not talking about good academic discourse and debate but about interpersonal negative behaviors. She reviews the sources of such conflict. Faculty, she says, are more different than they are alike. Faculty members have different responsibilities and spend their time in different activities. Individuals are rewarded differently; they have different values and personal lives. These differences create conflict. We need to be concerned about faculty conflict because students can be hurt by it. Copp suggests no easy answers but does indicate the solution. Morale, she says, is the key. The way to achieve a better work environment and decrease conflict is through more collegiality. Good colleagues support each other and rejoice in each others' successes. All faculty and potential faculty will benefit from reading this chapter. Furthermore, Copp's advice regarding collegiality is applicable to any setting.

Conflict and its resolution are the subject of Kritek's chapter. Kritek says that conflict is so endemic to nursing that it is often not even recognized as conflict. Her chapter is a personal philosophical reflection on the nature of conflict in nursing and the ways nurses handle conflict. She raises questions such as these: Why is it so pervasive? Do we like our solutions? She suggests some good reading materials and briefly overviews the philosophical viewpoints of Toulmin and Anderson. Nurses, she says, are multilingual at conflict management. We keep multiple perspectives about conflict alive and have good conflict management skills, but we often choose to act as codependents and smooth over or polarize conflicts instead of using the skills we have. Kritek wants nurses to think of themselves as people who can creatively and constructively assist in the resolution of conflicts. According to Kritek, the first step is to recognize that we are at an "uneven table" and that what we are doing now is harmful. Kritek says that conflict in health care will increase, and she wants nurses to transform their current behavior to that which is "beyond mere manipulation." This is a thoughtful, challenging chapter and should be read several times by many of us.

The last chapter in this section outlines the role transitions of women and nurses in Brazil. The history of nursing in Brazil is outlined by Chompré, Vas de Assis Medina, and Christofaro within the context of the history of the country. The authors show that nursing in Brazil was born linked to the domestic and undervalued activities of women. Early training schools for nurses had prerequisites, such as the requirements of a foreign language, which excluded women of lower classes. While some nurses in Brazil today have a university education, most health care is provided by a lesser-trained or undertrained workforce. The poor have no access to formal health care and rely (much as they did in the past) on mystical practices and healers. Recent economic and social transformations in Brazil include accelerating urbanization, increased schooling of women, increased participation of women in the labor force, and a decrease in family size. The history of nursing is linked to the history of women in all cultures. In Brazil, the past submissive status of women has shaped and severely handicapped the nursing profession. The authors challenge nurses in Brazil to refuse to accept their submissive role as natural. The recent changes in society and in women's roles will require a change in nursing in Brazil. This chapter and the authors' challenge have relevance to nurses in many countries.

Throughout the world, collaborative practice for nurses is closer to reality than it was in the past as a result of the changes in society and in health care delivery. But collaboration requires certain skills and a risk-taking attitude. And, in a sense, the opportunity for collaboration creates conflict. When we choose collaboration, we choose conflict. This realization may move us closer to a preferred future.

Collaboration between nurses and physicians: What is it? Does it exist? Why does it matter?

JUDITH GEDNEY BAGGS

COLLABORATION BETWEEN NURSES AND PHYSICIANS: WHAT IS IT?

To collaborate is to "work jointly with others or together," from the Latin *collaborare* ("to labor together") (*Webster's Ninth New Collegiate Dictionary,* 1989, p. 259). Indeed, this is the essence of the meaning of collaboration as we use it in nursing to describe a type of working relationship we value with physicians. Working together is not a specific enough definition, however. Working together could mean working in parallel, without communicating or planning together, or simply working in the same geographical area.

Thomas (1976) proposed that collaboration is a form of handling interpersonal interactions that combines cooperativeness (concern for the other's interests), with assertiveness (concern for one's own interests). In the nursing literature the critical attributes of collaboration include sharing in planning, decision making, problem solving, goal setting, and responsibility; working together cooperatively; coordinating; and communicating openly (Baggs & Schmitt, 1988). Based on the critical attributes and the Thomas Model, the definition of collaboration is "nurses and physicians cooperatively working together, sharing responsibility for solving problems and making decisions to formulate and carry out plans for patient care" (Baggs & Schmitt, 1988, p. 145).

Does collaboration mean the same thing to physicians as it does to nurses? The construct of collaboration is addressed more often by nurses than by physicians, as evidenced by an examination of the primary library indices for the professions. The *Cumulative Index to Nursing and Allied Health Literature* (CINAHL) has had a subject heading called "collaboration" since 1989. In the 1994 volume, that heading has two pages of citations. *Index Medicus* does not use "collaboration" as a subject heading; one must search under "interprofessional relations" or "patient care team," both of which also are found in the CINAHL.

Most of the literature about collaboration between physicians and nurses has been written by nurses (e.g., Barnum, 1991; Devereux, 1981a; England, 1986; Koerner & Armstrong, 1984; Lewis, 1991; McLain, 1988a; 1988b; Steel, 1986; Styles, 1984; Weiss & Davis, 1985), or by nurses and physicians together (Ames & Perrin, 1980; Dunbar & Bryan-Brown, 1988; Evans & Carlson, 1992). Physicians have occasionally written about the construct (Michelson, 1988).

Other articles by physicians have discussed collaboration, although it is not the primary focus of their work. For example, Stein, Watts, and Howell (1990) updated Stein's classic article on the "doctor-nurse game" (1967), noting that the earlier relationship between the professions has changed. In the past, nurses could only have input by convincing physicians that the physicians had initiated any decision making themselves (Stein, 1967). Stein et al. (1990) believe that nurses have become more highly educated and have a defined area of expertise, functioning more as autonomous health professionals. These authors characterize the new relationship between physicians and nurses as one of "mutual interdependency" (p. 547). They cite movement toward collaboration and collegiality, with a less hierarchical and more open relationship than in the past. They indicate the possible positive and negative aspects of this new relationship but generally approve of the direction it is taking. They appear to be speaking of collaboration with a definition comparable to the term used in the nursing literature.

Acknowledgment: I thank Madeline H. Schmitt, PhD, RN, FAAN, who reviewed this manuscript and offered helpful suggestions.

Despite this evidence of comparability of definition, there is also evidence of differences in implications and assessment of collaboration for the two professions. Styles (1984) noted that physicians often feel threatened when nurses discuss collaboration because they see the process as an invasion of their position of authority and power. Indeed, a secondary definition of collaboration is "to cooperate with an agency or instrumentality with which one is not immediately connected" (*Webster's Ninth New Collegiate Dictionary,* 1989, p. 259). Some physicians sense a collapsing hierarchy. In the past this impression may have been fueled by physicians collaborating with nurses. More recently it has been stimulated by concern about competition for patients with nurse practitioners, whom some view as physician substitutes. Stein et al. (1990), in their description of the negative aspects of collaboration, identify physicians' loss of the security of the old hierarchy and the potential for competition and disputes. Indeed, the movement toward interdisciplinary team care, a construct related to collaboration, has been described in part as a move by nurses to make interprofessional relations more egalitarian and less hierarchical (Brown, 1982).

Physicians who were comfortable with the older caste-like system (Wesson, 1966), in which nurses were subordinate, are not likely to welcome collaboration in practice (Campbell-Heider & Pollock, 1987; Prescott & Bowen, 1985). Fagin (1992) has noted that "physicians, more often than not, do not value or demonstrate collaboration in their work with nurses" (p. 295).

Nurses too may feel threatened by the increased responsibility and accountability involved in collaborative practice (Cape, 1986; Prescott, Dennis, & Jacox, 1987). For nurses to fulfill the assertive aspect of collaboration they will need to assume accountability and increased authority in practice areas. The different perceptions from nurses and physicians of areas appropriate for an increase in nursing authority were suggested by Katzman (1989), who asked nurses and physicians from a southwestern general hospital to rate their agreement as to whether specific nursing roles, functions and behaviors reflect the current status of nursing authority on a scale of 1 (strongly disagree) to 5 (strongly agree). She then asked them to rate the same behaviors in an ideal situation. The area of greatest difference between ratings from nurses and physicians in the current situation concerned the statement that nurses are not primarily physicians' assistants; the nurses agreed strongly (mean score 3.85) and physicians were neutral (mean was 2.53). In the ideal ratings the greatest difference concerned whether nurses should have equal say in health policymaking with physicians; the nurses' mean score was 4.46 while the physicians' mean score was 2.2. Some of the areas of greatest disagreement concerned nursing care, with physicians according nurses less authority in both current and ideal situations. In an ideal situation nurses rated their authority to decide standards of nursing care as 4.59, while physicians rated it 3.24; in determination of nursing care for patients, the nurses' rating was 4.64, while the physicians' score was 3.31. Perhaps in other settings and with other groups of providers some of these differences would diminish, but these disagreements about nursing authority suggest that we have to expect difficulties in moving to more collaboration in practice.

There is research evidence for different interpretations or observations of collaboration. In a medical intensive care unit (ICU), staff nurses and medical residents were given the same definition of collaboration and asked to report how much collaboration was involved in making decisions about transferring patients out of the medical ICU. The correlation between their reports of the amount of collaboration in making decisions was only $r = .10$ ($p = .10$) (Baggs, Ryan, Phelps, Richeson, & Johnson, 1992). In a more recent study, nurses and residents were questioned about collaboration in decisions about the level of ICU care to be provided. Despite agreement about important factors influencing such decision making and about who is involved, the correlation between reports of amount of collaboration was significant but still low ($r = .19$, $p = .04$) (Baggs & Schmitt, in press).

In ethical decision making too there is evidence of a lack of collaboration. Researchers in several studies have demonstrated nurse/physician differences about how aggressively patients should be treated (Farber et al., 1985; Frampton & Mayewski, 1987; Wolff, Smolen, & Ferrara, 1985). In three studies, nurses perceived ethical decision making as a problematic area in their interactions with physicians (Erlen & Frost, 1991; Gramelspacher, Howell, & Young, 1986; Holly, 1989). Nurses have been shown to perceive less communication about patient care decisions between the two professions than do physicians (Frampton & Mayewski, 1987; Webster, Mazer, Potvin, Fisher, & Byrick, 1991).

In a study involving interviews of administrators in medicine and nursing about interdisciplinary team care, the goals for team care differed for each profession. Physicians expected nurses to act as physician extenders, while nurses expected to use their knowledge to direct patient care (Temkin-Greener, 1983). Although there was agreement about the definition of a team (people with differing expertise working together to provide patient care), there was conflict about leadership and authority in decision-making and concern about territory.

The definitions of collaboration appear similar for nursing and medicine, but there appear to be differences in the implications of the term for each profession. Not too surprisingly, the loss of power by physicians and the gain of power by nurses that are inherent in collaboration in practice lead the two professions to approach such a move differently. Nurses and physicians also may observe or interpret interactions differently in assessing how much collaboration has taken place.

COLLABORATION BETWEEN NURSES AND PHYSICIANS: DOES IT EXIST?

One of the first groups to promote the notion of collaboration between physicians and nurses in practice was the National Joint Practice Commission (NJPC), which was established in 1971 "to make recommendations concerning the roles of the physician and the nurse in providing high quality health care" (NJPC, 1981, p. 1). The Commission, founded by the American Medical Association and the American Nurses Association, was composed of equal numbers of physicians and nurses. They proposed five guidelines for the development of what they termed joint or collaborative practice: establishment of a joint practice committee, primary nursing, encouragement of nurses' individual clinical decision making, integrated patient records, and joint patient care record reviews. Several model collaborative practice units were established implementing these five practices. Although data obtained were primarily subjective opinions of participants, increased quality of care, patient satisfaction, and nursing job satisfaction were reported (Devereux, 1981a; 1981b; 1981c; NJPC, 1981).

Currently, about 25 years after these guidelines were developed, many of them, particularly integrated patient records, have been implemented in various institutions. Does their implementation mean that collaborative practice is a reality? Work by Prescott et al. (1985) suggests that we are not yet at that point. In their study, they used the Thomas Model to classify the modes of handling disagreements reported by nurses and physicians in acute care settings. They found that only 14% of physicians and 7% of nurses reported using collaborative problem solving; the primary mode used by both providers was competition (Prescott & Bowen, 1985).

Further analyses of data from the same study suggest that the staff nurse role in clinical decision making about patient care is, at best, interdependent rather than truly collaborative, with physicians accepting nurses' input but handling final decision making themselves in most situations (Prescott et al., 1987). The nurses in the study were generally satisfied with this arrangement, provided they believed their input was listened to and valued by physicians. Many of the nurses did not want more responsibility for decision making. Physicians were willing to cede to nursing only decisions they considered unimportant. In fact, they did not view them as making decisions at all. This is less the new collaborative mode promoted in nursing and more the older "doctor-nurse" game, with the change being that nurses now may make suggestions openly.

Prescott believes we have not gone far enough toward collaboration, despite many nurses' satisfaction with the status quo. She sees collaboration as important in the development of professional practice and financially in the management of hospital care (Prescott, 1989; Prescott et al., 1987; Prescott, Phillips, Ryan, & Thompson, 1991). Professional practice is enhanced by nurses who have independence in some decision making, such as in decisions about administering analgesics for headache or changing diets as tolerated. Enabling nurses to make some decisions frees them from wasted and expensive time spent looking or waiting for physicians. Such decision making supports the assertive aspect of collaboration.

Collaboration in practice is not yet a reality for most nurses. Obstacles to collaborative practice come from both the nursing and medical professions. Collaboration is missing in some of the areas where we would most expect to find it, such as in primary care teams of nurse practitioners and physicians, in which the nurses are highly educated in their area of practice. Lamb and Napodano (1984) audiotaped interactions between team members on two teams. They found that only 23% of the interactions qualified as collaborative, although the providers rated themselves as collaborating 59% of the time. McLain (1988) said, "The research literature is strikingly devoid of studies that have demonstrated the actual existence of collaborative practice as a predominant pattern between nurses and physicians" (p. 391). She found that both physicians and nurses promoted distorted communication and nonmeaningful interactions that blocked collaboration (McLain 1988a; 1988b).

COLLABORATION BETWEEN NURSES AND PHYSICIANS: WHY DOES IT MATTER?

Several articles have summarized the reasons to support collaboration (Fagin, 1992; Miccolo & Spanier, 1993). Collaboration has been identified, along with primary nursing, as one of the two concepts from nursing and health care over the past 20 years that has been promoted as having a positive effect on patient care and provider satisfaction (Alpert, Goldman, Kilroy, & Pike, 1992). Christensen and Larson (1993) see collaboration as a way of maximizing the sharing of information unique to different professional participants and of creating the opportunity for each to learn more about the other's knowledge and talents—thereby improving future collaboration. McMahan, Hoffman, and McGee (1994) note that collaboration has become part of most quality improvement programs.

Prescott et al. (1991) note the importance of collaboration as a way of improving patient outcomes. There are a number of empirical studies that support such a belief. Studies of interdisciplinary teams in long-term care have demonstrated that team care leads to a slower rate of deterioration in patients with chronic diabetics (Feiger & Schmitt, 1979; Schmitt, Watson, Feiger, & Williams, 1981) and lower mortality in geriatric patients (Rubenstein et al., 1984). Outcomes of collaboration in acute care hospital general units include lower costs (Koerner & Armstrong, 1984) and increased patient satisfaction (Koerner, Cohen, & Armstrong, 1985). Investigators in ICUs have found collaboration to be associated with better-than-predicted mortality (Knaus, Draper, Wagner, & Zimmerman, 1986; Mitchell, Armstrong, Simpson, & Lentz, 1989), decreased risk of death or readmission to the ICU (Baggs et al., 1992), more provider satisfaction, and improved nurse retention (Baggs et al., 1992; Mitchell et al., 1989).

Collaboration between nurses and physicians may also support improved bioethical decision making in health care. Nurses' closeness to and communications with patients (Luce, 1990) and their support for patient autonomy (Davis & Jameton, 1987; Ott & Nieswiadomy, 1991; Ouslander, Tymchuk, & Rahbar, 1989; Zorb & Stevens, 1990) make their inclusion in ethical decision making important. Nurses tend to use a style of decision making that identifies the importance of personal relationships, while physicians are more concerned with rights and rules (Haddad, 1991). The combination of perspectives may enrich ethical decision making. In addition, Pike (1991) has proposed collaboration as a way to overcome the moral distress that arises when providers encounter institutional barriers to carrying out what they see as the morally appropriate action.

Critical care nurses have identified collaboration with physicians as their most important professional issue (Hartwell & Lavandero, 1991). For both ICU nurses and residents, collaboration is significantly associated with satisfaction with the decision-making process (Baggs & Ryan, 1990; Baggs et al., 1992; Baggs & Schmitt, 1995).

Some authors have developed new care models to promote collaboration (King, Lee, & Henneman, 1993). One example is a special care unit in Cleveland that was developed for treatment of the chronically critically ill (Daly, Phelps, & Rudy, 1991; Daly, Rudy, Thompson, & Happ, 1991). In this unit a nursing case management model using protocols for common patient problems, such as ventilator weaning, has decreased costs using a less hierarchical, more collaborative interdisciplinary approach to care. Care is organized around the patient, not around a physician team leader.

Another idea that has been proposed to improve physician/nurse collaboration is to begin with nursing and medical students to implement elements into the curriculum so that they learn together from the beginning (Kenneth, 1969; Mason & Parascandola, 1972; Shumaker & Goss, 1980; Yeaworth & Mims, 1973). Model programs have been described at New York University (Barnum, 1990) and Mount Sinai Hospitals (Anvaripour, Jacobson, Schewiger, & Weissman, 1991). Such programs could assist the two professions to have a better idea of each other's roles, supporting cooperation and promoting respect for assertion of the individual professional perspective in patient care situations.

There is support both conceptually and empirically for collaboration in practice between nurses and physicians, and there are examples of it. Some writers believe that collaboration is already occurring in practice, particularly in ICUs (Ames & Perrin, 1980), but there is still work to be done in understanding and promoting collaboration in practice. On the whole, it continues to be true that collaboration is not the usual mode of practice.

REFERENCES

Alpert, H.B., Goldman, L.D., Kilroy, C.M., & Pike, A.W. (1992). 7 Gryzmish: Toward an understanding of collaboration. *Nursing Clinics of North America, 27*(1), 47-59.

Ames, A., & Perrin, J.M. (1980). Collaborative practice: The joining of two professions. *Journal of the Tennessee Medical Association, 73,* 557-560.

Anvaripour, P.L., Jacobson, L., Schweiger, J., & Weissman, G.K. (1991). Physician-nurse collegiality in the medical school curriculum. *Mount Sinai Journal of Medicine, 58*(1), 91-94.

Baggs, J.G., & Ryan, S.A. (1990). Intensive care unit nurse-physician collaboration and nurse satisfaction. *Nursing Economic$, 8,* 386-392.

Baggs, J.G., Ryan, S.A., Phelps, C.E. Richeson, J.F., & Johnson, J.E. (1992). The association between interdisciplinary collaboration and patient outcomes in medical intensive care. *Heart and Lung, 21,* 18-24.

Baggs, J.G., & Schmitt, M.H. (1988). Collaboration between nurses and physicians. *Image: The Journal of Nursing Scholarship, 20,* 145-149.

Baggs, J.G., & Schmitt, M.H. (1995). Intensive care decisions about level of aggressiveness of care. *Research in Nursing and Health, 18,* 345-355.

Barnum, B.J. (1990). At New York University, the Division of Nursing develops a model for nursing and medical school collaboration. *Nursing & Health Care, 11*(2), 89-90.

Brown, T. (1982). An historical view of health care teams. In G.J. Agich (Ed.), *Responsibility in health care* (pp. 3-21). Dordrecht, Holland: D. Reidel Publishing Company.

Campbell-Heider, N., & Pollock, D. (1987). Barriers to physician-nurse collegiality. *Social Science and Medicine, 25,* 421-425.

Cape, L.S. (1986). Collaborative practice models and structures. In D.A. England (Ed.), *Collaboration in nursing* (pp. 13-26). Rockville, MD: Aspen.

Christensen, C., & Larson, J.R. (1993). Collaborative medical decision making. *Medical Decision Making, 13,* 339-345.

Daly, B.J., Phelps, C., & Rudy, E.B. (1991). A nurse-managed special care unit. *Journal of Nursing Administration, 21*(7/8), 31-38.

Daly, B.J., Rudy, E.B., Thompson, K.S., & Happ, M.B. (1991). Development of a special care unit for chronically critically ill patients. *Heart and Lung, 20,* 45-51.

Davis, A.J., & Jameton, A. (1987). Nursing and medical student attitudes toward nursing disclosure of information to patients: A pilot study. *Journal of Advanced Nursing, 12,* 691-698.

Devereux, P.M. (1981a). Essential elements of nurse-physician collaboration. *Journal of Nursing Administration, 11*(May), 19-23.

Devereux, P.M. (1981b). Does joint practice work? *Journal of Nursing Administration, 11*(June), 39-43.

Devereux, P.M. (1981c). Nurse/physician collaboration: Nursing practice considerations. *Journal of Nursing Administration, 11*(Sept.), 37-39.

Dunbar, S., & Bryan-Brown, C. (1988). Collaborative practice. In J. Boller (Ed.), *1988 International conference book* (pp. 153-154). Newport Beach, CA: American Association of Critical Care Nurses.

England, D.A. (1986). *Collaboration in nursing.* Rockville, MD: Aspen.

Erlen, J.A., & Frost, B. (1991). Nurses' perceptions of powerlessness in influencing ethical decisions. *Western Journal of Nursing Research, 13,* 397-407.

Evans, S.A., & Carlson, R. (1992). Nurse/physician collaboration: Solving the nursing shortage crisis. *American Journal of Critical Care, 1*(1), 25-32.

Fagin, C.M. (1992). Collaboration between nurses and physicians: No longer a choice. *Academic Medicine, 67,* 295-303.

Farber, N.J., Weiner, J.L., Boyer, E.G., Green, W.P., Diamond, M.P., & Copare, I.M. (1985). Cardiopulmonary resuscitation values and decisions. *Medical Care, 23,* 1391-1398.

Feiger, S.M., & Schmitt, M.H. (1979). Collegiality in interdisciplinary health teams. *Social Science and Medicine, 13A,* 217-229.

Frampton, M.W., & Mayewski, R.J. (1987). Physicians' and nurses' attitudes toward withholding treatment in a community hospital. *Journal of General Internal Medicine, 2,* 394-399.

Gramelspacher, G.P., Howell, J.D., & Young, M.J. (1986). Perceptions of ethical problems by nurses and doctors. *Archives of Internal Medicine, 146,* 577-578.

Haddad, A.M. (1991). The nurse/physician relationship and ethical decision making. *AORN Journal, 53,* 151-156.

Hartwell, J.L., & Lavandero, R. (1991). What's important to critical care nurses. *Focus on Critical Care, 18,* 364-371.

Holly, C. (1989). Critical care nurses' participation in ethical decision making. *Journal of the New York State Nurses Association, 20*(4), 9-12.

Katzman, E.M. (1989). Nurses' and physicians' perceptions of nursing authority. *Journal of Professional Nursing, 5,* 208-214.

Kenneth, H.Y. (1969). Medical and nursing students learn together. *Nursing Outlook, 17,* 46-49.

King, M.L., Lee, J.L., & Henneman, E. (1993). A collaborative practice model for critical care. *American Journal of Critical Care, 2,* 444-449.

Knaus, W.A., Draper, E.A., Wagner, D.P., & Zimmerman, J.E. (1986). An evaluation of outcome from intensive care in major medical centers. *Annals of Internal Medicine, 104,* 410-418.

Koerner, B., & Armstrong, D. (1984). Collaborative practice cuts cost of patient care: Study. *Hospitals, 58*(10), 52-54.

Koerner, B.L., Cohen, J.R., & Armstrong, D.M. (1985). Collaborative practice and patient satisfaction. *Evaluation and the Health Professions, 8,* 299-321.

Lamb, G.S., & Napodano, R.J. (1984). Physician-nurse practitioner interaction patterns in primary care practices. *American Journal of Public Health, 74,* 26-29.

Lewis, F.M. (1991). Consultation and collaboration among health care providers. In S.B. Baird, R. McCorkle, & M. Grant (Eds.), *Cancer nursing: A comprehensive textbook* (pp. 957-964). Philadelphia: Saunders.

Luce, J.M. (1990). Ethical principles in critical care. *Journal of the American Medical Association, 263,* 696-700.

Mason, E., & Parascandola, J. (1972). Preparing tomorrow's health care team. *Nursing Outlook, 20,* 728-731.

McLain, B.R. (1988a). Collaborative practice: A critical theory perspective. *Research in Nursing and Health, 11,* 391-398.

McLain, B.R. (1988b). Collaborative practice: The nurse practitioner's role in its success or failure. *Nurse Practitioner, 13*(5), 31-38.

McMahan, E.M., Hoffman, K., & McGee, G.W. (1994). Physician-nurse relationships in clinical settings: A review and critique of the literature, 1966-1992. *Medical Care Review, 51,* 83-112.

Miccolo, M.A., & Spanier, A.H. (1993). Making collaborative practice work. *Critical Care Clinics, 9,* 443-453.

Michelson, E.L. (1988). The challenge of nurse-physician collaborative practices: Improved patient care provision and outcomes. *Heart and Lung, 17,* 390-391.

Mitchell, P.H., Armstrong, S., Simpson, T.F., & Lentz, M. (1989). AACN demonstration project. *Heart and Lung, 18,* 219-237.

National Joint Practice Commission. (1981). *Guidelines for establishing joint or collaborative practice in hospitals.* Chicago: Author.

Ott, B.B., & Nieswiadomy, R.M. (1991). Support of patient autonomy in the do not resuscitate decision. *Heart and Lung, 20,* 66-72.

Ouslander, J.G., Tymchuk, A.J., & Rahbar, B. (1989). Health care decisions among elderly long-term care residents and their potential proxies. *Archives of Internal Medicine, 149,* 1367-1372.

Pike, A.W. (1991). Moral outrage and moral discourse in nurse-physician collaboration. *Journal of Professional Nursing, 7,* 351-363.

Prescott, P.A. (1989). Shortage of professional nursing practice: A reframing of the shortage problem. *Heart and Lung, 18,* 436-443.

Prescott, P.A., & Bowen, S.A. (1985). Physician-nurse relationships. *Annals of Internal Medicine, 103,* 127-133.

Prescott, P.A., Dennis, K.E., & Jacox, A.K. (1987). Clinical decision making of staff nurses. *Image: The Journal of Nursing Scholarship, 19,* 56-62.

Prescott, P.A., Phillips, C.Y., Ryan, J.W., & Thompson, K.O. (1991). Changing how nurses spend their time. *Image: The Journal of Nursing Scholarship, 23,* 23-28.

Rubenstein, L.Z., Josephson, K.R., Wieland, G.D., English, P.A., Sayre, J.A., & Kane, R.L. (1984). Effectiveness of a geriatric evaluation unit. *New England Journal of Medicine, 311,* 1664-1670.

Schmitt, M.H., Watson, N.M., Feiger, S.H., & Williams, T.F. (1981). Conceptualizing and measuring outcomes of interdisciplinary team care for a group of long-term, chronically ill, institutionalized patients. In J.E. Bachman (Ed.), *Interdisciplinary health care: Proceedings of the third annual conference on interdisciplinary team care* (pp. 169-181). Kalamazoo, MI: Center for Human Services Western Michigan University.

Shumaker, D., & Goss, V. (1980). Toward collaboration: One small step. *Nursing and Health Care, 1*(11), 183-185.

Steel, J.E. (1986). *Issues in collaborative practice.* Orlando: Grune & Stratton, Inc.

Stein, L.I. (1967). The doctor-nurse game. *Archives of General Psychiatry, 16,* 638-642.

Stein, L.I., Watts, D.T., & Howell, T. (1990). The doctor-nurse game revisited. *New England Journal of Medicine, 322,* 546-549.

Styles, M.M. (1984). Reflections on collaboration and unification. *Image: The Journal of Nursing Scholarship, 16,* 21-23.

Temkin-Greener, H. (1983). Interprofessional perspectives on teamwork in health care: A case study. *Milbank Memorial Fund Quarterly, 61,* 641-658.

Thomas, K. (1976). Conflict and conflict management. In M.D. Dunnette (Ed.), *Handbook of industrial and organizational psychology* (pp. 889-935). Chicago: Rand McNally College Publishing Company.

Weiss, S.J., & Davis, H.P. (1985). Validity and reliability of the collaborative practice scales. *Nursing Research, 34,* 299-305.

Webster's Ninth New Collegiate Dictionary (1989). Springfield, MA: Merriam-Webster Inc.

Webster, G.C., Mazer, C.D., Potvin, C.A., Fisher, A., & Byrick, R.J. (1991). Evaluation of a "do not resuscitate" policy in intensive care. *Canadian Journal of Anaesthesia, 38,* 553-563.

Wesson, A.F. (1966). Hospital ideology and communication between ward personnel. In R. Scott & E. Volkhart (Eds.), *Medical care* (pp. 458-475). New York: Wiley.

Wolff, M.L., Smolen, S., & Ferrara, L. (1985). Treatment decisions in a skilled-nursing facility. *Journal of the American Geriatrics Society, 33,* 440-445.

Yeaworth, R., & Mims, F. (1973). Interdisciplinary education as an influence system. *Nursing Outlook, 21,* 1973.

Zorb, S.L., & Stevens, J.B. (1990). Contemporary bioethical issues in critical care. *Critical Care Nursing Clinics of North America, 2,* 515-520.

Feminism and nursing

PEGGY L. CHINN

Passion, intellect, moral activity—these three have never been satisfied in woman. In this cold and oppressive conventional atmosphere, they cannot be satisfied. To say more on this subject would be to enter into the whole history of society, of the present state of civilization.
—Florence Nightingale (1979, p. 29)

This was written by Nightingale in 1852 just after she pursued her nursing training at Kaiserworth and appears in an essay entitled "Cassandra." For years during her young adulthood, Nightingale yearned to pursue a social calling to serve people, but as a Victorian woman her options were severely restricted. Her essay is an outcry against the plight of Victorian women like herself and reflects her strong conviction that women had many lost talents and abilities that could have been developed.

Nightingale's quote illustrates several aspects of feminism that remain pertinent today. "Passion, intellect, and moral activity" are three key aspects of women's experience that are addressed by feminists today. Her observation that these three "have never been satisfied in woman" is a fundamental premise of feminist activism. Feminist activists seek to right the wrongs and injustices that have been sustained against women, not only through equal opportunity but also through seeking to understand women's experiences in the world and to break down the barriers to valuing that experience. Finally, Nightingale's observation that "to say more on this subject would be to enter into the whole history of society, of the present state of civilization" summarizes precisely what feminist authors have set out to accomplish in the past several decades. In other words, feminism is not the singular, polemic, or fanatical movement that is portrayed in the media. Rather, it is a perspective that has entered the whole history of society and the present state of civilization.

Feminist thought and action are grounded in women's experiences and take a stance that assumes that women's experiences are real and valuable. Feminist thought and action are inherently political—they challenge the prevailing attitude of devaluing and discounting women. The actions and writings that come from feminist thinking are motivated by a desire to benefit women, with the underlying conviction that if something is not good for women, then it is not good. Because what affects women affects the world, and what affects the world affects women, feminist concerns are as broad as the world, even the universe.

Nursing and feminism, regardless of the definitions of either concept, are inextricably connected because of the presence of women. Not only are most nurses women, but nursing's social role—to care for the sick—is a role that has been historically assigned to women worldwide. Therefore, many of the actions and concerns that nurses assume in their day-to-day work are those that are associated with being female. The American Heritage Talking Dictionary (AHTD) gives the following as one definitions of "nurse:" "one that serves as a nurturing or fostering influence or means" (AHTD, 1994). Generally, those who nurture are women; and when men provide formal nurturing roles in society they usually enter social realms where women predominate. What are usually not associated with these roles are precisely the three concerns that Nightingale addresses—passion, intellect, and moral activity. Caring for others and fostering their growth is generally viewed as drudgery, lacking emotional or intellectual interest or ability. The ethical aspects of caring for others are prescribed by the dominant culture. Therefore, exercising independent moral activity is not presumed to be required. While the Western world has changed remarkably for women since Nightingale's time, women remain tied to their socially accepted "female" roles, and the roles associated with women are devalued. Even more striking is the fact that worldwide, not much has changed for women since the Nightingale's time.

In this chapter I explore feminist perspectives on passion, intellect, and moral activity and show how these perspectives can assist nurses to move toward changes that are consistent with what is good for nurses, for women, and for all people. Each of these concerns is interrelated with the others. Although they have distinct aspects, the suggested readings listed at the end of this chapter prove that they weave together to form a whole, a global concern.

PASSION

> When shall we see a life full of steady enthusiasm, walking straight to its aim, flying home, as that bird is now, against the wind—with . . . calmness and . . . confidence . . . ? (Nightingale, 1979, p. 36)

For Nightingale, the idea of passion included powerful emotion and even sexual desire, which were severely restricted for women in her time. However, her primary interest was what she termed "high sympathies," which in her view need to be fed and nurtured in order to serve society well. She said:

> If, together, man and woman approach any of the high questions of social, political, or religious life, they are said (and justly—under our present disqualifications) to be going 'too far.' That such things can be! (Nightingale, 1979, p. 28)

Activists and theorists of the feminist movement of the second half of the 20th century began to recognize the oppressive dynamic of being ridiculed with accusations of going too far (Morgan, 1968), when in fact they could see clearly that women had not gone far enough. And so women began, with an intensity and seriousness never before seen in human history, to approach the high questions of social, political, and religious life.

In speaking of passion, Nightingale (1979) stated that "poetry and imagination begin life" (p. 30). She believed that women begin life with vivid and rich imaginations, and that their dreams and imaginations hold a key to developing the intellect and moral activity that is required for meaningful social action. She speculated, however, that women learn very early to subdue their imaginations because they are so dangerous. Young girls receive messages early in life that society does not want, and that they cannot want, to fulfill their imagination and dreams.

Nightingale identified the daily circumstances of women's lives that restrict them from developing the seeds of social action that lie dormant in their imagination—lack of time, time consumed by service to the home, time constantly interrupted. Speaking of the constant demands made on women's time by anyone and everyone, Nightingale stated:

> Yet time is the most valuable of all things. If they had come every morning and afternoon and robbed us of half-a-crown we should have had redress from the police. But it is laid down, that our time is of no value. (Nightingale, 1979, p. 35)

Indeed, when the feminist movement of the second half of the 20th century began, women realized that they must gain control over their own time in order to begin to change the social and political structures that held control over their lives. They began to meet in small groups to foster the art and imagination that are necessary for social activism. The method of feminism—consciousness-raising—was developed in small group processes. In sharing stories of their lives, women began to discover patterns in and among their lives. They began to see that individual circumstances of women's lives began in the context of the social and political patterns that sustain their oppression. Thus was born the idea that the personal is political.

The insight that "the personal is political" represents a recognition of the interrelatedness of all things. It is an insight that is expressed in many forms, calling to join together what has been torn apart by centuries of patriarchal dominance. Passion, which is presumed to reside in the personal realm, is actually *in* all aspects of life. It is the necessary fire that gives energy to sustain action in the public world when all seems futile. It is through passion that the life of thought and the life of action can be brought together.

The enterprise of bringing together that which has been torn apart is a cultural and political enterprise. Culture in society teaches and reinforces the values that are held by its members to be good and right; politics is the ability to enact those values in a large social arena (e.g., the cultural norm that sustains different moral codes for the personal life from those of the public life). Undertaking to bring together a single moral code for all of life is a project of huge proportions, requiring enormous energy, vivid imagination, and commitment to action.

In nursing, the splits are many—mind-body splits, practice-theory splits, real-ideal splits, public-private splits, work-home splits. Feminist ideas and historical models provide a framework from which to begin to understand the origins of these splits, to understand how they are sustained, and to begin to form action to bring them together into one (Chinn, 1989).

INTELLECT

> What wonder if, wearied out, sick at heart with hope deferred, the springs of will broken, not seeing clearly *where* her duty lies, she abandons intellect as a vocation and takes it only, as we use the moon, by glimpses through her tight-closed window-shutters? (Nightingale, 1979, p. 37).

Nightingale reasoned that the sphere in which women were required to remain—the private sphere of home and family—was much too narrow a field for development of the mind. Speaking of the systematic ways in which women's lives and interests were curtailed, she said, "This system dooms some minds to incurable infancy, others to silent misery" (p. 37).

Nightingale had a strong conviction that women have the mental capabilities to achieve whatever they wish to achieve (e.g., compose music, solve scientific problems, create social projects of great importance). But the material limitations on women's lives robbed them not only of the time to devote to such activities but also of the development of the mental and physical skills required to achieve socially meaningful actions. Out of this conviction came her resolve and action to establish nursing as a profession wherein women could develop the intellectual abilities to contribute meaningful service to society.

Over a century later, as feminist thought and action developed, nursing began to be seen in different contexts. Feminists began to recognize the hazards of sustained sex segregation in occupations and the ways in which this social and cultural pattern sustained women's oppression (Greenleaf, 1980). Feminists also challenged the unquestioning acceptance by women of their nurturing and caring roles in society and often saw nurses as sustaining this unquestioning acceptance (Chinn & Wheeler, 1985). However, out of a commitment to value women and women's experience, feminist insights also began to give new meaning to the nature of nurturing and caring and to recognize the essential value of the attitudes, skills, and knowledge that are required to be in relation with others in a caring and nurturing way (Gilligan, 1982; Larrabee, 1993; Noddings, 1984).

Nursing as a profession did accomplish what Nightingale envisioned: It provided an avenue for nurses to leave the relatively restricted environment of home and family and to enter a broader world of social service. It has provided, worldwide, an avenue for women's education. For many women, becoming a nurse has been the only way to obtain an education and to develop their intellect. But has this been enough? What has been the nature of this education, and has it served women well?

Ashley, a feminist nurse historian, studied the history of nursing education in hospitals. She concluded that not only were nurses not served well by apprenticeship education, but that all nurses continue to suffer the remnants of attitudes and beliefs that continue to influence the content and processes of nursing education and of nursing (Ashley, 1976; 1980).

Consider, for example, the persistent language that sustains nursing's subservience to medicine. The phrase "physician's orders," which nurses are still legally responsible to follow, has not been changed or replaced since the earliest days of the nursing profession. There have been alternatives (e.g., physician prescription, medical treatments) that suggest the nature of physicians' work and relationship with their patients, and these contrast with the implications of the nurse-patient relationship in the phrase "physician's orders." Nurses have been educated (trained), however, in ways that differ little from the earliest days of nursing, to follow physicians' orders, and more importantly, not to question the terminology, the practices, or the orders themselves.

MORAL ACTIVITY

> Women dream of a great sphere of steady, not sketchy benevolence, of moral activity, for which they would fain [sic] be trained and fitted, instead of working in the dark, neither knowing nor registering whither their steps lead, whether farther from or nearer to the aim. (Nightingale, 1979, p. 38)

Nightingale has been criticized for her insistence on the moral character requirements that she imposed on the earliest nurses and for the heritage of emphasis on character that the profession inherited from her early views. Many of these criticisms are well founded from the perspective of more recent contexts; moral and ethical necessities change over time. However, it is now possible to also consider sustained values in her views on moral activity. Her essential concern in "Cassandra" was the social damage that results when what women valued, and how they would impact the world based on these values, was not realized. In addition, she decried the waste of human resources when women were denied the circumstances to develop and know their own moral sense of what is good and what is right.

For Nightingale, two circumstances are required to develop moral activity: time for learning and reflection (bringing together passion and intellect) and sustained experience in applying or acting on what is reflected on (experience). She states:

> Women . . . long for experience, not patch-work experience, but experience followed up and systematized, to enable them to know what they are about and *where* they are "casting their bread" and whether it is 'bread' or a stone. (Nightingale, 1979, p. 39)

She speculated how any profession or occupation could be developed at odd times, which is what women have generally been required to do in developing anything. She wondered how an art can be developed if it is only viewed as an amusement, which is how women's arts are typically viewed. She likened the situation of women's sketchy opportunities for development of the intellect and moral activity to starvation, and saw it as serious a situation as if we were physically starved of food. She viewed women's unquestioning acceptance of prescribed social roles as a moral problem:

> With what labour women have toiled to break down all individual and independent life, in order to fit themselves for this social and domestic existence, thinking it right! And when they have killed themselves to do it, they have awakened (too late) to think it wrong. (Nightingale, 1979, p. 42)

Ironically, Nightingale's criticism about women's unquestioning acceptance of their social and domestic existence applies today to the profession she founded. Consider how her words would read if revised to apply to nursing today:

> *With what labor nurses have toiled to break down all individual and independent life, in order to fit themselves for this social and professional existence, thinking it right! And when they have killed themselves to do it, they have awakened (too late) to think it wrong.*

Today, nurses do have models and frameworks with which to begin to judge what is right and what is wrong in their nursing practice (Fry, 1992). However, much of what is practiced in nursing is not questioned, and if it is questioned, it feels much too dangerous to act on the insight. So now we turn to the question: What is a nurse to do?

FEMINIST PERSPECTIVES ON BEING, KNOWING, AND DOING

> Nothing can well be imagined more painful than the present position of woman, unless, on the one hand, she renounces all outward activity and keeps herself within the magic sphere, the bubble of her dreams; or, on the other, surrendering all aspiration, she gives herself to her real life, soul and body. For those to whom it is possible, the latter is best; for out of activity may come thought, out of mere aspiration can come nothing. (Nightingale, 1979, p. 50)

Today, the choice of action does not require women to also surrender all aspiration. A multitude of possibilities for action have emerged out of the dreams and imaginations of the feminist activists and theorists of the past few decades. In fact, the disjunction between thought and action has been directly opposed by feminists, and healing that disjunction is a major enterprise of feminist activists and theorists. Feminist activists in the second half of this century struggled with the choice of whether to develop theory or to take social and political action. Not everyone did both, but the prevailing practice that emerged was to be sure that both theory (thoughtful reflection) and action always characterize feminist enterprises (Redstockings, 1975).

Table 70-1 summarizes definitions of feminism and the concerns—both in aspiration and in action—that feminism has developed in this century. The suggested readings at the end of this chapter provide classic and recent resources in which you can find additional information on each of these concerns. The following sections describe the various definitions linked with Nightingale's ideas of passion, intellect, and moral activity and provide a sketch of ways in which women have actually claimed places in society to exercise these three ideas.

Passion: feminism as a culture grounded in women's experience

Feminist writers, scholars, and activists have indeed entered the whole history of society and the present state of civilization. They have developed extensive cultural resources from which to change both women's experience and the patriarchal tendencies of the dominant culture. Consistent with other social movements, a major concern has been to reclaim women's heritage in history, in religion, in the arts, and in the emergence of civilization. Feminists have been persistent to ask "where were the women, and what were they doing" in every period of known human history. Out of this question has come new

Table 70-1 Definitions and Characteristics of Feminism

Definition	Characteristics
A culture grounded in women's experience	• Reclaims women's heritage in history, religion, and culture • Reclaims women's personal and social power • Reclaims women's wisdom • Celebrates women as healers, artists, creators, and statespersons
A political stance to right injustices against women and the earth	• Acts on the premise that the personal is political • Connects gender socialization and women's roles with larger political issues, including restoring the earth's ecology • Critiques the institutionalization of patriarchal norms • Seeks an end to private and public violence • Seeks balance of power in economic and political terms
A discipline seeking to give voice to women's experience	• Critiques patriarchal norms, practices, and theories • Relates the diverse experiences of women to social, political, philosophical, and scientific interests • Explores the dynamics by which women are silenced and the ways to end the silence and invisibility of women • Explores women's health and development • Revises criteria of worth for scholarship and for what counts as knowledge about women
An ethic of valuing women and women's experience	• Critiques "malestream" morality and ethics • Develops ethics of caring and relationship • Reunites as one the public/private ethic • Redefines meanings of responsibility, truth, right, justice, good, and beauty

appreciation of women as healers, artists, statespersons, creators, and inventors. From knowledge of women's heritage, women have reclaimed their personal power to create, to shape the values of the culture, and to bring women's wisdom to bear on the higher questions of society.

Passion: feminism as a political stance to right injustices

No other perspective has remained so persistent and broad-based in its concern for righting injustices. While women's well-being is a central focus, feminist insights link the rights and well-being of women with children, with all people (particularly other oppressed groups), and with the earth. The historical and current situation of women in the family and in society are linked with such far-reaching issues as economics, agricultural, industrial production, war and other forms of social violence, ecological health, and prevailing patterns of political violence. Feminist writers have shown how women's roles in the family and society are sustained by the larger political patterns and in turn sustain the nature of local, national, and global political patterns.

Feminist examination of political issues and the creation of new theories of politics have given new meanings to such political concepts as equality, justice, rights, peace, and diversity. For example, rather than merely accepting the prevailing notion that "equality" means "equal to white middle-class males," feminists seek to carefully construct meanings, criteria, and standards for "equality" that examine what is good for all. Out of these insights, and committed to bringing together the personal and the political, feminist activists have taken significant local, regional, national, and international stands.

Nurses and nursing have particularly benefitted from feminist political activism that demanded equitable pay for women's work. For example, in the 1970s nurses in Denver fought to be paid more than tree trimmers established the idea that work should be paid in accord with its educational and skill requirements, not with the gender of the person who typically performs it.

Intellect: feminism as a discipline seeking to give voice to women's experience

Feminism has developed as a discipline that seeks to give voice and understanding to women's experiences. One focus is the plight of women in the patriarchy and seeking ways for women to change their existence in the patriarchy, as well as ways to change the patriarchy itself or to create a different world order based on women's aspirations. Another aspect of feminism as a discipline is consideration of the biology-culture debate, that is, addressing questions concerning the extent to which women's experiences are shaped by biology and to what extent they are shaped by culture or experience.

Women's health and development are a large area of concern for feminist scholars. The questions posed by feminists include those as to how women's health and development—particularly mental health and development—have been defined, distorted, created, or shaped by the patriarchy. Redefining what health is, and what healthy development is for women, is a major feminist enterprise. This redefinition does not occur in an ivory tower vacuum; rather, it happens in conjunction with experience, with practice, and with action. An example of the redefinition of women's health and development is the work of the Boston Women's Health Book Collective, producers of many books for women about women's health.

Another important area of study for feminist scholars has been discovery of the ways in which women have been silenced, with their work rendered invisible in society, and exploring ways to change women's experience so that they know what it is to be valued, to be heard, and to be strong and courageous to act in the world. Work related to explorations of women's silence is directed toward revising the criteria by which something is judged to be worthy of scholarly attention, or worthy to count as knowledge. Feminist scholars have insisted that women's concerns can no longer be excluded as worthy of scholarly attention.

Moral activity: feminism as an ethic of valuing women and women's experience

Feminist ethics is both thought and action directed toward values that sustain life, well-being, peace, nurturing, and growth for all. Ethics includes critique of "malestream" morality and ethics, particularly the prevailing patriarchal morality that differentiates standards of ethical behavior at home and in the workplace. Feminist ethics seeks to reunite as one the public and private ethic.

Explorations of the relationship between gender and moral development have led to a better understanding and valuing of women's experience as well as a valuing of the perspectives that tend to emerge when women's values are taken into account. Women tend to value relationships, and they perceive personal and social obligations in terms of relationships and the well-being of significant others. This perspective redefines what it means to be responsible, to act justly, or to know what is good or right.

Much of the tension that nurses experience in their working lives involves difficult ethical dilemmas for which there are no resolutions if only the traditional patriarchal perspectives of justice and worth are considered. This is largely because patriarchal ethics does not take into account that which most concerns nurses—the quality of relationships and the meaning of caring. As nurses embrace more fully the perspectives of feminist ethics, it will be possible to embrace ethical sensibilities that more closely align with the fundamental values of nursing.

CONCLUSION

Contrary to popular perception, feminism is not an ideology. Feminism embraces many ways of viewing the world that bring women into focus. It is a perspective that values seeing clearly the diversity that exists among all women—not an attempt to define "woman." As you think about what I have presented, and as you explore some of the suggested readings, ask yourself the following questions:

- In what ways do I value women? Who am I in relation to women?
- Do my views and values benefit women and in turn all people?
- What do I know about women and nurses in history?
- Are my assumptions about women and nurses in history accurate and well conceived?
- What do I know about the experience of women who are not like myself in economic status, culture, ethnic background, or belief?

REFERENCES

American Heritage Talking Dictionary (Windows, Macintosh). (1994). Cambridge, MA: Softkey International.

Ashley, J. (1976). *Hospitals, paternalism, and the role of the nurse*. New York: Teachers College Press.

Ashley, J. (1980). Power in structured misogyny: Implications for the politics of care. *Advances in Nursing Science, 2*(3), 3–22.

Chinn, P.L., & Wheeler, C.E. (1985). Feminism and nursing. *Nursing Outlook, 33*(2), 74–77.

Chinn, P.L. (1989). Nursing's patterns of knowing and feminist thought. *Nursing and Health Care, 10*(2), 71–75.

Fry, S.T. (1992). The role of caring in a theory of nursing ethics. In H.B. Holmes & L.M. Purdy (Eds.), *Feminist perspectives in medical ethics* (pp. 93–106). Bloomington, IN: Indiana University Press.

Gilligan, C. (1982). *In a different voice: Psychological theory and women's development*. Cambridge, MA: Harvard University Press.

Greenleaf, N.P. (1980). Sex-segregated occupations: Relevance for nursing. *Advances in Nursing Science, 2*(3), 23–37.

Larrabee, M.J. (Ed.). (1993). *An ethic of care: Feminist and interdisciplinary perspectives*. New York: Routledge.

Morgan, R. (1968). *Going too far: The personal chronicle of a feminist* New York: Vintage Books.

Nightingale, F. (1979). *Florence Nightingale's Cassandra: An angry outcry against the forced idleness of Victorian women.* With an Introduction by Myra Start and Epilogue by Cynthia Macdonald. New York: The Feminist Press.

Noddings, N. (1984). *Caring: A feminine approach to ethics and moral education* Berkeley, CA: University of California Press.

Redstockings. (1975). *Feminist revolution: An abridged edition with additional writings.* New York: Random House.

SUGGESTED READINGS

Achterberg, J. (1990). *Woman as healer.* Boston: Shambala.

Alcoff, L., & Potter, B. (Eds.). (1993). *Feminist epistemologies.* New York: Routledge.

Allen, J. (1990). *Lesbian philosophies and cultures.* Albany, NY: State University of New York Press.

Bunch, C. (1987). *Passionate politics: Feminist theory in action.* New York: St. Martin's Press.

Cheatham, A., & Powell, M.C. (1986). *This way daybreak comes: Women's values and the future.* Philadelphia: New Society Publishers.

Chinn, P.L. (1995). *Peace and power: Building communities for the future.* New York: NLN Press.

Daly, M., & Caputi, J. (1987). *Websters' first new intergalactic wickedary of the English language.* Boston: Beacon Press.

Edwalds, L., & Stocker, M. (Eds.). (1995). *The woman-centered economy: Ideals, reality, and the space in between.* Chicago: Third Side Press.

Freeman, J. (Ed.). (1995). *Women: A feminist perspective* (5th Ed.). Mountain View, CA: Mayfield Publishing Co.

Frye, M. (1983). *The politics of reality: Essays in feminist theory.* Freedom, CA: The Crossing Press.

Hine, D.C. (1989). *Black women in white: Racial conflict and cooperation in the nursing profession: 1890-1950.* Bloomington, IN: Indiana University Press.

Holmes, H.B., & Purdy, L.M. (Eds.). (1992). *Feminist perspectives in medical ethics.* Bloomington, IN: Indiana University Press.

hooks, B. (1990). *Yearning: Race, gender, and cultural politics.* Boston, MA: South End Press.

Humm, M. (Ed.). (1992). *Modern feminisms: Political, literary, cultural.* New York: Columbia University Press.

Johnstone, M.J. (1994). *Nursing and the injustices of the law.* Philadelphia: Harcourt Brace & Co.

MacKinnon, C.A. (1989). *Toward a feminist theory of the state.* Cambridge, MA: Harvard University Press.

Rich, A. (1986). *Of woman born: Motherhood as experience and institution* 10th Anniversary Ed.). New York: W.W. Norton.

Roberts, J., Thetis, I., & Group, M. (1995). *Feminism and nursing: An historical perspective on power, status, and political activism in the nursing profession.* Westport, CT: Praeger.

Ruether, R.R. (1985). *Womanguides: Readings toward a feminist theology.* Boston: Beacon Press.

Spender, D. (1982). *Women of ideas and what men have done to them.* Boston: Routledge & Kegan Paul.

Stanley, L. (Ed.). (1990). *Feminist praxis: Research theory & epistemology in feminist sociology.* New York: Routledge.

Tong, R. (1989). *Feminist thought: A comprehensive introduction.* Boulder, CO: Westview Press.

Tuana, N. (1989). *Feminism & science.* Bloomington, IN: Indiana University Press.

Entering collegial relationships: The demise of nurse as victim

ADELE W. PIKE

Scholars of women's development have observed a uniqueness in women's ways of thinking, of knowing, of relating to others, and of being (Belensky, Clinchy, Goldberger, & Tarule, 1986; Gilligan, 1982; Miller, 1976). They refer to this uniqueness as "women's voice." Their metaphor of voice is borrowed here and applied to nurses. "Nurses' voice" thus refers to the unique perspectives and contributions that nurses bring to patient care. Disturbingly, this voice is often silent, and that silence is seriously demoralizing to nurses. For patients the consequences are more grievous because the silence denies them the integration of the nursing perspective into the care they receive.

The factors involved in silencing—in censoring—nurses affect the way nurses define their professional self-concept, often leading them to perceive themselves as helpless victims. Most of the factors are rooted in cultural and social mores that, despite being outdated and no longer applicable in present-day health care, are deeply etched in memory. Despite the persistence of their legend, the power of these traditions to silence nurses should be rendered invalid.

For this to occur, nurses must appreciate that they are presented with opportunities for choice: the choice to remain silent or to become equal colleagues in the health care team. This chapter presents an analysis of the factors that suppress nurses' voice and of the significance of the choice nurses make with regard to making their voices heard. In discussing the implications of this choice, critical incidents (Benner, 1984) depicting patients and families facing ethical dilemmas are used in order to contrast two divergent outcomes that result from the different ways in which nurses choose to exercise their voice.

SILENCING OF VOICE

Numerous forces affect nurses' voice. Many of these forces are external, such as the historical role of nurse as handmaiden, the hierarchical structure of health care organizations, the perceived authority and directives of physicians, hospital policy, and the threat of disciplinary or legal action. Alarmingly, the current restructuring of health care in this country renews a powerful external constraint to nurses' voice. Changes in health care financing and reimbursement have led to the closing of nursing units, displacement of nursing staff, and reductions in the labor force (Pike & Alpert, 1994). The very real threat of job loss, combined with the turmoil that accompanies downsizing of health care systems and institutions, can quickly and insidiously lure articulate, autonomous professionals into the perceived safety of being but a cog in a bureaucratic wheel.

Equally ominous and plentiful are the internal forces that constrain nurses' voice. Characteristics such as role confusion, lack of professional confidence, timidity, fear, insecurity, or sense of inferiority lead nurses to *choose* silence as often as external forces impose silence on them (Pike, 1991; Yarling & McElmurry, 1986).

These internal and external constraints inflict wounds on nurses' professional self-esteem. These wounds deepen and expand the innate capacity for self-doubt that nurses, like all individuals, have. Having been wounded,

---

The critical incidents published in this paper initially appeared in: Pike, A.W. (1991). Moral outrage and moral discourse in nurse physician collaboration. *Journal of Professional Nursing 7*, 351-363. Used with permission.

The author wishes to acknowledge the ideas and feedback of the nurses and physicians who worked on the former 7 Gryzmish (North), Beth Israel Hospital, Boston, MA, who were essential in the writing of this chapter.

nurses experience great difficulty believing in their own capacity, ability, and right to contribute to patient care as autonomous, vital, and equal professionals. Their ambitions and aspirations are stifled. Their vision grows myopic, and they fail to recognize both their opportunities and their obligation for self-advancement. Such an inclination establishes a pattern in which nurses perceive themselves as inferior and unable to change their lot (Steele, 1990).

This poor professional self-concept sabotages any possibility of collaboration between nurses and other care providers because it identifies nurses as embattled victims and customarily marks physicians as their antagonists. Such a relationship urges an adversarial stance in which the victims place the onus of responsibility for the problematic relationship on their perceived aggressors rather than accepting responsibility and accountability for who they are and what they want to be (Steele, 1990).

The stance of victimization is very seductive; and there are many incentives for maintaining this role. Victims are perceived as innocent, and by assigning the locus of their control to external forces they avoid responsibility and accountability. Victims are spared the stress of change, because in the matrix of victimization it is the oppressor who must change in order for the victim's condition to improve (Cooper, 1991; Steele, 1990).

There can be no argument that in the past nurses were the victims of oppression and were made to suffer the subjugation of physicians and hospital administrators. They had little choice but to be exploited as conveniences, as loyal and obedient servants. Today, nurses must grapple not only with the memory of this exploitation but also with the very real threat that the current crisis in health care economics will drive them back into a role of subservience. It will take tremendous courage and strength of professional character for nurses to maintain and further the success that advances in nursing practice, education, research, and administration have made toward unraveling the traditional socialization of health care providers and culture of health care organizations. Nurses are thus faced with a critical choice: to consider themselves helpless victims of past injustice and present-day economic threats or to define themselves as autonomous, equal, and essential members of the health care team (Pike & Alpert, 1994).

The choice is not easy given the unconscious incentives to remain victims (Cooper, 1991). Defining oneself as an equal and autonomous professional means being responsible and accountable, which are stressful, difficult, and frightening burdens. This definition obligates nurses to exercise their voice; to articulate their unique knowledge of patients and their responses to illness; and to participate with other health care professionals as colleagues rather than as subordinates. It means overcoming self-doubt and timidity and resisting the forces that threaten to corrupt nurses' obligations to patients. Overcoming the internal and external constraints that inhibit the voice, the aspirations, and the talents of nurses requires relentless effort. While the choice to exercise nurses' voice is risky, the choice to remain silent is an unacceptable alternative (Pike & Alpert, 1994).

BEING A COLLEAGUE

Part of the difficulty for nurses in defining themselves as colleagues of other health care professionals is that so little is known about how to best operationalize the role (Alpert, Goldman, Kilroy, & Pike, 1992; Petro, 1992; Prescott & Bowen, 1985; Stein, 1967; Stein, Watts, & Howell, 1990). Equal colleagueship involves entering into a collaborative relationship that is characterized by mutual trust and respect and an understanding of the perspective each partner contributes. Collaboration involves a bond, a union, a depth of caring about one another and about the relationship. The colleagueship this breeds obliges individuals to put aside their feelings of interprofessional competition and antagonism that are rooted in history so that the work and expertise of all participants may be integrated and patient care maximized (Alpert et al., 1992; Aradine & Pridham, 1973; Pike, 1991; Weiss & Davis, 1985).

Colleagues openly acknowledge that they share a common goal—the health and comfort of patients in their care. They recognize their interdependence and, accordingly, share responsibility and accountability for patient outcomes. Collegial relationships are safe. Each participant accepts the other as someone who is well-intentioned and trying to do his or her best. When conflict arises, it is addressed at its source and not escalated up a hierarchical chain of authority (Alpert et al., 1992; Mangiardi & Pellegrino, 1992; Pike et al., 1993).

Colleagueship has many characteristics of a caring relationship, as defined by the ethic of care. It dispenses with hierarchical habits of relating, replacing dominance and rank with mutual respect and shared decision making. As colleagues, individuals attend to each other's growth and development, protect each other from belittlement, and enhance each other's professional dignity (Gadow, 1985; Mayeroff, 1971; Noddings, 1984; Watson, 1988).

Incorporating the concept of colleague into one's professional identity is a developmental process that requires critical self-reflection. In order to collaborate with others, a nurse must understand and value the unique perspective that nursing offers. Being a colleague requires a breadth of clinical experience that solidifies professional confidence. Nurses who define themselves as colleagues must develop a language that allows them to articulate their unique perspective to nonnurses so that they will be understood. This definition of professional self also requires the maturity to recognize the incentives to remain victimized and to reflect on how one might be seduced by these incentives. Additionally, one must understand the historical and cultural roots to the internal and external constraints imposed on nurses and appreciate that their influence can quickly subjugate nurses at a time when patients can ill afford a silencing of nurses' unique perspectives. Nurses who choose to define themselves as colleagues must overcome these constraints and learn to manage their backward pull.

Operationalizing the concept of professional self as equal colleague frees nurses from the internal constraints that contribute to the silencing of their voice. Once the influence of these internal forces is curtailed, nurses can question, challenge, and overcome external constraints. Colleagueship is difficult work fraught with anxiety, confusion, and frustration; but it is also a very fruitful enterprise offering tremendous promise and benefits to both nurses and patients (Pike, 1991).

CONSEQUENCES OF CHOICE

The way in which nurses choose to construe their professional selves has significant implications for both patient care and nurses' role and satisfaction. The consequences of their choice are particularly dramatic in the care of patients and families in the throes of ethical uncertainty. Consider the following critical incident involving Mr. S. This incident describes a dilemma not unfamiliar to nurses, and it leaves powerful images of morally unacceptable care.

Mr. S. was a 72-year-old man admitted to the hospital from a nursing home as a result of his failure to thrive and a severe infection. On admission he was frail, cachectic, and minimally responsive. He had a temperature 101.8°F, heart rate 160 beats per minute in atrial fibrillation, respiratory rate of 28 breaths per minute, and unstable blood pressure. His blood tests suggested severe dehydration.

Mr. S.'s peripheral veins were small and fragile, and repeated attempts to start an intravenous line in his arms were unsuccessful. A line was finally established in his foot, and intravenous fluids and antibiotics were administered.

Long before his admission, Mr. S. had made it known that he did not want "heroic measures" taken to prolong his life in the event of a grave illness. It was documented and well known that "do not resuscitate" applied in his case.

We were unable to determine the source of his infection. Even gentle attempts to provide hydration exacerbated his congestive heart failure and atrial fibrillation. His kidneys failed, and his lungs, damaged by years of smoking, were barely able to meet the increased demands of his illness. It seemed clear that Mr. S. was dying. His nurses worked to minimize any pain or distress he might suffer during his terminal illness.

On his fourth hospital day, Mr. S.'s intravenous line infiltrated and another peripheral line could not be placed. On the following day, the physicians involved in Mr. S.'s care felt obligated to establish a central intravenous line, since, in the absence of peripheral access, Mr. S. was not receiving any fluid or antibiotics. At the time, no one openly questioned this decision, despite the fact that his nurses considered such an invasive, aggressive intervention to be wrong in the context of Mr. S.'s illness and wishes.

During the central line insertion Mr. S. suffered a pneumothorax, and an emergency chest tube was inserted. At this point he exhibited notable signs of pain and discomfort, which had been absent during the earlier days of his admission.

Mr. S.'s family was called, and they were distressed that invasive interventions had been carried out. They requested that no further aggressive treatment be used in his care.

Mr. S. was given oxygen and morphine for comfort. He died less than 2 days later, but continued to show signs of respiratory distress throughout this period.

The nursing staff agonized over the pain and suffering he experienced. We began to place blame and among ourselves spoke of the callousness, aggressiveness, and insensitivity of physicians . . . of their ability "only to cure, not to care." We felt anger, frustration, pain, remorse, and guilt.

The story of Mr. S. is one of moral failure and moral outrage that resulted in large measure from the silencing of nurses' voice. Mr. S.'s nurses encountered a moral dilemma while they cared for him about whether to place a central line and continue hydration or to forgo the line and allow him to die. Faced with this dilemma, the nurses reasoned that Mr. S. was at the end of his life and wanted to prevent his pain and suffering.

Mr. S.'s physicians, faced with the same dilemma, reached a different decision. Tragically, there was no discourse and the authority and directives of the physicians took precidence over the nurses' plan. The physicians' action was seen as unquestionable, and this perception served as a constraint to the nurses who had legitimate concerns about Mr. S.'s suffering. The physicians' response—and the nurses' willingness to subjugate their own moral reasoning—effectively censored the nursing perspective.

It is true that the physicians acted in an authoritative manner and never solicited nursing advice, but they had accomplices in this censorship. The nurses caring for Mr. S. chose to be silent: "No one openly questioned this decision." The words used by the nurse reporting this incident suggest that she and her peers were disturbed, even horrified, by the physicians' decision. Yet no nurse spoke up.

The nurses responded to their silencing with moral outrage. An emotional response to the inability to carry out moral choices or decisions, moral outrage is characterized by demoralizing frustration, anger, disgust, and a sense of powerlessness (Pike, 1991). The nurses were furious about the moral failure of Mr. S.'s care, yet they only blamed the physicians, failing to recognize their own contribution to this tragedy. Had any one of Mr. S.'s nurses defined herself as an equal colleague, instead of a helpless victim, a nurse's voice would have been heard, moral outrage would have been averted, and moral discourse would have ensued. In the end, Mr. S. most likely would have received more morally appropriate care.

In contrast, the following case illustrates the morally acceptable care that resulted from a nurse's choice to see herself as an integral and equal colleague of physicians.

> Mrs. H. had been a healthy, active 65-year-old woman until she suffered massive intracerebral bleeding. She showed severe neurological impairment, with only occasional and minimal responses to noxious stimuli. The prognosis for neurological recovery was grim. Mrs. H. had prepared a handwritten statement 2 years earlier, at the time of her husband's death from cancer. It was a request that her life not be sustained in the event of an irreversible illness or injury. A photocopy of this statement hung on the bulletin board in her room.
>
> Mrs. H's children, however, expressed their desire to pursue every treatment possible. They were adamant that they wanted their mother resuscitated in the event of a cardiac arrest. Mrs. H.'s physician felt obliged to comply with her children's wishes. I understood and respected his feeling of obligation, but found it morally conflicting. I suspect he did also.
>
> Mrs. H. was deteriorating daily. Aggressive, invasive care continued. I had to leave the room more than once during invasive procedures due to the assaultive nature of the treatments. I saw them [as being] clearly in opposition to Mrs. H.'s wishes.
>
> I spoke with her children and her physician each day. Although I could see and appreciate the agony they were experiencing in light of the massive ethical issues facing them, it was as if we were all speaking different dialects of the same language. We needed a three-way conversation to help us understand the perspectives each of us brought to the situation.
>
> I arranged a conference during which the patient's family, [the] physician, and I reviewed Mrs. H.'s condition and prognosis, and elaborated care plan options. Her family spoke of their grief and their feelings that they would be abandoning their mother if invasive treatments were discontinued. The physician and I explained that their mother would never be abandoned. We discussed how we could provide care for her in accordance with her wishes, and what the specifics of that care would be. In the end Mrs. H.'s family decided to change the aim of care and keep her comfortable until she died.

This is a difficult and poignant story. There was clearly a dilemma and clearly conflict. At an earlier point in her professional development, Mrs. H.'s nurse might have taken on the role of helpless victim and remained silent. The conflict would have simmered and bred moral outrage. Instead this nurse chose to see herself as an equal colleague who had the right, the duty, and the ability to facilitate discourse among all involved parties. In doing so she not only avoided her own moral outrage but also transformed the meaning of the situation from conflict to miscommunication. Her actions prompted a discussion that allowed all perspectives to be integrated into Mrs. H.'s care. Her exercise of nurses' voice changed the nature of care for this patient, making it more consistent with the patient's wishes and more comfortable for her family.

CONCLUSION

These critical incidents strongly suggest that the choice a nurse makes about how she defines her professional self affects not only her morale but also the nature of care her patients receive. When a nurse identifies herself as the victim of deeply rooted social and economic constraints, she increases the probability that her voice will be silenced. The stance of victimization can lead to feelings of moral outrage and denies patients the benefits of the nursing perspective. However, when a nurse makes the choice to define herself as a colleague, participating in patient care as an integral and equal member of the health care team, she seizes opportunities for professional fulfillment while affording patients the benefits of integrated care.

The responsibility and accountability for defining oneself as a colleague resides in individual nurses. Perhaps it does not seem fair that nurses, because they have inherited internal and external constraints to their professional identity, autonomy, and aspirations, now have to rescue themselves from subjugation. Perhaps it would seem fairer if those whose predecessors exploited nurses made concessions. Fairness aside, history shows that members of dominant groups do not generally offer restitution to those whom they have exploited (Steele, 1990). While growing numbers of physicians are to be commended for enlightened attitudes and behaviors, nurses will only grow increasingly frustrated by waiting for past injustices to be repaid.

While the issue of fairness will always linger, it is, ironically, fortunate that compensation is not forthcoming. For the possibility of compensation keeps the responsibility for collegiality with physicians and leads to the familiar slogan among nurses: "We're ready to be colleagues just as soon as the doctors change." Making colleageship dependent on changes among physicians maintains nurses as victims; it asks nonnurses to exercise nurses' voice. The only one who can declare herself an equal colleague is the individual nurse, and to do so she must emancipate herself from both internal and external constraints.

Nurses' choice to define themselves as colleagues, as full-fledged vital members of the health care team, holds great moral significance for nursing and for patient care. In making this choice, nurses take the opportunity to overcome subjugation and to assume a stance of empowerment. By defining themselves as equal colleagues, nurses initiate a move on their own behalf and on behalf of their patients to make their voice heard (Cooper, 1991). Such a professional self-concept is a prerequisite for, as well as a driving force in, the development of collaborative relationships with physicians, health care administrators, and, in this era of managed care, even with third-party payers. Collaboration unifies the contributions of all involved in patient care, making that care more efficient, effective, and comprehensive (Aiken, 1990; Knaus, Draper, Wagner, & Zimmerman, 1986; Pike, 1991; Prescott & Bowen, 1985). By choosing to make their voice heard, nurses afford patients not only the advantage of the nursing perspective but also the full benefit of integrated care. The promise this holds for advancing the care delivered to patients and families cannot be underestimated.

REFERENCES

Aiken, L.H. (1990). Charting the future of hospital nursing. *Image: The Journal of Nursing Scholarship, 22*(2), 72-78.

Alpert, H.B., Goldman, L.D., Kilroy, C.M., & Pike, A.W. (1992). 7 Gryzmish: Toward an understanding of collaboration. *Nursing Clinics of North America, 27*(1), 47-59.

Aradine, C.R., & Pridham, K.F. (1973). Model for collaboration. *Nursing Outlook, 21*(10), 655-657.

Belenky, M.F., Clinchy, B.M., Goldberger, N.R., & Tarule, J.M. (1986). *Women's ways of knowing.* Boston: Basic Books.

Benner, P. (1984). *From novice to expert.* Menlo Park, CA: Addison-Wesley.

Cooper, M.C. (1991). Response to moral outrage and moral discourse in nurse-physician collaboration. *Journal of Professional Nursing, 7*(6), 362-363.

Gadow, S.A. (1985). Nurse and patient: The caring relationship. In A.H. Bishop & J.R. Scudder (Eds.), *Caring, curing, coping: Nurse-physician-patient relationships.* (pp. 31-43). University, AL: University of Alabama Press.

Gilligan, C. (1982). *In a different voice.* Cambridge, MA: Harvard University Press.

Knaus, W.A., Draper, E.A., Wagner, D.P., & Zimmerman, J.E. (1986). An evaluation of outcome from intensive care in major medical centers. *Annals of Internal Medicine, 104*(3), 410-418.

Mangiardi, J.R., & Pellegrino, E.D. (1992). Collegiality: What is it? *Bulletin of the New York Academy of Medicine, 68*(2), 292-296.

Mayeroff, M. (1971). *On caring.* New York: HarperCollins.

Miller, J.B. (1976). *Toward a new psychology of women.* Boston, MA: Beacon Press.

Noddings, N. (1984). *Caring: A femine approach to ethics and moral education.* Los Angeles, CA: University of California Press.

Petro, J.A. (1992). Collegiality in history. *Bulletin of the New York Academy of Medicine, 68*(2), 292-296.

Pike, A.W. (1991). Moral outrage and moral discourse in nurse-physician collaboration. *Journal of Professional Nursing, 7*(6), 351-363.

Pike, A.W., & Alpert, H.B. (1994). Pioneering the future: The 7 North model of nurse-physician collaboration. *Nursing Administration Quarterly, 18*(4), 11-18.

Pike, A.W., McHugh, M., Canney, K., Miller, N., Reilly, P., & Seibert, C.P. (1993). A new architecture for quality assurance: Nurse-physician collaboration. *Journal of Nursing Care Quality, 7*(3), 1-8.

Prescott, P.A., & Bowen, S.A. (1985). Physician-nurse relationships. *Annals of Internal Medicine, 103*(127), 127-133.

Steele, S. (1990). *The content of our character.* New York: St. Martin's Press.

Stein, L.I. (1967). The doctor-nurse game. *Archives of General Psychiatry, 16*(6), 699-703.

Stein, L.I., Watts, D.T., & Howell, T. (1990). The doctor-nurse game revisited. *New England Journal of Medicine, 322*(8), 546-549.

Watson, J. (1988). *Nursing: Human science and human care.* New York: National League for Nursing.

Weiss, S.J., & Davis, H.P. (1985). Validity and reliability of the collaborative practice scales. *Nursing Research, 34*(5), 299-305.

Yarling, R.R., & McElmurry, B.J. (1986). The moral foundation of nursing. *Advances in Nursing Science, 8*(2), 63-73.

Collaboration between medical and nursing education in community-based settings

JOELLEN B. EDWARDS

Health care delivery in the United States, including the education of health professionals, is in an era of unprecedented change in all components of the system. Assumptions long held by the public, legislators, third-party payers, administrators, and health professionals themselves are being challenged daily. The acute care setting, once the nearly singular focal point for health professions education and practice, is giving way to the recognition that in order to meet the true health needs of populations, health professionals must go far beyond the walls of an institution to learn and to practice their disciplines.

The Pew Health Professions Commission (1993) provided a succinct statement of the competencies that will be needed by health professionals as the century turns (described in the box). In order to meet these competencies, educators and practitioners in all academic health professions must take a hard look at collective and individual values, beliefs, traditions, and structures. Our students become what we teach them, and our present system of educating nursing and medical professionals is fraught with barriers to facilitating the kinds of learning experiences that successful practitioners in the emerging delivery system will need. That education, however, holds the key to the realization of the kind of health care needed by people and envisioned in the Pew competency statements.

NURSING AND MEDICAL EDUCATION

Both nursing and medicine arose from the tradition of caring for the health and illness of people. However, as the disciplines became formally recognized, distinct differences in their educational patterns became institutionalized. After the Flexner Report in 1910, the medical profession organized university-based schools at the graduate level, creating the only path to the legal right to practice medicine. Nursing, even after the Goldmark Report in 1934, remained for many years closely aligned with hospital training schools. The autonomy and societal acceptance of medicine as a profession was readily established, while recognition of nursing as a profession was stifled until well into the 20th century. Medical schools fostered the development of autonomy and the idea that the physician was the decision maker and responsible party in all aspects of patient care. Until the relatively recent past, nursing schools fostered the development of subservience, strict adherence to policies and procedures, and support of the singular authority of the physician (Kalisch & Kalisch, 1977).

Separate courses of study created teaching patterns that remain largely discipline-specific. Historically, physicians have been accepted as teachers of nurses (Melosh, 1982), yet nurses are seldom called on to teach medical students. When nurses do teach physicians, it is often informal and disguised, as in the guiding of residents through their practice experiences (Prescott & Bowen, 1985). Nursing and medicine maintain different philosophical approaches to the education of students. Although there are more and more signs to indicate change, medicine has valued content, rationality, data, and assimilation of scientific information in their educational strategy over attention to the social and relational aspects of health care (Bloom, 1988; Greenlick, 1992). Nursing, on the other hand, values and teaches a more holistic and relational approach to caring for both well and ill persons (Lindeman, 1995). The values of the profession are transmitted through educational processes and approaches; a study by Wolf (1989) identifies the core values of nursing as centered on individuality of the person and a wholeness of mind, body, and spirit. Medicine's core values

COMPETENCIES FOR HEALTH CARE PROFESSIONALS

An ability to care for the community's health, including health-promoting activities appropriate to a diverse population

The provision of contemporary clinical care to meet public health needs

Participation in the emerging system with expanded accountability, especially with regard to innovative health care settings, interdisciplinary team arrangements, and responsiveness to the shape and direction of the health care system

Cost-effective and appropriate use of technology

Emphasis on prevention and healthy lifestyles

Patient and family involvement in decision making

Information management and dedication to lifelong learning

Note. From O'Neil, E. H. *Health Professions Education for the Future: School in Service to the Nation* (p. 8), by Pew Health Professions Commission, 1993; San Francisco, CA. Copyright 1993 by Pew Health Professions Commission. Adapted with permission.

were identified as responsibility for others and preservation of human life. These core values are reflected in the differing approaches to education, and consequently to practice, between the two disciplines.

One similarity between nursing and medical education stands out. The focus of educational experiences for both groups, since its emergence, has been the hospital as the predominant training site. Hospital care has made significant contributions over the years to the preservation of human life. While the acute care setting can offer ample opportunity for health professions students to learn to care for the extremely ill, it cannot introduce them to the ongoing needs of the majority of the population for health promotion, illness prevention, environmental health, and primary care services. Nor can it help the health professions student find his or her place in the larger world outside the hospital walls, as part of a community striving for the best possible environment for its citizens. The biggest difference in the lives of the most people can be made in the community.

COMMUNITY-BASED EDUCATION AND PRACTICE

Both medicine and nursing have begun approaching the challenge of community-based education and practice. Community-based education and practice tend to be perceived and defined differently by the two professions. Congruence with intraprofessional values is evident in the differences in approaches to defining and implementing community-based care. Nursing tends to view "community-based" as the incorporation of the whole of the community—homes, schools, shelters, stores, day care centers, primary care practices, and others—into the clinical education of nursing students and as sites for professional practice (Oermann, 1994).

Outside the community-oriented primary care movement (Nutting, Wood, & Conner, 1985), medicine more often views "community-based" as the incorporation into the medical school or residency curricula of precepted ambulatory care experiences in physicians' offices, and community-based practice as a physician enterprise outside the auspices of the university.

If the voice of prominent health care foundations, professional organizations, and national leadership is heard, community-based practice and education will evolve to be about far more than the site of clinical learning or care delivery. Community-based care is about a basic commitment by health professionals to come out of the ivory tower of academe and the hallowed hospital halls to work where the people are. The National League for Nursing (1993) discussed that commitment as "re-aligning our allegiance and accountability away from institutions and toward populations" (p. 7).

Community-based care requires a shift in power from institutions and expert professionals to community members in terms of creating accessible, affordable, and *acceptable* health services that will meet the needs of the population. People in communities, in partnership with professionals, define the health needs to be met and maintain control of the strategies for meeting those needs. This pattern is in direct opposition to the current system of education and practice, in which health care organizations and expert professionals decide what communities need and maintain control of the services offered.

In short, for students to emerge from health professions education programs ready to implement holistic, primary health care that meets population needs, significant changes in the approach to medical and nursing education that embrace and incorporate community-based philosophy will be necessary. Flexibility, creativity, and true collaboration among the disciplines and their communities will be the key to success.

COLLABORATION

Merriam-Webster's Collegiate Dictionary (1993) defines collaboration as "laboring together; working jointly, especially in an intellectual endeavor; cooperating with the enemy or opposing force; and cooperating with an agency with which one is not immediately connected" (Mish, 1993, p. 224). The American Nurses Association defines collaboration as follows:

> . . . a true partnership, in which the power on both sides is valued by both, with recognition and acceptance of separate and combined spheres of activity and responsibility, mutual safeguarding of the legitimate interests of each party, and a commonality of goals that is recognized by both parties. (American Nurses Association Social Policy Statement, 1995, p. 7)

Collaboration can also be viewed as a relationship in which individuals become increasingly invested in each other's success, to the benefit of all. Collaborators are willing to share information, alter their activities for the betterment of all concerned, share resources to accomplish a common goal, and willingly enhance the capacity of another to achieve a common purpose.

Several themes emerge from commonalities in these definitions and descriptions. First, collaboration is about empowerment. Empowerment is the ability of each involved party to find the strength from within to do what needs to be done for self or others. Empowerment is about mutual support of involved parties to find and exercise that power (Rappaport, 1984). It is *not* about coercive power over one another.

Second, collaboration is about relationships. Collaboration requires communication, and no communication exists outside the context of the relationship of the communicators (Coeling & Wilcox, 1994). Collaboration is only possible in relationships that are mutually respectful, open, direct, and assertive.

Third, collaboration is about synergy. Collaboration makes possible the achievement of a common goal in a way that is greater than the sum of the contributions made by each party. The knowledge and expertise of each person involved in the collaborative effort are recognized and valued and are freely given and accepted among the collaborators. Collaboration is not about competition, fragmentation, and condescension (Mariano, 1989).

Collaboration between nursing and medicine

Collaboration between medicine and nursing is an ideal long sought by many members of both professional groups. The idea that the two most predominant health professions would not collaborate is almost incomprehensible. Yet societal, professional, and economic forces mitigate against collaboration in education and practice.

Power relationships between the two disciplines have historically remained inequitable, with the clear balance of traditional forms of power in the hands of physicians (Doering, 1992; Kalisch & Kalisch, 1982). Nursing remains a predominantly female profession. Medicine is moving more rapidly to gender equity in terms of numbers entering the profession, yet socialization processes in medical school often "co-opt" women students into the traditional masculine approaches to power. The negative effects of traditional sex role stereotyping, despite efforts to equalize power between the genders, remain operational in relationships between the disciplines. Social class differences between nursing and medical career aspirants contribute to power differences as well. These differences, all of which are related to a form of power and influence, pose significant barriers to collaboration (Fagin, 1992).

There is evidence that traditional forms of physician power are eroding; physicians are acutely aware of threats to their autonomy and to the professional privileges they have enjoyed without question for so long (Friedman, 1994). Medical responses to this perceived threat that attempt to maintain the status quo, along with the slow but sure advancement of the legal and public recognition of nursing as a full partner in the health care system, may compromise collaborative efforts in the short term (Mowry & Korpman, 1987).

Relationships between nurses and physicians, expressed through communication, are also rooted in sex role stereotyping and development of the professions in inequitable patterns. Stein (1967) documented common communication styles between physicians and nurses, naming the dominant physician-deferential nurse pattern as "the doctor-nurse game." A follow-up study by Stein, Watts, and Howell (1990) revisited communication patterns and found that, to the dismay and frustration of some physicians, nurses had generally abandoned the submissive patterns of the past, moving to a more confrontational and direct style.

Other studies of communication that may directly affect the ability to develop effective collaborative relationships have been conducted. Kalisch and Kalisch (1977) identified sources of conflict in physician-nurse relationships that were roadblocks to effective communication. These included physician dominance and nurse deference, physician devaluation of nursing, lack of mutual knowledge about each profession, and different areas of emphasis by nurses and physicians in practice, among others. Prescott and Bowen (1985) found that the majority of nurses and physicians described their relationships as positive, yet when disagreements over patient care occurred, competition was most likely used to solve differences. Physicians frequently challenged the authority of nurses to make decisions and judgments, while nurses exhibited more accommodating and cooperating behavior than physicians.

Barriers to the synergy created through collaboration exist as well. The two professions are likely to differ in the areas of problem identification and mutual goal setting, which are two key elements of collaboration (Jones, 1994). The differing value systems of nursing and medicine contribute to disparity rather than cohesiveness in goal setting in patient care situations (Haddad, 1991; Wolf, 1989). Less valuing of nurses' opinions and judgments by physicians than vice versa has been documented, with nurses required to establish their credibility again and again (Prescott & Bowen, 1985). Physicians may confuse professional expertise with moral authority (Haddad, 1991) and may view themselves as holding ultimate authority and responsibility for every facet of health care (Friedman, 1994; Makadon & Gibbons, 1985; Steel, 1986). When outdated, stereotypical ideas of the omnipotence of physicians and the subservience of nurses are held by members of either profession, a significant barrier to effective collaboration is maintained.

Despite barriers, evidence of effective collaboration between the disciplines gives hope for success in the critical endeavor of changing the way health care is delivered through community-based, interdisciplinary education. Positive outcomes have been documented across many settings (Baggs, Ryan, Phelps, Richeson, & Johnson, 1992; Maguire, 1994; Middleton & Whitney, 1993; Pacheco et al., 1991).

One of the most effective national efforts to demonstrate collaboration between nursing, medicine, and other health professionals has come about as a result of the W. K. Kellogg Foundation's initiative to redirect health professions education toward interdisciplinary, community-based, primary care (Richards, 1996). In the seven sites selected to create and implement health professions education according to these principles, nursing, medical, and other health professions such as pharmacy, public health, and social work study and practice together outside hospital settings. Their learning is under the direction of an interdisciplinary faculty for significant portions of their professional education. The result has been increased levels of care in underserved communities, a deeper understanding and appreciation for the contributions of all health professionals to care, and significant empowerment of the community to define and meet their own health care needs.

Interdisciplinary collaboration between nursing and medicine is not only possible; it is working in some areas of practice. The beginning of adopting collaboration as the norm for health professionals rather than as the exception starts with the education of nursing and medical students as well as students from other health disciplines (Fagin, 1992; Forbes & Fitzsimons, 1993; McEwen, 1994).

Collaboration among health professions and the community

The establishment of a collaborative relationship between members of health professions and communities has remained as elusive as collaborative relationships among health professionals from various disciplines. Health professionals have been notorious for their domination of the planning and implementation of health care systems (Osborne & Gaebler, 1992). Health care services are organized on the turf of professionals; are offered at times convenient to professionals rather than users; and are often implemented without regard for the true needs of the population to be served. A narrow focus on illness and acute care, the area in which many health professionals are most comfortable, is more common than attention to the health promotion and illness prevention strategies sought by community members. The ability to pay is more often the driving force in availability of services than is true need.

Health professionals hold expert power in medicine or nursing and often hold positional power in society (Kalisch & Kalisch, 1982). Implementation of a power rather than the empowerment model has created an imbalance in the power relationships among health care providers and users of health care systems. Educational and economic gaps between health professionals and members of some communities pose an additional barrier to collaboration. Community members may believe they have nothing to offer or may feel helpless to influence highly educated experts in health fields.

Relationships among community members and health professionals, expressed through communicative processes, can be problematic. Health professionals maintain their own "language" that, sometimes unintentionally, excludes those who do not understand medical terminology. Professional jargon, or conversely, colloquial terminology, can lead to unshared or misinterpreted meanings among potential collaborators (Northouse & Northouse, 1985). The ability to understand each other effectively is critical to collaboration.

When community members and health professionals do come together to set goals for improving health and well-being, different perspectives often emerge. Values, beliefs, and priorities can be highly divergent (Cortes, 1986). Difficulty in valuing and appreciating the contributions of both community members and professionals can arise. Collaboration with community, like collaboration among professionals, is a process of sharing power and appreciating diverse expertise. Palmer (1990) defines community as "a gift to be received, not a goal to be achieved" (p. 4). The power of collaboration with the community can only be realized by the willingness of those who hold traditional power to give it away (Richards, 1993).

Collaboration between nursing and medicine in community-based settings: a case study

In 1990, the Colleges of Nursing and Medicine at East Tennessee State University were approached by business and governmental leaders from a rural mountain community for assistance in rebuilding their shattered health care system. Unemployment had skyrocketed to 35%. The small local hospital had closed due to financial distress after the loss of 9 of the county's 12 physicians. The need to re-create a viable health care system was identified by these leaders as essential to attracting new businesses and building tourism in the beautiful Blue Ridge Mountain setting. Their first priority was primary care for citizens who were isolated from health services by long distances and dangerous mountain roads. The Health Sciences Division of East Tennessee State University, whose mission encompasses a commitment to rural health care, was a natural ally in their quest to strengthen their community through better health.

The foundations for collaboration among the community, nursing, medicine, and public health sectors were laid. By September 1990, two clinics opened in Mountain City, Tennessee. One was a traditional medical clinic, operated by the Family Medicine Department of the Quillen College of Medicine, and the other was a primary care practice operated by nurse practitioner faculty from the College of Nursing (Edwards, 1994; Edwards, Lenz, & East-Odom). The nursing clinic was initially dedicated to evening and weekend primary care, to health promotion activities for the citizens of the county, and to the demonstration of nurse-managed primary care as an effective source of health services. An extensive longitudinal community assessment was conducted by multidisciplinary faculty from the Health Science Division and community members. Significant investment in the form of facilities, equipment, moral support, and advice and direction for the endeavor was extended by the community. Nursing and medicine made the first ventures toward collaboration through a bridge between the nursing and medical clinics created by the engagement of a family medicine physician as a preceptor for the nurse practitioners, by mutual referrals, and by involvement in community-based activities (Pullen, Edwards, Lenz, & Alley, 1994).

In 1991, the Health Sciences Division received a 5-year, $6 million W. K. Kellogg Foundation Community Partnerships grant to further develop the collaborative efforts among the community, medicine, nursing, and public health sectors, and to implement a model for rural, interdisciplinary, community-based primary care education for health professions students. Johnson County was selected as the first educational site, with Hawkins County scheduled to become operational 1 year later.

The first grant year was spent in building the primary care practices in Johnson County, learning to work together, documenting and analyzing with community members the need for health services, refining the administrative structure that would support the effort, and creating an interdisciplinary, rural, and community-based primary care curriculum. Twenty-five percent of all nursing and medical content was to be offered through this hands-on, community-based format. Interdisciplinary students would study and practice together in the community for 25% of their time for a minimum of 2 years, with activities continuing into a third year of guided interdisciplinary practice and community projects. Nursing chose to deliver the majority of its entire curriculum through the community-based approach for students enrolled at the Johnson County site, and later, at the Hawkins County site.

All disciplines sought and successfully attracted faculty who would live as well as work in the rural communities, thus increasing the deep human connections that are so critical to the success of this unique endeavor. Community boards, set up to guide and direct the project, were instrumental in attracting faculty and students. In 1992, the first cohort of nursing, medical, and public health students entered what became known as the Rural Primary Care track. In 1993, cohorts of interdisciplinary students were entered into both Hawkins and Johnson Counties; admissions of up to 25% of nursing and medical classes consistently enter the Rural Primary Care track today.

At times, the problems faced in interdisciplinary and community collaboration in the implementation of such a unique and challenging effort seemed overwhelming. Faculty who didn't know each other were thrown into an intense year of negotiation over what content would comprise a rural, community-based interdisciplinary curriculum that would meet the needs of nursing, medical, and public health students. Even the language that would be used to describe the same phenomenon had to be agreed upon. For instance, are the people who are offered health services called *patients* or *clients?* Are hands-on techniques for gathering data about the patient/client called physical *assessments* or physical *examinations?* Myths and stereotypes on all sides had to be given up. Some gave up the ghost easily, some died hard, and after 5 years of working together, some reappear from the grave to haunt us occasionally! A full range of emotions, from anger and mistrust to joy and elation, were encountered and had to be addressed.

Long-cherished stereotypes held by the community about academe and by academe about the community had to be given up on all sides as well. Myths about "ivory tower university types" came tumbling down as deans, faculty, and community members worked together intellectually and physically to prepare space and move equipment and supplies. Any idea that rural people were not interested in planning for the health of their community, or were too backward to state their needs, disappeared quickly. Respect and true friendship grew rapidly among representatives from the university and community members.

Outcomes at this point in time can be viewed through the lens of collaboration. Evidence of increasing empowerment, rather than "power-over," is clear. Community members are 51% of the voting members of the Executive Board. Leaders in the two communities have been instrumental in budget, recruitment, planning, teaching from a community perspective, caring for students, promoting legislative awareness of rural health needs, and most of all, building the health services needed by community members. Faculty have learned to trust, value, and actively seek the contributions of community members. The feeling of community members that they have indeed shaped their own health care system is strong.

Empowerment of faculty and students is evident as well. Over the years of the project, students have taken an increasingly active role in shaping their own experiences and those of the classes to follow, with their most recent formal activity being full participation in a curriculum planning retreat. At the retreat the students' ease in stating their views and ideas to administrators, faculty, and community members was apparent. Nursing, medical, and public health faculty have learned to value the contributions to the whole made by each discipline. Faculty who have been involved over time are as cognizant of the needs of each discipline's individual curriculum as they are of their own. The interdisciplinary curriculum is owned, influenced, and implemented by all.

Relationships, expressed through communication among participants, have changed over the years of working in close quarters. While all relationships are subject to individual idiosyncrasies, trust, respect, and friendship among most members are evolving. Interpersonal conflict still occurs, but conflict is more often attributed to individual styles rather than to a stereotypical "that's how that profession is" attitude, which occurred in the beginning of the endeavor. Competitive styles of handling conflict are used less frequently. The level of trust necessary for direct and open communication, rather than game playing, is increasingly present. Disagreements are resolved through compromise and negotiation whenever possible, whereas in the beginning of the project, appeal to a perceived higher authority was common.

Without question, the synergy created by collaboration among the disciplines and the community has facilitated a far greater set of achievements than any profession or community could accomplish alone. The most frequent value disagreement that still occurs is the belief, strongly held by some (not all) physicians, that he or she is the party ultimately responsible for all health care. Yet the adoption of core values for the project and mutual goal setting consistent with those values has afforded multiple accomplishments. The box depicts only a few.

SUMMARY

Community-based, multidisciplinary education and practice for health professions students is the wave of the future. It is the way the health needs of populations will be met. Health care economics, professional altruism, and the voices of the people who need accessible, affordable, and acceptable health care take away the choice to remain cloistered within hospital walls and isolated as professional groups. Entering into a commitment to collaborate

OUTCOMES OF EAST TENNESSEE'S COMMUNITY PARTNERSHIP PROJECT

Creation of a broad spectrum of primary care services in underserved areas

Development of academic, community-based, rural health systems

Completion of research projects in primary care

25% of nursing and medical curriculum taught together in the community for rural track students

Standardized test results of graduates and students equal to or better than those in traditional study

Ongoing community assessment and needs analysis by community members, faculty, and students

Increased valuing of wellness in partner communities

Creation of a direct state appropriation for rural, primary care education

Changes in traditional nursing and medical curricula based on the success of interdisciplinary, community-based activities

State policy changes that favor interdisciplinary care delivery

Development of further community/provider partnerships in areas such as teen pregnancy, childhood immunizations, cancer prevention, wellness activities, women's health, and others

to achieve this goal requires patience, persistence, communication skill, willingness to trust past opponents, incredibly hard work, and most of all, an unshakable inner belief that this is the right thing to do. When it works, the results are beyond the highest hopes.

REFERENCES

American Nurses Association (1995). *Nursing: A social policy statement,* 7, Washington, DC.

Baggs, J., Ryan, S., Phelps, C., Richeson, J., & Johnson, J. (1992). Collaboration in critical care: The association between interdisciplinary collaboration and patient outcomes in a medical intensive care unit. *Heart & Lung, 21*(1), 18-24.

Bloom, S. (1988). Structure and ideology in medical education: An analysis of resistance to change. *Journal of Health and Social Behavior, 29,* 294-306.

Coeling, H., & Wilcox, J. (1994). Steps to collaboration. *Nursing Administration Quarterly, 18*(4), 44-45.

Cortes, E., Jr. (1986, July 11). Organizing the community. *The Texas Observer* (10-16).

Doering, L. (1992). Power and knowledge in nursing: A feminist poststructuralist view. *Advances in Nursing Science, 14*(4), 24-33.

Edwards, J. (1994). Achieving FNP care for an Appalachian community. *NP News, 2*(1), 1, 4.

Edwards, J., Lenz, C., & East-Odom, J. (1993). Nurse-managed primary care: Serving a rural Appalachian population. *Family/Community Health, 16*(2), 50-56.

Fagin, C. (1992). Collaboration between nurses & physicians: No longer a choice. *Nursing & Health Care, 13*(7), 354-363.

Flexner, A. (1910). *Medical education in the United States and Canada.* D.B. Updike. Boston, MA: The Merrymount Press.

Forbes, E., & Fitzsimons, V. (1993). Education: The key for holistic interdisciplinary collaboration. *Holistic Nurse Practice, 4*(7), 1-10.

Friedman, E. (1994). The power of physicians: Autonomy and balance in a changing system. *National Health Policy Forum,* 1-9.

Greenlick, M. (1992). Educating physicians for population-based clinical practice. *Journal of the American Medical Association, 267*(12), 1645-1648.

Goldmark, J. (1923). *Nursing and nursing education in the United States.* New York: Macmillan.

Haddad, A. (1991). Ethics. *AORN Journal, 53*(1), 151-156.

Jones, R. (1994). Conceptual development of nurse-physician collaboration. *Holistic Nursing Practice, 8*(3), 38-53.

Kalisch, B., & Kalisch, P. (1977). An analysis of the sources of physician-nurse conflict. *Journal of Nursing Administration, 7*(1), 50-57.

Kalisch, B., & Kalisch, P. (1982). *Politics of nursing.* Philadelphia: Lippincott.

Lindeman, C. (1995). *Refocusing undergraduate nursing education.* Atlanta, GA: Southern Council on Collegiate Education for Nursing in affiliation with the Southern Regional Education Board.

Maguire, D. (1994). Multidisciplinary collaboration in neonatal intensive care. *Nursing Administration Quarterly, 18*(4), 18-22.

Makadon, H., & Gibbons, M. (1985). Nurses and physicians: Prospects for collaboration [editorial]. *Annals of Internal Medicine, 103*(1), 134-136.

Mariano, C. (1989). The case for interdisciplinary collaboration. *Nursing Outlook, 37*(6), 285-288.

McEwen, M. (1994). Promoting interdisciplinary collaboration. *Nursing & Health Care, 15*(6), 304-307.

Melosh, B. (1982). *The physician's hand: Work culture and conflict in American nursing.* Philadelphia: Temple University Press.

Mish, F. (Ed.). (1993). *Merriam-Webster's collegiate dictionary.* Springfield, MA: Merriam-Webster, Inc.

Middleton, E., & Whitney, F. (1993). Primary care in the emergency room; A collaborative model. *Nursing Connections, 6*(2), 29-40.

Mowry, M., & Korpman, R. (1987). Hospitals, nursing, and medicine: The years ahead. *Journal of Nursing Administration, 17*(11), 16-22.

National League for Nursing (1993). *A vision for nursing education.* New York: The National League for Nursing.

Northouse, P., & Northouse, L. (1985). *Health communication.* Englewood Cliffs, NJ: Prentice Hall.

Nutting, P., Wood, M., & Conner, E. (1985). Community oriented primary care. *Journal of the American Medical Association, 253*(12), 1763-1766.

Oerman, M. (1994). Reforming nursing education for future practice. *Journal of Nursing Education, 33*(5), 215-219.

O'Neil, E.H. (1993). *Health professions education for the future: School in service to the nation.* Pew Health Professions Commission. San Francisco, CA.

Osborne, D., & Gaebler, T. (1992). Community-owned government: Empowering rather than serving. In *Reinventing government: How the entrepreneurial spirit is transforming the public sector.* (pp. 49-75). Reading, MA: Addison-Wesley.

Palmer, P. (1990). Scarcity, abundance, and the gift of community. *Community Renewal Press, 1*(3), 1-5.

Pacheco, M., Adelsheim, S., Davis, L., Mancha, V., Aime, L., Nelson, P., Derksen, D., & Kaufmann, A. (1991). Innovation, peer teaching, and multidisciplinary collaboration: Outreach from a school-based clinic. *Journal of School Health, 61*(8), 367-369.

Pullen, C., Edwards, J., Lenz, C., & Alley, N. (1994). A comprehensive primary health care delivery model. *Journal of Professional Nursing, 10*(4), 201-208.

Prescott, P., & Bowen, S. (1985). Physician-nurse relationships. *Annals of Internal Medicine, 103*(1), 127-133.

Rappaport, J. (1984). Studies in empowerment: Introduction to the issue. *Prevention in Human Services, 3,* 1-7.

Richards, R. (1993). Observations on redirection of an iceberg: Leading educational reform in medical schools. *Annals of Community-Oriented Education, 6,* 207-217.

Richards, R. (Ed.). (1996). Building partnerships: Educating health professionals for the communities they serve. San Francisco, CA: Jossey-Bass.

Steel, E. (1986). *Issues in collaborative practice.* Orlando, FL: Grune & Stratton.

Stein, L. (1967). The doctor-nurse game. *Archives of General Psychiatry, 16*(6), 699-703.

Stein, L., Watts, D., & Howell, T. (1990). The doctor-nurse game revisited. *New England Journal of Medicine, 322*(8), 546-549.

Wolf, B. (1989). *Nursing identity: The nursing-medicine relationship.* Denver, CO: Denver Bookbinding Co., Inc.

Nurses and physician assistants: Issues and challenges

VIRGINIA KLINER FOWKES, JANET MENTINK

The concept of the profession of physician assistants (PAs) began in the mid-1960s as a response to widespread concern about the geographic and specialty maldistribution of health personnel, particularly physicians. There was a recognized need to improve access to primary care services for medically underserved rural and urban populations. The first training of PAs began at Duke University in 1965 when Eugene A. Stead, M.D. initiated a 2-year program with four ex-military corpsmen. Oddly enough, this followed a collaborative project in the late 1950s and early 1960s with a member of the nursing faculty, Thelma Ingles, who was training nurse practitioners (NPs) through the master's program. The National League for Nursing denied accreditation for the graduate program on three different occasions, suggesting that the assumption of medical tasks by nurses was inappropriate and potentially dangerous (Bliss & Cohen, 1977). Without accreditation, the NP training was discontinued. Unfortunately, considerable acrimony arose between medical and nursing leaders as a result of these decisions. Stead then turned his attention to another source of clinically experienced personnel—corpsmen who were returning from the Vietnam War and were interested in civilian roles in health care.

Stead's vision of a new role in primary care was shared by other medical and nursing leaders of the time. Their intent was to recruit individuals with patient care experience and prepare them with the skills necessary to practice primary care in rural settings or with medically underserved populations. NP programs began to develop shortly thereafter. As of 1995, there were approximately 25,000 PAs in active practice (Advisory Group on Physician Assistants and the Workforce, 1994). The American Academy of Physician Assistants (AAPA) has adopted the following definition of a PA:

> Physician assistants are health professionals licensed to practice medicine with physician supervision. Physician assistants are qualified by graduation from an accredited physician assistant educational program and/or certification by the National Commission on Certification of Physician Assistants. Within the physician/PA relationship, physician assistants exercise autonomy in medical decisionmaking and provide a broad range of diagnostic and therapeutic services. The clinical role of physician assistants includes primary and specialty care in medical and surgical practice settings in rural and urban areas. Physician assistant practice is centered on patient care and may include educational, research and administrative activities. (AAPA, 1995)

EDUCATION OF PHYSICIAN ASSISTANTS

Through the Health Resources Administration, Bureau of Health Manpower, the federal government provided funding for most of the initial PA training programs. The federal program did not restrict training to medical schools. Rather, to provide closer ties with ambulatory settings, programs were encouraged to offer the required basic and clinical sciences in other academic settings.

As of 1995, there were 80 PA programs throughout the United States offering a variety of academic options and different approaches to clinical training. The number of new programs is increasing to accommodate the demand for PAs in the marketplace. The majority of programs are affiliated with academic health centers, medical schools, or 4-year colleges and universities. A few others are sponsored by community colleges, the military, or hospitals. The majority of programs (61%) award a baccalaureate

The authors thank Nancy Hughes of the American Academy of Physician Assistants for her expert review of this manuscript.

degree, 19% a master's degree, 8% an associate degree, and 13% a certificate only (Simon et al., 1996).

The typical program is 24 months in length and includes instruction in basic and behavioral/social science; physical assessment and clinical medicine; and supervised clinical rotations, clerkships, and preceptorships. All programs teach an average of 70 hours of pharmacology. Basic science courses include anatomy, physiology, microbiology, biochemistry, nutrition, epidemiology, and others. Behavioral/social sciences typically include content about psychosocial aspects of care, health promotion, medical ethics, professional role development, human sexuality, health care systems, and multicultural needs, among other topics. Following this background, PA programs provide instruction in interviewing skills, patient education, and basic counseling techniques. Clinical instruction takes place in a variety of primary care specialties including family medicine, general internal medicine, obstetrics and gynecology, pediatrics, and geriatrics. Most of the primary care training is conducted in hospital outpatient clinics, community clinics, private physician practices, or other ambulatory settings where PAs learn to care for clients of all ages. Most PA programs in the western states have preceptorships based in community outpatient or office practice settings where students receive almost all of their clinical training. The preceptorships are often located in medically underserved areas, and some programs require a preselection student-preceptor match. The programs utilize a multidisciplinary faculty including PAs, physicians, basic and social scientists, pharmacists, and NPs.

BACKGROUNDS OF PHYSICIAN ASSISTANTS

Physician assistant education builds on students' academic, clinical, and life experiences. Over half (53%) have bachelor's degrees on program entry, 8% hold master's degrees, and 1% hold doctoral degrees. Others have associate degrees or other academic preparation. The vast majority have an average of 4.5 years of health care experience. PAs may have clinical backgrounds as nurses, emergency medical technicians, physical or respiratory therapists, pharmacists, laboratory technicians, health aides, or other occupations. Among the entering 1995 class, 60% were women and 40% were men; the majority (63%) were over 27 years of age. Twenty-two percent were ethnic minorities (Simon et al., 1996).

There are regional differences in both the background characteristics and training of PAs. For example, students in the central and western states tend to be older and to have more health care experiences than students in other areas (Simon et al., 1996; Fowkes & McKay, 1990). Most programs in the western states utilize community-based ambulatory settings as opposed to hospital inpatient areas for the majority of clinical training.

NATIONAL CERTIFICATION AND STATE LICENSURE

To qualify for PA licensure, almost all states require graduation from a program accredited by the Commission on Accreditation of Allied Health Education Programs and passage of the Physician Assistant National Certifying Examination. The examination is rigorous, with both written comprehensive and clinical practicum components. To maintain national certification, PAs obtain 100 hours of continuing medical education every 2 years and recertify by examination every 6 years. Some states have well-defined licensing procedures, whereas in others the process is more flexible, taking the form of a registry. State laws also vary in the provisions for PA practice. Most enable broad functions in any health care setting (Gara, 1989).

Physician assistants are supervised by physicians who delegate a broad range of medical tasks. The manner of supervision varies according to state law. Examples include one-to-one review of patient care; regular review of chart notes; remote supervision where the PA seeks consultation by telephone; and protocols or standardized procedures, where physicians and PAs establish in writing the procedures and plans necessary for the care of specific client problems.

ROLES OF PHYSICIAN ASSISTANTS

The PA functions as a member of the health care team. The 1994 survey by the AAPA of its 16,524 members (77% response rate) reveals that PAs practice in a variety of specialties (Fig. 73-1). Almost half (48%) practice in primary care, including family practice, general internal medicine, obstetrics and gynecology, and general pediatrics. Others are in surgery (17%), emergency medicine (9%), orthopedics (8%), industrial medicine (3%), or other subspecialties (15%) (AAPA, 1994-1995).

The practice settings of PAs also vary (Fig. 73-2). The vast majority (70%) practice in outpatient settings. Eighteen percent are employed in areas with a population of 10,000 or fewer, and 9% live in areas of 5,000 or less.

With the increasing proliferation of managed care systems, the services of PAs (and NPs as well) are in great demand. PAs can manage approximately 80% of health

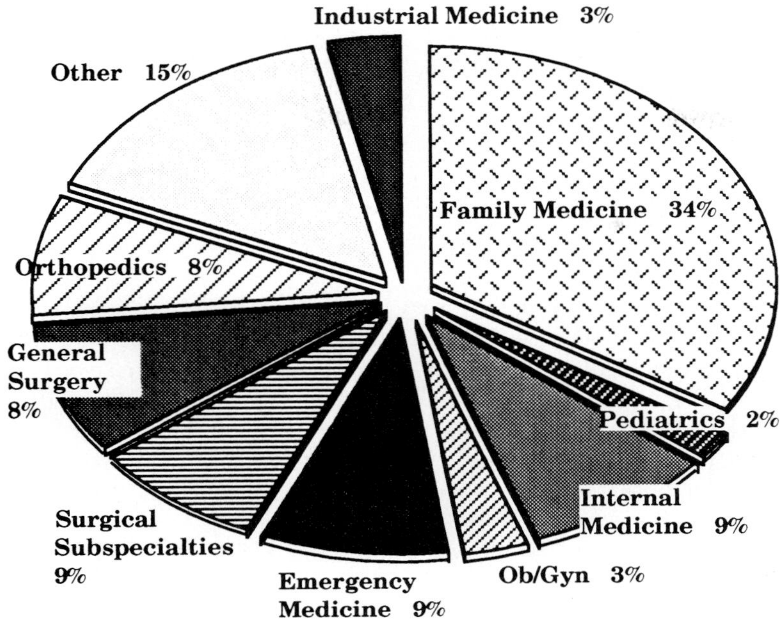

Fig. 73-1. Practice specialties of physician assistants. (From the American Academy of Physician Assistants. Used with permission.)

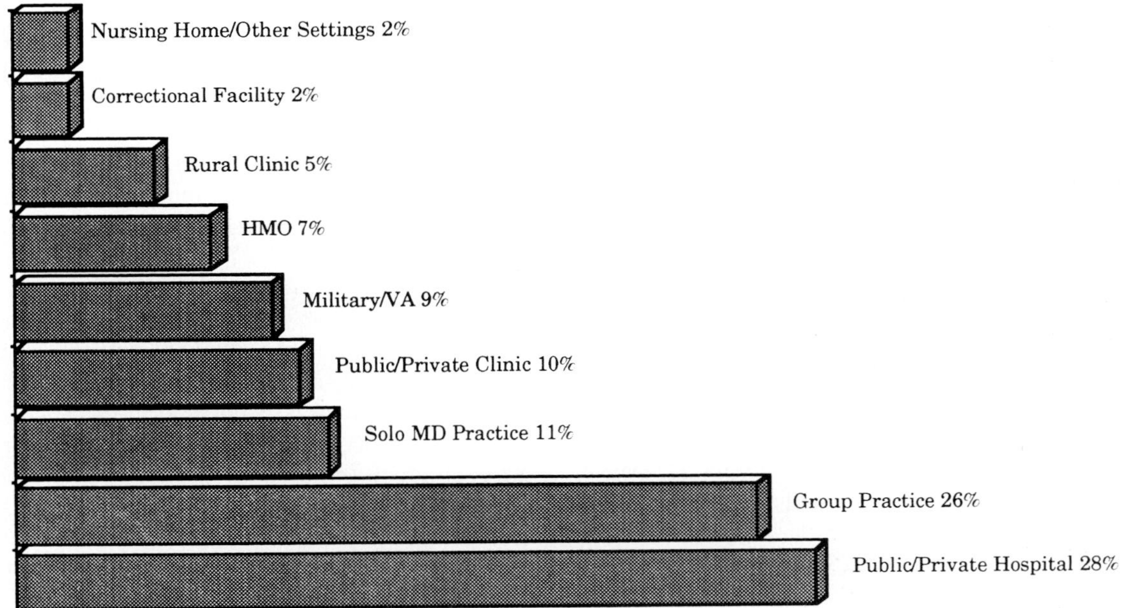

Fig. 73-2. Practice settings of physician assistants. (From the American Academy of Physician Assistants. Used with permission.)

care services required in ambulatory settings. PA clinical productivity is comparable to that of physicians, particularly in organized ambulatory settings where team approaches and structured division of staffing are present (Jones & Cawley, 1994).

A profession is sometimes defined as a unique body of knowledge, tasks, skills, or responsibilities. The PA profession overlaps with other professions, particularly physicians. PAs both substitute for and augment services customarily performed by physicians. They substitute for physicians by performing routine care such as health maintenance and by allowing physicians more time for complex problems. PAs expand the numbers of clients receiving care in the practice setting and often extend services for physicians in nursing homes, client homes, or satellite clinics. PAs augment physician services when their own clinical skills offer new services. PAs have considerable expertise in health education, and their former clinical backgrounds influence their practice. For example, a PA with a background in nutrition brings new knowledge and services in counseling to a practice. A female PA with a special interest in women's health may attract more women to a group practice of male physicians.

There are both nonnegotiable and negotiable aspects of the PA role. Nonnegotiable is that all PAs function under the supervision of physicians. The PA profession is dependent on the laws and regulations that govern practice and define the PA's relationship to the physician. However, the PA performs services independently or interdependently with the health care team. In other words, the PA has an independent role within a dependent practice arrangement (Schaft & Cawley, 1987).

The negotiable aspects of the PA role are numerous. PAs influence their duties and responsibilities by negotiating their own practice preferences and functioning as coordinators with clinical and management tasks interspersed or as case managers for a particular group of clients.

A role delineation study conducted by the AAPA in 1985 found distinct differences in practice characteristics among PAs in various specialties. However, nine clusters of activities were common to PAs in any practice: (1) gathering data, (2) seeing common problems and diseases, (3) conducting laboratory and diagnostic studies, (4) performing management activities, (5) performing surgical procedures, (6) managing emergency situations, (7) conducting health promotion and disease prevention activities, (8) prescribing medications, and (9) using interpersonal skills in patient education and counseling (Schaft & Cawley, 1987).

PHYSICIAN ASSISTANTS AND NURSE PRACTITIONERS

Physician assistants are often compared with NPs (discussed in Section 1), and it is useful to understand the similarities and differences between these two groups of professionals who often practice in the same settings. With regard to similarities, both the PA and NP professions were established in the mid- to late 1960s by their medicine and nursing counterparts in response to the needs for more primary care services. Studies of both PAs and NPs document that they increase access to care in rural areas and to underserved populations; provide high-quality care; decrease costs of medical care to employers and society; and provide care that is generally satisfying to patients, particularly the interpersonal aspects of care (U.S. Congress, Office of Technology Assessment, 1986).

Many settings employ both PAs and NPs, posting the same job descriptions and salary structure for both and utilizing the same mechanism for physician collaboration and supervision. The tasks and roles or *functions* of PAs and NPs within the same specialty (e.g., family practice) and in the same setting are very similar. Other similarities can be noted in the goals of some programs, particularly those targeting underserved populations, and in the components of curricula (e.g., management of patients with chronic disease or skills in taking a patient history or performing a physical examination) (Fowkes et al., 1979; Clawson & Osterweis, 1993). In California, two programs train PAs and NPs jointly with the same curriculum (Fowkes et al., 1979; Clawson & Osterweis, 1993).

There are also numerous differences among and within these professions, including practitioner backgrounds and educational, legal, professional, and political considerations. With regard to *background*, NPs are licensed registered nurses, whereas PAs enter training with a variety of backgrounds, some being nurses. The *educational preparation* of PAs was developed initially by physicians, and most training programs have been established with strong attachments to medical schools and academic health centers. The majority of programs provide baccalaureate degrees, although the number of master's programs is increasing. In contrast, educational programs for NPs are largely within schools of nursing. While a few certificate programs remain, the majority of NP education occurs at the master's level. NP students build on their skills in advanced nursing practice. The National Organization of Nurse Practitioner Faculties (NONPF) has developed guidelines for curriculum in several domains that include components in research and administration and set a useful national standard. This document recommends multiple pathways for attaining skills and advanced degree requisites (Zimmer et al., 1992).

There has been considerable discussion about differences in the educational preparation of PAs and NPs. One common, somewhat confusing comment refers to PA education as the "medical model" and NP education as the "nursing model." A careful examination of curricula for both types of programs reveals many similarities in content. For example, although different labels may be used, such as "behavioral science" in PA programs and "psychosocial" in NP programs, the emphasis within both of these components includes the development of sensitive skills in taking histories from clients, formulating plans, conducting education, and advocating empowerment. Any program at the master's level, whether PA or NP, has a research component. Nursing programs include nursing theory, whereas PA programs do not. In addition, PA programs tend to have a multidisciplinary faculty, while in most NP programs the majority of didactic and most clinical training is conducted by nursing faculty.

Other differences occur in specialty training within and across disciplines. All PAs are trained as primary care generalists. In addition, there are accredited postgraduate programs for PAs in women's health, neonatal, or surgical specialties. Similarly, there are numerous NP program specialties (e.g., family, adult, obstetrics-gynecology, pediatrics, and geriatrics).

Each discipline has its own educational organizations, accrediting body, and certification procedures. The Association of Physician Assistant Programs is the organization of PA educational programs. PA accrediting and certifying bodies have been discussed previously. For NPs, NONPF is the association of NP educators. The National League for Nursing is responsible for accreditation of nursing programs. The American Nurses Credentialing Center sponsors examinations in several specialties for individual NP national certification. In addition, some specialties have their own national certification examinations. However, states vary considerably in licensure requirements for NP practice, and some do not require national certification (Clawson & Osterweis, 1993).

There are *legal* differences in licensure requirements, reimbursement, and state practice acts. While these factors differ substantially from state to state, PAs generally practice under some provision of the states' medical practice acts and under the direct supervision of physicians. NPs practice under nursing licensure and provisions made in nurse practice acts for collaborative practice when the functions of nursing practice and medical practice overlap.

Professional differences are important to recognize. NPs identify with their nursing backgrounds. PAs and NPs have their own national professional organizations. The only national organization to represent PAs in all medical specialties is the AAPA; for NPs, there are multiple national organizations in the various specialties, all of which have representatives to the National Alliance of Nurse Practitioners.

Lastly, there are *political differences,* generated by the disparate origins and unfortunate beginnings in antagonism and conflict between organized medicine and nursing as well as by the assumptions of the educational programs. Political differences are accentuated locally where there is competition for employment sites or around state legislative issues, such as privileges for practice, reimbursement, or prescribing. Even within the PA or NP disciplines these sensitivities exist. An awareness of these sensitivities is critical in working with PAs and NPs in the same setting. Acknowledging similarities where they exist (e.g., in goals or purposes) and respecting differences are necessary parts of collaborative efforts.

In some regions, such as California, there is evidence of educational and professional collaboration between the two disciplines (Fowkes et al., 1979). For nearly a decade, the California Council on NP and PA Programs, an organization of all NP and PA program directors, met regularly to pursue common political interests toward improving legislation. Practicing PAs and NPs have developed local professional organizations for the purposes of continuing education, peer support, and local political strength. Recently, the PA and NP state professional organizations have agreed to exchange and publish information in each other's newsletters. Nationally, a group of PA and NP practitioners has collaborated to form a professional journal that sponsors a national conference.

AREAS OF ROLE CONFLICT

Nurses may be employed in any of the settings in which PAs practice—the most common of which are hospitals. The interaction between nurses and PAs in settings of common practice is either as parallel figures in patient care or in an assisting nurses function. Legally, PAs are agents of physicians; they order procedures, treatments, or prescriptions on behalf of physicians. Nurses, then, interact with PAs much as they would with physicians, as comembers of the health care team. Periodically, however, there is conflict in the intersection of their roles. The conflict may be the result of personalities, unclear institutional policies or state regulation and practice acts, or a misunderstanding of roles due to previous bias or lack of exposure. Role conflict can be related to issues associated with gender, competition for salaries or jobs, or confusion about local or state professional policies or laws.

Gender issues

The number of women entering the PA profession has increased substantially since its formative years, and today women represent a majority of PA student enrollment and graduate practitioners. The PA movement evolved along with a national women's movement characterized by many women reentering the workforce or broadening their career options. However, for the first decade, the PA profession was dominated by men. Thus both subtle and overt male-female issues are evident as their roles intersect. More subtle are issues about style. For example, the PA profession has its roots in medicine, a profession still dominated by men. Men tend to be more comfortable working or leading in a solo style. Women have typically learned a participatory, collaborative style in work and decision making. Such differences in style may create conflict when male PAs interact with female nurses over the care and management of patients. Perhaps as the gender gaps lessen in these health professions, such perceptions will be mitigated.

A more specific issue concerns salary differences. Some nurses are uncomfortable when PAs earn higher salaries than them. Because salary scales for any profession vary considerably based on geographic location, number of hours worked, after-hours responsibilities, amount of experience, amount of responsibility assumed in the practice, and other factors, issues about salary have been difficult to study.

In both the medical and PA professions, salaries for men have been higher than those for women. However, it is unclear whether this relates to a choice by women to work fewer hours or to actual gender discrimination. Salary discrepancies appear to have lessened as nurses have organized and advanced their issues and recognition within hospital systems.

Competition

Competition is usually the issue underpinning arguments against increased utilization of PAs. This issue is often veiled in arguments about concerns for patient safety or quality of care. When this occurs, the issues are often muddled and not substantiated by good data. Competition between professional interests can be manifested in many ways (e.g., in work settings or policies).

Because PAs and NPs are often hired in the same settings, either group of professionals may find themselves competing for jobs. This is particularly an issue if an area is dominated by one group, jobs are limited, and the other professional group seeks employment. Physicians and employers who indicate a strong preference for one group over another usually do so because they are more familiar with one than the other. In settings in which PAs and NPs have been trained together with common goals, a sense of mutual respect develops and competition is not a professional issue (Clawson & Osterweis, 1993; Fowkes et al., 1979).

The reimbursement system for health care services has contributed to competition between PAs and NPs as a result of a confusing array of policies. For example, the federal Medicare program developed separate policies for the reimbursement of PAs and NPs. There is also unevenness in the policies of individual states toward PAs and NPs in the implementation of Medicaid programs.

Local or state policies

The introduction of a new health professional or someone new to the role in an established health care system generates uncertainty and confusion unless there are clear policies within the institution and state practice acts. Both PAs and NPs have suffered from lack of policies that facilitate their practices. This creates confusion for nurses. For example, one state's nurse practice act specifies that nurses are to take orders from physicians, dentists, podiatrists, or clinical psychologists. Nurses who function in hospitals have thus questioned the authority of PAs to give orders. A number of states have clarified the issue by having attorneys general issue opinions about state regulations supporting PAs giving orders. In one state, the nurse practice act was revised and no longer lists the individual professions from which nurses can take orders.

Some nurses, particularly those in hospitals, view PAs as inhibiting their communication with physicians. Where there are good communications among PAs, nurses, and physicians and clearly defined protocols and institutional policies, these problems are less likely to occur.

CHALLENGES

Physician assistants are well established in our nation's health care system. PAs and nurses share common goals in the prevention of disease and the caring and curing of patients. In many regions, one group of nurses, the NPs, have recognized this and developed collaborative relationships in which common professional needs and interests are evident. Hopefully, conditions of mutual respect among these two health professions will continue to grow by each acknowledging and valuing the different perspectives and skills that the other can contribute to the health care team.

REFERENCES

Bliss, A., & Cohen, E.D. (1977). *The new health professionals: Nurse practitioners and physician's assistants.* Germantown, MD: Aspen Systems Corp.

Advisory Group on Physician Assistants and the Workforce. (1994). *Physician assistants in the health workforce/1994* [Final Report submitted to Council on Graduate Medical Education (COGME)]. Rockville, MD: Bureau of Health Professions, Health Resources and Services Administration, Public Health Service.

American Academy of Physician Assistants. (March, 1995). *Report of the Professional Practice Council.*

Simon, A., Link, M., & Miko, A. (1996, May). Twelfth annual report on physician assistant educational programs in the US. *Association of Physician Assistant Programs.*

Fowkes, V., & McKay, D. (1990). A profile of California's physician assistants. *The Western Journal of Medicine, 153,* 328-329.

Gara, N. (1989, July/August). State laws for physician assistants. *Journal of the American Academy of Physician Assistants, 2,* 303-313.

American Academy of Physician Assistants. (1994-1995). *General census data survey on physician assistants.* Alexandria, VA.

Jones, P.E., & Cawley, J.F. (1994, April). Physician assistants and health system reform: Clinical capabilities, practice activities, and potential roles. *JAMA, 271,* 1266-1272.

Schaft, G., & Cawley, J. (1987). *The physician assistant in a changing health care environment.* Rockville, MD: Aspen Publishers, Inc.

U.S. Congress, Office of Technology Assessment (1986, December). *Nurse practitioners, physician assistants, and certified nurse-midwives: a policy analysis.* Washington, DC: Author.

Fowkes, V., O'Hara-Devereaux, M., & Andrus, L.H. (1979, October). A cooperative education program for nurse practitioners/physician's assistants. *Journal of Medical Education, 54,* 781-787.

Clawson, D.K., & Osterweis, M. (Eds.). (1993). *The roles of physician assistants and nurse practitioners in primary care.* Washington, DC: Association of Academic Health Centers.

Zimmer, P.A., Brykczynski, K., Martin, A.C., Newberry, Y.G., Price, M.J., & Warren, B. (1992). *Advanced nursing practice: Nurse practitioner curriculum guidelines.* Final report: NONPF Education Committee. National Organization of Nurse Practitioner Faculties.

Conflict among nursing faculty

LAUREL ARCHER COPP

Faculty conflict can permeate the entire environment of a college, school, or department of nursing. Whether it be a faculty-to-faculty, faculty-to-dean, faculty-to-higher administration, faculty-to-clinical agency personnel, or even faculty-to-alumni disagreement, many people can be hurt by such conflict. Most vulnerable to lasting damage are the very students we are hired to teach—the consumers who, in part, pay our salaries.

CAN CONFLICT BE GOOD?

In a sense, academic discourse, debate, and practice in arguing first one side and then another are the stuff of which academia is made and on which scholars thrive. So this sonnet reminds us:

Trouble me with opposite opinions
Thought out ones, in-between and those off-slant
From usual, or what is au courant
But honest; or from dictator minions.

From this melee, let the necessary
Salvage work be done, and result in shaping
Of some new possibility, aping
Nothing and no one; if adversary

Turning, reaching, far out and above all
From loaned and common owned material
From considered content, and gestalt-cull
Find form; and let no furrow-thought forestall.

A jagged process, and with pain attached,
And often with new person's birth-time matched.

(Copp, 1995)

This "stuff of academia" is the rich and exhilarating exchange of *ideas!* Those trained in debate techniques know the zest of high adrenalin and congratulate their opponents on admired offensive or defensive tactics, combining the positions of established scholars with the boldness of the new "comers" in the field.

Unfortunately, we are concerned here with another type of conflict that is less appropriate and unbecoming to academia—faculty conflict on a *personal* level, between scholars and would-be colleagues. This type of conflict is a draining and demeaning process that pollutes the academic air of inquiry, intimidates others, damages the human spirit, and ruins careers.

HOW CONFLICT COMES ABOUT

How does conflict manifests itself in the faculty behavior? Behaviors, observable by outsiders and by the insider faculty members themselves, may be arranged on a continuum from positive to negative. These behaviors may range from collegiality, cooperation, and competition to the middle-position behavior of approach/avoidance (i.e., flirting with friction) to trying to stay out of it to avoiding those persons and cliques that fulminate conflict. The negative half of the continuum is manifested in enmity, conflict, and perhaps the most extreme—litigation (Copp, 1994a).

Perhaps at least one basic assumption should be challenged as we attempt to analyze how conflict comes about. We may assume that faculty members are much the same. In fact, there is worry in some settings that they are *too much* the same. We at least can challenge the fact that they have uncommon goals, spending their hours of work in different ways toward unlike ends. Priorities among faculty members are no doubt quite different. It is important to analyze whether this is true and note differences that sometimes not only generate conflict but also invest energies into sabotaging the projects of another. Let us consider differences that may lead from general grumbling to open conflict.

How we spend our time

Because they interact with faculty mainly in classroom or clinical settings, students have few ways of knowing how faculty members spend their time. Learning the scope of

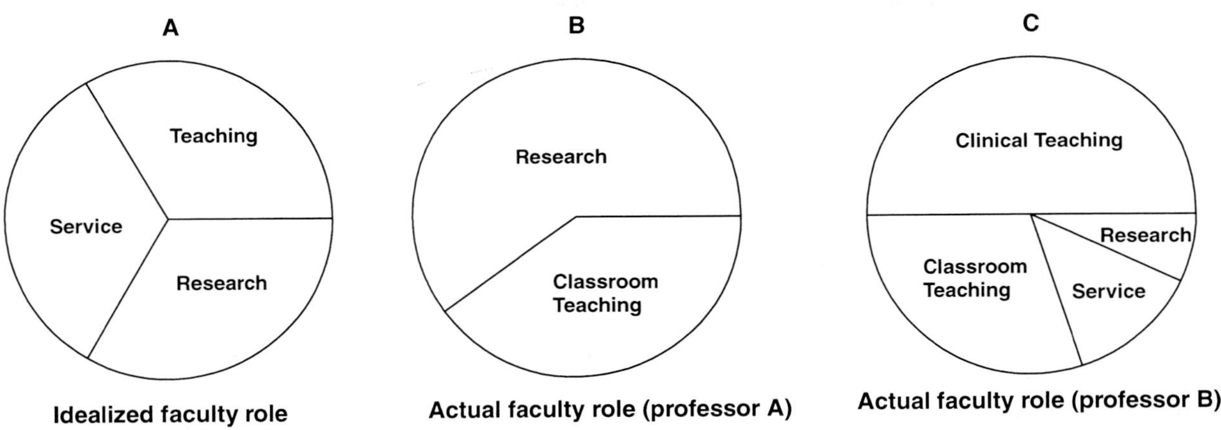

Fig. 74-1. Faculty responsibilities. **A**, Idealized faculty role. **B**, Actual faculty role (professor A). **C**, Actual faculty role (professor B).

faculty obligations is important in order to survive the curriculum and learn the realities of a potential future teaching position. Some faculty members assume they know what their colleagues do and how long it takes to complete their assignments. In reality, it can be revealing for students and faculty to study the variation on faculty assignments by probing deeper into annual reports of schools or departments, accreditation self-studies, or consulting and listening to colleagues.

The university mission characteristically states that the faculty role is one of teaching, research, and service. Simplistically, one imagines all faculty investing their time in an idealized way (Fig. 74-1). An equal distribution is rarely found, however. Professor A's time is divided between classroom teaching and research, with competing time pressures that include simultaneous obligations. Even with no "service" in the assignment, Professor A is not spared many meetings. Professor B, in an adjoining office, may have other obligations that more than fill the day. It is obvious that the more "pieces of the time pie" to which faculty members are assigned and the more diverse his or her activities are, the more fragmented is the resulting productivity and the more stretched and stressed Professor B may be. Professor A has the advantage of not being required to perform in all spheres of activity. Furthermore, the more congruent the teaching content is with the research activity the more focused the professor may be. These concepts do not have as much to do with clock hours as with stress and the vulnerability potential of feeling too little accomplishment with ensuing disillusionment.

Additionally, the endless and interminable meetings for which the academe is unfortunately famous frustrate all faculty with their disorganized agendas and ambling conversation, which steal time that may never be recaptured or represent the delayed work be done during evenings and on weekends. We have been affectionately considering two persons only—Professor A and Professor B. The dissonance between and among their assignments (teaching, research, and service) and those of colleagues is apparent.

How many members are on your faculty? Plotting the circles in Fig. 74-1 could be shown most graphically if we give a circle to each of your colleagues and then consider the overall impact on faculty morale, friction, and conflict. We asked the question "How does conflict come about?" Diverse assignments with too little time to complete them are bound to make a faculty member short on patience and prone to prolonging existing friction or initiating skirmishes that are counterproductive to all concerned. Olsen (1993) states that

> Findings thus confirm the pattern of stress related variables support the notion that role definition is in part prioritizing and allocating time and energy appropriately and effectively. (p. 470)

Terms of employment

We continue to consider sources of faculty conflict. *Why* faculty were hired, *when* they were hired, and even *by*

FACULTY TEACHING AND RESEARCH OBLIGATIONS	
Teaching obligations Class preparation Student conferences Grading assignments Knowledge renewal Travel	**Research obligations** Research tool selection or development Writing research proposal/protocol Grant application Subject recruitment/travel Institutional board compliance Data gathering and analysis Research team administration Report preparation/publication

OTHER FACULTY OBLIGATIONS	
Teaching obligations Classroom preparation Student conferences Grading papers/projects Knowledge renewal	**Clinical obligations** Clinical travel to site(s) Clinical assignments Clinical evaluation/conferences Learn new policies/procedures
Research obligations Project development All steps of inquiry Reports/publication	**Service obligations** Community meetings Elected to school offices Student services

whom they were hired hold seeds for potential dissension. Although most of us take seriously the basic contract of our employment and feel loyalty to the person with whom the contract was made, it is possible that neither the purpose nor the person contracting is still valid. In fact, neither may be relevant to the institution at a given time. If no one reconfirms or renegotiates, however, one has to work harder and harder to restate his or her role and interpret it convincingly to a new dean, department head, or those using business management techniques to set and monitor workload data. Feeling less and less valuable to the mission of the institution, the faculty member seems at a loss to know with whom to negotiate and about what. The "when" of reorientation and negotiation may become a trap, dividing old faculty from new, experienced from inexperienced, and institutionally aware from institutionally naive. All these counterpoints have potential for misunderstanding if not for conflict, because the bases for communication and relating are narrowed.

Terms of reward

How faculty are rewarded may be contentious. (Note that the word *contend* means to struggle, fight, compete, be in rivalry, argue) (Allport, Vernon, & Lindzey, 1951, pp. 3–5). This includes working conditions, tenure, promotion, salary, aspects of assignments (where, with what level learner, for what period of time), and perceived "scut work" or lack of it. *Scuttle* is a container for coal (*The Concise Oxford Dictionary,* 1929). Whereas nurses probably haven't refilled coal scuttles for several generations, faculty often feel that aspects of their work are low priority and demeaning and are opposite to reward. It may be of related interest to know that another definition of scuttle is to make holes in a ship for the purpose of sinking it (*The Concise Oxford Dictionary,* 1929). In faculty conflict and dissension, faculty and administration do manage to sink the very ship they depend on for their own survival!

The grumbling grows louder, and with it rises the problem of real or perceived inequity. Also present are grudges such as "I work twice as hard as she does and I get half the pay." Because the issues are either confronted in unhealthy ways or not at all, cross-perception between faculty peers is often inaccurate and based on assumptions; all too often the one with grievances does not wish to be confused with the relevant facts.

Rank differences

As in any setting there are differences in title, rank, and related terms of employment. Conflict can arise between tenure track and clinical track, tenured and nontenured, and full- and part-time faculty, many of whom may be perceived to be engaged in much the same activities. Intended or unintended, the nontenured, part-time faculty members whose contract is termed a clinical track or fixed-term appointment may perceive themselves as being alienated, unrecognized, and unrewarded, contributing to the success, promotion, and tenure of others but not themselves.

Some of these issues prompted Sommer (1994) to call on the academe to recognize "academe's other faculty." She calls for non–tenure-track faculty to be represented in college governance that would effect rewards, leaves, and professional development.

Tenure track is not the utopia that non–tenure-track faculty may perceive. Perceptions of life on the tenure track and pressures on junior faculty include those related to competition, peer relationships, publishing, performance feedback, social expections, and family life (Varrier, 1994). Both tenure track and non-tenure-track faculty often feel out of touch with the dean. Although the department head is all too often the person in the middle, between the policies of the dean from "above" and the dissatisfaction and complaints from the faculty constituency from "below," the department head is in a key and pivotal position to effect morale and, through sensitive responses to faculty instead of hostile reactions, to effect healthy discussion of the issues and employ steps of negotiation (Copp, 1994b).

Again, time plays a crucial role because most universities set a demanding "tenure clock," and unless readiness can be convincingly demonstrated to a panel of one's peers, there is an "up (promotion) or out" policy. Some female academicians are not at ease with what might be a countermanding tenure clock and a biological clock as well.

Personal differences

Faculty differ in gender, age, sense of humor, maturity, ethnic background, culture, sexual orientation, religious beliefs, and values. Some go home to a second job involving homemaking and child-rearing. Others have equally pressing home responsibilities with elderly and ill family members. Some faculty commute long distances. Some teach all day and go to school themselves on evenings, weekends, and during summers.

Study of Values
Allport-Vernon-Lindzey
Ranked Order

Actual faculty role (Professor A)	Actual faculty role (Professor B)
• Economic	• Theoretical
• Political	• Social
• Social	• Aesthetic
• Aesthetic	• Religious
• Theoretical	• Economic
• Religious	• Political

Aesthetic - form and harmony
Economic - interest in what is useful
Political - interest in power
Religion - unity
Social - love of people
Theoretical - discovery of truth

Fig. 74-2. Study of values: Allport-Vernon-Lindzey ranked order.

VALUE ORIENTATION

Perhaps even more differentiating is the value orientation among faculty members. Simply put, two faculty members taking the Study of Values (Allport, Vernon, & Lindzey, 1951) orient to vastly different priorities. Whereas we all maintain orientation in all of the values cited, it is worth consideration to wonder how dissimilar or similar we are related to our dominant values as compared with our faculty colleagues.

If all faculty rank values the same, then how we approach our assignments and each other might be more in tune. But of course this isn't true (see Fig. 74-2). Even Professor A and Professor B may differ sharply. Professor A for example may be oriented to the practical affairs of the business world, wanting education to be applicable and rewards to be tangible. Next ranked for Professor A would likely be a political orientation not necessarily limited to the world of politics but rather to one of power, competition, and struggle. Professor B is more likely to be oriented to the social and aspires to kindness, sympathy, and unselfishness. In some cases social values are combined with religious values, and whether or not institutional religion is embraced, this dominant value is held by those who seek to comprehend the cosmos as a whole and to relate themselves to its embracing totality.

Again, we are reminded that more people populate our faculty rosters than the hypothetical Professor A and B. When the reader is reminded of the number of colleagues in his or her environment, curiosity about the differences or consensus in value orientation is compelling. Faculty conflict related to values could be of a healthy type in the world of ideas and their application. Negatively, however, lack of appreciation and tolerance for values least like our own can result in stereotyping and personal attack in the folly of attempting to mold each colleague into our own (value) image.

We often hear the frustrated charge, "I just don't understand where you are coming from!" Indeed, we are "coming from" values long held, learned in culture and community, steeped in emotion and defended with conviction.

EFFECT ON STUDENTS

When conflict makes a faculty dysfunctional, students are immediately damaged. As they attempt to pick their way safely through a mine field of conflict on their path to graduation, students become wary, distrusting, defensive, bitter, and demeaned. For an already threatened and besieged faculty member, the student may be just another threat and may be treated as the enemy.

Students themselves suffer from assignment overload, conflict, family worry, time constraints, fatigue, and job expectations. In response, they: (a) try overfriendliness and humor; (b) bristle and nurse their wounds; (c) confront and argue; (d) cave in despite their principles; or (e) withdraw—sometimes in the psychological sense and in other cases in the literal sense of actually leaving school. In the heat of faculty battle, we lose our logic and behave as though we would still be employed if the students leave!

WHAT IS SATISFYING TO ACADEMICS?

Careers, like lives, have a shape, and different aspirations, needs, possibilities, and constraints shape them at different times. (Tinsley, 1984)

As faculty members, as with most humankind, we need to be valued. As we value ourselves we also value a work environment in which there is less conflict and more willingness to provide a listening ear, as well as increasing investment in the nature of the climate in which we spend more than one third of our working day.

If everyone had tenure, full-time employment, promotion, excellent working conditions, and the highest wages, there would be no conflict, right? Wrong. Poor morale, in fact, might persist. What more do faculty want? For a start they want more resources in the school, more flexible schedules, upgraded office and classroom facilities, a program of mentoring, and consultation/teaching access to those who can upgrade needed skills (e.g., professional writing, administrative know how, teaching and learning seminars, continuing education, and funding for the pursuit of degrees). It has a very familiar ring, indeed.

Olsen (1993) studied stress in faculty members in their first and third years of teaching. The ranked needs of what these faculty felt would lead to satisfaction (hence reduced conflict?) are representative of many of us, and only some of them are things that money can buy. We acknowledge that money can fix offices, pay for promotions, and hire services to help faculty. However, morale depends on more than these.

Faculty collegiality, if achieved, can help bring about the following for faculty: a true "company of scholars;" autonomy; an environment that is ethically responsible; a positive impact on others; a sense of accomplishment; fringe benefits; continuing learning; recognition by the university; expressions of appreciation for accomplishments; support for faculty scholarship; recognition in one's discipline; feedback; support for teaching; balance among research, teaching, and service; participation in decision making; opportunity to use present skills; increased time (formerly devoted to bickering) to do the work assigned; job security; support of the administration; salary; and support of colleagues. It seems particularly important to note those areas of satisfaction that are products of *the colleague relationship,* that by-product which is the opposite of faculty conflict. It is through faculty cohesion and collegiality that the following fruits are found:

- Impact on others
- Sense of accomplishment
- Recognition
- Feedback
- Participation in decision making
- Support of colleagues

Desperately needed is an academic environment in which we rejoice in the success of our colleagues, are generous in our admiration, engender health and maturity, and develop respectful reciprocal relationships that benefit all parties, especially students and those they care for.

REFERENCES

Allport, G.W., Vernon, P.E., & Lindzey, G. (1951). *Manual: study of values* (3rd ed.) (pp. 3–5). Boston, MA: Houghton Mifflin Company.

Copp, L.A. (1994a). Faculty behavior: Collegiality or conflict? *Journal of Professional Nursing, 10*(4), 195-196.

Copp, L.A. (1994b). In the middle: Department heads. *Journal of Professional Nursing, 10*(6), 329-330.

Copp, J.D. (1995). *Creativity.* Unpublished poem. Chapel Hill, NC.

Olsen, D. (1993). Work satisfaction and stress in the first and third year of academic appointment. *Journal of Higher Education, 64*(4), 453-471.

Sommer, B. (1994). Recognizing academe's other faculty. *Planning For Higher Education, 22*(4), 7-10.

The Concise Oxford Dictionary (1929). (p. 1074). Oxford Clarendon Press.

Tinsley, A. (1984). Career mapping in the professional development process. In A. Tinsley, C. Secor, & S. Kaplin (Eds.), *Women in higher education administration.* San Francisco, CA: Jossey-Bass Company.

Varrier, D.A. (1994). Perceptions of life on the tenure track. *Thought and Action, 9*(2), 95-124.

Some reflections on conflict resolution in nursing: The implications of negotiating at an uneven table

PHYLLIS BECK KRITEK

If one were to inquire among practicing nurses about their familiarity with conflict, the responses, ranging from anguish to hilarity, would document something so pervasive that nurses frequently fail even to call the presence by its name: conflict. They may tell you about their most recent experience with conflict, the difficulties they have experienced, and the outcomes they have achieved—charged alternately with chagrin or triumph. They would not, however, customarily open the dialog asking, "Have I told you about my latest conflict?" The presence of conflict in the work life of the practicing nurse is so endemic and integral it is simply not labeled as conflict. More often, it is simply perceived as a given, perhaps even a central fiber, in the tapestry of professional nursing activity.

Asked to document the locus of conflict, the list would be long and comprehensive: patients, families, other nurses, administrators, physicians, other health care providers, third-party payers, persons controlling access to services, alternative care institutions, professional organizations, the maintenance man in charge of light bulb replacement, the ambulance driver—the list can seem endless. If you ask nurses how they resolve these conflicts, their responses show equally rich variance, ranging from a serious reply about negotiation to descriptions of aggressive action or covert manipulation to a wink about who really knows "what's going on in this place!"

It is therefore not surprising that when you invite a group of nurses to learn more about conflict resolution, their eyes often glaze over and they drift to the next option on their menu. After managing conflict each day, as best one can, and feeling stressed or overwhelmed by the magnitude of the task, one does not welcome platitudinous advice that lacks awareness of the complexity of the problems nurses confront, or alternately, that provides a set of useful provisions that may disrupt the current carefully crafted and sustained practices of a given nurse. It is not a place where we go seeking advice, counsel, and the opportunity for transformative change.

These, too, are commonplaces that most nurses recognize when I describe them in workshops on conflict resolution: Nurses know what I mean and they readily see themselves in this picture. The commonplaces themselves warrant some reflection. More concretely, why is so much of a nurse's day focused on conflict; why are nurses expected and/or expecting themselves to resolve conflicts in their work environments; whose conflict is it; and why are nurses so reluctant to subject their models of conflict management to scrutiny? Do nurses manage conflict or resolve it? More subtly, are the models of conflict management that nurses use ones that deal with the temporary flare-up and fail in the long run to address more substantive issues? If this is true, even part of the time, what are the substantive issues nurses fail to address? Why do they fail to address them? Can or will any of this change? If so, how?

These are the questions that led me along a personal path that involved training in conflict resolution during a National Kellogg Leadership Fellowship, giving me an opportunity to study with some of the key national leaders in conflict resolution in the United States. This fellowship has resulted both in a book on conflict resolution that explores the nature of uneven tables (Kritek, 1994) and in the redirection of much of my energy toward the field of conflict resolution. It seemed to me then, as now, that the noble ideals and commitments of practicing nurses get twisted and sullied in the world of conflict management as they live it. I was in search of some tools that might help, and it was my hope to share those tools with other nurses. The journey has been instructive.

Part of the journey has involved interdisciplinary study, training, dialogue, writing, and collaboration, resulting in a second book with my collaborators (Marcus, Dorn, Kritek, Miller, & Wyatt, 1995). The experiences that resulted in that book have shaped me in myriad ways, taught me lessons that Walt Disney's Pocahontas would say "I never knew I never knew." I have also had the opportunity to teach my collaborators things they did not know. Together, we have struggled and celebrated our way through the morass of health care conflicts and wondered that we are able to do so much good in the midst of so much conflict. We have been able to bring diverse groups of health care providers together to resolve conflicts, to study conflict resolution, and to become negotiators of health care conflicts. It has been gratifying work and has unveiled for me the windows on conflict that others have—windows that in some ways are not unlike those nurses look through yet in other ways differ dramatically.

Part of the journey has, however, been more solitary and involved the reflective effort to think through the nature of conflict for the practicing nurse. I have listened to and studied the stories of nurses and have heard conflict descriptions from a variety of situations and perspectives. Some things seem consistent. A large number of practicing nurses see the management of conflict as a central dimension of their job. When it shows up, they feel obligated to do something about it; nurses do not ignore conflict. In addition, competent practicing nurses, if they create conflict, tend to have lengthy explanations for why they did so; they do not create conflict lightly and their reasons tend to tap into important values and passions. Most interesting to me, however, is that these same nurses accept that all sorts of other folks appropriately create conflicts for them to resolve. It is simply accommodated, like moon cycles and deciduous trees. It can leave the uncomprehending listener with the sense that the competent professional nurse is a conflict magnet. Concurrently, one senses that this conflict magnet is also fairly conflict-aversive, creating conflicts only as a last resort while identifying and busily smoothing over everyone else's conflicts as quickly and expeditiously as possible.

There are some tempting platitudes that emerge: It is because nurses are women, or socialized to be conflict-aversive, or essentially conservative, or primarily healers, or inherently nurturant. These seem to me to beg the question. Such platitudes are also further confounded by the recent emergence of nursing manager elites, nurses who perceive their role in nursing as leaders but who more often appear to struggle to achieve some identification with the control/management/success idiom of our culture, sometimes with a frenzy. Much as our histories of science, theory, education, and research have emerged from imitations of other groups we perceive as "correct" or "successful," we now have a generation of nursing manager elites who mimic the prevailing discourse of the organizational and business idiom. Many of the members of this elite group appear to be neither nurturant nor healing nor conflict-aversive. Indeed, they are increasingly identified by some practicing nurse groups as the locus of new, sometimes more pernicious conflicts.

A disclaimer may prove helpful here. These are observationally based generalizations, the musings of a thoughtful student of the culture of nursing in the United States. They are meant neither to condemn nor condone. I view neither as useful investments of my energy. Rather, they raise questions and activate my curiosity. Exactly what is nursing's relationship with conflict? Why is it so pervasive in our nursing culture? What do we intend to do about it? Do we like our solution?

The first and perhaps most difficult observation that compels me through this exploration is the honest recognition that the values, beliefs, hopes, and dreams of nurses and their convictions about what ensures health, wholeness, and healing for humans is not the prevailing world view guiding health care decision making in the United States, nor has it been for the life span of even the oldest among us. We have spent a good deal of time and energy as a health care subculture contesting this fact, trying to assure ourselves that someday our world view will prevail, or sneaking it in the back door, but the reality is that the world Nightingale envisioned is not the overriding perspective guiding health care decision making. An equally compelling honest recognition is the fact that as a collective of health care providers, while we are the group with the largest numbers, we are at least second and often third and fourth to other groups in health care when it comes to status, power to control outcomes, income, influence, and the freedom to exercise moral agency. Because these are measures of import in the larger social system, clearly knowing our position in the health care hierarchy (and it is a hierarchy, no matter how nervously we wish otherwise) is a critical insight.

These seem truisms to me, yet I am continually amazed at the number of nurses who become uncomfortable confronting them. They of course lead to the next worrisome observation: Given our scope of impact on health care and the critical role we play in people's lives, we would be wise to admit honestly that we are disadvantaged in negotiating health care conflicts, and that disadvantage is one that just about everyone but nurses consents to and intends to sustain. This, in short, makes us aptly described as a group that is systematically discriminated against. There are implications for this in the land of conflict and its resolution.

While much has been developed over the last 30 years on the behaviors that emerge from systematic discrimination, I think few writings capture the candor of Allport's (1958) early work on the theme. He noted that groups that are systematically discriminated against can become either intropunitive or extropunitive. It has seemed to me that nurse "smoother overs" are behaving in a fairly intropunitive fashion and nurse "elite controllers" are acting in an extropunitive fashion. This is an oversimplified distinction, but it helps one to begin to understand some of the most overt dimensions of nurse-managed conflict. The former use an array of manipulative tools to contain conflict and keep themselves in a state of relative, albeit compromised, safety from what they perceive as external threats. The latter become party to and members in the external threats to the best of their ability. In both cases, pleasing powerful others may be the most compelling motive. Likewise, the simple effort to diminish the discomfort associated with conflict is more compelling than some honest recognition of the nature of the conflict and some honest effort to responsibly identify, address, experience, explore, and resolve the conflict. Consequently it is sustained. Accommodation is not resolution, and it is not transformative.

It is not my interest, in confronting these givens in the world of nursing, to engage in the country's current inclination to blame some evil other or to excuse inappropriate personal behaviors with elaborate explanations of abuse by others. I further do not wish to be party to the trivialization of the real pain and struggle involved in systematic oppression. There is some tenuous path of balance in this exploration that is difficult to achieve, but it is my goal. I am convinced that the game victims and victimizers play is a dangerous and pathological one, and I am not interested in playing. I am interested in alternatives.

This returns me to my interest in conflict resolution, one of the few tools I have been able to locate that provides me with a potential pathway to an alternative. The first and most obvious option confronting nurses is to learn what experts in the field are doing these days. The literature is ample; workshops abound. For the curious reader who wants to begin the process, I can comfortably recommend those I find most useful and acceptable to nurses. Fisher and Ury's classic *Getting to Yes: Negotiating Agreement without Giving In* (1981) is always a good starting point. Moore's (1986) comprehensive and morally sensitive discussion of the mediation process is the one I find most congruent with nursing's values. Ury's more recent *Getting Past No: Negotiating with Difficult People* (1991) seems to have a particular appeal for the kinds of conflicts nurses confront. These are useful tools and can activate a learning process. They will guide you to more demanding texts if your curiosity peaks.

Merely absorbing the guidance from expert others, however, seems to me only a partial solution. Indeed, it can easily become one more case of imitating the "correct" or "successful" others without an honest scrutiny of fit with nursing's unique realities. None of the books I have studied in conflict resolution honestly confronts the issue of systematic discrimination and the intent to sustain it, the focus of my book. The struggle to find these alternative perspectives and articulating them is for me the more compelling and fascinating task in any honest exploration of conflict in health care.

Because I am by inclination and gifts a nurse philosopher, these alternatives are for me first embedded in philosophical discourse. Because the descriptor nurse is central to my approach to philosophy, these alternatives are necessarily focused on action, on the practical and the pragmatic meaning of my philosophical discourse, here and now, with real nurses doing real nursing today. Those two perspectives make me reluctant to be prescriptive for others without a basket of disclaimers, so the alternatives are for me personal ones I can elect to share with others in an honest fashion but without the presumptive hook that they must then change or elect to do things my way.

SOME REFLECTIONS OF THE PHILOSOPHER

When I slogged through my doctoral education in the late 1970s, Kuhn's (1970) insights had not yet infected the programmatic discourse, and I was left feeling assaulted by a picture of reality that was deeply incongruent with portions of the reality I knew. The received view was still alive and well in nursing, and those of us slow to embrace that view were a troublesome lot, resistive to the thrills of certitude and finality. As I prepared to develop a doctoral program, however, Kuhn came to my aid, along with Rorty (1979), Gale (1979), Laudan (1977), Reason and Rowan (1981), and a host of others. Postmodernism was edging its way into the nursing dialogue.

It is still edging, from what I can tell. Toulmin (1990) more recently has completed an analysis of the origins and potential future of modernity. He posits that the first phase of modernity was actually the Renaissance with its distinctively humanistic focus, and the second, the more familiar referent, the Cartesian era we call the Enlightenment. He posits that postmodernism can also be referred to as the third phase or modernism, where the promise of both the Renaissance and the Cartesian era will serve as a springboard to something new in the next millennium. The next generation of doctoral students in nursing will chew on this menu.

His analysis is noteworthy, however, because he delineates four distinct shifts that occurred during the transition from the Renaissance to the Enlightenment eras: from the oral to the written, from the particular to the general, from the local to the universal, and from the timely to the timeless. He then posits some bringing together of these perspectives in the future. In describing this future, one of his contentions is that "scientific inquiry will increasingly shift from abstract laws of universal application to particular decipherments of the complex structures and detailed processes embodied in concrete aspects of nature" (Toulmin, 1990, p. 204). I hope he's right. Certainly all the evidence says that's where we're headed, and that can only be good news for nurses since the unique world view they bring to our culture is not the prevailing one. The prevailing view is, of course, deeply Cartesian in character, even when it tries not to be. We are creatures of habit and we are having a good deal of difficulty letting go. Nurses intuitively seem to know that the Cartesian world view has served us well, and is also limited in its applicability to all that can be known.

Anderson (1995), who has compiled a wonderful collection of readings on postmodernism, attempts to draft an efficient map of the evolutionary path from premodernity through modernity and into postmodernity. With the arrival of postmodernity, he posits that there are now "at least four distinguishable worldviews," each with a distinct culture and an epistemology (p. 110). He describes them as follows: (a) the postmodern-ironist, which sees truth as socially constructed; (b) the scientific-rational, in which truth is "found" through methodical, disciplined inquiry; (c) the social-traditional, in which truth is found in the heritage of American and Western civilizations; and (d) the neoromantic, in which truth is found either through attaining harmony with nature and/or spiritual exploration of the inner self. Each of these views has its own set of truths and its own ideas about what truth is—where and how you look for it, how you test it, and how you prove it.

By now you may be wondering if I got lost in the philosophy section of the library; what has this to do with nursing and conflict? All of these world views are active in nursing in the United States today and shape our dialogue both among ourselves and with others who are equally diverse. Most of us, however, were neither educated nor trained to live in a pluralistic world without certainty, fraught with ambiguity, and awash in social constructs where we are unable to locate the social constructors and take them to task for their products. Indeed we are the constructors and the products, and this worries us some. Anderson (1995) posits that the postmodernists "are the wave of the future, the people you want to study to see where the world is going" (p. 115). He notes that "some people seem to be completely organized around one way of understanding truth, are deeply threatened by the others, and repress their own tendencies to wander into the forbidden worlds of postmodernism or neo-romanticism" (p. 115). He concludes that the optimal location, knowing we are all slowly becoming postmodernists, is multilingualism, being "able to think rationally and understand science, able to appreciate and draw on a social heritage, and able to drink from the well of ecological and spiritual feeling that is being tapped by new-romanticism" (p. 116).

As I noted, all of these perspectives abide in nursing. Indeed, the competent balanced nurse distinguishes him- or herself by being multilingual in exactly this way. In this sense we are a bit of a national resource because we have somehow been working at keeping all four of these perspectives concurrently alive in the body politic, with compelling reasons for all four. We seem un–self-conscious of the richness, unable to get enough distance from ourselves to think of ourselves as valuable. In addition, we often collapse before the pressure by one or another external authority to treat the four world views as if they were some sort of competition in which one must prevail. This propensity for edging backward is characteristic of humans dealing with monumental change. Indeed, Toulmin (1990) posits that the 1980s in this country were "a time for nostalgia rather than imagination" (p. 205), a longing look backward in search of an illusion of certainty that is no longer available. This requires a bit of compassion for us all.

This is the context for conflict in health care today. It is an attempt to provide an alternative forest, where the trees of managed care or the leaves of a physician or pharmacist do not distract us unduly from the actual process we are collectively experiencing and the reasons for its discontents. In particular, most of the humans cutting their path through this change were taught to believe that being right was imperative and that there was only one right answer. This equips us poorly for postmodernity. When the issues at stake are or seem to be life-and-death issues, the stakes go up. We would be wise to assume conflict will endure and even worsen on occasion as we struggle culturally through this morass to the future we are collectively birthing, sometimes against our will.

Pulling these threads together, it seems to me nurses would be wise to become a bit more conscious and self-aware about the global, national, local, and institutional contexts in which the conflicts they confront occur. We find an ease in the extremely local and personal aspects that make us lose contact with the bigger picture, which might serve us well. In addition, we might be startled to find that we are skillful at analyzing conflicts in part because we are a fairly multilingual lot, schooled through education and experience in all four world views and living out some nervous tension of them as best we can. We might further take the daring leap of thinking of ourselves not so much as persons who alternately smooth over or polarize conflicts to people uniquely equipped in some dimensions to creatively and constructively assist in the resolution of these conflicts. That could be good news for everyone.

SOME REFLECTIONS OF THE PRAGMATIST

Which raises the obvious question: if we have these gifts and insights, why aren't we using them more constructively? The postmodernists would have us survey the current language systems that inform our understanding of human behavior gone awry. Today in the United States, this idea is most often reflected in a body of literature that springs from the self-help movement. Any casual trip through a local bookstore will document this fact. While the established health care community flounders with regard to the vagaries of human behavior, hoping to reduce all manner of human vulnerabilities to simple physical phenomena, the public has crafted and implemented an enormous structure designed to address the real problems of real humans today. Where we have failed, self-help groups have done strikingly successful things. Using this paradigm for understanding our reluctance to solve our own struggles with conflict management might prove useful. Its most powerful voice is the twelve step types of program groups.

In November 1989, the *American Journal of Nursing* published an article by Hall and Wray entitled "Codependency: Nurses Who Give Too Much." The article did not cause a national moment of self-honesty, although it might have been good news if it had. I admire Hall and Wray for raising the issue so candidly. The codependency literature itself often identifies nurses as a specific group trained and reinforced to be codependent. It is unquestionably part of my education, and I find it unwise to ignore this fact. I also believe I have never worked in an organization among nurses where the insights of Shaef and Fassel (1988) describing the addictive organization didn't fit.

I bring up this topic with some trepidation. There are dimensions to this literature and to the proponents who espouse it that are deeply uncomfortable for me: too facile, too dogmatic, too simplistic, too prescriptive. As a good postmodernist willing to look at emerging neoromantic world views, however, I have elected to tackle this powerful voice-shaping public life. Whitfield (1991), one of my preferred authors on the topic, posits that multiple definitions of codependence are desirable but provides this description, among others, that has served me well: "We become codependent when we turn our responsibility for our life and happiness over to our ego (our false self) and to other people" (p. 3). I like this description because it highlights my sense of nursing's role in health care conflicts: All sorts of other people have the power and make the decisions; we just carry them out and smooth over the fracas created as necessary.

On September 22, 1989, a group of experts in the field generated the following consensus description or definition: "Co-dependency is a pattern of painful dependency on compulsive behaviors and on approval from others in an attempt to find safety, self-worth and identity. Recovery is possible" (Wegscheider-Cruse and Cruse, 1990, p. 8). While the latter statement in the definition is purportedly good news, it is surely of little worth and value if the presence of the problem is denied or ignored. In nursing we have fretted about our oppressed status without much willingness to look at the primary mechanisms we use to deal with this status. Those who study the phenomenon are not so reticent; most identify nurses as one of the groups that manifest and perpetuate codependency. This is worrisome news.

The community of practitioners and proponents of this world view is, like us all, evolving. For nurses struggling with the insights of this particular world view, Kasl (1992) provides a stabilizing antidote that may prove useful. In her critique of the pervasive mystique surrounding twelve-step programs and their related ideas about addiction and codependency, she examines both social and personal contexts with particular emphasis on internalized oppression. She encourages alternate pathways. What is useful is her clear-headed recognition of and willingness to tackle the problems that current solutions have engendered without escaping the original stimulus: the codependency and the addictions.

Once more pulling these threads together, it seems that for me as an individual (and for the vast majority of my colleagues), the socialization I have historically and even currently experienced as a nurse encourages me to engage in codependent behaviors. I can rebel against the program—and have—but it changes neither the system nor me. Rebellion is not resolution. Indeed, I have slowly learned it is merely a different face to entrapment. The critical key is questioning the system, beginning to understand better how it operates and what it asks of me. Co-optation wears many costumes and requires reasoned scrutiny. In engaging in such scrutiny, what I find is a system nostalgically looking backward more than forward, often hoping that the nurses will smooth over the inevitable conflicts that emerge from that incongruity. The repeated effort to find new ways to deal with this system was for me a significant impetus in writing a book about alternate ways of being at an uneven table. The first step in meaningful conflict resolution, however, is the willingness to see the uneven table, to know you are at one, and to make clear decisions about what you are now doing that is harmful and what you might do in the future that is more constructive.

In the book I call these "ways of being," and list 10 exemplars that I believe, interactively, can change how we negotiate as nurses. They presuppose that we will have climbed over the habits of the codependent heart, one way or another, and faced the way we "do" conflict now, usually with complex skill arrays of manipulations and maneuverings that serve to harm ourselves and others and keep the conflict and the source of conflict afloat. We have some choices to make here.

SOME OBSERVATIONS OF A PERSONAL NATURE

What I have written here is, in a good postmodernist fashion, a personal appraisal of the situation as it looks to me from where I am sitting. I have no corner on this market, nor do I purport to have one. What I have learned has stood me in good stead and may prove useful to some others. That would please me. What is clear to me is that the frequency and depth of conflict we will experience in health care settings and among nurses are likely to increase, not decrease, and we are ill prepared for that eventuality. It is equally clear to me that if nurses elected to tap into their considerable conflict management skills, transformed them with honesty and moral courage so that they move beyond mere manipulations, we could be a formidable force in enhancing the health care environments we inhabit and create. I have no wisdom on whether we will elect to do that, or to what degree. I love the imagination of it, however, and when I list my personal collection of rainbow-level hopes and dreams, I always include it with a smile.

REFERENCES

Allport, G.W. (1958). *The nature of prejudice.* Garden City, NY: Doubleday.

Anderson, W.T. (1995). *Four different ways to be absolutely right.* In W.T. Anderson (Ed.). *The truth about the truth, de-confusing and reconstructing the postmodern world* (pp. 115, 116). New York: G.P. Putnam's Sons.

Fisher, R., & Ury, W. (1981). *Getting to yes: Negotiating agreement without giving in* (2nd Ed.). New York: Penguin Books.

Gale, G. (1979). *Theory of science.* New York: McGraw-Hill Book Company.

Hall, S.F., & Wray, L.M. (1989). Codependency: nurses who give too much. *American Journal of Nursing, 89*(11), 1456-1460.

Kasl, C.D. (1992). *Many roads, one journey: Moving beyond the 12 steps.* New York: HarperCollins Publishers, Inc.

Kritek, P.B. (1994). *Negotiating at an uneven table: Developing moral courage in resolving our conflicts.* San Francisco, CA: Jossey-Bass.

Kuhn, T.S. (1970). *The structure of scientific revolutions* (2nd Ed.). Chicago, IL: The University of Chicago Press.

Laudan, L. (1977). *Progress and its problems, towards a theory of scientific growth.* Los Angeles, CA: University of California Press.

Marcus, L.J., Dorn, B.C., Kritek, P.B., Miller, V.G., & Wyatt, J.B. (1995). *Renegotiating health care: Resolving conflict to build collaboration.* San Francisco, CA: Jossey-Bass.

Moore, C.W. (1986). *The mediation process: Practical strategies for resolving conflict.* San Francisco, CA: Jossey-Bass.

Reason, P., & Rowan, J. (Eds.). (1981). *Human inquiry, a sourcebook of new paradigm research.* New York: John Wiley & Sons.

Rorty, R. (1979). *Philosophy and the mirror of nature.* Princeton, NJ: Princeton University Press.

Schaef, A.W., & Fassel, D. (1988). *The addictive organization.* San Francisco, CA: Harper & Row.

Toulmin, S. (1990). *Cosmopolis.* Chicago, IL: The University of Chicago Press.

Ury, W. (1991). *Getting past no: Negotiating with difficult people.* New York: Bantam Books.

Whitfield, C.L. (1991). *Co-dependence, healing the human condition.* Deerfield Beach, FL: Health Communications, Inc.

Wegscheider-Cruse, S., & Cruse, J. (1990). *Understanding co-dependency.* Deerfield Beach, FL: Health Communications, Inc.

Traditional roles for women and the impact on nursing services in Brazil

ROSENI ROSANGELA CHOMPRÉ, ANAMARIA VAZ de ASSIS MEDINA,
MARIA AUXILIADORA CARDOVA CHRISTOFARO

Throughout history, the work of women—considered by many societies as essential for the production of food and survival—has been invisible. Women's work was done behind the conspicuous activities of the highest levels of popes and kings, wars and discoveries, tyranny and defeat, as indicated by official history. Through their work, women wove the true screen of history that has yet to receive the attention it deserves (Miles, 1989).

With this in mind, it should be noted that the longer any society lives in a given situation, the less urgent or conflicting that situation will appear. It comes to be regarded more as a condition than a contradiction or problem. In the case of women, the lack of change in the division of labor for so many centuries and in different geographical settings has made reproduction and the care of people within and outside the context of the family their unquestioned responsibility (Medina, 1991). This activity consolidates itself as a traditional role because of women's biological capabilities of gestation, delivery, and breast-feeding. Women extend their actions of nutrition and care to other families and communities in the roles of midwives, faith healers, healers, and wet nurses.

Gestation and breast-feeding in particular create relations between women and the concepts understood in certain periods, societies, or social groups as limiting factors to their insertion in production and public space. As an example, the reduction of mobility—common during gestation, delivery, and breast-feeding—is seen in many societies as a "loss," inhibiting women from taking on certain roles and functions.

The hegemonic assumption that the family is the nuclear basis of organization, harmony, security, and development, both economically and morally, is intrinsically linked to women: To be "mother," "wife," and "housewife" becomes part of the social function of procreation, strengthening the ideal model in which the home becomes the power domain of women.

In addition to the roles of reproduction and caretaking, women also play the role of educator, transmitting beliefs, values, and knowledge about social dynamics and the functioning of the body. Even as women hold the function of perpetuating values and traditions, the very evolution of society exerts an influence over these traditions so as to change them. It must not be forgotten that there are complex interrelations between differentiated movements and tendencies at the heart of society that determine the coexistence of prevailing, residual, and emerging values. It is in this permanent process of change that there occurs the alteration of the traditional roles of women.

The passing from acceptance of the so-called "feminine condition" to an analysis of the problems of women only became relevant in the course of history when three basic factors appeared simultaneously. The first factor is a reality perceived by society as inadequate and unacceptable, that is, the status of women in society as a whole and male domination. The second factor is the existence of proposals to solve the questions considered problematic, and the third is a political climate that is favorable to change.

These factors are at the root of nursing's history in Brazil because of the strong link between the history of women and the significant repercussions of their traditional roles on the evolution of Brazilian nursing in the country as a whole.

WOMEN AND THE HISTORY OF NURSING IN BRAZIL

Earliest roots of nursing

In order to analyze the evolution of nursing in Brazil, it is first necessary to examine the different stages of development of Brazilian society and, within that society, the development of women. The origins of Brazil as a Western country are linked to the European trade expansion that began in the 15th century. The native culture of the precolonial period continues today to be marginalized and discounted in the power structure and organization of Brazilian society, in both its values and its social, political, and economic parameters.

Concurrent with the process of exploration of the natural resources of the new land, the process of "civilizing" the inhabitants—the so-called Indians—was carried out through the invasion and massacre of tribes, Jesuit catechism, and the enslavement of Indians and Africans. This resulted in the imposition of Portuguese culture and domination in a comprehensive way throughout the territory.

The issue of participation of women in this expansion is only gradually being revealed. The point of view of distinguished historians was usually more concerned with conquests than with colonial settlements. This left the impression that, in this great period of navigational exploration, there were in the world only a few women, mostly of the nobility (e.g., Isabel I of Spain; Catherine of Austria, wife to Dom João III of Portugal; and Elizabeth I of England).

However, when the subject of colonizing the new land was raised, the efforts of women rose in importance as a result of their traditional social roles. This was due to the fact that effective colonization was based on the formation of the family; working together and dividing functions among its members, families would do the work of production and reproduction.

Assimilating with native women in the new lands was considerably more common among the Portuguese than among other peoples. In addition, the mother country made various efforts to send local women to the colonies to establish families in order to lay down their habits and customs, including language and religion.

While the men opened new horizons, fought the natives, and advanced into new areas looking for Eldorados, the women usually produced the food, administered the goods and properties, had children, and then, very often, fought hard for their own survival and that of their children (Medina, 1992). In order to get white women to send to the new territories, a variety of methods were used, from recruiting volunteers to kidnapping and permanent removal.

In addition to the presence of both Portuguese and native women in the colonization of Brazil, the large-scale production activities of the plantation demanded the incorporation of large numbers of workers, comprised primarily of enslaved and transported Africans. In setting up Brazilian society, women of different ethnic origins became the object of commercial stimulus to the reproduction and occupation of land, together with the wish to spread the Roman Catholic faith. Each ethnic group, Native Brazilians, white immigrants, and African slaves, contributed its knowledge and specific cultural norms in shaping the Brazilian nation.

Portuguese women came from two classes: the noble (rich) families and the lower classes. Given the social concern with the division of goods and properties through inheritance, noble women were limited to the domestic arena or religious institutions. Keeping up the traditions of the home country, the rich Portuguese women only left their homes when accompanied by male relatives for religious ceremonies, or were restricted to convents. This same treatment of women, transported to Brazil, would result in the kind of family comprised of a "taciturn father, obedient mother and withdrawn children," as referred to in the famous phrase by Abreu (1934, p. 62).

Lower-class women, on the other hand, made up the great majority and included the poor Portuguese, the half-caste, the freed African slaves, and slaves. Many documents from the colonial period show them as unchaste women or libertines. The great concern of this social group, however, was their survival and that of their children. The high mortality rate of men and the instability of the relations between the sexes must not be forgotten. As a result of the circumstances at that time, most of the families were mother-centered.

Although they comprised the largest segment of the female population, the values, beliefs and modus vivendi of the lower class did not shape the predominant ideals of Brazilian society in terms of women's roles. It was always the poorest who took on the responsibility of feeding, caring for, and educating the children; caring for the sick and handling and administering medicine; and assisting in the delivery and feeding of other women's children, in addition to all the activities of cleaning. These activities would determine the informal process of health care, carried out by midwives, faith healers, and those who cared for the dying and the dead.

Institutionalization of health care and formal training

Given the nature of the work of women, they were permitted to join the workforce when health care was institutionalized. However, as this care was organized institutionally, it was not these women from the lower classes who would take on the nursing procedures in the hospitals. Given the living conditions and social organization at that time, the services were institutionalized under the responsibility of nuns, who came mainly from the higher classes.

The first health institutions in Brazil were the Santas Casas de Misericordia (Holy Houses of Mercy), which had been planned by the Portuguese monarchy from the earliest days of colonization. The first one in Brazil was the Santa Casa de Santos, established in 1543. Despite the almost immediate establishment of hospitals in Brazil after the arrival of the Portuguese (1500), there is no reference to any kind of systematic health care available to slaves and other lower classes. This remained true until the second half of the 19th century. Therefore, while nobility and those from the upper classes were cared for by doctors from Portugal, the other societal layers were cared for by the same poor women, very often considered transgressors against the dominant social norms by carrying out volunteer work. For Germano (1983), nursing in Brazil can trace its beginning to this context and virtually kept the same profile until the period of the so-called "Old Republic" (1930). From the early 18th century, the doctor became involved in a more active way with activities related to reproduction and women's health. He invaded rituals that were lived in an exclusively feminine community (e.g., the moment of delivery, when knowledge transmitted from mother to daughter brought together the pregnant woman, the midwife, and others (women friends and neighbors) in a warm meeting of public and private spheres).

It may be emphasized, therefore, that nursing as a social practice in Brazil is linked to domestic activities and the empirical practice of mothers, nuns, slaves, and even prostitutes. Silva (1986), in his study on medicine and nursing in the precapitalist period, states that these origins resulted in a lack of prestige for the continuing work in this field of knowledge, since it is seen as mere common sense.

In 1808 the royal family migrated to Brazil, fleeing the invasion of Portugal by French troops. They moved first to Bahia and later to Rio de Janeiro. This event, coupled with the opening of the ports to friendly nations, aided in the process of political, economic, and social transformation in Brazil in the 19th century. These changes stimulated other commercial links, especially with England, which demanded a new urban structure, mainly in the ports. In the same year, the first educational course of surgery, anatomy, and obstetrics was created in Bahia.

In 1832 the medical-surgical academies of Rio de Janeiro and Bahia were called schools or faculties of medicine, and a specific course for midwives was created. During the second half of the 19th century other faculties of medicine appeared, often created with midwifery, pharmacy, and dentistry courses. In 1854 a new statute for the schools of medicine was approved, in which prerequisites were established for courses in obstetrics, pharmacy, and "cirurgioes boticarios" (surgeons who could also mix their own medicines) as "annexes" to medical courses, again concentrated in Bahia and Rio de Janeiro. Only in 1890 was the first course for midwives established in the state of São Paulo.

The continuation and consolidation of the agricultural and exporting model meant that the imperial government that was established after independence from Portugal (1822) had to set up strategies of social action. Among these was health care, since endemic diseases such as yellow fever, smallpox, and plague threatened commercial relations with other countries. Among the measures adopted, priority was given to action directed at collective diseases, and a system of sanitary vigilance was established for the control of endemic diseases and hygiene in the cities. These measures meant new demands on health care at that time, including that carried out by women. This work was now done inside the hospitals and would later become nursing services.

The first nursing school in Brazil was created in 1890 as part of the Hospital Nacional de Alienados of Rio de Janeiro. Since the beginning, there were several prerequisites to enrolling in the institutionalized training of nurses. It was necessary, for example, to know a foreign language (French or English) as well as arithmetic and geometry. Previously, these had been relevant to male courses at the undergraduate level, available only to the social elite. Even in the teaching for women of the upper class, handicrafts was substituted for geometry. As a result, demands would not allow entry in the courses of nursing by women of lower classes, who continued to carry out a significant part of the formal and informal health work.

It is important here to highlight another relevant characteristic. Although efforts were made to include community health content based on the control of endemic diseases and other public health problems, the institutionalized training of nurses was done in the hospital setting and remained disconnected from the health needs of most of the population.

Modern nursing

So-called modern nursing, along the lines of the Nightingale system, was established in Brazil through English professionals recruited to organize the nursing services of the Hospital of the Foreigners' Association in Rio de Janeiro in 1892. The beginning of the 20th century saw the expansion of institutions for the training of nurses with the creation of the School of Nursing of the Hospital Samaritano (1901) and the School for Midwives (1902).

At the turn of the century there was also a serious crisis in commercial relations resulting from, among other causes, the reappearance of yellow fever in the main ports. The threat of having trading countries cut their relations with Brazil led the government to define tough measures for the control and eradication of endemic diseases, with the obvious consequences on health activities. Working on an emergency contract basis for the government, sanitary agent Cruz defined a very comprehensive program for the control of endemic diseases. This increased the demand for specialized nursing labor in order to carry out the Cruz Plan. Despite the existence of institutions responsible for the training of health professionals, the greater part of the nursing workforce, even at this time, did not have systematic training.

In order to respond to the lack of both quality and quantity of this workforce, international cooperation was invited to organize a model of training considered adequate. This resulted in the setting up of the School of Nursing by the National Department of Public Health in 1922. In 1926 this institution became the Ana Nery School of Nursing, which was a "model school" for the establishment of other schools in the country. Although the training was originally proposed as a strategy for collective health actions within the Cruz Plan, once again hospital care came to predominate in the training of nurses as a result of the methodology adopted in the teaching.

The continuity of the institutionalization and expansion of higher education nursing courses (currently about 100) did not eliminate the use of unqualified labor, which even today is the wide base of the workforce. On the other hand, the hospital has been kept as the main place for the practice of the nurses.

Today nursing work is performed by four distinct categories, created according to levels of qualification. The nurse, representing about 10% of nursing personnel, has university training (a minimum of 4 years beyond high school). The technical nurse and the nursing auxiliary, who have high school or equivalent training, comprise approximately 30% of nursing professionals. The fourth category is nursing attendants, helpers, and health auxiliaries, who make up 60% of the total, and its members have no specific training. The majority of these workers have only 4 years of basic schooling (Conselaho Federal de Enfemagem, 1995). In all of these categories, women comprise about 97% of the workforce. Their efforts not only represent work by women but also reflect the very depreciative nature of "women's work" in Brazilian society.

THE CURRENT AND FUTURE ROLE OF FEMALE NURSES IN BRAZIL

As in other Latin American countries, Brazil has experienced important economic and social transformations in the last decades that have produced significant results in health care. Médici (1994) suggests that in order to understand these effects, the first elements to be surveyed are those relating to the transformations that occurred in the relations between state and society in Brazil in recent decades. He suggests that the transformations in the work processes in the health sector were shaped according to the ways they were funded. In a period of democratic reconstruction, where the demand is for health services that are equitable and efficient, the challenge is to face the accumulated problems. The challenge is compounded by the tax crisis faced by the state and by expansion of privatization.

This picture will not be complete, however, if it is not placed within the context of the accelerating urbanization that has occurred in Brazil. It is estimated that 70% of the Brazilian population will be living in urban settings by the year 2020. This phenomenon occurred while there was a slow but constant expansion in basic infrastructure services, especially those of basic sanitation and preventive actions in health care, such as inoculation, treatment of water and waste, and an intense campaign to encourage natural breast feeding. A significant improvement, which will soon be in the social statistics, is the steady fall in the child mortality rate and the increase in life expectancy.

These processes did not occur in a uniform manner in all parts of the country, as some of these indicators suggest. There was an increase in regional differences between races and social classes to the point that some segments of the population have access to a state of social well-being that is equivalent to that of countries of advanced industrialization, while other areas or parts of the population are excluded from the basic benefits of development, sometimes unable to get daily meals.

All of these changes are occurring simultaneous to profound changes in the family structure and the role of women in Brazilian society. Among the most visible aspects of those alterations are the increase of schooling of the female population and their growing participation in the labor force (Machado, 1984). This aspect reveals deep changes in the role of Brazilian women both inside the family and in the public sphere as well as the accelerated voluntary reduction of fertility. This has, as a possible cause, the accelerated urbanization process mentioned previously. The number of children born to fertile women fell from 6.2 per woman at the beginning of the 1960s to 2.8 per woman in 1991, and household surveys on desired fertility foresee the continuation of this downward trend (Fundacáo Instituto Brasileiro de Geografia e Esátistica, 1994; Simões & Oliveira, 1988). Not very significant in terms of numbers and yet full of meaning is the greater participation of women in political life.

It is easy to infer that these highlighted transformations have consequences in the breakdown and composition of the workforce in nursing, opening new areas in the provision of health services in the country and demanding new models for the practice of nursing. An increase in the social role of nurses may be anticipated along with a corresponding increase in the degree of responsibility provided to sick individuals, spreading to a greater action with individuals or social groups outside the hospital setting. There is also the forecast of a greater participation of nurses at the various levels of decision making in health policy in both public and private institutions. These transformations in the current and future role of female nurses in Brazil are of fundamental importance, especially taking into account that nursing personnel represented more than 50% of the labor force in health care in 1995, of whom 96% are women.

In this positive and desirable scene, schools of nursing will have an important role in drawing up innovative proposals and qualifying leadership for their implementation. In order to meet this new scenario, innovative curricula and new teaching models directed at nursing personnel who are already working are needed. This will include continuing distance education through the use of educational methods based on critical participation. Nurses should therefore have the skills and commitment necessary to carry out a relevant role in the process of institutional innovation in the areas of teaching and health care.

Above all, these changing times demand that nurses take on leadership roles in the sense indicated by Lewis (1995, p. 14): "that she should always be seeking to expand or change her way of working, manifesting her dissatisfaction with the status quo, and making the most of opportunities that others do not perceive." In this way nurses will build new opportunities in Brazilian society both as women and as professionals.

CONCLUSION

Throughout history in Brazil, as in other parts of the world, access to all levels of schooling was limited for women, and this was particularly true with regard to university training. Adding the usual discrimination to this, the greater presence of women is in socially undervalued professions such as nursing and education.

A large part of the Brazilian population currently does not have access to health services. The poor continue to be left to the resources of informal care, carried out even today by housewives, midwives, faith healers, and popular healers. These practices are often associated with mystical values and esoteric prescriptions, which are deeply ingrained in Brazilian culture.

Social recognition of these practices is reinforced by their affective connotation and the sense of belonging to a group, which is generally missing in formal health care institutions. As in these institutions, however, informal health care also seeks to meet the demands of allopathic therapy presented by the population and predominant as the healing model. Therefore teas, potions, bottled homemade medicine, and ointments mix with prayers and medicine from the drugstore.

Despite the importance of women in terms of both quality and quantity in producing health and nursing services in the country, it must be highlighted that women and nursing care have been held back by many government policies of protection of family, maternity, and infancy. Among these policies, we emphasize those that are meant to control pregnancy, delivery, the neonatal period, and family planning, thereby controlling the woman's body. Therefore, by being the subjects and objects of formal and informal health care, the "docile bodies" of women (Foucault, 1984) are transformed into productive, consuming bodies, perpetuating a culture that, in spite of this, very often excludes them.

In the sphere of the health institutions and professions, this exclusion is even clearer in nursing, which is looked down on as "women's work" that has become institutionalized. It is clear, therefore, that nursing in Brazil is not only influenced by the traditional roles of women in society, but it has also incorporated and accepted these roles as inherent and necessary, derived from a conceptual framework of feminine submission.

In Brazilian society the submissive status of women has already begun to advance insofar as relevant issues are being raised and changes have begun. However, in the nursing arena this status is seen as a "natural" state of affairs and is not, therefore, something that must be overcome.

REFERENCES

Abreu, C. (1934). *Capitulos de historia colonial [Chapters from colonial history]*, 1500-1800. Rio de Janeiro: Briguiet.

Conselaho Federal de Enfemagem. (FEDERAL NURSING COUNCIL). (1995) Rio de Janeiro.

Foucault, M. (1984). *Vigiar e punir: Nascimento da prisao [Watching and punishing: The birth of prison]* (3rd ed.). Petrópolis, Brasil: Vozes.

Fundacáo Instituto Brasileiro de Geografia e Esátistica. (1994). *Censo.* Rio de Janeiro.

Germano, R.N. (1983). *Educacao e ideologia da enfemagem no Brasil [Education and nursing ideology in Brazil]*. São Paulo: Cortez.

Lewis, J. (1995). *Lideres de educacion a distancia: Intrepreneurs e in entrepreneurs.* Center for International Nursing Education, California State University: Carson, CA.

Machado, M.H. (1984). A mão do obra feminina no Brasil (Female labor in Brazil). In M. Eliana (Ed.). *Labra. Mulher, saúde e sociedade no Brasil.* Rio de Janeiro: Vozes.

Médici, A.C. (1994). *Economia e financiamento do setpr saúde no Brasil: e perspectivas do processo de descontralizaç (Economy and Financing of the health sector in Brazil: Figures and outlooks in the process descontralization).* São Paulo, Faculdade do Saúde Pública/USP.

Medina, A. (1991, April-June). Questoes e direitos relativos a mulher nas Constituicoes do Brasil e de Minas Gerais [Issues and rights relating to the woman in the fundamental laws in Brazil and Minas Gerais State]. *Revista de Informacao Legislativa, 28,* 181-198.

Medina, A. (1992). *Que faziam as mulheres portuguesas enquanto estavam a ver navios? [What did the Portuguese women do while they watched the ships?]*. Unpublished manuscript.

Miles, R. (1989). *A historia do mundo pela mulher [The woman's world history]*. Rio de Janeiro: Livros Tecnicos e Cientificos, Editora Ltda. and Casa-Maria Editorial.

Silva, G.B. (1986). *Enfermagem profissional: Analise critica [Professional nursing: A critical analysis]*. São Paulo: Cortez.

Simões, C.S., Oliveira, L.A. (1988). *Porfil estatístico do criançás e mães no Brasil: A situação da fecundidade, determinates gerais e caraterísticas da transição recente [Statistical profile of children and mothers in Brazil: The situation of fertility, general determining factors and aspects of the recent transition]*. Rio de Janeiro: FIBGE/UNICF/PHO.

Section Ten

CULTURAL DIVERSITY

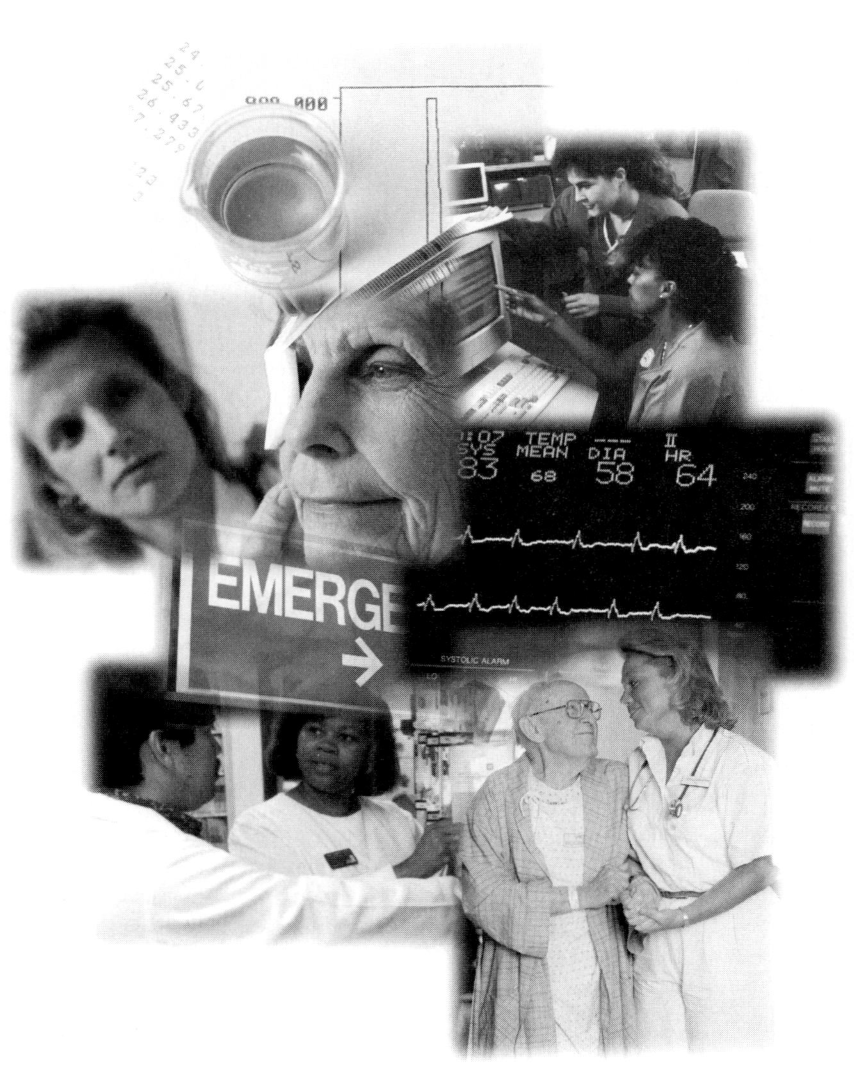

Diversity in nursing: A formidable challenge

JOANNE COMI McCLOSKEY, HELEN KENNEDY GRACE

Throughout history, nursing has been a pathway for social mobility, particularly for women, who in earlier times had relatively few options for advanced education or economic independence. Specifically, white women from rural backgrounds found in nursing a culturally acceptable field in which they might advance economically. Ironically, that has not been the case for women from minority groups. Women from underrepresented groups in this country have been relegated primarily to roles of servitude within the health care system, either as nursing aides or licensed practical nurses with limited access into the mainstream of nursing. Another irony is that in times of nursing shortages, nurses have been welcomed from other countries, particularly the Philippines, to fill the vacant slots. Because the traditions of nursing have been closely tied to women in society, the profession has not been a comfortable field for men either. As we move toward the 21st century the necessity for nursing to become more inclusive is more pressing than ever. This section examines some of the issues related to diversity within nursing and raises challenges that must be addressed by the profession.

Malone's opening debate chapter poses the question, "Why isn't nursing more diversified?" Noting that the logic underlying affirmative action was to "treat everyone the same," the "underlying principle of diversity is acknowledging, addressing, and managing the differences." Affirmative action ensured representativeness but then raised concerns over compromising quality to achieve that end. Nursing has always struggled with being the handmaiden of the physician; and stigmatized, nursing has in turn been reluctant to accept into its ranks people who by virtue of their race, culture, and gender are further stigmatized. This is at odds with the rhetoric of nursing. Ten percent of the workforce in nursing hails from minority groups. Blacks, Hispanics/Latinos, and Native Americans are particularly underrepresented in proportion to the population. Nursing leadership is challenged to engage fully the human resource potential that is represented in diverse groups and lead the profession confidently into the future rather than getting caught up in being gatekeepers in the interests of "maintaining quality."

In the first issues chapter, Castiglia looks at the quality of the pool of potential students. While it is predicted that by the year 2000 one third of the U.S. population will be minorities, only 10% of practicing nurses are from minority groups. Of the minorities entering nursing, nearly 50% of Hispanic and black nurses enter nursing through associate-degree programs, making the challenge of moving upward through advanced educational levels more difficult. Despite this difficulty, 10% of the black nursing population hold doctoral degrees, more than the percentage for white, non-Hispanic nurses. Hispanic nurses are the least represented in completing college and advanced degrees. Focusing on increasing the number of minorities in nursing, particularly those with advanced degrees, Castiglia speaks to the importance of both financial and social support systems. Increasing the numbers of faculty from minority groups is essential if we are to be successful in diversifying nursing to meet the challenges of the 21st century.

Turning to the question of gender equity in the field, Bullough recaps the historical development of nursing and the plight of men to enter and work in the field. Medieval hospitals were staffed primarily by men. The Crimean War was a turning point not only for nursing, but also for women in society. Nightingale became a heroine for all women. In American nursing, men were excluded in a number of ways, except from mental health nursing. Wartime further delineated the roles for men and women—men were to fight the war, and women were to nurse the injured. More recently, the "radical caring theorists" have taken up the cause, arguing that women are by their nature caring, and by inference that men are not caring. Fear that the small numbers of men in the profession will move into leadership roles and have undue influence is also a compounding factor.

Focusing on the challenges of diverse ethnic groups, the next three chapters address specific issues relevant to African Americans, Hispanics/Latinos, and Native Americans, respectively. Dennis speaks to the importance of understanding the cultural context in providing health care. Tracing the history of Africans in America, she examines the interrelationship between ethnicity and a specific set of health problems. The predominant Eurocentric model of nursing is inappropriate in addressing the health care needs of African Americans.

Addressing the underrepresentation of Hispanics/Latinos in nursing, particularly those prepared at the baccalaureate and graduate levels, Torres and Castillo relate this to the financial constraints of this group and the inflexibility of nursing programs, which are compounded by language barriers. Only 1.8% of all nurses and less than 1% of nurses holding doctoral degrees are of Hispanic/Latino origin. This severely limits the number of visible role models or of leaders that might work to rectify the situation. Career mobility is limited on the one hand by cultural, social, and educational barriers and on the other by a profession that has not reached out to be inclusive. These authors argue for systematic efforts beginning at the elementary school level and extending through higher education to develop a pipeline of students to enter and advance in nursing.

Turning to Native Americans in nursing, Crow relates her personal experience in moving from the Eurocentric nursing model to which she had been socialized to provision of care for a Native American community. The importance of understanding Native American traditions and the interplay between these traditions and Western medicine is underscored. The struggle of Native Americans to maintain their culture while federal policy has exerted all forms of pressure to integrate them into the mainstream is played out and needs to be understood by those engaged in providing health care.

In the final chapter in this section, Meleis and Aly turn to the issue of women's health from a global perspective. While there are differences in the cultural backgrounds of people around the world, there are also similarities. Women's health is a global concern. Noting a number of common problems related to women's health, the authors caution that the ways in which these problems are addressed must take into consideration the cultural context in which women live. The involvement of women in the design and management of health care programs worldwide would do much to improve women's health care.

Nursing has prided itself on being at the forefront of advocacy for people in receiving good health care. Yet ironically, nursing has been notably insensitive to the nuances of quality health care that relate to understanding the culture and values that are so much a part of the person. The diversification of the workforce, and celebrating this diversity as a part of nursing's contribution to improved health care for all, is a critical challenge that the profession must address if we are to continue to be a bridge between the "health care system" and the people.

Why isn't nursing more diversified?

BEVERLY L. MALONE

Diversity is a subject that lends itself to polarization. It reverberates with the often conflicting imperatives of pluribus (many) and unum (one) (Cortes, 1991). In a nation built on a multicultural ethos (diversity), but designed and led primarily by Americans of European descent (unum), the inclusion and exclusion of other ethnic groups remain debatable issues.

This is reflective of the debate regarding societal diversity (pluribus) and maintenance of the societal core (unum). Affirmative action is an excellent example of a national debate that continues within the opposing boundaries of the societal core versus societal diversity. The affirmative action programs were designed with a "right-the-wrongs" approach to rectifying the damages perpetrated by the societal core on those who were different. Differences were downplayed by promoting assimilation into the dominant culture of a workplace, school, or institution. There was an appreciation that specific groups had been systematically disadvantaged by the dominant culture. These groups were identified as women, blacks, Hispanics, Asians, and Native Americans. A basic fear of acknowledging differences prevailed because open discussions might immediately polarize the situation, resulting in judgments of right and wrong, superiority and inferiority, or normality and oddity (Thomas, 1990).

Early affirmative action programs in the 1970s were based on the following premises: 1) adult white men comprised the corporate world; 2) women, blacks, immigrants, and other minorities should have access to the mainstream of corporate America as a matter of public policy; 3) widespread racial, ethnic, and sexual prejudices were barriers that protected the corporate world from change; 4) legal and social mandates were necessary for change (Thomas, 1990); and 5) universities were designated points of entry for a rebalancing of opportunity in America.

As a resounding response to the affirmative action efforts (pluribus), in the intervening years between the late 1970s and early 1990s, Presidents Reagan and Bush pushed conservatism, or principles of the societal core (unum), even into the Office of Civil Rights of the Department of Education. More recently, in 1995, Governor Pete Wilson (R-CA) repealed all affirmative action programs that gave preferential treatment to women and members of minority groups in hiring and contracts for the state-supported university system of California. Wilson stated, "No one, in fact, envisioned that redressing two centuries of unfairness would launch a whole new era of unfairness. But it has" (Lively, 1995, p. A25). The tension between the societal core and societal diversity continues. But there is a new reality.

This new reality is framed by rapidly changing demographics—changing the color of the nation, creating a new economic necessity that requires a transformation of the corporate culture of industry into a mosaic of cultural diversity. By the year 2000, the U.S. Department of Labor projects that 85% of new entrants into the workforce will be minorities, women, and immigrants. However, the affirmative action policies that were assumed to be transitional vehicles to the new culture of diversity have produced only moderate results. They were based on treating everyone equally, whereas the underlying principle of diversity is acknowledging, addressing, and managing the differences (Allen, 1991).

The debate about affirmative action is not solely tied to its limitations as a transitional object to an organizational culture of diversity, however. The basic opposing argument is similar to that espoused by Wilson. For example, Genovese (1991) states that in response to diversity, organizations have become so politically correct that in educational institutions professors have been silenced for being insensitive by requiring students to read racist material. Furthermore, Genovese states that to right old wrongs, leading universities are attempting to buy, through scholarships and high salaries, black students and professors, some of whom may not even compete on merit. The crux of the argument against affirmative action is the lowering of standards for minority "protected" populations, which in turn penalizes those in the dominant "unprotected" culture. An article by Shipler (1995) in the *New York Times* describes the issue with this title: "My Equal Opportunity, Your Free Lunch."

These arguments abound in organizational literature and particularly within the liberal educational walls of academe. Yet the composition of corporate organizations continues to change into a more diverse constellation. Likewise, in academic settings student bodies are changing in color, requiring more diverse faculty and staff.

On the other side of the coin is the view that previous wrongs should be addressed. White privilege, which interestingly includes both white men and women, is a more powerful domineering force than any affirmative action plan. McIntosh (1989, p. 10) describes white privilege as "an invisible, weightless knapsack of special provisions, maps, passports, codebooks, visas, clothes, tools and blank checks." In further describing the concept of white privilege, racism is viewed by many whites as individual acts of meanness, not as invisible systems and patterns of interaction that silently confer dominance on a particular group.

From one's own original group experience—the family—to the larger community, the issues of difference as it relates to status, achievement, and recognition are primary, emotionally laden concerns of all people. Responses to diversity that provide some form of redress for prior and continuing disadvantages to one group may result in perceived and real disadvantages for members of another group.

Thus far, the discussion has centered on the national scene, representing a balancing act between pluribus (diversity) and unum (the societal core). Yet the initial question, "Why isn't nursing more diversified?" has not been addressed. The answer to this provocative question could either exonerate or indict the nursing profession. The reason that nursing is not more diversified is that the profession is a microcosm of this nation, constructed with the same building blocks of institutional racism, sexism, and other "isms" that destroy the fabric of a society. Similar to the national debate, nursing wishes to protect its societal core against societal diversity. The uniqueness of nursing is its gender makeup, which is predominantly female and very familiar with the harsh realities of oppression and victimization by others. Perhaps nursing deserves to be relieved of a microscopic examination of the diversity issue, for nursing itself is a victim (Malone, 1993).

A different perspective of an answer to the same question is that nursing, above others, should be held accountable. Nursing is the profession that philosophically cares for all people regardless of race, color, or creed. Nursing is the caring profession. Nursing has experienced the stigmatized pain of being perceived as only the physician's handmaiden, always under the supervision of the male doctor. Nursing knows the pain of exclusion. Yet statistically almost 90% of the 1.8 million employed nurses are white, and in the past 10 years this figure has not significantly changed. In other words, nursing has not increased its pace of diversification over the past 10 years. This resistance to change has been in the face of sweeping demographic changes that forecast a nation with a workforce of a new minority group—white men.

Using the discussion frame of debate, this section explores possible reasons for the lack of change in nursing's level of diversification. The areas of exploration include numbers, philosophy, professionalism, practice, and leadership strategies that could lead to increased diversification in nursing.

THE NUMBERS DEBATE

According to statistics, nursing might simply be described as a white, female profession. This description belies the complexity of the health profession with the highest representation of diversity in its ranks. The most recent survey of nursing (Moses, 1992) reveals that there were 2,239,816 registered nurses (RNs) in the United States in 1992, of whom 1,853,024 were employed in nursing. Of those employed in nursing, 186,000 (10.0%) were minorities. The employed RN workforce consisted of 79,980 (4.3%) Blacks, 27,900 (1.5%) Hispanic, 7,440 (0.4%) American Indians, 70,680 (3.8%) Asians; 11,160 (0.6%) others, and 1,655,704 (90%) whites. Men comprised 4.3% (80,000) of the employed RN workforce. These are highly respectable numbers in comparison with medicine, dentistry, and the allied health professions. For example, of 548,000 employed physicians, only 47,676 (8.7%) are minorities; dentistry reports 7.5% minorities, optometry 4%, and pharmacy 8.9% (U.S. Department of Health and Human Services, 1994). Nursing has excelled among the professions in providing a professional atmosphere that invites the participation of those who are different in culture, race, and ethnicity.

On the other hand, excluding men, when compared with the growth rate and the percentage of the U.S. population that is represented by these diverse ethnic and racial groups, the nursing profession is lacking in diversity. For example, while blacks comprise 11% of the population in the United States, only 4.3% of employed nurses are black. The only group that approaches a positive comparison or parity is the Asian population. Since 1980, the Asian population in the United States has grown by 107% to 7.3 million, or approximately 3% of the total U.S. population. This compares favorably with 3.8% employed Asian nurses. The Hispanic growth rate in this country (53%), although less than half that of the Asians, has resulted in the second largest minority group with 21.1 million (8.6%) in the U.S. population and 1.5% employed Hispanic nurses (Moses, 1992; U.S. Bureau of Census, 1990).

In 1980, one in five Americans was classified as a minority. In 1990, one in four has African, Asian, American Indian, or Hispanic ancestry. This change has been explained primarily by immigrants from Latin America and influxes from the Philippines, China, India, and Southeast Asia. By the year 2000, it is predicted that three out of five children will be children of color. Presently more than half the labor force is women and people of color (Waldrop, 1990). The use of the term *minority* to describe people of color must be reevaluated as a result of these changes in the complexion of the United States.

RHETORIC AND REALITY: THE DEBATE CONTINUES

Nursing has consistently been caught between rhetoric and reality (Church, 1990; Malone, 1993). The rhetoric associated with the high ideals of a newly birthed profession viewed with the reality of technical training sufficing as an acceptable avenue of entry into nursing is representative of the dialectical history of the profession. Another example is nursing's assertive commitment to the concept of autonomy, one of the critical components of a profession (Beletz, 1990), and the reality of a general acceptance and dependence on physicians, hospital administrators, and others in the field to define nursing's roles and functions.

Nursing's evolution into professional status has been a path beset by issues of women, power, and control. On entering the hospital, a male- and physician-dominated institution, nurses formed an alliance with the medical system. The parameters for nursing practice were more restrictive within the institutional walls of the hospital than outside in the community (Church, 1990). The initial alliance was based on submission to the philosophy that physicians were the primary reason for a hospital's existence. The hourly wage mentality rather than a fee or salary also attested to an assistive, piecework role for nursing that was subsumed within the physician's overall responsibility and that denied the primacy of the nurse-patient relationship. Perhaps nursing has been so focused on the injustices and inequities perpetuated throughout the years by a domineering medical model that nursing's own biases and fears of differences and the acknowledgement of the contributions of others who are different have been relegated to the shadows of obscurity. For example, Carnegie (1986) states:

> Despite there being many general books on the history of nursing, until recently only a few have mentioned or devoted more than a sentence or two to Black nurses and their contributions to health care. The one typical sentence found in nursing history texts is, "Mary Mahoney was the first trained Black nurse in America, having been graduated from the New England Hospital for Women and Children in 1879" (p. ix).

The invisible history of those who are different in nursing is reflected in the absence of Mary Seacole from the written nursing record. Seacole was a Black Jamaican woman who nursed the sick during the Crimean War along with Florence Nightingale. The invisibility and lack of respect for differences in nursing are captured as recognition for the first nursing program in a university setting. This honor is bestowed on the University of Minnesota, which initiated its program in 1909, rather than on Howard University in Washington, D.C., which established its program in 1893, 16 years earlier than its nearest contender. Nursing rhetoric values diversity, while nursing reality disregards it.

There is some indication that historical disregard for diversity in nursing is changing. In a recent work by Kalisch and Kalisch (1994), a chapter is devoted to minorities in nursing, with clear descriptive historical passages that reveal the "American dilemma" as so aptly outlined by Myrdal (1944). This dilemma suggest that rights and benefits due all Americans do not include Americans of color, specifically blacks. Myrdal observed a caste system based on entrenched beliefs about blacks that were demonstrably false but that provided the rationale and defense by whites that blacks belonged to a separate and lesser race of mankind, inferior in all important respects. As this was revealed in 1944, nursing scholars and professionals have had access to this information for more than 50 years. Why isn't nursing more diversified?

THE AMERICAN DILEMMA/NOT NURSING'S DILEMMA

One answer is that nursing does not own the "American dilemma" as "nursing's dilemma." If the American dilemma is also nursing's dilemma, then it could be said that nursing, like America, as an institution has systematically denied access to people of color in becoming members of the profession. Once again the rhetoric of high ethical and human rights principles would be compromised by the reality of nurses plagued by irrational human fears of differences and susceptible to a model of exclusion rather than one of inclusion (Malone, 1993). While the nursing profession speaks strongly to being responsive to differences by individualizing the caring process and tailoring theory-based, scientifically determined patient care principles to the needs of the individual community, the cloaked vestiges of early parental influence and bias lie unexplored and unidentified within the human heart of the institution of nursing.

NURSING/NURSES

Similar to rhetoric and reality, the same disparity may exist between the profession of nursing and nurses themselves. The ideals of inclusion that are valued and promulgated by the profession are often applied selectively in the daily interactions of the nurse. This selectivity may be based on biases, stereotypes, or preconceived ideas. In addition, there is a component of psychological and physical wear and tear on the nurse. With the majority of nurses having personal responsibilities that stretch from home into their clinical work settings, there may be a continual feeling of being on the edge of managing the dual roles of home and work. This edge behavior is not conducive to decision making that reflects a professional respect for differences. If the assumption is that when one becomes a nurse the cloak of professionalism neatly falls into place, nurses may not understand the need for a conscious, deliberate, systematic approach to including culturally competent care as a component of professional behavior. Being culturally and racially competent is an unnatural process that requires awareness and new learning with the resulting new behavior rewarded and valued by the health care institution. While the nursing profession has high ethical and human rights principles, it is comprised of individual nurses plagued by irrational human fears of differences who are susceptible to a model of exclusion rather than inclusion (Malone, 1993). Once the issues of differences are identified, strategic and appropriate solutions can be devised ranging from increased familiarity and knowledge of those who are different to intensive diversity training. This reflects an individual level of assessment, intervention, and evaluation.

ORGANIZATIONAL VALUING OF DIVERSITY: A LEADERSHIP ISSUE

There is also the organizational level of analysis of nursing's willingness or reticence to further diversify the profession. At the organizational level, the following processes need to be assessed: the philosophy, goal or mission statement, strategic plan, budget, and evaluation. The institutions and the nursing departments or schools should resonate with the profession's overall philosophy of providing care to all regardless of race, creed, or color. It is not at the philosophical level of the system that dissonance is visible within the profession of nursing. However, with the mission/goal statement/strategic plan, there may be a lack of any acknowledgment of the organization's standard of relating to groups who are different. The status of the institution's relationship with culturally diverse groups must be reflected in the organization's guiding principles (Malone, 1993).

The next system's process is the budget, which represents the most truthful indicator of an organization's priorities. The final organizational component is evaluation, which is a systematic method of matching intent with performance and outcome. It is evaluation that illuminates the path from a nursing department's or school's philosophy to the individual nurse's or faculty's performance. An evaluation line item addressing diversity on each staff member's evaluation form is one method to ensure that diversity is a systemwide responsibility. These organizational processes move the issue of diversifying nursing to an organizational and administrative level of responsibility. This does not nullify the individual's responsibility, but it does make diversifying nursing a collective endeavor and a leadership issue. Organizations must use a broad range of initiatives in their efforts to value and manage diversity. Valuing diversity is a task that requires individuals to let go of assumptions about the universal rightness of their own values (Carnevale & Stone, 1994).

GATEKEEPERS OF THE NURSING PROFESSION

Culturally blind gatekeepers

Faculty and nursing administrators are frequently the gatekeepers of the nursing profession. Lenburg (1995) states, "A fundamental issue for educators and administrators is the extent to which they will change essential components of educational programs in response to the transformation of society" (p. 7). Whether nursing educators and administrators will respond may be related to several factors identified by Cross, Bazron, and Dennis (1989): cultural destructiveness, cultural incapacity, and cultural blindness. *Cultural destructiveness* relates to the clear intent to destroy another's culture through dehumanization of the individuals within the group; whereas *cultural incapacity* refers to a void or inability to be receptive to culturally different people. For the nursing profession, however, the gatekeepers are more likely to be culturally blind than destructive or incapable. *Cultural blindness* is a condition that acknowledges only the values and norms established by the dominant culture (unum) as relevant and appropriate. An easily recognized symptom of cultural blindness is color blindness. The nursing faculty or administrators may enthusiastically announce that they see no difference between an American of European descent and an American of African or Asian descent. Yet the behavior of the faculty or administrators toward the dominant and diverse cultures portrays an incongruence between the rhetoric of nursing's gatekeepers and the reality of their behavior.

Gatekeepers: protecting quality

A different perspective of the gatekeepers' response relates to ensuring the consumer the delivery of competent nursing care. The gatekeeper's responsibility includes guarding the quality and safety of nursing care by controlling the admission of potential nurses who would be destructive or incapable of providing quality care. This concern for the lowering of standards resonates with the affirmative action example mentioned in the beginning of this chapter.

Brink (1994) states that nursing faculties prefer teaching a homogenous student body. She points out that the faculty can more easily determine the appropriate content, pace, clinical experiences, examinations, and level of reading assignments when students share a mean grade point average of 3.5 with generally the same cultural experiences. With a homogeneous, white middle class group of students, passing the licensing examination on the first attempt and successful entry into the profession are more clearly assured.

Castiglia (1994) addresses the issue of quality as a matter that must be considered carefully. The exceptions to admission criteria, once granted to minority students to sustain adequate enrollments, may no longer be necessary. She predicts that the pendulum may swing to quantitative measures such as American College Test and Scholastic Aptitude Test scores along with grade point averages. As a result, faculty may fill nursing classes with only the "brightest and the best," which according to traditional measures may exclude students of color. In deference to the delivery of quality care to patients, one can argue that only the "brightest and best" should become nurses.

SUMMARY

Nursing is at an interesting crossroads. The opportunity for the profession to move into a pivotal role within a reformed health care system is a revolutionary event. The opportunity to reform the nursing profession in terms of diversity is also revolutionary. These opportunities are inextricably linked by demographic changes, with resulting economic necessities that can only be addressed through increasing the diversity within nursing. Yet traditional wisdom of bygone eras whispers to gatekeepers, "Protect the societal core (unum)." The pluribus (diversity) is not worthy of consideration and inclusion. Nursing faculty, nursing administrators, staff nurses, community-based nurses, and advanced practice nurses must stand at the crossroads and consciously and deliberately choose.

While individual nurses in various roles can make individual decisions, the reality is that diversity has arrived and continues to reshape corporate and health care policies and principles of management. If nursing chooses to be a policy shaper and maker rather than only responding in a delayed time frame to changes, the profession must embrace the concept that managing diversity is not equivalent to lowering standards but rather to fully engaging the human resource potential of every member of the nursing workforce (Thomas, 1990). Nursing must first reach a level of increased diversity, which will require affirmative action to move from a homogenous leadership to a diverse leadership; from homogenous faculties to diverse faculties; and from homogenous advanced practice nurses to diverse advanced practice nurses. The ultimate goal is to move beyond affirmative action, but nursing must start with reality.

REFERENCES

Allen, G. (1991). Valuing cultural diversity: Industry woos a new work force. *Communication World, 8*(6), 14-17.

Beletz, E. (1990). Professionalization—a license is not enough. In Chaska, N. (Ed.), *The nursing profession turning points* (pp. 16-22). St. Louis, MO: Mosby.

Brink, P. (1994). Cultural diversity in nursing: How much can we tolerate? In J. Mcloskey & H. Grace (Eds.), *Current issues in nursing* (4th ed., pp. 658-664). St. Louis, MO: Mosby.

Carnegie, M.E. (1986). *The path we tread.* Philadelphia: Lippincott.

Carnavale, A. & Stone, S. (1994). Diversity beyond the golden rule. *Training and Development.*

Castiglia, P. (1994). Increasing the pool of minority students. In J. Mc-Closkey & H. Grace (Eds.), *Current issues in nursing* (4th ed., pp. 676-681) St. Louis, MO: Mosby.

Church, O. (1990). Nursing history: What it was and what it was not. In N. Chaska (Ed.), *The nursing profession turning points* (pp. 3-8). St. Louis, MO: Mosby.

Cortes, C. (1991). Pluribus & unum: The quest for community and diversity. *Change, 23,* 9-13.

Cross, T.L., Bazron, B.J., & Dennis, K. (1989). *Toward a culturally competent system of care.* Washington DC: National Institute of Mental Health, Child and Adolescent Service System Program.

Genovese, E. (1991). Heresy, yes—sensitivity, no. *The New Republic, 204,* 30.

Kalisch, P., & Kalisch, B. (1994). *The advancing of American nursing.* Philadelphia: Lippincott.

Lenburg, C.B. (editor). (1995). *Promoting cultural competence in and through nursing education. A critical review and comprehensive plan for action.* (p. 7). Washington, DC: American Academy of Nursing.

Lively, K. (1995, June 9). *Chronicle of Higher Education,* pp. A25-A28.

McIntosh, P. (1989). White privilege: Unpacking the invisible knapsack. *Peace and Freedom,* pp. 10-12.

Malone, B.L. (1993). Caring for culturally diverse racial groups: An administrative model. *Nursing Administration Quarterly, 17*(2), 21-29.

Moses, E. (1992). National sample survey of registered nurses. Washington, DC: U.S. Department of Health & Human Services, Division of Nursing.

Myrdal, G. (1944). An American dilemma. In *The negro problem and modern democracy* (p. ix). New York: Harper & Brothers.

Shipler, D. (1995, March 5). My equal opportunity, your free lunch. *The New York Times,* p. 15.

Thomas, R., Jr. (1990, March–April). From Affirmative Action to Affirming Diversity. *Harvard Business Review, 2,* 107-117.

U.S. Bureau of Census. U.S. Department of Health and Human Services. (1990). *Labor Statistics Dept,* Rockville, MD: Author.

U.S. Department of Health and Human Services. (1994). *Minorities and women in the health fields.* Rockville, MD: Author.

Waldrop, J. (1990). You'll know it's the 21st century when . . . *American Demographics, 12*(12), 22-27.

Minority representation in nursing educational programs: Increasing cultural awareness

PATRICIA T. CASTIGLIA

Since 1990, affirmative action programs, many of which were instituted in the 1960s, have been a subject of considerable continuous and escalating debate. Civil rights protests, including marches on Washington, did much to formulate more proactive policies to assist members of minority groups into schools and positions formerly closed to them. For 2 years Alexander, Education Secretary during the Bush administration, studied the legality of minority scholarships and developed a draft document of guidelines that would have barred them (Jaschik, 1993).

The current debate emphasizes the idea of reverse discrimination, that is, that qualified whites are being denied access to academic programs and jobs because they do not have minority status. The Bakke decision in 1978 (*Regents of the University of California v. Bakke*) endorsed the use of race as one factor in admissions decisions. In the case of Podberesky, a Hispanic student, the U.S. Court of Appeals for the Fourth District ruled that the University of Maryland at College Park had failed to meet the legal tests for offering a minority scholarship. This suit challenged a scholarship for black students at the University, and the decision made is the only one at the appellate level that deals with a minority challenge. The ruling stated that past discrimination was not sufficient cause for a race-based remedy, and that such discrimination must exert some present effect (Jaschik, 1993). The Adarand decision in June 1995 held that race could only be used for preferential treatment if it can withstand "strict scrutiny" by the federal courts (Michaelson, 1995). As it is interpreted, this decision affects higher education because all colleges and universities are, to some extent, governed by state and federal civil rights laws in order to receive federal and state money. Therefore, "strict scrutiny" would have a far-reaching effect. Both California and Michigan are currently engaged in legislative processes to ban or severely modify affirmative action in those states. In 1996, the Adarand decision was used when the federal Fifth Circuit court ruled on a suit brought by law students at the University of Texas at Austin regarding preferential treatment given to minority applicants. The ruling on this case, *Hopwood v. U.T. Austin Law School,* stipulates that universities in the Fifth Circuit jurisdiction cannot use race or ethnicity as factors in determining admission to the university, to special programs, or for scholarships or financial aid (Kauffman, 1996, August). Admissions can be made, for example, on the basis of economic disadvantage, bilingual ability, or regional or geographical needs. This legislation means that educational institutions must find new or additional ways to continue to improve diversity in our student bodies. The Hopwood case may have far-reaching effects in other states and on the federal level. The National Science Foundation (NSF) and other funding agencies have modified or are modifying their guidelines to encourage recruitment and selection strategies.

In relation to health care in the United States, it is obvious that minority populations are greatly underserved. Since the 1960s, the federal government has increased its efforts to provide accessible, cost-effective care to underserved populations: The Department of Health and Human Resources plays a major role in that effort. Among the programs that have been developed are the National Health Service Corps, the Health Careers Opportunity Program, Centers of Excellence in Minority Health, and Student Assistance Programs (U.S. Department of Health and Human Services [DHHS], 1991). The underlying assumption of these programs is that the recruitment and support of minority students in the health professions will assist in meeting the health care needs of underserved minority communities. By the year 2000, it is estimated that ethnic minorities will constitute 25% of the U.S. population, and that this number will increase to 51.1% by the year 2080 (Andrews, 1992). Curtailing affirmative actions might seriously impact on the ability to prepare minority students who have a vested interest in serving underserved minority communities.

MINORITY REPRESENTATION IN NURSING

Nursing can no longer sustain itself without incorporating, to a greater extent, diverse minority groups into the profession. Interwoven with the issues related to minorities in nursing are a number of issues that reflect societal views toward women, toward subcultures in our society, and toward demographic changes that have occurred over time. Although the number of men in nursing has increased, the profession remains predominantly female (approximately 96%). Therefore, gender socialization has played and continues to play a major role in both the continuation and the development of nursing. Stereotypes related to both gender and ethnicity cannot be separated artificially when examining the past, present, and future considerations of minorities in nursing.

Basic influences when selecting a career relate to one's beliefs about oneself. Where do I belong or fit? What is an acceptable career from the viewpoint of my family and my social group? Where can I find personal fulfillment? Financial reward? Advancement? Security? Ability to be mobile, yet permanence in a career?

All statistics related to minority status are self-reported. Students indicate their ethnic status as they perceive it. For federal government reports, the usual categories are black non-Hispanic, American Indian or Alaskan native, Asian or Pacific Islander, Hispanic, white, non-Hispanic, and race/ethnicity unknown (Borden, 1995). In 1992, there were 2,239,816 licensed reported registered nurses (RNs) in the United States. Of these, less than 10% (approximately 207,000) are identified as being of a minority background: blacks (90,600), Asian or Pacific Islanders (76,000), Hispanics (30,400), and American Indian or Alaskan Natives (10,000) (Moses, 1993). When these data are compared with data collected by the Division of Nursing in 1988 (U.S. Department of Health and Human Services [DHHS], 1990), it appears that the growth in the number of minority RNs has probably kept pace with the growth of the total number of nurses, but the proportions of minority nurses have not increased. The 10% minority population in nursing is less than the 25% representation of minorities found throughout the United States. The only equal representation appears with those of Asian or Pacific Island backgrounds (Moses, 1993).

It should be noted that there is a difference in the type of education for nursing for minority groups. Completion of associate-degree programs is the prevalent mode for 46% of Hispanic nurses and 42% of black nurses. Although baccalaureate programs have higher proportions of minority students than do associate-degree programs, because associate-degree programs tend to produce more graduates than do baccalaureate programs, the actual numbers of associate-degree graduates in the nursing population is greater (Moses, 1993). An analysis of educational levels for minority nurses also indicates that about 10% of black nurses have master's or doctoral degrees as compared with 8% of white nurses and 6% of Hispanic and Asian nurses (Justiz, 1995). It is important to note that Hispanics remain very underrepresented at the collegiate level. Only 2.9% of Hispanics are awarded baccalaureate degrees, and only 1.8% receive doctoral degrees (Justiz, 1995).

These figures must be related to what is occurring in nursing education. Obvious questions to be investigated include the following: Are members of minority groups attracted to nursing? Do they successfully complete programs of study? Do they remain in the profession? Why should we be concerned about the representation, or rather lack of representation, of significant numbers of minorities in nursing? What directions should we pursue?

CURRENT STATUS OF MINORITIES IN NURSING EDUCATION PROGRAMS

Nursing is not unique among the health professions, which have traditionally attracted predominantly white students. This trend has persisted despite efforts at equal opportunities for the culturally diverse segments of American society. It is indeed incongruous when one considers Hodgkinson's 1985 study of demographic trends and their impact on our educational system. That study concludes that by the year 2000, one in every three U.S. citizens will be nonwhite. Harris (1990) predicts that by the 21st century one third to one half of all students will be students of color. The nursing population is not a predominantly young group. In 1984, 20% of all graduates were younger than 30 years of age, and in 1988 this number decreased to 15.6%. The average age for all RNs is 43.1 years, with Hispanic nurses being somewhat younger (39.7 years) than other groups (Moses, 1993).

During the 1980s, declining enrollments in nursing education programs encourage schools to actively pursue minority candidates. The Nurse Training Act of 1964 and subsequent revisions provided special funding to increase the number of disadvantaged and minority students in schools of nursing. In 1965 the Sealantic fund (Rockefeller brother's fund) began sponsoring a program in nursing education for disadvantaged students. This project emphasized recruitment, counseling, summer enrichment programs, and financial assistance. The American Nurses Association Minority Fellowship program and the Kellogg Fellows program are other examples of attempts not only to improve the numbers of minority nurses but also to assist minority nurses to advance in the profession.

In 1963, the National Student Nurses' Association developed the Breakthrough to Nursing project, which focused on recruiting minorities into the nursing profession. Federal funding for this project was obtained in 1971 and again in 1974. The Breakthrough project emphasized the establishment of one-to-one relationships with prospective candidates and also included a planned tutoring-advocacy-counseling component (Carnegie, 1988). Despite this 25-year effort in nursing, the racial-ethnic composition in nursing education programs remained the same as that reported for all higher education students in 1988, with the number of blacks being marginally higher for nursing (11.4%) than for all students (10%). In 1990, Carter reported increases in the number of American Indian, Hispanic, and black students in 2-year institutions, while there were more Asians enrolled in 4-year institutions.

The tracking of nursing students by the National League For Nursing (NLN) clearly illustrates that the minority composition of nursing students varies across geographical areas of the country. A variety of sources verifies this geographical distribution. For example, approximately 73% of black RNs are employed in the Northeast and South, with about 47% of black nurses working in the South. Seventy percent of all employed RNs are found in the western or southern regions of the country (36% in the West and 33.5% in the South). Asian nurses are usually employed in the West (38%) and Northeast (32%) (Moses, 1993). As in earlier reports, the midwestern section of the country has the fewest number of minorities in all categories. In addition, the 1991 NLN report found that more Hispanics and American Indians graduated from licensed practical nurse (LPN) and licensed vocational nurse (LVN) programs than from RN programs. Men continue to represent only a small minority in nursing; and because the recruitment efforts in nursing focus on ethnic minorities, it is expected that this representation will continue. However, while the national average for male enrollment is reported as 3.3% by Moses (1990), enrollment in geographical areas varies. In west Texas, for example, men constitute anywhere from 15% to 18% of the student nursing enrollment. It may be that the increased enrollment of men in this region is a reflection of their viewing nursing as a route upward in the social and economic structure, the acceptance in these communities of men in a predominantly female profession, or the great need for nurses in this area.

Statistics related to minority enrollment in nursing programs become of even greater concern when considered in relation to the enrollment in specific types of nursing programs. At the baccalaureate level, for example, Hispanics constitute 2.9% of the total enrollment, but at the master's and doctoral levels their enrollments are only 1.7% each. Although blacks generally represent the largest minority in nursing, it is worth noting that of all black nursing students, 8.8% are enrolled in generic baccalaureate programs, 7.4% in RN baccalaureate programs, 5.2% in master's-degree programs, 4.3% in doctoral programs, and only 1 of 14 postdoctoral students was black (American Association of Colleges of Nursing [AACN], 1990).

Factors influencing the need to change minority ratios

A persistent decline in the number of young people eligible for college admission has been documented nationwide. Concurrently there has been an increase in the number of older students (those over 25 years of age) who are interested in pursuing college careers, including nursing.

Applications to nursing programs recovered from the 1980s slump as a result of the compounded impact of the nursing shortage, a lack of access to health care for many Americans, an aging population, a shift in emphasis to primary community health care, cost containment efforts by hospitals (including the use of diagnostic-related groups), and a movement to break down barriers between the health professions through expanded reimbursement by Medicaid, Medicare, and third-party insurers for specifically prepared nurses. These factors have forced the health care system to upgrade salaries and benefits for nurses. When adequate financial reimbursement occurs in a profession, members of that profession develop an increased sense of self-esteem, and colleagues in other professions develop an increased respect. The waiting lists for admission to many schools of nursing attest to the increased attractiveness of the nursing profession today. As health care moves to a managed care system, there has occurred a downsizing of beds and nursing staff in hospitals. Unfortunately, adequate remuneration has not extended to areas of need beyond hospital settings. Public health nursing salaries, school nursing salaries, and salaries in extended care facilities still lag. This is a serious manifestation of the blatant lack of provision for quality health care to the poor, to rural and urban underserved and underinsured citizens, and to minority populations, and particularly a diminished commitment to health promotion and disease prevention activities.

The question of quality in nursing practice continues to be a factor that must be considered carefully. In the past, nursing schools were tempted to make exceptions to admissions requirements in order to maintain programs through sustained enrollments. Now the pendulum may swing toward admitting only the most highly qualified applicants in relation to quantitative measures such as American College Test (ACT) scores, Scholastic Aptitude Test (SAT) scores, or grade point average (GPA). Because of the increased applicant pool, admissions committees may be tempted to fill classes with only the best students as measured by these traditional criteria. If efforts are not made on elementary, middle, and high school levels to better prepare minority students, we may find that the equal opportunity access has been thwarted. Most admissions evaluations cannot accommodate all minimally prepared applicants, so admissions committees seek to select the students with the most potential for success (Boyle, 1986). If this is carried to the extreme, minority students may suffer because they will not be afforded the opportunity to attempt to succeed.

Traditionally, minority students have been classified as high-risk students because they often experience higher attrition rates than white students. The most frequently used criteria on which admission to nursing schools is based include high school GPA, high school rank, interviews, health data, college GPA, ACT assessment scores, SAT scores, and autobiographical essays. There have been a number of conflicting studies regarding the usefulness of these criteria for the prediction of success in a nursing program. Dell and Halpin (1984) recommend the use of high school GPA, SAT scores, and National League of Nursing (NLN) scores as effective for use with all ethnic groups.

The Boyle (1986) study found that the ACT score was the strongest and most effective predictor of state board examination achievement and of final GPA. Entering GPA was the only variable that was found to account for program completion, but it did not accurately predict program dropouts. The higher the entering GPA, however, the greater the likelihood of program completion. The predictive power for blacks was less than that for other minorities, but an earlier investigator (Schwirian, 1977) maintained that less than 50% of attrition is really related to academic difficulty, and that attrition may rather be due to greater social and economic disadvantages. A study by Schmidt, Pearlman, and Hunter (1980) sought to evaluate the validity and fairness of employment and educational tests for Hispanics. The results of this study indicate that there is strong evidence that the tests are neither differentially valid for, nor unfair to, Hispanics. The validity and slope differences were found to be a result of chance as reported in an earlier study by Bartlett, Bobko, Mosier, and Hannon (1978) of blacks and whites.

In recent years, women have been attracted to professions other than the traditional occupations of nursing and teaching. The attractiveness of the nursing profession has been enhanced during the past 30 years, however, by the development of new and expanded roles in nursing. These new roles are characterized by increased autonomy and by increased appreciation and recognition from the public and from professional colleagues.

High school students today have a broad range of career choices. The AACN (1990) report dealing with enrollment management found that a large percentage of students cited nursing as a career objective and that parents exerted the most influence on student career choice. When students were asked why they had an interest in nursing, they cited the following desires: (1) to help others, (2) to work directly with people, and (3) to work with life-and-death situations. The reasons they lacked interest in nursing were related to the requirements to (1) work in high-pressure situations, (2) work in stressful situations, and (3) work different shifts. Parental goals for their children were reported as follows: (1) to be financially secure, (2) to do rewarding work, and (3) to have time to spend with family. These items were rated 11, 2, and 10, respectively, by parents in relation to the nursing profession (AACN, 1990).

The Hispanic student in nursing

The term *Hispanic* includes those of Spanish, Mexican-American, Puerto Rican, and Cuban descent. The greatest numbers of Hispanics in the United States are Mexican-Americans (Chicanos). Rojas (1994) cites data from the

Laredo Morning Times of December 5, 1992, that estimates that 33% of the U.S. population growth from 1992 through 2000 will be a growth in the Hispanic population. This growth is predicted to accelerate to 57% from 2030 to 2050. Hispanic students rely heavily on financial aid for college expenses because almost 25% of Hispanic students come from families with an annual income of less than $10,000. An additional 20% of Hispanic students come from families earning between $10,000 and $20,000 annually (Dutko, 1994). Despite this great need, the average financial aid award to Hispanic students ($3,466) is less than that for other groups, including Asians ($4,383), blacks ($3,788), and non-Hispanic white ($3,524) (Dutko, 1994). Over half of all Hispanic students attend 2-year programs, and almost half of all Hispanic students attend school part-time.

A study by Vasquez (1982) found that sex-role restrictions and low socioeconomic status rather than culture or language partially accounted for the relatively low number of Chicanas (Mexican-American women) in postsecondary education. Chicanas are no different than other people in wanting education as a means to socioeconomic mobility and independence. Unfortunately, these women, who are often the first in their families to attend college, experience dissonance in relation to their expected role in Mexican-American society as wife, mother, and subservient person to the man; all of these factors exert an influence to diminish professional career expectations. Unfortunately, Mexican-American students are often steered into taking noncollege preparatory courses in high school. This may be promulgated by the family as a means of keeping women in less demanding work, which in turn is perceived as having a less negative impact on the woman's traditional role. Such advice from family members may be reinforced by educators who often stereotype Mexican-American students as unable to prepare for more challenging careers. Most of these students need financial assistance because their parents are generally unable to contribute as much to their education as white parents can (Vasquez, 1982). Therefore, they generally rely heavily on scholarships and work-study programs and, to a lesser extent, on loans. Because of the difference in cultures and the difficulty in acculturation, many of these minority students feel more comfortable in smaller colleges or community colleges. Support systems such as associations and organizations that can recognize, promote, and reinforce cultural values are important for student adjustment regardless of the size of the educational setting.

Financial difficulty and discomfort in the setting, while problematic, are not the primary factors for leaving educational programs. A study by Cope and Hannah (1975) found that the motivation to finish college was influenced in great measure by the family's emotional support of the student. This may be a comforting fact to relay to parents who fear "losing" their child when she or he pursues higher education. Because parents do influence their child's choice of a career, some reassurance from an individual's ethnic group—such as continued inclusion in family and community activities—has been found to be a necessary positive component of adjustment and success in college. This finding may reassure Mexican-American parents of their continued important role. In fact, several researchers, including Ramirez and Castaneda (1974) have found that participating in two or more cultures may provide for a more flexible adjustment.

It would appear self-evident that Hispanic students, like other students, would tend to persist in their education when their parents have higher educations and when parental occupations result in higher incomes. Low family income, for many students, results in their dropping out of school. Because Mexican-American families generally have lower incomes, and either larger or extended families to absorb those incomes, their children are at risk for attrition. Efforts must persist, therefore, to obtain scholarships and grants to attempt to alleviate some of this financial pressure. In 1991, the DHHS instituted a new scholarship program called Scholarships for Disadvantaged Students. These scholarships recognize that the concept of being disadvantaged is not necessarily tied to ethnicity alone, but rather is linked to socioeconomic factors including deficits in a particular school district's ability to offer enriched programs for students.

The black student in nursing

Almost 15% of the graduates of LPN/LVN programs and only 9.1% of the graduates of RN programs are black (Rosella, Regan-Kubinski, & Albrecht, 1994). Only 7.1% of all RNs are black. This is significant because blacks, in terms of general health, tend to be sicker than the general population. While European-Americans have a life expectancy of 76.0 years, the average life expectancy of blacks is 69.2 years (National Center for Health Statistics, 1992). Blacks have 6.6 times as many homicide deaths as European-Americans, and hypertension occurs in 2% of the black population and 0.1% of European-Americans (Rosella et al., 1994). These statistics are important examples because the low numbers of black nurses present a barrier to treatment because of the lack of integration of the cultural beliefs, values, and practices of blacks. Thus, despite the fact that numerous studies have shown that compliance to treatment by blacks is affected by cultural values (Berg & Berg, 1989) there are few black nurses who impact positively on the integration of cultural values.

Nursing education has historically provided one of the few avenues for black women to acquire a respected profession. However, for many years that education was primarily obtained in black hospitals and colleges. New graduates worked only with blacks. As the nursing profession evolved, an elitist system developed in which most white schools had racial quotas. An early effort to recruit black nursing students was stimulated during World War II by the Cadet Nurse Corps program. Today the emphasis is on attracting black and other minority students—not to fill quotas but to develop a cohort of professional nurses who better represent the general population.

Between 1976 and 1982, the National Advisory Committee on Black Higher Education and Black Colleges and Universities studied the admission and retention problems of black students at seven predominantly white universities. Although this committee no longer exists, the problem it faced—the retention of black baccalaureate nursing students—persists (Allen, Nunley, & Scott-Warner, 1988).

Black students, like other minority students, often receive a poor secondary education. Their self-esteem has been low, and the university setting has generally been perceived as hostile to them. Not only have high school counselors failed in encouraging black students to pursue higher education, but university counselors have also not been able to effectively thwart the feelings of loneliness and alienation that black students frequently experience. Inadequate financial aid has been found to be a barrier to both the admission and the retention of black nursing students (Allen et al., 1988).

Graduate nursing education and the minority student

Almost 12% of the enrollees in master's programs are minorities: 5.3% black, 33.3% Hispanic, 2.6% Asian, and 0.5% Native American (Rosella et al., 1994). Graduate education in nursing continues to grow, as indicated by an 8.1% increase in master's-degree graduates from 1989 to 1990 (NLN, 1991). In addition, the number of doctoral programs in place rose to 50 in 1990 (NLN, 1991). The expansion of advanced educational preparation in nursing is related to increased specialization in the practice arena, necessitating increased preparation in terms of the complexity and competency needed to administer quality nursing care and to pursue relevant research.

Funding for students to attend graduate programs is always subject to the legislators' awareness of the importance of and need for such funding. Federal monies distributed as a result of the Nursing Education Act are primarily allocated for nurses pursuing advanced preparation as nurse practitioners, nurse-midwives, nurse anesthetists, and advanced clinical specialists.

As in undergraduate education, geographical distribution differences exist, with the largest number of graduate minority students being found in the South and the smallest number in the West (NLN, 1991). Almost two thirds of all master's graduates prepare for advanced clinical practice, 9% prepare for administration, and 12% prepare for teaching. Of those nurses prepared at the graduate level, 14.2% are members of minority groups: Almost 7% are black, 3% are Hispanic, 4% are Asian, and 1% are American Indian. The number of those who actually complete graduate programs is somewhat lower (NLN, 1991).

Between 1989 and 1990, the number of nursing doctoral degrees awarded in the United States dropped from 324 to 295. The NLN (1991) speculates that this may be a result of increased numbers of part-time students, decreased funding for dissertation research, and a lack of doctorally prepared faculty to work with students. Minority enrollment in doctoral programs has been reported as 1.1% or lower for American Indians or Alaskan Natives, 1.7% for Hispanics, and 4.3% for blacks. All minority groups are represented by lower percentages at the graduate level as opposed to the baccalaureate level. This is in contrast to the white students, who increase in percentage at the graduate level: Whites account for 81.9% of all baccalaureate students, 86.1% of all master's students, and 83.0% of all doctoral students. It should be noted that at the doctoral level 2.6% (more than Hispanics and Asian or Pacific Islanders) are nonresident alien students, and 5.3% are of unknown heritage (AACN, 1992).

What do these data mean? It is obvious that the numbers of minority students seeking higher education in nursing are not representative of the general population, especially in the case of Hispanics. Therefore, these nurses are not able to move within the profession to positions of leadership and power. Why does this happen? Once again a variety of factors interact. The following interpretation is a premise for those of Hispanic origin. Because of the low economic status of most Mexican-American families, when the student completes the basic nursing program, she or he is expected to go to work immediately, often the day after graduation, to contribute to the family's finances. In more than one instance, the graduate is expected to put the next child through college. In addition, at this stage in their lives, marriage and child-rearing become a focus. The Mexican-American family culture frowns on leaving children at day-care centers or in the care of non–family members. In addition, the basic cultural value of the dominant male figure often overrides a career drive. In other words, the nurse resumes life in a culture that generally does not encourage advanced preparation. Survival of the family unit is the primary motivator. This is not to judge that value but rather to acknowledge that it exists and that it may be a factor that discourages minority nurses from pursuing graduate education.

STRATEGIES TO IMPROVE THE ETHNIC MIX IN NURSING

If demographic trends persist, there will be an increase in Hispanic and Asian populations and a modest growth in the black population (NLN, 1991). Mexican-Americans comprise the second-largest minority group in the United States and can be found not only in the Southwest but also in urban areas throughout the United States. Therefore, increased representation of these minority groups must be a priority. As these populations grow, there will be an increased need for nurses who can relate to, understand, and be accepted by the community. Two important roles will be (1) assisting those who have been deprived of access to health care to participate in the existing health care system and (2) molding the future health care system to be responsive to their needs.

In order to accomplish these goals, federal, state, and local financial support must be available. Inequities in public education must be addressed. Local public school boards must direct resources toward the goal of quality educational opportunities for all children. Poor school tax districts must receive assistance from the state.

Factors inhibiting minority members from attaining a career in nursing include inadequate academic preparation, especially in the sciences; financial costs and the actual and projected decrease in financial aid; inadequate career counseling; and more and better recruitment strategies by other disciplines. At the postsecondary level, institutions must provide counseling and tutorial services as well as financial aid.

A major problem in nursing education is the few members of minority nursing faculty. Less than 9% of nursing faculty were minority members in 1992: 5.9% were black, 0.9% Hispanic, 1.6% Asian, and 0.3% Native American or Alaskan (NLN, 1993). The composition of nursing faculties must reflect an ethnic mix not only for token representation or to reflect a specific community, but also to become a living model of diversity in collaboration—a model that stresses competence, academic ability, caring, and true equality. Potential minority faculty members must be identified as early as possible in their academic careers and supported in their efforts to obtain graduate degrees. In one possible system, they could pay back the institution's financial support through a committed service period.

These young faculty members, like all junior faculty, must be nurtured through a mentoring program. They have the potential to serve as role models for minority students and, in time, can serve as mentors themselves. It is unfortunate that research by minority faculty members is often not only unappreciated but also denigrated. For example, colleagues in nursing may look despairingly at research concerning American Indian rites related to health or black nutritional practices. If culturally based research is not valued, minority faculty members may not be tenured. This prevents career advancement and limits contributions to that particular program (Campbell & Sigsby, 1994).

There is currently a greater proportion of black faculty members in nursing as compared with their representation in all other colleges. There is a smaller percentage, however, of all other minority groups in nursing as compared with that in all other colleges. Regional population differences exist, with more blacks in the South and more Asians and Hispanics in the West. Associate-degree programs appear to have more faculty diversity (NLN, 1991). This may be related to the minimal academic credential of a bachelor's degree that is required to teach in an associate-degree program. Additionally, less than 8% of the chief administrators of nursing programs are designated as members of a minority group (NLN, 1991). These figures are similar for all nursing administrative positions.

In recent years there have been philosophical discussions about whether or not there should be organizations for minorities in nursing, such as the Hispanic Nurses' Association or the National Black Nurses' Association. It would appear that these organizations provide support and networking for minority nurses who may not be able to take advantage of opportunities in the major nursing organizations because of their small numbers. Therefore, until the minority nurses themselves feel that a need no longer exists, local chapters of these organizations should be encouraged. Professional nursing success, which is necessary to advance in the profession, can be interpreted as psychological success whereby an internalized goal includes ego involvement. Psychological success increases self-esteem and strengthens commitment (Hall, 1976). A supportive social network is a means of minimizing the threat to one's sense of self-worth and fostering career enhancement.

Nursing education has a direct responsibility to educate practitioners for the future. The demographics of the United States have changed. Spanish has become a second language in many parts of the country, and we must educate our own to meet these changes.

SUMMARY

Health care reform issues mandate minority representation in all health professions. The new health care system must reflect the community, and as care moves into the community, health care provider-community partnerships are formed.

There is considerable literature on recruiting and maintaining minority representation in nursing. Some educational institutions recruit very heavily from minority institutions. They offer excellent financial assistance to students and woo faculty members with high salaries. The fact that many of these programs experience difficulty in retaining minority students and faculty members should send a message to everyone. The issue of minority representation in nursing is a complex one. Unless efforts are made to integrate the values, beliefs, and cultures of minority populations into the curricula and into support programs, there will be no success. Multiple strategies are required, and financial assistance, while very important, is not solely sufficient. Unless strategic planning for minority recruitment and retention is implemented, all efforts will be doomed. For example, hiring minority faculty members, without mentoring and assistance in the assumption of leadership roles, will not be successful as a long-term strategy. For both students and faculty, support services, formal and informal, can assist in resolving cultural dissonance. Such strategies must be incorporated throughout the curriculum. Content areas such as interpersonal skills, communication skills, leadership ability, and professionalism must be blended. It is amazing that we are still grappling with racial and ethnic issues as we head into the next century. If we do our job well, however, these issues will become extinct.

REFERENCES

Allen, M.E., Nunley, J.C., & Scott-Warner, M. (1988). Recruitment and retention of black students in baccalaureate nursing programs. *Journal of Nursing Education, 27*(3), 107-116.

American Association of Colleges of Nursing. (1990). *Enrollment management for programs in nursing education* (Publication No. 19-2419). Washington, DC: Author.

American Association of Colleges of Nursing. (1992). *1991-1992 Enrollment and graduations in baccalaureate and graduate programs in nursing* (Publication No. 91-92-1). Washington, DC: Author.

Andrews, M.M. (1992). Cultural perspectives on nursing in the 21st century. *Journal of Professional Nursing, 8*(1), 7-15.

Bartlett, C.J., Bobko, P., Mosier, S.B., & Hannon, R. (1978). Testing for fairness with a moderated multiple regression strategy. An alternate to differential analysis. *Personnel Psychology, 31,* 233-241.

Berg, J., & Berg, B.L. (1989). Compliance, diet and cultural factors among Black Americans with end-stage renal disease. *Journal of National Black Nurses' Association, 3*(2), 16-28.

Borden, V.M.H. (1995, June). Analysis of postsecondary degrees conferred to minorities. *Black Issues in Higher Education,* 38-73.

Boyle, K.K. (1986). Predicting the success of minority students in a baccalaureate nursing program. *Journal of Nursing Education, 25*(5), 186-192.

Campbell, D.W., & Sigsby, L.M. (1994). Increasing minorities in higher education in nursing: Faculty consultation as a strategy. *Journal of Professional Nursing, 10*(1), 7-12.

Carnegie, M.E. (1988). Breakthrough to nursing: Twenty-five years of involvement. *Imprint, 35*(2), 55-56, 59.

Carter, D.J. (1990). Racial and ethnic trends in college participation: 1976-1988. *Research Briefs* (American Council on Education), 1(3).

Cope, R.G., & Hannah, W. (1975). *Revolving college doors: The causes and consequences of dropping out, stopping out, and transferring.* New York: Wiley-Interscience.

Dell, M., & Halpin, G. (1984). Predictors of success in nursing school and on state board examinations in a predominantly black baccalaureate nursing program. *Journal of Nursing Education, 23*(4), 147-150.

Dutko, K. (1994). Enrollment rise: Will aid follow? *Hispanic, 16*(7), 14.

Hall, D.T. (1976). *Careers in organizations.* Pacific Palisades, CA: Goodyear.

Harris, R.L. (1990). Recruiting Afro-Americans into the graduate school pipeline. *Perspectives, 28*(1), 6, 11-12.

Hodgkinson, H.L. (1985). *All one system: Demographics of education, kindergarten through graduate school.* Washington, DC: Institute for Educational Leadership.

Jaschik, S. (1993, February). Supporters say threat to minority scholarship outlasts the Bush years. *The Chronicle of Higher Education,* p. A 25.

Justiz, M.J. (1995). Hispanics in higher education. *Hispanic 8*(5), 96.

Kauffman, A.H. (1996, August). The Hopwood Case—What it says, what it doesn't say, the future of the case and the rest of the story. *Intercultural Development Research Association (IDRA) Newsletter,* 7-8.

Michaelson, M. (1995, July 28). Building a comprehensive defense of affirmative action programs. *The Chronicle of Higher Education,* p. A 56.

Moses, E.B. (1990, June). The registered nurse population: Findings from the National Sample Survey of Registered Nurses, 1988. Rockville, MD: U.S. DHHS, PHS, HRSA, Bureau of Health Professions.

Moses, E.B. (1993). *Nurse leadership: Caring for the emerging majority. Empowering nurses through partnerships and coalitions* (pp. 15-26). Bethesda, MD: U.S. Department of Commerce.

National Center for Health Statistics. (1992, January 7). *Monthly vital statistics report* (Suppl. 2). Hyattsville, MD: Public Health Service.

National League for Nursing. (1991). *Nursing data review (1991)* (Publication No. 19-2419). New York: Author.

National League for Nursing. (1991). *Nursing datasource: Vol. 3. Leaders in the making: Graduate education in nursing* (Publication No. 19-2422). New York: Author.

National League for Nursing, Division of Research. (1993). *Nursing data review* (Publication No. 19-2529). New York: Author.

Ramirez, M., III, & Castaneda, O. (1974). *Cultural democracy, bicognitive development and education.* New York: Academic Press.

Rojas, D. (1994). Leadership in a multicultural society: A case in role development, *Nursing and Health Care, 15*(5), 258-20.

Rosella, J.D., Regan-Kubinski, M.J., & Albrecht, S.D. (1994). The need for multicultural diversity. *Nursing and Health Care, 15*(5), 242-246.

Schmidt, F.L., Pearlman, K., & Hunter, J.E. (1980). The validity of fairness of employment and education tests for Hispanic Americans: A review and analysis. *Personnel Psychology, 33*(4), 704-724.

Schwirian, P. (1977). *Prediction of successful nursing performance: Part 2. Admission practices, evaluation strategies and performance prediction among schools of nursing* (HEW Publication No. HRA 77-27). Washington, DC: U.S. Government Printing Office.

U.S. Department of Health and Human Services. (1990). *The registered nurse population: Findings from the national sample survey of registered nurses, March 1988.* Washington, DC: Author.

U.S. Department of Health and Human Services. (1991). *Nursing: Health personnel in the United States, 1991: Eighth Report to Congress* (Prepublication Report). Washington, DC: Author.

Vasquez, M.J.T. (1982). Confronting barriers to the participation of Mexican-American women in higher education. *Hispanic Journal of Behavioral Success, 4*(2), 147-165.

Men in nursing: Problems and prospects

VERN L. BULLOUGH

In 1994 there were 88,623 male registered nurses (RNs) in the United States (4% of all RNs). This was the highest percentage since 1910, when 6.98% of RNs were men. After 1910, the percentage of RNs in the United States declined, until reaching a low of 0.91% in 1960. Since 1960, the numbers have been rising slowly: 1.3% in 1970 to 2.7% in 1980 to 3% in 1980 to 3.3% in 1988. In 1994, 11% of first-time nursing students in bachelor's-degree nursing programs were men, and there was a much higher percentage of men in associate-degree programs (American Nurses Association [ANA], 1946, 1994; Hospital and Health Network, 1994).

BACKGROUND

American nursing is now and will be in the foreseeable future clearly a woman's profession, yet the dominance of women in nursing did not come about until almost the beginning of the 20th century. Although women have traditionally been the primary caregivers in the home, this was not the case outside the home. In the institutions set up to care for the sick, whether temple houses or hospitals, the attendants were likely to be men—priests, monks, physician's assistants, and in the military either tent companions or shipmates. Although in medieval times some of the women's religious orders did staff a few of the urban hospitals, most were staffed by members of male orders who were far more numerous than nuns. In the Byzantine or Eastern Roman Empire, during which secular hospitals were developed, women did work as nurses alongside men. The men remained most numerous, however, and those few women who did nurse were restricted to the women's ward (Bullough & Bullough, 1993a).

As a general rule, women in the past were always under the legal control of their husbands, fathers, brothers, or sons. Much of modern history can be interpreted as a story of women's efforts to break free of the limitations put on them by a male-dominated society; women struggled to be recognized as important individuals in their own right. As Wollstonecraft (1759-1797) put it in her 1792 manifesto, *Vindication of the Rights of Women,* which might be said to mark the birth of feminism:

> Men complain, with reason, of the follies and caprices of our sex, when they do not keenly satirize our headstrong passions and groveling vices. Behold, I should answer the natural effect of ignorance! The mind will ever be unstable that has only prejudices to rest on, and the current will run with destructive fury when there are no barriers to break its force. Women are told from their infancy and taught by the examples of their mothers, that a little knowledge of human weakness, justly termed cunning, softness of temper, outward obedience, and a scrupulous attention to a puerile kind of propriety, will obtain for them the protection of man, and should they be beautiful, everything else is needless, for at least twenty years of their lives. (Woolstonecraft, 1929, p. 23)

One reason a woman like Wollstonecraft could argue for and achieve an audience for change is that the Industrial Revolution was undermining traditional patterns of life. Although the emerging factories, first in England and then elsewhere, employed the village women, this only accentuated the problem of the middle class women, who lacked opportunities to make themselves useful. Greg, writing in 1853, complained that proper women

> . . . must not work for profit, or engage in any occupation that money can command, lest she invade the rights of the working classes. . . . Men in want of employment have pressed their way into nearly all the shopping and retail businesses that in my early years were managed in whole, or in part, by women. The conventional barrier that pronounced it ungenteel to be behind a counter, or serving the public in any mercantile capacity is greatly extended. The same in household economy. Servants must be up to their offices, which is very well; but ladies, dismissed from the dairy, the confectionery, the store room, the still

room, the poultry yard, the kitchen garde, and the orchard have hardly yet found themselves a sphere equally useful and important to the pursuits of trade and arts to which to apply their too abundant leisure. (Greg, 1969, pp. 315-316)

The problem that women faced was how to break through the barriers yet retain the proper feminine image. An obvious solution was to busy oneself with traditional women's activities in the home and somehow make them into a profession. These activities included caring for the sick, raising and educating small children, visiting and helping neighbors, raising the cultural consciousness of the men in their lives, and assisting their husbands in his or work or profession. It was from these housewifely tasks that nurses, primary school teachers, friendly visitors (who eventually came to be called social workers), librarians, and secretaries emerged, although the last case also coincided with the invention and widespread use of the typewriter.

The first efforts of women in of all these fields were essentially charitable ones, and only gradually did these tasks become paying jobs. One of the early efforts in nursing was the founding of the Sisters of Charity by St. Vincent de Paul (1576-1660). Organized originally to encourage lay women to visit the sick and the poor, some of the sisters went further and moved into the hospitals to help the nuns who did nursing tasks (Bullough & Bullough, 1978; 1984). Most other early efforts to raise the level of nursing also concentrated on either Protestant or Catholic religious orders, because it was often by receiving a "religious call" that women could break through the limitations imposed on their lives.

Whether consciously or unconsciously, women who wanted to challenge tradition seized on the 19th century notion that they constituted a special class, that they were different than men, somehow made of finer materials. Women were the guardians of culture and tradition, although few fit the stereotype of wan, ethereal, spiritualized creatures that some of the literature of the time tried to make them. In fact, such portrayals bore little resemblance to the real world of lower-class women who operated machines, worked the fields, washed clothes by hand, and took care of large households. Nonetheless, these portrayals were endorsed by the science and religion of the time, at least for middle- and upper-class women. Nightingale was in full-scale rebellion against such an image, and this is best illustrated by her essay "Cassandra," which was written before she visited Kaisersworth (Nightingale, 1979). She didn't want to marry and turn her fate over to some man; rather she wanted to be her own woman and still be socially useful. Nursing was her answer because it allowed her to fit the image of a proper woman, yet still be on her own.

Nightingale was of a class and economic background in which she was well acquainted with the important people in British society. When her friend, Minister of Defense Herbert, was attempting to overcome bad publicity about the dreadful care of the sick and wounded during the Crimean war, he (with prompting from his wife and from Nightingale herself) conceived of a public relations coup of sending a contingent of women to nurse the troops (Bullough & Bullough, 1978). Nightingale and her nurses became what in today's terms would be a media sensation and continued to be one because the female nurses proved to be extremely effective. The American poet Henry Wadsworth Longfellow made her a mythical heroine in his poem that included the following lines:

A lady with a lamp shall stand
In the great history of the land,
A noble type of good,
Heroic womanhood (Longfellow, 1922)

THE AMERICAN EXPERIENCE

Inevitably, Nightingale became a heroine for all young women, and her life became reading material (somewhat highly embroidered) for generations of girls who wanted to make something of themselves (Vicinus, 1990). During the American Civil War, many women seeking to emulate Nightingale's example became nurses, although men served as caretakers for the sick as well. In 1873, in the aftermath of the Civil War, groups of women in New York City, New Haven, Connecticut, and Boston organized training schools for women to become nurses, based on what they believed was the model Nightingale had established at St. Thomas Hospital in London. The organization of these schools coincided with a period of hospital expansion in the United States that resulted from the development of aseptic techniques and the need for institutional care of the poor and homeless in America's growing urban centers. Moreover, medicine itself was changing, and procedures formally reserved for the home, including childbirth, began to move into the hospital setting as physicians took over tasks formerly performed by midwives and other nonprofessional healers. Nursing made the growth of hospitals possible, especially when it became clear that nursing students were cheap labor because they could staff the hospitals in return for room and board and a modicum of education. Because the hospital administrators wanted the nurses available, they established homes for them, a concept that also fit in with the perceived need to protect women. This also meant that homes for nurses were restricted to women, and this made it more difficult for men to gain entry into nurse training.

Although there was no perceived struggle between male and female nurses, the majority of hospitals simply did not allow male nurses, with the exception of mental hospitals where it was believed nurses needed greater strength. This led to schools for men only such as that established by the Department of Mental and Nervous Diseases at Pennsylvania Hospital or the Mills School of Nursing for Men at Bellevue.

Although women in nursing did not necessarily object to the men in their ranks, it is clear that nursing was conceived of by most of them as a woman's profession where the role of men was limited. None of the male nursing schools was affiliated with the Associated Alumnae (which became the ANA), and when the ANA was reorganized between 1916 and 1922, no provisions were made for male nurses. It was not until 1930 that the membership bylaws were revised to include properly qualified male nurses (Nash, 1936). Male nurses existed but were on the fringe of mainstream nursing.

This borderline status was emphasized in 1901 by the organization of the U.S. Army Nurse Corps, which specifically excluded male nurses (Bullough & Bullough, 1978; Kalish & Kalish, 1978). Men were to fight, not nurse; and when male nurses were drafted into the military during World War I, they fought in the trenches and were excluded from staffing the hospitals. The military disregard of male nurses in World War I proved to be a crucial factor in the decline of men in the profession. At a time when nursing school enrollments were increasing radically, and the special army school was established to train nurses, enrollment of men almost disappeared.

This was also true in World War II. Concerned about the repetition of events in World War I, however, Leroy Craig, Director of the School of Nursing for Men at Pennsylvania Hospital, and his allies (both men and women), persuaded the ANA at its 1940 convention to set up a section for "men nurses." Although the section focused its attention on many issues such as upgrading patient care and raising salaries for nurses, they were not at all successful in changing treatment of male nurses in the military. For example, Luther Christman, a 1939 graduate of the Pennsylvania Hospital, was denied enlistment in the Army Nurse Corps at the onset of World War II. He found, much to his dismay, that male nurses were not even given priority enrollment in medical corpsmen schools—supposedly on the basis that their knowledge often intimidated their less well-educated teachers. Christman tried to bypass the issue by joining the Merchant Marines as a medical corpsman and then petitioning for appointment to the Army Nurse Corps and assignment to the front lines (where female nurses were not then assigned). He was unsuccessful. Enrollments of men in nursing schools during this period dropped even further, from 725 in 1939 to 169 in 1945 (ANA, 1946, 1994).

MEN BEGIN TO ENTER NURSING IN GREATER NUMBERS

Conditions for male nurses began to change following the end of World War II, and male enrollments in nursing schools slowly started to build. They did not climb very high, however, until the establishment of associate-degree programs and the decline of traditional hospital schools. One indication of change was the granting of military commissions to male nurses through legislation initiated by Bolton. This legislation led to Edward Lyon becoming the first male RN to be commissioned as a reserve officer in the Army Nurse Corps on October 6, 1955. The change in the military was rapid until by 1990 approximately 30% of the RNs in the various Military Nurse Corps were men—almost four times their ratio in civilian nursing. During the Vietnam War, more than 500 male nurses were drafted and given commissions in the various Military Nurse Corps.

In the long run, the most important factor in attracting men to nursing was the improvement in salaries and working conditions in the profession that took place during the 1950s and 1960s. Although census data indicate that male nurses generally were and still are paid much more than female nurses (Bullough & Bullough, 1978), part of this disparity is due to fact that a disproportionate number of men were nurse anesthetists, nurse administrators, or held other high-paying nursing jobs. This disparity was also due to the fact that men were often paid more than women for doing the same job, that there were more job alternatives open to men than to women, and that men could leave nursing if the salaries were not equal. It was only as the new wave of feminism of the 1960s and the demand for equal pay began that the salary gap between men and women lessened, both in and out of nursing. Undoubtedly, this inequality created some tension between male and female nurses, although many nurses encouraged men to enter the field because they felt that their own salaries might rise as a result.

Tensions came from other directions as well, and these

became more noticeable as growing numbers of men entered nursing. Nursing educators who traditionally had taught only female students found their male students behaving somewhat differently. They were not as submissive as female students. These problems required simple adjustments and were soon solved by most teachers (Bush, 1976; Schoenmaker, 1976).

MEN AND NURSING THEORY

More serious was the objection raised by men to the way that many female nurses regarded themselves and their profession, particularly as the new megatheories of nursing emerged (Bullough, 1994)—a development that coincided with a spurt in the number of men in nursing. Philosophers Dickoff and James worked with Wiedenbach, a nurse, at Yale University, to outline a process necessary for developing theories, which were regarded as an essential step to the professional growth of nursing theories. They argued that nursing theory was necessary to provide a bridge between practice and research, and that theory-based research was the key to broadening nursing knowledge (Dickoff, James, & Wiedenback, 1968). Contemporaries of the Yale group were a group of grand theorists of nursing who defined nursing in broad outlines; most of these theorists were centered at the University of California at Los Angeles and New York University.

Among the most troublesome theories to men were the caring theories, particularly those that emphasized caring as a particularly feminine trait. Although rooted in the work of Johnson, who distinguished between caring and curing (Johnson, 1959) others such as Kreuter contributed. Kreuter (1957) defined *caring* as a special task of a nurse clinician: "Care is expressed in tending to another, being with him, assisting, protecting . . . providing for his needs and wants with compassion—tenderness." (p. 303) Caring became a major part of the theory of Watson, and led her to establish an early caring center (Watson, 1979; 1985). The concept of caring was also given special sanction by the ANA in its 1965 position paper, *Educational Preparation for Nurse Practitioners and Assistant to Nurses,* in which the professional role of nurse was defined as social psychological support, teaching, and sustaining care (ANA, 1965).

There is nothing particularly wrong with emphasizing caring from a male point of view because caring is one of the fundamentals of nursing. The problem, however, was with the implementation. One faction of nursing interpreted caring as a uniquely feminine quality. By implication, caring was something that men (as males) were not especially qualified to do. Although nowhere is this thesis stated quite so baldly, it has certainly contributed to male uneasiness.

One male graduate student in nursing summed this up in a recent letter to the *Skeptical Inquirer* explaining the beginning of his graduate coursework:

> . . . there was a cohort of vehement feminists in the program. It became rapidly apparent to me that not only did these women have strong opinions about traditional science, but they also felt that men had no place in nursing.
>
> These feminists were critical of empirical methodologies and proposed that nursing science should be much more qualitative and based only on intuitive knowledge. It was the feminists' contention that traditional science was paternalistic and male-oriented and thus suspect at all levels. They stated that men's and women's minds operated in dramatically different ways. "Men's science" dissected an event and attempted to empiricize it and in the process lost the Gestalt that was essential to understanding the event. It was the feminists' contention that *only* women could understand a holistic viewpoint.
>
> The next stage of the feminists' argument was that nursing is an eclectic, and holistic science that requires an understanding of each individual patient's Gestalt. Because nursing practice required a holistic view of patients and men could not comprehend this view, nursing research and the knowledge base of nursing should be developed by women. Their next conclusion was that caring requires specific mental functions that men are not able to accomplish. Therefore, men are incapable of "caring." (Ross, 1995, p. 58, 60)

To the extent that such an attitude exists, and Ross is careful to state that the caring view he criticizes is not held by the majority of nurses, it is strongly held by many and makes male nurses uncomfortable. In my own experience, I have met a few female nurses who will not recognize me as a nurse because I am a man. The sad part is that most current research would indicate that caring is not particularly confined to women. Although men statistically tend to be more aggressive than women and seemingly have special mathematical skills, this shows up at the skewed end of the spectrum. The most interesting finding is the tremendous overlap in talents between most men and women (Bullough & Bullough, 1993b; Hyde, 1986). Moreover, some of the most obvious differences are as much or more cultural than biological.

WHAT DOES THE FUTURE HOLD?

Because there are little scientific data to back up the radical caring theorists, it might well be that they are misusing the theory because they feel the "invasion" of men in nursing is a threat to traditional nursing, and that nursing will change for the worse, losing those special qualities and aspects that have made it unique. There is little doubt that nursing will change—it is always changing—but hopefully it will guided by a joint effort of nurses of both genders.

It is not only American nurses who are concerned by the entrance of men into the profession. Our British counterparts are concerned as well, and the entrance of men into nursing is further along there than in the United States. Some see men in the profession a threat to the power of women. One study in the 1980s found that half of the top posts in nursing within the British National Health Service were held by men (Nuttal, 1983). Men were also found to hold disproportionate strength in the Royal College of Nursing, where 15 of the 31 elected members were men. One female nurse felt that once male power was established, it would tend to be self-perpetuating, making it very difficult for women to regain leadership (London, 1987). These British fears have carried over into American nursing (Ryan & Porter, 1993). Although there are unique factors in the British system that led to what might be called the "disproportionate" power of men, there is a real basis for these fears. I feel, however, that with the changing power relationships between men and women in American society, such fears are grossly exaggerated. As an academician for over 40 years, I have observed the rapid change in the role of women not only in American higher education but also in the business and professional world as well. There are still a few isolated campuses where the dean of nursing is the only woman in the higher ranks of administration, but this is rare and becoming rarer as women of all backgrounds hold major administrative jobs.

It might be, as one theory holds, that the problems faced by gender minorities tend to increase as their numbers in a particular occupation grow, until they reach a critical mass when the barriers more or less disappear. If this is the case, then it is important to determine this critical mass when the barriers collapse. Kanter (1977) estimated that this percentage in any group ranges between 20% to 40%. Testing this theory on nursing was a study comparing women in law enforcement and men in nursing (Ott, 1989). Ott's study supports the theory in law enforcement, where women tended to see increasing resistance to their presence, but not in nursing, where men found greater acceptance in their increasing numbers (Ott, 1989). This tends to illustrate that women, or at least female nurses, are more willing to share their domain with men than men in typically male professions such as law enforcement are with women. It would also indicate that those uncomfortable with men in the nursing profession constitute only a very small minority.

As women seek fields of employment other than the traditional women's professions, the major source of potential recruits in nursing in the future is from men. Those women who do enter nursing will be far more committed to it than those who once entered merely because there seemed to be no alternative. This will undoubtedly be true of the men as well, although every male nurse is conscious of the tremendous contribution that women have made to our profession.

Interestingly, although much of the empowerment of women in the marketplace has come through Title 9 of the Civil Rights Act, no similar provision exists for men. This only emphasizes that nursing is helping to change itself by recruiting men, which is a credit to the profession. Like any minority, men in nursing need occasionally to meet with some of their own. It was for this reason that Martin organized the National Male Nurse Association in 1971 to give support to male nurses. The objectives of the organization, as defined in 1981 when it was renamed the Assembly for Men in Nursing, are:

1. Men and boys in the United States are to be encouraged to become nurses and join together with all nurses in strengthening and humanizing health care for Americans.
2. Men who are now nurses are encouraged to grow professionally and to demonstrate to each other and to society the increasing contributions made by men within the nursing profession.
3. The American Assembly for Men in Nursing intends that its members be full participants in the nursing profession and its organizations and use their association to achieve these goals.

The association holds that every professional nurse position and every nursing educational opportunity shall be equally available to those meeting the entry qualifications regardless of gender (see various issues of *Interaction*). These are not particularly revolutionary goals, nor should they be. We went into nursing because we wanted to be nurses, and this is the way nursing should be. The nursing profession emphasizes the caring potential in both genders. It is quite a different profession than the one Nightingale first visualized, and women and men will continue to influence how it grows. This is what the men who are nurses want.

REFERENCES

American Nurses Association. (1946, 1994). *Facts about nursing*. Kansas City, MO: Author.

American Nurses Association. (1965). *Educational preparation for nurse practitioners and assistants to nurses.* Kansas City, MO: Author.

Bullough, B., & Bullough, V.L. (1975). Sex segregation in health care. *Nursing Outlook, 23* (January), 40-45.

Bullough, B. (1994). Nursing theory and critique. In Bullough, B., & Bullough, V.L. (Eds.), *Nursing issues for the nineties and beyond* (pp. 64-82). New York: Springer.

Bullough, V.L., & Bullough, B. (1978). *The care of the sick: The emergence of modern nursing.* New York: Prodist.

Bullough, V.L., & Bullough, B. (1984). *History, trends, and politics of nursing.* Norwalk, CN: Appleton-Century-Crofts.

Bullough, V.L., & Bullough B. (1993a). Medieval nursing. *Nursing History Review, 1,* 217-226.

Bullough, V.L., & Bullough, B. (1993b). *Cross dressing, sex, and gender.* Philadelphia: University of Pennsylvania.

Bush, P.J. (1976). The male nurse: A challenge to traditional role identities. *Nursing Forum, XV,* 390-405.

Dickoff, J., James, P., & Wiedenback, P. (1968). Theory in a practice discipline. *Nursing Research,* 17, 415-435, 545-554.

Greg, M. (1969). In *Women workers and the Industrial Revolution 1750-1850* (pp. 315-316). London: Frank Case.

Hospital and health network [computer database], (1994, October 5). 68(19), p. 78.

Hyde, J.S. (1986). Gender differences in aggression. In J.S. Hyde & M.C. Linn (Eds.), *The psychology of gender: Advance through meta-analysis* (pp. 51-56). Baltimore, MD: Johns Hopkins University.

Interaction. Newsletter of the American Assembly for Men in Nursing. Pensacola, Fl.

Johnson, D. (1959). A philosophy of nursing. *Nursing Outlook 7,* 198-200.

Kalish, P., & Kalish B.J. (1978). *The advance of American nursing* (2nd ed.). Boston: Little, Brown.

Kanter, R.M. (1977). *Men and women of the corporation.* New York: Basic Books.

Kreuter, E.R. (1957). What is good nursing care? *Nursing Outlook,* 5:302-305.

London, F. (1987). Should men be actively recruited into nursing? *Nursing Administration Quarterly, 12*(1), 75-81.

Longfellow, H.W. (1922). *The complete poetical works of Longfellow.* Boston: Houghton-Mifflin.

Nash, H.J. (1936, August). Men nurses in New York State. *Trained Nurse and Hospital Review,* 123.

Nightingale, F. (1979). *Cassandra.* M. Start (Ed.), Old Westbury, NY: Feminist Press.

Nuttal, P. (1983). British nursing: Beginning of a power struggle. *Nursing Outlook, 31*(3), 184.

Ott, E.M. (1989). Effect of the male-female ratio at work: Policewomen and male nurses. (1989). *Psychology of Women Quarterly, 13*(1), 41-57.

Ross, D. (1995, July-August). Letter. *Skeptical Inquirer,* 19 pp. 58-60.

Ryan, S., & Porter, S. (1993). Men in nursing: A cautionary comparative critique. *Nursing Outlook, 41*(6), 262-267.

Schoenmaker, A. (1976). Nursing's dilemma: Male versus female admissions choice. *Nursing Forum, XV,* 406-412.

Vicinus, M. (1990). What makes a heroine? Girls' biographies of Florence Nightingale. In V.L. Bullough, B. Bullough, & M.P. Stanton (Eds.), *Florence Nightingale and her era: A collection of new scholarship* (pp. 96-107). New York: Garland.

Watson, J. (1979). *The philosophy and science of caring.* Boston: Little, Brown.

Watson, J. (1985). *Nursing: Human science and human care. A theory of nursing.* Norwalk, CT: Appleton-Century-Crofts.

Woolstonecraft, M.A. (1929). *A vindication of the rights of women.* London: J.M. Dent.

Bridging cultures: African Americans and nursing

BETTY PIERCE DENNIS

When the United States enters the 21st century, it will no longer be a predominately white nation whose culture is rooted in Northern Europe. Nearly half of all Americans will be minorities. The increase in plurality will enhance the diverse and rich character of the United States.

African Americans,* who now comprise 12% of the population, are expected to account for 15% by the year 2000 (O'Hare, 1992). Unlike some immigrant groups of the past that were absorbed by the larger population and achieved full participation in society, African Americans did not assimilate. More than 300 years after arriving, African Americans are still only marginally represented in the important arenas of power and influence.

Nowhere are the effects of this marginality more evident than in health care. As a consequence of cultural and social interactions, health has become a surrogate, multifaceted measure of group status. Assignment of meaning to health in its social and cultural context necessitates nontraditional ways of understanding health behavior. These new ways begin with the conceptualization of health as a nonlinear, developmental process instead of as a "state" or point on a wellness-illness continuum. Typical descriptors of health focus on broadly applicable practices and observable behaviors. This custom obscures the prismatic patterns of experience in which health is but one interacting element within the larger cultural and social context. Even after working closely with African American clients, many nurses—regardless of race—fail to recognize how ethnohistory shapes the perceptions of health and the behaviors that relate to health.

*The terms *African American* and *black* are used interchangeably.

CULTURE AND CONTEXT

The cultural and social lives of blacks are interdependent constructs that emerge from history, education, income, and a host of other factors. Taken together, they form a contextual framework that is unique to the group. The philosophy of contextualism embraces the full range of conditions and motivations that are expressed through person-environment exchanges. The nurse and client may, and often do, behave out of dissimilar contexts or theoretical and empirical frameworks (Gergen, 1982). For this reason, interpretive perspective is always necessary. Interpretive perspective allows both the nurse and the client to identify points of divergence and, more importantly, points of convergence from their respective cultural perspectives. Without this process, genuine bonding between the black client and the nurse is either altogether elusive or in a permanent nascent state—very much as it is today. Therefore, the challenge to nursing is not only to see the worldview of the African American client but also to allow that vision to guide nursing practice. Three factors will hinder or facilitate the progress of nursing toward cultural competence: breadth of perspective, depth of commitment, and evolution of nursing systems.

In the care of African American clients, an approach that accepts differences and recognizes commonalities will call to question traditional nursing therapeutics. Usually, these therapeutic approaches are based on ahistorical, acontextual ways of knowing clients. Contrary to this emphasis on objectivity in nurse-client interactions, reaching out to other cultures requires subjectivity borne of shared experiences. As used here, *sharing* indicates acceptance of ethnopluralism without subscribing to a cultural hierarchy or ranking that places lesser or greater value or individual cultures. Myers (1991) contends that only through subjective experiences are we able to acquire knowledge that "deepens" what we know of another culture. The culturally competent nurse has to have more than a superficial understanding of other cultures. Being a stranger to black culture will not support an increase in levels of competence in the delivery of culturally sensitive health care to black clients. Ancient African systems of knowledge, Myers contends, were built on subjectivity. When substantive cultural knowledge is the basis of cultural competence, it bridges the chasm between African Americans and the health care system.

At its most basic level, *culture* is an expression of the lifeways of a collection of individuals in a group or community. Because culture is intelligible only within its own context, comparisons between cultures are neither informative nor valid. Unfortunately, comparisons are an all too common practice that often leads to stereotypical characterizations. Closely related yet distinct from culture is the social system in which that culture exists (Valentine, 1968). The dynamism of the two is implicit in Whitehead's (1992) description of culture as enmeshed in an ". . . ecological system, historically created, intergenerationally reproduced and moderated, to allow humans to meet their basic . . . needs . . ." (p. 95). Through a consideration of history it is possible to uncover the generative layer that is responsible for the attitudes, beliefs, and values unique to African Americans. History does, in fact, endow this and other cultures. History is the wellspring of many societal forces that promote or restrain, extend or limit the options available to black clients.

Explorations of African-American culture and nursing from the perspective of a construct/contextualism philosophy address the following questions: (1) Is the health of African Americans proscribed by their ethnohistorical legacy as well as by their contemporary reality? (2) How can nursing become a proactive force in bringing these facts together within a paradigm explicating culturally competent health care?

HISTORY AND HEALTH

History is a major component in understanding African-American culture. Africans arrived in America either before Columbus (Van Sertima, 1976) or before the Mayflower in 1619 (Bennett, 1982). Initially, the work obligations for these Africans and their conditions of freedom were like those for other indentured servants. However, the growth of colonial economics led to an escalation in the need for manpower and ultimately the creation of slavery. In 1661, Virginia was the first state to legally convert immigrant Africans from indentured servants to slaves (Johnson, 1982). Trade in humanity exploded. Although millions were captured trying to escape, an estimated one half to two thirds perished in transit, either dying by their own hands or succumbing to the rigors of the journey before reaching the endpoints in North America, South America, or the Caribbean (Bennett, 1982).

Before the mid-20th century, historians proposed two main theories about the culture of captured Africans in America. The first theory is that the African culture was destroyed by a repressive system that randomly disbursed them and continually disrupted their lives. It was hypothesized that these practices made order and stability impossible. Communication was hampered by the lack of a common language and the outlawing of the use of drums. The void caused by these circumstances was thought to have been filled by the English language and European culture. The second theory of this "peculiar institution" (Stampp, 1956) was that slaves had acceded to their fate, as evidenced by their tranquil deportment. They were depicted as healthy and robust despite severely deprived living conditions, exhaustive work requirements, and poor nutrition (Byrd & Clayton, 1992). Interpretation of the behavior of African Americans then, as now, was based on outward observations and objective versus subjective assessment.

After the mid-century, the institution of slavery was analyzed using actual documents of that era. The findings contradicted earlier writings. Several seminal works attested to the adaptability, resistance, and will to survive displayed by Africans. They were, after all, descendents of ancient societies with well-developed family and clan systems. Gutman's (1976) study of the black family from 1750 to 1925 described the transcendence of this heritage over slavery. Writers today detail how Africans were able to succeed in transmitting their beliefs, values, and social and familial behaviors and rituals from generation to generation. Because mothers and, more often, fathers were sold away from their families, children were socialized by the community in accord with the African adage that "it takes a whole village to raise a child." The few long and stable marriages that did exist provided role models for younger adults (Stampp, 1956). Finally, historians confirmed that the way of life within the slaves quarters not only had dimension but also purpose. In the slave quarters the designations of "field hand" or "house slave" were replaced by status based on the ability to contribute to community life. There were midwives, healers, teachers, nurses, and other contributors. This organized and supportive subterranean community, however, did not stem the many insurrections and almost daily incidence of runaways. Importantly, escape attempts at that time were not discouraged by harsh punishment like mutilation or whippings or death (Bennett, 1982). Many successful escapees joined the community of free blacks living in "free" states in the North. During the early 1700s, it is estimated that almost one in eight blacks was a free person (Franklin, 1956).

Creating one culture from many and preserving it against formidable odds was a major achievement. What this demonstrates about perceived meaning as a derivative of acontextual versus contextual exploration, however, is directly correlated to nursing care. For example, the music of slaves, objectively observed, was taken to mean that they were accepting, even happy, with their lot. From a subjective vantage point, however, the role of music was more of an expressive channel for the hopes, fears, sorrows, and dreams of the slaves, and, in essence, it was a way of communicating with one another. Just as history has refuted many myths about the meaning of the behavior of blacks, nursing must have the courage and audacity to question tradition and devise other ways of knowing and caring for black clients.

The ethnohistory of health issues reveals the germ layer of some current practices and attitudes about health among blacks. High rates of illness, injury, and death among slaves were recorded. Mortality reports from an 1850 Louisiana parish are typical (Rene, Daniels, Jones, & Moore, 1992). According to the 1850 census in Natchitoches parish, slaves accounted for 63.8% of mortality. The leading cause of death was helminthiasis due to geophagy or dirt eating. Fever, pneumonia, whooping cough, and cholera were also major causes of mortality. Exposure to new diseases like tuberculosis, syphilis, and measles drove mortality and morbidity figures up by estimates of 15% to 50% (Byrd & Clayton, 1992; Savitt, 1978). Along with society as a whole, the medical community ignored environmental causation and ascribed black mortality and morbidity to unalterable pathological differences. Treatment, therefore, when it was given, was differential. Slaves were, however, pressed into serving as subjects for many medical experiments and treatment trials, including repeated and unnecessary surgeries, starvation, and burning (Beardsley, 1987; Jones, 1981; Jordan, 1968; Savitt, 1982). Southern medical journals of the time carried reports of such experiments (Savitt, 1982). Once they learned what organized medicine offered, slaves either delayed or avoided reporting illnesses. Instead, there was a growing reliance on a cultural healing system in which root doctors, spiritualists, and priests ministered to the ill (Charatz-Litt, 1992).

Questions about the motive and intent of the organized health care system relative to African Americans remain unanswered for many, whose opinions and feelings are reinforced by suspect or unethical practices like the 40-year study of untreated syphilis in African-American men that was conducted by the U.S. Public Health Service (Jones, 1981) as well as studies at Johns Hopkins, Chicago Medical College, and Medical College of Virginia (Beecher, 1966; Newman, Amidei, Carter, Kruvant, & Russell, 1978). This persistent unease is reflected in a recent nationwide poll in which 61% of African Americans admitted being wary and distrustful of people of other races versus 30% unease in whites (Edwards, 1995). A sensitive critique and valuation of these patterns of experience in the African-American past must be factored into the development of a credible and reciprocal nurse-client relationship.

Following the end of the Civil War in 1865, the Reconstruction period opened a window of opportunity that altered the context of black life. During this time, clinics, schools, soup kitchens, and churches were opened. Blacks entered politics and bought land. Their health status improved. This progress ended abruptly after 10 years, however, when segregation or "Jim Crow" laws were passed (Bennett, 1982). These laws placed legal limits on the economic and social progress of blacks for nearly 100 years. The health status of blacks began to decline. The separate-but-equal doctrine actually fostered disparities in health outcomes between blacks and whites. These inequities are clearly seen in the infant mortality rates of 1929—they were 98.4 deaths per 1,000 live births for blacks and 60.2 per 1,000 for whites (Cooper & David, 1986; Reed, Darity, & Robertson, 1993).

Attracted by the economic boom of World Wars I and II, many blacks migrated from the South to the North; but in the North they were largely confined to ghettos. It soon became obvious that this northern separation yielded results similar to those of southern legal oppression. Infant mortality and life expectancy rates for blacks and whites offer verification. In 1950, infant mortality was 43.9 versus 26.8 per 1,000 live births, and life expectancy was 60.7 versus 69.1 years for blacks and whites, respectively (National Center for Health Statistics [NCHS], 1995).

In the 1960s, legislation initiated by the Civil Rights Movement led to improved access to health care for blacks. This was another window of opportunity that lasted a little more than a decade. Again, the upward trend in black health status reached a plateau and steadily worsened. Over a 30-year period, differences in life expectancy between blacks and whites changed from 8.0 years in 1960 to 6.9 years in 1980 to 8.2 years in 1990. In the same years, infant mortality rates were higher for blacks by 14.8%, 10.4%, and 10.7% (Haynes, 1975; NCHS, 1995).

Today, the excess death rate exemplifies the problem of health. "Excess death" is calculated as actual deaths before 70 years of age, minus the number of deaths that would be predicted when death rates of the white population in the United States are applied to the minority population. In 1990, the excess deaths for African Americans exceeded 59,000 (Thomas, 1992). McCord and Freeman (1990) studied mortality among blacks in Harlem and found rates double those of whites and 50% greater than those of other blacks in the United States. It was felt that the impact of urban ghetto life had an enduring effect.

CONTEMPORARY AFRICAN AMERICAN CLIENTS

African Americans are a heterogeneous group. Ten percent are in the upper socioeconomic class, 40% middle class, and 50% lower class (Johnson, 1982). In addition to those born in the United States, blacks emigrate from Haiti, Guyana, Brazil, the Caribbean, and Africa. A study by Cabral, Fried, Levenson, Amaro, and Zuckerman (1990) illustrates that these groups vary in language, history, culture, and health practices. Their investigation of perinatal outcomes between foreign-born and native-born black pregnant women found significant differences in the mother's nutrition, the babies' birth weights and perinatal outcomes.

The sense of self of all African Americans begins as an intragroup attitude but is finely and finally shaped by how the world sees them. The term "African American" is a cognitive construct with uncertain scientific merit. In other words, African Americans are African Americans because they are recognized and treated as such. Variation characterizes all racial and ethnic groups, and as a component variation is thought to move on a continuum through all racial groups and cannot be contained in neat racial boxes ("Biological Anthropologist," 1995). However, the nature–nurture or genetics–environment concept of disease causation persists as an expanatory model (Anonymous, 1983; Cooper & David, 1986; Langford, 1981; Thomas, 1992). It is this dichotomous perception that we must revisit.

Race is heavily weighted in perceived meanings of 'African American': Race is almost always an antecedent of diseases that are defined by genetics or environmental factors (Freeman, 1991). Variations such as income and education are combined with health measures to form comparative relationships. On the face of it, African Americans do exhibit differences in some morbid conditions. They have a low incidence of multiple sclerosis, cystic fibrosis, and skin cancer ("Biological Anthropologist," 1995) and a high incidence of hypertension, diabetes, and cancer of the prostate and cervix (NCHS, 1995). However, validation of genetic variation requires more than a counting of cases. When the aperture is widened to include nontraditional measures, a more complete picture appears. Genes, environment, and culture must be synergized to see how they affect health. The pseudoscience of writers like Jensen, Shockley, Herrnstein, and Murray, however, confuses issues by perpetuating flawed propositions about African Americans. Their works encourage theories of genetic deficits in blacks. They also support the repugnant practice of "blaming the victim," for illness or disease—which is reminiscent of some 17th and 18th century medical thinking (Charatz-Litt, 1992). Although unsubstantiated, these works preserve myths and act as barriers to the development of equitable, open, honest communications between black clients, nurses, and other health professionals.

About one third of black families have incomes below the poverty level, but blacks with higher incomes may have similar health problems. In other words, income is not a protective factor for African Americans. Thomas, Semenya, Neser, Thomas, and Gillum (1990) and Thomas et al. (1985) studied precursors of hypertension in a cohort of black physicians for over 25 years. The mortality of these physicians matched the mortality of low-income blacks rather than that of their white peers. Similarly, hypertension in men in low occupational classes increased when they remained in that status or moved to a lower status. Although blacks and whites experienced elevated pressures, increases in hypertension were greatest for blacks (Waitzman & Smith, 1994). Among blacks, hypertension develops earlier and with greater severity. Sixty-six percent of all cases of end-stage renel disease due to hypertension occurs among African Americans (Woodhandler et al., 1985; Reed et al., 1993).

When health data are partitioned according to factors like urban density, outcomes change. Used as a surrogate measure of socioeconomic status, urban density reduces differences in cancer risks between blacks and whites. High-population areas have higher incidences of cancer regardless of race. Some of the cancers (e.g., prostate) that have the highest prevalence in blacks are not correlated with either income or education (Baquet, Horn, Gibbs, & Greenwald, 1991).

In this society, violence is assumed to have a black face. Centerwall (1984) investigated this assumption by considering the prevalence of domestic homicides in Atlanta from 1970 to 1971. Using household crowding as a measure of socioeconomic status, the relative risk of blacks and whites was nearly identical. Findings like these suggest that there is a strong correlation between health outcomes and living conditions that is not related to race.

The two sources of causation of ill health coalesce more often than not, and teasing apart those inborn versus acquired characteristics is a complex process. For example, the unborn fetus is subject to the environment experienced by the mother. That environment, like exposure to noxious agents or a mother's nutritional state, is the source of elements that may or may not be detected, but the resultant health effects on the fetus are as decided and lasting as genetic inheritance.

Without improvement in the statistical picture of health in blacks, has the relationship improved between black clients and the health care system? Actually, the breach appears to be maintained with reports like "Mississippi appendectomies" or eugenic hysterectomies performed on black women (Chase, 1980; Weisbord, 1975), testing of women for sickle cell anemia without consent (Farfel & Holzman, 1986), and court-ordered surgical interventions (Kolder, Gallagher, & Parsons, 1987). Blacks delay entry into the health care system, and incidents like these are part of the reason. Added to this is the historical reliance of blacks on self-care or folk medicine (Bushy, 1992; Wilson-Ford, 1992). It is estimated that 70% to 90% of recognized illnesses in blacks are managed outside the formal health care system (Kleinman, Eisenberg, & Good, 1978).

One must ask how welcome clients are to share their self-care approaches? Does the health care system acknowledge that there is more than one right way to care? Most African Americans are reticent about sharing culturally derived treatment methods. Instead, they often use a technique called "impression management" (Whitehead, 1992) to project conforming behavior. Using impression management, the client responds as expected and avoids appearing self-destructive or unconcerned. The level of tolerance for divergent beliefs must be raised to eliminate the need for impression management.

Some of the messages currently sent by the health care system have a historical familiarity. Racial differences in drug response were recorded as early as 1929. However, recent studies show that while African Americans differ in drug response and disposition, they continue to be underrepresented in clinical trials of new drugs (Svensson, 1989). Heart disease is the number one cause of death in blacks, but whites use significantly more of the available treatments for heart disease, such as coronary angioplasty and coronary artery bypass grafting (Wenneker & Epstein, 1989).

If it is accepted that one of the roles of research is to inform, thereby improving nursing practice, then research outcomes must have reliability and validity. Some of the traditional approaches to methodology are unable to provide this, and change is imperative. Being unfamiliar with an ethnic group is a serious consideration in the study of that group. In conducting research among the poor, African Americans, and other minorities, the methodology and theoretical constructs used must be applicable and appropriate (Zambrana, 1991). Knowledge of the group should be more in-depth than a mere statistical profile because the data collection and data treatment techniques bear directly on the accuracy of outcomes (McGraw, McKinlay, Crawford, Costa, & Cohen, 1992). For example, the practice of combining ethnic minorities to generalize cultural variations makes results highly suspect, if not meaningless (Weitzel & Waller, 1990).

Nurses are uniquely positioned to offer culturally competent care to African-American clients. African Americans have high incidences of diseases that are preventable. Therefore, the probability of making a significant difference in the health of this group is exceptional. Since the 1960s, the nursing profession has encouraged the incorporation of culture into care. Achieving this, however, has been a slow and difficult process. In 1992, the American Academy of Nursing (AAN) Expert Panel on Culturally Competent Nursing Care concluded that, ". . . there are no excuses for continuing to provide care that is insensitive and [culturally] incompetent." (p. 277)

The Eurocentric model of nursing care has been applied to all who enter the health care system, but it has never been adequate. The limitations of the North American Nursing Diagnosis Association (NANDA) nursing diagnoses is a case in point. Two hundred forty-five nurses from eight countries rated the usefulness of the defining characteristics listed by NANDA for three nursing diagnoses. In each instance, the diagnosis had to be expanded and rewritten, a significant number of its diagnostic characteristics deleted, and others added (Geissler, 1991). From a cultural viewpoint, many NANDA terms have multiple meanings. Social dysfunction and social isolation are two of those labels that must be defined within their cultural context. Across cultures they are without meaning (Kelley & Frisch, 1992). Nursing diagnoses are a mainstay of the nursing process, but blacks and other culturally diverse clients may not be well served by their use.

Several cultural assessment tools have been proposed to capture relevant data. To date, most of these assessments are comprehensive but too lengthy and time consuming for clinical utility (Giger & Davidhizar 1991; Tripp-Reimer, Brink, & Saunders, 1984). A promising approach is the use of the client's own explanatory system. Included as a fundamental part of the nursing process, the client's cultural parameters can be assessed quickly through the use of open-ended questions, as suggested by Kleinman, Eisenberg, & Good (1978):

> What do you think caused this illness? What concerns you most about this illness? Why do you think it started when it did? How do you feel about it? What did you do about treating it before you came to the clinic? Hospital? What do you think your sickness does to you? How serious is this illness? What kind of treatment do you think you should receive? (p. 256)

These questions are amenable to time and circumstance. They may be asked early or late in a client's contact with the health care system. They are easily postponed until after the acute phase of an illness.

Heurtin-Roberts and Reisin (1992) found that among hypertensive African-American women, the patients' cultural beliefs about hypertension influenced their acceptance of treatment, and in turn, the control of their blood pressure. Data from Kumanyika et al. (1989) and Kumanyika, Wilson, & Guilford-Davenport (1993) strongly suggest that beliefs may not be modified by the health-promotion campaigns that are so widely used. They can be affected, however, when the message is delivered in a culturally sensitive format (Martin & Henry, 1989; Parks, 1988). The well-intentioned but culturally inappropriate message is apparent in the following two examples. First, African-American women in abusive relationships, states Campbell (1993), have concepts of independence and female strength that run counter to accepted ways of help seeking and resource utilization. These women are more likely to remain in their relationships and prefer assistance in working through the abuse problem. This is at odds with the Eurocentric model, which places emphasis on leaving the relationship. The deliberate capture of cultural content must precede real changes in nursing approaches. Second, ethnohistorical influences are basic to nurse-client relationships and, whether acknowledged or ignored, they frame the interaction. African Americans respond positively to culturally sensitive therapeutics. A pilot project in which music therapists used African-American music to open avenues of expression for psychiatric clients was remarkably successful when compared with programs using Eurocentric music (Campinha-Bacote & Allbright, 1992).

I believe that as nursing appreciates the impact of culture on practice, the need for expertise will advance. As we are encouraged to actively seek out cultural patterns, the inescapable importance of history and social context will become more apparent. Culture must be allowed to move up in the curricular hierarchy when students are being transformed into professional nurses. Culture must be as integrated as part of the nursing process with a permanent, prominent venue. Given the opportunity to identify their own attitudes, beliefs, and values, nurses can begin to explore ways in which their heritage affects their own behavior. Nurses are pivotal members of the health care team. They personify one culture (their own), convey another (nursing and health care), and arbitrate a third (the client's). They can either lead the way to cultural plurality or they can continue to display half-hearted attempts at change. It is a brave new world—similar to the old and familiar yet remarkably diverse and different. We may argue as to whether health care is a right or a privilege, but there is no disagreement that it is a choice. African Americans make that choice based on their perceptions of what nurses and the health care system offer. Health behaviors are retained because they are functional, but they do not stand alone. Health behaviors are embedded in social and economic arrangements (Pappas, 1994; Smith, 1995). When black clients are entirely validated by the health care system in all their sociocultural dimensions, a reciprocal relationship can develop that is built on mutual understanding and respect.

REFERENCES

AAN Expert Panel on Culturally Competent Nursing Care. (1992). *AAN Expert Panel Report: Culturally competent health care. Nursing Outlook, 40*(6), 277-283.

Anonymous. (1983). Genetics, environment, and hypertension. *Lancet, 1*, 681-682.

Baquet, C.R., Horn, J.W., Gibbs, T., & Greenwald, P. (1991). Socioeconomic factors and cancer incidence among blacks and whites. *Journal of the National Cancer Institute, 83*(8), 551-556.

Beardsley, E.H. (1987). *A history of neglect: Health care for blacks and mill workers in the twentieth century south.* Knoxville, TN: University of Tennessee Press.

Beecher, H.K. (1966). Ethics and clinical research. *New England Journal of Medicine, 274*, 1354-1360.

Bennett, L. (1982). *Before the Mayflower: A history of the Negro in America 1619-1964* (5th Ed.). New York: Penguin Books.

Biological anthropologist pursues her taste for the big picture. (1995, July 28). *The Chronicle of Higher Education*, pp. A11, A16.

Bushy, A. (1992). Cultural considerations for primary health care:

Where do self care and folk medicine fit? *Holistic Nursing Practice, 6*(3), 10-18.

Byrd, M.W., & Clayton, L.A. (1992). An American health dilemma: A history of blacks in the health system. *Journal of the National Medical Association, 84*(2), 189-200.

Cabral, H., Fried, L.E., Levenson, S., Amaro, H., & Zuckerman, B. (1990). Foreign-born and US-born black women: Differences in health behaviors and birth outcomes. *American Journal of Public Health, 80*(1), 70-71.

Campbell, D.W. (1993). Nursing care of African American battered women. *AWHONN's Clinical Issues, 4*(3), 407-414.

Campinha-Bacote, J., & Allbright, R. (1992). Ethnomusic therapy and the dual-diagnosed African American client. *Holistic Nursing Practice, 6*(3), 59-63.

Centerwall, B.S. (1984). Race, socioeconomic status, and domestic homicide, Atlanta, 1971-72. *American Journal of Public Health, 74*(8), 813-815.

Charatz-Litt, C. (1992). A chronicle of racism: The effects of the white medical community on black health. *Journal of the National Medical Association, 84*(8), 717-724.

Chase, A. (1980). *The legacy of Malthus: The social costs of the new scientific racism.* New York: Alfred A. Knopf.

Cooper, R., & David, R. (1986). The biological concept of race and its application to public health epidemiology. *Journal of Health Politics and Law II, 1* 97-116.

Edwards, A. (1995, October). Coming together. *Essence, 26*(6), 99-100, 102-103, 150-152.

Farfel, M.R., & Holtzman, N.A. (1986). Education, consent, and counseling in sickle cell anemia screening programs. *American Journal of Public Health, 74*(4), 373-375.

Franklin, J.H. (1956). *From slavery to freedom.* New York: Alfred A. Knopf.

Freeman, H. (1991). Race, poverty, and cancer. *Journal of the National Cancer Institute, 83*(8), 526-527.

Geissler, E.M. (1991). Nursing diagnoses of culturally diverse patients. *International Nursing Review, 38*(5), 150-152.

Gergen, K. (1982). *Toward transformation in social knowledge.* New York: Springer-Verlag.

Giger, J., & Davidhizar, R. (1991). *Transcultural nursing: Assessment and intervention.* St. Louis: Mosby.

Gutman, H.G. (1976). *The black family in slavery and freedom 1750-1925.* New York: Vantage Books.

Haynes, M.A. (1975). The gap in health status between black and white Americans. In R.A. Williams (Ed.), *Textbook of black-related diseases* (pp. 1-30). New York: McGraw-Hill Book Co.

Heurtin-Roberts, S., & Reisin, E. (1992). The relation of culturally influenced lay models of hypertension to compliance with treatment. *American Journal of Hypertension, 5,* 787-792.

Johnson, J.E. (1982). The Afro-American family: A historical overview. In B.A. Bass, G.E. Wyatt, & G.J. Powell (Eds.), *The Afro-American family: Assessment, treatment, and research issues* (pp. 3-11). New York: Grune & Stratton.

Jones, J.H. (1981). *Bad blood: The Tuskegee syphilis experiment.* New York: The Free Press.

Jordan, W.D. (1968). *White over black: American attitudes toward the negro 1550-1812.* New York: WW Norton & Co.

Kelley, J.H., & Frisch, N.C. (1992). A transcultural concept analysis of social isolation. In R.M. Carroll-Johnson & M. Paquette (Eds.), *Classification of nursing diagnosis: Proceedings of the tenth conference* (pp. 232-233) Philadelphia: Lippincott.

Kleinman, A., Eisenberg, L., & Good, B. (1978). Culture, illness, and care: Clinical lessons from anthropologic and cross-cultural research. *Annals of Internal Medicine, 88,* 251-258.

Kolder, V., Gallagher, J., & Parsons, M.T. (1987). Court-ordered obstetrical interventions. *New England Journal of Medicine, 316*(19), 1192-1196.

Kumanyika, S., Savage, D.D., Ramirez, A.G., Hutchinson, J., Trenino, F.M., Adams-Campbell, L.L., & Watkins, L.O. (1989). Beliefs about high blood pressure prevention in a survey of blacks and Hispanics. *American Journal of Preventive Medicine, 5*(1), 21-26.

Kumanyika, S., Wilson, J.F., & Guilford-Davenport, M. (1993). Weight-related attitudes and behaviors of black women. *Journal of the American Dietetic Association, 93*(4), 416-422.

Langford, H.G. (1981). Is blood pressure different in black people? *Postgraduate Medical Journal, 57,* 749-754.

Martin, M.E., & Henry, M. (1989). Cultural relativity and poverty. *Public Health Nursing, 6*(1), 28-34.

McCord, C., & Freeman, H. (1990). Excess mortality in Harlem. *New England Journal of Medicine, 322*(3), 173-177.

McGraw, S.A., McKinlay, J.B., Crawford, S.A., Costa, L.A., & Cohen, D.L. (1992). Health survey methods with minority populations: Some lessons from recent experiences. *Ethnicity & Disease, 2,* 273-285.

Myers, M.J. (1991). Expanding the psychology of knowledge optimally: The importance of world view revisited. In R.L. Jones (Ed.), *Black psychology* (pp. 15-32). Berkeley, CA: Cobb and Henry.

National Center for Health Statistics. (1995). *Health, United States, 1994.* Hyattsville, MD: Public Health Services.

Newman, D.K., Amidei, N.J., Carter, B.L., Kruvant, W.J., & Russell, J. (1978). *Protest, politics, and prosperity: Black americans and white institutions; 1940-1975.* New York: Pantheon Books.

O'Hare, W.P. (1992). America's minorities—The demographics of diversity. *Population Bulletin, 47*(4), Washington, DC: Population References Bureau, Inc.

Pappas, G. (1994). Elucidating the relationship between race, socioeconomic status, and health [Editorial]. *American Journal of Public Health, 84*(6), 892.

Parks, C.P. (1988). Development of a hypertension educational pamphlet for the black community: A model approach. *Health Education, 10,* 8-10.

Reed, W.L., Darity, W., & Robertson, N. (1993). *Health and medical care of African Americans.* Westport, CT: Greenwood Publishing Group, Inc.

Rene, A.A., Daniels, D.E., Jones, W., & Moore, F.I. (1992). Mortality in the slave and white population of Natchitoches Parish, Louisiana, 1850. *Journal of the National Medical Association, 84*(9), 805-811.

Savitt, T.L. (1978). *Medicine and slavery: The diseases and health care of blacks in antebellum Virginia.* Urbana, IL: University of Illinois Press.

Savitt, T.L. (1982). The use of blacks for medical experimentation and demonstration in the old south. *The Journal of Southern History, 48,* 331-335.

Smith, C.A. (1995). The lived experience of staying healthy in rural African American Families. *Nursing Science Quarterly, 8*(1), 17-21.

Stampp, K.M. (1956). *The peculiar institution: Slavery in the antebellum South.* New York: Alfred A. Knopf.

Svensson, C.K. (1989). Representation of American blacks in clinical trials of new drugs. *Journal of the American Medical Association, 261*(2), 263-265.

Thomas, J., Semenya, K., Neser, W.B., Thomas, J., & Gillum, R.F. (1990). Parental hypertension as a predictor of hypertension in black physicians: The Meharry Cohort Study. *Journal of the National Medical Association, 82*(6), 409-412.

Thomas, J., Semenya, K.A., Neser, W.B., Thomas, J., Green, D.R., & Gillum, R.F. (1985). Risk factors and the incidence of hypertension in black physicians: The Meharry Cohort Study. *American Heart Journal, 110*(3), 637-645.

Thomas, V.G. (1992). Explaining health disparities between African-American and white populations. Where do we go from here? *Journal of the National Medical Association, 84*(10), 837-840.

Tripp-Reimer, T., Brink, P.J., & Saunders, J.M. (1984). Cultural assessment: Content and process. *Nursing Outlook, 32,* 78-82.

Valentine, C.A. (1968). *Culture and poverty.* Chicago: The University of Chicago Press.

Van Sertima, I. (1976). *They came before Columbus.* New York: Random House.

Waitzman, N.J., & Smith, K.R. (1994). The effects of occupational class transitions on hypertension: Racial disparities among working-age men. *American Journal of Public Health, 84*(6), 945-950.

Wenneker, M.B., & Epstein, A.M. (1989). Racial inequalities in the use of procedures for patients with ischemic heart disease in Massachusetts. *Journal of the American Medical Association, 261*(2), 253-357.

Weitzel, M.H., & Waller, P.R. (1990). Predictive factors for health-promotive behaviors in white, Hispanic, and Black blue-collar workers. *Family and Community Health, 13*(1), 23-34.

Whitehead, T.L. (1992). In search of soul food and meaning: Culture, food, and health. In H.A. Baer & Y. Jones (Eds.), *African Americans in the South: Issues of race, class, and gender* (pp. 94-110). Athens, GA: University of Georgia Press.

Wiesbord, R.G. (1975). *Genocide? Birth control and the black American.* Westport, CN: Greenwood Press.

Wilson-Ford, V. (1992). Health-protective behaviors of rural black elderly women. *Health and Social Work, 17*(1), 28-36.

Woodhandler, S., Himmelstein, D.U., Silber, R., Bader, M., Harnly, M., & Jones, A. (1985). Medical care and mortality: Racial differences in preventable deaths. *International Journal of Health Service, 15,* 1-22.

Zambrana, R.E. (1991). Cross-cultural methodological strategies in the study of low income racial ethnic populations. In M. Grady (Ed.), *Conference Proceedings, Primary Care Research: Theory and Methods* (pp. 221-227). Washington: U.S. Department of Health and Human Services.

Bridging cultures: Hispanics/Latinos and nursing

SARA TORRES, HELEN CASTILLO

Hispanics/Latinos and the nursing profession will be faced with a tremendous challenge in the coming decade: to increase the representation of Hispanics/Latinos in the nursing profession at all levels.

The demographic browning of America poses both an issue and a dilemma, that is, meeting the health care needs of an ethnically diverse population in an infrastructure that is philosophically and economically unprepared to do so. Statistics indicate that 90% of all nurses are non-Hispanic whites from middle and working class backgrounds. It is posited that the only way for the nursing profession to increase the number of Hispanics who are needed to meet existing nursing service demands is to become more culturally diverse. Cultural diversity, however, includes many variables and is not simply a matter of making a choice.

Cultural diversity is not occurring in nursing. Baccalaureate and graduate degree nursing programs are especially challenged to increase the number of new student admissions and to facilitate the admission process for Hispanics. This challenge includes providing flexibility and allowing course credits for registered nurses (RNs) with associate degrees in nursing (ADN) who wish to pursue baccalaureate or master's degrees. The highest education credential of most Hispanic nurses is the ADN, with a significantly lower number of Hispanic nurses attaining baccalaureate, masters, and doctoral degrees than the rest of the RN population in the United States.

Given the financial limitations of Hispanics in this country, most are educated in 2-year ADN programs and in the few remaining 3-year hospital-based diploma schools of nursing. These programs attract students primarily because they provide earning power earlier than the 4-year (BSN) degree programs and have less stringent entrance criteria requirements. Thus the majority of Hispanics continue to enroll in 2-year programs, limiting their long-term mobility in the nursing profession unless they continue into baccalaureate education and beyond.

Hispanic nurses who attend 2- and 3-year nursing programs are not appointed to positions of nursing leadership and responsibility because of the lack of specialty preparation in these programs that is provided in higher education. Additionally lacking are Hispanic mentors in higher education and nursing leadership positions who can promote other Hispanics. Hispanics who do hold leadership positions are deluged with requests to participate in activities that demonstrate cultural diversity and visibility of the agency by including an academically prepared Hispanic nurse. Together, selective discrimination and family and financial responsibilities make it more difficult for Hispanics to continue their studies, often precluding them from attaining masters and doctoral degrees.

There has been only one Hispanic employed at the level of "dean" in the history of nursing in the United States. At present, approximately four Hispanics are positioned at the level of director of schools of nursing or nursing programs—one at the baccalaureate level, one each at the undergraduate and graduate levels, and two at the ADN level. The few visible Hispanics in leadership positions further limit opportunities for students to view Hispanics as role models in nursing.

Role modeling is the product of a complex set of social, economic, and educational factors. High dropout rates, poor academic preparation, and inadequate facilities and equipment in underserved communities, together with the low expectations by teachers of Hispanic students, contribute to the small pool of Hispanics who ultimately achieve professional careers and serve as role models. More significantly, these low numbers reflect an education system that remains ill prepared to develop Hispanic students to their fullest potential.

Why are Hispanics/Latinos not entering nursing in correlation to the growing population of Hispanics? According to demographic data, RNs in the United States numbered 2.3 million in 1988. Only 26,163 of these nurses were Hispanic, a meager 1.1%. Further, of the 5,400 nurses with doctoral degrees in the United States, approximately 50 are Hispanic, an even more dismaying 0.9%. These are dismal statistics considering that the number of Hispanic communities and their populations are increasing rapidly, while the increase in the numbers of Hispanic nurses is not occurring. From a nursing leadership perspective, two major questions arise. First, how aware are nursing leaders of this critical issue? Second, what steps are being taken to resolve this issue? Data from both national and state levels are disturbing illustrations that validate the underrepresentation of Hispanics in nursing education and practice. These data support expressed concerns at the baccalaureate and graduate levels, from which most nursing leadership evolves.

Nursing faculty and government agencies must address the recruitment, retention, and attrition problems in nursing schools from a Hispanic/Latino perspective. By the year 2000, the U.S. workforce is expected to be so diverse and complex that nursing must anticipate these effects and their long-term implications in order to prepare accordingly. Recruitment efforts need to be improved dramatically to reflect the cultural diversity of society within the nursing population. Although not consciously intended, health care agency recruiters often select nurses who appear similar to themselves instead of considering their patient population preferences or needs as the first priority. Thoughtful consideration of patients' needs must be brought to the awareness level of nursing staff members, including recruiters.

OVERVIEW OF THE HISPANIC/LATINO POPULATION IN THE UNITED STATES

The demographic profile of the Hispanic/Latino population is changing in the United States. According to the U.S. Bureau of the Census (1993), Hispanics are the fastest-growing minority group in the country. The Hispanic population grew by 61% between 1970 and 1980 and by 53% between 1980 and 1990. Hispanics now represent 9.6% of the total U.S. population, and by 2000 will comprise 11% (U.S. Bureau of the Census, 1993). By the year 2010, Hispanics are projected to make up 13% of the U.S. population, 17% by 2030, and 21% by 2050. In 1990, about one of every 10 Americans was Hispanic, and this number is expected to rise to one of every five by 2050. This tremendous Hispanic population increase since 1970 has been attributed to several factors. Among them are a higher birth rate than the rest of the population, substantial immigration, and improvements in census-reporting procedures.

The largest group of Hispanics/Latinos in the United States are Mexican Americans, followed by Puerto Ricans and Cubans. Although found in every state, nearly nine of every 10 Hispanics/Latinos live in just 10 states. California is the home of one of every three Hispanics; Texas has nearly one of every five, and other large concentrations reside in the Northeast states of New York, New Jersey, and Massachusetts. Florida, Illinois, Arizona, New Mexico, and Colorado round out the top 10 states with sizable Hispanic populations.

Hispanic Americans are more likely than non-Hispanics to live in metropolitan areas and central cities. Approximately 90% of Hispanics lived in metropolitan areas in 1990, according to the U.S. Bureau of the Census (1993), as compared with about 76% of non-Hispanics. In 1990, about 27% of Hispanic families lived below the poverty level compared with about 10% of non-Hispanic families. The poverty rate for Hispanics in 1990 was not statistically different from that in 1980, an indication that essential changes have not taken place. In 1990, nearly 32 million persons (14% of the population) 5 years of age and older spoke a language other than English at home. Of this number, about 6.7 million (less than 3%) did not speak English well or at all. Second to English, Spanish was spoken by over 17 million people (8%) 5 years of age and older. Among Spanish-speaking persons, 8.3 million could not speak English well or at all, and Spanish speakers represented 54% of all non-English speakers in the United States.

THE USE OF HISPANIC/LATINO TERM

The term Hispanic/Latino is used interchangeably. Label preferences seem to be geographic, that is, divided by locale. For example, the term Hispanic is often used in the Midwest and the East Coast, while Latino is preferred on the West Coast. Yet, Hispanics living along the 2,000 mile United States-Mexico border, prefer to self-report as Mexican American, Chicano, or Hispanic. It is important to distinguish between these terms as having a historical base from which negative or positive images and connotations arise. Because long standing cultural values and military conflicts such as the historical Battle of The Alamo between Mexico and the United States, Hispanic/Latino terms remain controversial and generate strong feelings and emotions. These labels are distinctive and arise partly from the period of history in which the ethno-cultural label was applied. Perhaps it is also a function of the age of the "labeled" and the stage of their acculturation. Throughout this chapter, Hispanic and/or Latino will be used interchangeably.

HISPANIC/LATINO WOMEN IN LEADERSHIP ROLES

The question arises, why so few Hispanic/Latino women aspire to leadership roles. In the Hispanic culture few women are in leadership roles because leadership has been viewed as a competitive male attribute especially in business and health care circles. Consider the traditional physician-nurse dyad where the physician has been male while the nurse has been female. Today, these roles are changing as more women enter male-dominated health care disciplines, law, and business careers. Conversely, more men are also entering nursing and other health care professions. In the past, Hispanic/Latino women were relegated to "ama de casa," which translates to "housewife." The independent, well educated, entrepreneurial woman has not been readily accepted in the traditional Hispanic family because men have been expected to provide financial and other supports for both wife and family, while the wife remains at home. In the past, Hispanic males were considered poor providers if they were unable to do so. As Hispanic women have initiated stronger leadership efforts and sought opportunities for higher education, their numbers are increasing. Far from representative of the Hispanic population, this group needs to grow significantly. Mentoring by peers and other women leaders is sorely needed, regardless of their ethnicity or culture. The new leadership role of the Hispanic/Latino woman is emerging and needs to be fully addressed.

PROBLEMS FACING HISPANICS/LATINOS IN NURSING

The deteriorating health status of our country's growing Hispanic population is disturbing. Hispanics are disproportionately affected by certain cancers, alcoholism and drug abuse, obesity, hypertension, diabetes, dental diseases, and HIV/AIDS. More Hispanic nurses are needed to care for the specific health and cultural needs of Hispanic patients.

There are few if any data on the career mobility of Hispanics in nursing. The term *career mobility* implies that an individual moves from one career level to another, either laterally or to a higher level. It is important to note that the problems of career development and mobility are applicable to the whole of nursing, and not to Hispanic nurses alone. Historically, however, career advancement in nursing has been difficult and limited for Hispanics, due primarily to their lack of advanced educational preparation in nursing. However, with the promotion of the BSN, master's, and PhD degrees in nursing, along with the major restructuring taking place in health care facilities today, an ever-increasing number of nurses are moving beyond basic ADN and BSN preparation.

The mobility of Hispanics in nursing has been limited for two basic reasons. First, although there has been an increase in the proportion of Hispanics enrolled in nursing schools during the past decade, the increase has been well below the Hispanic population parity. Second, Hispanics continue to enroll in ADN programs, limiting their future mobility and leadership opportunities in the profession. Certainly, while the many options in nursing do allow lateral career moves more easily, mobility into leadership positions is clearly restricted by a "glass ceiling" effect. Research studies (Hickey & Solis, 1990) show this to be true of women in general, specifically women in management and academia (U.S. Department of Health and Human Services [DHHS], 1990; Wilson & Flores, 1992).

As mentioned earlier, the problem of career mobility for Hispanic nurses is intensified by cultural, social, and educational differences. In addition, because Hispanic/Latino nurses lack contact with important professional role models, their opportunities to be socialized in the dynamics of self-advancement are fewer than for their non-Hispanic counterparts. New Hispanic nurses often do not look beyond the prospect of their first position. Instead, they view their "job" as a satisfying career of helping others rather than as a first step in the progression of a lifetime career as well. If we are to promote career mobility within the existing ranks of Hispanic nurses, we must initiate career development programs that include leadership skills development and provide a variety of resources to guide Hispanics through the educational process. These educational efforts need to begin early and continue through higher education in colleges and universities.

Hispanic nurses must prepare themselves academically and acquire the necessary experience and expertise in clinical areas of specialization. Additionally, Hispanic nurses must develop their leadership skills and other informal skills to increase their competitive edge and success in attaining leadership posts. They need to learn the unwritten rules of success and find out how they "fit" into the organization's culture. These skills are essential to command positions of responsibility and prestige in nursing. Institutions that espouse support need to assist Hispanic/Latino nurses in their career development and mobility by providing opportunities for career planning, addressing professional issues, rewarding nurses for direct patient care and other contributions, and facilitating their education. The nurse should have a personal plan for career development as well. In addition, mutually beneficial plans for career development should be jointly prepared by the nurse and the employing agency to achieve success for both.

Models of career mobility and professional advancement for Hispanic/Latino nurses need to be developed. Nursing organizations such as the American Nurses Association, the National League for Nursing, and the Association of Colleges and Universities must promote and support the advancement of underrepresented Hispanics/Latinos at all levels of nursing practice within the scope of their mission. Needed are strategies that will develop well-prepared leaders among the ranks of nursing practice at state, national, and international levels.

Role socialization is the process by which an individual comes to internalize certain knowledge, skills, behaviors, values, and attitudes that are integral to one's chosen profession. Role modeling is the method of teaching professional attitudes and behaviors by being the person students emulate; it becomes the process by which a person takes on the values and behaviors of another through identification. For Hispanics/Latinos, the dearth of visible role models is a major contributing factor to a lack of career orientation that exists among the Hispanic nursing population. Dissatisfaction, attrition from nursing, and limited career commitment have been linked to inadequate socialization into nursing as well as insufficient exposure to appropriate role models.

What potential currently exists for career development among Hispanic/Latino nurses in the United States? Hispanics/Latinos must be educated and socialized into professional nursing; their leadership potential must be encouraged through leadership opportunities. The supply of Hispanic/Latino nurses graduating from nursing programs continues to be disproportionately low compared with the representation of Hispanics in the general population (U.S. Bureau of the Census, 1993). In 1988, only 2.9% of all graduates of basic RN programs (including ADN, diploma, and baccalaureate programs) were Hispanic/Latino. Although increasing numbers of Hispanics/Latinos graduate from these programs every year, retention of these students is critical to maintain the number of qualified students eligible to progress into graduate studies. Only 1.6% of nursing graduates were Hispanic in 1978—too few to respond to the increasing need for Hispanic/Latino professionals as this population grows. Options are available for Hispanic/Latino nurses. The same factors that influence career development and mobility of Hispanics, such as culture, family support, diplomacy, bilingualism, risk taking, and personal goals, also restrict their leadership opportunities if they are lacking.

With the known available pool of young Hispanics/Latinos in the nation, it is time to capitalize on their abilities by facilitating financial aid and providing new opportunities for higher education. Innovative measures are needed to encourage Hispanic/Latino nurses to pursue graduate education and leadership opportunities that provide career mobility.

FUTURE DIRECTIONS

The factors that will promote successful career development and mobility among Hispanic nurses that have been discussed here include career counseling, career development models, mentoring approaches, networking systems among peers, and role modeling. Career development for Hispanic/Latino nurses should include incentives and recognition for practice, development of clinical and management ladders, and institutional support for their education and professional advancement. Additional incentives should include financial support for nursing faculty such as academic leaves of absence, paid sabbatical opportunities for further study and research, and release time to utilize new knowledge and gain clinical expertise. Institutions need to support the professional development of their members, including attendance at conferences and participation in professional organizational activities. Career development requires further support for participation in focused programs of personal development, personal financial management, and policy development. Career development also means the inclusion of Hispanic/Latino nurses in agency committees and on policy development boards.

The need to increase the number of Hispanics entering the profession of nursing remains. Educators must provide the basic preparation, information, and incentives to encourage Hispanic/Latino nurses to pursue higher education. Accelerated tracks, including RN options for licensed vocational nurses, BSN options for ADN nurses, and master's options (including specialty completion programs) will increase the opportunity for more Hispanic/

Latino nurses to achieve doctoral study. The retention of Hispanic/Latino nurses in generic nursing programs is also critical. Additionally, the voice of Hispanic/Latino nurses in the political arena needs to be heard in order to secure substantial grants for educational programs, stipends for students, faculty development, and curricular change in this time of economic cutbacks. State and federal governments need to develop databases that provide track record information about Hispanic students to appropriate agencies.

Strategies must be developed that inform the public at every level about the comprehensive needs of Hispanic/Latino nursing students in this country. Together, educators can develop strategies that provide pathways of opportunities for the success of Hispanic/Latino nursing students. Participative and cooperative endeavors between the private business sector and nursing schools must be fostered for the recruitment and retention of Hispanic/Latino nursing students in schools, especially in higher education. Additionally, networking systems among peers continue to be a priority for the development of information and centralized key group efforts.

Education has always been an important indicator of success in American society. Studies indicate that Hispanics have not attained an educational level sufficient to compete aggressively in the labor market, especially at the professional levels. Hispanics/Latinos and the nursing profession are faced with a tremendous challenge in the coming decade to increase the representation of Hispanics at all levels in nursing and to provide them with true opportunities for leadership. This leadership will affect the quality of health care delivery of culturally responsive health services, and in the process will enhance the continuing education of professional nursing staffs.

Issues relating to the supply and demand of nursing professionals in the United States continue to change dramatically as major shifts in financial and human resources continue to unfold. Nursing resources have been reallocated from hospitals to community-based facilities and to new structures such as mini-hospitals, elderly care centers, community nursing organizations, and health screening stations in malls and other centers of commerce. Additionally, the critical need is to respond to the growing underserved bilingual and culturally diverse Hispanic population—a need that has not yet been met and continues to be an elusive goal.

The dilemma of poor health care for Hispanics and underrepresentation of Hispanics in nursing is demonstrated by the following issues:

1. A disproportionate number of Hispanics are socioeconomically and educationally disadvantaged. As a result, there is a high attrition rate throughout the educational pipeline.
2. The present and future enrollment of Hispanic secondary education students will continue to represent a large prospective applicant pool for nursing. However, the pool is concentrated in school districts that traditionally have limited educational resources, give little attention to engendering goal-oriented students toward nursing careers, and lack culturally appropriate recruitment models for Hispanics.
3. Hispanic college enrollment is concentrated in community colleges. In the academic year 1986-87, 54% of all Hispanic college students were enrolled in community colleges versus 35% of white college students and 43% of black college students (Hickey & Solis, 1990). Nursing enrollment data also indicate that most Hispanics continue to enroll in ADN programs instead of baccalaureate programs.
4. Hispanic nurse professions employment data between 1980 and 1988 illustrate the substantial underrepresentation and general lack of progress in increasing employment numbers for Hispanics. Hispanic nurse enrollment and program completion trends between 1974 and 1987 also suggest the lack of significant progress in the representation of Hispanic nurses in the health professions. This continuing disparity is widening between Hispanic enrollments in nursing and degree completion and is not anticipated to increase given the school-age Hispanic student populations.
5. The literature is sparse and documented program interventions few in attempts made to increase opportunities for Hispanics in nursing. Inadequate leadership has been demonstrated by nursing representatives in addressing these important issues both in the public and private educational institution sectors.

Three central recommendations address these issues:

Recruitment: Increase the applicant pool of Hispanics/Latinos in higher education programs for prenursing and nursing students.

Retention: Retain Hispanics/Latinos in nursing education programs for prenursing and nursing students.

Career mobility: Promote the career mobility and leadership of Hispanic/Latino nurses.

Within the profession, there is a lack of understanding about cultural perspectives and needs, and this leads to conflict. Workforce and workplace conflicts are often silent. Anger that may be present may be difficult to verbalize and is exhibited in other ways, often increasing the intensity of individual and group conflicts. Discussions about cultural differences and similarities are needed to encourage nurses to work together effectively and constructively.

Communication patterns are learned and are culturally based. With Hispanics/Latinos, verbalization may be limited as a result of fear of conflict, reprisal, deference, or feelings of intimidation and violence. Communication and language barriers in health care settings must be recognized and discussed. With the insufficient number of bilingually prepared nurses, the few who are bilingual become overburdened with requests not only to serve as "translators" for an entire institution but also to assist in other similar or greater responsibilities. Language differences that should be viewed as assets often become barriers that serve to further isolate Hispanics/Latinos.

There is a natural affinity and commonality between groups of Hispanic/Latino nurses that draws them together. It is within these groups that they find support and guidance rather than from society as a whole. Likewise, insufficient emphasis is placed on the significant differences among various Hispanic/Latino cultural groups. The tendency is to place all cultural groups together and label them broadly as Hispanic/Latinos without allowing for these differences, especially socioeconomic differences. Institutional ethnocentrism exists. If nurses are to deliver culturally appropriate care, the unique differences among cultures, such as health care beliefs, sick role responses, and the meaning of illness, need to be addressed openly and nonjudgmentally. The institutional racism and discrimination that exist regionally need to be reassessed and eliminated by working together in collaborative environments that foster positive care and nursing outcomes.

Economic, familial, and many other societal factors interfere with the advancement of many Hispanic/Latino nurses. These and other barriers also prevent them from entering the nursing profession or preclude advancement in the profession. For the majority of Hispanic nurses attaining at least an ADN or BSN, this accomplishment is momentous indeed. Many are the first college or university graduates in their families. This accomplishment is equally important for the many obstacles that they have overcome during the completion of their degrees. Because of these constraints, many Hispanic/Latino nurses complete degree requirements as part-time students.

Hispanics are quickly becoming the largest culturally and linguistically different group in the United States. Hispanic cultural values and family experiences provide the foundation for research and for many positive, culturally based intervention models that can be integrated into efforts for increasing Hispanic student enrollment, retention, career mobility, and leadership in nursing.

The major strides expected of Hispanics were not achieved this decade, partly because systems have informally inhibited such progress with "glass ceilings." This obstacle is clearly evident in the lack of educationally prepared Hispanics in nursing and the absence of Hispanics in health care leadership positions regardless of their capabilities. On the other hand, qualified Hispanics may choose not to enter the subtle second-class status afforded them in acquired leadership roles assigned by non-Hispanics, some of whom condescendingly assume that Hispanics/Latinos achieved these positions for reasons of ethnicity alone.

Stronger links between academic and service settings must be established, such as the development of career ladders between hospitals and local colleges or universities. Hospitals and other health care agencies need to build mutually beneficial partnerships with schools and nursing programs via paid preceptorships, adjunct faculty roles, and other alternatives used to provide financial and other assistance to students and the academic programs. The new generation of professional nurses and educators has the tremendous responsibility of opening doors that will secure professional growth, development, and mobility for Hispanic/Latino nurses in education, practice, and research. The process of advocating for access to health care for Hispanics in the United States must continue, and the time for planning strategies has passed. The time for action is now.

REFERENCES

Hickey, C.A., & Solis, D. (1990). *The recruitment and retention of minority trainees in university affiliate programs—Hispanics.* Madison: University of Wisconsin-Madison.

U.S. Bureau of the Census. (1993). Hispanic Americans Today. *Current Population Reports* P-23,-183. Washington, DC: U.S. Government Printing Office.

U.S. Department of Health & Human Services. (1990, June). *Minorities & Women in the Health Fields.* HRSA-P-DV 90-3.

Wilson, J.M., & Flores, J.H. (1992). *First National Hispanic Nurse Symposium Proceedings: Strategy for Change: Recruitment, Retention, Career Mobility.* San Antonio, TX: Center for Health Policy Development, Inc.

Bridging cultures: Native Americans and nursing

SHELLY CROW

AN ACCEPTED APPLE IN AN INDIAN SETTING

An apple is red on the outside and white on the inside. This term is used by many full-blood Indians to refer to "thin-blood" Indians.

As a full citizen of the Muscogee (Creek) Nation but not a full-blood Indian, raised in a non-Indian environment, and working in the nursing profession for over 10 years in non-Indian institutions, it was quite a shock to work for the Cherokee Nation as a community health nurse based in an Indian health service hospital. I could not know that within 5 years I would be second in command of the Muscogee Nation as an elected official.

Working with clients in a private institution is quite different than working with clients in a government-run institution. In private institutions clients generally ask many questions concerning their health care and often demand to speak with their physicians about health issues related to their care. As a health educator in Tulsa, Oklahoma, and Houston, my clients were interested in learning about childbirth, parenting, breast feeding, and child safety.

There were many things that I was not prepared for in serving as a community health nurse for an Indian population. As I began to plan the health care with my Native American people, I assumed that they would be interested in learning the same things as non-Indians. One of the most important factors that I neglected in the implementation of care was my clients' Indian traditions. Community health nursing for a hospital serving 39 federally recognized tribes with differing cultures and traditions can be very challenging.

THEORETICAL FRAMEWORK

I know now that a well-versed community health nurse relies on the framework of a theorist. Leininger's (1991) theory of Cultural Care Diversity and Universality would have been very helpful to me. This theory gives structure to the process of learning the cultural and social dimensions that influence health and health care, including technological factors, religious and philosophical factors, kinship and social factors, cultural values and lifeways, and political and legal factors. Following this framework, nursing care involves an integration and balancing of cultural care or folk practices with professional nursing and health care systems. The ultimate goal of nursing is to provide care that is culturally meaningful, sensitive, and effective.

RELIGION

Although many Indians have been converted to European religions a majority still hold on to some of their traditional beliefs. Many "traditional Indians" still practice the religion of our forefathers. In the Indian health service facility where I worked, it was rarely known when the medicine man was around. He was paged by his English name, and his true identification was not given. He was not allowed an office nor did he attend any staff meetings.

The medicine person (most commonly a man) is the traditional health care giver of the community. On a daily basis, the medicine person is sought out for curative plants, minerals, songs for aches, pains, infections, contusions, disorientation, and any other aspect of personal well being. Throughout the religious cycles of a ceremonial ground, they are the preparers of sacred items which are used to "feed" the town's fire and potions shared by the town's members to guarantee their good health and behavior.

The first thing I learned and admired about my people was their spiritualism. I discovered that it is very important to my people, no matter what religion they practice, to be close to the Creator in order to get well.

Discussing what type of health care my Indian clients would like to receive was quite an eye opener. Many stated that they felt isolated in the hospital setting and became frustrated over their lack of control of the environment. They stated that Indians need to be a part of nature, and the hospital setting is far from nature.

KINSHIP

A hospitalized Indian expects his or her family to visit. My definition of family was much different than theirs. In a non-Indian hospital, 10 visitors would be a lot for a new baby or someone who is dying, but for Indians up to 50 visitors are not uncommon for these events. The extended family is very important to Indians, who gain strength from the family.

SOCIAL FACTORS

Traditional medicine versus western medicine

Most of my traditional Indian patients were willing to share with me why they preferred the medicine man to a physician. Indians consider the medicine man to be a physician with healing powers. Although the IHS physician has book knowledge concerning healing, Indians believe that the medicine man is in contact with the creator while the physician is not.

Lifeways

When a community health nurse is sent to the home to follow up on an Indian client's health status, it is not surprising to discover that the patient has begun practicing his or her own beliefs at home. The patient is no longer under the control of the institution's guidelines, and this is Indian territory. The community health nurse either learns the Indian's beliefs and designs care around both western medicine and Indian traditional medicine or walks away.

One of my clients referred me to a very special quote by Sitting Bull: "I have advised my people this way. When you find anything good in the white man's road, pick it up. When you find something that is bad, or turns out bad, drop it and leave it alone." This quote became very real to me several times during home visits when I found clients not taking prescribed medications for diabetes or high blood pressure. If the medicine prescribed by the physician hadn't worked in a few days, the patient would call the medicine man.

I remember my grandfather telling me that when his mother was dying of pneumonia a white doctor was present. Just to be safe, however, the medicine man was there for days as well. In interviewing a very great man within my tribe my eyes were opened to my people's beliefs. He stated,

> The Creator is the source of all living things. The plants are living things that are used for medicine. A person has to have a calling to practice the gift of healing. When you remove a plant from the Mother Earth you must thank her and replace it with something, another plant or tobacco to show her that you respect her and thank her for sacrificing this plant to help you heal another living thing.

It became easy for me to understand why some of my Indian clients believed that the non-Indian physician does not thank the Creator for the medicine or skills with which he or she has been blessed or has obtained through education. The physician's way of trying to help the Indian client is not favorable with the Creator and therefore will not work.

With this type of belief, nurses in Indian hospitals or private hospitals who serve Indians should understand that these patients interpret their stay in the hospital as a powerless situation. The people surrounding them are not blessed by the Creator and have no knowledge of Indian beliefs.

ECONOMIC FACTORS—TRADITIONAL EXCHANGE FOR MEDICINE VERSUS WESTERN MEDICINE FOR PAY

Another situation I encountered with Indian clients was their difficulty understanding payment to a physician whom they were referred to outside the Indian Health Service. Usually, if there were contract funds to cover the referral then indian health or tribal governments paid the bill, but if the funds were depleted the clients were told they would have to pay. At first I thought their thinking was a result of Indians always being taken care of by the federal government as a result of treaties, through which they expected every service to be free.

In reality, I was wrong in some cases. Some of my clients believe in giving gifts to their healer; there is no price attached to healing. Once an Indian client receives his or her healing, the medicine man is offered whatever that person wishes to give. Unlike Western medicine, in which physicians profit from their healing knowledge, Indian medicine men do not believe that profit should be gained by their practice.

The medicine man practices several rituals for his own purification. He tries to be pure in thought and in deed before performing a healing service. Indian clients are aware of the sacrifice that the medicine man has made in order to work with them. They cannot perceive of any sacrifices made by the non-Indian physician who is in charge of their care. It is consequently very hard for them to accept his or her advice.

Many Indians complain about having to wait for care in the indian health and tribal government health care systems, labeling their experiences as "cattle treatment." One Indian client stated that "the employees at these places work for the Indian, but they forget that. It's like we are lucky we have them to take care of us."

Some Indians do not use indian health and tribal facilities for health care because they feel that the private physicians and the private hospitals are not patient enough with them when explaining their care. They sometimes do not understand the terms used and need more time to translate from English to their native languages. There may not even be a native word for the translation.

POLITICAL ISSUES

Health care providers who wish to work with Native Americans may need to research the political infrastructure of the health care system available for the patient. The federal government has an obligation to provide health care to Indian people as a result of treaties. Many times the moneys are not available, however, and tribal governments may be allowed to contract these funds, which are then under the guidelines of that particular tribal government.

The nurse may become frustrated because he or she cannot carry out the health care plan in the hospital or community setting as a result of both federal and tribal politics. For example, clients may need further work-up for a certain diagnosis, but no funding is available; or, if they are properly diagnosed, no medications are available.

One of the Muscogee Creek leaders, Chief Pleasant Porter stated in 1896 that "My people are not dying due to disease, but due to the lack of hope" (Debo, 1968). This is still true today in Indian country; many have low-self esteem, are unemployed or underemployed, receive poor health care, and are stereotyped as lazy. Indian people express an overall lack of trust in the system of federal and tribal governments. Tribal health care systems are a form of rationed health care; the tribes are typically limited in the services they can provide. Contract health service funds only cover a small number of clients.

What is a tribal government to do in prioritizing the needs of its people? Should priorities be based on helping the greatest number of people or those with the most serious illnesses? Should priorities be based on age or concern for quality of life? Funding can only go so far.

Politics may have a tremendous impact on who receives services so that tribal officials may be elected. In addition, the qualifications of personnel in tribal government health care systems deserve close scrutiny. Are the best qualified people recruited, are those who can effectively help with a re-election recruited?

LEGAL ISSUES

The federal government issues guidelines for tribal governments to follow, but the tribal governments stand on sovereignty as their defense for employing less-qualified people. Assertive and committed health care providers (Indian or non-Indian) do not have the training to deal with all the intricacies of federal and tribal governments. Their main mission should be to assist the Indian community in becoming more self-sufficient and less codependent on the health care system.

EDUCATION

More of the history, culture, and language of Native Americans must be taught to all U.S. citizens in lower grades to build up cultural and political understanding of tribal governments. To prevent culture shock, the education of health care providers must be enhanced to include guidance in understanding federal and tribal governments' relationships, duties, and responsibilities. Health care providers for Indian people must be ready for resistance to change in the form of political barriers that may interfere with their efforts to ensure good health care outcomes for their Indian clients.

In educating health care providers, educators must instill in their students that they should never give up their own values while serving other cultures. However, they must plan health care that incorporates their clients' values and cultural beliefs.

Institutions of higher education in nursing have an obligation to research and improve their curricula to introduce to nursing students the problems of politics in all level of governments and how politics can impact health care delivery throughout this country.

Tribal governments must encourage and educate their people to network more effectively with other systems to help serve their people and provide better health care and a better quality of life. Tribal leaders must abandon the practice of using health care as a political pawn in their re-election plans.

CULTURAL SHOCK

It has been a cultural shock for this "Apple," being female in a cultural system that has changed from a matriarchal to a patriarchal one that is not intent on providing a better quality of life for our Indian people. My professional background is one in which everyone is served, not for a vote but to improve quality of life. This holistic approach is not always consistent with tribal goals. The tribal chief today is not elected through Indian traditions, but rather by the European style of government. This history of the Muscogee Nation, based upon the interrelationships of clans and patterns of both interrelationship and contrast between the towns of the confederacy, governed through participatory, consensual, and holistic politics instead of representation and conflict winning, has proven that the customs of the chiefs of our forefathers and their tribal towns (governed until recently by the leadership of the ceremonial grounds) were much better and worked for many years.

The history of the Muscogee Nation has proven that the customs of the chiefs of our forefathers (and the ceremonial grounds) were much better and worked for thousands of years. Imposing European style government has been used to destroy our Muscogean people and take their true government away from them. The real chiefs were trained from birth and knew what was expected of them. This is in contrast to today, when chiefs must play the political game at the expense of the best qualified people in their administration. The government has imposed not cultural-based values, but greed values.

In the 1898 debate on the Curtis Act to force allotment of tribal lands on the Muscogee (Creek), Cherokee, Chockasaw, Choctaw, and Seminole Tribes, Senator Dawes commented that, "We need to teach these Indians how to be greedy" (Debo, 1968; Foreman, 1932). Life is the most important matter, not playing politics to help only those chosen by those in power.

In working with Native Americans one must realize that the Indian people are descendants of the original inhabitants of this country and that many are striving to maintain their tribal heritage and cultural values in the face of strong pressures toward incorporation into the mainstream of American life. Our governments are really fairly new and not at all like the original governments of our forefathers. We have adopted non-Indian ways to establish our governments, and this has been a disaster because it limits our ability to retain our culture and beliefs.

REFERENCES

Debo, A. (1968). *And still the waters run: The betrayal of the five civilized tribes.* New Jersey: Princeton University Press.

Foreman, G. (1932). *Indian removal.* Norman, OK: University of Oklahoma Press.

Leininger, N.M. (Ed.). (1991). *Culture care diversity and universality: A theory of nursing.* New York: National League of Nursing.

Women's health

A global perspective

AFAF I. MELEIS, FERIAL A.M. ALY

The purpose of this chapter is to discuss global issues related to women's health. Several universal issues were selected for presentation to provide a context for understanding health care for women and to challenge readers to identify potential threats to quality care. In addition, principles that have been proposed for the development and implementation of a viable and comprehensive health care system for women are identified and discussed. The intent here is not to capture the situation and health experience of women in all parts of the world; nor is it possible to address all the contextual contingencies needed for addressing women's health. Rather, the intent is to provide a framework for understanding the neglect that women have encountered in all aspects of their lives, including health care. Furthermore, our aim is to provide those who have been committed to health care for women with support in their attempt to provide quality health care for other women. Finally, our goal is to raise the readers' consciousness of women's health needs beyond the United States. We fully realize that women's health issues cannot be understood in isolation from the specific sociocultural context of their situations; however, by highlighting some universals, perhaps we can underscore the need for global cooperation in taking a more coherent and coordinated approach to providing affordable and quality health care for women.

There are certain contextual patterns of the treatment of women that are global. There is a universal tendency to define women by their marital status, and there is an overall pressure on women to conform to certain global expectations that are considered normative and ideal. Women are expected to attach themselves to a father, a brother, a husband, or a son. Although the intensity and the quality of this normative ideal differs from one country to another, from one culture to another, and from one class to another, there is a general agreement that young girls are socialized to prepare themselves for spousal and maternal roles. These expectations decrease the potential for promoting and supporting educational or career goals and increase the potential for status and power issues.

Similarly, there is a global focus on reproductive health and on reducing women's health concerns to only the reproductive aspects of their life cycle. The focus on physical reproduction, as opposed to socially productive tasks of women, tends to decrease the potential for understanding and attending to the critical needs of women throughout the life cycle and beyond conceiving and delivering a healthy baby (National Council for International Health, 1991). The focus on reproductive aspects of women's health also tends to take these issues out of context and render the results unsatisfactory for both the planners and recipients of health care. Family planning programs that focus on birth control are a good example of how an important issue in women's lives that is bound to the family and society is reduced to the question of birth control methods. This in turn tends to decrease the potential success of these programs. McFarland (1988) reviewed the literature on development theory and women and made the following assertion:

> In the population policy and reproductive rights area, women's perspective has been ignored. Planners have had little understanding of women's mixed responses to family planning. The role of children as workers, old age security, and property inheritors has been ignored, as well as the fact that all or most of the birth control methods are unsafe or unsatisfactory. (p. 304)

Questions and studies about family planning that are inspired by such an approach, that is, one with a focus on women as defective reproductive beings, tend to center on (1) why women are unable to plan the size of their families and the spacing of their children (i.e., what is wrong with them?); (2) mortality and morbidity related to reproduction; (3) why women are not capable of taking advantage of the great services provided by the ministries of health in the various countries; and (4) how it is that all of the grant money that is being allocated for these purposes appears not to be effective in halting the frightening growth in the world population. These questions do not address the ways in which women are constrained from using the services provided, nor do they address the parts played by other important variables (such as roles, societal expectations, and spousal demands) that may be far more compelling in influencing women's options, choices, and decisions. In addition, a focus on reproductive health tends to promote neglect of other health issues that women confront and women who are neither pregnant nor in the process of childbearing.

Another universal trend centers on women's caregiving roles. Women tend to be the caregivers in most regions of the world. They are expected to be either the primary or the sole care providers for children, spouses, parents, and the elderly in their families, and they are expected to teach sound health practices to future generations. In addition, they are expected to provide similar caregiving services and education to their spouses' extended families. These responsibilities are additive instead of substitutive in nature, the result of which is overload and limited time, energy, and resources to attend to their own personal needs. This continues to be true whether women are working inside or outside the home and whether their work is visible and acknowledged or invisible and unacknowledged.

However, most of women's work is invisible and devalued. Women who work extended hours as spouses and mothers are labeled nonworking women or housewives. They may be the farmers who carry the major bulk of domestic work and are paid minimally for it. They also tend to be the nurses, teachers, and clerical workers, for which their income is incongruent with their worth and their work. These no- or low-income positions bring with them limited resources, a lack of regulatory policies to protect women as laborers, and inadequate enforcement of their rights. Furthermore, in many countries women's contributions are falsely reflected in labor statistics (Population Crisis Committee, 1988) because of the invisible nature of their work that in turn makes their contributions even more invisible. Invisibility brings with it neglect, neglect breeds abuse, and abuse renders women more vulnerable and powerless. The cycle then continues, with more violence against women.

Women also have other invisible roles that consume their time and energy and are equally ignored. An example is women's work in facilitating health care for family members. Women are consistently expected to be the first gatekeepers to preventive, promotive, and curative health care; they are the key providing access to and utilization of health care for others in the family and the community (Meleis & Rogers, 1987).

Despite the apparent involvement of women in productive work in or outside the home, and despite their needs for "development" and for better compensation, development programs have focused primarily on men. These programs are designed to make men's lives easier by developing the technology to support their work, whether that work is on a farm or in the business world. Even when development programs have considered women, they have tended to label their work as craftwork, which means that it is extra and not as central to a country's economy as other forms of productive work (McFarland, 1988). There is a growing discomfort with development programs in general because of the lack of clarity of their missions. Questions such as development of what, for whom, by whom, and for whose benefit need to be debated carefully and ethically. Exploitation of resources and labor in developing countries for the benefit of "first world" white males is being questioned and debated in both developing and developed countries.

HEALTH AND ILLNESS EXPERIENCES AND RESPONSES

Within this context, we describe and discuss some aspects of women's health related to the experience of and response to illness. In addition to the communicable diseases and other illnesses shared by both sexes, there are a number of illnesses and injuries that are primarily associated with women (Rodin & Ickovics, 1990). These nonreproductive health problems are less likely to be detected and treated because of the narrow framework used in considering health care for women that results from the lack of awareness of both the recipients and providers regarding the extent of women's health care needs and their need for comprehensive care. By and large, women are either not aware of such health care needs; they are aware but tend to ignore these needs because of their demanding role responsibilities, workload, and other caregiving activities; or they have been prevented from seeking health care and from maintaining their health by limited resources and structural constraints. Personal health hazards that make women more vulnerable thus remain obscured until the women show symptoms related to reproductive health, which makes their illness situation more legitimate. Or women seek health care later than they should, after their work becomes affected. Education of women in many countries influences their chances to obtain better jobs and affects their lifestyle and health practices (Population Crisis Committee, 1988). We have selected only six aspects of women's health to discuss here.

Eating disorders and nutritional problems

Women make up the bulk of the population who consume fewer calories than needed. Similarly, the death rate for female children is higher than that for their male counterparts in some parts of the world such as India and Egypt. One reason for this discrepancy is society-imposed eating conditions that increase the probability of nutritional deficiencies in women—"they eat last and least" (WHO, 1984; 1985).

In some developing countries, male and female children are fed differently, with boys getting more nutrients and larger quantities of food than girls. The pattern begins early in life: boys are breast-fed longer and given more solid foods after weaning than girls (Ojanuga & Gilbert, 1992). For example, in one country a study of intrafamilial sex bias in the allocation of food and health care showed that among children the caloric consumption was on average 16% higher for boys than for girls. This was reflected in a significantly higher prevalence of malnutrition among the female children–11% of them being severely malnourished compared with 5% of the male children (WHO, 1984). Moreover, girls start work early as helpers in household chores. Accordingly, the increased energy needs and deficient caloric intake affect girls' weights and heights. In addition, many of these girls start their reproductive lives early, which drains more of their energy reserves, leading to pregnancy-related complications. These nutritionally deficient women give birth to children with low birth weights, to start the vicious cycle again (WHO, 1985).

Nutritional anemias in women warrant special emphasis. Nutritional anemias are due to metabolic defects, hemorrhage, or chronic blood loss. However, they are also due to deficiencies in the diet that restrict the formation of new blood cells. Shortage of iron, folate, or vitamin B_{12} in the diet can contribute to anemia. Anemia occurs more commonly in women because of dietary restrictions and increased iron needs during reproductive years. It has been estimated that 47% of all women and 59% of all pregnant women in developing countries are anemic (Bruce, 1981).

Another nutritional deficiency of importance that affects these women is rickets. Rachitic osteomalacia and contracted pelvis—a condition that still occurs in developing countries—is almost extinct in the more economically advantaged countries. The same story is repeated in many other nutritional deficiency conditions that are aggravated by the maternal depletion syndrome. Studies have shown that poor nutritional status can lead to low–birth-weight babies, unfavorable reproductive histories, obstetrical complications, and increased susceptibility to infection (Bruce, 1981). Similar nutritional status is manifested in more economically advantaged countries, where they are labeled eating disorders. Examples are obesity, bulimia, and anorexia nervosa. These eating disorders can only be adequately understood when considered within the context of societal expectations of women and the myths surrounding women's figures and weight.

Infections

Infections and reinfections of the female organs are numerous, widespread, and increasing, and continue to be ignored. They are caused by viruses, yeasts, bacteria, and other agents that are acquired through poor hygiene around the menstrual period; through sexual intercourse, childbirth, or abortion; or through the use of intrauterine devices (IUDs). IUDs were introduced to help planners control family size and to help women gain control over their lives. However, limited long-term, careful research resulted in the creation of another menace to women's health and a threat to the quality of their lives; more infections resulted or were aggravated by the use of IUDs.

These genital infections, besides their effect on the general health of the woman, affect reproductive health by causing infertility or by forming the basis for later ectopic pregnancies and other problems such as low birth weights and congenital anomalies. Pelvic inflammatory disease (PID), which involves the fallopian tubes and/or the ovaries and uterus, follows genital infection, particularly gonorrhea. In many developing countries, endemic diseases such as schistosomiasis and filariasis weaken tubal tissue and make it more vulnerable to secondary infection, and may also affect the incidence of PID.

These genital infections are of serious consequence and may lead to infertility. It is estimated that 10% to 17% of all women who suffer from genital inflammatory disease become infertile because of blockage of fallopian tubes. In addition, in Central and West Africa it was estimated that 30% or more of these genital infections not only affect the women but also the offspring, with effects ranging from low birth weight to congenital deformity to death of the newborn (Bruce, 1981).

Women are also prone to communicable diseases that are acquired through their caregiving activities for the sick members of their families. In addition, during their household duties they are exposed to many unsanitary conditions that put them at risk. Predisposition to diseases is counteracted by resistance, but this is compromised by malnutrition and complications of pregnancy.

Violence against women

The lower status of women in the family in many cultures makes them more susceptible to violence (Russo, 1990). In some communities and nations, manliness and machismo tend to support a system in which the wife and the child are considered the property of the men in the family; such systems condone "disciplinary" actions through all forms of abuse. In wars and other upheavals, women are usually very susceptible to violence. For example, there are many chilling historical accounts of violence to, and abuse and rape of, women in the Pakistan-Bangladesh war, during the coup against Salvador Allende in Chile, and in the Persian Gulf War. Newspaper accounts in the United States included incidents of women in the military being abused by their colleagues and superiors. These women were afraid to discuss their abuse. Reporting of violent incidents is minimal for fear that exposure will bring dishonor to the woman and her family and for fear of reprisal.

Female circumcision is a practice that is carried out in some societies and is considered by many to be a form of violence. There are three types of circumcision: clitoridectomy, excision, and infibulation. Depending on the type, either the clitoris only is excised; the clitoris and the labia minora are excised; or the clitoris, the labia minora, and the labia majora are excised and stitched together, causing scar tissue (Koso-Thomas, 1987). All forms of female circumcision are done to diminish or prevent the sexual arousal of the female as a method of preserving her chastity before marriage. It is related to beliefs of purification and is called "Tahara," which means purification. It is reinforced by aggressive structural components in societies and by the matriarchal side of families (Baasher, Bannerman, Rushwan, & Sharas, 1982; Kaamel, 1987).

The origin of this custom is obscure. It is not a part of Islamic doctrine, but it is a part of the definition of rites of passage for women in many parts of Africa and the Middle East. This practice was alleged to have been based on religious practices, but it is now known beyond a doubt that this is not the case (Ahoyo & Kaamel, 1987). Female circumcision is against the law in most communities in the world but is still practiced, usually under unhealthy conditions, without anesthesia, and by practitioners who range from traditional birth attendants to so-called gypsies to health care providers. All forms of female circumcision have serious implications for female personal health in the form of shock, hemorrhage, infection, urine retention, and injury. There are still cases in the hospital records of developing countries of young girls being admitted in shock as a result of postcircumcision bleeding (WHO, 1979).

There are many other aftereffects of this practice, not the least of which is the psychological trauma for young girls. The effect on these women's sex lives is tremendously profound and shapes their view of sexuality and of their participation in the sexual encounter. These women are even blamed for their husbands' drug use, because it is claimed that men use drugs in order to derive sexual satisfaction from their "surgically mutilated frigid wives." Moreover, some of these extended circumcisions may have an effect on the process of childbirth, causing injuries and bleeding during labor. Contrary to popular belief, the custom of circumcision is carefully guided and supported by women in the family. Although men may condone it, they are not the ones who keep it in practice.

Circumcision is not the only form of violence against women. More compelling and more significant from the women's perspective are the laws that condone and support domestic violence under the pretense of men's obligation to preserve face or honor against women's so-called insubordination, infidelities, or freedoms. Women also consider the lack of regulatory laws to protect their rights in socially unequal societies and in systems that condone colonialism and patriarchy as aggressive acts that are invariably ignored. Nor are the Western or the "developed" countries immune from other forms of "circumcision" or "vaginal mutilation." Young women are socialized to deny early sexual abuse experiences (molestation and rape) in favor of adopting more sanctioned and socially acceptable roles that mirror purification and normative expectations. The influence of these experiences on women's mental health is well documented (Bickerton, Hall, & Williams, 1991; Orbach, 1986; Scott, 1992; Zimmerman, 1991).

Reproductive health

Reproductive and maternity health are an important aspect of women's health and are considered an element of primary health care, especially as they relate to maternal-child health. Also, women usually enter the health care system for reproductive care. In a number of countries, maternal mortality rates remain at alarmingly high levels, as does the low nutritional status of women throughout their reproductive cycles ("Family Planning Programs," 1984; WHO, 1991). It has been estimated that there are at least half a million preventable maternal deaths in the world each year (WHO, 1986). This maternal mortality is not evenly distributed in different parts of the world. For example, women in Bangladesh face a risk of dying that is 400 times greater than that of women in Scandinavia and 50 times greater than that of women in Portugal. The maternal mortality rate is as high as 900 per 100,000 in some countries, compared with a rate below 10 in 100,000 in developed countries (WHO, 1986). Moreover, according to a survey in India between 1974 and 1979, for each maternal death there were 16.5 illnesses related to pregnancy, childbirth, and the puerperium. Many authorities believe these figures to be underestimated (WHO, 1986).

The factors behind the immense difference in the effects of childbirth in developing versus developed countries have been widely examined. Some of them are health service factors while others are socioeconomic and medical; there are also reproductive factors that include pregnancy in girls younger than 18 years of age, pregnancy after age 35, pregnancy more than four times, and less than 2 years between pregnancies ("Family Planning Programs," 1984).

It has been estimated that the number of maternal deaths would decline by over 20% if the first through the fifth births were confined to women from 20 through 39 years of age (WHO, 1986). In addition, these changes would reduce the total number of births, lowering the general fertility rate by 25% (Trussell & Pebley, 1984). The number of maternal deaths would drop by one third and would decline even further if there were no births after age 35 or beyond the fourth child (Maine, 1982; Rochat, 1979). Women having more than four children are at risk; this is known as a *grand multigravida*. Different studies have shown that primigravidas have slightly higher mortality rates, which decrease during the second delivery and start rising again after the third, increasing with the number of pregnancies and the lack of adequate time between pregnancies. Not only parity and age, but also intervals between births, have an effect on maternal mortality. In Bangladesh and Indonesia, for example, the highest death rates are found in women under the age of 20 with three or more children (Chen, Geshe, Ahmed, Chowdhury, Mosely; Williams, 1973). There are, however, limited studies that have examined the effect of birth intervals independent of age and parity (Trussell & Pebley, 1984).

The other factor affecting the reproductive health of women and their general health is age at marriage. Early marriage is the norm in many parts of the world; for some, puberty marks a milestone for marriage. In Bangladesh, for example, two thirds of all women 19 years of age or younger are already married (Bangladesh Ministry of Health and Population Control, 1978), and in Afghanistan, Malawi, Mali, Nepal, North Yemen, and Egypt more than half of all women 19 or younger are married (Hassan, 1988). In the Middle East, South Asia and parts of Africa, marriages arranged by families are often between adolescent girls and considerably older men. These conditions increase women's risk of morbidity and mortality and decrease women's options for education and employment. In turn, decreased options may influence women's awareness of their health needs and their access to quality health care. Developed countries are not immune to adolescent pregnancy. In the United States, adolescent pregnancy has been linked to low birth weight and maternal complications (Zambrana, 1988). However, the availability of health care resources in the high-income countries acts as a buffer against these complications.

Abortion is an important factor that also affects women's health in general. Abortion is considered illegal in most of the Christian and Islamic doctrines and is viewed as a defiance of God's will. Religious law forbids the killing of innocent children, yet innocent mothers who are trying to exercise control over their own bodies become victims. Induced abortions, which are unregulated because of restrictive laws, expose women to another set of major risks. This is particularly problematic. In the majority of developing countries, abortion is illegal but is the most widely used method of fertility regulation. It is estimated that 35 to 55 million pregnancies worldwide are terminated each year through induced abortion (Blair, 1980). Infection, hemorrhage, and trauma are quite common. Tetanus is a serious danger accompanying criminal abortion. Its effect on the procedure, even if that procedure spares the woman's life, seriously affects her fertility and personal health later.

Even in those developing countries where laws are liberal, as in India, lack of facilities renders legal abortion unobtainable for most women; therefore, women resort to ways of ending their unwanted pregnancies that increase their health risks. Such ways include introducing plant stems or foreign bodies into the uterus through the vaginal canal or herbal pastes prepared by an herbalist.

Recently, developing countries have been watching the United States struggle as it attempts to resolve the issues surrounding abortion in a way that addresses and encompasses the rights of women as well as those of their unborn children. Limiting and regulating conception is considered a woman's problem in most of the world. Even when methods are developed to help women decrease the health problems related to reproduction, these methods are not carefully developed and monitored. Safety of contraceptive methods has been assumed more than proved, and not until recently have these methods been investigated through longitudinal research studies. As a result, a number of methods have been withdrawn from the market, after having been used for decades, because of new discoveries related to adverse long-term effects on women's health. For example, the relationship between smoking and contraceptive pills has promoted the issuance of new warnings (Population Crisis Committee, 1988). The interaction between contraceptives and other major lifestyle factors has been largely ignored. New discussions about the significance of these relationships are emerging in international conferences and in global agendas such as those at the recent United Nations Conferences in Cairo (1994) and Beijing (United Nations, 1995).

Occupational health

Women are equally exposed to the occurrence of health hazards as are men, whether in developed or developing countries. Some conditions, however, make women more vulnerable. For example, women's work at home exposes them to hazards that have been overlooked because women's work is either invisible (e.g., housework, farm work) or devalued (e.g., clerical work, domestic work, hospital work). Lane and Meleis (1991) reported that farmers' wives fall off roofs or are exposed to unwarranted illnesses and diseases while attending to their daily roles and responsibilities such as scooping manure with their bare hands.

Agricultural workers exposed to chemicals used in pesticides are at risk for cancer, and pregnant women tend to suffer additional consequences that affect the health of their children. They may suffer from pregnancy complications such as miscarriage, or their babies may show birth defects. This occurs more often in developing countries, where overspraying by untrained workers takes place and wearing of protective clothing is largely unknown. The toxic effect of the chemicals is passed to the infants through the mothers' milk. In addition, the effects of anesthetic gases that cause a higher incidence of miscarriage, congenital defects, and infertility among nurses working in the operating room have been inadequately studied and poorly regulated (Datta, Sharma, Razack, Ghosh, & Arora, 1980).

Women are also more vulnerable to overwork as an occupational hazard (Hibbard & Pope, 1991). Working women generally take care of their households and children in addition to their full-time jobs outside the home. The "double day," or second-shift phenomenon (Hochchild, 1989), in which there is a combination of economic and family responsibilities, results in fatigue and predisposes women to mental health problems. A 1988 study analyzed 2.3 billion women (92% of the world's female population) in an effort to determine and score their social status (Population Crisis Committee, 1988). Five aspects were included: health, education, employment, marriage and children, and equality. Fifty-one of the 99 countries included in the study fell into the lowest third of the ranking. The results further indicated that 60% of all women and girls in the world live under conditions that threaten their health, deny them a chance to bear children, limit their educational attainment, restrict their economic participation, and fail to guarantee them equal rights and freedom from oppression.

One of the interesting findings of this study was how the number of births is related to the status score. In countries with higher scores, indicating a higher status for women, the pregnancy rate is lower as compared with the rate in countries with poor or lower rankings in social status. The number of births in the countries with high ranking ("very good" to "good" categories) averages two per woman, while it is four or above in the "poor," "very poor," and "extremely poor" countries.

Better education and work that produces financial remuneration increase women's options and resources and enhance their power base. However, women seem to be disenfranchised even as they attempt to exercise these options. Sons are favored over daughters to receive education. Even when they enter the educational sector, girls get less time to study; and in some countries, their education is terminated at puberty under the false pretense of preserving their honor and their chastity. Education and employment, key in women's health, are both related to resources and to a level of consciousness. A unique situation is that, as health care providers, women often constitute a majority. Available statistics suggest that in most countries the labor force in the formal health care system tends to be predominantly female. But here again, women tend to feel underpaid, holding the less prestigious jobs rather than those with status and decision-making power.

Women also constitute the majority of the volunteers in hospitals, clinics, and other community health organizations. The unique predominance of women in the health care system makes them a major target of importance in primary health care. It is also the woman who is expected to be the health provider and educator in the family. She is the one who teaches sound health practices to future generations, creates a home environment conducive to better health through factors such as clean water and nutrition, and ensures that the children are immunized and cared for during the crucial years of their lives. A good share of the essential elements of primary health care fall almost exclusively in the woman's domain at the family level (WHO, 1982).

The woman's role as primary health provider could be enhanced by considering this role within the totality of her daily life experiences. For example, it is recommended that women who live in rural areas boil drinking water; and the implications of this seemingly simple act, which are far-reaching for an already overburdened woman, must be considered. To boil water, women have to carry water receptacles for long distances, search for and obtain burning fuel, and use different containers for boiling and for storing the water. Another example is breast-feeding. Breast-feeding for prolonged periods of time (2 years) has been proved to result in healthier babies, less time spent by women on sick children, and less money spent on formula (WHO, 1991). It also has a contraceptive effect (although this is questionable because of factors such as length of feeding and amount of milk). However, breast-feeding for a prolonged time has also been related to an increased likelihood of anemia in these women.

Limited access to health care

Although access issues are most often related to variables such as a country's socioeconomic level, the status of women in a particular culture, the position of women in the workforce, and a country's cultural and ethnic heritage, gender plays an equally important role in limiting access to health care (Puentes-Markides, 1992). Limitation of access may also be due to poverty, to a mismatching of the explanatory frameworks of both the provider and recipient, or to a general lack of comprehensiveness in health care services (Bernal & Meleis, 1995). Additionally, role overload and work responsibilities have also prevented women from seeking out health care and have promoted self-neglect (Walker & Best, 1991).

Other structural barriers exist for women, particularly in some developing countries. Women are generally not included in the planning and designing of health services; therefore, their issues and concerns may not be reflected in the resulting programs. Furthermore, these programs, which are developed by men, tend not to meet specific female health care needs as perceived by women. In these countries, young girls often face additional limitations placed on them by their families, who give preferential treatment to their male children when both children are sick (Chen, Huq, & D'Souza, 1981), or by the health care system through institutional discrimination (Gopalan & Naidu, 1972). It is vitally important to increase women's access to health care services in developing countries (Ojanuga & Gilbert, 1992), as well as to improve access of disenfranchised populations (including women) in developed countries (Stevens, 1993).

WOMEN'S HEALTH: A CHANGING AGENDA

Women's health issues have emerged at the top of the worldwide health care agenda. This global concern was evidenced during two milestone conferences that resulted in the Cairo Action Document (United Nations, 1994) and the Beijing Document (United Nations, 1995). The Cairo Action Document identified women, their status, and their development as central to population programs and to global development efforts, and the Beijing document emphasized attention to women's human rights. Both of these documents called for the strengthening of political commitments to population-related policies, to family planning programs, and to women's health and development in general. The heated debates related to the development of these documents attracted the interest of the international media, thereby focusing even more attention on women and their health care issues. The participants in each of the conferences recognized the importance of constructing a framework that was more congruent with women's specific health care requirements—requirements that were subsequently incorporated into these policy documents by their respective authors.

To enhance women's health globally, health care programs should be established within a framework that acknowledges women's perspectives, experiences, and contexts. The context of the totality of women's daily situations and daily experiences and role responsibilities as women themselves see them must be captured, described, and carefully integrated into health care plans (Meleis et al., 1990). It is through such an approach that groups of women who are most vulnerable to health risks may be identified and that appropriate resources that are more congruent with their needs may be developed (Stevens, Hall, & Meleis, 1992). To do these things, health care researchers, planners, and providers need to think of ways in which the women's different voices can be heard.

Gaps in knowledge related to women's situations should become a top priority. The ways in which women tend to integrate their roles on a daily basis and the patterns of management of the complex and intricate aspects of each of their daily roles need to be uncovered and addressed (Meleis & Bernal, 1995; Meleis & Stevens, 1992). Special attention should be given to how women perceive and enact their roles as providers, mothers, caregivers, spouses, daughters, and workers, and to experiences that render them vulnerable. *Vulnerability* is defined as "the process or state of persons being unprotected or open to damage in their interactions with a challenging or threatening environment" (Hall, Stevens, & Meleis, 1992, p. 755). A focus on women's roles, integrations, and vulnerabilities could help to identify women's critical needs.

Strategies are needed for the development of nursing therapeutics to empower women. A focus on empowerment is holistic, encompassing, and potentially fruitful. Empowerment does not only include increased understanding of women and their problems or enhancement of their education; more importantly, it means providing them with resources and a social structure that support them in carrying out their various roles. It also means providing them with accessible services. Health service accessibility includes cost, convenience, and compatibility. Cost involves not only the cost of the service but also the cost of transportation to the service for the mother and/or child. The convenience of the service, including the time schedule, should be compatible with the scheme of the mother's life. Women cannot easily leave their day-to-day chores and responsibilities. Compatibility of services includes compatibility with the woman's beliefs, her preferences, and her habits. The most outstanding example of incompatibility would be the discomfort of some women in dealing with an unfamiliar male health provider. In this respect, the use and upgrading of already existing services, such as traditional birth attendants, can be of great benefit. Careful analysis and consideration of laws that put women at risk, and of the gaps between the spirit of the law and its implementation, should be a context for any discourse related to women's health. Examples of relevant laws are those that govern age requirements for marriage, leaves of absence for domestic workers, and working with hazardous materials. Discourse about laws related to such issues as female circumcision should be handled within sociocultural and historical contexts. To have a viable women's health program, women need to think both locally and globally. The development of a united front is the single most powerful strategy to improve women's status and situation, which in turn could have a profound effect on women's health. Examples of the effects of a united front are the United Nations Decade of Women that started in 1975 in Mexico City and ended in 1985 at the world conference in Nairobi, and the review of accomplishments that occurred in Copenhagen in 1980. These brought women from around the world together to address women's issues (Pietila & Vickers, 1990). These international meetings were powerful in enabling women to initiate more local changes.

Involvement of women's organizations at different levels in the upgrading of women's health has been continually suggested. This approach has been followed in some parts of the world and proved to be effective—for example, in Indonesia. Involvement of other sectors of the community in programs to ensure better health for women is mandatory. Participation by members of the grass roots in each community should be promoted. The framework to guide women's health care should attempt to capture all the work that is defined as nonwork and thus goes unreported, undocumented, unrewarded, and unregulated. Therefore, a crucial role for governments is providing priority social supports for women in all their roles, instead of relying on the informal social support of their extended families (Leonard, 1989).

Finally, a commitment to women's health is needed at all levels to advance the development of policies to protect and promote it. Action agendas similar to those provided by the U.S. National Council for International Health (NCIH, 1991) are significant in providing local frameworks. However, policies and international aid programs that are developed without careful consideration of the diversity of women and without recognition of their critical needs and the extensiveness of their tasks and responsibilities ignore their contributions, stifle their potential, and decrease the likelihood of their long and active participation.

REFERENCES

Ahoyo, V., & Kaamel, A. (1987, April 6-10). *Islam in the face of traditional practices affecting mothers and children* (p. 70). [Report on the regional seminar on traditional practices affecting the health of women and children in Africa] Addis Ababa, Ethiopia: International African Committee on Traditional Practices Affecting the Health of Women and Children.

Baasher, T., Bannerman, R., Rushwan, H., & Sharas, I. (Eds.). (1982). *Traditional practices affecting the health of women and children: Female circumcision, childhood marriage, nutritional taboos.* [Background papers to the WHO seminar. Technical Publications, 2(2)] Alexandria, Egypt: World Health Organization.

Bangladesh Ministry of Health and Population Control. (1978). *Bangladesh fertility survey (1975-1976).* Dacca, Bangladesh: Author.

Bernal, P., & Meleis, A. (1995). Self care action of Colombian por día domestic workers on prevention and care. *Women and Health, 22,* 77-95.

Bickerton, D., Hall, R., & Williams, A.L. (1991). Women's experiences of sexual abuse in childhood. *Public Health, 105,* 447-453.

Blair, P. (1980). *Programming for women's health.* [Report prepared for the office of women's development of the U.S. agency for international development] Unpublished report.

Bruce, J. (1981). Women oriented health care: New Hampshire feminist health center. *Studies in Family Planning, 12,* 353-363.

Chen, L.C., Geshe, M.C., Ahmed, S., Chowdhury, A.I., & Mosely, W.H. (1974). Maternal mortality in rural Bangladesh. *Studies in Family Planning, 5,* 334-341.

Chen, L., Huq, E., & D'Souza, S. (1981). Sex bias in the Bangladesh. *Population Development Review, 7,* 55-70.

Datta, K.K., Sharma, R.S., Razack, P.M.A., Ghosh, T.K., & Arora, R.R. (1980). Morbidity pattern amongst rural pregnant women in Alwar, Rajasthan—a cohort study. *Health and Population Perspectives and Issues, 3,* 282-292.

Family planning programs, healthier mothers and children through family planning (Population information program, Series 1, No. 27). (1984, May-June). Baltimore: Johns Hopkins University.

Gopalan, C., & Naidu, N.A. (1972). Nutrition and fertility. *The Lancet, 2,* 1077-1079.

Hall, J.M., Stevens, P.E., & Meleis, A.I. (1992). Experiences of women clerical workers in patient care areas. *Journal of Nursing Administration, 22,* 11-17.

Hassan, E.O. (1988). *Safe motherhood—efforts and the role of professional societies in Egypt.* Paper presented at the World Health Organization workshop "Role of Obstetricians and Gynecologists in Promoting Women's Health and Safe Motherhood." Alexandria, Egypt: World Health Organization.

Hibbard, J.H., & Pope, R.P. (1991). Effect of domestic and occupational roles on morbidity and mortality. *Social Science and Medicine, 32,* 805-811.

Hochchild, A.R. (1989). *Second shift: Working parents and the revolution at home.* New York: Viking.

Kaamel, A. (1987, April). *Activities against female circumcision in Egypt.* Reports on the regional seminar on traditional practices affecting the health of women and children in Africa. Addis Ababa, Ethiopia: International African Committee on Traditional Practices Affecting the Health of Women and Children.

Koso-Thomas, O. (1987, April 6-10). *Female circumcision and related hazards* (p. 65). Reports on the regional seminar on traditional practices affecting the health of women and children in Africa. Addis Ababa, Ethiopia: International African Committee on Traditional Practices Affecting the Health of Women and Children.

Lane, S., & Meleis, A.I. (1991). Roles, work, health perceptions and health resources of women: A study in an Egyptian delta hamlet. *Social Science and Medicine, 33,* 1197-1128.

Leonard, A. (Ed.). (1989). *Seeds: Supporting women's work in the Third World.* New York: Feminist Press.

Maine, D. (1982). *Family planning, its impact on the health of the women & children.* New York: Columbia University Press.

McFarland, J. (1988). The construction of women and development theory: A review essay. *Review of Canadian Sociology and Anthropology, 25,* 299-308.

Meleis, A.I., & Bernal, P. (1995). The paradoxical world of "muchacha de por dia" in Colombia. *Human Organization, 59* 393-400.

Meleis, A.I., Kulig, J., Arruda, E.N., & Beckman, A. (1990). Maternal role of women in clerical jobs in southern Brazil: Stress and satisfaction. *Health Care for Women International, 11,* 369-382.

Meleis, A.I., & Rogers, S. (1987). Women in transition: Being versus becoming or being and becoming. *Health Care for Women International, 8,* 199-217.

Meleis, A.I., & Stevens, P.E. (1992). Women in clerical jobs: Spousal role satisfaction, stress and coping. *Women and Health, 18,* 23-40.

National Council for International Health. (1991). *Women's health—The action agenda.* The 18th Annual International Health Conference of the National Council for International Health, Arlington, VA.

Ojanuga, D.N., & Gilbert, C. (1992). Women's access to health in developing countries. *Social Science & Medicine, 35,* 613-617.

Orbach, I. (1986). The insolvable problem as a determinant in the dynamics of suicide behavior in children. *Journal of American Psychotherapy, 40,* 511-520.

Pietila, H., & Vickers, J. (1990). *Making women matter: The role of the United Nations.* London: Zed.

Population Crisis Committee. (1988). In S. Kemp, M. Barberis, & C. Lasher (Eds.), *Country ranking of the status of women: Poor, powerless, and pregnant.* (Population Briefing Paper No. 20). Washington, DC: Author.

Puentes-Markides, C. (1992). Women and access to health care. *Social Science and Medicine, 35,* 619-626.

Rochat, R. (1979). Effect of declining fertility on maternal and infant mortality. In W.P. McCreevey & A. Shelfield (Eds.), *Guatemala: Development and population* (Working Paper No. 4, pp. 21-43). Washington, DC: Battele Population.

Rodin, J., & Ickovics, J.R. (1990). Review and research agenda as we approach the 21st century. *American Psychologist, 45,* 1018-1033.

Russo, N.F. (1990). Overview: Forging research priorities for women's mental health. *American Psychologist, 45,* 369-373.

Scott, K.D. (1992). Childhood sexual abuse: Impact on a community's mental health status. *Child Abuse and Neglect, 16,* 285-295.

Stevens, P.E. (1993). Who gets care? Access to health care as an arena for nursing action. In Barbara Kos-Munson (Ed.), *Who gets health care? An arena for nursing action* (pp. 11-26). New York: Springer Publishing Company.

Stevens, P.E., Hall, J.M., & Meleis, A.I. (1992). Examining vulnerability of women clerical workers from five ethnic/racial groups. *Western Journal of Nursing Research, 14,* 754-774.

Trussell, J., & Pebley, A.R. (1984). *The impact of family planning programs on infant, child and maternal mortality.* Unpublished manuscript, World Bank Staff Working Paper.

United Nations (1994). *Report of the international conference on population and development,* Cairo, 513.

United Nations (1995). *Platform for action.* Preparatory committee for the fourth World Conference on Women for Beijing. People's Republic of China.

Walker, L.O., & Best, M.A. (1991). Well-being of mothers with infant children: A preliminary comparison of employed women and homemakers. *Women and Health, 17,* 71-89.

Williams, I.I. (1973). Some observation on maternal mortality in Jamaica. *West Indian Medical Journal, 22,* 1-14.

World Health Organization. (1979). *Traditional practices affecting the health of women and children: Female circumcision, childhood marriage, nutritional taboos, etc.* (Technical Publication No. 2). Geneva: Author.

World Health Organization. (1982). Report of the second WHO consultation on women as providers of health care, Geneva, August 16-20. Unpublished WHO document HMD/82.10.

World Health Organization. (1984). Report on women, health and development activities in WHO's programs 1982-1983. Unpublished WHO document LHG/84.1.

World Health Organization. (1985). Report on women's health and development. Report by the Director General, WHO Offset Publication No. 90. Geneva: Author.

World Health Organization. (1986). Maternal mortality: Helping women off the road to death. *WHO Chronicle, 40,* 175-183.

World Health Organization. (1991). *Strengthening maternal and child health programs through PHC* (WHO Regional Office for the Eastern Mediterranean, Technical Publication No. 18). Alexandria, Egypt: Author.

Zambrana, R.E. (1988). A research agenda on issues affecting poor and minority women: A model for understanding their health needs. *Women and Health, 12,* 137-160.

Zimmerman, J.K. (1991). Crossing the desert alone: An etiologic model of female adolescent suicidality. *Women and Therapy, 11,* 223-240.

Section Eleven

ETHICS AND LEGAL ISSUES

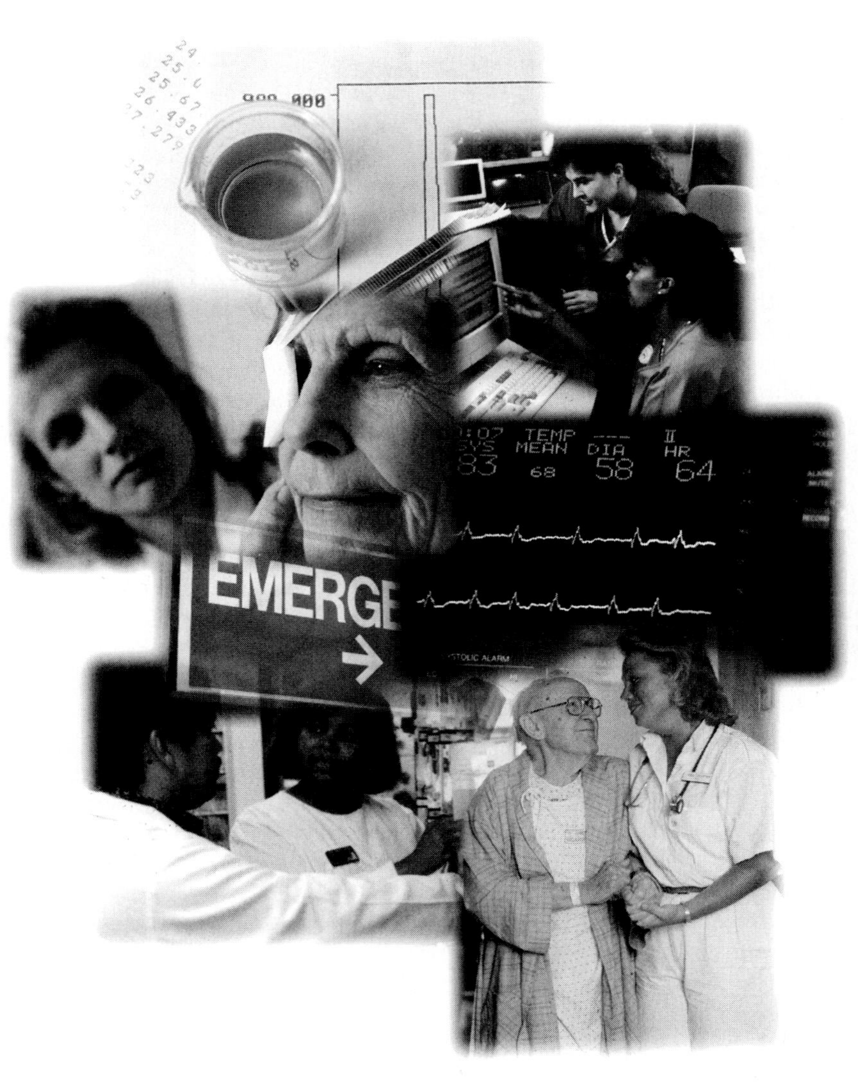

OVERVIEW

Ethical and legal concerns in a changing health care world

JOANNE COMI McCLOSKEY, HELEN KENNEDY GRACE

As the world of health care changes and the concerns for cost control escalate, it is increasingly difficult to keep a focus on the needs of people and the underlying ethical and legal issues that surround health-care decision making. As the debates over the future of health care continue, much of the discourse is based on an assumption that the problem is one of lack of resources, and therefore rationing in some form is the only solution. This basic assumption requires examination. Is the problem one of lack of resources, or is it rather how these resources are deployed? Is it fair and just that 25% of health-care costs are tied to processing the paperwork necessary to keep the providers paid? And whose problem is it? While this final section does not address some of the more basic assumptions, it does call attention to some of the critical ethical issues that must be addressed as the system changes. As you read these chapters, we encourage you to keep in mind some of the broader questions. Are our problems a result of lack of resources? Or do they stem from the lack of will to redirect the system so that the health-care needs of all in our society can be addressed?

In the opening debate chapter, Fry addresses the question of the ethics of targeting the elderly for health-care rationing. After describing three means of rationing, market rationing (based on the ability to pay), implicit rationing (setting limits on the available options), and explicit rationing (making administrative decisions about limits), the pros and cons of targeting the elderly for explicit rationing approaches are debated. Fry concludes by arguing that the debate needs to be refocused on the aims of health care. If caring is the focus, a moral obligation is created by the special human relationship that brings together the one who needs assistance or is ill and the one who offers to help. The moral base for care then is on the obligations that are inherent in being a caregiver. The chapter concludes with the observation that "if the aims and goals of the health professions were changed, rationing might not even be viewed as an acceptable way to contain health care costs."

In the first issues chapter, Weiler turns the focus to the legal implications of nursing. She makes the observation that the nursing issues addressed throughout this book demonstrate "that law and nursing are intimately intertwined." After a careful explanation of critical terminology, Weiler goes on to explicate some of the commonalities between nursing and the law: licensure and scope of practice; malpractice; and education and the importance of including the legal aspects of nursing care in the curriculum. By examining the legal implications of nursing care measures, nurses are able to ensure that the focus remains on quality patient care.

While individual nurses need to maintain a focus on the ethical and legal dimensions of practice, ethics committees at the institutional level are increasingly pressured to play a more active role in setting some boundaries for overall practice. Zink and Titus raise the question of the function of institutional ethics committees as distinct from nursing ethics committees. While institutional ethics committees address the broad purposes of education, policy development, and clinical consultation, they usually do not address issues specific to nursing. The authors argue for the importance of nursing ethics committees and outline a set of functions. Noting the gap in nursing education in teaching ethics, a major function of these committees is self-education for nurses in the practice setting. As nurses become increasingly informed about the ethical considerations of care, they can become more vocal advocates for their patients in the overall institutional setting.

The next four chapters turn to specific issues. Aiken

addresses the issue of sexual harassment. After carefully outlining the specific conditions defining sexual harassment, Aiken provides information about courses of action that might be taken. The importance of sexual harassment policies and procedures at the institutional level is stressed.

Turning to a specific nursing-care problem, Hughes, MacLeod, and Boyd address the issue of working with drug users and the various approaches that are used in the field. Differentiating two major approaches, abstinence versus harm reduction, the authors argue for harm reduction as the better alternative. Arguing that harm reduction is more feasible, the authors explain the compatibility of this approach with public health and nursing approaches. Harm reduction allows for nurses to be advocates for their patients as decision makers. "Nurses using this model will be able to more fully engage in prevention and rehabilitation based on real client needs and participation."

Child maltreatment is another issue of major concern to nurses. Cowen provides a comprehensive overview of the types of child maltreatment and the dimensions of the problem in the United States today. Approaches to family assessment are outlined, and signs and symptoms that are indicators of abuse are described. Cohen stresses the importance of nurses working in a preventive mode and being alert to the conditions that are conducive to this form of destructive behavior. Nurses have key roles to play in multidisciplinary treatment teams and in being alert for early signs and symptoms of child maltreatment. This chapter concludes with the mandate from child abuse legislation that all cases of suspected child abuse be reported—an area of great ethical and legal concern.

Noting this fundamental value of individualism in the United States, Kjervik addresses the issue of advance directives as a means of empowering patients. After describing the main types of advance directives, the author clarifies their ethical aspects. The value of a living will is that it is a clear way of stating what the patient values at a point prior to a crisis. Kjervik details the pros and cons of advance directives and then speaks to how nurses can use them as a base for face-to-face encounters that build mutual understanding. They believe through this process comes more effective decision making about health-care choices.

In the next issues article, Zoloth-Dorfman turns the focus to managed care and the ethical obligations attendant to this system, noting that "at stake are the deepest ethical decisions about the meaning and intent of medicine itself, and the responsibility of the nurse toward his or her patient." As the ones "standing at the gate in the organization," nurses are particularly torn in a system built on "negative rewards." Zoloth-Dorfman argues that "if we are to take the dominance of medicine by the managed-care system as a first premise, we are then obligated to create a system in which a strong moral agency is encouraged and supported, and patient advocacy is a normative structure of the nursing role." Using a case example she describes the nurse advocacy role.

In the closing chapter in this section, Smith describes in detail the current political and economic situation in Russia, and within this context, health care and the role of nursing. Despite the general oppression of women in Russian society, and of nursing as a women's profession, nursing is making some advances. Nursing organizations are beginning to develop, and nursing educational programs are being strengthened. As we view the struggles in Russia, our ethical concerns need to extend to nurses in that part of the world. East-West collaboration is encouraged, and nurse-to-nurse exchanges are advocated. Smith concludes that, "nurses, once docile and subservient, are finding new political and professional savvy as they confront worn traditions of medical authority."

Nurses do stand in the gap between patients and the health-care system. As pressures build from all sides, the profit-making motives of "big business" at the expense of humane and quality patient care, the escalation of a wide array of social problems inextricably intertwined with health (such as drug abuse and child maltreatment), and the plight of nurses and patients around the world, nurses are obliged to examine the moral, ethical, and legal dimensions that govern their practice. Never have the challenges been greater, but with these challenges comes great opportunity for nurses to rise to the forefront in their role of advocacy.

The ethics of health care reform: Should rationing strategies target the elderly?

SARA T. FRY

It is not surprising that health care costs have risen sharply in recent years. The growth of medical knowledge, development of new technologies, public demands and expectations concerning health issues, and other matters have led to a spiraling escalation of private and public costs for available health-care services. In 1989, approximately $550 billion was spent on health care in the United States, and it is projected that by the year 2000, this amount may triple to $1.5 trillion (Callahan, 1990). Given these figures, economists, legislators, and health-care insurers are all urging various types of health care reform aimed at controlling and reducing health-care costs. Elderly citizens are finding themselves vulnerable as proposals to specifically reduce Medicare coverage are debated in the public arena (McGrory, 1995). At issue are the appropriate amounts of government spending for health care, restrictions for some health-care services, and the ethical implications of health-care rationing strategies to large segments of our society, such as the elderly.

Ethicists argue that the ethical implications of various actions and their alternatives should be considered before a particular course of action is chosen and put into practice (Beauchamp & Childress, 1994). It is appropriate, therefore, if not prudent, for the ethical implications of various cost-containment measures in health care to be considered before limitations on government spending for health care are decided and some health-care goods and services are rationed. When a decision is made that some persons will receive an available but scarce medical resource that cannot be provided to everyone who needs it, a *rationing* decision is made (Beauchamp & Childress, 1994). A cautious approach to these matters is very important because limiting health care resources often has serious implications for both health professionals and consumers.

In this chapter, several methods of health-care rationing are presented. The general pros and cons of health-care rationing are discussed, and the ethical implications of various rationing strategies are described. A proposal for the provision of nursing care under conditions of rationing is also considered.

The goal of this chapter is to emphasize how rationing strategies pose significant challenges to professional ethics. Rationing of health-care resources has the potential to dramatically affect how nurses in particular view their professional responsibilities as mandated by society. As demonstrated in a recent survey, nurses consider cost-containment strategies that jeopardize patient welfare to be one of the most frequently occurring ethical issues confronting them in practice today (Scanlon, 1994). How practicing nurses should respond ethically to such issues is a subject of great professional concern and interest.

CURRENT RATIONING STRATEGIES

It is widely understood that current cost-containment measures in health care use a mixture of rationing methods that affect access to health care (Mechanic, 1985). These methods are designed to influence the behavior of the consumer (market rationing), the behavior of the health professional (implicit rationing), or the administration of health-care services (explicit rationing).

Market rationing

In the market rationing system prior to the 1950s, health care was rationed by the consumer's ability to pay for services, the availability and distribution of medical personnel and services, and professional decisions about the allocation of professional services (Mechanic, 1980). This essentially fee-for-service system was gradually eroded by social forces resulting from the rapid rise in medical knowledge and technology as well as government subsidy of health care. The market system then shifted slowly to a system dominated by a variety of third-party payments for health-care services. As the new system grew, however, the availability of health resources to all consumers became a genuine problem. Other methods for rationing health care were needed.

Cost sharing for health care, in the form of coinsurance and deductibles, was one method that promised to help alleviate the problem of resource availability. Its initial success as a method of rationing indicated that consumers tend to use services more wisely if they share in the cost of their health care. The result, of course, would be reduced utilization of services, depending on the specific cost-sharing arrangements agreed on and the economic status of the persons involved.

Unfortunately, in living up to its promise to reduce utilization of services, cost sharing reduces medical consultation for less serious problems or for those conditions that can be treated more adequately if appraised early. It is also recognized as a method that differentially affects low-income rather than high-income groups and results in inequities in the distribution of health care (Mechanic, 1985). Although it is not the best of rationing strategies and not the most popular method among consumers, cost sharing remains a feature of many health care programs.

Implicit rationing

Implicit rationing is another method that is frequently used to limit health resources. Its aim is to set limits on providers' decisions without interfering with clinical judgments for individual consumers. In other words, health professionals, rather than health administrators, make decisions about the allocation of professional time and resources among client populations. When limitations on provider decisions occur, they are imposed by capitation payments for clients, limitations on available hospital beds, limitations on available specialists, and, in some cases, fixed budgets for health-care resources. This type of rationing is seen most often in prepaid health-care or group practices such as health maintenance organizations (HMOs).

Implicit rationing is initially attractive to practitioners because their clinical judgments are in theory not hampered by outside forces. Providers are simply encouraged, through various incentives, to be conservative in their use of health care resources. These incentives, however, may exert a strong influence on the clinical practitioner. It is well known that if professionals contracting with HMOs or prepaid group practices overuse available resources for clients, they may be dropped from employment with the organization (Luft, 1982).

This method of rationing also carries certain disadvantages for the consumer. For example, the way in which health professionals allocate their time can always be influenced by personal tastes and professional interests. If individual practitioners spend more time with disorders or ailments that are of greater interest to them than others, an unjust distribution of professional resources for all persons might result. Furthermore, as long as practitioners do not overutilize their resources, it is unlikely that their use of resources will ever be questioned. This rationing method allows the individual practitioner either to work at a comfortable and leisurely pace or to give disproportionate time to some patients in comparison with others (Mechanic, 1985). Obviously, implicit rationing can be exploited by health-care professionals and may lead to inequities in the distribution of health care. However, it is a rationing strategy that is firmly established in the U.S. health-care system.

Explicit rationing

As an alternative to market or implicit rationing, explicit rationing is frequently employed as a cost-containment method and a means to limit resource consumption. Explicit rationing involves administrative decisions about coverage within health-care plans, the limitation of health-care visits (including specific resources or procedures), and the setting of required intervals between certain services (Mechanic, 1985).

Explicit rationing is used in federally supported health programs such as Medicare and in some private and nonprofit health insurance programs. This method is well liked by health administrators because it allows for direct control over health-care allocations. It is not as well liked by health-care practitioners because administrative control of health-care decisions often interferes with clinician decision making and professional autonomy. As a result, practitioners often seek ways to "beat the system" or otherwise manipulate the administrative rules regulating the allocation of health resources, including the use of themselves.

This method of rationing also has the undesirable side effect of overlooking individual consumer health needs. Administrative decisions on resource allocations are typically made on the basis of aggregate data about health-care needs, consumption, and available resources. By setting limits on the amount of available health resources, this kind of decision making acts against individual health needs and usurps provider decisions about individual care. These undesirable effects are especially pronounced when explicit rationing strategies are used in limiting health-care resources to the elderly.

RATIONING HEALTH CARE AND THE ELDERLY

Faced with the fact that market, implicit, and explicit rationing strategies have done little to reduce either health care costs or resource consumption during the past 50 years, new strategies are being explored. The most provocative of these strategies targets certain segments of the population for reduced health-care attention and resource consumption because of the high costs of providing them. In recent years, the elderly is one such population group that has received a great deal of attention with regard to rationing health care. Should explicit rationing of health-care resources really start with widescale restrictions on resources to the elderly, especially Medicare reductions? Should age be a criterion for the use of certain health care resources?

Pro argument

It can be argued that the elderly should be targeted for health-care rationing for several reasons. First, rationing in this group is inevitable, given the high cost of providing the elderly with needed health care. According to Callahan (1987), the cost of health care for persons who are in their last year of life amounts to about 1% of the gross national product. Their needs in the last year of life usually require the use of costly technology, and the length of time that care is needed is often protracted. All of this amounts to enormous quantities of money spent trying to forestall death—money that could have been used to prevent health-care problems in younger populations.

Second, the number of people over 65 years of age in the United States is rapidly increasing, and this trend is expected to continue over the next 20 years (U.S. Bureau of the Census, 1984). Indeed, those over 85 years of age comprise the most rapidly growing age group in our society today (Davis, 1986). Given the high rate of consumption of health-care resources by the elderly, this means that depletion of health-care resources will occur at a rapid rate over a very short time. It is imperative that some limitations of health-care consumption be implemented to ensure that those in their thirties and forties will have the necessary health-care services when they become elderly.

Third, there are some health-care resources that the elderly should not expect to receive after a certain age. As argued by Callahan (1987), the proper role of the elderly in society is to care for the young and future generations, *not* to concentrate on their own welfare. After all, it is possible to experience a meaningful old age that is limited in time and in health-care support—in other words, to live a natural life span. This view of the life cycle supports health as a wholeness of the body combined with the wholeness of a human life. This view sees the life cycle followed by "a tolerable death" that occurs when one's moral obligations have been fulfilled, the majority of life's possibilities have been accomplished, and it will not seem offensive to others if one dies (Callahan, 1987). Death is then viewed as a sad but relatively acceptable event that occurs when life's possibilities have, on the whole, been achieved. This view of aging focuses on the ends and the meaning of aging and promotes individual acceptance of one's mortality.

Fourth, rationing health care to the elderly would support a needed change in the goals and aims of medicine and nursing. No longer would the goal be to cure the elderly of underlying disease or to extend life. The goal would be to provide an honorable and viable life in later years and to provide humane, sensitive care that is appropriate to the special needs and dignity of the individual elderly person. This would allow changes in medical and nursing education that would focus on supportive care and the needs of elderly and dying patients rather than saving lives at all costs.

Finally, if rationing strategies are *not* targeted toward particular age groups, then the decision of who gets what health-care resources may be made in an ad hoc, situation-dependent manner that will, in the long run, seem unfair to all health-care consumers rather than just to one group. If restrictions on available resources based on age are made in advance, then expectations will change over time, and the system will not seem unfair as long as all those who are the same age experience the same restrictions. Using age as a criterion is a fair approach that recognizes that consumption of resources is high, yet there is little hope of benefit in providing them to the elderly.

For these reasons, health care resources to the elderly should be rationed. It is reasonable, just, and pragmatic.

Con argument

Others might argue that health-care rationing strategies should *not* target the elderly for the following reasons. First, age should not be a criterion for the use of certain health-care services. Resource allocation decisions should be based solely on need. Age-based decision making will inevitably disadvantage the healthy elderly. If one has taken care of his or her health, exercised, eaten the right foods, lived moderately, and so forth, then that person should expect no restrictions on health-care resources if he or she should experience a major health-care crisis in later years. In fact, a healthy 70-year-old person might fare better if treated than an unhealthy 50-year-old suffering from the same disorder. If a certain treatment has been shown to benefit a condition, it should be available to whomever has need of that treatment regardless of the person's age.

Second, the elderly have contributed more to society than younger people. Because the elderly have had a longer working history and have made significant contributions to the harmony and stability of society, they are actually more deserving of treatment than those who have not contributed as much. If rationing must occur, it should be targeted toward younger members of society rather than the elderly because the young have not contributed as much to the accumulation of health-care resources.

Third, health-care rationing strategies should be aimed at restriction of the very costly technologies used in providing health care to all age groups, and not at restriction of resources by the elderly. Many very costly technologies have few benefits or are used in treatments for individuals who have little potential to contribute to society even with the treatment. It is these technologies that should be targeted for rationing schemes, not the elderly.

Fourth, rationing of resources to the elderly is potentially disrespectful to our older members of society and may characterize our society as inhumane. Most societies throughout the world honor their older members and feel special responsibilities toward older citizens. If our country treated the elderly differently, our moral standing among many other countries would be lowered and others would regard the United States as an undesirable place to live. In addition, if they do not see themselves as reaping some special benefits from their contributions as they become older, younger citizens might be discouraged from contributing as much as they can to society.

Finally, health professionals would find it extremely difficult to limit health-care resources to the elderly given their codes of professional ethics. Physicians and nurses are mandated to provide care to individuals regardless of religion, culture, race, economic circumstances, or the nature of the disease. Health professionals would find age as a criterion for receiving health-care services as discriminatory and contradictory to their ethical obligations. They would refuse to limit resources to the elderly, and the rationing strategy would not work.

For these reasons, health-care rationing strategies should not be targeted to the elderly in our society.

AN ALTERNATIVE TO RATIONING HEALTH CARE IN THE ELDERLY

What is needed in any plan for health-care reform and the reduction of health-care costs is a refocusing on the goals and aims of health care. As Callahan (1990) points out, the disciplines of medicine and nursing must refocus their efforts away from the cure of disease and the extension of nonmeaningful life for any person. Instead, they should focus on *caring* as the central goal of health care. It is the ideal of caring that promises to unite the health professions in their efforts to resolve ethical dilemmas posed by cost-containment measures and health-care rationing strategies.

A number of caring-focused approaches are beginning to appear in the health-care literature. Gadow (1985), for example, argues that the value of caring provides a foundation for a professional ethic that will protect and enhance the human dignity of patients receiving health-care services. Viewing caring in the nurse-patient relationship as a commitment to certain ends for the patient, Gadow analyzes existential caring as demonstrated in the actions of truth-telling and touch. By telling the truth to a patient, the nurse assists him or her in assessing both the subjective and objective realities in illness and in making choices based on the unique meaning of the illness experience for that person. Through touch, the patient is affirmed as a person rather than an object, and the value of caring as the basis for nursing actions is communicated.

This approach identifies a moral foundation for a professional ethic that is supported by others (Cooper, 1988; Fry, 1989; Huggins & Sclazi, 1988; Packard & Ferrara, 1988). Caring is viewed as a natural state of human existence and as one way that individuals relate to the world and other human beings. Caring is also viewed as occurring in society to serve human needs. As an ideal for health-care professionals, caring actually gains moral significance when it is formally adopted by those who have the responsibility to serve the needs of others.

Another model of caring with important implications for health-care practices under rationing strategies is Watson's (1985) Model of Human Care. In this model, "caring calls for a philosophy of moral commitment toward protecting human dignity and preserving humanity" (p. 31).

Not only is caring a value and an attitude that eventually manifests itself in concrete acts, but it is also an ideal that transcends the act of caring itself to influence the collective acts of the professional group. Such human caring is transcribed into a philosophy of action and is based on moral notions of needs and considerations for the welfare of others.

Pellegrino (1985) offers a third approach to human caring that focuses on the relationship between caregiver and care receiver and promises to enhance the carrying out of moral obligations to vulnerable individuals in the health-care system. Four senses of care are essential to Pellegrino's approach. The first sense is care-as-compassion, or being concerned for another person's welfare. This is a feeling, either a sharing of someone's experience of illness and pain or just being touched by the plight of another person. To care in this sense is to see the ill individual not only as the object of our ministrations but also as a fellow human.

The second sense of caring is doing for others what they cannot do for themselves (Pellegrino, 1985). This type of caring entails assisting the individual with activities of daily living that are compromised by illness. It is the type of caring that nurses have traditionally been recognized for, but that is in danger of being lost during this time of transition.

The third sense of caring is caring for the health problem experienced by the patient (Pellegrino, 1985). It includes inviting the patient to transfer to the caregiver responsibility for and anxiety about what is wrong. It is a type of caring that ensures that knowledge and skill will be directed to the patient's problem. It also recognizes that patient anxiety needs a specialized type of caring that is best provided by the professional caregiver.

The fourth sense of caring is taking care of or carrying out the necessary procedures (personal and technical) in patient care with conscientious attention to detail and with perfection (Pellegrino, 1985). Not entirely separable from the third sense of caring, this is what most professionals understand as *competence*.

When joined together, the above four senses of caring comprise a moral obligation for the health professional. Such caring is not an option that can be exercised or interpreted idiosyncratically within the health-care system. As Pellegrino (1985) claims, the moral obligation to care in this manner is created by the special human relationship that brings together the one who needs assistance (or is ill) and the one who offers to help. It requires an understanding of the professional ethic as something that attends to the concept of caring in the broad sense and that makes caring a strong moral obligation between caregiver and care receiver.

These approaches to caring can assist in refocusing the aims and goals of health care toward more equitable and judicious uses of health-care resources without the employment of rationing strategies. When combined with traditional moral obligations (such as curing), caring is a necessary aspect for a nursing ethic (Omery, 1995). It provides an acceptable alternative to rationing aimed at the elderly and is more consistent with all other professional obligations toward members of society. Indeed, if the aims and goals of the health professions were changed, rationing might not even be viewed as an acceptable way to contain health-care costs.

SUMMARY

Since market, implicit, and explicit rationing strategies have not proved successful in reducing health-care costs or resource consumption during the past 50 years, an age-based rationing strategy is being explored. This strategy is aimed at the elderly and will limit their access to some health-care resources after they have attained certain ages. Arguments in favor of this rationing scheme emphasize the high cost of providing care, especially in the last year of life; the increasing numbers of elderly citizens who expect to need costly health-care services; faulty expectations of the elderly with regard to their own welfare rather than the care and sustenance of the young; support for changes in the aims and goals of providing health care; and the fact that it is a more equitable method of reducing health-care costs than ad hoc decision making.

Arguments against rationing of resources to the elderly emphasize the unfairness of limiting health-care access for one age group in society; the fact that the elderly are entitled to all health-care resources because they have already contributed more than younger groups in society; the idea that rationing should be aimed at the technologies and their costs rather than at a population group; the belief that targeting the elderly is disrespectful and may have serious political and cultural implications for our society; and the belief that rationing strategies are contrary to codes of professional ethics and difficult to implement.

As an alternative to rationing health-care resources and their consumption by the elderly, it is proposed that the health professions refocus their aims toward caring rather than curing and its associated high costs. If models of caring were used in planning for the distribution of health-care resources, then discussion of a rationing strategy aimed at the elderly might be moot.

REFERENCES

Beauchamp, T.L., & Childress, F.F. (1994). *Principles of biomedical ethics* (4th. Ed.). New York: Oxford University Press.

Callahan, D. (1987). *Setting limits: Medical goals in an aging society.* New York: Simon & Schuster.

Callahan, D. (1990). *What kind of life?: The limits of medical progress.* New York: Simon & Schuster.

Cooper, C.C. (1988). Covenantal relationships: Grounding for the nursing ethic. *Advances in Nursing Science, 10*(4), 48-59.

Davis, K. (1986). Aging and the health-care system: Economic and structural issues. *Daedalus, 115,* 234-235.

Fry, S.T. (1989). The role of caring in a theory of nursing ethics. *Hypatia, 4*(2), 88-103.

Gadow, S. (1985). Nurse and patient: The caring relationship. In A.H. Bishop & J.R. Scudder (Eds.), *Caring, curing, coping: Nurse, physician, patient relationships* (pp. 31-43). Birmingham, AL: University of Alabama Press.

Huggins, E.A., & Sclazi, C.C. (1988). Limitations and alternatives: Ethical practice theory in nursing. *Advances in Nursing Science, 10*(4), 43-47.

Luft, H.S. (1982). Health maintenance organizations and the rationing of medical care. *Milbank Memorial Fund Quarterly, 60,* 268-306.

McGrory, B. (1995, November 9). Elderly describe fears of medicare curbs. *Boston Globe, 248*(132), pp. 1, 12.

Mechanic, D. (1980). Rationing of medical care and the preservation of clinical judgment. *Journal of Family Practice, 11,* 431-433.

Mechanic, D. (1985). Cost containment and the quality of medical care: Rationing strategies in an era of constrained cost. *Milbank Memorial Fund Quarterly, 63,* 453-475.

Omery, A. (1995). Care: The basis for a nursing ethic? *Journal of Cardiovascular Nursing, 9*(3), 1-10.

Packard, J.S., & Ferrara, M. (1988). In search of the moral foundation of nursing. *Advances in Nursing Science, 10*(4), 60-71.

Pellegrino, E.D. (1985). The caring ethic: The relation of physician to patient. In A.H. Bishop & J.R. Scudder (Eds.), *Caring, curing coping: Nurse, physician, patient relationships* (pp. 8-30). Birmingham, AL: University of Alabama Press.

Scanlon, C. (1994). Survey yields significant results. *American Nurses Association Center for Ethics and Human Rights Communique, 3*(3), 1-3.

Watson, J. (1985). *Nursing: Human science and human care.* Norwalk, CN: Appleton-Century-Crofts.

U.S. Bureau of the Census. (1984). *Current population reports. Series P-25 No. 952. Projections of the population of the United States by age, sex, and race: 1983-2080.* Washington, DC: U.S. Government Printing Office.

Legal implications for professional practice

KAY WEILER

Although the author suspects it was not intended, this book affirms the assertion that the law and nursing are intimately intertwined. The table of contents for this book reflects the issues facing the nursing profession in the late 1990s; and these issues mirror the broad impact that the law has had on nursing practice.

Some examples of legal implications of nursing practice are identified in the initial section of this book that debates the question, "What is nursing?" To answer this question, the nursing profession, both currently and historically, reviews or drafts state statutes to assist in examining or defining different aspects of nursing practice (Section One). In addition to the impact of state statutes in defining nursing practice, nursing practice is influenced by government and private-sector decisions regarding which health-care interventions will receive payment, who will pay for the health care, and how much will be paid for the health-care services (Section Eight). In response to the decisions regarding health-care payments, modifications in the health-care system may be made to access the available health-care dollars (Section Seven), which then precipitates changing practice settings for nursing care (Section Four) and provides an increased demand for quality care in exchange for the expended health-care dollar (Section Five).

All of these reactions to the legislative determination of delivery and payment for health-care services raise questions regarding the following: (1) nursing's role in its own professional governance in the changing health-care arena (Section Six); (2) the new nursing role expectations and transitions that will occur in the workplace (Section Nine); (3) the new educational needs of current practitioners and students entering this changing profession (Section Three); and (4) additional legal and ethical implications for nursing practice (Section Eleven). By presenting the issues currently facing the nursing profession, this book also presents the multiple aspects by which the law has had and continues to have a significant impact on the nursing profession.

INTRODUCTION TO THE LAW

A careful exploration of the legal implications for professional nursing practice demands that an initial description of the law be presented and then applied to selected aspects of nursing practice. The law is a system of principles and processes by which the people in a society attempt to control each other's conduct in an effort to minimize the use of force in conflict resolution (Burton, 1995a).

The law governs the relationships between individuals and between individuals and government entities. The term *law,* however, has more than one discrete meaning. The law that governs the relationships between individuals is *private law* and includes contract and tort law. Contract law involves either the enforcement of specific promises or agreements between individuals or the determination of whether compensation is due to an individual because another failed to provide the agreed on goods or services (Burton, 1995b). Tort law involves the enforcement of rights and duties between individuals based on societal standards of behavior (Speiser, Krause, & Gans, 1983).

The law that governs the relationships between individuals and government entities is *public law.* Criminal law is perhaps the most well-known realm of public law. Criminal law is aimed at identifying behavior that is prohibited and, if violated, has associated penalties (Scheb & Scheb, 1994).

SOURCES OF LAW

The government of the United States creates the sources of law and the resulting balancing of power among the different entities. All three branches of government—judicial, legislative, and executive—have an interactive role in the development, execution, and modification of the law.

The *judicial branch* of the law is responsible for the adjudication of disputes. This adjudication is based on the specific parties involved in the lawsuit and the specific issues or questions that have been raised by the suit. The court system is organized into several categories. Each state has its own court system that functions independently of the other states and includes trial and appellate courts. The trial courts receive the information from the specific parties to the case, review the evidence offered to support each position, and render a decision in the case. The appellate courts are then involved with appeals related to cases that have been heard at the trial court level. Most states have a system in which the state supreme court is the final authority for the resolution of a dispute involving state-related questions or statutes (Nowak & Rotunda, 1995).

The Constitution of the United States establishes that all of the federal judicial power will be placed in one supreme court and lower courts as Congress may establish (U.S. Constitution, 1787). The federal courts may not issue advisory opinions, respond to moot issues, or answer hypothetical questions. Instead they are limited to hearing cases or controversies involving (1) individuals or parties who have "standing" or a personal stake in the case and (2) issues that have developed or are "ripe" and not merely hypothetical. In addition to having the proper parties and issues before the court, federal courts may only hear cases that involve proper subject matter jurisdiction (i.e., federal questions or diversity jurisdiction). A federal question involves issues that evolve out of federal statutes, the U.S. Constitution, federal treaties, or federal regulations. Diversity jurisdiction means that a case involves a lawsuit between citizens in different states or a suit between a citizen of one state and a foreign citizen or country; and the suit must meet the jurisdictionally required amount of money in controversy (Nowak & Rotunda, 1995).

The parties to the lawsuit and the actual question under dispute determine which court system (state or federal) is the appropriate venue for the case. The highest level of judicial review is the U.S. Supreme Court. The U.S. Supreme Court may review appeals from federal and state supreme courts in limited circumstances (Nowak & Rotunda, 1995).

The *legislative branch* at the federal level is composed of two houses, the House of Representatives and the Senate. Most state legislative branches are also composed of two houses. Much of the work of the legislature is done by committee members from the houses who are responsible for listening to their constituents' concerns, examining the issues, drafting new bills or reviewing old legislation, and voting to enact new or revised bills into law (Northrop & Kelly, 1987).

The *executive branch* is responsible for approving or vetoing the legislative proposals. Without express or implied executive approval, the legislation becomes moot. If the legislation is vetoed by the executive branch, the proposed bill may only become law if the legislature is able to override, with the appropriate majority, the executive veto (Northrop & Kelly, 1987).

In addition to the three branches of the government, a fourth source of law is administrative law. Administrative agencies are created by the legislature and given delegated power to operate within their defined areas. *Administrative law* refers to the delegated power that may be exercised by the agency, the principles that have been established to govern the agency's exercise of that delegated power, and the legal remedies that individuals aggrieved by the agency may pursue to have their complaints heard (Schwartz, 1983).

An example of an administrative agency is a state board of nursing. The board of nursing is responsible for proposing revisions to the nurse practice acts; supervising the licensing of individual nurses; establishing and monitoring nurses' compliance with mandatory continuing education requirements; and reprimanding, suspending, or revoking the license of a nurse who fails to meet the statutory requirements. The public, via the legislature, holds the state boards of nursing responsible for protecting the public by ensuring that only qualified individuals are licensed, represent themselves as qualified nurses, and then practice as nurses in various health-care settings.

EXAMPLES OF THE RELATIONSHIP BETWEEN THE LAW AND NURSING

As identified earlier, this book is a testimony to the multiple examples of legal issues of nursing practice. The intent of this chapter is to provide an overview of two areas of nursing practice that have been influenced by the legal system and are currently receiving considerable attention—the scope of nursing practice and malpractice litigation. The third area, educational preparation of current and future practitioners in legal aspects of nursing practice, has received minimal attention from the profession and may be the greatest failure of the profession in examining the legal implications of professional nursing practice.

Licensure and scope of practice

In 1888, the U.S. Supreme Court held that national licensure laws were not an appropriate use of federal power, but that states could exercise their police powers by enacting medical licensure laws and accompanying criteria for the practice of medicine (*Dent v. The State of West Virginia,* 1889). This decision opened the door for state legislatures to enact statues, and in 1903, four states (North Carolina, New Jersey, New York, and Virginia) enacted state nursing licensure laws (Acts and joint resolutions passed by the general assembly of the State of Virginia during the extra session of 1902-3-4, 1902 [sic]; Acts of the one hundred and twenty-seventh legislature of the state of New Jersey and fifty-ninth under the new constitution, 1903; Laws of the State of New York passed at the one hundred and twenty-sixth session of the legislature, 1903; Public laws and resolutions of the State of North Carolina, passed by the general assembly at its session of 1903, 1903). These licensure laws had a direct impact on the nursing profession by defining who could hold a nursing license and, therefore, who could legally use the title of nurse. The statutes were not ideal and did not prevent a lay person from receiving payment for nursing services; they merely prevented the lay person from providing care and using the title of nurse. The statutes included minimal educational requirements, and only New York and Virginia created a nurse examining board composed exclusively of qualified nurses. Despite the limitations of the initial nurse practice acts, however, it is clear that these interactions between the law and nursing had a significant role in the emerging definition and recognition of nursing practice (Shannon, 1975).

In 1938, New York enacted the first licensure statute that made it mandatory for persons practicing nursing to have a license. The New York statute was also the first nurse act to identify the role of the practical nurse and provide definitions of the roles of the professional and practical nurses (Laws of the State of New York passed at the one hundred and sixty-first session of the legislature begun January fifth and ended March eighteenth, 1938). This statute, combined with efforts of the American Nurses Association (ANA) to define professional and practical nursing practice, served as the model for the next generation of nurse practice acts ("ANA Board Approves," 1955).

The current professional definition of nursing practice and the legislative parameters of an expanded scope of practice are the products of multiple professional, legal, and social factors. The Federal Professional Nurse Traineeship Program originated in 1959 and has been expanded over the years to include financial assistance for individuals pursuing a nursing career, including nurses pursuing education in advanced clinical practice areas (U.S. Department of Health, Education and Welfare, 1967; 42 USCS §297, 1991).

In conjunction with the expanding scope of this federal nursing education legislation, state nurse practice acts have been modified to recognize advanced nursing practice. One legislative approach that has been used allows state nursing boards to develop rules and regulations regarding specific advanced nurse practice areas. The second legislative approach recognizes specific acts by defined nurse practitioners (e.g., nurse midwives). The third legislative approach recognizes responsibilities delegated by physicians to nurses as the nurses' valid exercise of advanced practice. The fourth legislative approach is to create a broadly phrased nurse practice act that seems to convey an authorization for all nursing functions (Greenlaw, 1985).

The ANA acknowledges that each state has responsibility for statutorily identifying the minimum requirements for nursing practice. The ANA, then, is responsible for developing the standards and guidelines for competent nursing practice and for describing the competent level of professional behavior (ANA, 1995). In 1980, the ANA proposed the following model definition of nursing practice: "the diagnosis and treatment of human responses to actual or potential health problems" (ANA, 1980, p. 9). This broad definition is designed to provide for flexibility and expansion of nursing practice. This broad, expansive language, however, may leave nurses uncertain regarding which actions or interventions are within the realm of nursing practice and which lie outside the professional boundaries (Greenlaw, 1985).

The uncertainty associated with a broad definition of nursing practice was specifically the problem that arose with the Missouri nurse practice act in *Sermchief v. Gonzales* (1983). In *Sermchief,* two nurses were employed in a nonprofit clinic providing family planning health services to the general public. The obstetrics and gynecological services provided to low-income clients and included taking patient histories, performing breast and pelvic examinations, taking Pap smears, and providing contraception information. No action by either nurse at this clinic was alleged to have caused harm to any patient. The nurses and physicians in the clinic initiated a suit asking the court to declare that the acts performed by the nurses were indeed nursing practice, and included in the broadly stated nurse practice act, and not the practice of medicine. The court refused to declare that the actions were nursing practice, and the case was appealed to the Missouri Supreme Court.

The Missouri Supreme Court reviewed the state nurse practice act, the physician practice act, and the documented legislative intent in writing both of those statutes. Although the court was not bound by the nurse practice acts in other states or judicial decisions based on those practice acts, the court did review several other revised nurse practice acts. The Missouri Supreme Court concluded that the nurses in the family planning clinic were practicing within the scope of the Missouri nurse practice act and were not participating in the unauthorized practice of medicine (*Sermchief v. Gonzales,* 1983).

Another legal implication of broadening the definition of nursing to include advanced practice is the question of which standard of care should be used to assess the competency of an advanced nurse practitioner—the standard of care that a nurse should meet or the standard of care that a physician should meet? This question was addressed by the court in *Fein v. Permanente Medical Group* (1981). In February 1976, Mr. Fein, a 34-year-old attorney, was riding his bicycle to work and experienced brief chest pain. The pain quickly subsided, and Mr. Fein continued with his daily activities. He continued to experience intermittent chest pain during exertion over the next several days. After experiencing chest pain while sitting at his desk, Mr. Fein called the Permanente Medical Group, a subdivision of the Kaiser Health Foundation. He could not get an appointment with his regular physician but was able to get a clinic appointment with a nurse practitioner. After examining Mr. Fein and consulting with the supervising physician, the nurse practitioner told Mr. Fein that he was having muscle pain and gave him a prescription for Valium that the supervising physician had written.

That night Mr. Fein awoke with severe chest pain. His wife drove him to the Kaiser emergency room, where a physician examined him and ordered a chest radiograph. Based on the physical examination and the results of the chest radiograph, the physician concluded that Mr. Fein was having severe muscle spasms and gave him narcotics for the pain. Mr. Fein continued to have intermittent chest pain and returned to the emergency room the next day. A different physician examined Mr. Fein and again concluded that the problem was muscle pain. However, when narcotics failed to relieve the pain, an electrocardiogram was obtained and a diagnosis of acute myocardial infarction was made. Mr. Fein was transferred to the cardiac care unit (*Fein v. Permanente Medical Group,* 1985).

When Mr. Fein sued the Permanente Medical Group, one of the questions that arose was whether a standard of care for nurses or for physicians should be used to determine whether the nurse practitioner in the clinic provided the minimum standard of care. The trial court instructed the jury that the nurse practitioner should be held to the physician's standard of care because she was performing skills traditionally performed by physicians (*Fein v. Permanente Medical Group,* 1981). The California Supreme Court cited extensively the California nurse practice act and the documented legislative intent that accompanied the revisions to the California nurse practice act. The California Supreme Court concluded that the trial court had erred and that the nurse should be responsible for meeting the standard of care expected of other nurse practitioners and not a physician's standard of care (*Fein v. Permanente Medical Group,* 1985).

Although *Sermchief* (1983) and *Fein* (1981; 1985) do not represent widespread litigation regarding the expanded definition of nursing practice, they do demonstrate that the expanded scope of practice may be examined by the courts for various reasons. These cases also illustrate that the expanded definition of nursing practice that is supported by the ANA, state legislatures, state boards of nursing, and judicial decisions has precipitated new questions and legal issues for the nursing profession.

Malpractice

Unfortunately, the interrelationship between the state licensure laws, nursing's professional definitions of scope of practice and standards of care, and nursing practice is explored most frequently in the context of nursing malpractice litigation. Malpractice is a form of tort law that includes two very similar forms of negligent acts—negligence and malpractice. *Negligence* is the failure to do something that a reasonable and prudent person would do under similar circumstances or performing an action that a reasonable and prudent person would not do under similar circumstances (Beckmann, 1995). *Malpractice* is professional misconduct or lack of skill. It is the failure to perform professional skills that a reasonable and prudent professional would perform in a similar situation or performing actions that a reasonable and prudent professional would not perform under similar circumstances (Beckmann, 1995).

Four elements must be established to prove negligence or malpractice: (1) a duty owed to the person, (2) a breach of duty or the standard of care by the professional, (3) a causal link between the breach and the harm or injury that has occurred, and (4) that the person bringing the claim has actually been harmed (Aiken, 1994). The critical difference between negligence and malpractice is the role of a person in his or her ordinary daily life as compared with the performance of the same person in his or her professional capacity.

Combined with the question of whether nurses' conduct is personal or professional is the issue of whether the nurses were exercising independent judgments. In many lawsuits, the employing agency (usually a hospital) has been liable for the nurses' conduct under the doctrine of respondeat superior, which means "let the master answer" (Aiken & Catalano, 1994). The respondeat superior doctrine, developed from English common law, means that the master or employer is vicariously responsible for the actions of the employees. The elements of respondeat superior are a negligent act of an employee during the employment relationship and within the scope of employment. If these three elements are established, the hospital or health care employer may be responsible for the negligent actions of a nurse (Aiken, 1994).

One special application of respondeat superior is the "borrowed servant" rule. The borrowed servant rule means that not only is the nurse an employee of a healthcare facility, but the nurse is also responsible to a second "master" who is usually a physician. This rule has been applied in some lawsuits involving operating room nurses who are employees of a hospital and are placed "on loan" for the duration of a surgical case to another "master," who is usually a surgeon. The borrowed servant doctrine indicates that the hospital had employed the operating room nurse but was not directly supervising her conduct. The physician or surgeon in the operating room assumed control of all of the personnel and events in the room. Therefore, if a nurse failed to meet a prevailing standard of care, the surgeon, as the second master, and not the hospital could be held liable to the patient for the nurse's negligent acts (Speiser, Krause, & Gans, 1987).

In 1929, one court addressed the question of whether nurses were professionals or if they practiced the skills of a trade. In this action, a hospital-employed nurse applied a hot water bottle to a patient's limbs while the patient was unconscious. The patient suffered severe burns and more than 2 years later sued the hospital for the nurse's negligence. The main issue in the case was whether the nurse should be considered a professional. If the nurse were a professional, the lawsuit had been filed after the 2 year statute of limitations for bringing a malpractice action had expired. If the nurse were not a professional, however, then the patient had 3 years to file a negligence action and the lawsuit was within the three year time frame (*Isenstein v. Malcomson,* 1929).

The court did not recognize the nurse's conduct as professional; therefore, the nurse's actions were classified as negligence, not malpractice, and the patient could continue with the law suit (*Isenstein v. Malcomson,* 1929). This case identified that, at the time of this suit, only physicians and lawyers were considered professionals with the 2 year statute of limitations applicable to their actions, whereas the 3 year statute of limitations applied to actions by all others.

In a 1964 lawsuit, the same question arose. In *Richardson v. Doe* (1964) it was alleged that two nurses cared for the plaintiff after the delivery of her child and allowed her to hemorrhage for 8 hours before contacting the attending physician. As a result of the hemorrhaging, the patient received a blood transfusion and developed hepatitis from the transfused blood. Under the doctrine of respondeat superior, the patient sued the nurses and the hospital for negligence.

In *Isenstein* (1929), the suit was brought against the nurse for her actions that resulted in burning the patient. In Richardson (1964), the suit was brought against the nurses for their own actions and the hospital on the basis of vicarious liability. The court in both cases determined that the nurses were not professional, did not exercise independent judgment, and therefore were held to the statute of limitations for the filing of negligence, not malpractice, suits. In comparing these two lawsuits, Weiss (1995) identifies that, "The poignant message of the Richardson case was that by the 1960s the issue of whether nurses made independent judgments was not firmly established. Nursing was not yet universally recognized as a profession" (p. 27).

Clearly, the intent of the ANA in expanding the scope of nursing practice, the various state legislatures in broadening the statutory definitions of nurses to include nursing practice in expanded roles, and the extension of funding via the federal Nurse Training Act for nursing students in specialty areas all indicate that nursing is moving into roles in which independent nursing judgment will be expected. It is hoped that as more specialized education is sought and nurses assume increased responsibilities for patient care, future litigation involving nursing practice will recognize nursing practice as professional, not merely skilled, labor, and many instances of expanded practice will describe nurses' independent judgments. With increased autonomy, nurses must realize that there may be an accompanying recognition that the nurse is independently responsible for nursing care and that there may not be an employer who shares the responsibility.

Education

In 1873, the first formal nursing education programs were founded in the United States. These programs, the Bellevue Training School in New York City, the Connecticut Training School in New Haven, and the Boston Training School, were modeled after the Nightingale program in England (Donahue, 1995). These and subsequent training programs, focusing on the physical needs of patients, did not address the legal aspects of nursing practice. The first book on the legal aspects of nursing, *Jurisprudence for Nurses,* was published in 1931 (Scheffel, 1931), with later editions in 1938 and 1941. The preface to the first edition identifies that a nurse of the day was able to find texts to assist in learning about

> bacteriology, chemistry, clinical medicine, therapeutics, and a number of other subjects of a scientific nature which will help her to become more proficient as a nurse. But when it comes to enabling her to learn something concerning how jurisprudence affects her most intimately every day of her professional life, the field has been left notoriously barren. (preface)

In the second edition, Scheffel was joined by McGarvah (Scheffel & McGarvah, 1938), who is credited with being the first American nurse attorney (Northrop & Kelly, 1987).

Today, increased recognition of the legal aspects of nursing care has prompted many nurses to extend their education into the legal arena and bring that knowledge back into nursing practice. The American Association of Nurse Attorneys (TAANA) was formed in 1982 by nurse-attorneys to provide a common forum for the discussion and analysis of legal aspects of nursing practice. TAANA currently has over 650 members who represent diverse areas in which expertise in nursing and law may have a significant impact on the nursing profession by providing leadership in the following areas: nursing professional organizations; legal counsel in health-care risk-management divisions; legal representatives for plaintiffs and defendants in nursing or health-care malpractice litigation; and preparing and presenting educational courses or seminars in colleges of nursing and law to examine legal aspects of nursing and health care (TAANA, 1995). One of the most significant contributions TAANA has made to nursing practice is the development of a model curriculum of legal issues for inclusion in undergraduate nursing education (TAANA, 1992). TAANA members are currently developing a model curriculum for graduate nursing education.

Given the multiple ramifications of the law on the nursing profession and the lack of information available to early nursing students, an obvious question arises: Do undergraduate and graduate nursing curricula today have legal issues courses or seminars? Despite the dozens of interfaces that have emerged between the law and the nursing profession, the answer is that very few nursing curricula have a specific course designated for the legal aspects of professional nursing practice. Reasons given for this lack of legal content are: (1) The National League for Nursing (NLN) guidelines do not require that legal content be included in the basic educational curricula; (2) The nursing programs do not have anyone qualified to teach these courses; and (3) The National Council Licensing Exam (NCLEX) does not include legal aspects content.

The NLN does not require that legal aspects of practice be integrated into nursing curricula (NLN, 1992). However, required qualities of nursing curricula that are evaluated by the NLN as outcome criteria include the students' skills in critical thinking and communication. Critical thinking is described as the "students' skills in reasoning, analysis, research, or decision making relevant to the discipline of nursing" (NLN, 1992, p. 26). Certainly students need to apply principles of legal aspects of nursing practice, including the scope of practice as defined by the relevant nurse practice act, the professional definition of nursing practice, the prevailing standards of care, the impact of third-party payment for services or lack of adequate health-care coverage, and the possibility that the patient or the nurse's colleague is chemically dependent. All of these legal aspects of professional nursing practice are accepted as a portion of the information that should be incorporated in the nurse's reasoning and analysis in patient-care decision making. However, these aspects of critical thinking are rarely taught explicitly as identifiable components of nursing curricula.

The NLN identifies the communication outcome as "the students' abilities in areas such as written, oral and nonverbal communication, group process, information technology and/or media production" (NLN, 1992, p. 27). Students need to recognize multiple legal aspects of professional practice in communicating with patients, including the need to document the care that has been provided, the obligation to listen for and question circumstance that may indicate potential patient neglect or abuse, or the obligation to support the patient's need to discuss whether to accept or reject life-sustaining treatment. These two NLN criteria demonstrate how nursing education could legitimately integrate legal aspects of care into the undergraduate curriculum. However, the nursing profession must make a commitment to teaching legal aspects of nursing practice before that integration can occur consistently at a national level.

Nursing programs fail to provide identifiable legal content in the curriculum because there is a lack of qualified faculty members to teach the legal aspects of nursing. The ideal faculty preparation for teaching legal aspects of nursing practice would be a nurse attorney with clinical-nursing and health-law practice experience. This preparation would provide the faculty person the opportunity to apply health-law principles to clinical-nursing practice. For the best integration of legal aspects into nursing curriculum, TAANA has identified that full-time faculty members are needed to teach legal aspects and be involved with curriculum development, integration, and evaluation (TAANA, 1992). The number of nurse-attorneys in the United States is unknown; however, TAANA is currently collaborating with the American Bar Association and the ANA to develop a comprehensive database that would identify all nurse-attorneys in the country. Once identified, nursing programs could search this database to identify potential faculty members for teaching the legal aspects of professional practice.

Finally, the NCLEX does not integrate legal aspects into the final certification examination. As identified earlier, the nursing profession is responsible for identifying essential definitions of nursing practice and standards of care. The impetus for explicit and recognized integration of legal aspects content into nursing curricula must be based on the students' need to master this information and not the content included in the final examination. It is illogical and unprofessional that the curriculum content would be or should be driven by the content of the final examination.

CONCLUSION

In examining the extensive impact of legal aspects of nursing practice, the author was challenged to narrow this chapter to a manageable scope of content. The author was continually reminded, however, that no single chapter could hope to present the depth and breadth of this issue. The sections on scope of practice and malpractice litigation were chosen because these topics have received recent attention with the expanded areas of nursing practice. The third topic, education, was selected because it is a vitally important component of all nursing education and yet has received only scant consideration by the profession.

In all aspects of developing this chapter, the author was consistently faced with the question of which, if any, aspect of nursing practice does *not* have legal implications. In voicing this question to a colleague, one response that was particularly notable was, "I view legal aspects as a form of universal precautions." This colleague identified that she needed to recognize the legal implications of every practice setting, patient, and nursing intervention. She recognized that she needed to always be alert to the legal implications of practice, not just in the situations that seemed to be laden with the potential for malpractice litigation, administrative review or reprimand, or the violation of state statute. By examining the legal aspects of each patient interaction—whether it takes place in the home, industrial, long-term care, or acute-care setting, or whether it occurs with infants, pregnant women, young athletes, middle-aged workers, elderly retirees, or any person who is physically or mentally challenged—nurses are able to recognize, implement, or avoid the legal consequences that may be attendant to the situation.

REFERENCES

Acts and joint resolutions passed by the general assembly of the State of Virginia during the extra session of 1902-3-4. chapter 191. 1902(sic).

Acts of the one hundred and twenty-seventh legislature of the state of New Jersey and fifty-ninth under the new constitution. 1903. Chapter 109.

Aiken, T.D., & Catalano, J.T. (1994). *Legal, ethical, and political issues in nursing.* Philadelphia: F.A. Davis Company.

American Nurses Association. (1980). *Nursing a social policy statement.* Kansas City, MO: Author.

American Nurses Association. (1995). *Implementation of nursing practice standards and guidelines.* Washington, DC: American Nurses Publishing.

ANA board approves a definition of nursing practice. (1955). *American Journal of Nursing, 55*(12), 1474.

Beckmann, J.P. (1995). *Nursing malpractice: Implications for clinical practice and nursing education.* Seattle, WA: University of Washington Press.

Burton, S.J. (1995a). *An introduction to law and legal reasoning* (2nd ed.). Boston: Little, Brown, and Company.

Burton, S.J. (1995b). *Principles of contract law.* St. Paul, MN: West Publishing Co.

Dent v. The State of West Virginia, 129 U.S. 114 (1889).

Donahue, M.P. (1995). *Nursing the finest art: An illustrated history.* (2nd ed.). St. Louis: Mosby–Year Book.

Fein v. Permanente Medical Group, 175 Cal. Rptr. 177 (1981).

Fein v. Permanente Medical Group, 211 Cal. Rptr. 368 (1985).

Greenlaw, J. (1985). Definition and regulation of nursing practice: An historical survey. *Law Medicine & Health Care, 13*(3), 117-121.

Isenstein v. Malcomson, 236 N.Y.S. 641 (1929).

Laws of the State of New York passed at the one hundred and twenty-sixth session of the legislature. 1903. chapter 293. §§ 206-209.

Laws of the State of New York passed at the one hundred and sixty-first session of the legislature begun January fifth and ended March eighteenth. 1938. Article 52 §§ 1374-1386.

National League for Nursing. (1992). *Criteria and guidelines for the evaluation of baccalaureate and higher degree programs in nursing.* New York: National League for Nursing Press.

Northrop C.E., & Kelly, M.E. (1987). *Legal issues in nursing.* St. Louis: Mosby.

Nowak, J.E., & Rotunda, R.D. (1995). *Constitutional law* (5th ed.). St. Paul, MN: West Publishing Co.

Public laws and resolutions of the State of North Carolina, passed by the general assembly at its session of 1903, begun and held in the city of Raleigh on Wednesday, the seventh day of January, A.D. 1903. (1903). c. 359, §§ 1-11.

Richardson v. Doe, 199 N.E.2d 878 (1964).

Scheb, J.M., & Scheb, J.M., II, (1994). *Criminal law and procedure* (2nd ed.). St. Paul, MN: West Publishing Co.

Scheffel, C. (1931). *Jurisprudence for nurses.* New York: Lakeside Publishing.

Scheffel, C., & McGarvah, E. (1938). *Jurisprudence for nurses* (2nd ed.). New York: Lakeside Publishing.

Schwartz, B. (1983). *Administrative law: A casebook* (2nd ed.). Boston: Little, Brown, and Company.

Shannon, M.L. (1975). Our first four licensure laws. *American Journal of Nursing, 75*(8), 1327-1329.

Sermchief v. Gonzales, 660 S.W. 2d 683 (Mo. banc 1983).

Speiser, S.M., Krause, C.F., & Gans, A.W. (1983). *The American law of torts* (Vol. 1.). New York: The Lawyers Co-operative Publishing Co. and San Francisco: Bancroft-Whitney, Co.

Speiser, S.M., Krause, C.F., & Gans, A.W. (1987). *The American law of torts* (Vol. 4.). New York: The Lawyers Co-operative Publishing Co. and San Francisco: Bancroft-Whitney, Co.

The American Association of Nurse Attorneys. (1992). *Model curriculum of legal content in nursing education.* Baltimore, MD: Author.

The American Association of Nurse Attorneys. (1995). *Inside TAANA.* Baltimore, MD: Author.

42 USCS §297 (1991).

U.S. Constitution. (1787).

U.S. Department of Health, Education, and Welfare. (1967). *Nurse training act of 1964: Program review report* (Public Health Service Publication No. 1740). Washington DC: U.S. Government Printing Office.

Weiss, J.P. (1995). Nursing practice: A legal and historical perspective. *Journal of Nursing Law,* 2(1), 17-36.

Nursing ethics committees: Do we need them?

MARGO R. ZINK, LINDA TITUS

Never before in the history of health-care delivery have we experienced as many bioethical challenges as we do today. Medical technology has mushroomed, providing an ever-increasing array of diagnostic and interventional modalities that can diagnose and treat illnesses deemed lethal only a few years ago. Life can be sustained, often precariously, for long periods, frequently utilizing an intensive-care environment, or more often simply through artificial fluid and nutrition or sophisticated pharmacology. Likewise, the explosion of genetic information has created concerns of confidentiality.

A push for cost containment finds us fearful for those without financial access to service and suspicious of the clinical decisions made by for-profit managed-care organizations. Support of the patient's right to self-determination includes scrutiny of informed-consent policies, the quality of objective information sharing with patients and families, truthtelling, and a vigorous avoidance of paternalistic care.

The increased recognition of bioethics as an important aspect of health-care management has led to the development of institutional ethics committees (IECs) within many health-care settings. These committees were first spawned in the early 1980s when clinicians needed a forum in which to address difficult patient choices or clinical dilemmas concerning what "could" be done versus what "should" be done.

Loewy (1993) poses the need for ethics committees to have a sense of what is involved in what would be considered a "good resolution" to these issues. The members of an ethics committee need a conceptual framework from which to base decisions and a body of knowledge related to ethics and ethical decision making.

With the broadly held purposes of education, policy development, and clinical consultation, these committees have provided a forum in which to address difficult patient choices. Staff education and the establishment of clear policies with regard to areas such as informed consent and limitation of treatment have been typical committee activities. Clinical consults are routinely available to health-care teams and patients to assist with ethical dilemmas. Nurses have been highly visible among the membership, bringing a strong clinical voice and patient-focused approach to committee activity.

> As patient advocates, nurses are in an excellent position to stimulate the development of ethics committees and participate in them. . . . Ethics committees can help patients and families reach well-balanced decisions, reduce the burdens of healthcare providers, avoid litigation, and enhance a healthcare institution's control by reviewing past decisions and suggesting future policies and procedures. (Feutz-Harter, 1991, p. 11)

The IEC has the authority to provide a more systematic and principled approach to decision making that can link ethical and social values as well as medical technology. "Ethics committees are a necessary resource for all healthcare settings—home health, long-term care, psychiatric institutions, clinics, private practices, and hospitals" (Feutz-Harter, 1991, p. 44).

THE NEED FOR NURSING ETHICS COMMITTEES

With nurses well positioned on IECs, one might sense that there is no clear need for a separate nursing ethics committee (NEC). This is a dangerous misconception because NECs are needed now more than ever! Let's examine why.

Institutional ethics committees do not consistently address the specific concerns of nurses. Dilemmas such as the allocation of decreasing resources and changing delivery systems are seldom discussed in IECs. Hospital downsizing and managed-care mergers have led to reductions and reallocations of professional staff, creating yet another nurse-focused ethical issue of rationing their skills among many patients.

Institutional ethics committees have a limited membership; they are able to offer a forum for only a few nurses. In most settings, this leaves the majority of nursing staff without an opportunity to participate.

Nurses are not prepared educationally to deal effectively with ethical concerns. Aroskar (1977) found that only 7% of the accredited bachelor of science programs in nursing require a course in ethics. The preliminary findings from a recent study on ethical issues found similar results in the 1990s (Zink & Titus, 1994; Titus, 1995). "The real tragedy with regard to ethical dilemmas in nursing practice is not that nurses do not recognize that such dilemmas exist; rather it is their lack of preparation to solve these dilemmas using ethical principles" (Fromer, 1982, p. 20).

Daily nursing practice problems are seldom appropriate topics for discussion at a hospital-level ethics committee because other discipline representatives may not be prepared or interested in nursing concerns (Scanlon & Fleming, 1990). Edwards and Haddad (1988) found that the unique concerns of nurses, such as nursing dilemmas related to increasingly high-tech care, the allocation of decreasing resources, and changing delivery systems were not felt to be appropriately addressed within IECs. While there has been some criticism that NECs compete with hospital ethics committees, it is generally recognized that NECs provide an important forum for nursing-specific issues and also prepare nurses to become involved effectively in IECs (Donovon, 1983; Ross, 1991).

Erlen (1993) related how emerging economic restrictions, increased technology coupled with more limited resources, and fragmentation of the overall health-care delivery system have created more intense ethical issues, none of which have easy solutions. Nurses do not always have a clear understanding about their role in ethical deliberations or even in the way ethical decisions are made. Nurses frequently feel powerless in these situations.

Bosek (1993) asserts that medical-surgical nurses face ethical issues daily and call on either clinical or theoretical resources to solve these issues. Nurses in one study indicated that they often did not know that an IEC existed and that this source would not be their first avenue in dealing with clinical ethical issues (Hoffman, 1991). When they need more information, nurses may consult theoretical resources, including institutional resources, journals, reading groups, and professional publications as available (Bosek, 1993). However, these avenues do not provide a strong opportunity for discussion of ethical concerns.

Efforts to articulate nurses' involvement in ethical issues is evident in the literature and within professional organizations. Dalby (1993) outlines the beginning of nursing ethics in the description as cited in Robb in her 1900 publication *Nursing Ethics from Hospital and Private Use.* The American Nurses Association (ANA) Code of Ethics "provides general moral principles based on ethical principles that inform nursing practice and serve as tools in evaluating nursing's goals. The *Code for Nurses with Interpretive Statements,* published by the American Nurses Association, expresses nursing's moral concerns, goals, and values, rather than announcing a set of laws that dictate nursing behavior" (ANA, 1988, p. 1). Although this code has been revised through the years, it continues to contain statements from the original 1926 code (Dalby, 1993). The ANA created the Center for Ethics and Human Rights in 1991 with the objectives of developing a body of knowledge concerning ethics and human rights, disseminating information, and advocating for patients' rights. These mechanisms serve as broad sources of guidance but do not sufficiently meet nurses' needs for support and direction in resolving ethical dilemmas in everyday practice.

In an attempt to address the specific needs of nurses, nursing professionals began establishing NECs in the early 1980s. Several objectives were targeted. First, nurses needed preparation in ethical concepts, decision-making, and pertinent legal standards. This knowledge was necessary in order to participate articulately in interdisciplinary discussions of an ethical nature. Second, many issues relating to the nurse's role as a patient advocate required a forum in which these issues could be clarified. Appropriate nursing development of the advocacy role has emerged as a crucial element of nursing practice.

Surveys are cited in the literature that assess the existence of NECs. Scanlon and Fleming (1987) surveyed 121 hospitals in five boroughs of New York City and Westchester County and found only one that had an NEC. A later survey in 1989 found only two such committees (Mason, Johansson, Fleming, & Scanlon, 1989).

A survey in 1991 by the Connecticut Nurses Association (CNA) Ethics and Human Rights Committee found six NECs in the state, all within acute-care hospitals. Subsequent activities, however, have led to interest in NECs in 23 other agencies, several of which have developed a functioning committee. These results suggest that at this time NECs are still relatively rare and are not the predominant method of addressing nurses' ethical concerns.

Earlier surveys have revealed the extent to which nurses feel a lack of education in bioethics. The CNA survey showed that 24 of the 44 agencies that responded thought that continuing-education programs on topics related to ethical dilemmas and concerns were needed in the state. Suggestions of topics included restraints/seclusion practices, do-not-resuscitate orders, right-to-die issues, advance directives with implications for nursing, nutrition and hydration issues, neonatal care, and workshops on establishing ethics committees.

A survey conducted by the ANA's Center for Ethics and Human Rights in June 1994 at the ANA Convention polled 934 convention participants from across the country (Scanlon, 1994). The majority of respondents (79%) reported confronting ethical issues daily or weekly in practice. The 10 most frequently occurring ethics and human rights issues confronting these nurses are outlined in Table 86-1. These ten issues have been incorporated, with permission, into another survey currently under way that will pilot a new tool to assess nurses' ethical issues in acute- and home-care settings. The specific aims of this study are to do the following:

1. Develop and pilot the Nursing Ethics Issues Survey (NEIS)
2. Survey registered nurses in practice and management in select acute-care facilities in New England to assess their preparation, the ethical issues they encounter, and the resources they utilize to resolve them
3. Survey registered nurses in practice and management in select home-care agencies in New England to assess their preparation, the ethical issues they encounter, and the resources they utilize to resolve them

The research questions will examine whether the NEIS has validity and reliability in testing nurses' preparation for the ethical issues they encounter in their practice settings. The study will also determine whether there is a difference in the responses of the nurses in acute-care and home-care settings in relation to their preparation and the ethical issues they encounter. One resource that will be considered are NECs (Zink & Titus, 1995).

An examination of nursing staff educational and experiential background in ethics is an essential first step before establishing NEC goals. A random survey at Mount Sinai Medical Center in New York City evaluated this issue. The majority of the nurses surveyed indicated that they had read the ANA Code of Ethics, although only 42% recalled any specifics of the document, and 23% were not sure when they had read it. It was also found that nurses with less than 1 year in practice (38%) had fewer problematic ethical situations than nurses in practice for longer than 1 year (NEC, 1989). The four problematic ethical concerns identified in this survey are cited in Table 86-1.

Table 86-1 Frequently cited ethical issues

American Nurses Association Center for Ethics and Human Rights	Mount Sinai Center Ethics Survey
Cost issues that jeopardize patient welfare	Giving care to an offensive patient
End-of-life decisions	Using life-support systems on terminally ill patients
Breaches of patient confidentiality	Giving care to noncompliant patients
Incompetent, unethical, or illegal practices	Providing care that poses risk to nurses' health (Nursing Ethics Committee, 1989)
Pain management	
Use of advance directives	
Informed consent for procedures	
Access to health care	
Issues in the care of HIV/AIDS persons	
Providing "futile" care (Scanlon, 1994)	

Such compelling survey results demand a serious look at nursing curricula. Close communication between the clinical and academic domains can facilitate identification of course content and student exposure, which will develop an understanding of both ethical principles and practice application.

What about the millions of today's practicing nurses in both inpatient and community environments? How can their acquisition of core skills and continued education in bioethics be ensured? This critical need can be met, in part, by the development of NECs. Their usefulness need not be confined to the hospital setting; rather, they can serve to build skills in bioethics for nurses in many settings such as long-term care, home care, clinics, health maintenance organizations, and other emerging sites of health-care delivery. Newer delivery sites can, in fact, present their own special areas of ethical concern and drive the discussion of ethics to new dimensions.

Nurses are patient advocates, and resolution of ethical concerns is vital to the nurse-patient relationship. This advocacy role requires nurses to seek an understanding of their patients' values and ensure that they are honored in all phases of decision making. Paramount are articulate, assertive contributions from nurses to health-care team case management—an activity that can be actualized through an active NEC.

NURSING ETHICS COMMITTEE FUNCTIONS

A review of the limited publications (Donovon, 1983; Edwards & Haddad, 1988; Fowler, 1988; Fromer, 1982) on starting an NEC summarized the functions of such a committee as follows:

1. *Identification, exploration, and resolution of ethical issues in nursing practice.* Nursing ethics committees allow nurses to open up dialogue and provide a mechanism for them to take action when a sense of distress or concern about ethical dilemmas occurs. This committee structure also provides nurses with the ability to follow a defined model of critical thinking and activity toward resolution. In a sense, NECs legitimize nurses' concerns.
2. *Education of nurses in bioethics and nursing ethics.* A basic understanding of ethical principles and moral reasoning is essential for nurses in identifying, articulating, and resolving dilemmas in clinical practice. Discussion and understanding of the nurse's role in an interdisciplinary environment encourages a broad consideration of bioethics as well as those issues of ethics within the nurse-patient relationship.
3. *Preparation of nurses for participation in interdisciplinary decision making about ethical issues.* With a well-grounded understanding of ethical principles and resolution methods, nurses can strengthen their role as patient advocates. Clear articulation of issues as well as a willingness to work toward their consentual resolution with other health-care team members is essential in today's environment. Most ethical conflicts involve the whole team and demand communication among all.
4. *Service as a resource group.* Once an NEC matures, staff are aware that if an ethical concern arises, committee members can be contacted for assistance. Informal consults are often helpful for individual clinical issues. The committee can also undertake a wide variety of educational activities to increase staff knowledge in this area.
5. *Review of nursing ethics materials.* Many committees assign members to follow particular journals and bring pertinent articles forward for general discussion, thus keeping current with the vast array of information now being published. Committees can also recommend the purchase of books and audiovisual materials for establishment of an ethics reference center within a facility.
6. *Review of departmental policies related to ethics.* Many policies have an ethical component, such as those involving patient abuse, questioning the care a patient is receiving, the nurse's role in informed consent, the impaired nurse, and care of the HIV-infected patient. Policies related to these issues can benefit from review by the NEC.
7. *Involvement with nursing ethics research.* An NEC can serve a role in encouraging research in nursing ethics or even in developing a research study as part of committee activity. Review of proposed research in nursing ethics by students or staff would also be appropriate.
8. *Preparation of nurses to serve on IECs.* Institutional ethics committees must have nursing membership in order to be effective and to meet Joint Commission on Accreditation of Healthcare Organizations requirements. A strong preparation in bioethics, group process, and decision making is crucial for nurses who sit on these committees. Membership of NECs can provide this preparation and increase a nurse's awareness of the clinical issues that are most problematic to his or her discipline.

Fowler (1988) included an additional function of an NEC as addressing practice issues, such as nurse staffing patterns, allocation of nurses' time for patient care, nurse refusal of assignment, and admissions without sufficient staff coverage, which are not normally within the realm of IECs. Edwards and Haddad (1988) went on to state that NECs assist nursing personnel in assuming ethical responsibilities, which is done through education, support, development, and consultation.

Activities of NECs should first focus on self-education (Fowler, 1988). Self-education can take up to a year, requiring commitment, attendance, and the use of adult learning techniques. Inservice education, printed material, audiovisual materials, and the use of an ethics consultant can all provide successful educational opportunities. Agencies should identify resources within the institution who can be tapped for education and support of the group, such as physicians, clergy, social services, legal counsel, and psychologists. Members should select a decision-making model to utilize in discussing ethical issues in a systematic fashion. Numerous models can be found in the literature (Curtin, 1982). The case-study approach, using an identified model for decision making, has been found to be a successful tool in nurses' understanding of ethical dilemmas (Veatch & Fry, 1987). Including ethics materials, such as a copy of the ANA Code of Ethics, would also be an initial step in new staff orientation to ethical involvement.

Membership considerations for NECs include the nurses' willingness to invest in self-education, complete a sustained term, have excellent interpersonal and group process skills, have the ability to set aside personal values and focus on patient advocacy, serve as role models, and be comfortable with public speaking. Representation from many patient care areas and nursing roles, predominantly from the staff level, is optimal. Some NECs strive to have staff members from every patient care unit in order to maximize the impact within the institution and facilitate access to the committee for ethical problems.

Yale–New Haven Hospital, an institution surveyed by the CNA, has had an operating NEC for over 12 years under the leadership of Donovon, a nationally known nurse ethicist. It consists of a unit-based ethics resource member and includes inservice courses on ethics that deal with such topics as principles of ethics, models of ethical decision making, nurse-patient relationships, principle versus autonomy, informed consent, life support, nursing research in ethics, resource allocation, and confidentiality (C.T. Donovon, personal communication, November 26, 1991).

"An essential prerequisite to [NEC] program development is clarification of key facilitating and inhibiting factors that seem to influence the staff nurse's ability to make ethical decisions and deliberately act on those decisions" (Donovon, 1983, p. 56). Donovon goes on to say that the overall purpose of the NEC is to facilitate nurses' participation "in interdisciplinary decision making regarding ethical matters" (Donovon, 1983, p. 58).

FUTURE DIRECTIONS

It is of great concern to note that so many practicing nurses feel unprepared to cope with the ethical issues they encounter. Concerns are further heightened by the knowledge that nurses are facing ethical challenges more frequently and in a wide range of practice settings. Future challenges will only intensify the array of ethical dilemmas to be managed. Here are but a few of them.

Genetic information

The ANA Center for Ethics and Human Rights has issued a comprehensive document entitled, *Managing Genetic Information: Implications for Nursing Practice* (Scanlon & Fibison, 1995), which provides a full discussion of ethical issues related to genetics such as consent, privacy, confidentiality, truthtelling, disclosure, and nondiscrimination. These issues require nurses to be prepared to respond appropriately in safeguarding patients' rights amid the explosion and utilization of genetic information (Smith, 1989).

Informed consent

The right to full disclosure of health-care information has become a key patient right that creates ethical dilemmas in practice. What is full disclosure? When has valid informed consent been given? When is truthtelling secondary to other ethical principles? What is the role of the nurse in the informed-consent process? Who is entitled to give information to patients?

Reproductive issues

It is clear that our collective social fabric is divided on the moral and ethical issues entwined in reproduction. Nurses are at the forefront of many of these issues, including birth control, abortion, artificial insemination, in vitro fertilization, and fetal tissue utilization. Selective abortion for multiple pregnancies and embryo implantation in postmenopausal women also raise many new questions. Is it ethical to give birth control information to minors? Should nurses participate in abortions? How should fetal tissue be obtained or utilized for medical research or treatment? Should any social or sexual condition limit the availability of artificial insemination for an individual? When six fetuses are created by medical manipulation, is it ethical to selectively reduce the number in order to enhance the chances for survival of those remaining? Should a 60-year-old woman be implanted with an embryo?

Transition from inpatient to outpatient care

Nurses working in hospital settings are caring for patients with higher acuity, more social stressors (e.g., homelessness, violence, isolation, poverty, illiteracy) and reduced hospital lengths of stay. These conditions provoke enormous ethical concerns in the area of beneficence. Can effective patient education occur with a short hospital stay? When is a patient ready for discharge? What are the institutional obligations to ensure patient safety after discharge? What if a patient has no financial means for needed posthospital care?

Community practice

As hospital nurses are experiencing ethical issues related to shortened length of stay, nurses in the outpatient and community settings are facing their own challenges. Access to health care, homelessness, abuse, issues of teenage confidentiality, violence, and crime are frequent concerns of nurses, who must have the training and resources to respond to these and other issues in an ethical manner.

End-of-life decisions

An understanding of the multiple variables in end-of-life decisions requires ongoing education and practice for nurses. What constitutes quality of life? When is cost a factor? Are clinical goals clear and achievable? Do the patient and family have sufficient understanding to make decisions? What role does the nurse have in discussing end-of-life discussions? How does the nurse serve as a patient advocate?

CONCLUSIONS

While IECs serve a vital role within the broad areas of education, policy, and consultation, they do not provide a broad forum for the educational and practice issues faced daily by nurses. Significant data show that nurses are inadequately prepared to address the burgeoning complexities of bioethics.

Nursing ethics committees are one means of empowering nurses in their role as advocates as they prepare for more effective ethical deliberations with other health-care professionals. NECs enhance nurses' empowerment, thus enabling them to have full participation in ethical decision making. If indeed nurses are to become more actively involved with ethical decision making, they must see themselves as authorities with resources available to them, such as membership in an NEC. IECs are only one forum, and a limited one, for nurses to participate in ethical decision making. IECs should not function in isolation of the NEC. "Nursing ethics groups are yet another way to help health care professionals reflect upon their own experiences and to learn from the experience of others, as well as to participate in shaping the ethical environment of hospitals . . ." (Ross, 1991, p. 7).

Nursing ethics committees are a means for nurses to develop their base of power when dealing with ethical situations. They provide a forum for nurses to verbalize viewpoints without infringing on the views of others. Ethical power comes from clarifying one's purpose, which must be persistent (Holly & Lyons, 1993). "Nurse ethics committees will help nurses to make decisions based on knowledge, rather than intuition and personal values" (Dalby, 1993, p. 610).

Nursing ethics committees serve to empower nurses in their vital role within the health care team. As primary care providers, nurses have their fingers on the pulse of the patient's total experience. They are often the first discipline to sense an ethical issue. NECs assist nurses to identify the issues and take action to ensure their resolution, thereby fulfilling the vital role of patient advocate.

REFERENCES

American Nurses Association. (1988). *Ethics in nursing: Position statements and guidelines.* Kansas City, MO: Author.

American Nurses Association. (1985). *Code for nurses with interpretive statements.* Kansas City, MO: Author.

Aroskar, M.A. (1977). Ethics in the nursing curriculum. *Nursing Outlook, 25,* 260-264.

Bosek, M. (1993). A comparison of ethical resources. *MEDSURG Nursing, 2*(4), 332-334.

Curtin, L. (1982). *Nursing ethics: Theories and pragmatics.* New York, NY: Prentice-Hall Publications.

Dalby, J. (1993). Nurse participation in ethical decision making in the clinical setting. *AWHONNS- Clinical Issues in Perinatal Women's Health Nursing, 4*(4), 606-610.

Donovan, C. (1983). Towards a nursing ethics program in an acute care setting. *Topics in Clinical Nursing, 5*(3), 55-62.

Edwards, B., & Haddad, A. (1988). Establishing a nursing bioethics committee. *Journal of Nursing Administration, 18*(3), 30-33.

Erlen, J. (1993). Empowering nurses through nursing ethics committees. *Orthopaedic Nursing, 12*(2), 69-72.

Feutz-Harter, S. (1991). Ethics committees: A resource for patient care decision-making. *Journal of Nursing Administration 21*(4), 11-12, 44.

Fowler, M. (1988). Nursing ethics committees. *Heart & Lung, 17*(6), 718-719.

Fromer, M. (1982). Solving ethical dilemmas in nursing practice. *Topics in Clinical Nursing, 4*(1), 49-56.

Hoffman, D.E. (1991). Does legislating hospital ethics committees make a difference? A study of hospital ethics committees in Maryland, the District of Columbia, and Virginia. *Law, Medicine, & Health Care, 19,* (1-2), 105-119.

Holly, C., & Lyons, M. (1993). Increasing your decision-making role in ethical situations. *Dimensions of Critical Care Nursing, 12*(5), 264-270.

Loewy, E. (1993). An inquiry into ethics committees' understanding: How does one educate the educators? *Cambridge Quarterly of Healthcare Ethics, 2,* 551-555.

Mason, D., Johansson, E., Fleming, C., & Scanlon, C. (1989). Ethics committees in health care institutions in the New York City metropolitan region: A report of two nursing surveys. *Journal of the New York State Nurses Association, 20*(4), 13-16.

Nursing Ethics Committee, Dept of Nursing, The Mount Sinai Medical Center, New York City. (1989). The ethics survey: An important step in promoting nursing ethics. *Journal of the New York State Nurses Association, 20*(4), 4-8.

Ross, J. (1991). Ethics committees for nurses. *Ethical Currents, 25,* 1-2, 7.

Scanlon, C. (1994). Ethics survey looks at nurses' experiences. *The American Nurse, 26*(10), 22.

Scanlon, C. & Fibison, W. (1995). *Managing genetic information: Implications for nursing practice.* Washington DC: American Nurses Publishing.

Scanlon, C., & Fleming, C. (1990). Confronting ethical issues: A nursing survey. *Nursing Management, 21,* 63-65.

Scanlon, C., & Fleming, C. (1987, December). Nurses come together to face ethical issues. *Health Progress,* 46-52.

Smith, J. (1989). Ethical issues raised by new treatment options. *Maternal-Child Nursing, 14,* 183-186.

Titus, L. (1995). CNA ethics survey published. *Connecticut Nursing News, 66*(4), 1.

Veatch, R., & Fry, S. (1987). *Case studies in nursing ethics.* Philadelphia: Lippincott.

Zink, M., & Titus, L. (1994). Nursing ethics committees: Where are they? *Nursing Management, 25*(6), 70-76.

Zink, M., & Titus, L. (1995). *Validity and reliability testing for the nursing ethical issues survey.* Unpublished study in process.

Sexual harassment

TONIA D. AIKEN

Sexual harassment is a form of sex discrimination; it is a violation of the Civil Rights Act of 1964. Until the 1970s, the term *sexual harassment* was not acknowledged by most people. During the 1970s, sexual harassment started to gain attention but was not seen as a form of sex discrimination under Title VII of the Civil Rights Act. The focus was on male/female work interactions and not on same-sex violations. In the late 1970s, the term was broadened to include any behavior that required sexual favors in exchange for promotions, advancements, or better benefits. Because this broader definition considered sexual favors a condition of employment, sexual harassment fell under the laws and statutes dealing with sex discrimination.

In the 1980s, sexual harassment was defined in more detail. In 1980, the Equal Employment Opportunity Commission (EEOC), defined sexual harassment in its guidelines as (1) unwelcomed sexual advances, (2) requests for sexual favors, (3) verbal conduct of a sexual nature, or (4) physical conduct of a sexual nature. These advances, requests, and types of conduct were considered sexual harassment when they (1) acted as a term or condition of employment, (2) were a criterion for employment decisions, (3) interfered with the victim's job performance, or (4) created a hostile, intimidating, or offensive work environment.

In the mid-1980s, lawsuits began to surface. One notable suit was *Meritor Savings Bank v. Vinson* (1986). In June 1986, the U.S. Supreme Court affirmed sexual harassment as a cause of action under Title VII. The Supreme Court also held that economic losses were not required for a sexual harassment claim. In *Meritor,* the victim alleged that her supervisor made repeated demands for sexual favors, fondled her in front of other employees, forcibly raped her on numerous occasions, and exposed himself to her. The Court in *Meritor* held that the following were true: (1) The allegations were sufficient for a case of sexual harassment based on a quid-pro-quo theory; (2) Even if a victim engages in sexual relations with a supervisor, the person can still have a claim for harassment if the conduct was *unwelcome;* (3) The "totality of circumstances" rule will be used to determine if there is evidence of sexual harassment; and (4) Employers are not necessarily liable for the sexual harassment acts of their supervisors.

WHO SEXUAL HARASSMENT AFFECTS

Sexual harassment affects many people, not just the victims. Employers can lose not only valuable employees as a result of harassment, but they can also lose the trust and productivity of other employees and monetary awards from such lawsuits and litigation costs. Employees can lose dignity, trust, promotions, monetary gains, jobs, and self-esteem. These factors not only affect the employee victims but also their families and coworkers.

Sexual harassment is against the law. Many more claims have been filed since the early 1970s because people are becoming more educated about sexual harassment and are no longer afraid, embarrassed, or intimidated to bring forth such claims.

TYPES OF SEXUAL HARASSMENT

Quid pro quo

As mentioned earlier, since the 1970s the definition of sexual harassment has been broadened to include more than just sexual demands for preferential treatment at work. Sexual harassment also includes unwelcomed sexual advances; requests for sexual favors, and nonverbal, verbal, or deliberate physical behavior of a sexual nature by the offender. With quid-pro-quo sexual harassment, submission to the above conduct is made implicitly or explicitly a condition of the person's employment; employment decisions are based on whether the employee submits to or rejects the offender's conduct. Following are a few examples:

- A supervisor requires sexual favors of an employee in order for the employee to be promoted, hired, or receive raises.
- A male supervisor promises a new male nurse a promotion if he has a sexual relationship with him.
- A hospital administrator tells a nursing supervisor that she looks great in tight dresses and he likes good looks and brains. The nursing supervisor just walks away after the comment and doesn't acknowledge him. The administrator then "finds fault with her work" and fires her.

In the last example, all of the elements of sexual harassment are present: The employee is a member of a protected group. The sexual remarks and advances were unwelcomed. The harassment was sexually motivated. The employee's reaction to the administrator's advances affected an aspect of her employment (e.g., she was fired). The courts have held that "unwelcomed conduct" is conduct that the employee did not solicit or incite and the employee regards as undesirable or offensive.

Causal connection

To prove sexual harassment, employees must show a causal connection between the harassment and the job benefit in question. They must show that they were qualified for the job benefit in the absence of harassment. The harasser must also play a role in the benefit decision of the alleged victim (*Neidhardt v. D.H. Holmes, Co.*, 1979).

Hostile environment

The second type of harassment falls under the Hostile Environment Theory. If the offender or the employment conditions create a hostile environment that unreasonably interferes with a person's job performance or creates an intimidating, offensive, or hostile working environment, a claim of sexual harassment can be made. "Hostile environment" can include unwelcomed sexual advances; requests for sexual favors; verbal conduct of a sexual nature; physical conduct of a sexual nature; sexually explicit jokes; offensive language, gestures, or comments; or sexual pictures, calendars, or objects.

More subtle examples of sexual harassment include the following:

- Requesting a person to have dinner after work
- Requesting a person to have drinks after work
- Requesting a person to participate in other social activities after work

The EEOC will determine if the conduct was unwelcomed by examining the totality of circumstances of each case. Factors that the EEOC will focus on and that should be reviewed by the company or institution include the following:

- Conduct (verbal, physical, or both)
- Frequency of conduct
- Type of conduct (hostile or offensive)
- Category of offender (coworker, supervisor, or other)
- Others who assisted or were a part of the harassment
- Direction of harassment (focused on one or several individuals)
- Consistency of the victim's conduct

Sexual harassment may consist of only one incident if, for example, an employee is denied a promotion because of refusal of a sexual advance by an employer (Quid-Pro-Quo Theory). Under the Hostile Environment Theory, the single incident or series of incidents usually has to be quite severe to create a hostile environment. Although the incident may not fall under hostile environment, it may be covered by Title VII as a violation.

Verbal sexual harassment

Verbal remarks can constitute sexual harassment. Several factors are examined to determine whether the remarks can be classified as harassment:

1. Were the remarks derogatory?
2. Were the remarks hostile?
3. Did the alleged harasser single out the victim?
4. Did the victim participate in any exchanges with the alleged harasser?
5. What is the relationship between the parties involved?

Sexual harassment of men

Title VII protects both men and women. For example, a male general manager pressures two male employees to participate in and observe sex with his secretary. He threatened to blackball them, eliminate medical benefits, and fire them if they refuse to participate in the ménage à trois. The court held the employer liable for quid-pro-quo and hostile environment sexual harassment (*Showalter v. Allison Reed Group, Inc.*, 1991).

Homosexual harassment

Title VII prohibits sexual harassment by homosexuals against members of the same sex. In an Alabama case (*Joyner v. AAA Cooper Transportation*, 1983), a male employee sued for sexual harassment based on unwelcomed homosexual advances by the terminal manager. The employee was laid off and the employer refused to recall him when a position became available. The employee was entitled to be reinstated with back pay.

Examples of offensive conduct

Offensive conduct can be sexual in nature, demeaning, threatening, or hostile. Case examples of conduct that were found by the courts to be "welcomed" include:

1. An employee tells dirty jokes or makes dirty remarks, and the discussions are never complained about by the employee.
2. The employee participates in sexual innuendoes or vulgar story telling.
3. The employee flirts and behaves provocatively and asks the alleged harasser to have dinner at his or her home despite repeated refusals by the harassed.

Conduct does not have to be directed at the victim. It can either be observed, or the victim can have knowledge of incidents involving other employees that affects the plaintiff's psychological and emotional status and well-being. For example, an environment would be considered hostile if a female nurse has to listen to remarks about her anatomy and physical characteristics while she is in the operating room. If a sexually explicit joke about men is shown and passed around the emergency department by female coworkers, and a male nurse is offended and embarrassed by it, the requirements for a hostile environment have been met. If a victim is aware that those employees who have sex with the supervisor receive more benefits, then a hostile environment exists.

WHY PEOPLE SEXUALLY HARASS OTHERS

Power is one reason for sexual harassment. It is an abuse of authority by someone (usually in a supervisory position) who uses power, force, and authority over someone in a lower position. Harassers can be supervisors, subordinates, customers, patients, suppliers, friends, acquaintances, relatives, business associates, or strangers. Harassers are found at all levels and in all occupations. Harassment also takes place among both genders: male to female, female to male, male to male, and female to female.

Dominance

The need to dominate also lends itself to influencing or controlling others. Harassers use dominating behavior to get what they want or need. Some dominate to prevent from being dominated by others. Dominating individuals look for weak traits or spots they can use to control the other individual.

Insecurity is another reason why individuals harass. By harassing or "bullying" others, these people hide their insecurities. Power, dominance, and insecurity needs result in the type of harasser seen in the workplace.

EMPLOYEE/EMPLOYER ACTIONS FOLLOWING HARASSMENT

If you are being harassed, do something about it. Many employers have developed sexual harassment policies and procedures that include guidelines on the administrative process, who should be notified, and penalties for the harasser.

The procedures for a complaint should be confidential and fair to both parties. These policies and procedures should apply to employees, management and men and women alike. Confidentiality is crucial because of the nature of the complaint. If the complaint is false it could ruin both the private life and public life and career of an individual.

If the victim knows that confidentiality will not be maintained, he or she is less likely to come forward because of the implications and effects on his or her public and private life. This is not how a program should be structured. Harassment programs must encourage complaints.

Complaints should be handled promptly, seriously, and sensitively. Programs may provide such things as counseling to victims, publication and publicizing the complaint process, and training employee support groups to aid victims. Employers must maintain an environment that continues to show support and respect for victims after complaints are made.

If you are a victim of sexual harassment, the following actions are crucial:

1. Do not accept your position as a victim.
2. Do something about the harassment.
3. Respond promptly and assertively toward the problem.
4. Make your feelings and position known to the harasser.
5. Communicate directly to the harasser that his or her conduct is unwelcome either through a face-to-face confrontation or through conduct that demonstrates to the harasser that the conduct is unwelcome.
6. Document the times and places of harassment, the people having knowledge of the incidents, and your

reactions to and comments about the behavior of the harasser.
7. Document what you have said to the harasser.
8. Report continuing harassment to the appropriate person in your company or institution. If the harasser is your supervisor and the person to whom you report, notify the person with authority over the supervisor.
9. Be assertive and follow through with the process.
10. Do not allow harassment to continue.
11. If these methods are ineffective, contact your local EEOC office as soon as possible.

If you know someone who is being harassed, be supportive and encourage that person to pursue the complaint process. As an employee, know and understand sexual harassment; know how to respond to the harassment and know the process for making a formal complaint. You can also function as a teacher, informing your coworkers about the types of sexual harassment and what to do if harassed.

If you are an administrator, be sure that your institution or company has an effective complaint program and reasonable policies and procedures that can be followed to handle such matters as quickly and confidentially as possible. However, prevention is the best tool. A statement about sexual harassment should be in the institution's policy manual and in the employee handbook.

All personnel in supervisory positions should be notified about the procedures for handling sexual harassment problems. Emphasis should be placed on disapproval of harassers and sanctions for victims. Keep communication lines open with the victim and witnesses. Do not ostracize the victim or make the claim public. Lack of communication and attention given to a claim sends out a message that sexual harassers shouldn't worry because the company or facility does not place such problems high on its priority list. If an employer can prove that the harassment has been eliminated, the victim has been made "whole" again, and future preventive measures have been taken, the EEOC will usually close the case.

EMPLOYER PROBLEMS

Employers face multiple problems when harassers are in the workplace. Following are just a few of the ramifications:

1. Turnover costs of rehiring, recruiting, and retraining employees
2. Dehumanization of employees—humiliation, embarrassment, and physical problems such as headaches or gastrointestinal upsets
3. Increased absenteeism
4. Loss of productivity
5. Inability to concentrate
6. Attorneys' fees
7. Settlement of damage awards

LAWS AFFECTING EMPLOYER LIABILITY

Several state and federal laws pertain specifically to the employer's liability in cases of sexual harassment. These include Title VII of the Civil Rights Act of 1964 and its interpretation by the EEOC; state and local sexual discrimination laws and regulations; and federal/state courts/administrative agency decisions on sexual harassment claims.

PREVENTION OF SEXUAL HARASSMENT IN THE WORKPLACE

To prevent sexual harassment, employers should develop and adopt a strong sexual harassment policy; communicate the policy to all employees; and train supervisory personnel to handle harassment problems in a professional and sensitive manner. The employer can be held liable if the employer knew or should have known of the harassment and failed to take appropriate and immediate action to correct it.

How to discourage sexual harassment

To discourage sexual harassment, every complaint should be investigated. A written policy and procedure specifically prohibiting sexual harassment should be developed. Likewise, a policy and procedure for employee complaints should be developed.

How the policy can be communicated to employees

The following venues can be used to let employees know about the sexual harassment policies:

1. Posting information (bulletin boards)
2. Newsletters
3. Institution or company papers
4. Memos (sent out at least once a year)
5. Employee committees/employee meetings
6. Personal communications
7. Employee evaluations

8. Employee disciplinary proceedings
9. Case decisions in court
10. Personnel policy and procedure manuals
11. New employee orientation and training meetings
12. Questionnaires and surveys

Developing a sexual harassment policy

A sexual harassment policy should include the following information:

1. How to lodge a complaint
2. Where to lodge a complaint
3. Whom to speak to about potential complaints or harassing conduct

Developing policies for the managerial level

Procedures for managerial personnel should be developed on the following:

1. How to spot harassment
2. What to do when harassing conduct is detected
3. How to dissolve the problems
4. How to prevent potential lawsuits

Policies for this level should include the following:

1. Types of conduct that constitute sexual harassment
2. Managerial obligations for identifying and handling harassment
3. What is acceptable and unacceptable behavior
4. The complaint process (where to go, whom to see, what to do, and when to do it)
5. The potential for liability and exposure to the employer for such claims

To prevent a breach of contract suit (e.g., do not guarantee absolute confidentiality), nothing should be guaranteed in this policy that cannot be accomplished. Disclaimers may be used (e.g., this policy is not to be construed as a contract between the employer and employee).

Developing the complaint procedure

Oral complaints. Some companies make sexual harassment complaint procedures separate from the usual grievance procedure, while others do not. Here are some guidelines:

1. Allow both oral and written complaints.
2. The employer's representative must put the oral complaint in writing.
3. Have the victim read and verify it for accuracy.

Pros and cons.

1. Grievance procedures may take too long.
2. Confidentiality may be diminished because of the structure of the routine grievance procedure.
3. Harassment claims should be given immediate attention by the upper echelon of a company or facility.
4. Policy language must emphasize that there will be prompt investigation of complaints and appropriate actions taken against persons guilty of harassing.
5. The employer must maintain all information regarding complaints as confidential as possible for both victims and witnesses.

EQUAL EMPLOYMENT OPPORTUNITY COMMISSION (EEOC)

The EEOC provides guidelines that are neither law nor binding in court but do carry considerable weight.

Filing a charge with the EEOC

A victim can file a charge at any filed office located in cities throughout the country. The offices are usually listed under U.S. Government in the phone book. Victims can call (800) 669-4000 for the information on the office closest to them. The EEOC also offers sexual harassment information by calling (800) 669-EEOC, TTD number (800) 800-3302; FAX (202) 663-4912. The EEOC's address is Office of Communications and Legislative Affairs, 1801 L. Street, N.W., Washington, D.C. 20507.

Time limits for filing. A sexual discrimination charge must be filed with the EEOC within 180 days of the alleged discriminatory act *or* within 300 days if there is a state or local employment practices agency that enforces a law prohibiting such discriminatory practices. It is best to contact the EEOC as soon as you believe discrimination has taken place so that you can file a claim in a timely manner.

Laws enforced

The EEOC enforces Title VII of the Civil Rights Act of 1964, which prohibits discrimination based on race, color, religion, sex, or national origin. It also enforces the Age Discrimination in Employment Act, the Equal Pay Act, and sections of the Civil Rights Act of 1991. Other acts covered include Title I of the Americans with Disabilities Act, which prohibits discrimination in the private sector, state and local government. The ADA prohibits discrimination against disabled persons in the federal government.

Legal remedies

Actual damages. With Title VII, the victim can receive actual damages such as promotions, lost benefits, hiring, reinstatement, and back pay that were lost as a result of the harassment.

Injunctive relief. Injunctive relief is obtained through the courts and orders the employer to stop the alleged harassment and to take steps to prevent such conduct in the future.

Attorney's fees. Attorney's fees are usually allowed in these cases.

Punitive damages. Punitive damages are intended to punish the defendant for the egregious nature of the tort. The defendant's actions must be willful and wanton, and the damages are not based on the plaintiff's actual monetary loss. The award is usually doubled or tripled to "punish" the defendant economically in order to deter this type of behavior in the future. Punitive damages may be awarded if the employer acted with reckless indifference or malice.

Other damages. Compensation may be given for future pecuniary losses, mental anguish, and inconvenience.

Lawsuit against employer. A lawsuit can also be filed directly against the employer and the harasser based on a breach of contract or tort law. Awards can include compensatory damages, economic damages, and actual damages. Tort suits may allow punitive damages.

Intentional tort suit. Victims may also sue for such intentional torts as assault, battery, wrongful termination, and intentional infliction of emotional distress.

Criminal suits. In some cases, the harasser may be charged with a criminal offense such as assault, battery, rape, and attempted rape. The employer usually has no liability under criminal statutes although civil liability still exists.

Many states now have laws that deal with sexual harassment. Victims may use the state court system, claiming a violation of state fair employment laws and are entitled to a jury trial in most states. However, under Title VII there is no jury. In the state courts, awards can include punitive damages, compensatory damages, back pay, and legal fees.

15 women will share $1.2 million for ordeal. NEW YORK—Fifteen women who accused their former boss of lewd behavior, including grabbing their breasts and buttocks, going to the bathroom with the door open and conducting business with his fly down, will share a nearly $1.185 [million] settlement.

The $1.185 million sum is more than twice the biggest previous settlement ever obtained by the EEOC in a sexual harassment case.

The women worked as secretaries or executive assistants for a chief executive of Del Laboratories of Farmdale.

As part of the settlement, the company agrees to hold training sessions for its 1,600 employees.

REFERENCES

Meritor Savings Bank v. Vinson, U.S. Sup Ct, No. 84-1979, June 19, 1986.

Niedhardt v. D.H. Holmes, Co., 21 Fair Empl. Prac. Employment Practice CAS.BNA 452 (E.D. La. 1979), aff'd 624 F. 2d 1097 (5th Cir.)

Showalter v. Allison Reed Group, Inc., 767 F. Supp. 1205 (DIR. 1991)

Joyner v. AAA Cooper Transportation, (D.C. Ala. 1983)

BIBLIOGRAPHY

Aiken, T.D. (Contributor/Editor). (1994). *Legal, ethical, and political issues in nursing.* Philadelphia: FA Davis Company.

How to recognize and prevent sexual harassment in the workplace. (1992). Madison, CT: Business and Legal Reports, Inc.

Howard, J., & Myers, M.S. (1992). *Countering sexual harassment: A handbook for self-defense.* Florida: Choctaw Publishing.

Lloyd, K.L. (1992). *Sexual harassment: How to keep your company out of court.* New York: Panel Publishers, Inc.

Working with drug users: Is abstinence the best policy?

TONDA L. HUGHES, CYNTHIA MacLEOD, CAROL J. BOYD

Views of drug* use and addiction have varied markedly across time as well as across social and cultural groups. In the early part of this century, Americans' views on drug use and drug users differed substantially from the majority view of today. At that time, although having a "drug habit" was not approved or encouraged, it was regarded as neither criminal nor heinous. For example, opium and its derivatives were openly used in this country for a wide variety of human ills until the early 20th century, and in fact were considered by many as less offensive than cigarette smoking (Clausen, 1977). It is estimated that there were 200,000 narcotics addicts in the United States in the early 1920s, two thirds of whom were women (Ogur, 1986).

Following the Harrison Narcotic Act of 1914 and prohibition (1920-1933), and especially since the 1970s "war on drugs," drug use and addiction have been treated primarily as crimes or moral failings and only secondarily as public health problems. Recently, however, another major transformation in the way we think about and respond to drug-related problems has been occurring. The advent of the AIDS epidemic has forced us to review our current perspectives and practices related to drug-use intervention. In particular, harm reduction—a strategy for addressing a variety of public health problems, including HIV/AIDS and other drug-related problems—is growing in recognition and use. This chapter reviews the tenets of the Harm Reduction Model (HRM) and provides specific examples of how this model can be used to address problems related to drug use. The current focus on abstinence as the primary goal of drug intervention and treatment is questioned, and harm reduction as an alternative approach is suggested. Advantages of this model, including its potential for application in addressing a broad range of drug-related health risks, are discussed.

*Although we have chosen to use the generic term "drug" in our discussion, we wish to emphasize that we view this term as inclusive of a variety of psychoactive substances including alcohol and nicotine as well as illegal drugs.

WHAT IS HARM REDUCTION?

Harm reduction—sometimes referred to as harm minimization or risk reduction—is a social policy or perspective that uses a common-sense approach to decrease the harmful effects of drug use. It represents a more realistic balance between an "ideal" drug policy, such as "drug-free America," and a pragmatic acceptance that drug use will not go away regardless of the restrictions on it or the consequences associated with its use. HRMs assume a community-based philosophy. The operating principle of harm reduction is any positive change; the goal is ego building, not ego breaking, and strategies aim to increase self-esteem and self-efficacy (Harm Reduction Working Group [HRWG], 1993).

An alternate approach to the current medical model of treatment for drug users is important because a significant proportion of persons who use drugs are unable or unwilling to stop. Furthermore, many who do want to stop do not have access to formal treatment. In 1992 approximately 2.8 million people in the United States needed drug treatment, yet there were fewer than 600,000 slots available in treatment programs (Office of National Drug Control Policy, 1992). Many of the hospital-based programs for drug treatment are well beyond the economic reach of most street addicts, with some of the widely advertised and readily available programs costing $10,000 to $20,000 for one detoxification regimen (Bellis, 1993).

TENETS OF A HARM REDUCTION PHILOSOPHY*

- To recognize the intrinsic value and dignity of all human beings
- To seek to maximize social and health assistance, disease prevention, and education while minimizing repressive and punitive measures
- To recognize the right to comprehensive, nonjudgmental medical and social services for and the fulfillment of the basic needs of all individuals and communities, including users, their loved-ones, and the communities affected by drug use
- To emphasize the necessity for a comprehensive and holistic understanding of and approach to drug use that addresses the isolation, survival needs, and drug use of the user
- To not judge licit and illicit drugs and drug use as good or bad, but rather to looks at peoples' relationship to drugs and emphasize the reduction of drug-related harm and the encouragement of safer drug using
- To recognize the competency of users to make choices and changes in their lives, including those about their drug use
- To provide options in a nonjudgmental, noncoercive way and acknowledge the impossibility of controlling the outcomes whose determination is the legitimate realm of the client
- To demand that the individuals and communities affected by drug use be involved in the organization and cocreation of strategies for harm-reduction interventions and programs
- To recognize the diversity of users and drug use and the necessity for outreach and services to reflect and address every user's needs
- To expect accessible, flexible, nonjudgmental drug treatment, including methadone maintenance, on demand
- To support accessible, legal syringe exchange and the supply of sterile drug using and safer sex equipment
- To challenge current drug policies and their consequences, such as misrepresentations of drug users and misinformation about drug use

*From the Harm Reduction Working Group, P.O. Box 77240, San Francisco, CA 94107. Reprinted with permission.

The National Institute on Drug Abuse (NIDA) estimates that approximately 6.3% of the American population currently uses some form of illegal drugs, and that there are between 1.1 and 1.5 million injecting drug users in the United States (NIDA, 1991). Further, it is estimated that about one third of reported cases of AIDS are related directly or indirectly to injection drug use, with the majority of HIV-positive women being infected either by injecting drugs or through sexual contact with injecting drug users. The transmission of HIV, hepatitis B virus, and other communicable diseases to the sexual partners and children of injecting drug users perpetuates drug-related harm far beyond the drug-using population. Relying solely on the medical or criminal-justice approach to drug use is to abandon the health needs of millions of Americans. By providing information and the means to alter behaviors that are not solely aimed at abstinence, individual drug users are empowered to make the incremental changes that lead, over time, to improved health for themselves and their communities.

The relationship between the harm reduction model and public health

The box lists the tenets of the HRM agreed on by the HRWG (1993). Harm reduction has much in common with more familiar models of health-care delivery. For example, public-health approaches to drug-related harm also focus broadly on the community's experience with drug use. These experiences include, but are not limited to, infectious and chronic disease; mental health effects of drug use such as neglect, abuse, isolation, and depression; socioeconomic antecedents to and consequences of drug addiction such as poverty, unemployment and homelessness, and violence facilitated by drug use; and the drug economy and the war on drugs.

The war on drugs embodies policies that criminalize possession or distribution of illicit drugs or drug paraphernalia. The working premise of this drug-control policy is that by institutionalizing forceful interdiction of drugs and tools for drug use, the overall desire for and use of drugs will diminish more rapidly than by any other means. Although this policy may limit the ease with which drugs are distributed and acquired for personal use, its primary effect appears to be supporting and encouraging the illegal drug market and forcing drug users further "underground" into the illegal drug subculture. Discussion of the ineffectiveness, and often harmful repercussions, of this policy is beyond the scope of this paper but is available elsewhere (Drucker, 1992; Reuter, 1992).

Public-health and harm-reduction approaches challenge the dominant medicolegal drug-control policy that seeks to create a scarcity of drugs (other than alcohol and cigarettes) and drug-injection equipment and to punish the drug user. Public-health and harm-reduction approaches emphasize the necessity for a comprehensive and holistic understanding of approaches to drug use and employ a broad range of creative and innovative strategies that are reflective of the complexity and individuality of users' lives (HRWG, 1993). Drug use is viewed as existing on a continuum of the use and abuse of legal (e.g., alcohol and nicotine), prescription, and illegal drugs. Rather than perpetuating an "all-or-nothing" approach to drug-use intervention, risk is recognized and accepted as an inherent part of life and is viewed within the context of the user's life (HRWG, 1993). Unlike most services that are designed for those who seek treatment (and who accept the goal of abstinence), these approaches meet drug users wherever they are and move at the pace of the individual. They offer at-risk populations a variety of simple strategies that can reduce the danger associated with high-risk behaviors. For example, a nurse using a harm-reduction approach might discuss with injecting drug users the importance of not sharing injection equipment or the benefits of switching from injectable to oral or inhalable drugs. Other examples of harm-reduction strategies include reducing the quantity of alcohol or other drugs consumed or switching to a less harmful drug.

Harm reduction does not require that the provider support all behavior, but it recognizes that people are not defined by behavior alone and that all people deserve respect, dignity, and support. Advocates of this point of view consider addiction to be a health problem rather than a criminal activity. Because habitual drug use compromises personal judgment, the responsibility of users for their actions is also reduced. Thus, the drug user is viewed as a person in need of help—not punishment. Instead of judging drug use as good or bad, harm reduction focuses on the individual user's relationship to drugs—as defined by the user. Abstinence is not seen as the only clinically desirable endpoint or the only morally acceptable measure of success in providing services (Sorge, 1991). For some drug users who are attempting to reduce drug-related harm, the desired endpoint might well be abstinence. However, like the development of addiction, the process of stopping drug use happens over time and within a particular context. For users seeking to stop use as well as those who are unable or unwilling to stop, intermediate steps can be taken toward that endpoint that are valuable and sometimes life preserving.

Advocates of these models acknowledge that an individual's drug use, be it nicotine, alcohol, heroin, or crack, can have profound and persistent effects on both personal and community health. Public health, in synchrony with many facets of the HRM, recommends practical risk-reduction measures and expansive treatment options for the benefit of drug users, their families, and their communities. Although there is conflict and controversy among many health-care providers regarding some tenets of the HRM, a number of health practitioners have joined with affected communities to research, develop, and implement innovative and effective harm-reduction strategies.

HISTORY OF HARM REDUCTION

New jargon often disguises the fact that what is described is not new. Although the term "harm reduction" has only recently become more widely used and recognized, the philosophy, and many harm-reduction approaches, have been advocated and practiced for some time.

Methadone maintenance treatment programs (MMTPs), begun in the 1960s, were one of the earliest formalized examples of harm reduction. Methadone is a synthetic narcotic, and "methadone maintenance" involves providing methadone (also an addictive drug) to heroin addicts as a substitute for heroin. These early programs were viewed very much as harm reduction because drug users involved in MMTPs typically demonstrated substantial improvement in a number of areas, including emotional stability, improved work records, and retention in drug treatment. In addition, MMTPs also helped to reduce drug-related crime and assisted in the social reintegration of drug users. After a relatively brief period of popularity in the late 1960s and early 1970s, methadone maintenance became (and remains) a controversial form of treatment for drug addicts. Much of the controversy resulted from misleading and incorrect early publicity, which described methadone as a "cure for addiction" (Moss, 1977).

The more contemporary HRM has its roots in programs initiated in the Netherlands and the United Kingdom in the 1970s and early 1980s. One of the earliest needle-exchange programs began in Amsterdam in 1984. The primary goal of this program was to prevent the spread of hepatitis B. In order to accomplish this goal, workers in the program sought to facilitate contact with a broad range of drug users, to provide information on a personal level, and to produce attitudinal and behavioral change through the use of condoms, drug-free treatment with short waiting lists, methadone maintenance, and needle exchange. Similar programs have become increasingly prevalent in both the Netherlands and the United Kingdom as well as in other parts of Europe and Australia.

The discovery of HIV as a blood-borne pathogen has been the impetus for the greater acceptance of the HRM over the past several years in many parts of the world, including the United States. Harm reduction in the context of HIV/AIDS prevention began as a result of strategizing about how to create the minimal behavior change necessary to prevent HIV transmission among injecting drug users. A simple, easy-to-teach procedure was the outcome: using bleach, which kills the virus, to clean syringes between uses. This bleach protocol was first introduced in 1986 in San Francisco by trained community health outreach workers and since then has been adopted in numerous cities across the country (Aldrich, 1990).

More controversial in the United States have been the needle/syringe exchange programs (NEPs). First initiated publicly in Tacoma, Washington in 1988, NEPs currently operate in about 77 locations across the country. NEPs have as a primary focus the reduction of the spread of HIV infection by giving injecting drug users clean equipment in exchange for their used, often contaminated, needles and syringes. In addition to new hypodermic syringes, drug users are also provided with clean cotton balls, aluminum bottle caps, and vials of bleach and water—all the equipment necessary for preparing and injecting drugs such as heroin or cocaine. Because possession of drug paraphernalia is illegal, changes in or waivers of these laws have been instituted in many cities where NEPs operate.

Needle-exchange programs, characterized by a nonjudgmental, immediate response to participants' needs, represent one of the clearest examples of the harm-reduction philosophy. These programs offer a variety of services to a high-risk population that is unlikely to seek help in more traditional settings. For example, many NEPs provide free condoms and nonoxynol 9 (a spermicide that may kill the AIDS virus on contact), as well as written information and verbal reinforcement about safer-sex practices. Some programs provide HIV testing, and all provide drug treatment referral information. In addition to the above tangible services, these programs also offer participants a sense of acceptance, self-worth, and empowerment—all critically important in the first steps toward recovery.

Opponents of NEPs argue that supplying drug-injecting equipment fosters increased drug use and facilitates illegal behaviors. Recent studies conducted in the United States have found no evidence that needle exchange programs contribute to drug use or encourage young people to begin injecting drugs (Bowersox, 1994). For example, the results of a recent study sponsored by the Centers for Disease Control and Prevention show that NEPs are effective in reducing HIV infection, do not increase drug use, and may in fact decrease drug use (Marwick, 1995).

Although the federal government has refused to fund these programs, a wide range of professional groups and organizations (e.g., the American Academy of Pediatrics, the American Society of Addiction Medicine, and the American Public Health Association) publicly support NEPs. In December 1994, the American Medical Association (AMA) House of Delegates approved a resolution that unambiguously supports NEPs (AMA, 1994). Such advocacy from organizations like the AMA and the American Public Health Association will likely have a substantial impact in increasing awareness and acceptance of the HRM.

Other examples of drug-related harm reduction

A number of other successful (and less controversial) examples of harm-reduction strategies related to drug use can be cited. The "designated driver" program, the reduction in hard liquor consumption, and the growing popularity of "lite beers" and low-tar cigarettes are all well-known examples of harm reduction. Further, like these less controversial examples, the three primary areas in which the harm-reduction approach appears most promising in reducing drug-related harm are (1) the prevention of the transmission of HIV through needle exchanges and safer-sex condom use programs; (2) the treatment of ongoing addictive behaviors including methadone maintenance for heroin addicts and nicotine replacement therapy for tobacco users; and (3) the control of addictive behaviors such as heavy drinking through strategies that have moderate or controlled drinking as an alternative to abstinence.

IMPLICATIONS FOR NURSES

Nurses encounter drug users on a daily basis. Indeed, it is estimated that 10% to 50% of all clients admitted to general hospitals in the United States have alcohol-related problems (Moore et al., 1989). A similar percentage of clients (approximately 30%) in primary health-care settings have been found to misuse or be dependent on alcohol (Fleming & Barry, 1991). Furthermore, given that approximately 14.5 million Americans use illicit drugs (NIDA, 1991), a substantial number of clients with whom nurses come into contact likely have problems related to these drugs.

Despite the large numbers of drug users encountered in practice, nurses (like other health-care providers) are reluctant to address clients' drug use. The reasons for this reluctance are complex and are complicated by negative societal attitudes toward drug use and drug users (Hughes, 1989). Nurses may perceive that drug users do not want to help themselves or that they deserve the harm that comes their way as a result of drug use. Also complicating the recognition of and response to drug-using clients are health-care professionals' frustration at not being able to "cure" drug addiction. Like many other chronic, relapsing behavioral disorders, drug addiction forces health-care providers to acknowledge the limitations of the medical model in guiding strategies for intervention.

Despite the limitations of many of the current policies and approaches to drug use, health-care practitioners and policymakers have been reluctant to embrace less restrictive methods such as the HRM. It is likely that many nurses may feel a certain degree of conflict when planning strategies to address the health needs of drug users and their communities.

The duty to advocate for clients' autonomous decision-making is fundamental to the HRM and to many nursing models. In contrast, the medical model has traditionally taken a restrained paternalistic approach, which claims a special moral capacity and authority for physicians and certain health-care providers. In recognizing the drug user as a health-care consumer and stakeholder and accepting that the drug user is the expert on her or his own life, nurses can sidestep some of the obstructive stereotypes that inhibit health promotion and care. Through greater awareness of the full personhood of the drug user, the nurse communicates the essential caring nature of nursing. Genuine advocacy for autonomous decision making occurs when the nurse assists drug users to clarify personal values within current life contexts such that decisions derive from their own, rather than the provider's, values (Gadow, 1980). This presupposes a collaborative approach, the goal of which is to support the client's informed achievement of self-determined health outcomes.

In addition to the legal, ethical, and moral issues inherent in some harm-reduction approaches (such as NEPs), other aspects of the HRM are likely to create tension or discomfort for health practitioners accustomed to working within the traditional medical model. For example, harm reduction challenges the traditional asymmetrical power dynamic between health-care providers and clients. It replaces a hierarchial structure with an egalitarian model that encourages mutual exchange of information. Harm reduction is structured in a manner that empowers individuals, for example, by recognizing drug user's expertise and by respecting their rights to make health and behavioral choices. While providers have resources that the users want, the users have the power in their willingness to take (or reduce) risk. In addition, if the goal of the provider is to give drug users tools with which they are able to reduce the risks to themselves and their communities, then ultimately the success of any harm-reduction effort lies in the ability to create a structure in which egalitarian relationships can be developed in a way that produces trust and change and that maximizes users' participation and ownership. This requires options to be presented in a nonjudgmental, noncoercive way, respectful of the competence of drug users to make choices and changes in their lives. The goal is to educate drug users to become more conscious of the risks involved in their drug use and sexual behaviors (HRWG, 1993).

SUMMARY

The war on drugs has succeeded in creating a frightened and cynical nation—a country whose preoccupation has been with drugs instead of drug users. Casualties of this "war" have too often been drug users and their communities. As nurses would treat casualties in any war, their acknowledged duty to offer care extends to drug users. This care is motivated by strong moral and professional convictions (American Nurses Association, 1985) that emanate from empirical and theoretical foundations but also encompass realistic, creative, and compassionate approaches. Because the HRM reflects the experience of successful secondary prevention initiatives for a broad range of risk behaviors, nurses using this model will be able to engage more fully in prevention and rehabilitation based on real client needs and participation.

REFERENCES

Aldrich, M.R. (1990). Legalize the lesser to minimize the greater: Modern applications of ancient wisdom. *The Journal of Drug Issues, 20*(4), 543-553.

American Medical Association. (1994, December). *Resolution 231 adopted by the House of Delegates at the 1994 Interim meeting.* Chicago: Author.

American Nurses Association. (1985). *Code for nurses with interpretive statements.* Kansas City, MO: Author.

Bellis, D.J. (1993). Reduction of AIDS risk among 41 heroin addicted female street prostitutes: Effects of free methadone maintenance. *Journal of Addictive Diseases, 12*(1), 7-23.

Bowersox, J. (1994). Needle-exchange programs show promise for AIDS prevention. *NIDA Notes, 9*(3), 8-9.

Clausen, J.A. (1977). Early history of narcotics and narcotics legislation in the United States. In E. Rock (Ed.), *Drugs and politics* (pp. 7-22). New Brunswick, NJ: Transaction Books.

Drucker, E. (1992). US drug policy. Public health versus prohibition. In P.A. O'Hare, R. Newcombe, A. Matthews, E.C. Buning, & E. Drucker (Eds.), *The reduction of drug-related harm* (pp. 71-81). New York: Routledge.

Fleming, M.F., & Barry, K.L. (1991). The effectiveness of alcoholism screening in an ambulatory care setting. *Journal of Studies on Alcohol, 52*, 33-36.

Gadow, S. (1980). Existential advocacy: Philosophical foundation of nursing. In S. Spicker & S. Gadow (Eds.), *Nursing: Images and ideals* (pp. 79-107). New York: Springer Publishing Co.

Hughes, T.L. (1989). Models and perspectives of addiction. *Nursing Clinics of North America, 24*(1), 1-12.

Harm Reduction Working Group. (1993, October). *Working Paper from the National Harm Reduction Working Group Meeting*. San Francisco, CA: Author.

Marwick, C. (1995). Released report says needle exchanges work. *Journal of the American Medical Association, 273*(13), 980-981.

Moore, R.D., Bone, I.R., Geller, G., Mamon, J.A., Stokes, E.J., & Levine, D.M. (1989). Prevalence, detection, and treatment of alcoholism in hospitalized patients. *Journal of the American Medical Association, 261*(3), 403-407.

Moss, A. (1977). Methadone's rise and fall. In E. Rock (Ed.), *Drugs and politics* (pp. 135-153). New Brunswick, NJ: Transaction Books.

National Institute on Drug Abuse. (1991). *National Household Survey on Drug Abuse: Population estimates 1991*. Rockville, MD: Author.

Office of National Drug Control Policy. (1992). *National drug control strategy: A nation responds to drug use*. Washington, DC: U.S. Government Printing Office.

Ogur, B. (1986). Long day's journey into night: Women and prescription drug use. *Women and Health, 11*, 99-115.

Reuter, P. (1992). *Hawks ascendant: The punitive trend of American drug policy*. Santa Monica, CA: Rand.

Sorge, R. (1991). Harm reduction. A new approach to drug services. *Health/PAC Bulletin, (Winter)*, 70-75.

Child maltreatment: Nursing's changing role

PERLE SLAVIK COWEN

If our American way of life fails the child, it fails us all.
PEARL BUCK
THE CHILD WHO NEVER GREW

The first legal intervention in a case involving child maltreatment occurred in the United States in 1874 and involved a child who was malnourished, regularly beaten, and kept in rags by her adoptive parents. Ironically, the case was brought to the public's attention by the American Society for the Prevention of Cruelty to Animals. At that time, protective services for Mary Ellen Wilson could only be invoked on the basis that she belonged to the animal kingdom and was therefore entitled to protection (Helfer & Kempe, 1987).

Today, most states mandate that nurses report child abuse and neglect; others encourage or authorize them to do so (Krietzer, 1981). For nurses to fulfill their professional responsibilities in reporting suspected child maltreatment, they must have knowledge of the indicators that are manifested before, during, and after its occurrence. Early recognition and intervention with high-risk families is fundamental to treatment, and primary prevention is the ultimate goal of those involved in the well-being of all children and their families. That nurses are the most prevalent group of providers to have early, direct contact with families has placed them in a strategic position for early assessment and treatment of child abuse and neglect (Campbell & Humphreys, 1984). Their roles as autonomous practitioners, child and family advocates, and members of multidisciplinary teams require them to demonstrate an understanding of the current problems and issues in child maltreatment, including ethical, legal, and social ramifications.

It is becoming increasingly difficult in the current political climate for nurses to fulfill their professional roles in the prevention and intervention of child maltreatment. The current array of programs and services that address the health-care and preventive needs of at-risk families are often underfunded and poorly integrated, and many are now at risk of dissolution. Distinctly different doors are opened or closed based on how families intend or can afford to pay. Poor families face an imposing jungle of conflicting requirements and application procedures to establish service eligibility, while families with private coverage face care restrictions based on cost-containment or profit motives. Congress is currently hearing testimony from families whose infants died following the combination of early postpartum discharge and the failure of nurse home visitation services to materialize.

Nurses practicing in the perinatal and pediatric arenas face the daily frustration of deciding, often in a matter of hours, who is at risk and how to mobilize services for those most at risk. There are not enough community or institutional outreach nurses strategically positioned and/or allowed to fulfill their role in meeting the needs of America's most vulnerable children and their families. The shift to more community-based nursing is occurring at a time when many collaborating human service agencies are experiencing downsizing and reorganization. This often results in a static and sometimes chaotic environment that undermines the case management of at-risk families and places vulnerable children in a precarious position with inconsistent safety nets. The proposed shift of federal human service monies to state block grants will add immense pressures to this situation as agencies attempt to assimilate and accommodate changes that are intended to restrict resources for at-risk families (Kogan, Mann, & Super, 1995). As other resources dry up or become fragmented, nurses will experience an expanded role in directing and providing care and locating re-

Table 89-1 Types of child maltreatment

Type	Definition	Characteristics
Physical abuse	Nonaccidental injury of a child	Physical injury that is typically at variance with the history given of it, suffered by a child as the result of the acts or omissions of a person responsible for the care of the child; repeated patterns of physical punishment with short- or long-term effects
Neglect	Failure to provide a child with basic necessities of life when financially able to do so or when offered financial or other reasonable means to do so	Child is not provided with adequate food, clothing, shelter, supervision, assistance with hygiene, or medical care
Sexual abuse	Use of a child for sexual purposes including incest, rape, molestation, prostitution, or pornography	Perpetrator is usually someone in the child's family or known to the child; nonabusing parent or other family members are often aware of the abuse
Emotional abuse	Nonphysical, often verbal assault on a child, usually critical, demeaning, and emotionally devastating	Parent or other adult blames, belittles, rejects, or persistently demonstrates lack of concern for the child's welfare.

sources for at-risk families and their children. Nursing leadership continues to advocate with other health and human service professionals for an integrated system that provides access to basic health care and preventive services for all those in need.

BACKGROUND

Kempe coined the term *battered child syndrome* in 1962 to describe a "clinical condition in young children who have received serious physical abuse, generally from a parent or foster parent" (Kempe, Silverman, Steele, Drogmeuller, & Silver, 1962, p. 17). This description was further delineated in 1974 when Congress passed PL 93-247, which defines child abuse and neglect as

> the physical or mental injury, sexual abuse, negligent treatment or maltreatment of a child under the age of eighteen by a person who is responsible for the child's welfare under the circumstances which indicate that the child's health or welfare is harmed or threatened thereby. (Child Abuse Prevention and Treatment Act, 1974, p. 4)

This general definition actually encompasses four distinct types of child maltreatment, including physical abuse, neglect, sexual abuse, and emotional abuse (Table 89-1). Traditionally, there has been a singular approach to assessing, diagnosing, and treating each of these types of child maltreatment. However, current clinical thinking suggests that maltreated children are likely to be subjected to multiple forms of abuse and neglect (Burgess, Hartman, & Kelley, 1990).

Child maltreatment is a complex, destructive phenomenon that cuts across all sectors of society. Results of the Annual Fifty State Survey (42 states actually provided data) indicate that 3.1 million cases of child maltreatment were reported in 1994, up 4.5% from 1993 (Wiese & Daro, 1995). The average substantiation rate was 33%, with 16 of every 1,000 U.S. children found to be victims of child maltreatment following investigation. Child neglect continued to represent the most common reported and substantiated form of maltreatment. The distribution of substantiated cases included neglect (49%), physical abuse (21%), sexual abuse (11%), emotional maltreatment (3%), and other (16%) (Fig. 89-1). Increasingly, cases have been noted as "other," which may indicate a tendency of workers to use this classification when multiple forms of maltreatment are present or when the family is involved in substance abuse (Wiese & Daro, 1995).

An estimated 1,271 children died from abuse or neglect in 1994, with the rate of fatalities for children under 5 years of age at 6.6 per 100,000 (Wiese & Daro, 1995). Data from annual surveys between 1992 and 1994 indicate that 42% of the child victims died as a result of neglect, 54% died from abuse, and 5% died as a result of both forms of maltreatment. When data from 3 years of annual surveys were examined, it was found that 88% of maltreatment fatalities involved children who were under 5 years of age, while 46% involved infants under the age of 1. These figures most likely represent the lowest esti-

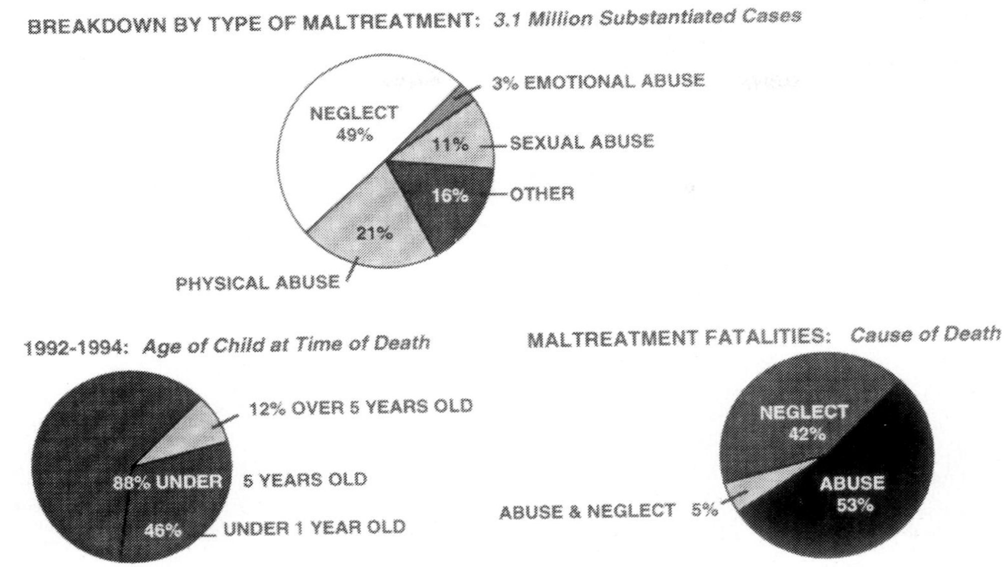

Fig. 89-1. 1994 substantiated cases of child maltreatment in the US. (Statistics from: Wiese D and Daro D [1995]. *Current trends in child abuse reporting and fatalities: The results of the 1994 annual fifty state survey.* Chicago: National Committee to Prevent Child Abuse. Working Paper Number 808.)

mate of the problem because they depend on the level of involvement of child protective services, the varying levels of comprehensive investigation into child mortality cases by local authorities, and classification variances among the states in reporting deaths due to child abuse (Mitchell, 1987).

The increased use of drugs and alcohol by caregivers has been noted as a primary factor in the increase in child maltreatment levels, with an average of 35% of substantiated cases involving substance abuse (Wiese & Daro, 1995). A well-known result of increased substance abuse by women is the growing number of infants born exposed to illegal substances that were ingested by their mothers during pregnancy. Estimates on the scope of this problem vary substantially depending on the type of substance ingested. One to three infants per 1,000 live births are afflicted with fetal alcohol syndrome (Petrakis, 1987). Nine thousand infants per year are born to opiate addicted women with well over 300,000 children exposed to heroine or methadone in utero, and an additional 375,000 infants are born to cocaine users each year (Hoegerman & Schnoll, 1991). In the 1994 annual survey, 14 states reported a total of 7,469 drug-exposed infants. While no state requires the uniform testing of infants for drug exposure, as of 1994 at least 27 states require health-care professionals to report drug-exposed newborns (Wiese & Daro, 1995).

The economic and human costs of maltreatment in America are astronomical. It is likely that billions of dollars are spent in treatment and social-service costs and lost in lessened productivity for a generation of maltreated children (Cicchetti & Carlson, 1989). The human costs include a litany of death, morbidity, and psychological tragedies. For many of the victims, the emotional damage due to maltreatment lasts a lifetime.

Theoretical perspectives on the causes and correlates of child abuse are many and varied (Cicchetti & Carlson, 1989). The inability of the one-dimensional models to address the known characteristics of child abuse adequately has resulted in multidimensional models of child maltreatment. One such attempt in this direction has been proposed by Garbarino (1977; 1980) in his Ecological Model of Child Maltreatment, which in turn derives from Bronfenbrenner's (1977) Ecological Model of Human Development. Garbarino's model is a paradigm for examining the complex interactions among parental and child characteristics, intra- and extrafamilial stressors, and the social and cultural systems that affect families. The model offers a framework for considering available supports and resources in relation to a topology of four levels that have

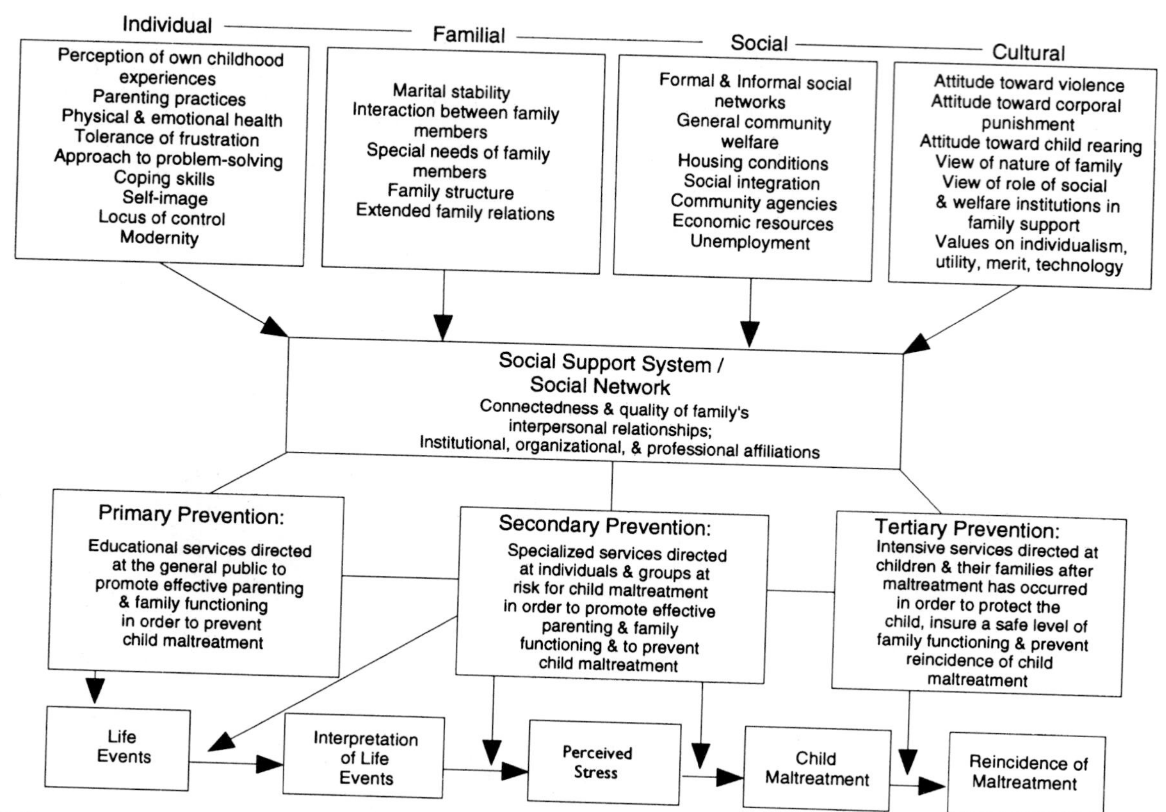

Fig. 89-2. The ecological model of child maltreatment: implications for prevention. (Adapted from Howze DC and Kotch JB [1984]. *Disentangling life events, stress, and social support: implications for the primary prevention of child abuse and neglect.* Child Abuse and Neglect, 8(4), 401-9. Reprinted with permission of Pergamon Press Ltd., Oxford, UK)

been adapted to include individual, familial, social, and cultural (Howze & Kotch, 1984). In addition, the model provides a framework for understanding the relationships among stress, social support systems, and child maltreatment and is here adapted to provide guidance to child abuse prevention efforts (Fig. 89-2). According to Garbarino and Sherman (1980), it is the unmanageability of the stress which is the most crucial factor, and this unmanageability is a product of a mismatch between the level of stress and the availability and potency of social support.

NURSING'S ROLE

The nurse's role in assessment of at-risk families

Maternal-child nurses, pediatric nurses, community nurses, emergency-room nurses, and school nurses have the direct opportunity to identify at-risk families. Thus, nurses should be aware of the high-risk indicators that signal potential child maltreatment. Equally important, they must have enough confidence in their assessment findings to take responsibility for translating their assessments into interventions that may involve a host of other specialties and agencies. Their role as advocate for the child and family is often the critical determinant of whether at-risk families are identified and receive the services they need.

The importance of early identification and intervention lies in its potential for reducing or preventing the occurrence of child abuse. Variables describing particular families at risk have been reported in the literature and can be classified into four separate domains: sociocultural, family, parents, and child characteristics (Garbarino, 1977; Garbarino & Sherman, 1980) (Table 89-2). Stress arising from these domains may be situational, acute, or chronic in nature. While some variables within each domain may appear entrenched, there are two fundamental

Table 89-2 Risk factors associated with child maltreatment

Socio-cultural	Family	Caretaker	Child
Acceptance of corporal punishment of children Depletion of economic resources in the community Economic stress, poverty, underemployment Homelessness Inadequate support and educational services Lack of or restricted access to health care Lack of respite and crisis child care Limited or unavailable prevention services in the community Low priority for parenthood education and training programs	Geographical or social isolation from family and friends Harsh discipline strategies and lack of positive parenting behavior Life stress and distress Low rate of positive interaction among family members Marital discord, conflict, or domestic violence Negative family interactions and problems Poor problem-solving abilities Unequal burden on one parent for childrearing, typically the mother	Depression Fears, disturbances of affect, poor peer relationships, and other symptoms associated with victimization as a child Lack of knowledge of normal growth and development Limited or dysfunctional coping skills Limited financial and household management skills Low self-esteem, poor motivation, poor impulse control, or limited social competencies Poor physical health Psychological problems associated with being abused or rejected as a child (excessive hostility, anger, unhappiness, rigidity, distress, flattened affect) Role reversal, expectations that the child will meet the caretakers needs Stress-related symptoms that affect emotional or physical health Substance abuse Unrealistically high expectations of the child	A child engaged in protracted crying Children 5 years of age or younger, particularly children younger than 1 year Children with significantly more major and minor health problems in the first year of life Children with subtle developmental abnormalities, such as attention deficits Infants or children with feeding problems Preterm, low-birth-weight, or handicapped infants Seriously ill newborns Teenagers 15 to 17 years of age, particularly boys Twins

truisms to remember: (1) multifaceted problems require multidisciplinary interventions (i.e., you're not in this alone), and (2) even slight remediation of stressors may change the individual's perception of those stressors (i.e., you're doing more good than you know). As nurses we not only provide assessment and treatment for at-risk families, but we also offer valuable consultation on the physical and psycho-emotional indicators and effects of child maltreatment, parent-child interactions, a parent's ability to care for his or her child, and parenting stress levels.

Several tools are available to assist nurses in assessing and evaluating at-risk families. However, it should be noted that to date research has not indicated that there are any factors that are present in all abusing parents and absent in all nonabusing parents (Wolfe, 1987). The Child Abuse Potential Inventory is a 160-item, client-administered screening device that was determined to correctly classify 82.7% of known abusive parents in a retrospective study (Milner, Gold, & Wimberley, 1986). Abidin's (1990) Parenting Stress Inventory consists of 101 items that measure the amount of stress experienced by the parent as a result of the parenting role, and it also includes a life stress scale. The Nursing Child Assessment by Satellite Training assessment tool consists of 73 items that were developed to evaluate critical features in parent-infant interactions (Barnard & Bee, 1984). The Checklist for Child Abuse Evaluation (Petty, 1995) is a 264-item tool used for investigation and evaluation of children and adolescents who may have been maltreated. Clinicians may use the entire checklist or only applicable sections, including emotional abuse, sexual abuse, physical abuse, neglect, and treatment recommendations and issues. Mc-Coy's (1995) Sexual Abuse Screening Inventory is a 61-item checklist within eight behavior categories that can be very helpful in routine screening of children entering day camps, group homes, or emergency shelters.

Browne (1989) developed a 13-item checklist based on known risk factors and conducted a retrospective study involving a matched sample of 62 known abusing families and 124 known nonabusing families. Nurse Health Visitors, in conjunction with professional colleagues, completed the checklist for both groups. Interestingly, while the tool could correctly classify 86% of the cases, the best predictor of child maltreatment was the health visitor's perception of whether the parent was indifferent, intolerant, or overanxious. The author concludes that perinatal screening for child maltreatment should have at least three stages: (1) screening for stressful social and demographic characteristics resulting in identification of a target group for further screening, (2) screening of the target group 3 to 6 months after birth for their perception of the newborn and their perceived parenting and life stress, and (3) assessment of the infant's attachment to the primary caregiver and parental sensitivity to the infant's behavior 9 to 12 months after birth.

The nurse's role in recognizing child maltreatment

Nurses who work with children and their families have a unique role in detecting child maltreatment, particularly with regard to the physical and developmental manifestations of the child and the interaction patterns between the parent(s) and the child. Nurses can often identify maltreatment during their initial physical examination of the child or their history interview with the child and parent(s). Their background in child growth and development is superior to that of most social workers, and thus it is their expertise that often forms the basis for questions that arise related to the child's behavior or the parent-child interaction patterns.

Although the physical indicators of child maltreatment may be mild to severe, they are usually readily observable to the experienced practitioner. Nurses are knowledgeable of the range of developmentally appropriate behavior expected of children, and they are quick to notice behaviors that fall outside of this range. Behavioral indicators of maltreatment may exist alone or may accompany physical indicators. They may appear as subtle clues that something is amiss, or they may raise questions that leave one with the "something is not right here" mindset. The role of the informed inquisitor is absolutely fundamental to the assessment of child maltreatment.

The list of physical and behavioral indicators displayed in Table 89-3 is not intended to be exhaustive; many more indicators exist and can be included. Although a single indicator does not necessarily prove that child maltreatment is occurring, the repeated occurrence of an indicator, the presence of several indicators, or the appearance of serious injury or suspicious death should alert the nurse to the possibility of maltreatment.

The involvement of the nurse is typically initiated because of the child's need for acute or preventive health-care services. When it is necessary to interview the child concerning possible maltreatment, nurses must keep in mind that the child may be hurt, in pain, fearful, or confused and may have been threatened not to say anything. Because children vary in their linguistic and interactive competence, it cannot be assumed that interviewing methods suitable for adults will work with children (Garbarino et al., 1989). Additional factors that must be considered include the child's cognitive development, psychological competence, language development, level of socialization, and cultural background. In general, it is important to start with openness, a good basis in child development, and an empathetic approach. Basic techniques include using sentences with only three to five more words than the number of words in the child's average sentence, using names rather than pronouns, using the child's terms, asking the child to repeat what you have said, rephrasing questions that the child does not understand, avoiding asking young children questions involving a time sequence, not responding to every answer with another question, and being careful in interpreting responses to very specific questions because children are apt to be very literal (Garbarino et al., 1989).

The parents' behavior and attitudes and the history of the injury can offer valuable clues to the presence of child maltreatment and can provide direction for interventions that address the family's needs (Table 89-4). In discussing suspicions of child maltreatment with the parents, the point of departure will most likely be the presenting problems of the child. The tone of the discussion should be professional, nonjudgmental, and supportive. Some common guidelines include: (1) conducting the interview in private with everyone sitting down; (2) being professional, direct, and honest and never displaying anger, repugnance, or shock; (3) being attentive and supportive; (4) collecting information and not trying to prove maltreatment by making accusations; (5) explaining that you must make a referral to Child Protective Services and explaining the process; (6) documenting in detail your assessment of the child, your observations of the parents, and your conversation with the parent; and (7) making the referral.

The nurse's role in preventive interventions

Nursing interventions in child maltreatment cover a broad spectrum of roles and approaches throughout the family lifespan. Different levels of family functioning require adaptations in the nursing role, therapeutic approach, and helping activities (Table 89-5). Primary pre-

Table 89-3 Physical and behavioral indicators of child maltreatment

Type of maltreatment	Physical/environmental indicators	Child behavioral indicators
Neglect	*Abandonment* or *emotional neglect:* Inadequate age-appropriate emotional support; parents emotionally distant or unavailable; bald patches on infant's scalp; physical delays *Nutritional neglect:* Inadequate age-appropriate food and fluids; inadequate growth or failure to thrive; dehydration; starvation; wasting of subcutaneous tissue *Health care neglect:* Inadequate basic preventive care during illnesses, timely visits to health professional, and/or maintenance of professionally prescribed health care routines for acute and chronic illnesses; indicators include: • Lack of immunization documentation; contraction of a preventable disease • Failure to seek dental treatment for visually untreated caries, oral infections, and pain • Failure to seek vision, hearing, or speech assessment when indicators of problems are present • Repeated failure to keep appointments for routine and follow-up care • Advanced stage of acute illness related to failure to seek initial treatment • Persistence or worsening of a symptom that should improve with treatment or medication • Failure to administer medications or infrequent administration as evidenced by laboratory testing, lack of a known side effect of medication, delay or failure to fill a prescription, lack of request for medication refills, and unused medications • Incomplete dietary records or medication journals for children with chronic diseases such as diabetes or phenylketonuria • Frequent exacerbations in chronic illness that are not consistent with the severity of disease pathology • Worn out or lack of wear of special shoes or braces • Reports from home visitors of children who are technology-dependent that needed equipment is dirty, frequently contaminated, not used, or used infrequently • Reports from siblings that caretakers either refuse or inconsistently provide prescribed treatment such as chest physical therapy, dietary regimens, medications, or dressing changes • Mortality related to aspiration, asthma, dehydration, diabetic ketoacidosis, hemorrhage, meningitis, pneumonia, or sepsis *Physical neglect:* Chaotic family lifestyle; deterioration in most areas of family functioning; indicators include: • Substandard housing; homelessness • Practically nonexistent housekeeping; living areas littered with rotting food, garbage, and animal feces; environmental hazards present and accessible • No routine for ADL's; emotional indifference to child's well-being • Children sleeping on floor mattresses without sheets/blankets; • Children bathed on an irregular basis; may be encrusted with dirt and have foul odors • Dirty, ragged, ill-fitting children's clothes that are inappropriate for extreme weather conditions • Children left unattended; inadequate supervision even when caretakers are present	• Apathy, watchfulness, or wariness • Assuming adult roles and responsibilites • Begging; stealing food • Cognitive and social developmental delays • Constant fatigue or listlessness • Extended stays at school in young children (early arrival/ late departure) • Inappropriate affection seeking; needy personality • Infants with stiff body position; resistance to being held • Truancy in older children • States there is no caretaker • Substance abuse; delinquency; criminal activity

Table 89-3—cont'd. Physical and behavioral indicators of child maltreatment

Type of maltreatment	Physical/environmental indicators	Child behavioral indicators
	• Injuries and fatalities related to falls; corrosive, hydrocarbon, and lead poisonings; prescription or illegal drug/alcohol ingestions; burns related to playing with matches; deaths due to drowning, electrocution, poisonings; burns and smoke inhalations associated with house fires; strangulation; choking; falls from windows; and gun accidents *Supervision neglect:* Inadequate guidance and protection of children, including protection from environmental hazards such as poisons, electrical sockets, guns, and standing water; parent may be in the home but impaired due to substance abuse, physical or mental illness, low intelligence, or immaturity, or may delegate their children's care to an inadequate caretaker	
Physical abuse	*Unexplained bruises and welts:* Located on eyes, mouth, lips, torso, buttocks, genitalia, thighs, and calves; injuries might be in shape of object used to produce them (e.g., sticks, belts, hair brushes, buckles); regularly appear after absence, weekend, vacation *Unexplained lacerations or abrasions:* To mouth, lips, gums, eyes, genitals; in various stages of healing; human bite marks of adult size *Burns* *Pattern burns:* Suggest object used (e.g., iron, stove grate, electric burner) *Circular burns:* On feet, face, hands, chest, or buttocks suggestive cigar/cigarette *Immersion burns:* "Socklike, glovelike or donutlike" appearence from area being immersed in very hot water or oil, typically arms, legs, buttocks *Friction burns:* Result from rope friction on legs, arms, neck, or torso *Unexplained fractures* Of skull, face, nose, long bones; multiple or spiral fratures caused by twisting motion; shaft fractures from direct blows; fractures in various stages of healing *Head injuries* Blows to head typically causing intracranial, subdural, and intraventricular hemorrhaging; whiplash-shaken infant syndrome typically causing intracranial, subdural, & intraoccular hemorrhaging; child presented nonresponsive or apneic *Munchausen syndrome by proxy* Illness simulated or produced by parent or someone in parental role; acute symptoms abate when child is separated from perpetrator; disease that is resistent to treatment and signs and symptoms are changing	• Afraid to go home • Apprehensive when other children cry • Behavioral extremes: aggressiveness/withdrawal • Capable of only superficial relationships • Feels deserving of punishment • Frightened of parents • Inappropriate or precocious maturity • Indiscriminately seeks affection; needy personality • Lies very still while surveying surroundings • Manipulative behavior to get attention • No age-appropriate separation anxiety • Nonreactive to painful procedures • Poor self-concept • Reports injury by parents • Responds to questions in monosyllables • Vacant or frozen stare • Wary of adult contacts
Sexual abuse	Acquired sexually transmitted diseases Difficulty in walking or sitting Dramatic change in previously well-managed chronic illness Genital or anal injuries or lacerations Masked complaints: genital symptoms, straddle injuries, constipation Poor sphincter tone Pregnancy Recurrent urinary tract infections Reddened or traumatized genitals Psychosomatic complaints Torn, stained, or bloody underclothing	• Betrayal feelings: anger, grief, depression, dependency; impaired ability to trust others • Poor peer relationships • Sense of powerlessness/hopelessness: anxiety, fear, phobias, nightmares, insomnia, hypervigilance, aggressive behavior; change in school performance; delinquency or running away

Table 89-3—cont'd. Physical and behavioral indicators of child maltreatment

Type of maltreatment	Physical/environmental indicators	Child behavioral indicators
		• Sophisticated sexual knowledge; sexualization; prostitution • Stigmatization: feelings of guilt, shame, isolation, low self-esteem, suicidal idealization; self-injurious behaviors; substance abuse • Sudden massive weight loss or gain • Unwilling to change for gym • Withdrawal and fantasy
Emotional abuse	Nonorganic failure-to-thrive Lags in physical development Physical developmental delays Speech disorders	• Attempted suicide • Behavior extremes • Cognitive developmental lags • Conduct/learning disorders • Habit disorders • Neurotic traits/psychoneurotic reactions

Table 89-4 Caretaker behavioral indicators of abuse on admission

Unexplained injury	Caretakers can't explain the injury; their explanation of the injury is vague or evasive; or their explanation is at variance with the child's actual injury.
Alleged self-inflicted injury	Caretakers allege that a very young child deliberately injured him- or herself or was injured because he or she engaged in behavior inappropriate for the child's developmental level.
Alleged third-party injury	Caretakers blame the child's injury on someone else, such as a neighbor, friend, or relative; a common allegation is that a sibling or another child caused the injury.
Delay in seeking medical attention	Caretakers do not immediately obtain medical care for the child following injury.
Discrepant history of injury	Caretakers explanations of the child's injury conflict in terms of date, time, or cause. There is discrepancy between physical findings and the date of the injury or between the injury and the child's developmental level. Parent's explanation of injury conflicts with the child's explanation of injury (if the child is verbal).

vention of child maltreatment includes all interventions that prevent the maltreatment of children, while secondary preventive interventions are focused on at-risk families and their children, and tertiary interventions are directed at preventing further injury or harm to children who have been maltreated. As health and social resources continue to be eliminated, more children are likely to be identified for the first time at the tertiary level.

Community-wide prevention efforts that are directed at each phase of the family life cycle, beginning with the prenatal period and continuing through a child's school years, have been identified as the most promising child maltreatment preventive interventions (Cohn, 1983). Two national research conferences on child abuse prevention, sponsored by the National Committee for Prevention of Child Abuse, identified several key life cycle child abuse prevention approaches: (1) support programs for new parents such as home health visitor and adolescent parenting programs, (2) parenting education programs, and (3) child care opportunities such as respite care services and crisis nurseries (Cohn, 1983).

Both home-based and center-based programs have demonstrated a wide range of positive client outcomes. Studies have identified gains that included improved mother-infant bonding and maternal capacity to respond to the child's emotional needs (Affholter, Connell, & Nauta, 1983; Dickie and Gerber, 1980; Field, Widmayer, Stringer, & Ignatoff, 1980; O'Connor, Vietze, Sherrod, Sandler, & Altemeier, 1980); demonstrated ability to care for the child's physical and developmental needs (Field

Table 89-5 Nursing roles and therapeutic approaches in supporting families at risk for child maltreatment

Family levels	*Infancy:* Chaotic family, barely surviving, inadequate provision of physical and emotional supports; alienation from community, deviant behavior, distortion and confusion of roles, immaturity, child neglect, depression, failure	*Childhood:* Intermediate family, slightly above survival level, variation in economic provisions, alienation but with more ability to trust; child neglect not as great, defensive but slightly more willing to accept help	*Adolescence:* Normal family but with many conflicts and problems, variation in economic levels, greater trust and ability to seek and use help; parents more mature, but still have emotional conflicts; family has successes and achievements and is more willing to seek solutions to problems, future oriented	*Adulthood:* Family has solutions, is stable and healthy with fewer conflicts or problems, very capable providers of physical and emotional supports; parents mature and confident, fewer difficulties in training children, able to seek help, future-oriented, enjoy the present	*Maturity:* Ideal family, homeostatic balance between individual and group goals and activities; family meets its tasks and roles well and is able to seek appropriate help when needed
Nurse's role	*Nurturing* to provide for health and safety needs of children and family	*Collaborating* to identify and plan to meet health needs	*Facilitating* family to follow through on health concerns	*Enabling* family to maintain health	*Consulting* with families to resolve problems/ crises as they arise
Therapeutic approach and helping activities	Establishment of a trusting relationship using acceptance, patience, warm support, consistency, clarification of role, and limit setting • Constant evaluation of relationships and progress; child safety, growth, and development, and family violence • Mobilization of community resources that address basic needs • Multidisciplinary team coordination	Based on trusting relationship; uses counseling and interpersonal skills to help family begin to understand itself and define problems; uses honesty, genuineness, and encourages self-evaluation • Frequent monitoring of child safety, growth and development; presence and level of family violence • Referrals to community agencies to address specific needs identified (i.e., substance abuse, marriage counseling) • Monitoring of family compliance with basic-needs referrals	Anticipatory guidance and assistance; provide information and teaching, coordinate referrals and teamwork; help family make decisions and find solutions to problems • Monitor child safety, growth and development, and family functioning on an enhanced schedule • Initiate preventive health services for all family members • Make referrals to community agencies that provide specialized services, such as home visitation, parenting education, respite and crisis child care, family counseling, and job training	Preventive teaching that identifies needs and anticipated problem areas and provides information and teaching • Monitor child safety, growth and development, and family functioning during routine care • Schedule preventive health maintenance for all family members • Provide information on how to access available resources	Assist families to identify relevant factors, potential solutions, and resources for facing situational crises and restoring equilibrium • Continue scheduled preventive health maintenance • Monitor child safety, growth and development, and family functioning during routine care

et al., 1980; Gabinet, 1979; Gray, 1983; Gutelius, Kirsch, MacDonald, Brooks, & McErlean, 1977; Larson, 1980; Love, Nauta, Coelen, Hewett, & Ruopp, 1976; Olds, Chamberlin, & Tatlebaum, 1982; Travers, Nauta, & Irwin, 1982); fewer subsequent unintended pregnancies (McAnarney et al., 1978; Badger, 1981; Olds et al., 1986); more consistent use of health-care services and job-training opportunities (Powell, 1986); and decreased welfare use, higher school completion rates, and higher employment rates (Gutelius et al., 1977; Badger, 1981; Seitz et al., 1985; Powell, 1986). In identifying the types of parents most likely to benefit from these educational and supportive services, several investigators have noted particular success with young, relatively poor mothers (Gabinet, 1979; Badger, 1981; Olds et al., 1986) and with mothers who felt confident in their lives prior to enrolling in the program (Powell, 1986).

A recent extensive study of the effectiveness of home health visitor programs reviewed randomized trials of prenatal and infancy home-visitation programs for socially disadvantaged women and children (Olds & Kitzman, 1990). The results of this study indicated that some home-visitation programs were effective in the following areas: (1) improving women's health-related behaviors during pregnancy, the birth weight and length of gestation of babies born to smokers and young adolescents, parents' interaction with their children, and children's developmental status; (2) reducing the incidence of child maltreatment, childhood behavioral problems, emergency department visits and hospitalizations for injury, and unintended subsequent pregnancies; and (3) increasing mothers' participation in the workforce (Olds & Kitzman, 1990).

The authors noted that home-visit programs with the greatest chances of success have the following three characteristics: (1) They are based either explicitly or implicitly on ecological models; (2) They are designed to address the ecology of the family during pregnancy and early childbearing years with nurse home visitors who establish a therapeutic alliance with the families; and (3) They are targeted toward families at greater risk for maternal and child health problems by virtue of their poverty and lack of personal and social resources (Olds & Kitzman, 1990).

A review evaluating studies that were undertaken from 1978 through 1988 concluded that three primary issues must be addressed in future studies if we are to expand our knowledge of prevention. These issues included formal evaluation of impact including who it benefited, evaluation of change in the rate of occurrence, and assessment of the efficacy of program interventions directed at preventing child maltreatment versus their role in meeting broader societal needs (Fink & McCloskey, 1990).

The continuity of nursing care between and among care settings is essential for effective nursing intervention with at-risk families. Many care-mapping and case-management models of care have been developed in response to cost-containment measures. If these models functioned to organize and integrate available services on behalf of at-risk families, they could provide structure to continuity efforts. However, some delivery systems are precipitously moving families between acute and community settings without regard to the continuity of nursing care needed between these modalities. Advanced nurse practitioners who coordinate their clients' care have the ability to follow their clients' progress across settings. Unfortunately, there are currently not enough of these practitioners strategically placed to address the fragmented care that is a current professional issue.

In order to link knowledge about diagnoses, treatments, and outcomes and to facilitate the ability of nurses to articulate their professional activities, nurses must become adept at contributing to and using the Nursing Intervention Classification system (Bulechek & McCloskey, 1992). The continued evolution of this system offers hope to nurses working with at-risk families in all practice settings that their care activities can be communicated, linked, mandated, and reimbursed.

The nurses' role on the multidisciplinary team

The multidisciplinary approach to diagnosing, evaluating, and planning the treatment of victims of child abuse and neglect has been widely advocated and adopted by hospitals and community-based protective service teams (National Center on Child Abuse and Treatment, 1975). One of the primary purposes of this approach is to reduce the fragmentation of the service delivery system through coordination of professional activities both within and between agencies and organizations. Additional services typically include consultation, case management, and provision of current information concerning child abuse to other professionals or agencies.

The team is typically composed of representatives from nursing, pediatric medicine, psychology, psychiatry, social work, and child life, with each discipline providing a unique perspective and specialized interventions. Traditionally, the coordinator of these interventions has been the representative from pediatric medicine. However, the professional nurse is in a prime position in most instances to initiate, coordinate, and evaluate the multidisciplinary approach to the care of violent families (Campbell & Humphreys, 1984). Nurses are in a much less threatening position to elicit information because they are generally perceived by the family as helpful rather than bureaucratic or authoritative. The case management that forms the basis of the multidisciplinary approach is an extension of the coordination and advocacy that is paramount to the nursing role. Clinical specialists with a background in maternal-child, pediatric, family, or community nursing are well suited to assume a leadership position in this area.

The nurse's role as a mandatory reporter

Child abuse legislation in each state mandates the reporting of suspected child maltreatment and broadly sets forth the process through which reporting occurs. In general, these processes describe the conditions for reporting, who reports, where reports are filed, and the legal protection afforded the reporter. Most states currently mandate that nurses report child maltreatment. However, because of the diversity in laws, particularly with regard to definitions, nurses should obtain a copy of their particular state's reporting statute and study its provisions carefully.

Typically, most state statutes require reports to be filed when there is "reason to believe" or "reasonable cause to suspect" that maltreatment may be occurring. While no state requires the reporter to have proof that maltreatment has occurred, most require that the report be made "in good faith" (McKittrick, 1981). To encourage reporting, all states provide at least qualified immunity or protection from legal liability for persons filing a child maltreatment report.

Failure to report suspected child maltreatment may result in civil or criminal penalties. The basis for criminal liability varies among states, and some states impose criminal penalties regardless of whether the failure to report is deliberate or a case of negligence. Other state statutes base liability on a "knowing" or "willful" failure to report and may hold liable the reporter who suspects maltreatment yet deliberately refuses to file a report (Krietzer, 1981). Regardless of the basis for this liability, the criminal charge for failure to report is generally a misdemeanor, and the possible penalties for conviction include fines, imprisonment, or both (Allen & Hollowell, 1990).

Civil liability can be brought for damages proximately caused by failure to report. The landmark case of civil liability for failure to report was a 1976 decision of the California Supreme Court, which held that a physician who fails to report suspected child maltreatment can be exposed to liability for subsequent injuries to the child on the theory of medical malpractice (*Landeros v. Flood*, 1976). This case involved a California physician who failed to report the injuries of an 11-month-old child, including a spiral fracture of her tibia and fibula, bruises over her entire back, superficial abrasions on other parts of her body, and an earlier, nondepressed linear skull fracture. Several months later the child sustained further injury, and a different physician reported these injuries as suspected child maltreatment. Following this second incident, the child brought an action against the initial examining physician for failure to diagnose the battered child syndrome properly and to report that diagnosis to the proper authorities. Under the law, a nurse having a similar opportunity to observe suspected child maltreatment would be equally liable for failure to report (Krietzer, 1981); and in child maltreatment cases, a successful malpractice claim would not be covered by malpractice insurance (Allen & Hollowell, 1990).

Record keeping or the documentation of evidence is vital because it substantiates the basis for reasonable belief and provides the legal basis for state intervention on behalf of the child. Nursing history, assessments, interventions, and referrals are considered germane to the diagnosis and treatment of the child and therefore qualify as admissible during a court hearing. Entries should be recorded immediately following contact with the family because they are admissible evidence only if they are recorded at or near the time of the event (Krietzer, 1981). Documentation should reflect accuracy, timeliness, and objectivity and should be devoid of feelings or conclusions that are made without documented evidence.

Nursing's role in specialty tracks in family abuse

Although a great deal of information related to child maltreatment has been compiled over the past 30 years, it is generally reported that academic training for professionals such as nurses, physicians, psychologists, attorneys, and social workers has not kept pace with the demands for expertise (Alpert & Paulson, 1990; Polk & Brown, 1988; Sevel, 1989). In response to the lack of university graduate programs in child abuse and neglect, the National Center on Child Abuse and Neglect (NCCAN) initiated a national effort to institutionalize interdisciplinary graduate training in child maltreatment (Gallmeier & Bonner, 1992). In 1987, 10 universities were selected by the NCCAN to receive $150,000 per year for 3 years to establish interdisciplinary graduate training programs in child abuse and neglect. These universities included Indiana University, New York University, Ohio State University, Temple University, University of California at San Diego, University of Michigan, University of Oklahoma, University of Pittsburgh, and University of South Carolina.

The training programs are designed for graduate and postgraduate students sufficiently trained in their own disciplines to benefit from interdisciplinary education in child maltreatment. The programs have collaborated to achieve consistency in the didactic portion of the training and have reached a general consensus regarding the body of information that is necessary for professionals in the field of child maltreatment. All 10 of the universities offer student stipend funds that range from $531 to $7000 per academic year, with an average stipend of $1,959 (Gallmeier & Bonner, 1992). To date a total of 418 students have graduated from this program representing the following disciplines: social work (n = 114), psychology (n = 97), law (n = 56), medicine (n = 36), nursing (n = 29), education (n = 20), and combined others (n = 66) (Gallmeier & Bonner, 1992).

It is generally accepted that child maltreatment is a multifaceted problem that requires multidisciplinary efforts. By virtue of its nature, the variety of its practice settings, and the sheer numbers of its practitioners, nursing can provide leadership in these important efforts.

REFERENCES

Abidin, R.R. (1990). *Parenting stress index.* Charlottesville, VA: Pediatric Psychology Press.

Affholter, D., Connell, D., & Nauta, M. (1983). Evaluation on the child and family resource program: Early evidence of parent-child interaction effects. *Evaluation Review, 7,* 65-79.

Allen, J., & Hollowell, E. (1990, June). Nurses and child abuse/neglect reporting: Duties, responsibilities, and issues. *The Journal of Practical Nursing,* 56-59.

Alpert, J., & Paulson, A. (1990). Graduate-level education and training in child sexual abuse. *Professional Psychology: Research and Practice, 21,* 366-371.

Badger, E. (1981). Effects of a parent education program on teenage mothers and their offspring. In K.G. Scott, T. Field, & E. Robertson (Eds.), *Teenage parents and their offspring* (pp. 283-309). New York: Grune & Stratton.

Barnard, K.E., & Bee, H.L. (1984). The assessment of parent-infant interaction by observation of feeding and teaching. In T.B. Brazelton & H. Als (Eds.), *Behavioral assessment of newborn infants* (pp. 199-218). Hillsdale, NJ: Lawrence Erlbaum Associates.

Bronfenbrenner, U. (1977). Toward an experimental ecology of human development. *American Psychologist, 32,* 513-531.

Browne, K. (1989). The health visitor's role in screening for child abuse. *Health Visitor, 62,* 275-277.

Bulechek, G., & McCloskey, J. (1992). Nursing diagnoses, interventions and outcomes. In G. Bulechek & J. McCloskey (Eds.), *Nursing interventions: Essential nursing treatments.* Philadelphia: Saunders.

Burgess, A., Hartman, C., & Kelley, S. (1990). Assessing child abuse: The TRIADS checklist. *Journal of Psychosocial Nursing & Mental Health Services, 28*(4), 6-8, 10-14.

Campbell, J., & Humphreys, J. (1984). *Nursing care of victims of family violence.* Reston, VA: Reston Publishing Co.

Child Abuse Prevention and Treatment Act of 1974. (1974). Public law 93-247, *U.S. Statutes at Large, 88,* 4-8.

Cicchetti, D., & Carlson, V. (Ed.). (1989). *Child maltreatment: Theory and research on the causes and consequences of child abuse and neglect.* New York: Cambridge University Press.

Cohn, A.H. (1983). *An approach to preventing child abuse.* Chicago: National Committee for the Prevention of Child Abuse.

Dickie, J., & Gerber, S. (1980). Training in social competence: The effects on mothers, fathers, and infants. *Child Development, 51,* 1248-1251.

Field, T., Widmayer, S., Stringer, S., & Ignatoff, E. (1980). Teenage, lower-class, black, mothers and their preterm infants: An intervention and developmental follow-up. *Child Development, 5,* 426-436.

Fink, A., & McCloskey, L. (1990). Moving child abuse and neglect prevention programs forward: Improving program evaluations. *Child Abuse & Neglect, 14,* 187-206.

Gabinet, L. (1979). Prevention of child abuse and neglect in an inner-city population: II. The program and the results. *Child Abuse and Neglect, 3,* 809-817.

Gallmeier, T., & Bonner, B. (1992). University-based interdisciplinary training in child abuse and neglect. *Child Abuse & Neglect, 16,* 513-521.

Garbarino, J. (1977). The human ecology of child maltreatment. *Journal of Marriage and the Family, 39,* 721-735.

Garbarino, J. Stott, F., and the faculty of Erikson Institute. (1989). *What children can tell us.* San Francisco: Jossey-Bass.

Garbarino, J., & Sherman, D. (1980). High-risk neighborhoods and high risk families: The human ecology of child maltreatment. *Child Development, 51,* 188-198.

Gray, E. (1983). *Final report: Collaborative research of community and minority group action to prevent child abuse and neglect, Vol. 1: Perinatal interventions.* Chicago: National Committee for Prevention of Child Abuse.

Gutelius, M., Kirsch, A., MacDonald, S., Brooks, M., & McErlean, T. (1977). Controlled study of child health supervision: Behavioral results. *Pediatrics, 60,* 294-304.

Helfer, R., & Kempe, R. (1987). *The battered child* (4th Ed.). Chicago: The University of Chicago Press.

Hoegerman, G. & Schnoll, S.H. (1991). Narcotics use in pregnancy. *Clinical Perinatol, 18*(1), 57-76.

Howze, D.C., & Kotch, J.B. (1984). Disentangling life events, stress, and social support: Implications for the primary prevention of child abuse and neglect. *Child Abuse & Neglect, 8,* 401-409.

Kempe, H., Silverman, F., Steele, B., Drogmeuller, W., & Silver, H. (1962). The battered-child syndrome. *Journal of the American Medical Association, 181,* 17-24.

Kogan, R., Mann, C., & Super, D. (1995, April 20). *The impact of federal Medicaid cuts: How can states be protected?* Washington, DC: Center On Budget And Policy Priorities.

Krietzer, M. (1981). Legal aspects of child abuse. *Nursing Clinics of North America, 16,* 149-160.

Landeros v. Flood, 17 Cal. 3d 399, 551 P.2d 389 (131 Cal Rptr. 69, 1976).

Larson, C. (1980). Efficacy of perinatal and postpartum home visits on child health and development. *Pediatrics, 66,* 191-197.

Love, J., Nauta, M., Coelen, C., Hewett, K., & Ruopp, R. (1976). *National home start evaluation: Final report, findings and implications.* Ypsilanti, MI: High Scope Educational Research Foundation.

McAnarney, E., Roghmann, K., Adams, B., Tatlebaum, R., Kash, C., Coulter, M., Plume, M., & Charney, E. (1978). Obstetric, neonatal, and psychosocial outcome of pregnant adolescents. *Pediatrics, 61,* 2.

McKittrick, C. (1981). Child abuse: Recognition and reporting by health professionals. *Nursing Clinics of North America, 16,* 103-115.

McCoy, D. (1995). *Sexual abuse screening inventory (SASI).* Odessa, FL: Psychological Assessment Resources, Inc.

Milner, J., Gold, R., & Wimberley, R. (1986). Prediction and explanation of child abuse: Cross-validation of the Child Abuse Potential Inventory. *Journal of Consulting and Clinical Psychology, 54,* 865-866.

Mitchell, L. (1987). *Child abuse and neglect fatalities: A review of the problem and strategies for reform.* Chicago, IL: National Committee for Prevention of Child Abuse.

National Center on Child Abuse and Treatment. (1975). *The community team approach to case management and prevention: Child abuse and neglect, the problem and its management* (Publication #OHD 75-30075). Washington, DC: Department of Health, Education & Welfare.

O'Connor, S., Vietze, K., Sherrod, K., Sandler, H., & Altemeier, W. (1980). Reduced incidence of parenting inadequacy following rooming-in. *Pediatrics, 66,* 176-182.

Olds, D., Chamberlin, R., & Tatlebaum, R. (1986). Preventing child abuse and neglect: A randomized trial of nurse home visitation. *Pediatrics, 78,* 65-78.

Olds, D.L., & Kitzman, H. (1990). Can home visitation improve the health of women and children at environmental risk? *Pediatrics, 86,* 108-116.

Petrakis, P.L. (1987). *Alcohol and birth defects: The fetal alcohol syndrome and related disorders.* [DHHS Publication Number (ADM) 87-1531]. Rockville, MD: U.S. Department of Health and Human Services.

Petty, J. (1995). *Checklist for child abuse evaluation.* Odessa, FL: Psychological Assessment Resources, Inc.

Polk, G., & Brown, B. (1988). Family violence: Development of a master's level specialty track in family abuse. *Journal of Psychosocial Nursing, 26,* 34-37.

Powell, D. (1986). Parent education and support programs. *Young Children, 11,* 47-53.

Seitz, V., Rosenbaum, L., & Aptel, N. (1985). Effects of family support interventions—ten year follow-up. *Child Development, 56,* 376-391.

Sevel, F. (1989). Interprofessional approaches to public policy issues: Graduate program in child abuse and neglect. *Family and Community Health, 12,* 80-82.

Tapia, J.A. (1972). The nursing process in family health. *Nursing Outlook, 20,* 267.

Travers, J., Nauta, M., & Irwin, N. (1982). *The effects of a social program: Final report of the child and family resource program's infant and toddler component.* Cambridge, MA: ABT Associates.

Wolfe, D.A. (1987). *Child abuse: Implications for child development and psychopathology.* Newbury Park, CA: Sage Publications Inc.

Wiese, D., & Daro, D. (1995, April). *Current trends in child abuse reporting and fatalities: The results of the 1994 annual fifty state survey* (Working Paper Number 808). Chicago: NCPCA Publications.

Advance directives—empowerment for patients

DIANE K. KJERVIK

One of the fundamental values of citizens of the United States is an orientation to individualism (autonomy). Individual freedom is seen as the hallmark of a democratic political system. Soldiers have fought and died for freedom from government oppression and for freedom of individuals to say and do what is desired. The Bill of Rights of the U.S. Constitution ensures Americans the freedom to speak their mind, to associate with persons and groups as desired, the right to practice their own religions, and the right to privacy.

Concomitant with the orientation to individual freedom is a corresponding right to make decisions about where one lives, what one does with one's property, and in terms of health care, what one will allow to be done with one's body. As Justice Cardozo stated, "Every human being of adult years and sound mind has a right to determine what shall be done with his own body; and a surgeon who performs an operation without his patient's consent commits an assault, for which he is liable in damages" (*Schloendorff v. Society of New York Hospital*, 1914, pp. 129-130). Assumed in this statement of the law is the necessity of a "sound mind" and the belief that without an affirmation to the opposite, consent is not present. Interestingly, the health-care system assumes more often than the legal system that consent is present unless refusal is noted in "do not resuscitate" orders, advance directives, and communications with providers.

The concept of informed consent has become widely accepted in health-care and legal circles as the standard for entering into a patient–health-care provider contract for services. Part of the reason for implementing informed consent in health care is to empower the patient by providing information about services to be given so that the patient is able to make a more meaningful choice among the available options (Kjervik & Grove, 1988). With knowledge of the options presented in a clear and consistent fashion, the patient becomes aware of his or her ability to participate actively and with authority in the decision-making process. In this way the patient is empowered as an active participant in the decision-making process, and the power imbalance created by the lack of information is redressed (Katz, 1984). A corollary of the right to consent to treatment is the right to refuse treatment (*Cruzan v. Director, Missouri Department of Health*, 1990). Advance directives in the health-care context usually state what the patient does not want done and, in effect, refuses to have done. Nurses are now influencing patients and their families about the use of advance directives and are encouraging patients to use this form of empowerment (Silverman, Fry, & Armistead, 1994).

TYPES OF ADVANCE DIRECTIVES

Advance directives are legal mechanisms that enable a person to make decisions about financial arrangements or health-care services before the occurrence of a situation in which the person is unable to make such decisions. Advance directives enhance individualism by providing a written document signed by the person that indicates what he or she wants done under certain specified circumstances. When properly legally executed, these documents serve as a valid statement of the person's wishes and cannot be invalidated without compelling reasons.

Advance directives include those relating to financial affairs such as wills, trusts, representative payeeships, powers of attorney, and joint tenancy (Weiler, 1989). These financial advance directives provide that a substitute decision maker, such as a personal representative in the case of a will or a trustee in the case of a trust, is empowered to act on behalf the person who executed the document. The purpose of articulating these wishes in advance is that the individual's wishes will predominate, rather than the wishes of persons who are likely to receive direct benefit from the estate of the individual. These legal arrangements have been available for some time to handle financial matters. Directives can also be given to a third party about care for oneself rather than one's property, such as those relating to health care (i.e., the living will and the durable power of attorney for health care).

The *living will* is a document that states that under certain circumstances, such as terminal illness, an individual prefers to have certain choices exercised on his or her behalf. In 1976, California became the first state to enact legislation that allowed advanced decision making for end-of-life situations (Fade, 1995). The typical direction of the living will is that life-sustaining activities such as the provision of food, fluid, and cardiopulmonary respiration are to be withheld so that the person may die a peaceful death. Without this kind of direction, a hospital or independent health-care provider would feel obligated to maintain life for fear of a lawsuit alleging wrongful death. Recently, the New York Office of Mental Health issued a policy encouraging the use of written statements by psychiatric patients who would identify the types of treatments they prefer to receive during crises ("18 Deaths," 1994). A psychiatric crisis can precipitate life-and-death consequences as with other illnesses, and many patients who have been through emergency episodes can identify what works well for them.

The *durable power of attorney for health care* document enables the person to name another person to be a substitute decision maker under the circumstances of impaired functioning on the part of the person executing the document. If the person is impaired to the point of being unable to make decisions, then the substitute decision maker can do so. Most states have enacted laws that provide for the living will and durable power of attorney for health care (Cate & Gill, 1991; "Choice in Dying," 1992). All states except Massachusetts, Michigan, and New York have laws governing living wills, and all states but Alaska and Alabama have statutes that allow appointment of a durable power of attorney for health care (Fade, 1995). The usefulness of these advance directives in assisting clinical decision making is not yet clear. One team of researchers concluded that advance directives were irrelevant to decision making regarding resuscitation of seriously ill patients (Teno et al., 1994).

ETHICAL ASPECTS OF ADVANCE DIRECTIVES

While advance directives are legal mechanisms to support substitute decision making, ethical principles underlie the development of the statutes and the practice related to advance directives. The concept of autonomy, which is a fundamental ethical principle, is closely related to the freedom of the individual to choose what is to be done with his or her body. Likewise, as Faden and Beauchamp (1986) have pointed out, the principles of justice and beneficence are also served by the implementation of informed consent. Katz (1984) discusses the history of silence between physicians and patients that has led to the doctrine of informed consent. Nurses and patients have not experienced the same degree of silence in relation to nursing care. This could be because nursing care involves patient participation and discussion about the implementation of nursing tasks. In addition, nurses have long espoused the importance of mutuality between nurse and patient.

Caring for patients (beneficence) is manifest in the concern for the individual's decision-making capability and the importance of empowering the individual to be part of the decision-making process. To give patients a voice in what happens with their health care is a beneficent act that respects varying human values and recognizes differences among human beings regarding life-and-death matters. To feel compassion for the person who is facing difficult choices exemplifies the ethic of care, a new orientation to ethics that attends to feelings that hold relationships together (Beauchamp & Childress, 1994).

The principle of justice is served by giving all individuals a fair share of attention to their wishes about the prolongation of their lives. Whether a person is rich or poor, black or white should make no difference in the decision about whether or not to end that person's life. Deontologically, the rules to be served by advance directives are those relating to the freedom of the individual to choose what will be done with his or her own body and the value of the individual's life and death. Teleologically, the goal to be served is that of peaceful and dignified death for all patients within the health-care system.

Empowerment is also an ethical concern from the vantage point of coerciveness by a more powerful party in the decision-making process. Coercion or manipulation makes the choices of less powerful individuals meaningless. Cooperation and conflict resolution among human beings is enhanced by empowering all persons in the relationship. In the case of advance directives for health care, empowerment of both nurse and patient is an ethical matter. If the nurse has far more power than the patient in the interactions, the decisions made by the patient are suspect as lacking autonomy. Therefore, the patient must be empowered to speak his or her mind with the nurse as they discuss the decisions to be made. Responsible assertiveness is a communication technique that can assist and empower a client to speak. As Lange and Jakubowski (1976) point out, "responsible assertion means not deliberately using personal power to manipulatively overpower weaker people in conflict situations" (p. 58). Therefore, the more powerful individual has the responsibility to encourage and teach assertive behavior to a less powerful person. An advance directive can strengthen the patient's ability to speak her or his own mind by providing a visible, concrete form of the statement of preference. Nurses are also empowered by advance directives because information is made available to them about the patient's orientation to life and death. This information assist nurses to implement the nursing process. In a recent study, nurses indicated that helping patients with advance directives promoted communication among patients, families, and health-care providers and increased staff knowledge about advance directives (Silverman et al., 1994).

The living will is a clear way of stating what the patient values at a point in time that is outside the time of crisis (i.e., when a patient is admitted to a hospital or nursing home). It is under the circumstances of these critical admissions to a health-care facility that decisions often must be made by the staff and the patient's family without benefit of prior consideration and decision by the patient. Effective December 1991, federal law mandated that hospitals and other health-care facilities inform patients of their rights under state law to have living wills and durable powers of attorney for health care (*Patient Self-Determination Act,* 1990). While it is useful for incoming patients to be informed of these rights, the time of admission is generally not the most fruitful time for development of this thought- and emotion-provoking document. However, the federal mandate to agencies and health-care workers raises their awareness of the importance of these documents to patients, families, and society, and the effect of this attitudinal change is presumably passed on to patients.

Another fundamental ethical issue underlying advance directives is the value placed by society on life. In *Cruzan v. Director, Missouri Department of Health* (1990), it became apparent that U.S. Supreme Court justices were divided on the importance that could be attached to life per se in relation to quality of life. The majority of justices in *Cruzan* believed that life itself was worth preserving and that a state had the right to set the parameters for using advance directives. The minority opinion emphasized quality of life and the right of an individual to determine when that quality of life had deteriorated to the point that intrusive measures were no longer justified.

Considerations of quality of life must always address the question of whom is to determine quality of life. Living wills and durable powers of attorney for health care are premised on the belief that the patient determines what quality of life means to him or her. Others who are willing to be more paternalistic in their orientation believe that quality of life should be determined by either health-care providers or the government. In reality, the quality of one's life can only be ascertained clearly by oneself based on an evaluation of whatever criteria the individual decides constitutes "quality." One's values are a critical element in ascertaining the quality of one's life and can be evaluated with a values history such as that developed by the Center for Health Law and Ethics at the University of New Mexico (Cate & Gill, 1991). A recent study showed that older persons often continue to rely on others to make decisions and so lack enthusiasm about creating advance directives even when they receive written information about them (High, 1993). The recent trend toward surrogate decision-making laws (Fade, 1995) responds to the need some persons have to rely on others to make difficult choices.

OBJECTIONS TO ADVANCE DIRECTIVES

There are several arguments in opposition to advance directives. The first is the paternalistic belief that the health-care provider, usually a physician, knows what is best for the patient. This notion is being eroded by consumer activism and by other health-care providers who are interested in sharing power with other members of the health-care team and their patients. Even the designation of "patient" is undergoing challenge and revision because of its emphasis on a one-up/one-down position between doctor and patient. As consumers become more active and interested in their own health care, they expect to be part of the decision-making process and ultimately to make their own decisions. Certainly, there are rare cases in which individuals do not want to be bothered with decisions about their own health care. However, these cases are less frequent as consumers become more sophisticated about health-care alternatives and therefore more interested in asserting their own voice or relying on a relative who is aware of their preferences. One reason they are interested in asserting their own voice is their experience with inadequate diagnostic and treatment decisions by health-care providers that have resulted in injury to patients and corresponding large medical malpractice awards.

Another argument against living wills asserts that these directives do not reflect an incompetent patient's interests accurately. Because these documents are formulated when the person is competent and presumably has different interests, it is argued that when the person actually becomes incompetent, his or her best interests are served in entirely different ways than what the patient long ago envisioned (Robertson, 1991). Following this line of reasoning, one's will and choice would have to be recorded continuously for a living will or any other form of advance directive to be considered valid. Contracts, wills, and trusts would all have to be invalidated because they were developed before the time that they are acted on. Clearly this is an absurd result that would create tremendous dysfunction in several areas of the law.

A third argument points to research that shows that patients are willing to grant their surrogates leeway in the way the living will is interpreted and do not expect strict adherence to the wishes they have stated in their living wills (Sehgal et al., 1992). The response to this argument is that specification as to which areas of leeway and which principles to be followed can be enumerated, and indeed should be enumerated in the living will itself. Alternatively, the proxy decision maker acting under the durable power of attorney for health care can be instructed orally by the patient as to the leeway to be given. Decisions of the surrogate thus can reflect an accurate and full discussion with the patient.

Probably the most vociferous argument against living wills has been raised in legislative sessions in which opponents warn of a slippery slope between living wills and murder or genocide. This argument can be rebutted by the realization that, as with any other legal contract, the law examines carefully any coercion or manipulation involved with living wills. Therefore, only documents that are the will of the patient are to be followed. No independent judgment by health-care professionals that a given patient or a given group of patients should die would control a situation in which a living will is in effect. The law would not want to reach the absurd result that no contract or other legal document could be entered into if there were any possibility of coercion or manipulation. Ethical and legal rules must be adopted based on their ability to organize human behavior. These rules cannot be controlled by the fear of numerous possibilities of human evil. As far as coercion and manipulation are concerned, to not allow a person to determine what will be done with his or her body during a terminal illness is a form of coercion as well, one in which the outside person decides that the life of another should be preserved at all costs. This argument against living wills also overlooks the fact that some persons indicate in their living wills that they wish every possible means to be used to keep them alive. A slippery slope in the other direction could be imagined in which a patient's wish overrules resource allocation decisions—an equally absurd result.

ADVANCE DIRECTIVES IN RELATION TO NURSING PRACTICE

The nursing process can be enhanced by the use of advance directives. As part of the assessment of the patient's goals in relation to severity of health-care status, the nurse can discuss the provisions of the patient's living will or durable power of attorney for health care. Because members of the health-care team need to respond to provisions of the living will, they must understand the meaning of the document to the patient as well as what the law within their state requires for the document to be considered valid. In a much publicized 1992 case in Texas, the patient and his family were distraught when the patient's living will was not followed by the facility because state law requires that two physicians certify the patient as terminally ill and only one physician had done so (Gamino, 1992). Close work with the attorney for the facility is necessary to make the legal mandates clear to staff and administrators. For example, a values history can give a picture of the patient's beliefs about organ donation, respirators, and independent functioning. If the patient has no advance directive, discussion of personal values may assist the patient in making a choice to execute a living will. Knowing the patient's belief about artificial extension of life, the nurse can plan and implement care that is respectful of the patient.

Care can be evaluated according to standards developed by the patient in addition to those imposed from the outside that have to do with technical choices such as which antihypertensive drug to prescribe. If the patient chooses to have no heroic measures exercised, the nurse will be present to assist with comfort measures. Interventions in the direction of this goal, rather than the goal of preserving life, might create moral conflict for some nurses. In the future, nurses may be called on to take a more active role in assisting with death (Johnson &

Weiler, 1990). Nursing must take an active part in the debate about aid in dying, because without doubt, nurses will be called on to play a close, active role in the process. The American Nurses Association (ANA) recently released a statement about nurse-assisted suicide in which it makes clear that direct assistance with suicide is not an accepted standard in nursing (ANA, 1994). Interestingly, however, carrying out the patient's wishes for withdrawal of treatment as specified in a written advance directive is legally and ethically acceptable.

Nurses are moral agents who are responsible for their own conduct. As Theis (1990) notes, "To conceive of the nurse as one who simply follows directives without moral reflection concerning the treatment being rendered fails to recognize the moral status of the nurse as an individual with standards of personal conscience and professional ethics" (pp. 445-450). The nurse cannot assist the patient to examine values without having a sense of his or her own values. Therefore, part of the process of caring for patients involves self-reflection and decision making about how one views one's own life and death. Nurses can act as role models for behaviors considered valuable for their patients (e.g., by having their own living wills) (Weber & Kjervik, 1992). Because the range of persons with advance directives ranges from less than 10% of the general public to 28% of AIDS patients (Crisham, 1990; Teno et al., 1994), nurses' role modeling is especially important.

Patients who have advance directives demonstrate health-promoting behaviors. By stating their values and preferences in writing, they show the strength to be active participants in the maintenance of their health rather than passive observers and recipients of the preferences of others. In the process of preparing an advance directive, the patient imagines his or her own possible incapacitation. Through the use of this imagery, the patient is able to consider all alternatives, including the opportunity to have a choice over life and death options. The act of imagining and then creating a written statement of choice is strengthening to patients, who often feel like victims in the health-care setting.

Advance directives also act as preventive measures. Just as primary prevention in health care means the practice of health-promoting and disease-preventing behaviors, risk management in the law means preventing legal difficulties. Advance directives prevent legal problems when the viewpoint of the patient may be at issue. Economically, respecting the patient's choice may reduce escalating health-care costs by ruling out a number of expensive procedures. As Katz (1984) suggests, "first patient opinions" may be less costly than "second medical opinions" (p. 228).

The encouragement of advance directives may also provide an opportunity for nurses to apply a relational ethic of care. Parker (1990) describes this ethic as a process of sharing relational stories of caregiving. This process is based on reciprocity and interconnectedness among human beings. To talk with patients about their stories of the meaning of life and death assists them to make decisions about advance directives. Self-disclosure by the nurse enriches the process and contributes to mutual understanding and concern.

An important foundation on which the realization of an ethic of care, the principles of justice, beneficence and autonomy, and the legal goal of self-determination are based is the relationship between the nurse and patient. Trust is imperative to this relationship and can be enhanced by the execution of advance directives. Katz (1984) poses several assumptions that are part of a trusting, mutual relationship in the context of informed consent:

1. There is no single right or wrong answer for how life, health, and illness should be lived. Numerous treatment options exist, and suffering can be alleviated in a variety of ways.
2. Health-care providers and patients both have vulnerabilities, conflicting motivations, interests, and expectations. Sameness of interests cannot be presumed; it must be confirmed in conversation.
3. Both parties relate to each other as equals and unequals. Professionals share professional expertise and patients their personal expertise. At the outset, neither knows what each can do for the other.
4. Human behavior contains both rational and irrational elements that must be accepted in health care providers and patients. Incompetence should not be presumed for either when signs of irrationality appear.

The assumptions enumerated by Katz indicate that physicians must engage in dialogue with patients about health-care choices, options, and decisions. While nurses do not demonstrate the silence referred to by Katz, the assumptions still are important for nurses to consider. Nurses should recognize the variety of "right" answers available to patients, should be aware of their own vulnerabilities and be able to discuss these with patients, should recognize their equalities and inequalities with patients, and should become comfortable with their own irrational sides. As Katz (1984) states, "Trust must be earned through conversation" (p. xiv). It is in face-to-face encounters with the patients that mutual understanding develops. With understanding comes more effective decision making about health-care choices.

CONCLUSION

Nurses play a key role in the development and implementation of advance directives. Nursing values of mutuality, open and direct communication, and caring and health promotion and prevention support the use of advance directives in health care. The skills nurses have in developing trusting relationships with patients can be used as a model for other health-care professionals who are burdened with silence or unsupportiveness in their relationships with patients. The Patient Self-Determination Act of 1990 provides the impetus for nursing involvement with patients on the topics of living wills and durable powers of attorney for health care.

We help our patients speak.
We help them look deep within
For truth, conflict and decision.
Then we accept their paths
As we accept our own.

REFERENCES

American Nurses Association. (1994). *Position statement on assisted suicide.* Washington, DC: Author.

Beauchamp, T.L., & Childress, J.F. (1994). *Principles of biomedical ethics* (4th ed.). New York: Oxford University Press.

Cate, F.H., & Gill, B.A. (1991). *The patient self-determination act: Implementation issues and opportunities* (pp. 65-73). Washington, DC: Annenberg Washington Program of Northwestern University.

Choice in dying: Right-to-die case and statutory citations. (1992, March 17). New York: Choice in Dying.

Crisham, P. (1990). Living wills: Controversy and certainty. *Journal of Professional Nursing, 6*(6), 321.

Cruzan v. Director, Missouri Dept. of Health 110 S. Ct. 2841, 111 L. Ed. 2d 224, 58. USLW 4916 (US Mo., June 25, 1990).

18 Deaths in NY psychiatric facilities instigate changes: Ethical concerns about restraints apply equally to mental patients. (1994). *Medical Ethics Advisor, 10*(12), 162-163.

Fade, A.E. (1995). Advance directives: An overview of changing right-to-die laws. *Journal of Nursing Law, 2*(3), 27-38.

Faden, R.R., & Beauchamp, T.L. (1986). *A history and theory of informed consent.* New York: Oxford University Press.

Gamino, D. (1992, May 15). A living will fails to ensure dignified death. *Austin American-Statesman,* pp. A-1, A-12.

High, D.M. (1993). Advance directives and the elderly: A study of intervention strategies to increase use. *The Gerontologist, 33*(3), 342-349.

Johnson, R.A., & Weiler, K. (1990). Aid-in-dying: Issues and implications for nursing. *Journal of Professional Nursing, 6*(5), 258-264.

Katz, J. (1984). *The silent world of doctor and patient* (pp. xiv, 28-29, 47, 102-103, 228). New York: Macmillan.

Kjervik, D.K., & Grove, S. (1988). A legal model of consent in unequal power relationships. *Journal of Professional Nursing, 4*(3), 192-204.

Lange, A.J., & Jakubowski, P. (1976). *Responsible assertive behavior: Cognitive behavioral procedures for trainers* (p. 58). Champaign, IL: Research Press.

Parker, R.S. (1990). Nurses' stories: The search for a relational ethic of care. *Advances in Nursing Science, 13*(1), 31-40.

Patient Self-Determination Act of 1990, 42 U.S.C.A. § 1395 cc (f) (1) (A) (I)(1991 Supp. pam.), PL 101-508 § 4206, 104 Stat. 1388-115 (1990).

Robertson, J.A. (1991). Second thoughts on living wills. *Hastings Center Report, 21*(6), 6-9.

Schloendorff v. Society of New York Hospital 211 N.Y. 125, 129-30, 105 N.E. 92, 93 (1914).

Sehgal, A., Galbraith, A., Chesney, M., Schoenfeld, P., Charles, G., & Lo, B. (1992). How strictly do dialysis patients want their advanced directives followed? *Journal of the American Medical Association, 267*(1), 59-63.

Silverman, H.J., Fry, S.T., & Armistead, N. (1994). Nurses' perspectives on implementation of the Patient Self-Determination Act. *The Journal of Clinical Ethics, 5*(1), 30-37.

Teno, J.M., Lynn, J., Phillips, R.S., Murphy, D., Youngner, S.J., Bellamy, P., Connors, A.F., Jr., Desbiens, N.A., Fulkerson, W., & Knaus, W.A. (1994). Do advance directives affect resuscitation decisions and the use of resources for seriously ill patients? *The Journal of Clinical Ethics, 5*(1), 23-30.

Theis, E.C. (1990). Life-sustaining technologies: Ordinary of extraordinary? *Focus on Critical Care, 17*(6), 445-450.

Weber, G., & Kjervik, D.K. (1992). The Patient Self-Determination Act: The nurse's proactive role. *Journal of Professional Nursing, 8*(1), 6.

Weiler, K. (1989). Financial abuse of the elderly: Recognizing and acting on it. *Journal of Gerontological Nursing, 15*(8), 10-15.

Just managing: Ethical obligations and the managed health-care marketplace

LAURIE ZOLOTH-DORFMAN

As the American health-care system moves toward the dramatic reorganization known as managed care, nurses are faced with ethical conflicts that range far beyond the familiar ethical dramas of withholding and withdrawing life support (Krieger, 1995). At stake are the deepest ethical decisions about the meaning and intent of medicine itself and the responsibility of nurses toward their patients. When we speak of a health-care system that is just, what is the place for advocacy? When we call for a health-care system that is effective, what is the cost of compassion? How do ethical principles and precepts help when nurses feel that instead of managing with justice, they are just managing? At the heart of this question is a search for the values that ought to guide the provision of medical care in the new world of health-care delivery. What are the mechanisms that will be necessary both to protect patients and to articulate provider standards in a health-care system increasingly regulated by the marketplace? How can the development of such ethical standards help to define parameters in the evolving health-care system?

This chapter makes reference to such core issues as how the necessity for justice, the creation of desire, the construction of need, and the historical formulation of a basic demand for health-care services have driven the present structure of health care.[1] The main focus, however, is on how specific ethical issues are created in a system of "negative reward." This system, employed to contain costs in a managed care health-care delivery system creates special problems for the nurse who often is the one "standing at the gate" in the organization. This chapter argues that only a robust and publicly accessible discourse prior to the onset of a crisis can create a just encounter over the issue of health-care intervention, and that as part of such a system, all participants must have access to the truthful data, the lucid process, and the clarity of the financial relationships that are suggested by each medical choice. The burdens and benefits of such a system must be mutually borne. It is only by opening the process up to such disclosure that the power differential can begin to be equalized and that both infinity of desire for medical care and the capacity for fiduciary abuse can be examined. This chapter argues that if we are to take the dominance of medicine by the managed-care system as a first premise,[2] we are then obligated to create a system in which a strong moral agency is encouraged and supported, and patient advocacy is a normative structure of the nursing role.

THE CASE

"The case has brought the unit nearly to a standstill," said Sheila, the clinical nurse specialist in the cardiac care unit, shaking her head slowly at the ethics committee meeting. The other nurses from the unit watched her quietly, their arms folded, waiting for their turn to present their side of the story. "Mr. McGill is a 27-year-old laborer from a poor rural family in the dusty California coastal range. He drifted down to Los Angeles for a construction job about 4 years ago, got on our health maintenance organization (HMO) plan, and then got sick. He tried to keep working, but finally he came home so his family could take care of him, which is how he landed up here, since our hospital

[1] For the best account of the current construction of healthcare, see Walzer, M. (1983). *Spheres of justice.* New York: Basic Books.

[2] This is not the only system, of course, but it is the one that is clearly dominant in the current health care marketplace in many areas of the country. This change in health care delivery is documented the scholarly literature and the popular press. See for example Zoloth-Dorfman and Rubin (1995, Winter). The patient as commodity: Managed care and the question of ethics. *The Journal of Clinical Ethics,* (6)4.

was just bought by his HMO. He was really sick—advanced endocarditis—and because he had insurance, the university hospital was only too happy to give him a transplant. But our HMO will only pay for 4.5 days of inpatient care, and they sent him home. His wound was not even closed—the drains were still in. Now 'home' is his parent's trailer on 15 acres of scrub land. So he got a massive wound infection. He needs twice daily sterile dressing changes, antibiotics, and still his wound is not healing. But here is the dilemma. His wound infection care is not covered by his HMO. The heart transplant is, but not the 4×4s he needs every day." She turns to her colleagues, some of whom are looking at their laps, while others look defiantly at the committee. "Mr. McGill has begun to show up on our floor, since he knows us, and ask for 4×4's. Sometimes his mother or his sisters come. Some of the nurses have even done a few changes themselves in the treatment room." One of the other nurses interrupts. "But some of us feel that it is just not fair to do this for him, *and not for the rest of our patients!" she says. "I am always sending home frail elderly women with no one to care for them! How can we use resources this way—steal them, really—for one patient and not for all?" Another nurse raises her voice. "I snuck McGill into the treatment room," she admits. "One day on the afternoon shift. You could see that snazzy new heart beating underneath a mass of necrotic tissue. How can you ignore the needs of your patient just because he can't pay? Have we really come to that?"*

Sheila is silent. She is facing an irony of her own. This is the last case she will bring to the ethics committee as a clinical nurse specialist: the hospital, in another cost-containment measure, has elected to phase out all clinical nurse specialist positions next month, and she will be looking for work. She used to be an unequivocal advocate for her patients, at whatever cost; now she wonders if the sum of this attitude has finally come home to roost.

DESIRE AND THE PRODUCTION OF HEALTH-CARE SERVICES

Fundamental ethical questions about the dynamics that drive the desire for good health-care services and the corresponding health system are partly historical and partly cultural (Daniels, 1985). We need to ask what are the ethical justifications for resolving the conflict between explicable desire and just health-care delivery, and to what moral appeals are we obligated to be accountable as institutions and as citizens of a good society?

One can think of a variety of ways in which to describe such a society. Many of the measures are descriptions of what we mean by fairness in the allocation of basic social goods such as health care (Menzel, 1990). In reflecting on how nurses committed to caring ought to describe a just allocation, several contending perspectives emerge. At the heart of each lies a theory of justice. Traditional ways to describe a theory have been based in libertarianism, utilitarianism, and egalitarianism. Each of these positions depends on giving different weight to the importance of such issues as desert, equality, or desire.

American health care is based on an amalgam of these different theories. Institutions develop and provide for their participants a particular narrative that is rooted in a belief structure based in these theories (Moreno, 1995). Yet because these narratives attempt to reconcile significantly different vantage points, there is a discrepancy in their underlying themes.

Hence, while we have a commitment to the relationship between hard work and rewarding outcomes, we are troubled by stark differences in the quality of health care for the poor and health care for the wealthy (Aaron, 1991; Daniels, 1985; Rhodes, 1992). While we speak of autonomy and consent as centrally important, we are concerned about our ability to set limits when the needs of one patient threaten to obscure the needs of many. While we retain a concern for the vulnerable, we are uneasy in an open-ended commitment, and we are troubled by the links between "lifestyle" and disease.

Into this theoretical confusion has been thrust central cultural myths of the late 20th century: Anything that is created can be repaired, all problems have a solution, and medical power and progress are infinite. The rewards for this promise have been lucrative for physicians, for pharmaceutical companies, and for the vast network of subsidiaries (Aaron, 1991). Even the insurance companies, despite the rising costs of medical care, have made substantial profits. In fact, one of the cautionary impulses that mitigated against reform is the fear of upsetting this powerful and robust industry.

After the recent failure of Congress to resolve the much-discussed health-care system crisis, in many states the market forces have already stepped in to reconstruct the health-care marketplace. In these states, the majority of the population (both private payers and Medicaid beneficiaries) is moving into managed care organizations (MCOs), physicians are organizing into networks, and hospital and health-care systems are consolidating into ever-larger health-care conglomerates every week.

What does this all mean for the clinical nurse? One thing is certain. It means that nurses and their patients are participating in a vast social experiment (albeit without prior consent) on how a population is served by such a medical care delivery system. How is this experiment faring, and is such a system fair? As the case mentioned earlier shows, the answer to this question depends on one's position in the power relationship.

CONFLICTS OF INTEREST

Ethical conflicts between stakeholders are inherent in any system of health-care delivery that relies on relationships between strangers as the basis of a contract for care (Arras & Steinbock, 1995). This is not a new feature of American health care. While the provision of health care is a compassionate and necessary gesture, it is also a business, a way that millions earn their living, and a product that is sold in a marketplace. In the current climate of economic downturn, nurses are being told about the marketplace with greater vigor. Ethics raises the questions: What of the older organizing principles of nursing and medicine? In a marketplace-driven system, what protection is there for the vulnerable, the frail, the patients without the ability to compete as "customers?"

In fee-for-service plans, ethical conflicts arose in the structure that asked a third party to pay for medical care in an unregulated relationship. The more medical interventions, the more money third-party payers have to throw toward the problem: overtreatment and overtesting were rewarded in such a system. In fact, the earliest cases in the clinical ethics literature reflect the need to protect patients (e.g., the Quinlans, the Cruzans) from burdensome overtreatment in situations that their families considered hopeless.

In a sense, the fee-for-service system has "taught" a generation of patients and staff that more was better, that the best medicine was the most expensive medicine. Health insurance, once the complexities of access could be ensured, allowed most patients, most of the time, to have a generous stay, tertiary care, and a recovery that included robust teaching, progressive ambulation, and at least a few days of bedbaths (Daniels, 1985). Hence, most patients did what they were told, accepting whatever the doctor said was needed for recovery. The doctor and the nurse had a fiduciary interest in the most abundant treatment plan. The third-party payer had an interest in paying out less, of course, but in a system in which most health-care dollars were generated by union contracts, huge premiums were ensured.

THE PATIENT AS CUSTOMER

Managed care has changed this model. Conflicts of interest between the patient and the physician are structured into the essential relationships of managed care. It is how the system creates incentives for providers in a capitated plan. The providers—doctors and hospitals—are either paid a capitated, fixed amount per patient or a salary that is influenced by their behavior. In such a system, the more treatment that is given out and paid for, the less the providers will take home to their families. Imagine a fixed pile of money, paid by patients (now called "customers") when they buy their health care every year. Now imagine that every time a visit is made, a computed tomography scan taken, or a drug provided, a few coins are taken away from the pile. If that money is now your own, and if there will be no more added until next year, and if the third-party payers are being told by the people who buy health care for their workers that next year they want premiums to go down 5%, then you have a picture of how managed care works. Each provider's interest in retaining the pile is in conflict with the patients' interest in using more services to support his or her health. Patients are seen in this system as revenue centers. This is not new but is more stark in the system of managed care, where the fewer care gestures that a capitated physician offers and that a nurse provides, the more profit is generated.

At this juncture in the nursing literature a new language emerged: the language of the patient as customer. The image of the healthy, immunized, bran-eating (or soy-eating) purchaser of health care replaced that of the needy ill person as the object of interest. (Efficient telephone advice replaced pm skin care as the expectation.) The goal, and it is not a bad goal, was reformulated as keeping people healthy. It is a goal that keeps people paying into the system, rather than taking from the system. No ethical conflicts emerge until the payee is struck by illness or accident. Then, as a vulnerable person, a patient and not a customer, his or her needs must be fully and truthfully met by the system that he or she has in essence supported, or a violation of an essential promise will have been made. It is a promise made not only by the physician, but by every nurse who works in the system, whose wages are paid in advance, as it were, by our patient, in trust for the time when he or she will need our care.

The case described here develops the themes of the moral meaning and the moral worth of our medical interventions. Any concrete cases of allocation will raise issues of the role and the duty of the health-care provider and the nursing leadership of the health-care institution (Menzel, 1990). Should the role of the nurse be one of gatekeeper, visionary, businesswoman, or citizen? Because the provision of this particular social good is so critical, does the provider stand outside the normative concerns of the marketplace or of justice considerations, or is this just a business relationship like any other? Do nurses have to be accountable to considerations of justice for a whole society, or just to their patients? Is the ethical choice that is required by a nurse to remain a part of an MCO an ethical compromise of her promise to serve the patient selflessly?

Beyond complaint

The problem changes, however, when the autonomous wishes of the patient, the real health needs of the patient, and the medical teams beneficent acts all suggest a costly treatment and the cost will directly affect the income or working conditions of the very team that is recommending its use. When the costly treatment is denied, the team rightly has mixed responses. Is the assertation of "good business practice" merely one way of preserving the income of the health plan at the expense of the patient? All of the nurses involved in the McGill case, however, had a keen sense of the crisis in private fee-for-service medicine. (That was in large part why they were committed to managed-care models in the first place.) All agreed that "too much is spent on medicine" in general, and all were strong proponents of alternative solutions to high technology. In the case they brought to the ethics committee, all reported feeling as though they were being coerced to act wrongly, even unethically. What is distinctive about such admissions is not that they are unique instances of patients not getting what they need, but that there were no checks and balances for what the patient needed in the new system. No one told Mr. McGill that the recovery phase of his surgery would be unsupported. No one told the nurses the limited parameters of available care until after the fact, and there was no plan for involving either the patient or the nurses in how such limits are set.

Patients are not presented with the consequences of their health-care choices as customers; most in fact have no idea of the compromises that their practitioners are agonizing over. While a story of grotesque abuse is occasionally revealed in public testimony (on *60 Minutes, Frontline,* or in *The New York Times*, for example),[3] it is impossible to monitor every detail of one's own plan. Patients expect that if a serious compromise is being made about their bodies, they would, of course, be made aware of such a problem. This is the essential trust relationship of the gesture of "stranger" medicine, made morally coherent and physically safe only by a reliance on the oaths and obligations of the physician and the role-specific duties of the nursing professional.

Who should decide about the limits of care if the traditional Hippocratic oath is no longer the keystone of medical practice, and to whom do such decision makers answer, to what code of honor?[4] Many nurses in the McGill case spoke of the need to advocate for the patient in this system but were frustrated about whom to turn to. In the past, the care could theoretically be given long past efficacy, but not long past desire, because it is only a fringe number of patients who would eagerly seek appendectomies capriciously. Hence patients themselves often decided on the medical question in a treatment plan. The traditional conflict had the patient and provider allied against a third party (e.g., the government, the employer, or the insurance company). This new era creates stranger bedfellows, more uneasy allies, leaving the patient not only in practice, but by theoretical design as the one who is structured out of the decision-making process by virtue of his prepayment status.

The organization of managed care in California is in an early stage, despite the presence of well-developed HMOs that have been in practice since the 1940s.[5] Now operating in anticipated advance of health-care reform, the system according to those who brought this case is capricious: serving many well and many poorly, marketplace-driven and subject, especially in the smaller MCOs, to the possibility of abuse. At issue is how to act fairly in the actual present, and how to operate more justly in an unjust world.[6]

RATIONING IN BROAD DAYLIGHT: THE ETHICAL OBLIGATIONS OF THE NURSE AS CITIZEN

One solution to such problems begins with the promise of absolute full disclosure to patients as they face medical crises. If cost-cutting mechanisms are to be employed, the true cost—that is, the social cost to all—must be explained publicly, and the burdens and the benefits shared jointly. According to this argument, then, the one who

[3] September 1, 1994. Television documentary that revealed that cost cutting had caused lab "speed-up" that seemed to be causally related to an 83% to 95% false-negative rate in the reading of Pap results. See also Herbert, B. (1994, September 11), Profits before patients, *The New York Times*, p. 19. In this article, Herbert relates the story of Karin "Smith," who won a lawsuit of $6.3 million after all but her last five Pap smears were misread over a 6-year period.

[4] There is no equivalent oath for the newly graduated MBA (master's in business administration), for example, no pledge to do the best for the customer. In the starkest terms, in fact, because it is not consumers who fund MBA training, there might be a curriculum basis in favor of protection of corporate profits over consumer interest should the two come into conflict.

[5] Most of the egregious conflicts of interests are most visible in small MCO systems, but theoretically all could be directly felt in personal income.

[6] LeBacqz, K. (1987). *Justice in an unjust world.* Minneapolis: Augsberg Publishing House.

bears the brunt of the burden is entitled to the bulk of the financial benefit. For such choices, all of which involve some elements of risk, the patient could elect to save the money, pay for his or her own care with it, or choose another social good. If sending the patient home days earlier than has been the case saves money for the plan ($3200 to $1000 per day), then that money may rightly belong back in the hands of the patient, who could then use it to buy his or her own 4×4s. One could argue that there would be some secondary social gain as a result of such a process. It would be perhaps true that earlier forms of care would reappear at the American sickbed: family, neighbors, and the like would again have to function as primary caregivers, with a corresponding increase in general lay knowledge about illness, childbirth, and death and a corresponding sense of the limits of the medical enterprise. After all, the notion that one's health-care insurance company, whose revenues are wielded by the hands of physicians, can and ought to solve the social as well as the medical facts of illness is a relatively recent concept in American society. It is most assuredly not a useful one. It must be noted that this solution is occurring, but with the considerable cost savings being passed on elsewhere. It is occurring with only provider incentive and patient burden, which is hardly an ethical solution. In several large MCOs, outpatient mastectomy is becoming standard, and childbirth stays are normally only 6 to 12 hours postpartum. Yet the process is sold and delivered as a "new standard of care," not as the cost-saving (and hence revenue-generating) move that it truly is.

The plan suggested here, however, is fraught with the familiar potential horrors of all stark marketplace schemes: when any individual is given the brunt of choice, in the context of all that surrounds such a choice, that individual has a bogus "liberty" based now fully on his or her socioeconomic status (measured by housing, food, and clothing). The wealthy will be able to contend for elaborate care, while the poor will merely have the ability to "freely" choose inadequate care.

There is of course an alternative model of a full social and a priori discourse that affects all equally (Danis & Churchill, 1991). Rather than the model of car salesmanship (full disclosure, individual incentive), this model more closely parallels the model of the public-police or library system (full disclosure, citizen response).[7] In this case, all members of an MCO can debate the reasonableness of limits and the allure of benefits gained by strict adherence to such limits. Just as taxes are intended to reflect a democratic assessment of what is just for citizens to pay, insurance premiums and the rationing of health-care benefits could reflect such shared democratic decision making. Such decision making would have to occur in a widely publicized public discourse, with the first premise being that care is being rationed covertly now, and that such rationing would be made visible and debatable. The conversations that seek to answer such ethical dilemmas must take place before the clinical bedside decisions raised by actual cases can be made. Such conversations must be face-to-face and specifically focused. Such discourse needs to begin at all levels and will have to include testimony about the widest range of outcome measures in addition to the full range of costs and the etiology of such costs. It will be critical to ensure that all outcome measures of such subjective factors as "utility" or "satisfaction" be applied equally to both physicians and patients. Any determination of the outcome of such a plan needs to resist efforts that ground success in merely instrumental terms of cost containment or utilization, although such measures will surely have their place. One of the early epistemic problems that any evaluative tool will have to address is who sets the criteria for the evaluation itself.

Not only patients but also nurses and physicians will need to expand the fullness of the informed-consent process to include honest disclosure of the fiduciary responsibility that is at stake.[8] It is only through a thorough and comprehensive reflection on the significant desire that undergirds the meaning of health care that reform can be constructed that is both comprehensible and congruent with our deepest social values. In such a system, the

[7] This model is based on the work of Churchill and Danis described in the *Hastings Center Report 21* "Autonomy and the Commonweal," January, 1991: 25-31. See also *Community and conscience*, an unpublished dissertation by Zoloth-Dorfman (1993). One such model for such discourse is the Oregon Health Care reform project, but the scope of the discourse could be smaller, based in one MCO or one community.

[8] In California, one state in which managed care is virtually hegemonic, a pilot grant project has begun that will design a curriculum to address the ethical conflicts that practitioners face in such bedside delivery. The author is a consultant ethicist for this grant. The project, funded by the Pew Charitable Trust (principle investigators Marten and Sommers of the Center for the Development of the Health Care Professions), could function as a much-needed support system if the curriculum is fully implemented, but the primary goal would be to address the main issues for the clinician: the problem of limits, the new reality of external limits, and the increasingly understood structural limits in the practice itself. In the interviews that I conducted for this grant I was moved by the depth of despair that the clinicians expressed in their work. The subjective feeling that I heard expressed was of new responsibility for that which had not been their problem: the issues of justice and allocation on a public scale. There is no flight from this, of course. A curriculum must teach the tools of the honest discourse.

nurse will have to address the ethics of managed care not only as "citizen" but also as a citizen with special knowledge. Such a role ought to buy access not to more privilege, but to more responsibility.

Such discourse is based on the language of the common good rather than the language of need-based or liberty-based autonomy (Danis & Churchill, 1991). The language of the common good is based on the premise that there is a basic decent minimum of social goods that is owed to all and that such a just share should be democratically arrived at. In addition, such language presumes that societies exist in large measure to bear the burden of the vulnerable who cannot obtain such social goods on their own. In any system like this, it is true that in any one individual case the person before you may not get what he or she needs to be well. The point of such conjunct responsibility, however, is that, given the tenuous equilibrium of the current era, such choices would even out over the long term. Unlike a strictly marketplace, liberty-based solution, such a priori discourse would create open reflection on the meaning of such choices long before they were made.

WHAT IS NEEDED FOR ETHICAL PRACTICE: TRUTHTELLING AND INDEPENDENT MORAL AGENCY

For such a citizen-based program to work, nurses must pursue a clear course of moral agency and the straightforward adherence to the principle of veracity. Patients must be told the truth not only about their diagnosis and prognosis, as in all informed-consent relationships, they must also know whether the treatment options they are offered are influenced by financial considerations. All conflicts of interests must be fully disclosed (Veatch, 1991). Nursing staff who witness such conflicts must be supported to uncover and open the process of true informed consent to the patient without any fear of reprisals. Nurses must be counted on to identify conditions of unsafe practice—areas in which the drive to cut costs endangers the health and safety of patients, in which the teaching role of the nurse is compromised, and in which the standard of care is unacceptably altered. Such objections must be documented and reported, and it must be a part of ethical professional practice to refuse to work without objection in such venues. Patients may well be unaware of previous standards, and may simply accept situations that are untenable; the role of nurses as moral agents must be to reflect on all aspects of current practice and insist on the maintenance of standards that are defensible.

The uncovering of financial considerations and the explicit dynamics of the marketplace as metaphor and social construct will have profound implications for the most privatized of relationships—that of physician and patient. Such a shift, or rather such an overt naming of the centrality of the need for considerations of social justice, is at the heart of the need for reflections on the competing moral appeals and theories of justice that underlie health-care reform.[9]

At stake in such a discourse will be the reframing of the methodology and the power in the medical decision-making process. Bioethics has stressed the necessity of the informed-consent relationship, but it does not as yet have a robust theory of informed consent in a time of scarcity. The model of autonomy is itself strained by the necessity to make public policy based on more generalized notions of the good. This underlying philosophy will have to be carefully examined to be clear about a number of troubling ethical issues.

First among these issues are the justice considerations concerning the place of the powerless, the vulnerable,

[9] Such discourse must also make a commitment to the full and frank exploration of the ethical implications of managed-care environment without undue hesitancy about problems of external judgments. The development of such curriculum is key.

Over the last several years my colleague Susan Rubin and I have taught the theory and practice that surround the ethical issue of distributive justice in the clinical setting. We have used several models, the most successful of which was based on the encounter between physician–direct care providers and administrators and utilization personnel over the issue of scarce resources. We have developed a curriculum that teaches intensive review of classic justice theory, challenges to these theories, and extensive case review of cases that involve explicit rationing. Included in this curriculum is a prioritization project based on the Oregon Health Care Model that uses the work of Churchill as a theoretical frame. Our experience, based on provider reports, is that such sessions have been extraordinarily useful in the clinical arena.

We have also developed a teaching module that examines in depth the issue of medical futility from a broad theoretical overview of the topic to detailed case review, which has been offered to ethics committees throughout our practice. In actual clinical case reviews we have observed, we have seen a rapid learning curve about this information affect the way case reviews are conducted. Our experience is that success with this model is based on the strongest possible theoretical ground and the consistent use of case review in the work. Another feature that is uniquely successful is the opportunity to directly address the concerns of a multidisciplinary group in an academic rather than an adversarial setting.

A third important part of the ethics curriculum that we have recently developed is a research project and teaching tool that examines the problem of truthtelling in the physician-patient relationship. Based on a model that stresses a strong theoretical base and focus on actual case encounters, the over 150 initial respondents have reported the immediate usefulness of the curriculum in their practice.

and the disenfranchised (Zoloth-Dorfman, 1994). Here the issues of power and rationality will have to be addressed clearly. Secondly, the use of outcome data as a tool carries with it all the complexities of unilateral decision making by the health-care provider, a particularly problematic history, and serious epistemological problems as well. At issue in many uses of outcome data will be not only the choice of instrument, but the community that sets the goals for the evaluative standards. Finally, the discourse must reflect on the reality of significant ethical and value conflicts over such questions as the ultimate worth of a human life, the meaning of quantitative assessment of life quality, and the plurality of religious and cultural perspectives on the goal and meaning of the person in health and in illness.[10]

Such a conversation held prior to the passion and loss of the bedside will not forestall all despair in the world, any more than after-the-fact remorse over poor social choices is avoided entirely by public discourse. But the patient in such a system can at least be assured of one thing: whether for harm or for good, the rationing that all such choices represents will be done in broad daylight, with all the goods bartered for and beckoned for on the table between us all.

Nurses in the new era of managed care will confront ethical dilemmas that will test the limits of their courage (McClinton, 1995). Moral agency is hard to maintain in a climate in which nurses themselves feel threatened. Layoffs and diminishing contractual benefits have been some of the subsidiary effects of cost cutting in the clinical setting, and nurses will have to remember that in many situations they must act despite their fear. Ultimately, moral responsibility in the system of managed care rests where it has always resided: in the heart and hands of the clinical provider.

[10] Many of the new strategic emphases in medicine are, in fact, geared to changing conceptions of the human person. These include the use of genetic research, the imperatives of technology, and the uses of pharmacological therapeutics. Such directions could be fruitfully explored in this model.

REFERENCES

Aaron, H. (1991). *Serious and unstable condition: Financing America's health care.* Washington DC: The Brooklings Institution.

Arras, J., & Steinbock, B. (1995). *Ethical issues in modern medicine.* Mountain View, CA: Mayfield.

Daniels, N. (1985). *Just health care.* Cambridge, MA: Cambridge University Press.

Danis, M., & Churchill, L. (1991, January–February). Autonomy and the common weal, *Hastings Center Report,* 12-19.

Krieger, L. (1995, January 17). Family doctors are disappearing. *San Francisco Examiner,* p. A1.

McClinton, D. (1995, June). Balancing the issue of ethics in case management. *Continuing Care,* 13-16.

Menzel, P. (1990). *Strong medicine: The ethical rationing of health care.* New York: Oxford.

Moreno, J. (1995). *Deciding together: Bioethics and moral consensus.* New York: Oxford.

Rhodes, R. (1992). *Health care politics, policy and distributive justice: The ironic triumph.* Albany, NY: State University of New York.

Veatch, R. (1991). Allocating health resources ethically: New roles for administrators and clinicians. *Frontiers of Health Services Management* 8, 3-44.

Zoloth-Dorfman, L. (1994, December). Standing at the gate: Managed care and daily ethical choices. *Managed Care Medicine,* 1-7.

Nursing in Russia: Impact of recent political changes

LINDA S. SMITH

UPHEAVAL IN RUSSIA

The Independent Republic of the Russian Federation became a reality on December 25, 1991, and its constitution purported a health-care system free of charge to all citizens (Fleischman & Lubamadrov, 1993). As Russia struggles now to enact social reforms and a market-driven economy, inflation, poverty, crime, and a disintegrating infrastructure are destroying hope for its people (Plant, 1993).

Many problems exist. When Gorbachev, former President of the Soviet Union, returned from forced exile after the aborted coup in August 1991, he returned to a changed nation. Soviet Union republics declared their independence, and the communist party disintegrated (Ryan, 1992). Deeply ingrained social strongholds, such as the lack of respect and acknowledgment for the contributions of health-care professionals, continued. Salaries for health-care workers were—and continue to be—dreadful (Curtis, Petukhova, & Taket, 1995). Health care was a centrally ordered, hierarchical system (Curtis et al., 1995) in which patients did not pay directly for care, and health-care professionals became state employees. This status permitted little autonomy or authority.

Although between 1970 and 1989 the number of hospital beds in Russia increased from 30 to about 48 per 10,000 population (Curtis et al., 1995), health-care concerns were given a lower priority than other industrial and military endeavors, the gross domestic product for health care spending was about 2.4%. This low rate leads to chronic underfunding and rationing. Because the purpose of all health care was to increase worker productivity, the elderly and disabled became vulnerable. Long waits and medical supply shortages impaired access. To circumvent these problems, informal methods of bribing and tipping were common, and separate elitist facilities developed. Primary health-care principles weakened, and individual patient needs were of little concern.

The author wishes to acknowledge the assistance of Louise M. Omdahl, MSN, RN.

Politics

Since prices for almost all goods and services have skyrocketed, police are considered corrupt, and safety at night—especially for women—is a major concern. In September 1994, a loaf of bread cost 650 rubles, milk 700 rubles, a Big Mac 2,000 rubles, and a new suit for a woman 190,000 rubles. Pensioners needed to pay these prices with a meager income of 70,000 to 100,000 rubles per month (L. Svirenko, personal communication, September 16, 1994).

Few Russians wish to turn back Glasnost reforms and return to a totalitarian regime. Since 1993, however, quiet legislation has rolled back some of Russia's most important and hard-won human-rights changes. Searches and seizures can be conducted without warrants, and the media was again restricted. The response of the government was that these rights had to be modified as a result of the increased crime, pornography, and business fraud in Russia ("Russian Parliament Is," 1993).

Fed by fear, food hoarding continues. Debts among businesses in Russia have increased to $45 billion, causing factories to lay off workers, skip payrolls, or pay employees with goods such as glassware and tampons. The concern now is that Russian nationalism will force a change. Russians report a hunger for the days when they experienced collective pride and identity (Cooperman, 1994). Older Russians, raised on Soviet ideals that are now destroyed, find their savings and pensions worthless. These Russians are too old to retrain for new careers and too disillusioned not to hold tight to past glories. Streets once clean, ordered, bright, and safe are now filthy, dark, and dangerous. Democratic dreams fade as crime runs rampant (Carpenter, 1994a). When *U.S. News and World Report* asked Russians, "Who really runs things in Russia today?" 32% responded "the Mafia," and only 10% identified democratically elected Russian President Yeltsin (Cooperman & Thoenes, 1995). In December 1995, communists and nationalists won a majority of seats during parliamentary elections. Their next goal is to overtake the presidency in 1996 (Cooperman & Thoenes, 1996).

Crumbling infrastructure

In 1993 and 1994, the U.S. State Department warned Americans not to fly on Russian domestic airlines (Groff, 1994a) because of widespread reports of safety problems. Passengers are faced with unpredictable schedules, difficult conditions, deteriorating maintenance systems, and overbooked flights (Groff, 1994b). Further evidence of the crumbling infrastructure occurred in June 1995 ("Aid comes too slowly," 1995) when a 7.5 earthquake hit Neftegorsk. Hundreds of people could have been saved were it not for the unpaved roads and insane bureaucracy that kept rescuers away. Russian communications, with about 12 phone lines per 100 people (in the United States there are 56 lines per 100 people), makes using a telephone in Russia difficult. Connections are uncertain or full of static, and there is no directory assistance, phone books, or call waiting. Nor has education been spared. Russian teachers are less qualified and have an average pay of $46 per month—less than half of the average Russian salary (Carpenter, 1994b). The police are also victims. Ridiculed by the public and the politicians, they must contend with aging police cars, gas shortages, tremendous physical dangers, and shrinking paychecks. Fourteen-year veterans earn about $80 per month, while the average wage in Russian is about $100 per month ("Russia: Little Gas," 1994).

In May 1995, the ruble hit an all-time low of 5,130 rubles per dollar (in July 1989, one ruble equaled $6). This inflation often means that the elderly must either sell their most prized possessions or beg in order to live. The Russian elderly are also vulnerable to crime and fraud. Russian police report that at least 5,600 organized crime groups and gangs are nearly immune to retribution ("Crime wave sweeps Moscow," 1994). Thus, crime has doubled between 1990 and 1994 yet laws remain outdated and courts ill prepared and ill funded. Police answering distress calls must carry automatic weapons and wear bullet-proof vests ("Moscow Cops Feeling Blue," 1995; Nelan, 1995). This growing violence has led to growing pessimism over democratic reforms. It seems likely that Russians will follow any politician who can guarantee law and order, regardless of the loss of civil rights.

Pollution

Russian industries, unable and unwilling to install quality water- and air-treatment devices, continue to pollute the environment. Based on old Soviet ideology, industry intends to survive at any cost. Untreated waste is commonplace, and only 15% of all Russians breathe air of acceptable quality ("Environment Still Bleeds," 1993). Russian women downwind from industrial plants are encouraged not to breast feed due to high levels of dioxin in breast milk. With the loose Russian standards, 20% of the drinking water is unfit for consumption. Thus, Russian people have endured ever higher rates of respiratory disease, mental retardation, and congenital deformities. New laws impose fines on polluters, but Russia's environmental inspectors remain impotent ("Environment Still Bleeds," 1993). Nuclear accident cover-ups, nuclear smuggling, and nuclear-safety violations have also led to increases in environmental disasters. These safety problems are blamed on the failing Russian economy ("Yeltsin's Secret Nuclear," 1995).

Ever-increasing pollution, crime, inflation, and unemployment and the virtual collapse of the Russian health-care system have led to increasing morbidity and mortality rates. In 1994, Russia's death rate was 15.6 per 1000 people, with only 9.4 live births per 1000. In contrast, mortality in the United States is about 5 per 1,000 (National Center for Health Statistics, 1995). In addition, fewer women are bearing children. In 1993, life expectancy figures showed male life expectancy to be 59 years of age and female life expectancy 72 years of age, lower than all other industrialized countries ("Russian Longevity Figures," 1995).

Russia's youth have also suffered. Without safety matches or flame-retardant clothing, burns are common among children. Domestic violence and suicide rates are also rising dramatically. A destabilized Russian society has led to aggressiveness, anxiety, despair, and hopelessness (Smirnov & Beznosuk, 1995). Increased numbers of two-generation single-child families, cramped living space, and state-run day-care programs (Stanley, 1993) have caused young Russians to have little understanding of privacy, motivation, or responsibility.

RUSSIA'S DISORDERED HEALTH-CARE SYSTEM

As mountain factories encase downwind cities in soot, diseases such as whooping cough, diphtheria, cholera ("Life is Shorter," 1994), rabies, polio, tuberculosis, and AIDS are rising. Childhood diseases are increasing as a result of malnutrition (especially in the first year of life and evidenced by rickets, stunted growth, and obesity) and the fear parents have regarding immunizations. Parents have seen evidence that diseases such as AIDS and hepatitis are transmitted through contaminated needles and vaccines. Therefore, only about one third of all infants stay healthy through their first year of life (Ryan, 1993), and 60% of all school-age children suffer from at least one chronic disease (Komarov, 1994).

In the past 10 years, viral hepatitis morbidity in Russia doubled largely as a result of contaminated blood transfusions (Komarov, 1994). Tuberculosis spread rapidly among prisoners, alcohol and drug abusers, the homeless, and Russian mountain dwellers. Scabies and lice infestations have also increased (Komarov, 1994). In addition to these disease-related statistics, 12 million Russians are injured or poisoned each year. In 1992, losses from traffic accidents (22% of all accidental deaths) were greater than losses from cancer or cardiovascular disorders. Adult mental health also fares poorly. Nearly 30% of Russian workers abuse alcohol, and suicides and homicides outrank losses from ischemic heart disease (Komarov, 1994). In 1992, according to unofficial investigations, infant mortality reached 22 per 1000 newborns.

Substance abuse is a concern for Russian youth, who abuse chemicals such as alcohol, homemade drugs, opiates, and cannabis (Stanley, 1993). Aftercare is rare for children and adults discharged from acute-care institutions. Clean laundry is a problem for hospitals. Poorly paid laundry workers have shortages of laundry detergents, causing hospitals to wait as long as 2 months for clean linen only to find it damp, moldy, and dirty (Plant, 1993). Painkillers and sterile dressings are unavailable or scarce.

Industry is divided into four categories, and salaries are paid accordingly. The first and highest paid are the workers in heavy industry, metallurgical endeavors, and machine manufacturing. The second level includes light industry and textile workers. Health-care workers, educators, and entertainers are in the third class (L. Filatova, personal communication, September 28, 1995). Additionally, physicians are divided into three categories, with the highest-paid physicians receiving about $80 per month (D. Chikh, personal communication, September 18, 1995).

Below physicians are middle-level workers, including feldshers (who receive 4 years of training beyond the 10th grade), pharmacists, and medical nurses. Nurses with the most training and status earn $35 to $40 per month. In 1995, only about 1% of Russia's gross national product (GNP) was devoted to health care (D. Chikh, personal communication, September 18, 1995). The Duma, Russia's lower parliament, has promised to make health and education top priorities. But will salaries for nurses improve? The Duma will need to move quickly because medical specialists, scientists, artists, educators, and highly skilled workers (including physicians and nurses) are leaving Russia and taking with them the contributions they could have made to Russian life.

Medications are out of reach for the poor. Russian production of medications is down 50% to 70%, forcing some hospitals to purchase foreign pharmaceuticals with precious hard currency because rubles have little foreign value (Monks, 1994). Physicians write prescriptions in the charts, and nurses document them as a received order, but the patients never get them. If patients receive any medications at all, it is likely due to efforts of their families to buy the medications on the black market. In 1994, when a typical pensioner received 14,000 rubles per month, a packet of aspirins cost 1000 rubles.

There is chaos in Russian hospitals. The Russian government has refused to change the time-honored communist practice of dictating to hospitals and health-care professionals. Therefore, hospitals are operating at only a 20% efficiency level (Carey, 1992). Doctors making referrals to hospitals or specialty centers (e.g., for needed surgery) must pay for those referrals from their budgets. Therefore, presents or bribes for treatments are common (Monks, 1994). Nurses make their own intravenous solutions by following chemical recipes and sterilizing recapped glass bottles in antique autoclaves. These intravenous solutions are often safer and more readily available than blood transfusions. Almost half of the rural hospitals in Russia (one third of the population lives in rural areas) have no sewer connections, and 80% have no hot water (Feshbach, 1993). The incidence of HIV has increased as a result of contaminated blood and unsterile needles. Up to six intensive care unit patients can be placed in one room, and the patient:nurse ratio can reach as high as 60:1 (Carey, 1992).

Each Russian hospital has two parts. The first part or corridor is for people without money or insurance. Their care is free, but they receive no medications and limited attention. The second corridor is reserved for patients who can pay for their care. Paying new mothers are in semi-private rooms, hold and feed their babies at will, receive care by the physician of their choice, and have televisions, telephones, and family visits. On the other side of the doors rest eight women to a room as they wait for a physician they have never met to deliver their babies. Babies are fed on a rigid schedule. Women have no contact with their husbands or families until they are discharged. This side of the facility is dirty but free—as guaranteed in the new Russian Constitution (Kunstel & Albright, 1994).

EVIDENCE OF REFORM

The first generation of children in decades is learning lessons without Soviet ideology. They are no longer taught to venerate Lenin, as new history curricula acknowledge his cruelty. Students have more choices, wear nail polish, and ask challenging questions (Carpenter, 1994b). Spiritually, the once atheist nation of Russians is having a revival of monumental proportions ("Study Shows More," 1993).

OPPRESSED RUSSIAN WOMEN

Gender discrimination is a powerful force in Russia. Under Soviet rule, most employees in nonindustry categories were women, and thus women received lower wages. This difference expanded even further after the collapse of communism as inflation rose (Ryan, 1992). Although the majority of physicians and teachers in Russia are women, these women lack authority and responsibility. Women are denied opportunities and continue to be relegated to menial labor (Boe, 1993), especially in the home. Western conveniences such as garbage disposals, dishwashers, microwave ovens, large-capacity washers and dryers, and even electric irons are scarce (Zagalsky, 1994).

Life is hard for Russian women. This is especially true for women working for state enterprises (such as nurses, teachers, and doctors), where salaries have not increased in proportion to prices. Russian men, generally loathe to participate with child care and housework, become lazy. Additionally, many Russian families break apart as Russian men look for younger, more attractive wives—an easy task due to the proliferation of young, unattached Russian mothers (L. Filatova, personal communication, September 28, 1995).

As Russian women seek men who will stay employed, avoid alcoholism, and assist with children, they turn to foreign marriage brokers in hopes of finding love and stability. Unfortunately, many are being lured into prostitution and exploitation as a result. Foreign men want beautiful subservient wives and may be surprised by the independence of Russian women ("Russian Women Want," 1994) caused by years of fending for themselves and surviving in hostile conditions. They have been called "drill sergeants" by men seeking fragile femininity.

Russian women also have pregnancy, labor, and delivery concerns Russian men never face. Two of every three pregnancies in Russia are aborted, and 75% of pregnant Russian women have pathologies during pregnancy that are related to poor health and poor nutrition (e.g., deficiencies in protein, vitamins, and minerals) (Feshbach, 1993; Komarov, 1994). Poor Russian women cannot get contraceptives (only 18% use them); condoms are unpopular and difficult to obtain; and sex education does not exist in Russia (Plant, 1993). The average Russian woman has between three and eight abortions.

Abortion as a right became popular when the Soviet state needed women in the workforce. Now, very few women have the time, money, social support, or living space to care for more than one child. However, under new health-care changes, abortions for fetuses beyond 5 weeks are no longer free, and Russian women are often told to go to private or regional clinics that are too costly for many. In response, women's groups in Russia are now drafting a law that would guarantee affordable abortions ("Abortions Rampant," 1995). Not surprising, Russian maternal mortality is four to five times greater than that in other developed countries. These deaths are due to abortions, gestational toxemia, and hemorrhage, but nearly 60% are avoidable. With 90% of Russian women in the workforce, workplace conditions become health risks. Nearly 39% of night-shift workers (including nurses) are women (Komarov, 1994).

OPPRESSED RUSSIAN NURSES

Hard physical labor and shift work are familiar burdens to Russian nurses. In many hospitals, nurses work double shifts and take increased patient loads just to bring their wages up enough to survive (Monks, 1994). Nursing is a female-based (about 2% male), physician-dominated, task-oriented profession, and as such Russian physicians believe that nurses have precious little to contribute (Fleischman & Lubamadrov, 1993). They believe fervently that physicians, not nurses, are best able to assess patients and plan care. Nurses often carry out the roles of respiratory, dietary, laboratory, cleaning, and clerical personnel, and "all nurses must follow physicians orders exactly as written, without exceptions" (Fleischman & Lubamadrov, 1993, p. 136).

CHANGES FOR RUSSIAN NURSING

Nursing education

Before the Russian Revolution of 1917, nursing practice blended the physical, social, psychological, and spiritual aspects of human life and death. However, after the rise of communism, nursing education moved to procedure-oriented technical schools (referred to as medical schools) with little attention paid to the social sciences and humanities (Edwards, 1994; Picard & Perfiljeva, 1995). Nurses are thus considered middle-level health-care workers (Kinsey, 1992) under the direction and authority of physicians. As the assistants of physicians, nurses function under a simplified medical model (Picard & Perfiljeva, 1995).

Russian nursing education generally takes place in 2-year programs, with candidates entering after the completion of the 10th grade (high-school graduate). Feldsher education also takes place in technical schools, where they learn advanced techniques such as suturing and birthings and may apply these techniques without physician presence. Feldshers ride in ambulances and work in polyclinics (Edwards, 1994).

Physicians receive 6 years of education after the 10th grade, generally studying an additional year in preparation for a specialty examination. Physicians earn their education in medical universities and obtain an additional diploma on completion of their specialty work (D. Chikh, personal communication, September 18, 1995). Post-graduation specialty training for nurses includes periodic continuing education for 1 to 4 months, after which a certificate is awarded and, depending on the specialty, additional salary. Salary for the best educated chief nurse position can equate to the salary of the lowest level of physician (second doctor) about $35 to $40 per month. (The chief nurse position in Russia is equated to a U.S. nurse vice president or director of nursing.) This pay is preset by the Russian government (A. Alekseyevna, personal communication, September 16, 1995; D. Chikh, personal communication, September 18, 1995). Even with additional education, nursing theory, nursing diagnosis, and the nursing process are not emphasized (Barron, 1994; Edwards, 1994).

Before 1991, Russian nurses had little hope of advancement other than becoming physicians. For decades, nursing journals were authored, edited, and directed by physicians. Nurse educators were physicians (Barron, 1994); supervisors of patients and nurses were physicians, and government standards for nurses were set by physicians. Today this physician dominance may be changing. Through the vision of Perfiljeva in 1991, the Moscow Medical Academy initiated a master's program in nursing. This prestigious educational facility also collaborated with Nursing College #1 to offer a baccalaureate in nursing program (Picard & Perfiljeva, 1995). Presently, 45 baccalaureate nursing programs exist within the Russian Federation, but these programs remain medical-model based. The master's program, in contrast, is fashioned after U.S. bachelor of science programs, emphasizing nursing theory, leadership, research, and education (Picard & Perfiljeva, 1995). In June 1995 the first class graduated from this program. The hopes of a national nursing system developed and implemented by nurses rather than physicians rests on these graduates, who have been taught to write, speak, and teach about the values of nursing (Picard & Perfiljeva, 1995).

At the Mytischi Medical College (nursing school) there is only one nurse on faculty. This nurse teaches clinically and holds a position equal to those of other physician-faculty (G. Karpova, personal communication, September 14, 1994). This change resulted directly from the efforts of the United States–Russian Nurse Exchange Consortium. Through this Consortium (established in 1989) and other efforts around the United States, nursing faculty from Russia and the United States have shared problems, solutions, ideas, and dreams.

Nursing practice

It has been said that Russian nurses must carry the health-care burdens of their country with their bare hands. Despite almost overwhelming oppression by physicians, Russian nurses continue to struggle for authority and dignity within their practice. They are trying now to improve the quality of the care they provide, but there is very little time (about 30 patients per nurse) and very little equipment with which to do so. In 1995, nurses wrote an application to the Russian Ministry of Health asking for enough equipment (e.g., gloves, disposables, and goggles) to remain safe from blood-borne pathogens. Russian nurses believe that the quality of patient communication has improved since the influences of nurse exchanges. They have seen the benefits of American nurses spending time listening to their patients, and they hunger to use these skills if given the time and resources.

Changes in Russian nursing practice include the additions of patient blood-pressure monitoring (a task formerly reserved for physicians) as well as screenings for glaucoma, vision, height, weight, and strength. Russian nurses in polyclinics such as those in the Pavloski-Posad region now may refer patients to higher-level facilities when needed. When physicians leave emergency care facilities at 2:00 P.M., nurses are in charge because they discovered that they could think for themselves, proclaiming that, "We can make minor decisions without the help of the doctor" (A. Alekseyevna, personal communication, September 16, 1995). With the Russian Ministry of Health, Russian nurses have shared numerous accounts of how and when their independent decision making made a difference. This Ministry is perceived to be progressive and responsive to the idea of independent nursing practice (A. Alekseyevna, personal communication, September 16, 1995).

In addition to independent practice, Russian nurses yearn for improved working conditions in hospitals—especially with regard to the problems of high nurse:patient ratios. They look for ways to finance medical equipment and pharmaceuticals in order to avoid shortages and maldistributions. Lastly, they wish to impose employment standards for hospitals so that only dedicated, qualified, hard-working nurses receive positions. Recently, hospitals have been forced to hire "bad" people without training or experience in hospital work. As in the United States, Russian nurses love their profession and care deeply for their patients (Barron, 1994). They know that the lack of knowledge, skill, and dedication demonstrated by these untrained assistants has hurt health care and the image of nursing (A. Alekseyevna, personal communication, September 16, 1995).

Nursing research

Although the master's in nursing program at the Moscow Medical Academy includes nursing research as a studied and supported endeavor, funding is precarious. Faculty at this federally funded academy received no salary for 4 months due to budget constraints (Picard & Perfiljeva, 1995). As a result, publishers of U.S. nursing research journals have been encouraged to donate subscriptions to the Academy.

As professional nursing journals and texts arrive in Russia, nurses will need to learn from them. Therefore, the School of Nursing Dean at the Moscow Medical Academy has facilitated English language classes for her students (Picard & Perfiljeva, 1995). Russian technology can also help nursing research efforts. Computer technologies are available that promote the diagnosis and treatment of physical as well as psychological impairments. Data gathering and analysis systems, with the intent of prevention, are realized goals for medicine (Smirnov & Beznosuk, 1995). Why not for nursing?

Nursing organizations

Several nursing organizations have surfaced in Russia. One strong and growing organization is the Association of Medical Nurses of the Moscow Region. The charter of the organization, complete with listings of officers, was officially registered and recognized in Moscow on June 8, 1994. Those original charter and nursing practice standards documents were generously shared with U.S. nurses and reflect the incorporation of U.S. practice principles. Following are some of the primary goals from this organization's charter:

- Defense of professional interests of medical workers and specialists working in the health field, independent of their place of employment
- Improvement of the professional and civil standing of all people in health care
- Contribution to theoretical knowledge and professional skills
- Information dissemination of health and healthy lifestyles for the population
- Encouragement of a basis for the preventive health care of the region, enhancing the quality of medical service
- Defense of rights and interests of all patients as customers of medical services in the region

Another young, private nursing group, titled Salvet, believes that an independent organization has more ability to make changes in health and nursing care than a government-sponsored association. Its leader warns that nurses cannot ignore physician/administrator groups because these groups hold the power and control. Nursing will not change as easily without their cooperation (L. Svirenko, personal communication, September 12, 1995).

The Ministry of Health of Russia also has an "Initiative Group" composed of the chief nurses of the regions. This group drafts normative documents and working rules relative to nursing. For these tasks, all regions of the country interact (G. Karpova, personal communication, September 21, 1995). With greater numbers joining nursing organizations, Russian nurses have greater power and opportunity to make needed changes. The largest nursing organization in Russia is the Moscow Nursing Association, to which 70% of Russian nurses belong (Picard & Perfiljeva, 1995).

I have had two opportunities to speak before the Moscow Nurses Association. On both occasions I was struck by the strength and fortitude of this visionary group. Love for our beloved profession remains as the binding force for us all. Watching these nurses struggle with almost overwhelming obstacles—yet making progress both politically and professionally—was inspirational.

Early in 1990, each Soviet republic sent nurses to a Ministry of Health–sponsored meeting to discuss the perceived need to standardize nursing education and practice throughout the Soviet Union (Picard & Perfiljeva,

1995). The breakup of the Soviet Union slowed some of these efforts. However, in 1993 I met with regional representatives from over 36 Russian districts. Representative regions are loosely connected subgroups of this national organization. Members of these groups are the leaders of nursing in Russia, at the forefront of nursing education, practice, and administration. They were willing to come together to explain their problems and their concerns for the purpose of improving nursing care. These colleagues asked wonderfully challenging questions regarding nursing practice models, theories, and decision-making tools. Knowledge and information that has been shared with Russian nurses from the United States have been utilized significantly.

EAST-WEST COLLABORATION

What we will learn

Many Western nurses lack the knowledge of our Russian colleagues regarding holistic, homeopathic health care, including herbal medicines and leach therapy. Russian nurses understand the art and science of massage therapy, contactless massage, acupuncture, and acupressure. With advanced training, they perform these techniques to promote patient relaxation and noninvasive pain relief. Russian nurses have truly learned to treat with their hands.

What we will teach

The Russian health-care system gives patients a passive, subordinate position in the health-care culture. This dependency presents problems regarding patient rights and responsibilities (Curtis et al., 1995). Additionally, palliative care concepts for the treatment of terminally ill patients are new and doubted philosophies (Novikov et al., 1995). One reason for this reluctance is the concern medical professionals have for honesty with their dying patients. Nurses are taught that under no circumstance should patients be told of an incurable disease, especially a malignant tumor. Because Russian nurses must express optimism to their patients (Kinsey, 1992), most were alarmed during discussion sessions that stressed openness with dying patients. Additionally, dying patients are often feared so much that families and health-care workers abandon them. To further complicate the problem, analgesia is either severely restricted or nonexistent (Swett, 1992).

Western nurses share with their Russian colleagues research-based nursing care that is sensitive to patients' physical and psychological distress. Besides formal lectures, Russian nurses seek one-to-one learning sessions at the patient's bedside (Fleischman & Lubamadrov, 1993).

Because Russian nurses have no authority unless given to them by physicians of power and position, bringing physicians over to the United States for nursing-exchange efforts will enhance Russian nursing practice (F. Petrick, personal communication, September 29, 1995). Western nurses need to teach physicians about the abilities of nurses. An example of this was seen in September 1995 in the Pavlovski-Pasad region where physicians who had been to the United States implemented some independent practices for nurses.

The aid-to-Russia controversy

Russian citizens ask for medical help, begging for supplies, knowledge, and medications (L. Svirenko, personal communication, September 14, 1995). Russia has received humanitarian aid from the United States–Russian Nurse Exchange Consortium, and this aid is in evidence just 1 year later. However, Russian financial and health-care problems can lead Westerners to believe that giving aid to Russia is like pouring money into a huge black hole. Doubts remain over the efficacy of such endeavors. A report by the U.S. Senate Foreign Relations Committee concluded that the average Russian is unaware "of or affected by international assistance or the reforms that it is supposed to foster" ("U.S. Aid Trickles," 1994, p. 1a). Few Russians witness any U.S. help even though Congress approved $2.5 billion in aid in 1993. Russian bureaucrats, black market racketeers, and inefficiency are blamed ("U.S. Aid Trickles," 1994).

Many believe that no amount of foreign aid will help until Russia can put inflation, unemployment (20% of Russia's workforce), the budget deficit (twice that of the United States), and crime in check ("What We'll Give," 1993). The frightening side of Russia's economic turmoil is the tendency for high-level underpaid Russian scientists to leave the country for more lucrative positions or to supplement meager salaries by selling sensitive knowledge and materials. Russian weapons spending has been cut 50% to 70%, leaving nuclear researchers poverty stricken and desperate (Cooperman & Belianinov, 1995). This Russian "brain drain" is a threat to world peace efforts.

Health care is inextricably linked to all other social concerns in Russia, and foreign intervention is essential (Vaile, 1993). For example, mass-media teaching projects that would convince Russians to immunize their children need to be funded. These aid benefits would be tangible and far reaching. The U.S. Congress battles over sending more money to Russia, however. Esoteric ideas of the United States as a world leader have little sympathy in the face of the national budget-cutting mentality of the 104th Congress (Doherty, 1995).

NURSE-TO-NURSE EFFORTS

The thrust of help given to Russian nurses by their American colleagues must be in education (Fleischman & Lubamadrov, 1993). This is and will continue to be accomplished through the efforts of many nursing groups such as the United States–Russian Nurse Exchange Consortium. With members in seven United States states and Russia, the consortium has hosted United States–Russian exchanges of health-care professionals since 1989 ("US/Russian Nurse," 1993).

Russian health professionals propose that education scholarships, people-to-people exchanges, and quality health-care research be financially supported (Komarov, 1994). Russian nursing education can be supported through the LEMON (Learning Education Materials on Nursing) Project, which is a World Health Organization (WHO)–sponsored activity designed to enhance generic and continuing-education efforts in nations of the former Soviet Union as well as Central and Eastern Europe. With the help of foreign money, nursing materials are translated, packaged, printed, and distributed to each country (Picard & Perfiljeva, 1995).

Nurse-to-nurse efforts must focus on teaching the teachers and leaders so they may teach each other. This is easy. Russian nurses are hungry to learn from their Western peers. They are well educated, quick to grasp concepts, and creative in their attempts to implement new knowledge. It will be a "domino effect" of understanding (Barron, 1994, p. 59).

RUSSIA'S FUTURE

Russia's new national charter reflects a nation trying to overcome a history of oppression and human rights violations. Within this document, Russia ensures citizens the right to refuse medical treatment and experimentation. For the first time in decades, Russians have the right to secret correspondence, telephone discussions, mail, and other forms of electronic communications. Freedom of speech is guaranteed ("Russia's New Freedoms," 1993).

These new freedoms will help nurses and other health-care professionals identify and track health-care issues and indices without forced data embellishment. Computer systems are in place that will restore the true health-care picture in Russia. With Russian health deteriorating, these freedoms and technology applications will be the impetus for change (Komarov, 1994). Especially important will be the Russian government's budget prioritization so that more than 1% of Russia's GNP can be devoted to the health and welfare of its people. Computer databases would also coordinate the disjointed efforts of foreign medical groups, tracking current and planned activities as well as educational needs and approaches. Collaboration of all Western efforts will be essential (Vaile, 1993). For example, a proposal has been sent to the WHO Department of Nursing, Midwifery, and Social Work (Euro-Division) to add the specialty of psychiatric nursing (Stanley, 1993). New human rights laws professing a new dignity for Russian citizens will dramatically change psychiatric nursing in Russia (Kinsey, 1994). Yet this future is uncertain. Difficult changes will need to be made within diverse structures of Russian law and medicine (Kinsey, 1994).

Nurses, once docile and subservient, are finding new political and professional savvy as they confront worn traditions of medical authority. They are showing officials that nursing decision making and independent practice can and will move Russian health care forward—affecting the very life and death of this great nation (Ryan, 1992). "Join us now as we struggle for our identity," Russian nurses seem to be saying. "We are strong and we will survive these difficult times. Our profession is our hope and our voice."

It is with the greatest admiration that I dedicate this chapter to my nursing friends and colleagues in Russia. On a daily basis, they show all of us the ideals for which our beloved profession stands. Let us share of ourselves toward one goal and purpose—international health, love, and peace.

REFERENCES

Abortions rampant in Russia. (1995, July 23). *The Journal Times* (Racine, Wis., AP), p. 2A.

Aid comes too slowly, quake survivors say. (1995, June 4). *The Journal Times* (Racine, Wis., AP), p. 12A.

Barron, S. (1994). A nursing experience in Russia. *Neonatal Network, 13*(2), 59.

Boe, B. (1993). Boe knows Russia. *The Carthaginian, 72*(4), 6.

Carey, T.E. (1992, April 17). Russian health care system in critical condition. *The Atlanta Constitution*, p. A7.

Carpenter, D. (1994a, November 20). Change is slow in Russia's heartland. *The Journal Times* (Racine, Wis., AP), p. 4C.

Carpenter, D. (1994b, September 4). New textbooks finish Soviet debunking. *The Journal Times* (Racine, Wis., AP), p. 6B.

Cooperman, A. (1994, September 26). From under the rubble: Yeltsin's summit message is that Russia's economy is on the mend. *US News and World Report, 117*(12), 65-66.

Cooperman, A., & Belianinov, K. (1995). Moonlighting by modem in Russia: Hard-up scientists sell skills abroad. *US News and World Report, 118*(15), 45, 48.

Cooperman, A., & Thoenes, S. (1995). Here's Russia's new face of communism. *US News and World Report, 119*(24), 50-54.

Cooperman, A., & Thoenes, S. (1996). The race for the top. *US News and World Report, 120*(1), 14.

Crime wave sweeps Moscow. (1994, June 17). *The Journal Times* (Racine, Wis.), p. 5A.

Curtis, S., Petukhova, N., & Taket, A. (1995). Health care reforms in Russia: The example of St. Petersburg. *Social Science and Medicine, 40*(6), 755-765.

Doherty, C.J. (1995, March 4). Top leaders' paths diverge on UN, aid to Russia. *Congressional Quarterly, 53*(9), 698.

Edwards, D.J. (1994). Transcultural nursing: A view of the Russian health care system. *Orthopaedic Nursing, 13*(2), 47-51.

Environment still bleeds in Russia. (1993, August 29). *The Journal Times* (Racine, Wis., KR), p. 2A.

Feshbach, M. (1993, September). The Russian health crisis: Declining mortality rates. *Current, 355,* 21-22.

Fleischman, C., & Lubamadrov, V. (1993). Heart to heart: Teaching pediatric cardiology and cardiac surgery to nurses in St. Petersburg, Russia. *Journal of Pediatric Nursing, 8*(2), 133-138.

Groff, D.D. (1994a, December 18). Russian airlines being punished for safety violations. *The Journal Times* (Racine, Wis., KR), p. 7.

Groff, D.D. (1994b, August 14). State department advises against flying domestic Russian airlines. *The Journal Times* (Racine, Wis., KR), p. 4E.

Kinsey, D. (1992). The moral and professional role of the Russian nurse. *Nursing and Health Care, 13*(8), 426-431.

Kinsey, D. (1994). The new Russian law on psychiatric care. *Perspectives in Psychiatric Care, 30*(2), 15-19.

Komarov, Y.M. (1994). Quality assurance in health care: Lessons for others. *International Journal for Quality in Health Care, 6*(1), 27-30.

Kunstel, M., & Albright, J. (1994, May 9). Gap widening in Russian health care. *Atlanta Constitution,* p. A8.

Life is shorter for a Russian. (1994, February 3). *The Journal Times* (Racine, Wis., AP), p. 7A.

Monks, P. (1994). Go private or die: Healthcare rationing, Russia. *Nursing Times, 90*(25), 46-48.

Moscow cops feeling blue. (1995, March 25). *The Journal Times* (Racine, Wis., AP), p. 2A.

National Center for Health Statistics. (1995). *Health United States 1994.* (DHHS Publication No. [PHS] 95-1232). Washington, DC: U.S. Government Printing Office.

Nelan, B.W. (1995, March 20). Crime and punishment. *Time, 145*(11), 54.

Novikov, G.A., Osipova, N.A., Starinsky, V.V., Prokhorov, V.M., Benenson, L.I., & Gazizov, A.A. (1995, October). Prospects in the development and improvement of palliative care of cancer patients. *Russian Medical Journal, 1*(1), 13-17.

Picard, C., & Perfiljeva, G. (1995). Nursing education in Russia: Visions and realities. *Nursing and Health Care: Perspectives on Community, 16*(3), 126-130.

Plant, F. (1993). Next stop Moscow. *Nursing Times, 89*(34), 44-45.

Russia's new freedoms reflect past repressions. (1993, June 30). *The Journal Times* (Racine, Wis., AP), p. 7A.

Russia: Little gas, lots of gripes. (1994, November 12). *The Journal Times* (Racine, Wis., AP), p. 6A.

Russian longevity figures dwindle. (1995, February 8). *The Journal Times* (Racine, Wis.), p. 7A.

Russian Parliament is quietly rolling back recent human rights guarantees. (1993, August 28). *The Journal Times* (Racine, Wis., AP), p. 6A.

Russian women want foreign men. (1994, January 6). *The Journal Times* (Racine, Wis., KR), pp. 1A, 9A.

Ryan, M. (1992). Russian report: Perspectives on strikes by health care staff. *British Medical Journal 305*(6848), 298-299.

Ryan, M. (1993). Russian report: Personalia and the current health crisis. *British Medical Journal , 306*(6882), 909-911.

Smirnov, I.V., & Beznosuk, Y.V. (1995). Prospects in the solution of problems in psychoecology and psychohygiene. *Russian Medical Journal, 1*(1), 30-35.

Stanley, S. (1993). Bringing mental health care to Russia. *American Nurse, 25*(2), 12,14.

Study shows more Russians turning to religion. (1993, December 10). *The Journal Times* (Racine, Wis., AP), p. 4A.

Swett, E. (1992). The health care crisis in Russia. *Caring Magazine, 11*(10), 46-48.

U.S. Aid trickles down to ordinary Russians. (1994, March 28). *The Journal Times* (Racine, Wis., AP), p. 1A, 7A.

U.S./Russian nurse group to host program. (1993). *The Journal Times* (Racine, Wis.), p. 1.

Vaile, M.S.B. (1993). Health and health care in the former Soviet Union. *The Lancet, 341*(8840), 310-311.

What we'll give Russia. (1993, April 5). *The Journal Times* (Racine, Wis., AP and KR), p. 1A, 7A.

Yeltsin's secret nuclear survey finds problems, reveals cover-ups. (1995, August 7). *The Journal Times* (Racine, Wis., AP), p. 3A.

Zagalsky, L. (1994, August). Lifestyles of the not-so-rich. *Popular Science, 245*(2), 42-44, 70, 72.

Concluding notes and future directions

JOANNE COMI McCLOSKEY AND HELEN KENNEDY GRACE

As we have stated in previous editions, there is no "ending" for a book on issues in nursing. Given the purpose of the book—to provide a forum for knowledgeable debate on today's nursing issues so that intelligent decision making can occur—an ending is, in fact, inappropriate.

An issue is an issue for one of two reasons: either what is known is not well understood or there is not enough known. What is needed is debate on what is known in order to foster understanding and ongoing search for knowledge about what is unknown. Thoughtful debate and research are the keys to understanding a professional issue.

Yet research and debate are not enough for continued growth. Decision making also has to occur, sometimes in the absence of full knowledge. In such cases, it is even more important to understand what is known and to be able to put this knowledge into a broader perspective.

The broader perspective requires that one keep current with the changes in the nursing profession and the entire health-care field. Many things have changed since the first publication of this book in 1981. Recent changes in nursing include the downsizing of hospitals, expansion of ambulatory and home care, more use of nurse practitioners, replacement of nurses with unlicensed assistants, a decline in applicants to nursing programs following a period of high enrollments, more use of computers and recognition of a standardized nursing language for documentation, more concern with costs and delivering a quality product, movement to a managed-care environment, more nurses desiring participation in policy making, more concern by all nurses with the care of the elderly and those with chronic illnesses, more inclusion of consumers in health-care policy making, more community-based care, and more interest in nursing and health care in other parts of the world.

Despite the many changes today's nurses face, the dilemmas remain much the same as in the past. Stating them in the debate format, the dilemmas are:

- Unity versus diversity
- Standards versus access
- Quality versus cost
- Independence versus dependence
- Collaboration versus competition
- Inside control versus outside control
- Safety versus risk

Our previous recommendations to aid in the resolution of these dilemmas have been expanded somewhat. In alphabetical order they are to:

- Become more involved professionally and politically
- Become more proactive
- Celebrate our successes
- Concern ourselves with costs
- Conduct and use nursing research
- Document our care with nursing's standardized languages
- Learn how to work in teams
- Make ethical decisions
- Perform our jobs well
- Produce more and better-prepared leaders
- Promote flexibility and diversity
- Realign education and service
- Support each other
- Take some risks and initiate needed changes
- Widen our horizons to include relevant issues outside the profession

Although our authors report that we are making progress on many of these suggestions, the general tone of this edition is not as positive as that of the fourth edition. The changes in the practice environment for nurses as a result of the widespread introduction of managed care have introduced a worried note. While we have made a good deal of progress in many areas, there are new challenges that threaten to confuse and overwhelm us. Financial cutbacks threaten to undo or at least slow recent gains. We must continue to identify and work to resolve the important issues facing our profession. We must also recognize when an old issue is no longer an issue and turn our energies to new issues.

We believe that continuous thought and debate on important issues can lead to effective decision making and professional growth, for both the individual and the profession. With our learning and growth will come important benefits for our patients and, we believe, for society in general. This book, now in its fifth edition, has been our contribution to that process.

Index

D

E

Q

R

V

W